James
Patho

MW00973844

BLADDER PATHOLOGY

BLADDER PATHOLOGY

LIANG CHENG, MD

Professor of Pathology and Urology
Chief of Genitourinary Pathology Division
Director of Fellowship in Urologic Pathology
Director of Molecular Pathology Laboratory
Indiana University School of Medicine
Indianapolis, Indiana, USA

ANTONIO LOPEZ-BELTRAN, MD, PhD

Professor of Anatomic Pathology
Department of Surgery
Cordoba University School of Medicine
Cordoba, Spain

DAVID G. BOSTWICK, MD, MBA

Medical Director
Bostwick Laboratories
Glen Allen, Virginia, USA

WILEY-BLACKWELL

A JOHN WILEY & SONS, INC., PUBLICATION

Wiley Blackwell is an imprint of John Wiley & Sons, formed by the merger of Wiley's global Scientific Technical and Medical business with Blackwell Publishing.

Published by John Wiley & Sons, Inc., Hoboken, New Jersey.
Published simultaneously in Canada.

For general information on our other products and services or for technical support, please contact our Customer Care Department within the United States at (800) 762-2974, outside the United States at (317) 572-3993 or fax (317) 572-4002.

Wiley also publishes its books in a variety of electronic formats. Some content that appears in print may not be available in electronic formats. For more information about Wiley products, visit our web site at www.wiley.com.

Library of Congress Cataloging-in-Publication Data:

Cheng, Liang.
  Bladder pathology / Liang Cheng, Antonio Lopez-Beltran, David G. Bostwick.
      p. ; cm.
  Includes bibliographical references.
  ISBN 978-0-470-57108-8 (cloth)
  I. Lopez-Beltran, Antonio. II. Bostwick, David G. III. Title.
  [DNLM: 1. Urinary Bladder—pathology. 2. Neoplasm Staging. 3. Urinary Bladder Diseases—pathology. 4. Urinary Bladder Neoplasms—pathology. WJ 500]
  616.6'2071—dc23
                                                            2011044251

Printed in Singapore

10 9 8 7 6 5 4 3 2 1

Contents

Preface

The urinary bladder is subject to a unique and extraordinarily diverse array of congenital, inflammatory, metaplastic, and neoplastic abnormalities. The objective of *Bladder Pathology* is to provide contemporary, comprehensive, and evidence-based practice information for pathologists, urologists, and medical oncologists. A full spectrum of pathologic conditions that afflict the bladder and urothelium are described and illustrated. The book is aimed especially at the practicing pathologist, with an emphasis on diagnostic criteria and differential diagnoses. It is our hope that this very comprehensive book, consisting of 34 chapters, 754 pages, 112 tables, and 1741 full color photographs, will aid in the pathologist's recognition, understanding, and accurate interpretation of the light microscopic findings in bladder specimens.

This is an age of enlightenment in surgical pathology. The emergence of personalized medicine with new understandings of cancer genetics has created a paradigm shift in our practice. Greater weight continues to be placed on an evidence-based approach to diagnosis and patient management. This includes an emphasis on the scientific validation of our diagnostic methods and their meaningful application in practice. This is especially true in the management of patients with medical conditions involving the urinary bladder. Cancer of the bladder represents the fifth most common cancer in the human body, with more than 60,000 new carcinoma diagnoses annually in the United States. Many patients with bladder cancer have a prolonged survival, necessitating long-term followup, including the procurement of numerous subsequent cystoscopic biopsies and urine samples for histologic and cytopathologic evaluation. This, in turn, has generated a considerable diagnostic burden for the pathologist and cost to the health care system. It is our hope that continuing advances in the urinary bladder field can lessen the impact of these burdens on both practitioners and patients.

In the text we strive to provide a comprehensive resource for practicing surgical pathologists and their clinical colleagues so that they may better meet the daily demands and challenges of this ever-evolving field. We hope that this volume has captured our sense of excitement as we strive to stay on the cutting edge of these advances in medical practice. We have incorporated recent advances in molecular genetics of the urinary bladder with discussion of their current or potential impact on patient care. It is our intent to provide a framework by which diagnostic criteria can be compared, evaluated, and integrated with molecular and other ancillary test data.

We are indebted to many people who have been involved in the preparation of this book. We are grateful to our mentors, colleagues, and trainees who have challenged and inspired us. They include Drs. George M. Farrow, John N. Eble, David G. Grignon, Thomas M. Ulbright, Michael O. Koch, Gregory T. MacLennan, John F. Gaeta, Rodolfo Montironi, and many others. Our special thanks go to Ryan P. Christy from the Multimedia Education Division of the Department of Pathology at Indiana University, who edited the illustrations, and to Tracey Bender for her assiduous assistance in the editorial process. We also thank the staff at Wiley-Blackwell, including Thomas H. Moore, Ian Collins, Angioline Loredo, and Sheeba Karthikeyan for their invaluable support throughout the project. Finally, we earnestly solicit feedback and constructive criticism from readers so that the book may be improved in future editions.

LIANG CHENG
ANTONIO LOPEZ-BELTRAN
DAVID G. BOSTWICK

March 2012

Chapter 1

Normal Anatomy and Histology

Bladder Pathology, First Edition. Liang Cheng, Antonio Lopez-Beltran, David G. Bostwick.
© 2012 Wiley-Blackwell. Published 2012 by John Wiley & Sons, Inc.

Embryology

Early in fetal life, when cloacal dilation first appears and the hindgut ends in a blind sac, an ectodermal depression develops under the root of the tail.[1] This depression, known as the proctoderm, deepens until only a thin layer of tissue, the cloacal membrane, remains between the gut and the outside of the body. The division of the cloaca results from development of the urorectal fold that closes caudally toward the cloacal membrane. As the urorectal fold cuts progressively deeper into the cloaca, a wedge-shaped mass of mesenchyme accompanies it and forms a dense septum between the urogenital sinus anteriorly and the rectum posteriorly. This separation of the cloaca is completed before the cloacal membrane ruptures, so that its two parts open independently. When it first opens to the outside, the urogenital sinus, which is the ventral division of the cloaca, is tubular and continuous with the allantois. At this stage, it can be divided into a ventral or pelvic portion, which will become the bladder proper, and a urethral portion, which receives the mesonephric and fused müllerian ducts and later becomes the prostatic and membranous urethra in the male and the entire urethra in the female.[2]

After 8 weeks, the ventral part of the urogenital sinus expands to form an epithelial sac, the apex of which tapers into an elongated narrowed urachus. The splanchnic mesoderm surrounding both segments differentiates as interlacing bands of smooth muscle fibers and an outer fibroconnective tissue coat. By 12 weeks, the layers of the adult urethra and bladder can be recognized. This sequence of events indicates that the detrusor muscle and the urethral musculature have the same origin, constituting one uninterrupted structure.[2] This arrangement is easily observed in the female, in that the bladder and urethra form one tubular unit with expansion of the upper part. However, in the male, the structure is complicated by simultaneous development of the prostate gland. The developmental sequence is the same in both genders, and the structural arrangement in the male is only slightly more complex than that in the female.[2]

Anatomy

Gross Anatomy

The bladder is a hollow muscular organ whose main function is that of a reservoir. When empty, the adult bladder lies behind the symphysis pubis and is largely a pelvic organ. In infants and children, it is more cephalad than in adults. When full, the bladder rises above the symphysis and can readily be palpated or percussed. When overdistended, as

in acute and chronic urinary retention, it may cause the lower abdomen to bulge visibly and is easily palpable in the suprapubic region. The empty bladder has an apex (superior surface), two infralateral or anterolateral surfaces, a base (posterior surface), and a neck. The apex extends a short distance above the pubic bone and ends as a fibrous cord derivative of the urachus. This fibrous cord extends from the apex of the bladder to the umbilicus between the peritoneum and the transversalis fascia. It raises a ridge of peritoneum called the median umbilical ligament. There is a peritoneal covering at the apex in both sexes that also covers a small part of the base in men.[2,3]

The apex of the bladder is apposed to the uterus and ileum in the female and to the ileum and pelvic portion of the colon in the male. The base of the bladder faces posteriorly and is separated from the rectum by the uterus and vagina in the female, and by the vasa deferentia, seminal vesicles, and ureters in the male. The anterolateral surface on each side of the bladder is apposed to the pubic bone, levator ani, and obturator internus muscles, but the central anterior bladder is separated from the pubic bone by the retropubic space, which contains abundant fat and venous plexuses. The neck of the bladder, its most inferior part, connects with the urethra. When the bladder is distended with urine, the neck remains fixed and stationary, whereas the dome rises above the pelvic cavity into the lower abdomen, touching the posterior aspect of the lower anterior abdominal wall and the small and large bowels.[3]

Beneath the urothelial lining of the inner bladder, there is loose connective tissue that permits considerable stretching of the mucosa. As a result, the urothelial mucosal lining is wrinkled when the bladder is empty but smooth and flat when distended. This arrangement exists throughout the bladder except at the trigone, where the mucous membrane adheres firmly to the underlying muscle; consequently, the trigone is always smooth, regardless of the level of distension (**Figs. 1-1** and **1-2**).

Blood Supply and Lymphatic Drainage

The bladder is supplied by the superior, middle, and inferior vesical arteries, all of which are branches of the anterior division of the hypogastric artery. Between the bladder wall proper and the outer adventitial layer, there is a rich plexus of veins that ultimately terminate in the hypogastric veins after converging in several main trunks.

The bladder lymphatics drain into the external iliac, hypogastric, and common iliac lymph nodes. There are rich lymphatic anastomoses between the pelvic and genital organs.[4-6]

Nerve Supply

The bladder is richly innervated by divisions of the autonomic nervous system.[2,7] Sympathetic nerves originate

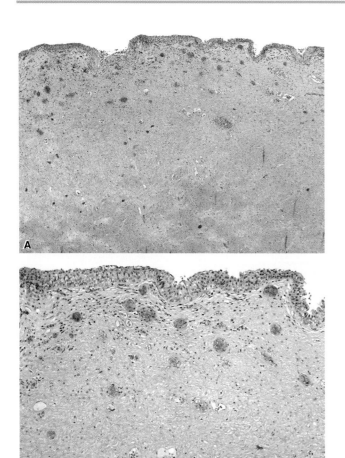

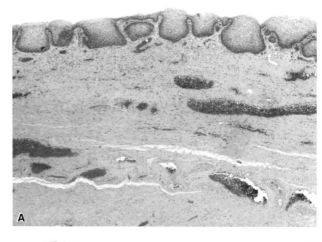

Figure 1-1 Normal trigone (A and B).

Figure 1-2 Normal trigone in a woman during the reproductive years. Note the squamous mucosa and closely packed underlying muscle (A and B).

from the lower thoracic and upper lumbar segments, mainly T11–T12 and L1–L2. These sympathetic fibers descend into the sympathetic trunk and the lumbar splanchnic nerves, connecting with the superior hypogastric plexus, an inferior extension of the aortic plexus. The latter separates into the right and left hypogastric nerves, and these extend inferiorly to join the pelvic plexus of the pelvic parasympathetic nerves. Parasympathetic nerves arise from sacral segments S2–S4, and these form the rich pelvic parasympathetic plexus. This plexus joins the sympathetic hypogastric plexus, and vesical branches emerge from this plexus toward the bladder base, innervating the bladder and urethra.[7,8]

Normal Histology

Urothelium

The urothelium is a unique stratified epithelium of variable thickness (**Figs. 1-3** to **1-6**). The number of cell layers

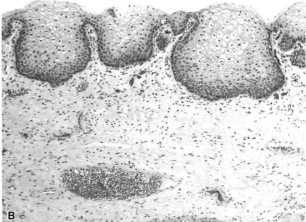

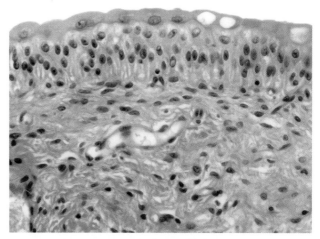

Figure 1-3 Normal urothelium. The thickness of urothelium is variable, up to seven cell layers in normal urothelium. Note the prominent superficial umbrella cells.

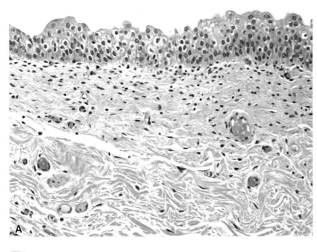

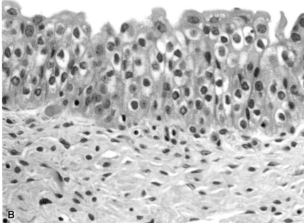

Figure 1-4 Normal urothelium (A and B). Cytoplasmic vacuolization is observed. In this preparation, the urothelium is up to seven cells in thickness (B).

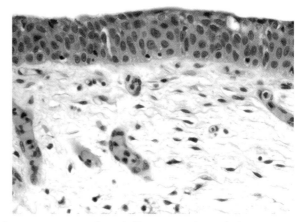

Figure 1-5 Normal urothelium. Note the orderly arrangement of the urothelial cells. The long axis of urothelial cells is often perpendicular to the mucosal surface. The superficial cells are less distinct. Prominent nuclear grooves are noted in some cells.

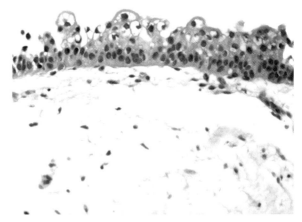

Figure 1-6 Normal urothelium. Note the variable thickness of urothelium in this preparation. The superficial cells have prominent cytoplasmic vacuolization.

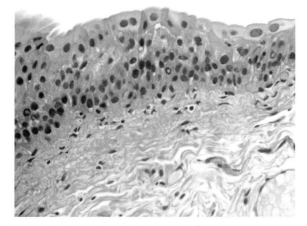

Figure 1-7 Normal urothelium. Note the prominent superficial cells. Nuclear vacuolization is occasionally seen in intermediate cells. Some variation of cell size and shape can be observed in normal urothelium and should not be interpreted as dysplasia.

depends on the degree of distension of the bladder, usually varying from three to seven layers. When distended, the bladder is three to six cell layers thick, although the typical biopsy contains about five layers; in the contracted state, it consists of six to eight layers.[9] For practical purposes, urothelium composed of more than seven cell layers is considered abnormal unless this finding can be attributed to tangential cutting of tissue.[10,11] In addition, the urothelium is thought to be monoclonal in origin, with some features of mosaicism.[12]

The normal urothelium contains a layer of large superficial cells that are frequently multinucleated, often referred to as umbrella cell thickness (**Figs. 1-7** to **1-9**). These cells have abundant eosinophilic cytoplasm, with large nuclei whose long axes are perpendicular to those of the smaller cells of the underlying basal and intermediate cell layers. The superficial cells vary in size and configuration according to the degree of bladder distension and angle

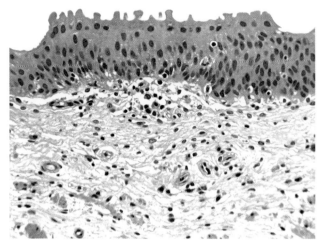

Figure 1-8   Normal urothelium. Note the prominent superficial cells.

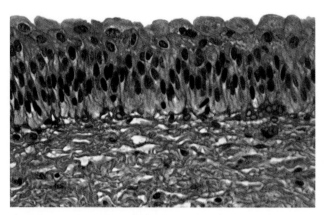

Figure 1-9   Normal urothelium. Basal and intermediate cells are located between the basal lamina and the superficial cells. Occasional prominent nuclear grooves may be seen. Note the binucleated superficial umbrella cells.

of tissue section; they may appear cuboidal in the distended bladder, but are often flattened. In addition, superficial cells are loosely attached to the underlying cells despite being interconnected with each other by extensive junctional complexes[13] and may be absent from otherwise normal urothelium in routine biopsies. Superficial umbrella cells express uroplakins and cytokeratin 20 with immunohistochemistry. The apical plasmalemma is thickened, with stiff plaques, unlike the short microvilli seen in the underlying intermediate cells.[13] However, the trigonal superficial cells of women during the reproductive years have a cobblestone pattern with long clubbed microvilli.[14] Superficial cells may persist on the surface of papillary urothelial carcinoma, particularly low grade carcinomas—a finding of

potential importance in pathologic grading of bladder cancer (see also **Chapter 9**).

Basal and intermediate cells are located between the basal lamina and the superficial cells (**Figs. 1-8** to **1-10**). These cells are morphologically identical to each other, and are distinguished only by their position in the mucosa.[13] They are regularly arranged, with distinct cell boundaries and oval, round, or fusiform nuclei with occasional prominent nuclear grooves. The nuclei are located centrally in the cells and contain finely granular chromatin that often accentuates the nuclear borders. Nucleoli are usually small and difficult to detect. Mitotic figures are rare in the normal urothelium. The basal layer of epithelial cells expresses Bcl-2, while the intermediate cells express RB1 and PTEN at varying intensities. HER2 and p53 are not expressed by normal urothelial cells. Ki67, indicating proliferation, may not be expressed in a single field. The long axis of the basal and intermediate cells is perpendicular to the basement membrane. The basement membrane is usually not visible in routine hematoxylin and eosin or periodic acid–Schiff stained sections, but appears as a razor-thin layer beneath the mucosa when present. Basement membrane markers such as laminin and type IV collagen may be useful diagnostically in select cases to define the basement membrane, but are not employed routinely.[15] Delicate capillaries of the muscularis mucosae are in intimate association with the basement membrane, and invaginations or tangential cutting may create the factitious appearance of intraepithelial extension.

The urothelium is able to respond to thermal, mechanical, and chemical stimuli ("sensor functions") and has the ability to release chemicals ("transducer functions").[16] Urothelial basal cells express certain receptors and ion channels (e.g., vanilloid receptor-1), similar to afferent

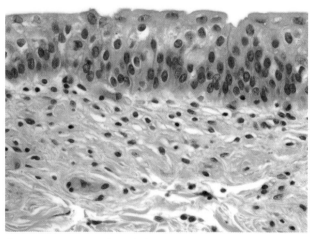

Figure 1-10   Normal urothelium. Basal and intermediate cells are more densely packed with a higher nuclear cytoplasmic ratio than that of superficial cells.

nerves.[16] The presence of afferent nerves adjacent to the urothelium suggests that these cells may be targets for transmitter release from bladder nerves or that chemicals released by urothelial cells may alter afferent excitability.

Bladder Wall

The lamina propria, located beneath the basement membrane, consists of a compact layer of fibrovascular connective tissue (**Figs. 1-11** to **1-13**). It may contain an incomplete muscularis mucosae composed of thin delicate smooth muscle fibers that may be mistaken for muscularis propria in biopsy specimens (**Figs. 1-14** to **1-16**).[17–23] The muscularis mucosae is an important diagnostic pitfall in evaluating bladder carcinoma because the management of cancer invading the muscularis propria is different from that of tumors limited to the lamina propria and surrounding the

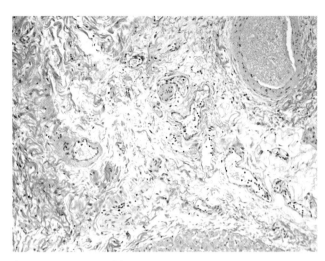

Figure 1-13 Normal lamina propria.

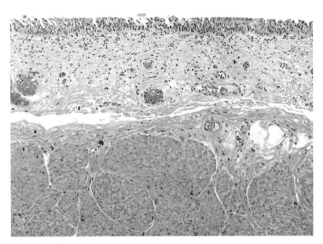

Figure 1-11 Normal lamina propria.

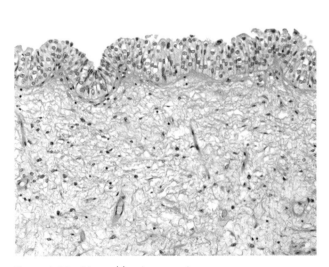

Figure 1-12 Normal lamina propria.

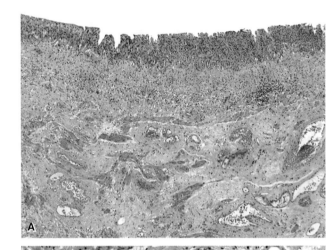

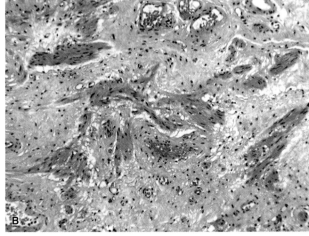

Figure 1-14 Muscularis mucosae in the lamina propria (A and B). The muscularis mucosae consists of scant delicate muscle bands interspersed with blood vessels and connective tissue stroma.

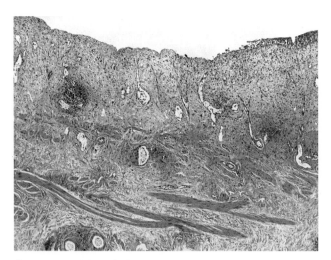

Figure 1-15   Muscularis mucosae.

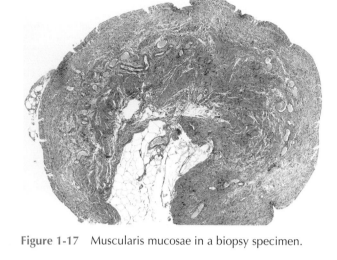

Figure 1-17   Muscularis mucosae in a biopsy specimen.

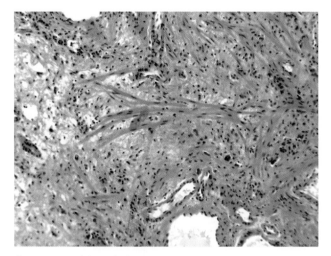

Figure 1-16   Muscularis mucosae.

muscularis mucosae. Therefore, it is important for pathologists to be aware of the existence of delicate muscle bundles within the lamina propria.[21,22,24] In biopsy specimens, these smooth muscle fibers may appear as a continuous layer, a discontinuous or interrupted layer, or as scattered thin bundles of smooth muscle fibers that do not form an obvious layer (Fig. 1-17).[22,25] These thin muscle fibers lie parallel to the mucosal surface, midway between the urothelium and the underlying muscularis propria.

Moderate-sized or large thick-walled blood vessels are a constant feature of the lamina propria, running parallel to the surface urothelium, in close association with the smooth muscle fibers of the muscularis mucosae (Fig. 1-18). However, these vessels are variable in distribution and may be close to the superficial lamina propria (Figs. 1-19 and 1-20). Therefore, large vessels cannot be used as a substitute for muscularis mucosae, as in some studies. It may be difficult to distinguish muscularis mucosae from muscularis

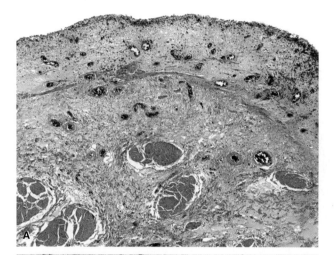

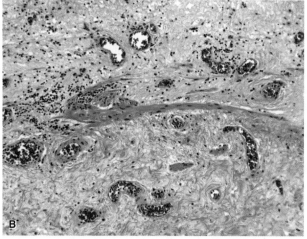

Figure 1-18   Musularis mucosae in close proximity to large vessels (A and B).

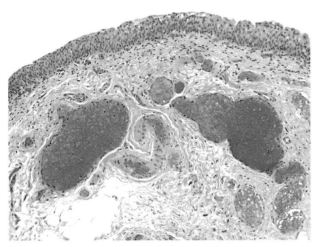

Figure 1-19 Large vessels may be seen in the superficial lamina propria and may or may not be associated with the muscularis mucosae. Therefore, large vessels cannot be used as a substitute for the muscularis mucosae.

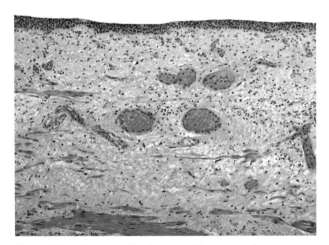

Figure 1-20 Variable distribution of large vessels and variably sized muscularis mucosae bundles.

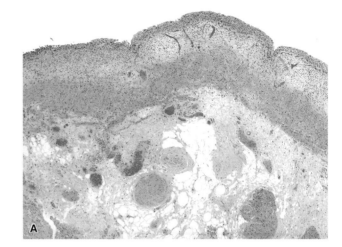

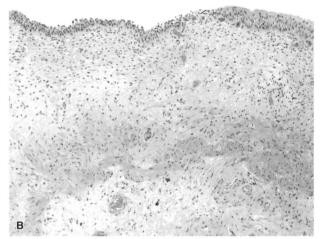

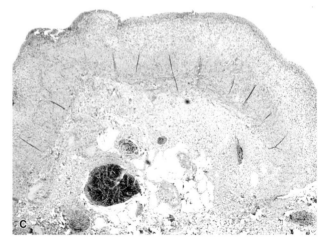

Figure 1-21 The muscularis mucosae is negative or shows weaker staining than the muscularis propria (A to C). Smoothelin usually stains strongly in the muscularis propria (detrusor muscle) (C).

propria (detrusor muscle). Trichome staining may be useful to resolve difficult cases.[26] Recent studies suggest that smoothelin can be a marker of interest in differentiating muscularis mucosae (negative or weak) from muscularis propria (positive and intense) (**Fig. 1-21**).[27–29]

To avoid overstaging bladder cancer, it is also important for the pathologist to be aware of the existence of fat within the lamina propria and the muscularis propria (**Figs. 1-22** and **1-23**).[30] Occasional bizarre stroma cells may be seen in the lamina propria and can be mistaken for invasive cancer cells. In difficult cases, immunostaining for cytokeratins is helpful. These bizarre stroma cells are negative for cytokeratin staining (**Figs. 1-24** and **1-25**).

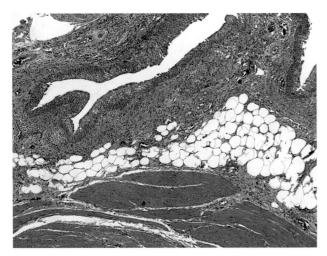

Figure 1-22 Adipose tissue can be seen in the lamina propria.

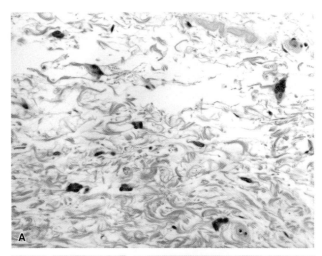

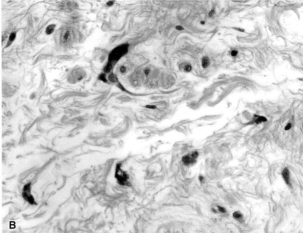

Figure 1-24 Bizarre stromal cells in the lamina propria (A and B).

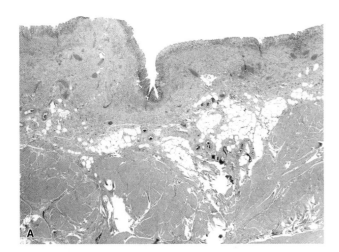

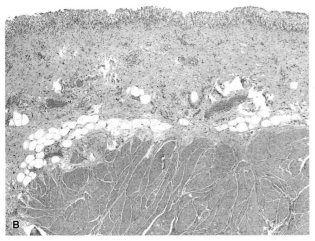

Figure 1-23 Adipose tissue is present in both the lamina propria and the muscularis propria (A and B). The presence of fat invasion in transurethral resection specimens does not indicate extravesical extension.

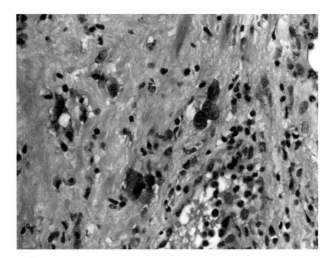

Figure 1-25 Bizarre stromal cells in the lamina propria.

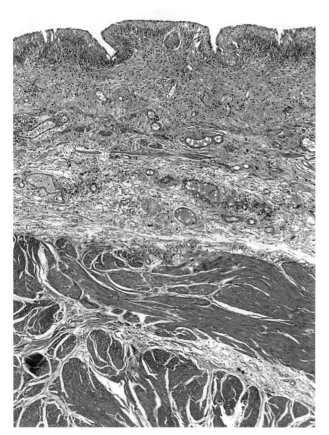

Figure 1-26 Muscularis propria (detrusor muscle). Note the contrast between the detrusor muscle and the muscularis mucosae in the lamina propria.

The muscle proper (detrusor muscle) of the bladder, the muscularis propria, is moderately thick and consists of an inner longitudinal layer, middle circular layer, and outer longitudinal layer (**Fig. 1-26**). It spirals around each ureteral orifice and increases in thickness around the internal urethral orifice, forming the internal sphincter of the bladder. The muscularis is surrounded by a coat of fibroelastic connective tissue, the adventitia, and perivesical fat.

Paraganglionic Tissue

Paraganglia are rarely found in routine sections of the urinary bladder.[31] Their presence in a bladder biopsy may be confused with neoplasm. Distinguishing features that are useful include the distinctive arrangement of cell nests, sinusoidal vascular pattern, monotonous benign cytology of the cells, and the absence of a stromal reaction.[32] Paraganglionic tissue typically demonstrates immunoreactivity with neuroendocrine markers such as chromogranin, synaptophysin, and neuron-specific enolase. The sustentacular cells exhibit immunostaining for S100 protein.

The Urachus

The urachus is an intraabdominal embryonic remnant. It contains the allantois, connecting the apex of the urinary bladder to the body wall at the umbilicus. The allantois originates in the portion of the yolk sac that gives rise to the cloacal portion of the hindgut. As the embryo grows, the urachus elongates to maintain its connection with the bladder dome and the body wall. At birth, the dome of the bladder and the umbilicus are closely opposed, and the urachus is only 2.5 to 3 mm long, with a diameter of 1 mm throughout most of its course and 3 mm where it joins the bladder.[33] The urachus lies in a space anterior to the peritoneum, bounded anteriorly and posteriorly by the umbilicovesical fascia.[34] Laterally, it is bounded by the two umbilical arteries, which, in turn, are surrounded by umbilicovesical fascia. Inferiorly, the umbilicovesical fascial layers cover the surface of the dome of the bladder. This space, the space of Retzius, is roughly pyramidal, and fascial planes separate it from the peritoneum and other structures. At the junction with the urinary bladder, the adult urachus is 4 to 8 mm wide, narrowing to about 2 mm at its superior end.

The urachus has three segments: supravesical, intramural, and intramucosal.[33] Tubular urachal remnants are found within the wall of the urinary bladder in approximately one-third of adults and are evenly distributed between men and women. There are three architectural patterns of intramural urachal canals, varying from simple tubular canals to complex branching canals (**Fig. 1-27**).[35] The mucosal portion of the urachus may have a wide diverticular opening, papilla, or a small opening flush with the mucosal surface. The majority (70%) of intramural urachal remnants are lined by urothelium; the remainder are lined by columnar epithelium, occasionally with small papillae or, rarely, mucous goblet cells or mucus-secreting columnar epithelium in women (**Figs. 1-28** and **1-29**).[35–37]

The Renal Pelvis and Ureters

The ureter and renal pelvis develop from the ampullary bud, which arises from the distal mesonephric duct during the fourth week of development. As the ureter elongates, there is a period of luminal obliteration followed by recanalization in the fifth week. Recanalization begins in the middle of the ureter and extends proximally and distally with the ureteropelvic and ureterovesical junctions; these are the last segments to recanalize. The mesonephric duct distal to the ampullary bud (the common nephric duct) is incorporated

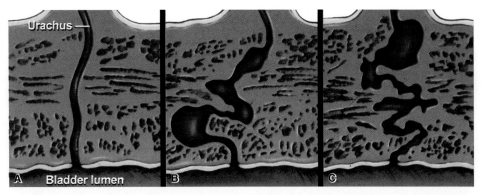

Figure 1-27   Patterns of intramural urachal canals: (A) type I, tubular canal without complexity; (B) type II; tubular canal with marked segmental dilatation and variable curvature; (C) type III, tubular canal with marked tortuosity and distortion, including segmental dilatation.

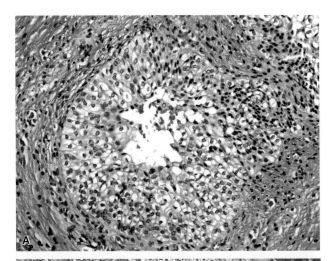

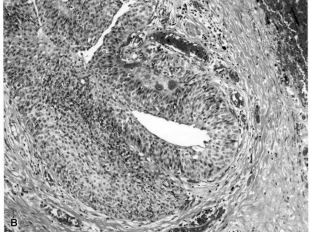

Figure 1-28   Normal urachus lined by stratified urothelium.

into the developing urogenital sinus, while the ureteral orifice migrates to the trigone and contributes to the prostatic urethra in the male.

Concomitant development of the male and female reproductive tract forms the mesonephric (wolffian) and müllerian ducts, respectively; division of the cloaca into bladder and hindgut occurs as the ureter and kidney develop. As a consequence, multiple malformations in these areas often occur together.

The lumen of the renal pelvis and ureter is lined by urothelium, which rests on a basement membrane (**Fig. 1-30**). The urothelium is composed of three to five layers of cells in the pelvis and four to seven layers of cells in the ureter. The pelvis and ureter have a continuous muscular wall that originates in the fornices of the minor calyces as small interlacing fascicles of the smooth muscle cells. The muscularis propria is not divided into distinct layers. Near the bladder, the ureter acquires an external sheath from the detrusor muscle, and the muscle fascicles become oriented longitudinally. The longitudinal fibers continue through the wall of the bladder and into the submucosa, where they surround the ureteral orifice and contribute to the trigone muscle.

The Urethra

The epithelium of the urethra is derived from the urogenital sinus, which is formed when the endodermal cloaca divides into the rectum dorsally and the urogenital sinus ventrally, separated by the urorectal septum. In women, the epithelium of the urethra is derived from endoderm of the urogenital sinus, while the surrounding connective tissue and smooth muscle arise from splanchnic mesenchyme. In men, the epithelium is also derived from the urogenital sinus except in the fossa navicularis, where it is derived from ectodermal cells migrating from the glans penis. As in women, the connective tissue and smooth muscle surrounding the male urethra is derived from splanchnic mesenchyme.

The male urethra is 15 to 20 cm long and is divided in three anatomical segments (**Figs. 1-31** and **1-32**). The

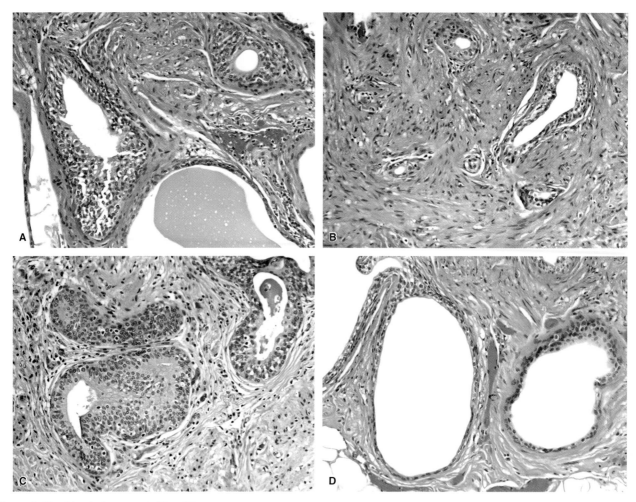

Figure 1-29 Urachal remnants (A to D).

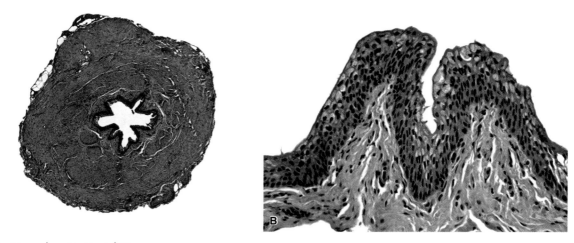

Figure 1-30 Normal ureter (A and B).

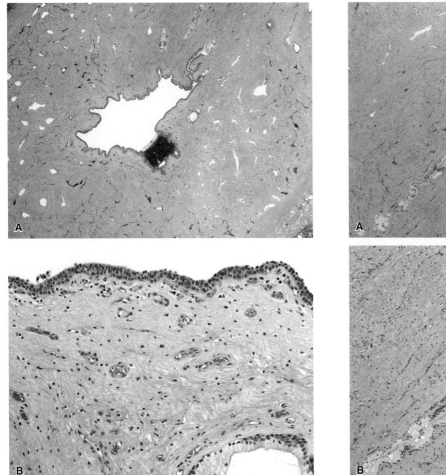

Figure 1-31   Normal urethra in a male patient (A and B).

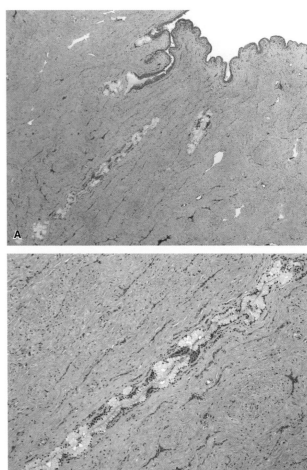

Figure 1-32   Normal urethra and periurethral glands (A and B).

prostatic urethra begins at the internal urethral orifice at the bladder neck and extends through the prostate to the prostatic apex. In the central part of the urethral crest is an eminence called the verumontanum. The verumontanum contains a slit-like opening that leads to an epithelium-lined sac called the prostatic utricle, a müllerian vestige. The ejaculatory ducts empty into the urethra on either side of the prostatic utricle. The membranous urethra extends from the prostatic apex to the bulb of the penis. Cowper glands are located on the left and right sides of the membranous urethra and their ducts empty into it. The penile urethra extends from the lower surface of the urogenital diaphragm to the urethral meatus in the glans penis. Bulbourethral glands are located in the proximal (bulbous) portion of the penile urethra. In addition, scattered mucus-secreting periurethral glands (Littre glands) are present at the periphery of the penile urethra except anteriorly (**Fig. 1-33**). The majority of unmyelinated nerve fibers penetrate the smooth muscle layers at 5 o'clock and 7 o'clock, whereas the majority of myelinated nerve fibers penetrate the striated muscles of the

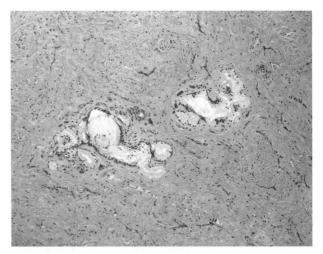

Figure 1-33   Littre glands are lined by mucus-secreting columnar cells.

fibers enter the smooth muscle part of the sphincter at 4 o'clock and 8 o'clock, whereas most myelinated fibers enter the sphincter at 3 o'clock and 9 o'clock. The female urethra is approximately 4 cm long, and, at its periphery, contains paraurethral Skene glands.

Immunohistochemical Findings

The urothelium has a characteristic immunophenotype. It expresses cytokeratins of both low and high molecular weights, including cytokeratins 7, 8, 13, and 19; cytokeratins 18 and 20 are present in the superficial cells.[38–41] This pattern of expression differs from that of normal stratified squamous epithelium, which shows predominantly high molecular weight cytokeratin immunoreactivity and from endometrium, endocervix, colorectum, and prostate, which demonstrate a preponderance of low molecular weight cytokeratin. High molecular weight cytokeratin immunoreactivity is restricted to the basal cell layer of the urothelium and squamous mucosa of the trigone. This can also be readily stained with antikeratin MAC387, which is not present in basal cells but in squamous cells of the trigone.[42] Other epithelial markers, such as epithelial membrane antigen, carcinoembryonic antigen, and LeuM1, are found on the surface of the urothelium. The normal urothelium synthesizes blood group isoantigens A, B, and H(O) as well as Lewis blood group antigens.[43] As mentioned above, the basal layer of urothelial cells expresses Bcl-2 while the intermediate cells express RB1 and PTEN at varying intensities. HER2 and p53 are not expressed by normal urothelial cells. Ki67, indicating proliferation, is uncommon in the normal urothelium. Prostate-specific antigen (or human glandular kallikrein 3), prostatic acid phosphatase, prostate-specific membrane antigen, and human glandular kallikrein 2 are not produced by the urothelium.

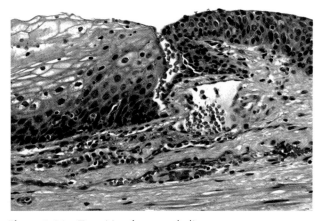

Figure 1-34 Transition from urothelium to squamous epithelium in the urethra.

prostatic capsule and of the urethral sphincter at 9 o'clock and 3 o'clock.

The type of epithelium lining the urethra varies along its length (**Fig. 1-34**). In general, urothelium lines the prostatic urethra, pseudostratified columnar epithelium lines the membranous segment and most of the penile urethra, and nonkeratinized stratified squamous epithelium lines the fossa navicularis and external urethral orifice. In females, the proximal one-third of the urethra is lined by urothelium and the distal two-thirds by nonkeratinized stratified squamous epithelium. The proximal one-third consists of a circular smooth muscle sphincter, the middle one-third of two circular layers of smooth and striated muscle fibers, and the distal one-third of a circular layer of smooth muscle fibers surrounded by an omega-shaped layer of striated muscle fibers. In the proximal one-third of the urethral sphincter, myelinated fibers run with unmyelinated fibers from the pelvic plexus. These fibers are closely related to the lateral and anterior aspects of the vagina. Unmyelinated

REFERENCES

1. Young RH. Non-neoplastic disorders of the urinary bladder. In: Bostwick DG, Cheng L, eds. Urologic Surgical Pathology, 2nd ed. Philadelphia: Elsevier/Mosby, 2008;215–58.

2. Tanagho EA. Anatomy of the urinary tract. In: Walsh PC, Retik AB, Stamey TA, Vaughan ED, eds. Campbell's Urology, 6th ed. Philadelphia: W.B. Saunders, 1992;40–54.

3. Chevallier JM. The bladder. Surgical anatomy. Cystectomy. *Soins Chir* 1994;41–3.

4. Poggi P, Marchetti C, Tazzi A, Scelsi R. The lymphatic vessels and their relationship to lymph formation in the human urinary bladder. *Lymphology* 1995;28:35–40.

5. Ravery V, Chopin DK, Abbou CC. Surgical anatomy of the lymphatic drainage of the bladder. *Ann Urol (Paris)* 1993;27:9–11.

6. Scelsi R, Scelsi L, Gritti A, Gozo M, Reguzzoni M, Marchetti C. Structure of the lymphatic microcirculation in the human urinary bladder with different intraluminal pressure and distension. *Lymphology* 1996;29:60–6.

7. de Groat WC. Anatomy and physiology of the lower urinary tract. *Urol Clin North Am* 1993;20:383–401.

8. Takenaka A, Kawada M, Murakami G, Hisasue S, Tsukamoto T, Fujisawa M. Interindividual variation in distribution of extramural ganglion cells in the male pelvis: a semi-quantitative and immunohistochemical study concerning nerve-sparing pelvic surgery. *Eur Urol* 2005;48:46–52.

9. Konishi T. Architectural ultrastructure of the urinary bladder epithelium. II. Changes in the urine-blood barrier in the contracted and distended state in the normal and inflammatory bladder. *Hinyokika Kiyo* 1988;34:23–31.

10. Montironi R, Mazzucchelli R, Scarpelli M, Lopez-Beltran A, Cheng L. Morphological diagnosis of urothelial neoplasms. *J Clin Pathol* 2008;61:3–10.

11. Montironi R, Lopez-Beltran A, Scarpelli M, Mazzucchelli R, Cheng L. Morphological classification and definition of benign, preneoplastic and non-invasive neoplastic lesions of the urinary bladder. *Histopathology* 2008;53:621–33.

12. Tsai YC, Simoneau AR, Spruck CH, 3rd, Nichols PW, Steven K, Buckley JD, Jones PA. Mosaicism in human epithelium: macroscopic monoclonal patches cover the urothelium. *J Urol* 1995;153:1697–1700.

13. Congiu T, Radice R, Raspanti M, Reguzzoni M. The 3D structure of the human urinary bladder mucosa: a scanning electron microscopy study. *J Submicrosc Cytol Pathol* 2004;36:45–53.

14. Davies R, Hunt AC. Surface topography of the female bladder trigone. *J Clin Pathol* 1981;34:308–13.

15. Wilson CB, Leopard J, Nakamura RM, Cheresh DA, Stein PC, Parsons CL. Selective type IV collagen defects in the urothelial basement membrane in interstitial cystitis. *J Urol* 1995;154:1222–6.

16. Birder LA, Kanai AJ, de Groat WC, Kiss S, Nealen ML, Burke NE, Dineley KE, Watkins S, Reynolds IJ, Caterina MJ. Vanilloid receptor expression suggests a sensory role for urinary bladder epithelial cells. *Proc Natl Acad Sci U S A* 2001;98:13396–401.

17. Anderstrom C, Johansson S, Nilsson S. The significance of lamina propria invasion on the prognosis of patients with bladder tumors. *J Urol* 1980;124:23–6.

18. Dixon JS, Gosling JA. Histology and fine structure of the muscularis mucosae of the human urinary bladder. *J Anat* 1983;136:265–71.

19. Keep JC, Piehl M, Miller A, Oyasu R. Invasive carcinomas of the urinary bladder. Evaluation of tunica muscularis mucosae involvement. *Am J Clin Pathol* 1989;91:575–9.

20. Cheng L, Weaver AL, Neumann RM, Scherer BG, Bostwick DG. Substaging of T1 bladder carcinoma based on the depth of invasion as measured by micrometer. A new proposal. *Cancer* 1999;86:1035–43.

21. Cheng L, Montironi R, Davidson DD, Lopez-Beltran A. Staging and reporting of urothelial carcinoma of the urinary bladder. *Mod Pathol* 2009;22 (Suppl 2):S70–95.

22. Ro JY, Ayala AG, el-Naggar A. Muscularis mucosa of urinary bladder. Importance for staging and treatment. *Am J Surg Pathol* 1987;11:668–73.

23. Younes M, Sussman J, True LD. The usefulness of the level of the muscularis mucosae in the staging of invasive transitional cell carcinoma of the urinary bladder. *Cancer* 1990;66:543–8.

24. Cheng L, Bostwick DG. Progression of T1 bladder tumors: better staging or better biology. *Cancer* 1999;86:910–2.

25. Paner GP, Ro JY, Wojcik EM, Venkataraman G, Datta MW, Amin MB. Further characterization of the muscle layers and lamina propria of the urinary bladder by systematic histologic mapping: implications for pathologic staging of invasive urothelial carcinoma. *Am J Surg Pathol* 2007;31:1420–9.

26. Aydin A, Uçak R, Karakök M, Güldür ME, Koçer NE. Vascular plexus is a differentiation criterion for muscularis mucosa from muscularis propria in small biopsies and transurethral resection materials of urinary bladder? *Int Urol Nephrol* 2002;34:315–9.

27. Paner GP, Shen SS, Lapetino S, Venkataraman G, Barkan GA, Quek ML, Ro JY, Amin MB. Diagnostic utility of antibody to smoothelin in the distinction of muscularis propria from muscularis mucosae of the urinary bladder: a potential ancillary tool in the pathologic staging of invasive urothelial carcinoma. *Am J Surg Pathol* 2009;33:91–8.

28. Council L, Hameed O. Differential expression of immunohistochemical markers in bladder smooth muscle and myofibroblasts, and the potential utility of desmin, smoothelin, and vimentin in staging of bladder carcinoma. *Mod Pathol* 2009;22:639–50.

29. Miyamoto H, Sharma RB, Illei PB, Epstein JI. Pitfalls in the use of smoothelin to identify muscularis propria invasion by urothelial carcinoma. *Am J Surg Pathol* 2010;34:418–22.

30. Bochner BH, Nichols PW, Skinner DG. Overstaging of transitional cell carcinoma: clinical significance of lamina propria fat within the urinary bladder. *Urology* 1995;45:528–31.

31. Honma K. Paraganglia of the urinary bladder. An autopsy study. *Zentralbl Pathol* 1994;139:465–9.

32. Young RH. Non-neoplastic epithelial abnormalities and tumor-like lesions. Pathology of the Urinary Bladder. New York: Churchill Livingstone, 1989:1–63.

33. Begg RC. The urachus: its anatomy, histology and development. *J Anat* 1930;64:170–83.

34. Gearhart JP, Jeffs RD. Urachal abnormalities. In: Walsh PC, Retik AB, Stamey TA, Vaughan ED, eds. Campbell's Urology, 6th ed. Philadelphia: W.B. Saunders, 1992;1815–21.

35. Schubert GE, Pavkovic MB, Bethke-Bedurftig BA. Tubular urachal remnants in adult bladders. *J Urol* 1982;127:40–2.

36. Eble JN. Abnormalities of the urachus. In: Young RH, ed. Pathology of the Urinary Bladder. New York: Churchill Livingstone, 1989.

37. Tyler DE. Epithelium of intestinal type in the normal urachus: a new theory of vesical embryology. *J Urol* 1964;92:505–7.

38. Alonso A, Ikinger U, Kartenbeck J. Staining patterns of keratins in the human urinary tract. *Histol Histopathol* 2009;24:1425–37.

39. Hodges KB, Lopez-Beltran A, Emerson RE, Montironi R, Cheng L. Clinical utility of immunohistochemistry in the diagnoses of urinary bladder neoplasia.

Appl Immunohistochem Mol Morphol 2010;18:401–10.

40. Lopez-Beltran A. Immunohistochemical markers in evaluation of urinary and bladder tumors. *Anal Quant Cytol Histol* 2007;29:121–2.

41. Yildiz IZ, Recavarren R, Armah HB, Bastacky S, Dhir R, Parwani AV. Utility of a dual immunostain cocktail comprising of p53 and CK20 to aid in the diagnosis of non-neoplastic and neoplastic bladder biopsies. *Diagn Pathol* 2009;4:35.

42. Lopez-Beltran A, Requena MJ, Alvarez-Kindelan J, Quintero A, Blanca A, Montironi R. Squamous differentiation in primary urothelial carcinoma of the urinary tract as seen by MAC387 immunohistochemistry. *J Clin Pathol* 2007;60:332–5.

43. Witjes JA, Umbas R, Debruyne FM, Schalken JA. Expression of markers for transitional cell carcinoma in normal bladder mucosa of patients with bladder cancer. *J Urol* 1995;154:2185–9.

Chapter 2

Inflammatory and Infectious Conditions

Bladder Pathology, First Edition. Liang Cheng, Antonio Lopez-Beltran, David G. Bostwick.
© 2012 Wiley-Blackwell. Published 2012 by John Wiley & Sons, Inc.

Table 2-1   **Inflammatory Conditions**

Acute and chronic cystitis
  Follicular cystitis
  Interstitial cystitis
  Eosinophilic cystitis
  Encrusted cystitis
  Emphysematous cystitis
  Gangrenous cystitis
  Hemorrhagic cystitis
  Viral cystitis
  Cystitis with atypical giant stromal cells
  Denuding cystitis

Granulomatous cystitis
  Postsurgical
  Suture granuloma
  BCG-induced
  Schistosomiasis
  Malakoplakia
  Tuberculosis
  Xanthoma
  Other

Other infection cystitides
  Fungal
  Actinomycosis
  Miscellaneous cystitides

A wide variety of nonneoplastic inflammatory conditions may involve the bladder primarily or secondarily (**Table 2-1**).[1]

Acute and Chronic Cystitis and Their Variants

Acute and Chronic Cystitis

Most cases of acute and chronic cystitis result from infection with gram-negative coliform bacteria such as *Escherichia coli (E. Coli)*.[2,3] The most common portal of entry is the urethra. Predisposing factors include structural abnormalities of the urinary bladder, diverticula, calculi, any process or lesion that causes outflow obstruction, and systemic illnesses such as diabetes. Infectious causes of cystitis include bacterial, viral, fungal, and protozoal agents. Irritative agents that cause cystitis include trauma from instrumentation and catheterization, radiation therapy, chemotherapy, bladder calculi, and chemical irritants such as formalin, turpentine, and ether (chemical cystitis).[4,5] Some cases of cystitis are of unknown etiology. Other forms of cystitis include interstitial, eosinophilic, and follicular cystitis.[6]

In early acute bacterial cystitis, there is vascular dilatation and congestion, erythematous and hemorrhagic

mucosa, and moderate to severe edema. With time, polypoid or bullous cystitis may develop, sometimes with ulceration. The urothelium may be hyperplastic or metaplastic, and, when ulcerated, is often covered by a fibrinous membrane with neutrophils and bacterial colonies (**Figs. 2-1** and **2-2**). Stromal edema and chronic inflammation gradually become more pronounced, particularly in the lamina propria (**Fig. 2-3**). If the acute inflammation persists, chronic cystitis usually develops, sometimes with prominent mural fibrosis.

In chronic cystitis, the mucosa may be thin, hyperplastic, or ulcerated, often with changes of reactive atypia (**Figs. 2-4** to **2-6**). Granulation tissue is typically conspicuous in the early stages, and may be replaced by dense scarring, particularly in the late healing stages. Edema may also be present (**Fig. 2-7**). This process may be transmural and involve

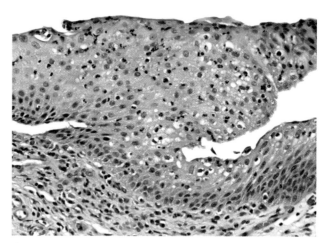

Figure 2-1   Acute cystitis. Numerous neutrophils are seen in the urothelium.

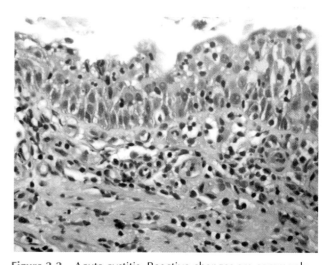

Figure 2-2   Acute cystitis. Reactive changes are commonly seen in the setting of acute cystitis and should not be mistaken for dysplasia or carcinoma in situ.

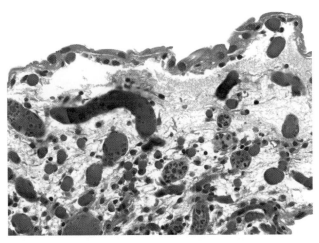

Figure 2-3   Acute cystitis. Note the stromal edema.

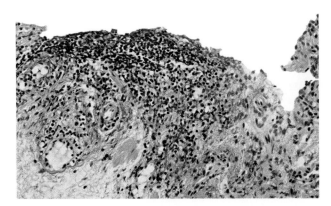

Figure 2-5   Chronic cystitis with mucosal erosion.

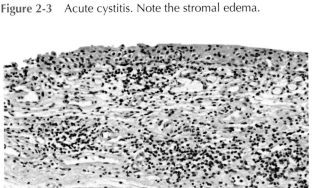

Figure 2-4   Chronic nonspecific cystitis. The mucosa is intact but thinned, and the lamina propria contains a mixed chronic inflammatory infiltrate.

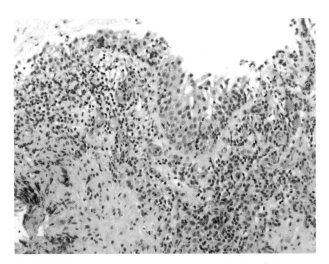

Figure 2-6   Chronic cystitis with reactive epithelial changes.

perivesicular tissue. Squamous metaplasia may develop at a later stage (**Fig. 2-8**).

Papillary–Polypoid Cystitis (Papillary Cystitis; Bullous Cystitis)

Polypoid cystitis may be clinically and microscopically mistaken for papillary urothelial carcinoma.[7-9] Polypoid cystitis refers to lesions with edematous and broad-based papillae (**Figs. 2-9** to **2-12**); the designation papillary cystitis is used when thin finger-like papillae are present (**Figs. 2-13** and **2-14**). In both, there is typically abundant chronic inflammation in the stroma, accompanied by prominent and often ectatic blood vessels. Sometimes the inflammation is not prominent, and the appearance varies from papillary or polypoid cystitis to bullous cystitis, depending on the amount of stromal edema. In bullous cystitis, the lesion is wider than lesions of polypoid or papillary cystitis.[10] On cystoscopy, the lesion frequently suggests papillary urothelial carcinoma.

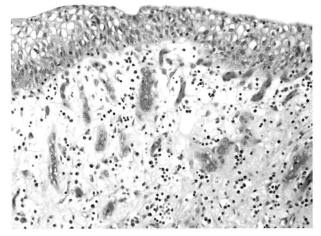

Figure 2-7   Chronic cystitis with mucosal edema. The overlying urothelium is metaplastic.

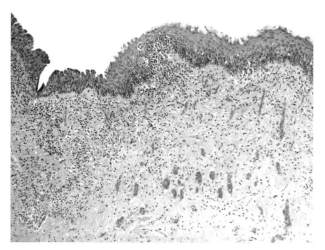

Figure 2-8 Chronic cystitis. Note the transition of normal urothelium to squamous epithelium (squamous metaplasia).

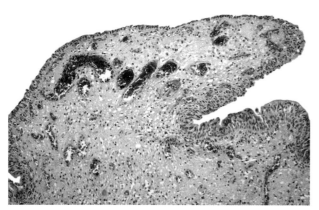

Figure 2-9 Polypoid cystitis with a broad frond of mucosa with prominent blood vessels and benign urothelial lining.

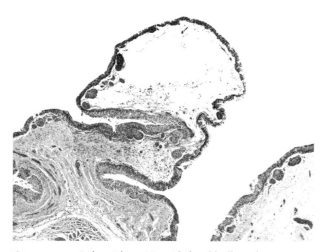

Figure 2-10 Polypoid cystitis with focal bullous formation.

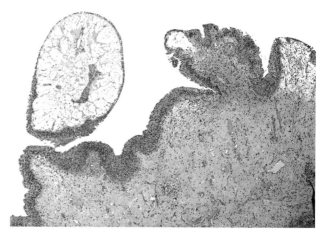

Figure 2-11 Polypoid cystitis.

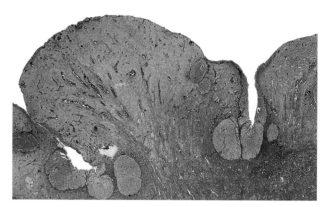

Figure 2-12 Polypoid cystitis. Broad polypoid growth that imparts a cobblestone appearance cystoscopically.

Exophytic growth of polypoid and papillary cystitis can be confused with carcinoma.[7,10] Occasionally, papillary–polypoid cystitis may be associated with reactive and metaplastic changes in the overlying or adjacent urothelium, with squamous metaplasia being the most common. The urothelium may be hyperplastic, but it lacks cytologic atypia. Less commonly, florid polypoid cystitis may suggest inverted papilloma.[10] Two clinical settings suggest that an exophytic bladder lesion is reactive or inflammatory—patients with an indwelling catheter[11,12] and those with vesical fistula.[10] Polypoid and bullous lesions are usually less than 0.5 cm in diameter, but larger, macroscopically visible lesions may involve the dome or posterior wall. The entire bladder is sometimes involved when a catheter has been present for more than six months.[10,13–15] Long-standing cases of polypoid cystitis may have a fibrous rather than an edematous stroma. The mucosal changes associated with vesical fistula may have the characteristics of reactive urothelium similar to what is seen in nonspecific chronic or acute cystitis.

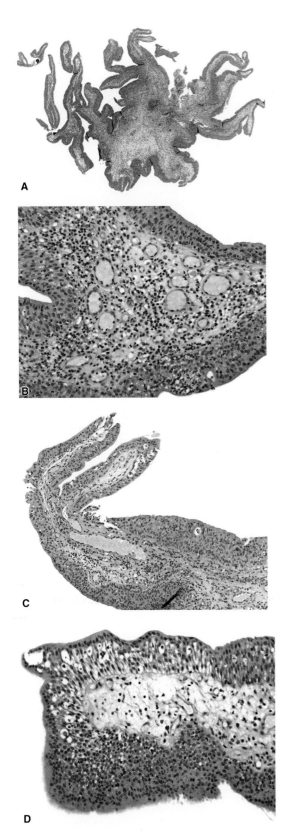

Figure 2-13 Papillary cystitis (A and D). Note the finger-like projections and prominent inflammatory infiltrates in the stroma.

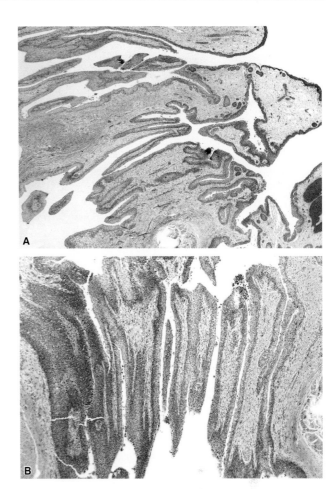

Figure 2-14 Papillary cystitis (A and B).

Papillary–polypoid cystitis should be differentiated from low grade papillary urothelial carcinoma.[7,16] Important distinguishing features include the clinical history of catheterization and the presence of broad fronds in polypoid cystitis. Of greater difficulty are the thin papillae of papillary cystitis, although the urothelium is usually not as thick as in carcinoma, umbrella cells are more common, and there are frequent reactive changes in the urothelium. The fibrovascular cores of the papillae of urothelial carcinoma typically have less inflammation and edema than polypoid cystitis, but exceptions are observed (**Fig. 2-15**).[17] The urothelium adjacent to papillary carcinoma is often hyperplastic; significant cytologic abnormalities within a papillary lesion or the adjacent urothelium favor the diagnosis of carcinoma.[10]

A recent report based on 155 consultation cases of polypoid cystitis identified 41 cases that were misdiagnosed as papillary urothelial neoplasms by contributing pathologists.[9] The original diagnoses included noninvasive low grade papillary urothelial carcinoma ($n = 23$), noninvasive high grade papillary urothelial carcinoma ($n = 6$), papillary urothelial neoplasm of low malignant potential ($n = 5$), papilloma ($n = 3$), urothelial neoplasia ($n = 2$),

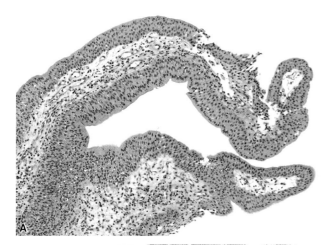

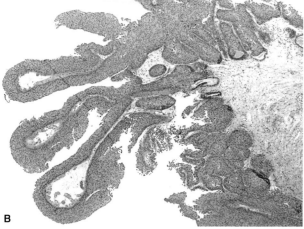

Figure 2-15 Comparison of papillary cystis (A) and low grade noninvasive papillary urothelial carcinoma (B). The stroma in papillary cystitis contains dense inflammatory cells (A). In contrast, papillary cores in urothelial carcinoma are finely vascular and less cellular (B).

carcinoma in situ ($n = 1$), and squamous carcinoma ($n = 1$). Architecturally, 31 cases had isolated papillary fronds, with branching papillary structures in one case. The base of the papillary stalks were characterized as both broad and narrow ($n = 24$), only broad ($n = 9$), and only narrow ($n = 3$). The overlying urothelium of polypoid cystitis was diffusely and focally thickened in eight cases and five cases, respectively. Occasionally, the overlying urothelium can take the appearance of a pseudocarcinomatous epithelial hyperplasia. Umbrella cells were identified in 32 cases. Mild to moderate acute and chronic inflammation was present in 28 cases. Eleven cases showed mild to moderate chronic inflammation. Reactive urothelial atypia was noted in 26 cases, with mitotic figures present in 22 cases (frequent in three and rare in 19 cases). Stroma edema was seen in 32 cases, with fibrosis within the polypoid stalks seen in 16 cases. The key to correct diagnosis of papillary–polypoid cystitis is to recognize

at low magnification the reactive nature of the process with an inflamed background that is edematous or fibrous with predominantly simple, nonbranching, broad-based fronds of relatively normal thickness urothelium, and not focus at higher power on the exceptional frond that may more closely resemble a urothelial neoplasm either architecturally or cytologically. Pertinent clinical history is also helpful in confirming the diagnosis.

Follicular Cystitis (Cystitis Follicularis)

Follicular cystitis is present at least focally in 40% of patients with bladder cancer and 35% of those with urinary tract infection.[18] Macroscopically, it typically consists of one or more small nodules of pink, white, or gray tissue, often with erythema, and may be mistaken for urothelial carcinoma. Microscopically, there are numerous lymphoid follicles within the lamina propria, usually with germinal centers, often slightly elevating the overlying intact or attenuated urothelium (Fig. 2-16).[19]

Malignant follicular-type lymphoma is the most important differential diagnostic consideration for follicular cystitis, particularly in small biopsy specimens. However, patients usually have a history of lymphoma elsewhere, and the infiltrate in lymphoma is usually extensive and monomorphic. Immunohistochemical studies are particularly helpful in distinguishing lymphoma from benign lymphoid infiltrates.

Interstitial Cystitis

Interstitial cystitis is a chronic idiopathic inflammatory bladder disease of unknown cause and pathogenesis (Fig. 2-17).[20–26] The diagnosis is based on a combination of symptoms, cystoscopic findings, and clinical findings that exclude other bladder diseases; biopsy is useful but often not necessary. The main indication of bladder biopsy

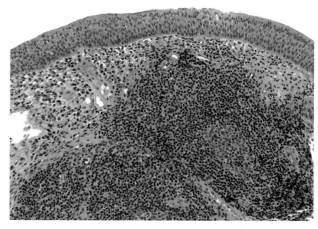

Figure 2-16 Follicular cystitis. Benign urothelium overlies a lymphoid follicle.

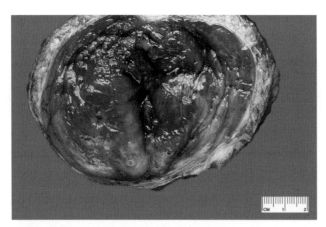

Figure 2-17 Interstitial cystitis. Grossly, there are scattered mucosal erosions and erythema.

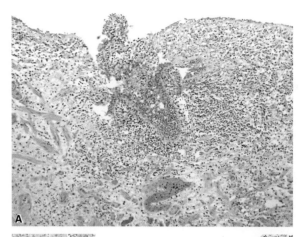

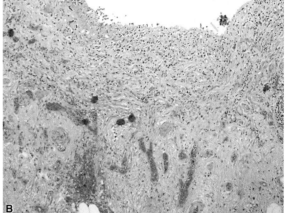

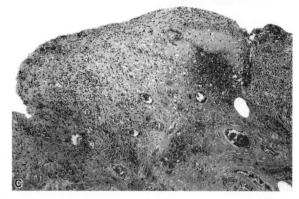

Figure 2-18 Interstitial cystitis, ulcer pattern. Note the wedge-shaped erosion with adjacent inflammation (A and B). The erosion is accompanied by prominent hemorrhage in the lamina propria (C). This young woman had typical clinical features of interstitial cystitis.

in these patients is to exclude urothelial carcinoma in situ, which usually presents with overlapping symptoms. Patients with interstitial cystitis suffer from urgency, frequency, and bladder-associated pain. At least 90% of the patients are women.

High pressure cystoscopy, up to 80 cmH$_2$O, reveals two patterns of cases: ulcerative (classic or Hunner ulcer) and nonulcerative interstitial cystitis. Patients with ulcerative interstitial cystitis (also known as Hunner ulcer[27]) develop large irregular ulcers, whereas nonulcerative interstitial cystitis patients have multiple strawberry-like petechial hemorrhages, referred to as glomerulations. The trigone is usually not involved in interstitial cystitis.[28]

The utility of bladder biopsy in patients with interstitial cystitis is controversial. In situ and invasive carcinoma of the bladder may be mistaken clinically for interstitial cystitis.[29–31] Some authors contend that the histopathologic findings are nonspecific and of limited value except to rule out carcinoma in situ.[30–32] Others believe that the histopathologic findings are useful in confirming the diagnosis.[33]

The majority of patients with the ulcer pattern of interstitial cystitis have ulcerations, marked inflammation, and granulation tissue (**Fig. 2-18**; **Table 2-2**). The inflammatory changes are almost always limited to the lamina propria.[34,35] The ulcerations are wedge-shaped and frequently filled with fibrin. Adjacent tissue may show marked chronic inflammation, composed principally of lymphocytes and plasma cells, often with germinal centers. In ulcer-type interstitial cystitis, mast cells are significantly increased in number in the lamina propria and the detrusor muscle. The urothelium is frequently denuded, detached, or floating above the surface. Mucosal denudation is more common in ulcer-type interstitial cystitis than in nonulcer interstitial cystitis, but is rare in patients without cystitis (**Fig. 2-19**).[33] Denudation may result from instrumentation, but the urothelium in interstitial cystitis is particularly

fragile, perhaps resulting from a type IV collagen defect in the urothelial basement membrane.[36] The lamina propria is edematous and contains dilated venules (**Fig. 2-20**). In about one-third of cases, abundant neutrophils in the venules show margination and involvement of the wall of the vein. Hemorrhage of the lamina propria is more marked in ulcer patients than in nonulcer patients

Table 2-2   Histologic Findings in Interstitial Cystitis

Classification of Interstitial Cystitis	No. Patients	Ulcer	Granulation Tissue	Mucosal Hemorrhage	Mucosal Rupture	Mononuclear Infiltrate				Perineural Infiltrate
						+	+	++	+++	
Ulcer (classic)	146	96%	89%	86%	0	0	11%	48%	41%	81%
Nonulcer (early)	64	0	0	89%	83%	77%	14%	9%	0	0

Source: Modified from Ref. 37.

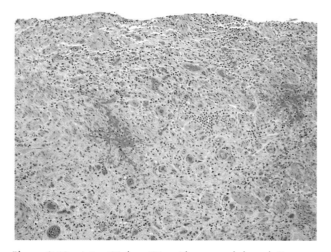

Figure 2-19   Interstitial cystitis with mucosal denudation.

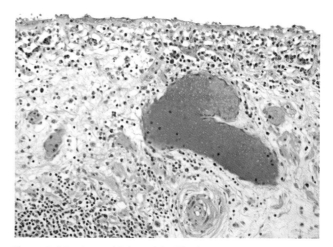

Figure 2-20   Interstitial cystitis. The lamina propria is edematous and vascular.

(**Fig. 2-21**). Eighty percent of patients have perineural inflammation, but this is also frequently seen in those with bladder cancer and is not specific for interstitial cystitis.[37] Granulation tissue probably results from rupture of the bladder mucosa during normal filling, with formation of reparative tissue. Significant fibrosis of the detrusor muscle is present in only 10% of cases, but is virtually never seen in nonulcer patients. One report described fibrosis with collagen distribution in a characteristic fashion within the muscle fascicles in interstitial cystitis, but this finding has not been confirmed.[38]

In contrast to ulcerative interstitial cystitis, nonulcerative interstitial cystitis shows very mild histopathologic changes. About 90% of cases display hemorrhage corresponding to the glomerulations.[37] This is usually focal, but may be extensive, sometimes with hemorrhage into the urothelium. Up to 83% of cases have mucosal rupture that only superficially involves the lamina propria and is not associated with inflammation. Rupture is associated with suburothelial hemorrhage and probably represents a defect in the urothelial lining.[37] The majority of nonulcerative interstitial cystitis patients have little or no inflammation, although edema and vascular congestion are frequently seen.

Mast cells are considered by some as a marker for interstitial cystitis,[39] but this has been refuted.[33,37] One study suggested that 28 mast cells per square millimeter in

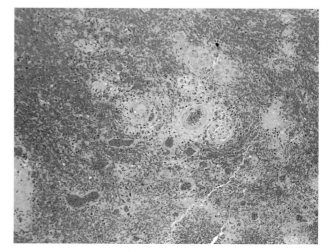

Figure 2-21   Interstitial cystitis with stromal hemorrhage.

the detrusor muscle was diagnostic of interstitial cystitis.[38] However, other authors found that control patients without interstitial cystitis had higher values.[33,37] Conventional toluidine blue stains and Giemsa stains are not adequate to identify all mast cells, according to some investigators, and they contend that it is necessary to fix tissues in isoosmotic formaldehyde/acetic acid.[40] This prevents initial aldehyde blocking, and subsequent staining with toluidine blue reveals a second population of mast cells, the so-called mucosal mast cells.[37]

In contrast with ulcerative (classic) interstitial cystitis, nonulcerative interstitial cystitis shows only mild histopathologic changes (**Fig. 2-22**). About 90% of cases display some urothelial hemorrhage corresponding to the glomerulations.[37] This is usually focal but may be extensive, sometimes with hemorrhage into the urothelium. Up to 83% of cases have mucosal rupture that only superficially involves the lamina propria and is not associated with inflammation; rupture is associated with suburothelial hemorrhage and probably represents a defect in the urothelial lining.[37] The majority of nonulcer cases have little or no inflammation, although edema and vascular congestion are frequently seen. Some patients with the nonulcer form of interstitial cystitis have a discontinuous uroplakin immunohistochemical staining at the level of superficial/umbrella cells of the urothelium, a finding of suggested diagnostic value that awaits confirmation. Uroplakin III-δ4, a splicing variant of uroplakin III, was significantly upregulated in interstitial cystitis, suggesting

that uroplakin III-δ4 is a potential marker for identifying nonulcerative interstitial cystitis.[41]

Tamm–Horsfall protein may be deposited in the epithelium and submucosa in patients with interstitial cystitis, indicating a barrier defect in this disease.[36,42–44]

Eosinophilic Cystitis

Eosinophilic cystitis is classified as allergic or nonallergic, depending on the likelihood of allergic etiology.[45] Other causative factors include atopic diseases, parasitic infection, systemic and topical agents such as mitomycin C,[46] and food allergy. Allergic eosinophilic cystitis occurs at any age, although more than 30% of cases occur in children. It is twice as likely in females. Patients typically have episodes of frequency, dysuria, and hematuria; many have a history of asthma or other allergic diseases, often with peripheral eosinophilia.[47] However, eosinophils are not always present in significant numbers in the urine or blood. The occasional polypoid growth may be cystoscopically mistaken for carcinoma[48] or, in a child, for sarcoma botryoides pattern of rhabdomyosarcoma.[49–54] Nodular and sessile growth with or without ulceration may also occur.[55] Microscopically, the lamina propria is typically edematous and chronically inflamed, with numerous eosinophils. Giant cells and granulomatous inflammation are occasionally present (**Figs. 2-23 and 2-24**).[52,56,57] The eosinophilic infiltrate is often transmural. Giemsa stain is useful for quantitating eosinophils.

In nonallergic eosinophilic cystitis, patients often have a history of transurethral resection with or without topical chemotherapy, but no history of allergy.[58] The typical patient is an elderly man with another urologic disorder, such as prostatic nodular hyperplasia or bladder cancer, who sustains bladder injury from instrumentation.[59,60] The cystoscopic findings are similar to those in allergic eosinophilic

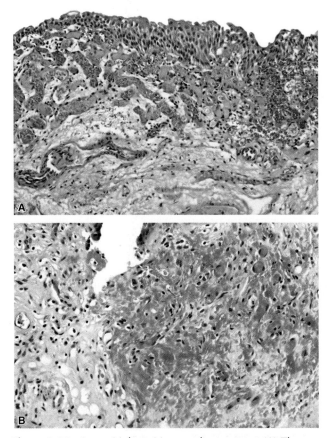

Figure 2-22 Interstitial cystitis, nonulcer pattern. (A) The urothelium is reactive, and there is prominent vascular congestion. (B) Glomerulation of the submucosa. Both have typical clinical features of interstitial cystitis.

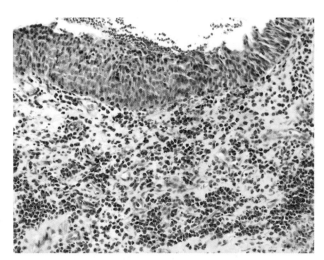

Figure 2-23 Eosinophilic cystitis. Note the prominent eosinophils in the urothelium and lamina propria.

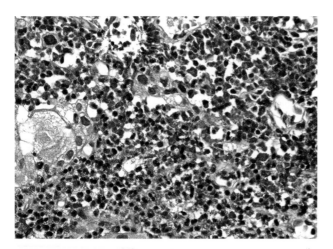

Figure 2-24 Eosinophilic cystitis.

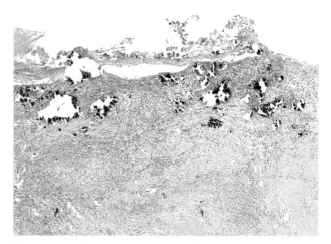

Figure 2-25 Encrusted cystitis. The histologic section is distorted by the mineralized debris.

cystitis, and the histologic pattern may be identical. Microscopically, necrosis and fibrosis of muscle are more common than in the allergic form.[61] The clinical significance of eosinophilic cystitis following transurethral resection of the bladder is uncertain.

Encrusted Cystitis

Encrusted cystitis is an uncommon condition that occurs when urea-splitting organisms alkalinize the urine, creating superficial deposits of inorganic salts.[62] Encrusted cystitis is more common in women and is associated with inflammatory or traumatic urothelial damage. Patients usually complain of urinary frequency, dysuria, and, commonly, of hematuria, associated with passage of gritty material, blood, mucus, and pus in the urine. In extensive cases in which salts are rich in calcium, encrusted cystitis may be detected radiographically.[62]

Macroscopically, there are single or multiple discrete exophytic or flat mineral deposits that are characteristically gritty. It is most common at the bladder base. In rare instances, encrusted cystitis may mimic a neoplasm.

Microscopically, calcified deposits are mixed with fibrin and necrotic debris on the mucosal surface or submucosa; muscle involvement is uncommon (**Figs. 2-25** and **2-26**). In early lesions, there may be prominent chronic inflammation, but the infiltrate is usually scant and there is a variable amount of fibrosis. Encrustation may also occur on the surface of a necrotic tumor or on necrotic tissue after a tumor has been fulgurated, sometimes masking the neoplasm, a critical factor in evaluating such cases.[63] Encrusted cystitis may be found in combination with malakoplakia.[64]

Emphysematous Cystitis

Emphysematous cystitis is an uncommon condition characterized by the presence of gas-filled vesicles that are visible

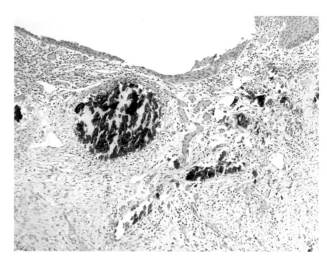

Figure 2-26 Encrusted cystitis. Note the thin overlying urothelium.

cystoscopically or on gross examination.[65] It is more common in women than in men, and 50% of patients are diabetic. Emphysematous cystitis is associated with a wide variety of infectious agents, including bacteria such as *E. coli* or *Aerobacter aerogenes*, and occasionally the fungus *Candida albicans*.[66,67] Macroscopically, these are small, thin-walled vesicles measuring between 0.5 and 3 cm in diameter that rupture easily and are most commonly seen within the lamina propria. Microscopically, these are small vesicular cysts lined by flattened cells surrounded by thin connective tissue septa in the lamina propria that may extend into the muscularis propria.[68] Frequently, there is an associated foreign body giant cell reaction.

Gangrenous Cystitis

This uncommon type of cystitis is typically found in elderly or debilitated patients, including those with compromised circulation and systemic infection.[69] There is often a urinary tract infection that progresses to diffuse gangrenous cystitis. No specific pathogen has been identified consistently, and the most likely cause is ischemia of variable severity or duration in combination with infection.[70,71] Virtually all of the bladder urothelium is necrotic and ulcerated, with blood clots and fibrinopurulent debris forming a membranous cast of the bladder lumen. The depth of necrosis into the bladder wall is variable but often involves the muscularis propria. Necrosis of blood vessels results in intramural and intraluminal hemorrhage.[72]

Hemorrhagic Cystitis

The classic cause of hemorrhagic cystitis is cyclophosphamide irritation (see also **Chapter 24**).[73-76] This chemotherapeutic agent was introduced in 1957 for the treatment of select types of leukemia but is now widely used for numerous malignancies as well as autoimmune disorders and organ transplantation.[73-76] Other causes include adenovirus type II and papovavirus, particularly in children.[77-80]

Patients note the sudden onset of dysuria and hematuria that is occasionally massive and intractable. There is no gender or age predominance, and it appears to be independent of the dose of cyclophosphamide administered. The histologic changes in hemorrhagic cystitis include severe edema, vascular telangiectasia, and hemorrhage within the lamina propria, usually associated with mucosal ulceration (**Figs. 2-27** and **2-28**). Intramural fibrosis is present in 25% of cases examined at autopsy. These reversible cytologic reparative abnormalities of the urothelial cells may be mistaken for malignancy, and a history of cyclophosphamide exposure is useful in avoiding this pitfall.[81] Hemorrhagic cystitis also occurs in patients treated with busulfan.[82]

Viral Cystitis

Human papillomavirus infection and condyloma acuminatum

Occasional cases of viral cystitis are associated with human papillomavirus infection (**Figs. 2-29** and **2-30**),[83] but, in our experience, this is extremely uncommon (see also **Chapter 14**).[84]

Viruses other than human papillomavirus

A variety of RNA and DNA viruses have been identified in bladder specimens. Patients are usually immunosuppressed or suffer from herpes genitalis.[85] The most commonly isolated viruses include adenovirus and papovavirus (hemorrhagic cystitis), herpes simplex virus type II, herpes zoster, and cytomegalovirus (**Figs. 2-31** to **2-33**), particularly in immunosuppressed children.[86-90] Polyomavirus infection may mimic high grade urothelial carcinoma of the bladder

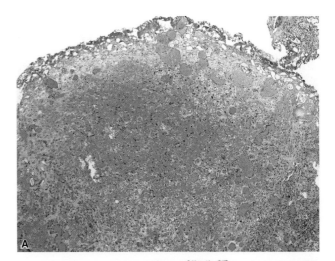
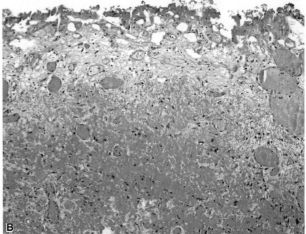

Figure 2-27   Hemorrhagic cystitis. This patient had bone marrow transplantation and chemotherapy for acute myeloid leukemia (A and B).

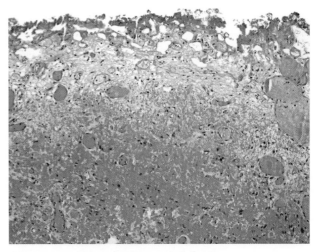

Figure 2-28   Hemorrhagic cystitis following cyclophosphamide therapy.

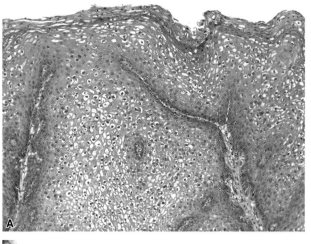

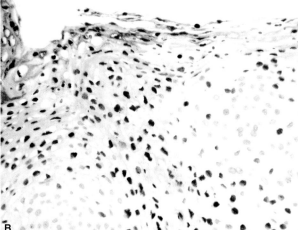

Figure 2-29 Condyloma acuminata of the urinary bladder (A). The infected cells are positive for human papillomavirus virus (B).

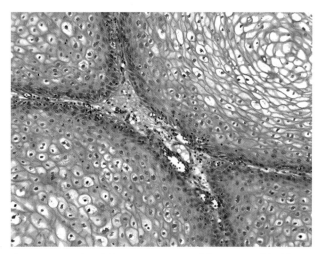

Figure 2-30 Condyloma acuminata of the urinary bladder. Note the koilocytic atypia.

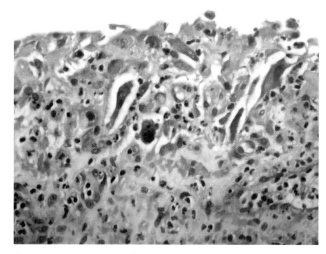

Figure 2-31 Cytomegalovirus cystitis.

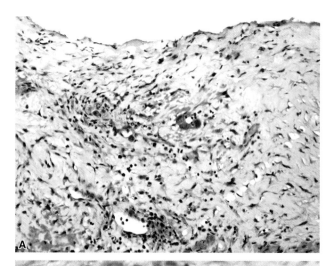

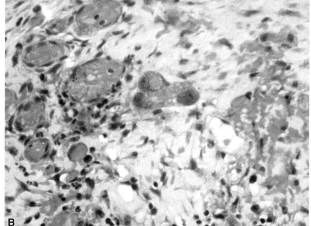

Figure 2-32 Cytomegalovirus cystitis (A and B).

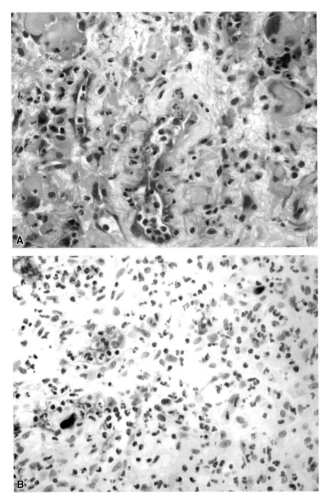

Figure 2-33   Cytomegalovirus cystitis (A and B). Scattered stromal cells are infected and positive for CMV immunostaining (B).

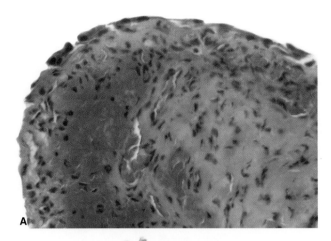

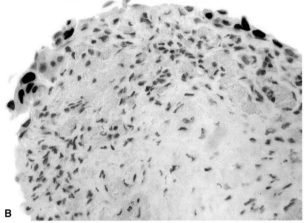

Figure 2-34   Polyomavirus infection in a 69-year-old renal transplant patient. This patient also has hemorrhagic cystitis (A). Immunostaining for BK virus is positive (B).

(**Figs. 2-34** and **2-35**).[91] Despite the frequency of viruria in patients with viral infections involving other organs or systemically, clinically significant viral infections of the bladder are rare, and histologic descriptions are sparse.[92]

Cystitis with Atypical Giant Stromal Cells

Giant cell cystitis should not be considered to be a distinct type of inflammation, but merely cystitis with a noticeable number of stromal giant cells (**Figs. 2-36** to **2-38**). Atypical mononucleated or multinucleated stromal cells are common in the lamina propria of the bladder, particularly in patients following instrumentation. These cells are also common in routine biopsies without obvious evidence of cystitis, and, when present in large numbers, may cause diagnostic difficulty.[17] The atypical cells may be stellate or elongate, with tapering eosinophilic cytoplasmic processes that simulate smooth and skeletal muscle cells. The nuclei are typically hyperchromatic and often irregular in size and

shape, but mitotic figures are not present. Similar cells are seen in patients treated with chemotherapeutic agents or radiation.

Denuding Cystitis

Denuding cystitis refers to a bladder lesion with extensive loss of the surface epithelium. It is often associated with urothelial carcinoma in situ.[93] Denuded epithelium also occurs frequently in association with many inflammatory conditions, including interstitial cystitis[94] or may be associated with instrumentation. Recognition of the denuding pattern of carcinoma in situ is important and should be considered in the differential diagnosis of any urinary bladder biopsy in which the urothelium is absent or fragmented (see also **Chapters 6** and **7**).[17,93,95,96]

Radiation Cystitis

A variety of abnormalities may be seen in the bladder as a result of radiation.[97–102] The earliest change, usually seen after 3 to 6 weeks, consists of acute cystitis

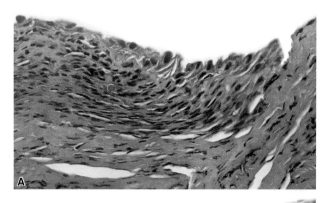

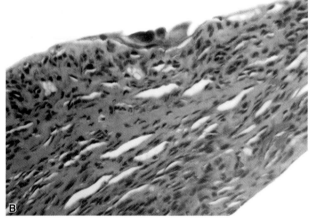

Figure 2-35 Polyomavirus infection (A and B).

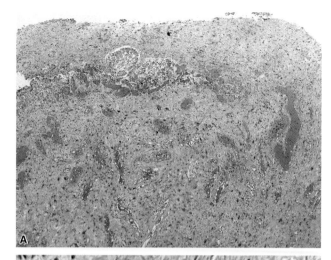

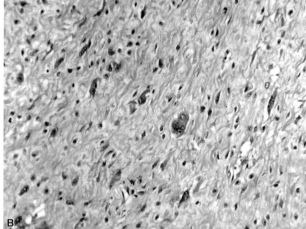

Figure 2-37 Giant cell cystitis (A and B).

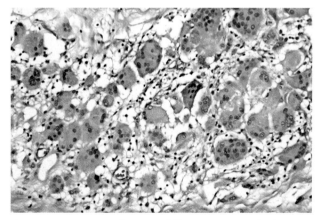

Figure 2-36 Giant cell cystitis following transurethral resection of the bladder for low grade papillary carcinoma.

with desquamation of urothelial cells and hyperemia and edema of the lamina propria (**Fig. 2-39**).[98] The urothelial cells show varying degrees of atypicality, including cytoplasmic and nuclear vacuolization, karyorrhexis, normal nuclear-to-cytoplasmic ratio, edema, prominent telangiectatic vessels, hyalinization, thrombosis of blood vessels, and atypical mesenchymal cells similar to those seen in giant cell cystitis (**Fig. 2-40**) (see also **Chapter 24**).[98–100]

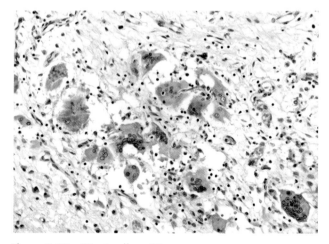

Figure 2-38 Giant cell cystitis.

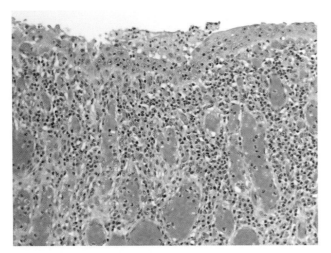

Figure 2-39 Radiation cystitis with acute inflammation, vascular congestion, and reactive atypia.

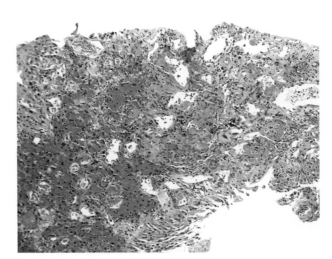

Figure 2-41 Radiation cystitis with pseudocarcinomatous epithelial proliferation.

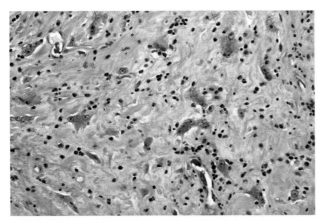

Figure 2-40 Radiation cystitis. Note the atypical stromal cells after radiation therapy.

A reactive, tumor-like epithelial proliferation, also called "pseudocarcinomatous epithelial proliferation," is seen in late phase of radiation cystitis, usually becoming evident months or years after radiation therapy. There is fibrosis of the lamina propria and/or muscularis propria, arteriolar mural thickening and hyalinization, and atypical and sometimes multinucleated stromal cells are features (**Fig. 2-41**) (see **Chapters 3** and **24** for further discussion).

Chemical Cystitis

See **Chapter 24** for further discussion.

Diverticulitis

A diverticulum may develop in the urinary bladder. It is invariably associated with chronic inflammation (**Fig. 2-42**) (see **Chapter 18** for further discussion).

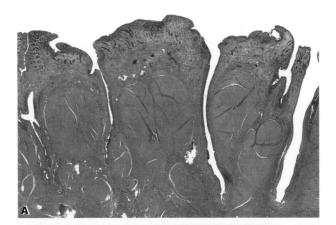

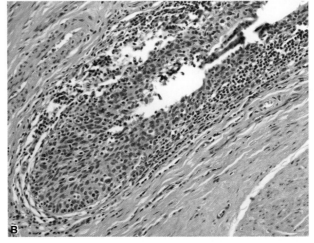

Figure 2-42 Chronic diverticulitis (A and B).

Granulomatous Cystitis

Postsurgical Necrobiotic Granuloma (Granuloma after Transurethral Resection)

Necrotizing palisading granulomas resembling rheumatoid nodule and foreign body-type granulomas commonly occur after biopsy or transurethral resection of the bladder, present in 13% of second resection specimens (**Figs. 2-43** and **2-44**).[103] The frequency with which granulomas occur increases with the number of surgical procedures. Necrotizing granulomas may be oval, linear, or serpiginous, often with a prominent infiltrate of eosinophils.[104] Granulomas may extend from the overlying ulcerated mucosa into the muscularis propria, eventually resulting in fibrous scarring and occasional dystrophic calcification.[103] Diathermy may induce antigenic changes in the collagen of the subepithelial connective tissue, inciting the granulomatous host response.[104]

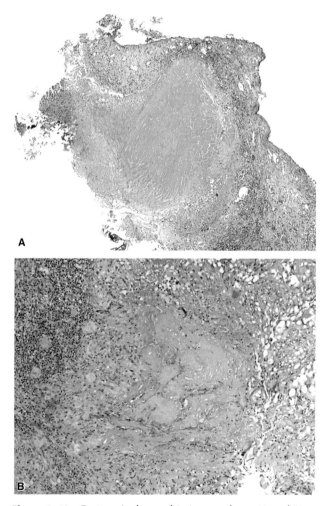

Figure 2-43 Postsurgical necrobiotic granuloma (A and B).

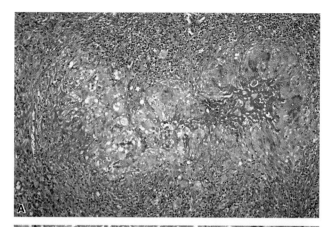

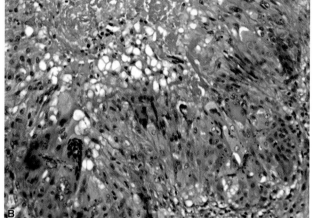

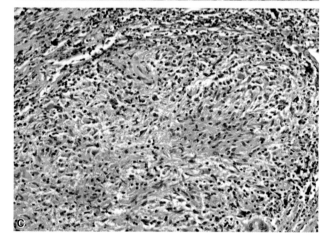

Figure 2-44 Granuloma after transurethral resection. The granulomas may be tightly cohesive (A and B) or poorly defined (C), invariably mixed with adjacent inflammation.

See **Chapter 24** for further discussion on treatment effects.

Suture Granuloma

Granulomas occasionally arise in response to silk sutures introduced at the time of herniorrhaphy or other surgical

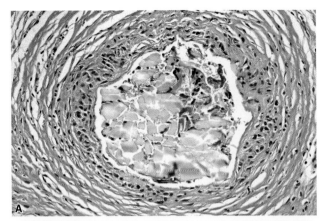

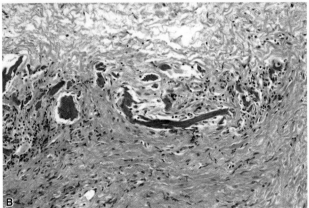

Figure 2-45   Suture granuloma, with residual foreign material eliciting a granulomatous response (A and B).

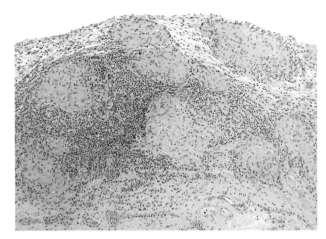

Figure 2-46   BCG-induced granuloma.

procedure, producing a mass in or adjacent to the bladder (**Fig. 2-45**).[105] In such cases, the herniorrhaphy is usually complicated by wound infection. The interval between herniorrhaphy and the appearance of the bladder mass was as long as 11 years in one case. Bladder neoplasm is the clinical impression in most of these cases, and the patients present with urinary symptoms, including hematuria, frequency, and dysuria.[106] The process primarily involves the bladder wall and perivesical tissue, producing an intraluminal mass visible at cystoscopy. Microscopically, there is a histiocytic reaction to suture with foreign body giant cells and varying degrees of fibrosis and chronic inflammation. We observed a case with prominent fibrosis associated with silk suture granuloma following diverticulectomy.

BCG-induced Granulomatous Cystitis

Bacillus Calmette–Guèrin (BCG), an attenuated strain of tubercle bacilli, is an effective topical therapeutic agent for noninvasive bladder cancer.[107–110] Indications for the use of BCG are similar to those for topical drugs, but this regimen is especially beneficial in patients with carcinoma in situ.

Pathologic changes associated with BCG are similar to those of tuberculous cystitis, including superficial ulceration with acute and chronic inflammation surrounding noncaseating granulomas (**Figs. 2-46** and **2-47**). A granulomatous reaction appears to correlate with BCG activity and may be an important indicator of tumor response. BCG may also produce a pattern of reactive epithelial atypia in association with denudation and ulceration of the urothelium.

See **Chapter 24** for further discussion.

Schistosomiasis (Bilharziasis)-associated Cystitis

Schistosomal disease of the urinary bladder induces a wide spectrum of histologic changes, including urothelial polyposis, ulceration, hyperplasia, metaplasia, dysplasia, and carcinoma (**Fig. 2-48**; **Tables 2-3** and **2-4**).[111–116] Schistosomal polyposis consists of multiple large inflammatory pseudopolyps resulting from heavy localized egg deposition during active disease. These lesions usually regress in the inactive stage of the disease. When polypoid, they may obstruct the urethral or ureteral orifices or may bleed, producing large obstructive clots and anemia. Approximately 30% of schistosomal polyps are found in inactive disease (**Figs 2-49** and **2-50**; **Table 2-4**) and appear as fibrocalcific outgrowths representing the remains of granulomatous polyps.[117] Five percent of schistosomal polyps are composed of hyperplastic epithelium. However, almost 60% of polypoid lesions of the urinary bladder in patients with schistosomiasis are due to causes other than egg deposition of the parasite, including nonspecific cystitis and edema (polypoid or bullous cystitis).

In the schistosomal bladder, ulcers occur in the active and chronic stages. Those that form during the early active stage are rare, occurring when a necrotic polyp sloughs into the urine. Those that form in the chronic stage are more common, and heavy infection produces constant, deep, "hard" pelvic pain, owing to the presence of greater than

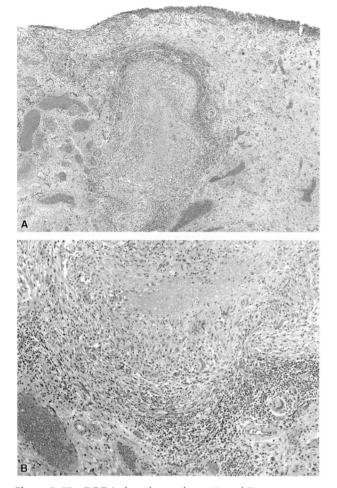

Figure 2-47   BCG-induced granuloma (A and B).

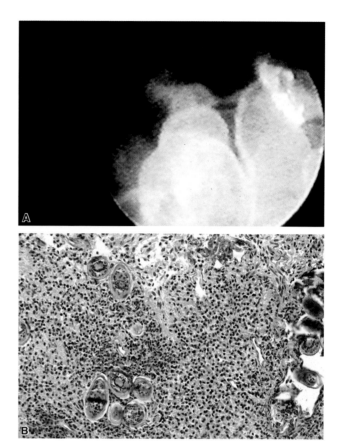

Figure 2-48   Schistosomiasis of the bladder. Cystoscopic appearance of urothelial polyposis in a 9-year-old boy (A). Characteristic eggs are present in association with prominent chronic inflammation (B).

250,000 eggs per gram of bladder tissue. Chronic ulcers are located at or near the posterior midsagittal line of the bladder and may be stellate or ovoid. They usually occur in young patients, with a mean age of 29 years, suggesting that they result from rapid accumulation of eggs.

The spectrum of urothelial proliferation includes hyperplastic squamous epithelium that is often keratinized. Hyperplasia associated with severe urinary schistosomiasis is seen in all stages of disease, although most commonly in the late stages. Dysplastic changes may accompany squamous metaplasia similar to the uterine cervix, but this is inconstant.

Urinary schistosomiasis may also cause bladder cancer. In endemic regions, schistosomiasis-induced bladder cancer is the most common malignant tumor. This cancer is found in a younger age group than that of other forms of bladder cancer (mean age, 46 years), is more common in women than in men, and is rare in the trigone.[118] Gross hematuria is less frequent than in patients with typical bladder cancer. Irritative symptoms are common, and white flakes of keratin may be passed in the urine; bladder calcification

Table 2-3   **Histopathologic Grading of Schistosomal Urinary Bladder Disease**

Grade	Criteria
I	Occasional eggs in lamina propria
II	Lamina propria filled with eggs; no involvement of detrusor muscle
IIIa	Lamina propria filled with eggs; involvement of superficial one-third of detrusor muscle
IIIb	Lamina propria filled with eggs; involvement of external two-thirds of detrusor muscle

is sometimes seen on radiographs. These patients have a higher frequency of squamous cell carcinoma and adenocarcinoma than do patients without schistosomiasis; the remaining patients who do not have squamous cell carcinoma or adenocarcinoma have urothelial or undifferentiated carcinoma. Squamous cell carcinoma in these patients is usually low grade, may be verrucous, and has a better

Table 2-4 Comparison of Active and Inactive Schistosomiasis[a]

Feature	Active	Inactive
Adult worm pairs	+	−
Oviposition	+	−
Urinary egg excretion	+	−
Important in transmission	+	−
Granulomatous host response	+	−
Polypoid lesions	+ (Possibly obstructive)	Very rare
Sandy patches	+ (In late active)	+ (Possibly obstructive)
Cause of obstructive uropathy	Polypoid lesions	Sandy patches
Schistosomal ulceration	Uncommon	Common
Treatment	Chemotherapy	Surgical repair

[a]+, present; −, absent.

prognosis than non—*Schistosoma*-induced squamous cell carcinoma, which is often high grade.[118]

Malakoplakia

Malakoplakia is an uncommon inflammatory condition that usually affects the urinary tract, with a predilection for the urinary bladder.[119,120] The term "malakoplakia," derived from the Greek, means "soft plaque." Urinary tract malakoplakia primarily affects women (75% of cases), with a peak incidence in the fifth decade; in men, it peaks in the seventh decade. There is a strong association with infection by coliform organisms, particularly *E. coli*, with impairment of intracellular capacity of mononuclear cells to kill bacteria.[121] Patients with vesicular malakoplakia present with symptoms and signs of urinary tract infection, and hematuria is also common. Occasionally, it appears in patients receiving immunosuppressive therapy.[122] Urine cultures most often yield *E. coli*, but *Proteus vulgaris*, *Aerobacter aerogenes*, α-hemolytic streptococci, *Klebsiella pneumoniae*, and other organisms have also been isolated. Intracellular bacilliform organisms have been found by transmission electron microscopy.[110,111]

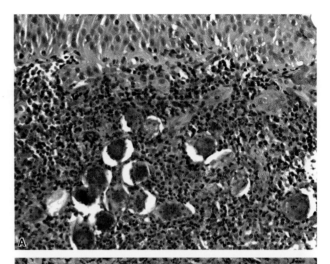
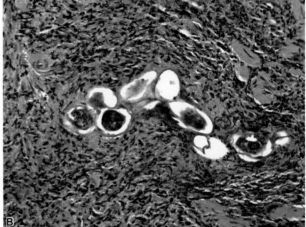

Figure 2-49 Schistosomiasis of the bladder (A and B).

Macroscopically, malakoplakia consists of multiple soft yellow or yellow-brown plaques, nodules, or papillary or polypoid masses usually measuring less than 2 cm in diameter (**Fig. 2-51**). Central umbilication and a hyperemic rim are common. When large and necrotic, malakoplakia may be mistaken for carcinoma.[123]

Microscopically, it is characterized by submucosal accumulation of macrophages with eccentric nuclei and granular eosinophilic cytoplasm (von Hansemann cells) (**Fig. 2-52**).[124] Diagnostic intracytoplasmic inclusion bodies, Michaelis–Gutmann bodies, consist of round targetoid ("bull's-eye") calcospherites, 5 to 8 μm in diameter. Frequently, these bodies are basophilic, but sometimes they are pale and difficult to see in routine preparations. Michaelis–Gutmann bodies are brilliantly periodic acid–Schiff positive and diastase resistant, and contain calcium and, frequently, iron salts; consequently, they give positive reactions with the von Kossa technique and Perls Prussian blue stain.[125] Michaelis–Gutmann bodies are not always conspicuous, particularly in the early stages of malakoplakia, and aggregates of macrophages without

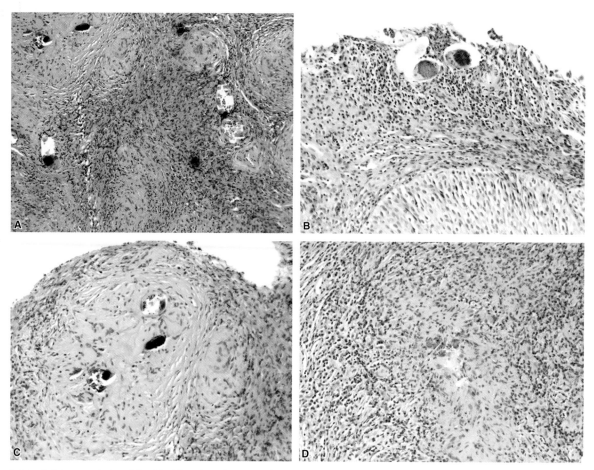

Figure 2-50   Schistosomiasis of the bladder (A to D). Note the prominent eosinophils and granulomatous inflammation (D).

Michaelis–Gutmann bodies may represent a prediagnostic phase. In some cases, there is granulation tissue, extensive fibrosis, and marked acute inflammation that may obscure the histiocytic nature of the process.[123] Malakoplakia may also contain foreign bodies or Langhans-type giant cells and lymphoid follicles at the edge.[121] The main differential diagnostic considerations are carcinoma with inflammatory stroma and xanthogranulomatous cystitis.[27,115]

Tuberculosis

Tuberculous cystitis is usually caused by *Mycobacterium tuberculosis*, although *Mycobacterium bovis* accounts for up to 3% of cases.[126] Bladder involvement is a secondary event, occurring in 1% of patients with genitourinary tuberculosis and in about 65% of patients who undergo nephrectomy for renal involvement. Patients characteristically have frequency, dysuria, hematuria, and urgency. The organisms implant in the vesical mucosa, often around the ureteral orifices via infected urine from the upper urinary tract. The initial microscopic changes occur around the ureteral orifices, and the earliest mucosal abnormality is marked hyperemia, sometimes with edema. The lesions progress to

form discrete tubercles measuring up to 3 mm in diameter that may ulcerate and become covered with friable necrotic debris. Occasionally, there is exuberant granulation tissue forming polypoid excrescences that macroscopically may be mistaken for carcinoma. The tubercles are sharply circumscribed and initially firm and solid; as they enlarge, they often coalesce and undergo central ulceration.

Microscopically, the tuberculous granuloma consists of an aggregate of epithelioid histiocytes with central caseous necrosis and variable numbers of multinucleated giant cells, plasma cells, lymphocytes, and circumferential fibrosis. Occasionally, caseating necrosis is absent, and the granulomas are not well formed; despite this, tuberculosis should still be strongly suspected with granulomatous inflammation, and efforts made to demonstrate mycobacteria.[63]

Xanthoma and Xanthogranulomatous Cystitis

Idiopathic cystitis consisting chiefly of sheets of vacuolated or foamy histiocytes is referred to as xanthoma or xanthogranulomatous cystitis, depending on the amount of associated inflammation (**Figs. 2-53** to **2-55**). This lesion

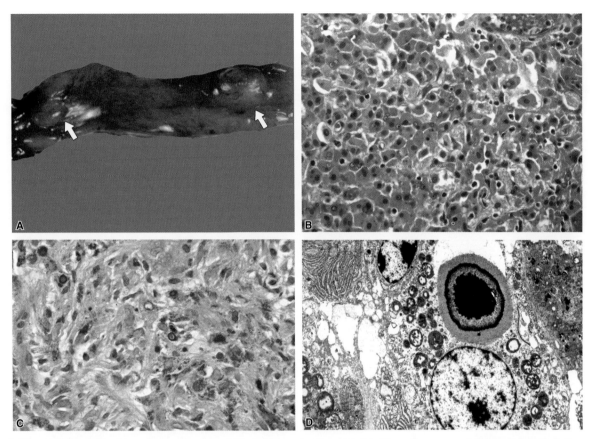

Figure 2-51 Malakoplakia. Note the mucosal nodules in the ureter (arrows) (A). The submucosa contains a chronic inflammatory infiltrate with abundant Michaelis–Gutmann bodies (B). The periodic acid–Schiff stain highlights the mineralized and nonmineralized targetoid bodies (C). Ultrastructure with a large round laminated mineralized cytoplasmic body (D).

is rare, and may occur in patients with recurrent urinary tract infections. Transmural involvement was described in one case.[127]

Xanthogranulomatous cystitis may represent an early phase of malakoplakia. It should be noted that large numbers of xanthoma cells may rarely be seen in association with bladder cancer.[128–130] Foamy histiocytes often accumulate within the fibrovascular cores of papillomas and low grade papillary carcinomas of the bladder. Xanthomas can be identified by cold-cup biopsy (**Figs. 2-56** and **2-57**),[131] and stromal aggregates of xanthoma cells have rarely been described in a fibroepithelial polyp of the ureter.[132]

Other Forms of Granulomatous Cystitis

Chronic granulomatous disease of childhood rarely affects the bladder, consisting of sheets of histiocytes, foreign body giant cells, and neutrophils.[133]

The bladder is occasionally involved in autoimmune diseases such as systemic lupus erythematosus, Wegener granulomatosis, Steven–Johnson syndrome, pemphigus vulgaris, lichen planus, and rheumatoid arthritis (**Fig. 2-58**).[134] Patients with BCG instillation following

bladder cancer have florid granulomatous inflammation in bladder biopsies.[107,135,136] Granulomas were found in the bladder wall fistula in a patient with Crohn disease. Sarcoidosis may involve the urinary bladder.[137] Periurethral and submucosal bladder neck injections of Teflon paste (polytetrafluoroethylene), used to treat urinary incontinence, sometimes result in an exuberant foreign body giant cell reaction with granulomas and stromal fibrosis.[138] Histologically, refractile aggregates of Teflon are readily identified, particularly with polarization.[139]

Other Infectious Cystitides

Fungal Cystitis

Candida albicans is the most common fungal cause of cystitis, but *Candida* cystitis is relatively uncommon.[140] Bladder involvement may occur from urethral spread or as part of hematogenous spread. Infection is usually restricted to the trigone. *Candida* cystitis usually occurs more in debilitated or immunocompromised patients than in those on

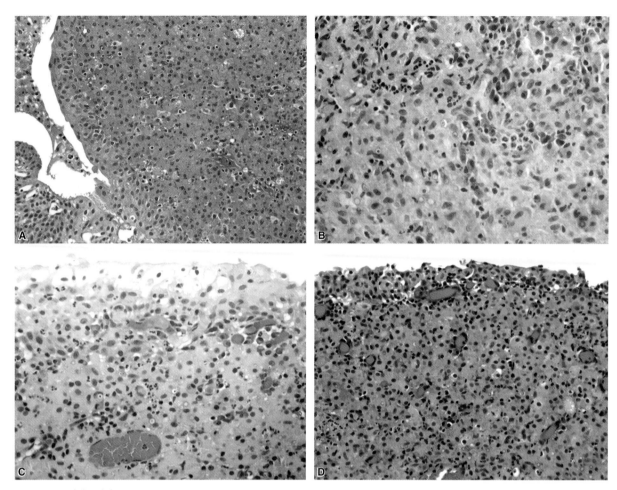

Figure 2-52   Malakoplakia (A to D).

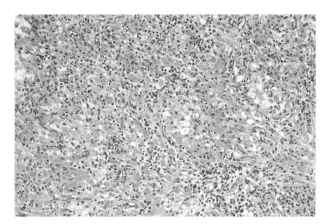

Figure 2-53   Idiopathic xanthogranulomatous cystitis in a transurethral resection specimen.

antibiotic therapy. Also, it is more frequent in patients with diabetes mellitus, particularly women.

Symptoms of *Candida* cystitis include nocturia, unremitting pain or discomfort, and increased frequency. The urine is often turbid or bloody. Macroscopically, the mucosa is irregular and slightly elevated, with sharply demarcated adherent white plaques that bleed when removed. Diffuse erythema is occasionally present. Large luminal fungus balls are rarely observed.[141]

Microscopically, the urothelium is ulcerated, and the submucosa is inflamed. Some patients have emphysematous or gangrenous cystitis. Typical fungal spores and hyphae are present within fibrinopurulent debris, often in large numbers. Other rare forms of fungal cystitis are caused by *Torulopsis glabrata*, *Aspergillus* species, and *Coccidioides immitis*.[142]

Actinomycosis

Actinomycosis of the bladder is rare and usually results from extension from adjacent organs such as the fallopian tube or ovary. Infection can also descend from the upper urinary tract or spread hematogenously.[143] Macroscopically, the bladder wall is usually focally or diffusely thickened. A localized mass simulating a bladder tumor or urachal tumor may be present.[144,145] The mucosa is often ulcerated and edematous. Transmural necrosis

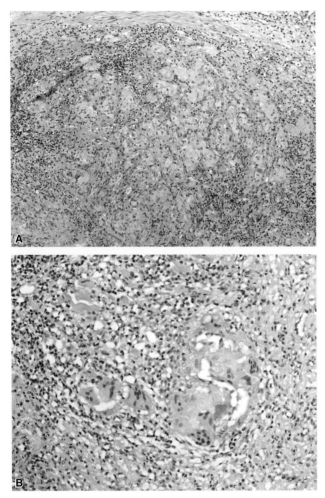

Figure 2-54   Xanthogranulomatous cystitis (A and B).

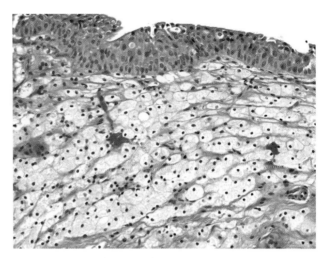

Figure 2-56   Xanthoma of the urinary bladder.

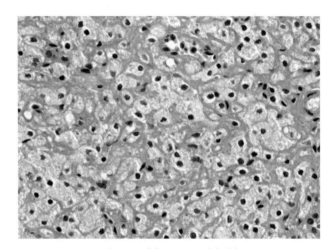

Figure 2-57   Xanthoma of the urinary bladder.

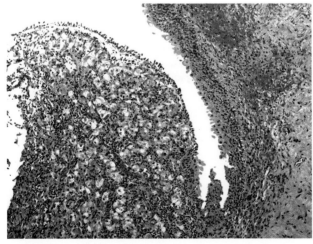

Figure 2-55   Xanthogranulomatous cystitis with polypoid configuration, mimicking cancer.

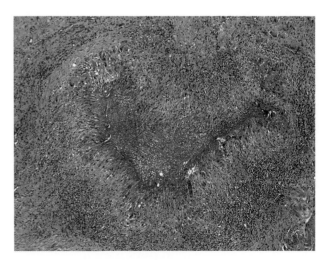

Figure 2-58   Necrotizing palisading granuloma.

often creates fistulae. Microscopically, the submucosa and muscularis propria contain abundant granulation tissue and numerous abscesses of variable size. "Sulfur granules" are present, consisting of masses of filamentous bacteria with a peripheral array of swollen eosinophilic "clubs." Periodic acid–Schiff and silver stains are helpful in recognizing these distinctive organisms.

Miscellaneous Infectious Cystitides

Uncommon infections of the bladder include trichomonal cystitis, hydatid cystitis, syphilis, and amebiasis. Trichomonal cystitis, due to *Trichomonas vaginalis* infection, is usually limited to the trigone and results from retrograde extension from the posterior urethra in women. In hydatid disease, the upper urinary tract becomes infected with the ova of *Echinococcus granulosa* during hematogenous spread, and typical cysts form. Rupture of these cysts leads to the discharge of their contents into the lower urinary tract and subsequent infection of the bladder.

Syphilis of the urinary bladder is extremely rare and may occur in secondary or tertiary syphilis. The gummas are usually located near the urethral orifice and are typically single.

Infection of the bladder by *Entamoeba histolytica* (amebic cystitis) is rare, usually following colonic involvement in which the trophozoites perforate through the colonic wall and invade contiguous structures. Hematogenous spread typically involves the liver and rarely involves the urinary bladder, where lesions are concentrated in the trigone. Microscopically, there are varying degrees of chronic inflammation. The diagnosis is based on recognition of trophozoites in tissue sections, and this is facilitated by using the periodic acid–Schiff stain.

Early experimental studies suggested that *Helicobacter pylori* may be a pathogen in the urinary bladder and renal pelvis, but this has not been confirmed in human studies.[146]

Pseudomembranous trigonitis, a curious disease that presents in women with the urethral syndrome, consists of vaginal-type glycogenated squamous metaplasia of the trigone associated with edema and vascular dilatation, but no significant inflammation.[147,148] It remains unclear if pseudomembranous trigonitis exists as an entity or if it represents a nonspecific reactive finding.

Extremely uncommon lesions of the bladder may be caused by microfilariae (*Wuchereria bancrofti*), myiasis (infestation with fly larvae), or Candiru, a tiny catfish living in the Amazon river.[149]

REFERENCES

1. Young RH. Non-neoplastic disorders of the urinary bladder. In: Bostwick DG, Cheng L, eds. Urologic Surgical Pathology, 2nd ed. Philadelphia: Elsevier/Mosby, 2008; 215–58.
2. Fukushi Y, Orikasa S, Kagayama M. An electron microscopic study of the interaction between vesical epithelium and *E. coli*. *Invest Urol* 1979;17:61–8.
3. Parsons CL, Mulholland SG. Bladder surface mucin. Its antibacterial effect against various bacterial species. *Am J Pathol* 1978;93:423–32.
4. Menon EB, Tan ES. Urinary tract infection in acute spinal cord injury. *Singapore Med J* 1992;33:359–61.
5. O'Neill GF. Tiaprofenic acid as a cause of non-bacterial cystitis. *Med J Aust* 1994;160:123–5.
6. Marsh FP, Banerjee R, Panchamia P. The relationship between urinary infection, cystoscopic appearance, and pathology of the bladder in man. *J Clin Pathol* 1974;27:297–307.
7. Algaba F. Papillo-polypoid cystitis. Focal cystitis with pseudoneoplastic aspect. *Actas Urol Esp* 1991;15:260–4.
8. Buck EG. Polypoid cystitis mimicking transitional cell carcinoma. *J Urol* 1984;131:963.
9. Lane Z, Epstein JI. Polypoid/papillary cystitis: a series of 41 cases misdiagnosed as papillary urothelial neoplasia. *Am J Surg Pathol* 2008;32:758–64.
10. Young RH. Papillary and polypoid cystitis. A report of eight cases. *Am J Surg Pathol* 1988;12:542–6.
11. Delnay KM, Stonehill WH, Goldman H, Jukkola AF, Dmochowski RR. Bladder histological changes associated with chronic indwelling urinary catheter. *J Urol* 1999;161:1106–8; discussion 1108–9.
12. Milles G. Catheter-induced hemorrhagic pseudopolyps of the urinary bladder. *JAMA* 1965;193:968–9.
13. Ekelund P, Johansson S. Polypoid cystitis: a catheter associated lesion of the human bladder. *Acta Pathol Microbiol Scand [A]* 1979;87A:179–84.
14. Ekelund P, Anderstrom C, Johansson SL, Larsson P. The reversibility of catheter-associated polypoid cystitis. *J Urol* 1983;130:456–9.
15. Johnson DE, Lockatell CV, Hall-Craggs M, Warren JW. Mouse models of short- and long-term foreign body in the urinary bladder: analogies to the bladder segment of urinary catheters. *Lab Anim Sci* 1991;41:451–5.
16. Cheng L, Bostwick DG. Overdiagnosis of bladder carcinoma. *Anal Quant Cytol Histol* 2008;30:261–4.
17. Grignon DJ, Sakr W. Inflammatory and other conditions that can mimic carcinoma in the urinary bladder. *Pathol Annu* 1995;30 (Pt 1): 95–122.

18. Sarma KP. On the nature of cystitis follicularis. *J Urol* 1970;104: 709–14.

19. Santamaria M, Molina I, Munoz E, Lopez A, Toro M, Pena J. Identification and characterization of a human cell line with dendritic cell features. *Virchows Arch B Cell Pathol Incl Mol Pathol* 1988;56:77–83.

20. van de Merwe JP, Nordling J, Bouchelouche P, Bouchelouche K, Cervigni M, Daha LK, Elneil S, Fall M, Hohlbrugger G, Irwin P, Mortensen S, van Ophoven A, Osborne JL, Peeker R, Richter B, Riedl C, Sairanen J, Tinzl M, Wyndaele JJ. Diagnostic criteria, classification, and nomenclature for painful bladder syndrome/interstitial cystitis: an ESSIC proposal. *Eur Urol* 2008;53:60–7.

21. Erickson DR, Simon LJ, Belchis DA. Relationships between bladder inflammation and other clinical features in interstitial cystitis. *Urology* 1994;44:655–9.

22. Hukkanen V, Haarala M, Nurmi M, Klemi P, Kiilholma P. Viruses and interstitial cystitis: adenovirus genomes cannot be demonstrated in urinary bladder biopsies. *Urol Res* 1996;24:235–8.

23. Koziol DE, Saah AJ, Odaka N, Munoz A. A comparison of risk factors for human immunodeficiency virus and hepatitis B virus infections in homosexual men. *Ann Epidemiol* 1993;3:434–41.

24. MacDermott JP, Charpied GC, Tesluk H, Stone AR. Can histological assessment predict the outcome in interstitial cystitis? *Br J Urol* 1991;67:44–7.

25. Ratliff TL, Klutke CG, Hofmeister M, He F, Russell JH, Becich MJ. Role of the immune response in interstitial cystitis. *Clin Immunol Immunopathol* 1995;74:209–16.

26. Ratliff TL, Klutke CG, McDougall EM. The etiology of interstitial cystitis. *Urol Clin North Am* 1994;21:21–30.

27. Hunner GL. A rare type of bladder ulcer in women: report of cases. *Southern Med J*. 1915;8:410.

28. Messing EM, Stamey TA. Interstitial cystitis: early diagnosis, pathology, and treatment. *Urology* 1978;12:381–92.

29. Lamm DL, Gittes RF. Inflammatory carcinoma of the bladder and interstitial cystitis. *J Urol* 1977;117:49–51.

30. Utz DC, Zincke H. The masquerade of bladder cancer in situ as interstitial cystitis. *J Urol* 1974;111:160–1.

31. Moloney PJ, Elliott GB, McLaughlin M, Sinclair AB. In situ transitional carcinoma and the non-specifically inflamed contracting bladder. *J Urol* 1974;111:162–4.

32. Van de Merwe J, Kamerling R, Arendsen E, Mulder D, Hooijkaas H. Sjogren's syndrome in patients with interstitial cystitis. *J Rheumatol* 1993;20:962–6.

33. Lynes WL, Flynn SD, Shortliffe LD, Lemmers M, Zipser R, Roberts LJ 2nd, Stamey TA. Mast cell involvement in interstitial cystitis. *J Urol* 1987;138:746–52.

34. Bohne AW, Hodson JM, Rebuck JW, Reinhard RE. An abnormal leukocyte response in interstitial cystitis. *J Urol* 1962;88:387–91.

35. Lynes WL, Flynn SD, Shortliffe LD, Stamey TA. The histology of interstitial cystitis. *Am J Surg Pathol* 1990;14:969–76.

36. Wilson CB, Leopard J, Nakamura RM, Cheresh DA, Stein PC, Parsons CL. Selective type IV collagen defects in the urothelial basement membrane in interstitial cystitis. *J Urol* 1995;154:1222–6.

37. Johansson SL, Fall M. Pathology of interstitial cystitis. *Urol Clin North Am* 1994;21:55–62.

38. Larsen S, Thompson SA, Hald T, Barnard RJ, Gilpin CJ, Dixon JS, Gosling JA. Mast cells in interstitial cystitis. *Br J Urol* 1982;54:283–6.

39. Sant GR, Theoharides TC. The role of the mast cell in interstitial cystitis. *Urol Clin North Am* 1994;21:41–53.

40. Christmas TJ, Rode J. Characteristics of mast cells in normal bladder, bacterial cystitis and interstitial cystitis. *Br J Urol* 1991;68:473–8.

41. Zeng Y, Wu XX, Homma Y, Yoshimura N, Iwaki H, Kageyama S, Yoshiki T, Kakehi Y. Uroplakin III-delta4 messenger RNA as a promising marker to identify nonulcerative interstitial cystitis. *J Urol* 2007;178:1322–7.

42. Fowler JE Jr, Lynes WL, Lau JL, Ghosh L, Mounzer A. Interstitial cystitis is associated with intraurothelial Tamm-Horsfall protein. *J Urol* 1988;140:1385–9.

43. Bushman W, Goolsby C, Grayhack JT, Schaeffer AJ. Abnormal flow cytometry profiles in patients with interstitial cystitis. *J Urol* 1994;152:2262–6.

44. Neal DE Jr, Dilworth JP, Kaack MB. Tamm-Horsfall autoantibodies in interstitial cystitis. *J Urol* 1991;145:37–9.

45. Rubin L, Pincus MB. Eosinophilic cystitis: the relationship of allergy in the urinary tract to eosinophilic cystitis and the pathophysiology of eosinophilia. *J Urol* 1974;112:457–60.

46. Ulker V, Apaydin E, Gursan A, Ozyurt C, Kandiloglu G. Eosinophilic cystitis induced by mitomycin-C. *Int Urol Nephrol* 1996;28:755–9.

47. Gregg JA, Utz DC. Eosinophilic cystitis associated with eosinophilic gastroenteritis. *Mayo Clin Proc* 1974;49:185–7.

48. Constantinides C, Gavras P, Stinios J, Apostolaki C, Dimopoulos C. Eosinophilic cystitis: a rare case which presented as an invasive bladder tumor. *Acta Urol Belg* 1994;62:71–3.

49. Barry KA, Jafri SZ. Eosinophilic cystitis: CT findings. *Abdom Imaging* 1994;19:272–3.

50. Goldstein M. Eosinophilic cystitis. *J Urol* 1971;106:854–7.

51. Hansen MV, Kristensen PB. Eosinophilic cystitis simulating invasive bladder carcinoma. *Scand J Urology Nephrol* 1993;27:275–7.

52. Ladocsi LT, Sullivan B, Hanna MK. Eosinophilic granulomatous cystitis in children. *Urology* 1995;46:732–5.

53. Littleton RH, Farah RN, Cerny JC. Eosinophilic cystitis: an uncommon form of cystitis. *J Urol* 1982;127:132–3.

54. Rosenberg HK, Eggli KD, Zerin JM, Ortega W, Wallach MT, Kolberg H, Lebowitz RL, Snyder HM. Benign cystitis in children mimicking rhabdomyosarcoma. *J Ultrasound Med* 1994;13:921–32.

55. Peterson NE. Eosinophilic cystitis. *Urology* 1985;26:167–9.

56. Antonakopoulos GN, Newman J. Eosinophilic cystitis with giant cells. A light microscopic and ultrastructural study. *Arch Pathol Lab Med* 1984;108:728–31.

57. Brown EW. Eosinophilic granuloma of the bladder. *J Urol* 1960;83:665–8.

58. Choe JM, Kirkemo AK, Sirls LT. Intravesical thiotepa-induced eosinophilic cystitis. *Urology* 1995;46:729–31.

59. Castillo J Jr, Cartagena R, Montes M. Eosinophilic cystitis: a therapeutic challenge. *Urology* 1988;32:535–7.

60. Mitas JA 2nd, Thompson T. Ureteral involvement complicating eosinophilic cystitis. *Urology* 1985;26:67–70.

61. Hellstrom HR, Davis BK, Shonnard JW. Eosinophilic cystitis. A study of 16 cases. *Am J Clin Pathol* 1979;72:777–84.

62. Estorc JJ, de La Coussaye JE, Viel EJ, Bouziges N, Ramuz M, Eledjam JJ. Teicoplanin treatment of alkaline encrusted cystitis due to *Corynebacterium* group D2. *Eur J Med* 1992;1:183–4.

63. Young RH. Non-neoplastic epithelial abnormalities and tumor-like lesions. Pathology of the Urinary Bladder. New York: Churchill Livingstone, 1989:1–63.

64. Berney DM, Thompson I, Sheaff M, Baithun SI. Alkaline encrusted cystitis associated with malakoplakia. *Histopathology* 1996;28:253–6.

65. Bailey H. Cystitis emphysematosa; 19 cases with intraluminal and interstitial collections of gas. *Am J Roentgenol Radium Ther Nucl Med* 1961;86:850–62.

66. Bartkowski DP, Lanesky JR. Emphysematous prostatitis and cystitis secondary to *Candida albicans*. *J Urol* 1988;139:1063–5.

67. Maliwan N. Emphysematous cystitis associated with *Clostridium perfringens* bacteremia. *J Urol* 1979;121:819–20.

68. Hawtrey CE, Williams JJ, Schmidt JD. Cystitis emphysematosa. *Urology* 1974;3:612–4.

69. Moncada I, Lledo E, Verdu F, Hernandez C. Re: Gangrenous cystitis: case report and review of the literature. *J Urol* 1994;152:492.

70. Dao AH. Gangrenous cystitis in chronic alcohol abuse. *J Tenn Med Assoc* 1994;87:51–2.

71. Devitt AT, Sethia KK. Gangrenous cystitis: case report and review of the literature. *J Urol* 1993;149:1544–5.

72. Stirling WC, Hopkins G, A. Gangrene of the bladder, review of two hundred seven cases; report of two personal cases. *J Urol* 1934;31:517–25.

73. Cox PJ, Abel G. Cyclophosphamide cystitis. Studies aimed at its minimization. *Biochem Pharmacol* 1979;28:3499–502.

74. deVries CR, Freiha FS. Hemorrhagic cystitis: a review. *J Urol* 1990;143:1–9.

75. Marshall FF, Klinefelter HF. Late hemorrhagic cystitis following low-dose cyclophosphamide therapy. *Urology* 1979;14:573–5.

76. Stillwell TJ, Benson RC Jr. Cyclophosphamide-induced hemorrhagic cystitis. A review of 100 patients. *Cancer* 1988;61:451–7.

77. Ambinder RF, Burns W, Forman M, Charache P, Arthur R, Beschorner W, Santos G, Saral R. Hemorrhagic cystitis associated with adenovirus infection in bone marrow transplantation. *Arch Intern Med* 1986;146:1400–1.

78. Arthur RR, Shah KV, Baust SJ, Santos GW, Saral R. Association of BK viruria with hemorrhagic cystitis in recipients of bone marrow transplants. *N Engl J Med* 1986;315:230–4.

79. Numazaki Y, Shigeta S, Kumasaka T, Miyazawa T, Yamanaka M, Yano N, Takai S, Ishida N. Acute hemorrhagic cystitis in children. Isolation of adenovirus type II. *N Engl J Med* 1968;278:700–4.

80. Shindo K, Kitayama T, Ura T, Matsuya F, Kusaba Y, Kanetake H, Saito Y. Acute hemorrhagic cystitis caused by adenovirus type 11 after renal transplantation. *Urol Int* 1986;41:152–5.

81. Koss LG. Errors and pitfalls in cytology of the lower urinary tract. *Monogr Pathol* 1997:60–74.

82. Pode D, Perlberg S, Steiner D. Busulfan-induced hemorrhagic cystitis. *J Urol* 1983;130:347–8.

83. Shibutani YF, Schoenberg MP, Carpiniello VL, Malloy TR. Human papillomavirus associated with bladder cancer. *Urology* 1992;40:15–17.

84. Lopez-Beltran A, Munoz E. Transitional cell carcinoma of the bladder: low incidence of human papillomavirus DNA detected by the polymerase chain reaction and in situ hybridization. *Histopathology* 1995;26:565–9.

85. Mininberg DT, Watson C, Desquitado M. Viral cystitis with transient secondary vesicoureteral reflux. *J Urol* 1982;127:983–5.

86. Goldman RL, Warner NE. Hemorrhagic cystitis and cytomegalic inclusions in the bladder associated with cyclophosphamide therapy. *Cancer* 1970;25:7–11.

87. Masukawa T, Garancis JC, Rytel MW, Mattingly RF. Herpes genitalis virus isolation from human bladder urine. *Acta Cytol* 1972;16:416–28.

88. Londergan TA, Walzak MP. Hemorrhagic cystitis due to adenovirus infection following bone marrow transplantation. *J Urol* 1994;151:1013–4.

89. McClanahan C, Grimes MM, Callaghan E, Stewart J. Hemorrhagic cystitis associated with herpes simplex virus. *J Urol* 1994;151:152–3.

90. Murphy GF, Wood DP Jr, McRoberts JW, Henslee-Downey PJ. Adenovirus-associated hemorrhagic cystitis treated with intravenous ribavirin. *J Urol* 1993;149:565–6.

91. Seftel AD, Matthews LA, Smith MC, Willis J. Polyomavirus mimicking high grade transitional cell carcinoma. *J Urol* 1996;156:1764.

92. Hanash KA, Pool TL. Interstitial and hemorrhagic cystitis: viral, bacterial and fungal studies. *J Urol* 1970;104:705–6.

93. Levi AW, Potter SR, Schoenberg MP, Epstein JI. Clinical significance of denuded urothelium in bladder biopsy. *J Urol* 2001;166:457–60.

94. Elliott GB, Moloney PJ, Anderson GH. "Denuding cystitis" and in situ urothelial carcinoma. *Arch Pathol* 1973;96:91–4.

95. Williamson SR, Montironi R, Lopez-Beltran A, MacLennan GT, Davidson DD, Cheng L. Diagnosis,

evaluation and treatment of carcinoma in situ of the urinary bladder: the state of the art. *Crit Rev Oncol Hematol* 2010;76:112–26.

96. Hodges KB, Lopez-Beltran A, Davidson DD, Montironi R, Cheng L. Urothelial dysplasia and other flat lesions of the urinary bladder: clinicopathologic and molecular features. *Hum Pathol* 2010;41:155–62.

97. Antonakopoulos GN, Hicks RM, Berry RJ. The subcellular basis of damage to the human urinary bladder induced by irradiation. *J Pathol* 1984;143:103–16.

98. Marks LB, Carroll PR, Dugan TC, Anscher MS. The response of the urinary bladder, urethra, and ureter to radiation and chemotherapy. *Int J Radiat Oncol Biol Phys* 1995;31:1257–80.

99. Hietala SO, Winblad B, Hassler O. Vascular and morphological changes in the urinary bladder wall after irradiation. *Int Urol Nephrol* 1975;7:119–29.

100. Fajardo LF, Berthrong M. Radiation injury in surgical pathology. Part I. *Am J Surg Pathol* 1978;2:159–99.

101. Pazzaglia S, Chen XR, Aamodt CB, Wu SQ, Kao C, Gilchrist KW, Oyasu R, Reznikoff CA, Ritter MA. In vitro radiation-induced neoplastic progression of low grade uroepithelial tumors. *Radiat Res* 1994;138:86–92.

102. Chan TY, Epstein JI. Radiation or chemotherapy cystitis with "pseudocarcinomatous" features. *Am J Surg Pathol* 2004;28:909–13.

103. Spagnolo DV, Waring PM. Bladder granulomata after bladder surgery. *Am J Clin Pathol* 1986;86:430–7.

104. Eble JN, Banks ER. Post-surgical necrobiotic granulomas of urinary bladder. *Urology* 1990;35:454–7.

105. Helms CA, Clark RE. Post-herniorrhaphy suture granuloma simulating a bladder neoplasm. *Radiology* 1977;124:56.

106. Pearl GS, Someren A. Suture granuloma simulating bladder neoplasm. *Urology* 1980;15:304–6.

107. Bassi P, Milani C, Meneghini A, Garbeglio A, Aragona F, Zattoni F, Dalla Palma P, Rebuffi A, Pagano F. Clinical value of pathologic changes after intravesical BCG therapy of superficial bladder cancer. *Urology* 1992;40:175–9.

108. Barlow LJ, Seager CM, Benson MC, McKiernan JM. Novel intravesical therapies for non-muscle-invasive bladder cancer refractory to BCG. *Urol Oncol* 2010;28:108–11.

109. Chiong E, Esuvaranathan K. New therapies for non-muscle-invasive bladder cancer. *World J Urol* 2010;28:71–8.

110. Cheng L, Davidson DD, Maclennan GT, Williamson SR, Zhang S, Koch MO, Montironi R, Lopez-Beltran A. The origins of urothelial carcinoma. *Expert Rev Anticancer Ther* 2010;10:865–80.

111. Khafagy MM, el-Bolkainy MN, Mansour MA. Carcinoma of the bilharzial urinary bladder. A study of the associated mucosal lesions in 86 cases. *Cancer* 1972;30:150–9.

112. Nash TE, Cheever AW, Ottesen EA, Cook JA. Schistosome infections in humans: perspectives and recent findings. NIH conference. *Ann Intern Med* 1982;97:740–54.

113. Raziuddin S, Masihuzzaman M, Shetty S, Ibrahim A. Tumor necrosis factor alpha production in schistosomiasis with carcinoma of urinary bladder. *J Clin Immunol* 1993;13:23–9.

114. Rosin MP, Anwar WA, Ward AJ. Inflammation, chromosomal instability, and cancer: the schistosomiasis model. *Cancer Res* 1994;54:1929s–33s.

115. Rosin MP, Saad el Din Zaki S, Ward AJ, Anwar WA. Involvement of inflammatory reactions and elevated cell proliferation in the development of bladder cancer in schistosomiasis patients. *Mutat Res* 1994;305:283–92.

116. Smith JH, Christie JD. The pathobiology of *Schistosoma haematobium* infection in humans. *Hum Pathol* 1986;17:333–45.

117. Von Lichtenberg F, Edington GM, Nwabuebo I, Taylor JR, Smith JH. Pathologic effects of schistomiasis in Ibadan Western State of Nigeria. II. Pathogenesis of lesions of the bladder and ureters. *Am J Trop Med Hyg* 1971;20:244–54.

118. Koraitim MM, Metwalli NE, Atta MA, el-Sadr AA. Changing age incidence and pathological types of schistosoma-associated bladder carcinoma. *J Urol* 1995;154:1714–6.

119. Dubey NK, Tavadia HB, Hehir M. Malacoplakia: a case involving epididymis and a case involving a bladder complicated by calculi. *J Urol* 1988;139:359–61.

120. Long JP Jr, Althausen AF. Malacoplakia: a 25-year experience with a review of the literature. *J Urol* 1989;141:1328–31.

121. Callea F, Van Damme B, Desmet VJ. Alpha–1-antitrypsin in malakoplakia. *Virchows Arch A Pathol Anat Histol* 1982;395:1–9.

122. Biggar WD, Keating A, Bear RA. Malakoplakia: evidence for an acquired disease secondary to immunosuppression. *Transplantation* 1981;31:109–12.

123. Baniel J, Shmueli D, Shapira Z, Sandbank Y, Servadio C. Malacoplakia presenting as a pseudotumor of the bladder in cadaveric renal transplantation. *J Urol* 1987;137:281–2.

124. Feldman S, Levy LB, Prinz LM. Malacoplakia of the bladder causing bilateral ureteral obstruction. *J Urol* 1980;123:588–9.

125. Damjanov I, Katz SM. Malakoplakia. *Pathol Annu* 1981;16:103–26.

126. Cos LR, Cockett AT. Genitourinary tuberculosis revisited. *Urology* 1982;20:111–7.

127. Walther M, Glenn JF, Vellios F. Xanthogranulomatous cystitis. *J Urol* 1985;134:745–6.

128. Ash J. Epithelial tumors of the bladder. *J Urol* 1940;44:135–45.

129. Bates AW, Fegan AW, Baithun SI. Xanthogranulomatous cystitis associated with malignant neoplasms of the bladder. *Histopathology* 1998;33:212–5.

130. Skopelitou A, Mitselou A, Gloustianou G. Xanthoma of the bladder associated with transitional cell carcinoma. *J Urol* 2000;164:1303–4.

131. Nishimura K, Nozawa M, Hara T, Oka T. Xanthoma of the bladder. *J Urol* 1995;153:1912–3.

132. Elson EC, McLaughlin AP 3rd. Xanthomatous ureteral polyp. *Urology* 1974;4:214–6.

133. Cyr WL, Johnson H, Balfour J. Granulomatous cystitis as a manifestation of chronic granulomatous disease of childhood. *J Urol* 1973;110:357–9.

134. Orth RW, Weisman MH, Cohen AH, Talner LB, Nachtsheim D, Zvaifler NJ. Lupus cystitis: primary bladder manifestations of systemic lupus erythematosus. *Ann Intern Med* 1983;98:323–6.

135. Betz SA, See WA, Cohen MB. Granulomatous inflammation in bladder wash specimens after intravesical bacillus Calmette-Guèrin therapy for transitional cell carcinoma of the bladder. *Am J Clin Pathol* 1993;99:244–8.

136. Jufe R, Molinolo AA, Fefer SA, Meiss RP. Plasma cell granuloma of the bladder: a case report. *J Urol* 1984;131:1175–6.

137. Tammela T, Kallioinen M, Kontturi M, Hellstrom P. Sarcoidosis of the bladder: a case report and literature review. *J Urol* 1989;141:608–9.

138. Kaczmarek A. Unusual complication of foreign body in the bladder. *Br J Urol* 1985;57:106.

139. McKinney CD, Gaffey MJ, Gillenwater JY. Bladder outlet obstruction after multiple periurethral polytetrafluoroethylene injections. *J Urol* 1995;153:149–51.

140. Goldberg PK, Kozinn PJ, Wise GJ, Nouri N, Brooks RB. Incidence and significance of candiduria. *JAMA* 1979;241:582–4.

141. Patel B, Khosla A, Chenoweth JL. Bilateral fungal bezoars in the renal pelvis. *Br J Urol* 1996;78:651–2.

142. Sakamoto S, Ogata J, Sakazaki Y, Ikegami K. Fungus ball formation of *Aspergillus* in the bladder. an unusual case report. *Eur Urol* 1978;4:388–9.

143. King DT, Lam M. Actinomycosis of the urinary bladder: association with an intrauterine contraceptive device. *JAMA* 1978;240:1512–3.

144. Guermazi A, de Kerviler E, Welker Y, Zagdanski AM, Desgrandchamps F, Frija J. Pseudotumoral vesical actinomycosis. *J Urol* 1996;156:2002–3.

145. Ozyurt C, Yurtseven O, Kocak I, Kandiloglu G, Elmas N. Actinomycosis simulating bladder tumour. *Br J Urol* 1995;76:263–4.

146. Isogai H, Isogai E, Kimura K, Fujii N, Yokota K, Oguma K. *Helicobacter pylori* induces inflammation in mouse urinary bladder and pelvis. *Microbiol Immunol* 1994;38:331–6.

147. Henry L, Fox M. Histological findings in pseudomembranous trigonitis. *J Clin Pathol* 1971;24:605–8.

148. Jost SP, Gosling JA, Dixon JS. The fine structure of human pseudomembranous trigonitis. *Br J Urol* 1989;64:472–7.

149. Herman JR. Candiru: urinophilic catfish. Its gift to urology. *Urology* 1973;1:265–7.

Chapter 3

Urothelial Metaplasia and Hyperplasia

Bladder Pathology, First Edition. Liang Cheng, Antonio Lopez-Beltran, David G. Bostwick.
© 2012 Wiley-Blackwell. Published 2012 by John Wiley & Sons, Inc.

von Brunn Nests

von Brunn nests are round to oval aggregates of benign urothelial cells in the superficial lamina propria that arise by invagination of the overlying urothelium (**Fig. 3-1**).[1] The term "Brunn buds" is sometimes used when attachment to the urothelium is still apparent.[2] von Brunn nests are a common finding, present in virtually all serially sectioned bladders at autopsy, present in all age groups, and are frequently associated with cystitis cystica and glandularis. They occur most commonly in the trigone and are thought to represent a normal variant of bladder mucosa. The etiology is uncertain, and the link with inflammation is disputed by some authors. Early reports suggested that von Brunn nests are precancerous, but that view is no longer accepted.

von Brunn nests are typically round circumscribed nests of urothelial cells usually devoid of atypia, located immediately beneath the urothelium, and may contain luminal eosinophilic secretions (**Figs. 3-2** and **3-3**; **Table 3-1**). Squamous metaplasia is uncommon. Occasionally, urothelial carcinoma may extend into von Brunn nests, causing bulbous expansion that may be misinterpreted as lamina propria invasion. Useful distinguishing features for invasive carcinoma include irregular infiltration of the stroma by nests of cells and single cells with cytologic abnormalities, often accompanied by a stromal response.[2,3] Diagnostic difficulty occurs when von Brunn nests are present deep within the lamina propria, often resulting from tangential cutting or mucosal invaginations; this deep separation from the overlying epithelium may result in the overdiagnosis of carcinoma.[4] Exuberant (florid) von Brunn nest proliferation may be observed, mimicking inverted papilloma, inverted urothelial carcinoma, and nested variant of urothelial carcinoma (see **Chapters 12** and **17**). The benign cytologic

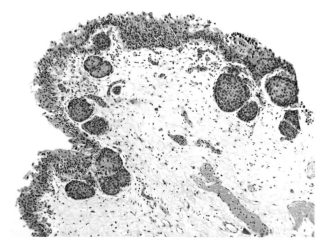

Figure 3-2 von Brunn nests.

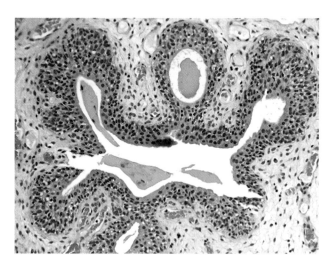

Figure 3-3 von Brunn nests. Note the luminal eosinophilic secretions.

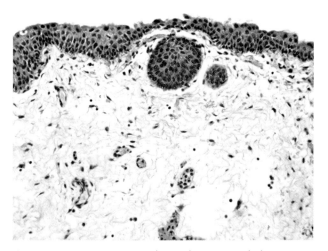

Figure 3-1 von Brunn nests beneath intact urothelium.

findings in von Brunn nests usually stand in contrast to the changes in urothelial carcinomas, but the epithelium in florid von Brunn nests, similar to the surface urothelium, may exhibit hyperplasia and reactive atypia, including the presence of occasional mitotic figures. In contrast to the nested variant of urothelial carcinoma, florid von Brunn nests in the bladder generally show larger nests with more regular shapes and regular spacing (**Figs. 3-4** and **3-5**; **Table 3-2**). In addition, Volmar and colleagues utilized immunohistochemical markers, including Ki67 (MIB1), p53, p27, and cytokeratin (CK) 20 in an attempt to differentiate florid von Brunn nests fom nested urothelial carcinoma.[5] They found that although some differences in staining with these markers do exist, they are generally slight and may not be useful in routine practice, proposing that careful application of histopathologic criteria is of the highest importance.

Table 3-1 Differentiating Histopathologic Characteristics of Cytologically Bland-appearing Glandular and Gland-like Lesions of the Urinary Bladder

von Brunn nests	Solid nests of urothelial cells; extension to a uniform depth in the lamina propria; lobular architecture (especially in the upper urinary tract); lack of muscularis propria involvement
Cystitis cystica	Central cystic degeneration of von Brunn nests without apical glandular differentiation; extension to a uniform depth in the lamina propria; lobular architecture (especially in the upper urinary tract); lack of muscularis propria involvement
Cystitis glandularis	Apical glandular differentiation in von Brunn nests; cuboidal or columnar central lining surrounded by urothelial cells; extension to a uniform depth in the lamina propria; lobular architecture; lack of muscularis propria involvement
Intestinal metaplasia	Glandular proliferation within lamina propria; abundant mucin-producing goblet cells, sometimes Paneth cells; extension to a uniform depth in the lamina propria; lobular architecture; lack of muscularis propria involvement
Microcystic variant of urothelial carcinoma	Characteristic variation in cyst size, up to 2 cm; infiltrative growth pattern throughout the bladder wall; lumen containing necrotic debris, PAS-diastase-positive mucin, or empty
Urothelial carcinoma with small tubules	Predominance of small tubules; extensive invasion of bladder wall; lack of nephrogenic adenoma features (tubulopapillary architecture, cuboidal epithelium, hobnail cells); negative for PSA and PSAP
Nested variant of urothelial carcinoma	Infiltrating nests of urothelial cells with a variable proportion of small tubular lumens, resembling von Brunn nests; focal significant atypia present in deeper aspects of infiltrative tumor (enlarged nucleoli and coarse nuclear chromatin); disorderly proliferation; jagged tumor stroma interface; focal myxoid or desmoplastic stroma; extensive infiltration of bladder wall out of proportion to histologic grade

PAS, periodic acid-Schiff; PSAP, prostate-specific acid phosphatase

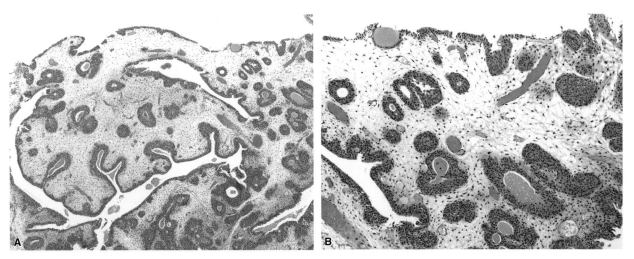

Figure 3-4 von Brunn nest proliferations (A and B).

Table 3-2   Key Morphologic Features Distinguishing Nested Variant of Urothelial Carcinoma from Florid von Brunn Nests

	Organization	Lumen Formation	Cytologic Atypia	Infiltrative Growth	Muscle Invasion
Nested variant	Crowded, irregular glands	Variable	Present	Present	Yes, frequent
Florid von Brunn nests	Large, regularly spaced, rounded nests	Variable	Absent	Absent	No

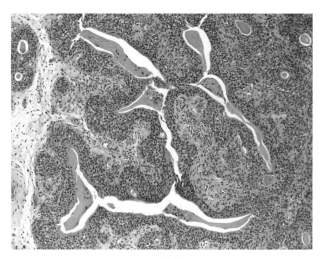

Figure 3-5   von Brunn nest proliferations.

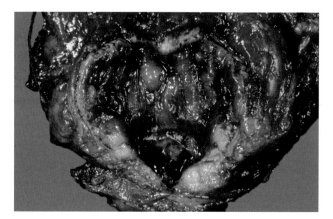

Figure 3-6   Gross appearance of cystitis cystica.

In bacillus Calmettc–Gruérin (BCG)-treated bladders, it is important to keep in mind that residual carcinoma in situ might be present only in von Brunn nests[6–8] (see Chapter 7).

Cystitis Cystica

Cystitis cystica probably results from central cavitation of von Brunn nests (**Figs. 3-6** to **3-8**). Not uncommonly, these nests demonstrate central cystic degeneration, resulting in a gland-like lumen termed "cystitis cystica." It is found in up to 60% of serially sectioned bladders[2,9] and is most common in adults, but it often occurs in children. Like cystitis glandularis, it occasionally simulates a neoplasm.[2,10–12]

Grossly or at cystoscopy, cystitis cystica consists of one or more discrete translucent, 2 to 5 mm in diameter, submucosal beads or cysts, varying from pearl white to yellow-brown (**Fig. 3-6**).[2,13,14] It contains clear or slightly yellow fluid, is lined by cuboidal or flattened urothelium,[2,13] and is often filled with eosinophilic fluid. Cystitis cystica is not premalignant.

Histologically, the nests are composed of layers of urothelial cells without significant atypia and, in the case of cystitis cystica, without true glandular differentiation.

Although these lesions are quite common and of a benign nature, occasionally there is the possibility for confusion with the nested variant of urothelial carcinoma, a deceptively benign histologic appearance of invasive urothelial carcinoma with clinical behavior more similar to that of a high grade tumor. The rare microcystic bladder carcinoma also enters the differential diagnosis in selected cases of cystitis cystica. Particularly, this challenge may be of greatest concern in limited biopsy specimens. Generally, histologic features that aid in this differential diagnosis include extension of the urothelial nests to a uniform depth in the lamina propria rather than an infiltrative appearance. In the bladder, large cystic spaces are frequently present, while extension of the proliferative process into the muscularis propria is absent. Although mild nuclear atypia is sometimes seen, significant atypia is not. This may be suggestive of an alternative process, such as involvement of the cystitis cystica by urothelial carcinoma in situ. The nested or microcystic variants of urothelial carcinoma may also show a moderate degree of nuclear atypia in deeper aspects of the tumor. Similarly, the microcystic variant of urothelial carcinoma, although rare, may be an even greater source of diagnostic difficulty. By definition, this variant of urothelial carcinoma is composed of variably sized tubular and cystic structures with bland cytology. Confinement of the cystic proliferative process to the superficial aspect of the bladder mucosa may be a helpful diagnostic feature of cystitis cystica; although, in a superficial biopsy specimen, this distinction may be challenging indeed.

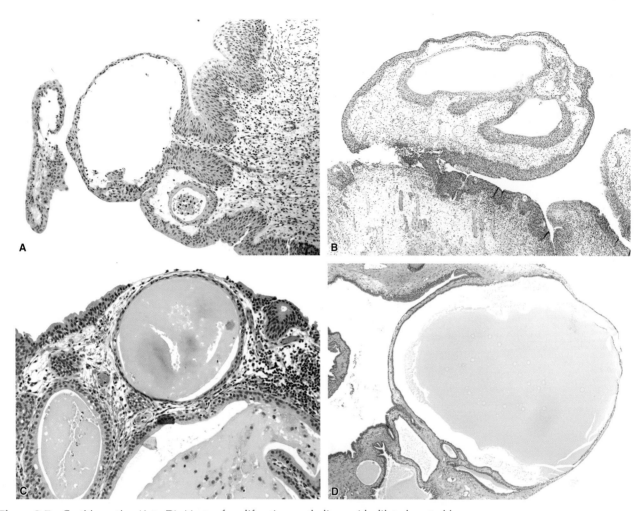

Figure 3-7 Cystitis cystica (A to D). Nests of proliferative urothelium with dilated central lumens.

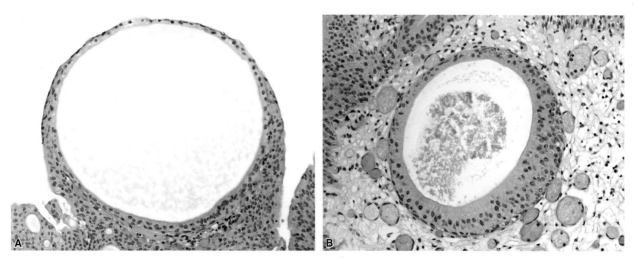

Figure 3-8 Cystitis cystica (A and B). Note the pink proteinaceous secretions in the lumens.

Cystitis Glandularis and Intestinal Metaplasia

Cystitis Glandularis, Usual (Typical) Type

Cystitis glandularis is thought to arise from von Brunn nests, similar to cystitis cystica, and is frequently associated with voiding symptoms (Fig. 3-9).[2,9] Cystitis glandularis is characterized by a central lining of cuboidal or columnar cells surrounded by layers of urothelial cells (Figs. 3-10 and 3-11). Some authors believe it to be a metaplastic change of the urothelial lining in response to chronic inflammation or irritation. It is present in 71% of serially sectioned bladders and, like von Brunn nests, is most common in the trigone. It may be responsible for unusual bladder masses in children,[2,15] and rare cases are associated with pelvic lipomatosis.[2,16,17] Cystitis glandularis is present in some patients with neuropathic bladder and chronic indwelling urinary catheter.[2,18]

Two forms of cystitis glandularis may coexist: usual (typical) type and intestinal type, the latter based primarily

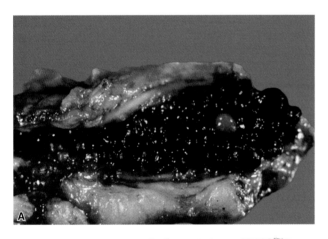

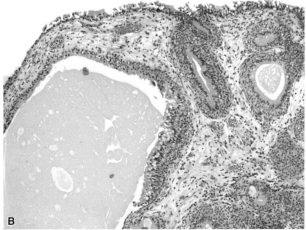

Figure 3-9 Cystitis cystica glandularis. Gross (A) and microscopic appearance (B).

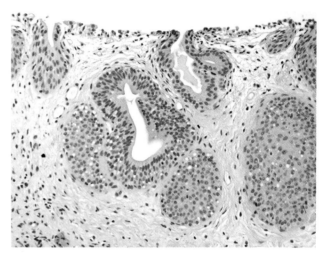

Figure 3-10 Cystitis glandularis.

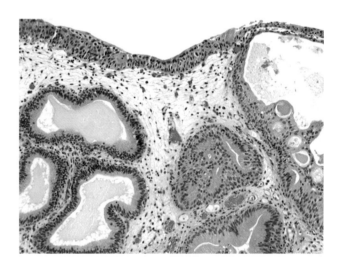

Figure 3-11 Cystitis glandularis.

on the presence of abundant, mucin-secreting goblet cells. The usual form is most common, consisting of acini lined by cuboidal to columnar cells often surrounded by layers of urothelial cells. Sung et al. demonstrated that these lesions have characteristic immunostaining with CK7, similar to normal urothelium, and absence of expression for CDX2 and CK20, markers associated with intestinal differentiation.[19]

Occasionally, a prolonged history of diffuse cystitis glandularis of intestinal form precedes adenocarcinoma.[2,20,21] In such cases, the bladder often contains a variety of abnormalities, including glandular dysplasia and adenocarcinoma in situ.[2,6] Intestinal metaplasia and the intestinal form of cystitis glandularis are not strong risk factors for bladder adenocarcinoma, although this remains controversial.[2,22–28] Occasionally, the cystoscopic appearance of cystitis glandularis suggests malignancy, particularly with polypoid cystitis glandularis. In this context, the microcystic variant of urothelial carcinoma may again be challenging to exclude from the differential diagnosis, as the characteristic cysts and tubular structures exhibit a great deal of variability in size and morphology. Traditionally, the term "cystitis cystica et glandularis" has been used when cytitis cystica and cystitis glandularis coexist in the same patient.

Intestinal Metaplasia (Cystitis Glandularis, Intestinal Type)

The intestinal form of cystitis glandularis consists of tall columnar and goblet cells with prominent mucin production resembling colonic epithelium.[2,27,29-31] Paneth and neuroendocrine cells are present. The intestinal form of cystitis glandularis has the same histochemical profile as that of colonic epithelium. Atypia and mitosis are not common features of intestinal metaplasia of the bladder.

Some authors tend to separate cystitis glandularis, intestinal type (as described above) from intestinal metaplasia, a lesion similar to the intestinal form of cystitis glandularis, but the term "metaplasia" is restricted to cases in which the surface urothelium contains columnar cells with goblet cells.[2,32,33] We, and others, now use the term "intestinal metaplasia" instead of "cystitis glandularis, intestinal type," suggesting a more technically accurate description of these interesting proliferative processes.

Grossly, it is often seen coexisting with cystitis cystica and cystitis glandularis (Fig. 3-12). Microscopically, intestinal metaplasia is composed of glandular proliferations within the lamina propria similar to those of typical cystitis glandularis; however, rather than a cuboidal or columnar lining surrounded by urothelium, the nests contain abundant mucin-secreting goblet cells (Figs. 3-13 and 3-14). In contrast to cystitis glandularis of the usual type, Sung et al. found these lesions to have positive immunohistochemical staining with CDX2 and CK20, coupled with absence of

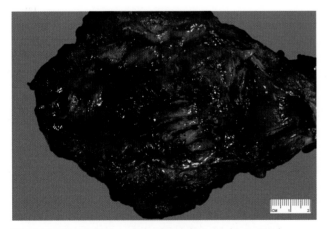

Figure 3-12 Cystitis cystica glandularis and intestinal metaplasia (gross).

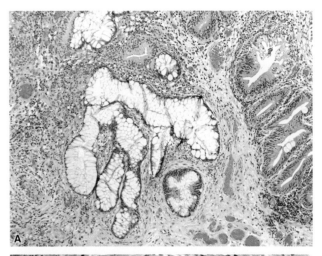

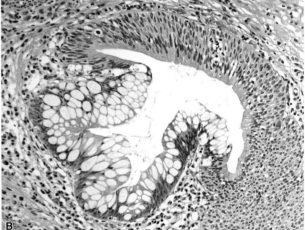

Figure 3-13 Intestinal metaplasia involving cystitis glandularis.

staining for CK7, suggesting genuine intestinal differentiation (Fig. 3-15).[19] Occasionally, a significant component of extracellular mucin may be present,[34] adding to the challenging differential diagnosis of primary adenocarcinoma and urachal adenocarcinoma. These cases have been called "florid cystitis glandularis of intestinal type with mucin extravasation" (Figs. 3-16 and 3-17).

Although intestinal metaplasia has been implicated in the development of bladder adenocarcinoma due to frequent coexistence of the two entities, a definitive premalignant link has been difficult to identify. As telomere shortening has been recognized in the development of epithelial cancers, Morton et al. studied telomere length via fluorescent in situ hybridization (FISH) and found that bladder intestinal metaplasia is associated with significant telomere shortening relative to adjacent normal urothelial cells (Fig. 3-18).[35] A subset of cases with telomere shortening also demonstrated chromosomal abnormalities common to urothelial carcinoma by FISH analyses. These findings suggest that

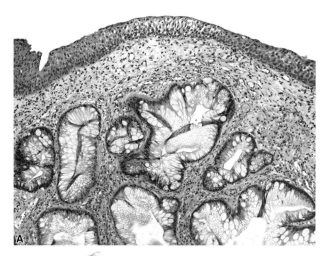

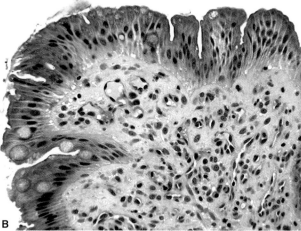

Figure 3-14 Intestinal metaplasia (A and B). Note the surface urothelium involvement by intestinal metaplasia (B).

intestinal metaplasia of the urinary bladder may indeed be a precursor in the development of adenocarcinoma. The authors therefore proposed complete resection of the areas affected, elimination of any inflammatory stimulus, and continued endoscopic surveillance in the management of such lesions. In contrast, however, Smith et al. found that both cystitis glandularis and intestinal metaplasia are seen relatively frequently in conjunction with both bladder cancer and benign bladder specimens, suggesting that there is no future risk of malignancy.[36]

Florid Cystitis Glandularis

Florid cystitis glandularis is usually an incidental finding and is distinguished from adenocarcinoma by the lack of stromal infiltration and the absence of marked cytologic abnormalities.[2,20,34,37,38] Cases in which there are distorted glands in the stroma or deep within the lamina propria, particularly with cytologic abnormalities (even if minor), should be evaluated carefully to exclude malignancy.

Patients may present with irritative obstructive symptoms or hematuria; florid cystitis glandularis has no malignant potential.

Grossly, it may be a nodular or polypoid lesion, with predilection for the trigone and bladder neck. On microscopic examination, there is involvement of von Brunn nests by glandular metaplasia, resulting in an exuberant proliferation of glands lined by columnar cells, with or without goblet cells characterized by proliferation of glands in the lamina propria, some with the appearance of cystitis glandularis of the usual type (**Figs. 3-19** to **3-21**). Most glands are lined by tall columnar cells with basally located nuclei lacking cytologic atypia; Paneth cells may be seen. Lesions are confined to the lamina propria and lack significant cytologic atypia, but some may be difficult to differentiate from adenocarcinoma, particularly when submitted for frozen section evaluation. The situation may be further confounded by the finding of acellular dissecting mucin pools in the lamina propria and muscularis propria.[2,34,39] In these cases, distinguishing well-differentiated adenocarcinoma from florid cystitis glandularis relies on the greater degree and extent of these atypical features in cancer.

The differential diagnosis of florid cystitis glandularis includes adenocarcinoma, which has significant cytologic atypia, infiltrative growth, invasion into muscularis propria, and frequent mitoses. Metastatic prostatic adenocarcinoma may also mimic florid cystitis glandularis (**Fig. 3-22**; see also **Chapters 23** and **26**). Endocervicosis and müllerianosis may involve both the muscularis propria and lamina propria, but the greater portion of the lesion is in the muscularis propria. Florid cystitis glandularis frequently recurs and may require aggressive therapy.[2,40] Metaplastic bone and cartilage may rarely appear in the stroma of florid cystitis glandularis.[2,41]

Squamous Metaplasia

Squamous metaplasia can be divided into nonkeratinizing and keratinizing types. It is a frequent finding in patients with *Schistosomiasis haematobium* infection, nonfunctioning bladder, exstrophy, or severe chronic cystitis.[18,42–45] It is more common in women than in men, and often occurs on the anterior wall.[2,3,46] Some studies suggest that keratinizing squamous metaplasia may be a malignant precursor lesion.[2,47]

At cystoscopy, the mucosa is thickened and typically white or gray-white. The appearance may be striking, with irregular flaky keratinizing material (**Fig. 3-23**).[2,48] Microscopically, there is squamous mucosa of variable thickness that is often covered by a layer of keratin (**Figs. 3-23** to **3-27**). Cytologic atypia is uncommon but may include dysplasia or carcinoma in situ, raising the

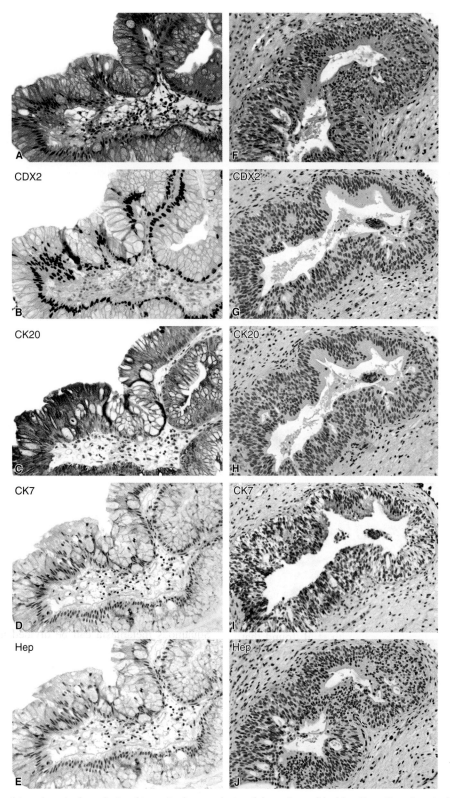

Figure 3-15 Immunohistochemical analysis of intestinal metaplasia of the urinary bladder (A to E) and typical cystitis glandularis (F to J). Intestinal metaplasia (A) demonstrates positive nuclear staining for CDX2 (B), positive cytoplasmic staining for CK20 (C), and negative staining for CK7 (D) and Hep (E). Typical cystitis glandularis (F) demonstrates negative staining for CDX2 (G), CK20 (H), and Hep (J), and positive cytoplasmic staining for CK7 (I).(From Ref. 19; with permission.)

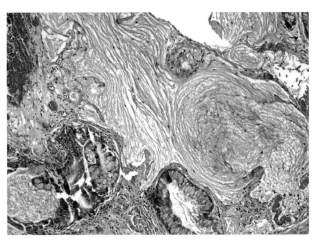

Figure 3-16 Florid cystitis glandularis of intestinal type with mucin extravasation.

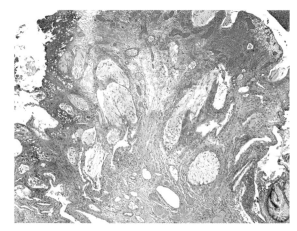

Figure 3-17 Florid cystitis glandularis of intestinal type with mucin extravasation.

possibility of invasive carcinoma elsewhere in the specimen.[2,3,49] The relationship of squamous metaplasia and squamous cell carcinoma is a matter of debate with contradictory findings.[2,44,50–52] In a series from the Mayo Clinic, 22% of patients with squamous metaplasia had synchronous carcinoma, and another 20% subsequently developed carcinoma when followed for as long as 30 years.[2,53] The mean interval from the diagnosis of squamous metaplasia to the development of carcinoma was 11 years. The high frequency of squamous metaplasia and squamous cell carcinoma in patients with schistosomiasis supports this association.[2,54] A recent review, based on 54 years of experience, found keratinizing squamous metaplasia to be more frequent in men (80%), with a mean age of 50 years (range, 13 to 80 years).[47] Keratinizing squamous metaplasia of the bladder was considered a significant risk factor for bladder contracture, ureteral obstruction, and carcinoma.[2,47] In Khan et al.'s study, eight (of 30) cases (27%) developed cancer.[47] The authors divided the cases into "limited" and "extensive" squamous metaplasia based on cystoscopic examination. Patients with "extensive" squamous metaplasia had a much higher rate of developing cancer (42%) than did those with "limited" squamous metaplasia (12%).[47]

Squamous metaplasia should be distinguished from nonkeratinizing glycogenated squamous epithelium, similar to that of the vaginal type, which is a normal finding in the trigone and bladder neck in up to 86% of women during the reproductive and menopausal years (**Figs. 3-28** and **3-29**).[2,55,56] Some authors, in older literature, referred to the finding of trigonal glycogenated squamous epithelium as "pseudomembranous trigonitis," a term no longer recommended. Epithelium of this type rarely occurs in men, except in patients receiving estrogen therapy for prostatic carcinoma. Glycogenated squamous epithelium in the trigone may be very thick in rare cases (**Fig. 3-29**).[2,3]

Nephrogenic Metaplasia (Nephrogenic Adenoma)

Nephrogenic metaplasia (nephrogenic adenoma) is most common in the bladder (55% of cases) but may also involve the urethra (41%) and ureter (4%).[2,57–64] It usually occurs in adults (90% of cases),[2,65,66] and male predominate (2:1 ratio). Symptoms and endoscopic features of nephrogenic metaplasia are not specific and may include hematuria, frequency, and dysuria.[2,67] Most patients have a history of an operative procedure or one or more irritants, including calculi, trauma, cystitis, and tuberculosis.[2,68,69] About 8% of patients have undergone kidney transplantation; in these patients, cells of nephrogenic adenoma derive from tubular cells of the renal transplant and are not metaplastic proliferations of the recipient's bladder urothelium.[2,62–64]

The terms "nephrogenic metaplasia" and "nephrogenic adenoma" have been used interchangeably, probably reflecting the interesting pathogenesis of these lesions. Nephrogenic adenoma is probably nonneoplastic and represents a metaplastic change of the urothelium in response to a stimulus (nephrogenic metaplasia), as these lesions are commonly seen in association with mucosal irritation of various etiologies. However, in the setting of renal transplant recipients with an opposite-gender donor, the lesional cells have been found to demonstrate the sex chromosomes of the donor by FISH, suggesting that the proliferative cells may have a true renal origin.[64] In this context at least, nephrogenic adenoma appears to be derived from shed renal tubular epithelial cells that migrate, implant, and proliferate in the urinary tract mucosa in a setting of mucosal injury, such as that induced by implantation of the donor ureter into the recipient's bladder, and the presence of an intravesical catheter in the immediate postoperative period.

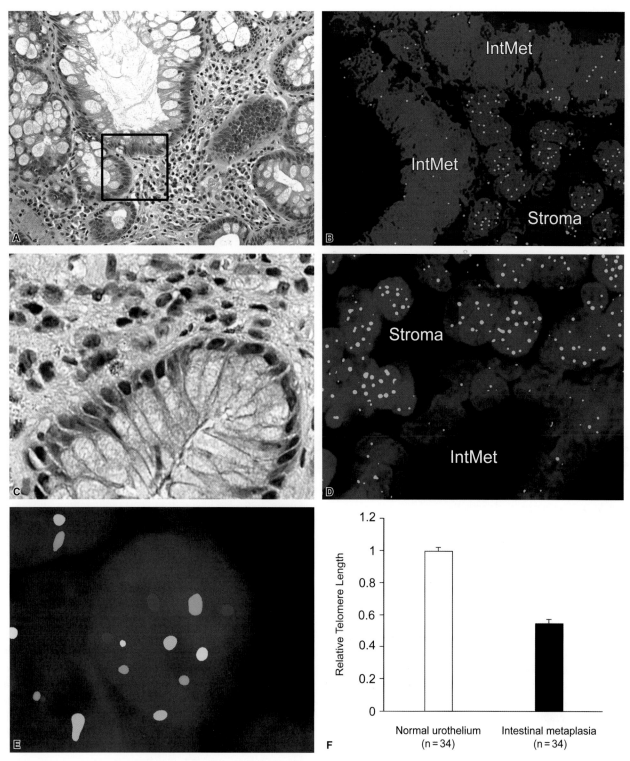

Figure 3-18 Telomere shortening in intestinal metaplasia of the urinary bladder. (A) H&E staining of intestinal metaplasia characterized by glandular structures in the lamina propria, lined by columnar epithelium, including goblet cells. (B) FISH with telomere-specific probe of inset in (A) showing reduced telomere signal intensity in metaplastic cells compared to the adjacent stromal cells. Another example of intestinal metaplasia demonstrating similar findings (C and D). (E) Representative hybridization in a case of intestinal metaplasia using the UroVysion probe set containing centromeric probes (CEP) 3, 7, and 17 and locus-specific probe (LSI) 9p21. The metaplastic cell shows three CEP3 (red), three CEP7 (green), two CEP17 (aqua), and two LSI 9p21 signals, indicating a gain of chromosomes 3 and 7. (F) Comparison of telomere length between normal urothelium and intestinal metaplasia. (From Ref. 35; with permission.)

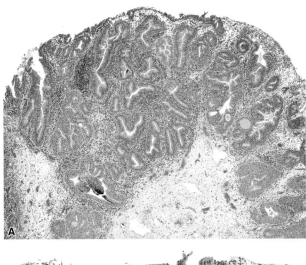

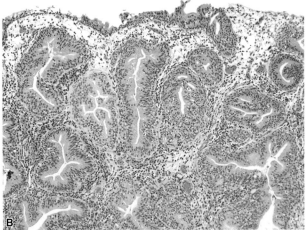

Figure 3-19 Florid cystitis glandularis.

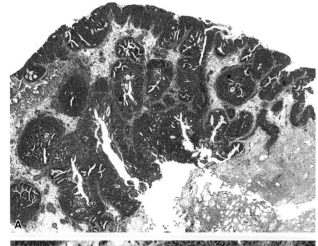

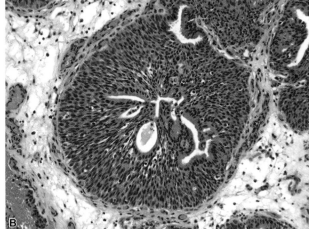

Figure 3-20 Florid von Brunn nest proliferations and cystitis glandularis (A and B).

Typically, nephrogenic metaplasia is 1 cm or less in diameter and single, but exceptions occur.[2,70] Microscopically, tubules are the most common histologic finding,[2,71] but the proliferation may also be papillary, tubular, cystic, tubolocystic, polypoid, and, rarely, diffuse and solid (Figs. 3-30 to 3-37). Mixed growth patterns are often seen in the same lesion. The papillary component of nephrogenic adenoma may mimic urothelial neoplasm; however, the lining of the papillary structures by a single layer of cuboidal cells favors a diagnosis of nephrogenic adenoma. The tubules of nephrogenic metaplasia appear as small, round, hollow acini reminiscent of renal tubules.[2,72] They are occasionally solid and surrounded by a prominent basement membrane that is highlighted by periodic acid–Schiff stain.[2,73] The tubules frequently become dilated and cystic, but may also appear as nearly solid nests. The lumens often contain eosinophilic or basophilic secretions that are weakly mucicarminophilic. Most of the cells lining the tubules, cysts, and papillae are cuboidal or low columnar with scant cytoplasm; occasionally, the cells have abundant clear cytoplasm.[2,74] Hobnail

cells line the tubules and cysts in up to 70% of cases, and large cysts may be lined by flattened cells. Signet ring cells may be seen in nephrogenic adenoma (Fig. 3-37).

Small amounts of mucin may be present in the cells of nephrogenic metaplasia, but glycogen is usually scant or absent. Nuclear abnormalities are uncommon and, when present, appear reactive or degenerative.[75] Mitotic figures are rare or absent. The stroma is typically described as edematous with a variable infiltrate of inflammatory cells, sometimes prominent. Other stromal features sometimes include dilated vessels, calcification, amyloid-like plaque, or multinucleate giant cells. There is often marked chronic cystitis, which may partially obscure nephrogenic metaplasia; squamous and glandular metaplasia may coexist with nephrogenic metaplasia. Rare cases of nephrogenic metaplasia are associated with prominent stromal calcification, malakoplakia, or cytomegalovirus infection.[2,76,77] Nephrogenic metaplasia is diploid[2,78] and associated with an abundance of mucosal mast cells, a finding related to immunoglobulin E–mediated allergy.[2,79]

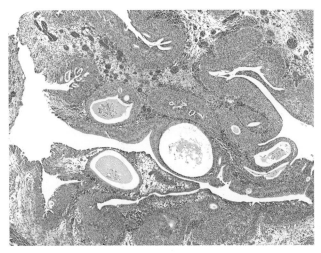

Figure 3-21 Florid von Brunn nest proliferations and cystitis glandularis.

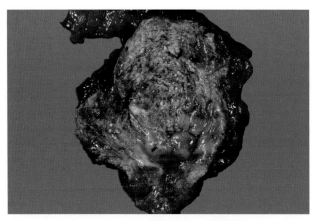

Figure 3-23 Keratinizing squamous metaplasia of the bladder. The mucosal surface is thickened, leathery, and gray-white (clinical history of extrophy).

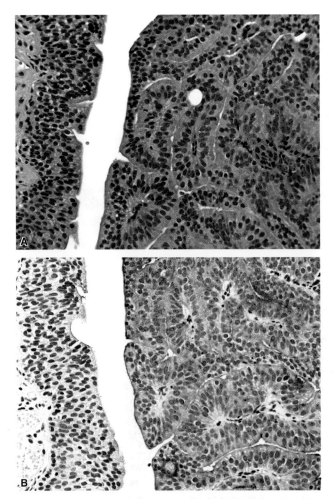

Figure 3-22 Metastatic prostatic adenocarcinoma mimicking florid cystitis glandularis (A). Immunostaining for prostate-specific antigen (PSA) is strongly positive (B). The urothelium (left side) is negative for PSA staining.

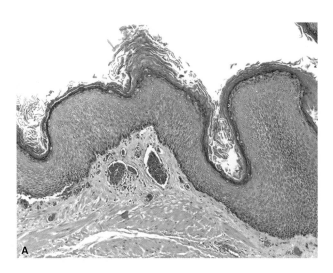

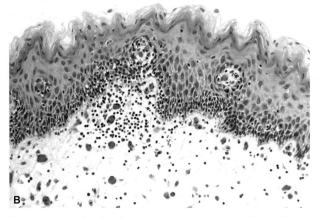

Figure 3-24 Keratinizing squamous metaplasia (A and B).

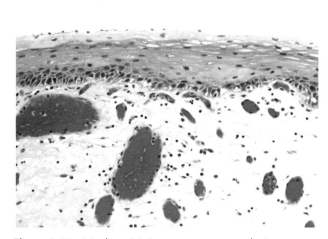

Figure 3-25 Nonkeratinizing squamous metaplasia.

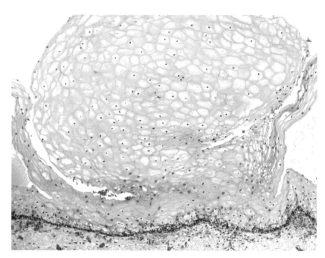

Figure 3-28 Glycogenated squamous epithelium in the normal trigone of a women during the reproductive years. The vaginal-type nonkeratinizing glycogenated squamous epithelium should not be mistaken for squamous metaplasia.

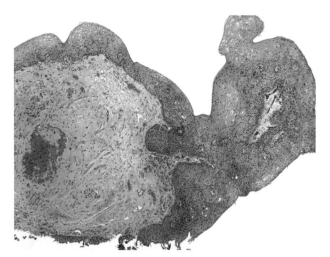

Figure 3-26 Nonkeratinizing squamous metaplasia in a bladder biopsy specimen.

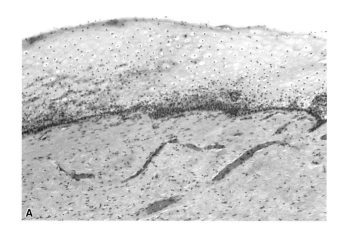

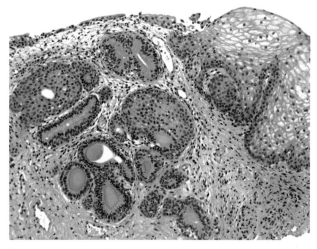

Figure 3-27 Transition of urothelium to squamous metaplasia. von Brunn nests and cystitis glandularis are also present.

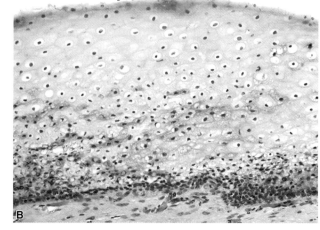

Figure 3-29 Glycogenated squamous epithelium. The epithelium is thickened (A and B).

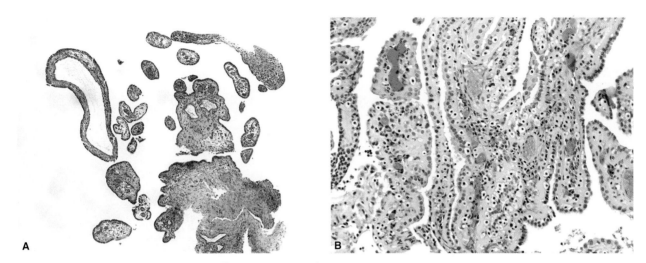

Figure 3-30   Nephrogenic metaplasia, papillary pattern (A and B).

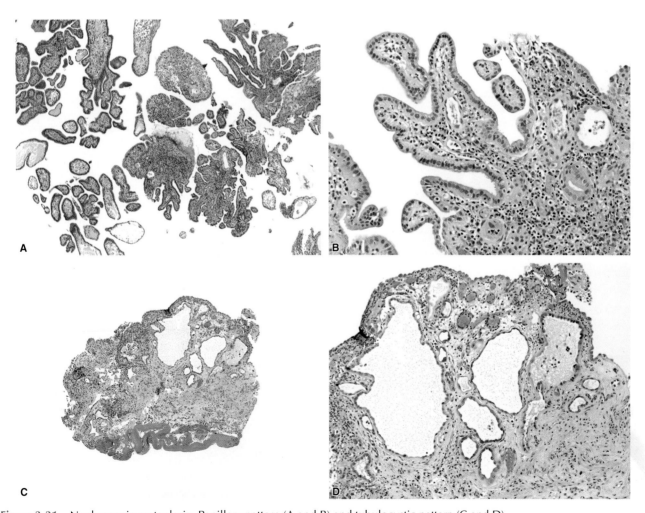

Figure 3-31   Nephrogenic metaplasia. Papillary pattern (A and B) and tubulocystic pattern (C and D).

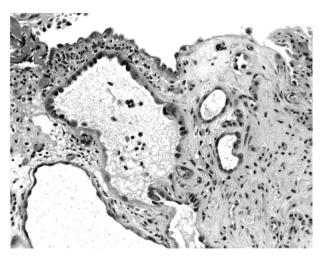

Figure 3-32 Nephrogenic adenoma, tubulocystic pattern. Dilated tubules are lined by hobnail cells.

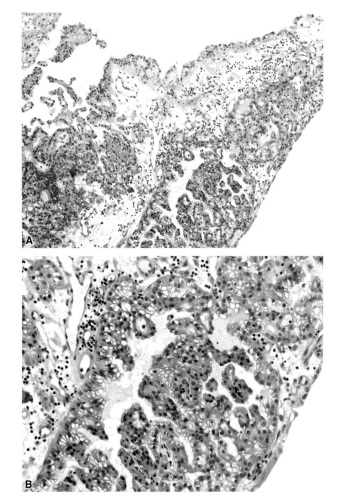

Figure 3-33 Nephrogenic adenoma, polypoid pattern (A and B).

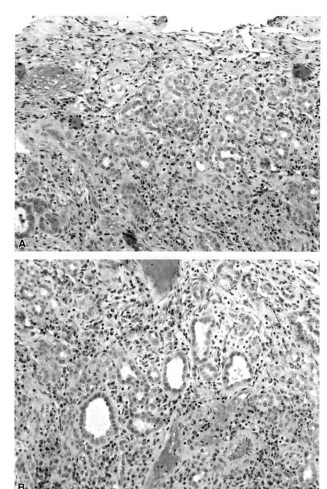

Figure 3-34 Nephrogenic adenoma, solid and tubular pattern (A and B).

The most common differential diagnostic considerations of nephrogenic metaplasia are adenocarcinoma and urothelial carcinoma with pseudoglandular differentiation (**Table 3-3**; see also **Chapter 13**).[2,12,80-84] The papillary component of nephrogenic adenoma may mimic urothelial neoplasm; however, the lining of the papillary structures by a single layer of cuboidal cells favors a diagnosis of nephrogenic adenoma. The proliferation of tubules may raise concern for adenocarcinoma, but the lack of significant cytologic atypia or mitotic activity, the presence of a mixture of tubular and papillary components, and the edematous/inflammatory stroma are features more in keeping with nephrogenic adenoma than with adenocarcinoma, especially in a pediatric patient with a history of prior bladder surgery. Nonetheless, significant cytologic atypia may also be seen in nephrogenic adenoma (**Fig. 3-38**). These lesions are termed "atypical nephrogenic metaplasia."[83] Despite cytologic atypia, these lesions are benign, and additional treatments are not necessary.[83]

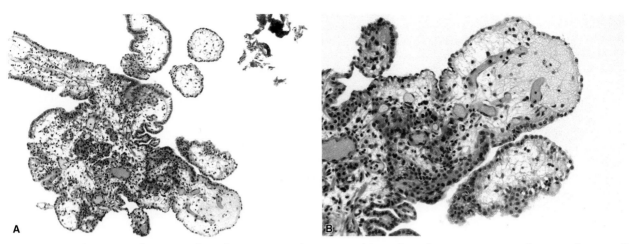

Figure 3-35 Nephrogenic adenoma, polypoid pattern (A and B). It resembles polypoid cystitis. However, there is only one cell layer lining. The stroma is edematous and vascular with scant inflammatory cells.

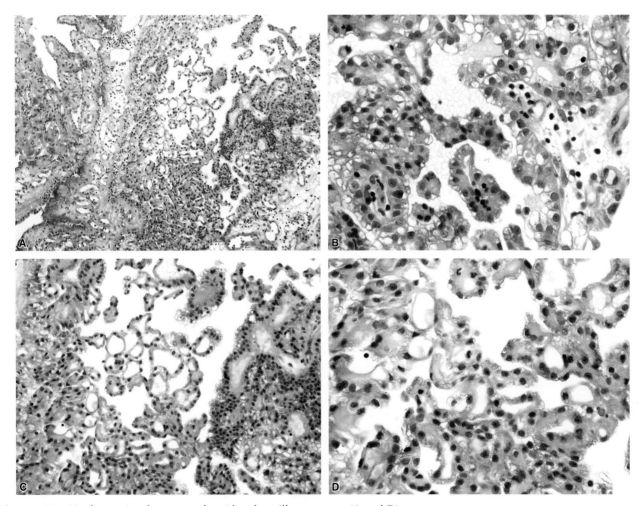

Figure 3-36 Nephrogenic adenoma, polypoid and papillary patterns (A and D).

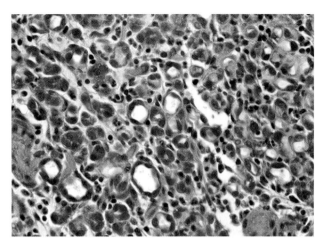

Figure 3-37   Nephrogenic adenoma with signet ring cell feature.

Based on the proposed origin of nephrogenic adenoma from renal tubular epithelial cells,[64] Tong and colleagues examined the expression of PAX2, a renal-specific transcription factor, in cases of nephrogenic adenoma as well as normal prostatic epithelium, urothelium, prostatic adenocarcinoma, and urothelial carcinoma.[85] They found positivity in all nephrogenic adenoma cases, while the counterpart normal epithelium and prostatic/urothelial neoplasms were negative, suggesting that PAX2 may also be a useful marker for challenging cases.

Another differential diagnostic consideration of nephrogenic adenoma is clear cell adenocarcinoma (see also **Chapter 13**).[12,82–84] In 1986, Young and Scully noted that hobnail cells, similar to those of clear cell carcinoma of the cervix and vagina, may be seen in up to one-third of cases.[86] However, differentiating features of nephrogenic adenoma include a minimum of cytologic atypia, infrequency of mitotic figures, male predilection (as opposed to female for clear cell adenocarcinoma), small to microscopic size, and infrequency of abundant clear cytoplasm. In some cases, nephrogenic metaplasia is composed of minute mucin-containing tubules lined by single cells with compressed nuclei that simulates signet ring cell carcinoma.[2,87] Hobnail cells suggest the possibility of clear cell carcinoma of the bladder, but such cells are focally present in 70% of cases of nephrogenic metaplasia. Solid tubules with cells containing clear cytoplasm also suggest clear cell carcinoma,[2,88] but this is an uncommon and focal finding in nephrogenic metaplasia.[2,87,89] Histopathologic features that favor clear cell adenocarcinoma over nephrogenic metaplasia include a predominance of clear cells, severe cytologic atypia, high mitotic rate, the presence of tumor necrosis, high MIB1 count, and strong staining for p53 (**Table 3-3**).[2,90] At present, the greatest difficulty in separating nephrogenic metaplasia and clear cell carcinoma arises in small specimens and biopsies of urethral diverticula. When present in the prostatic urethra, nephrogenic metaplasia may be mistaken for prostatic adenocarcinoma. In the differential diagnosis of adenocarcinoma, Skinnider et al. noted that as nephrogenic adenoma may be positive for α-methylacyl-CoA racemase (AMACR or P504S), it might be confused with prostatic adenocarcinoma, particularly when involving the prostatic urethra.[91] Similarly, lesions frequently show the absence of high molecular weight cytokeratin and p63, which may falsely confirm this impression. Gupta et al. demonstrated similar findings, leading the authors to conclude that careful examination of traditional hematoxylin and eosin–stained sections and application of morphologic criteria may be the most critical element in resolving the differential diagnosis.[92] Notable distinguishing features of nephrogenic adenoma include lack of significant cytologic atypia/mitoses or the presence of mixed tubular and papillary components, hobnail cells, or an edematous/inflammatory stroma. The absence of prostate-specific antigen in nephrogenic adenoma is a helpful diagnostic feature.

Further complicating this issue, Cheng and colleagues discussed 18 cases of nephrogenic adenoma with cytologic atypia (atypical nephrogenic metaplasia).[83] Defined as the presence of nuclear enlargement, hyperchromasia, and prominent nucleoli, these lesions may be highly concerning for malignancy; however, none of the patients studied developed bladder carcinoma over a followup period of 3.5 years. These authors cite circumscribed growth; confinement to the lamina propria; small size; absence of mitotic figures, necrosis, or nuclear pleomorphism; and the presence of inflammation and stromal edema as distinguishing features of nephrogenic adenoma.

Hansel and colleagues described an unusual variant of nephrogenic adenoma with areas of recognizable nephrogenic adenoma admixed with fibromyxoid areas composed of spindled cells resembling fibroblasts or small vessels and a fibromyxoid extracellular matrix (**Fig. 3-39**).[93] These lesions, termed "fibromyxoid nephrogenic adenoma," may closely mimic an infiltrating mucinous adenocarcinoma. Of the patients studied, the majority had a clinical history of treatment for prior prostate or bladder carcinoma, while one patient had no such history, and one patient had an associated adjacent carcinoma with extracellular mucin. The authors suggest that awareness of this unique appearance, coupled with the presence of typical nephrogenic adenoma histology and immunohistochemical features, may prevent misdiagnosis of this interesting lesion as a mucinous carcinoma.

Finally, nephrogenic adenoma should be differentiated from urothelial carcinoma with small tubules/acini, a rare variant of urothelial carcinoma that demonstrate a marked predominance of small tubules and acini.[94] In such cases, confusion with prostatic adenocarcinoma or nephrogenic

Table 3-3   **Differentiating Clinicopathologic Characteristics of Nephrogenic Adenoma, Clear Cell Adenocarcinoma, and Prostatic Adenocarcinoma**[a]

Nephrogenic adenoma	Male predilection; minimal cytologic atypia (limited to nuclear enlargement/hyperchromasia and prominent nucleoli in atypical NA); absence of pleomorphism; edematous, inflammatory stroma; infrequent mitotic figures; small to microscopic size; circumscribed growth (may be intermixed with superficial muscle fibers); confinement to lamina propria; absence of necrosis; less frequent abundant clear cytoplasm; minimal, focal p53 staining (up to 20% in atypical NA); Ki67 count < 14 per 200 cells; PAX2 positive; negative for PSA
Clear cell adenocarcinoma	Female predilection; significant tumor size; greater cytologic atypia; necrosis; significant mitotic rate; strong p53 staining; Ki67 count > 32 per 200 cells; lack of PSA or PSAP staining
Prostatic adenocarcinoma	Male; positivity for PSA and/or PSAP; lacking mixed tubulopapillary components of NA (except in ductal-type prostatic adenocarcinoma); negative for PAX2

[a]NA, nephrogenic adenoma; PSA, prostate-specific antigen; PSAP, prostate-specific acid phosphatase.

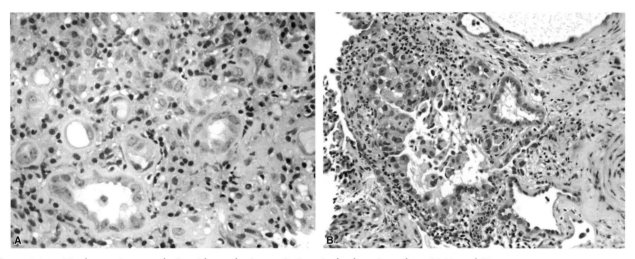

Figure 3-38   Nephrogenic metaplasia with cytologic atypia (atypical sclerosing adenosis) (A and B).

adenoma may be possible. The negativity of tumor cells for prostate-specific antigen and prostatic-specific acid phosphatase may be a helpful feature in such circumstances. In differentiation of this lesion from nephrogenic adenoma, morphologic evaluation for the characteristic tubular and papillary components, cuboidal to low columnar epithelium, and occasional hobnail appearance of nephrogenic adenoma may be helpful. Also, urothelial carcinoma with small tubules/acini may show extensive invasion of the bladder wall in opposition to its bland histology.

Urothelial Hyperplasia

Flat (Simple) Urothelial Hyperplasia

Flat (simple) urothelial hyperplasia is associated with a wide variety of inflammatory disorders, lithiasis, and vesical neoplasms, particularly those with papillary growth.[2,95,96]

This unusual finding may represent an early stage in the development of papillary urothelial neoplasms. The true incidence of flat hyperplasia is not known, due to a lack of large-scale screening studies.[2,96–98]

Histologically, urothelial hyperplasia is usually focal and consists of an increase in the number of cell layers, usually 10 or more (Figs. 3-40 and 3-41). However, it is not necessary to count the number of cell layers for the diagnosis. There are few or no significant cytologic abnormalities, although a slight nuclear enlargement may be present. Morphological evidence of maturation from base to surface is generally evident.[2,99] Hyperplasia may occasionally be associated with dysplasia or carcinoma in situ in the adjacent mucosa, but this is uncommon. Pseudopapillary growth is uncommon in flat hyperplasia and characteristically lacks well-formed vascular cores.

Mimics of flat urothelial hyperplasia include urothelial compression artifact and tangential sectioning of the mucosa.[2,96] It should be distinguished from urothelial

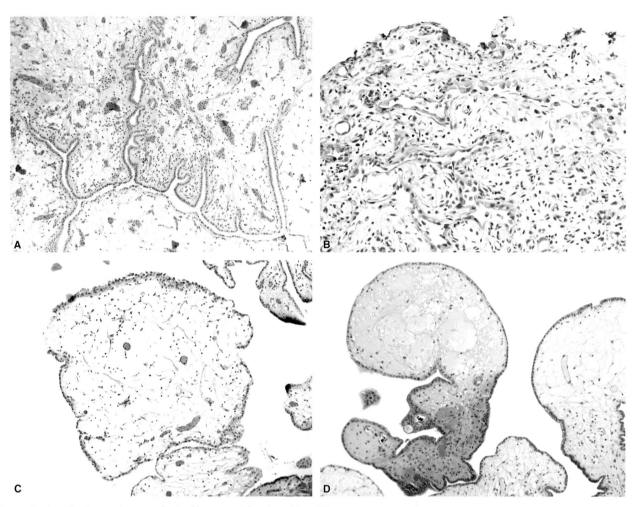

Figure 3-39   Nephrogenic metaplasia, fibromyxoid variant (A to D).

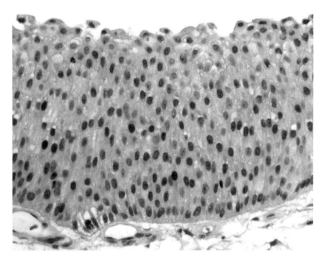

Figure 3-40   Simple urothelial hyperplasia. The urothelium displays normal maturation without papillae, uniform cell spacing, and no nuclear abnormalities; however, it is substantially thicker than normal.

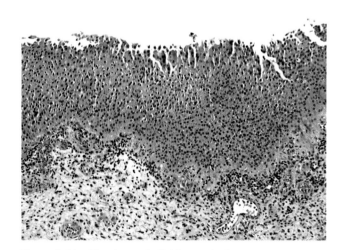

Figure 3-41   Simple urothelial hyperplasia.

dysplasia and carcinoma in situ (see **Chapters 6** and **7** for further discussion).

Molecular evidence suggests that flat urothelial hyperplasia is a putative precursor. Studies have shown that 71% of cases of flat urothelial hyperplasia had the same chromosome 9 deletions that exist with concurrent low grade papillary urothelial carcinoma.[2,97,98] FISH studies for 9q22 (FACC) and 9p21 (p16/CDK12) have shown the same chromosome 9 deletions in hyperplasia and normal urothelium when there are coexisting low grade papillary tumors. Also, 17p13 deletions were found in 8% of cases of urothelial hyperplasia and low grade carcinoma. In that study, the same chromosomal anomalies were present in the adjacent "normal-looking" urothelium. Also, a clonal relationship between flat urothelial hyperplasia and concomitant papillary carcinoma was observed in 50% of cases.[2,97] A possible genetic relationship between flat hyperplasia and low grade papillary tumors has been supported further by recent molecular studies showing chromosome 9 deletions and mutations in the fibroblast growth factor receptor 3 *(FGFR3)* gene in both urothelial hyperplasia and low grade papillary neoplasia. Recently, Majewski et al. found additional loss of heterozygosity at 3q22–q24, 5q22–q31, 10q26, 13q14, and 17p13 in benign hyperplastic lesions from bladders with urothelial carcinoma.[100]

Taken together, these molecular data indicate preneoplastic potential of flat lesions regardless of cellular phenotype and suggest a role for flat hyperplasia in the pathogenesis of low grade papillary urothelial carcinoma. However, when flat urothelial hyperplasia is seen in isolation, there is no evidence of premalignant potential.[2,99]

Papillary Hyperplasia

Within the spectrum of urothelial hyperplasia, papillary architecture may be present; most of these patients have concomitant papillary urothelial neoplasia. The term "papillary urothelial hyperplasia" remains controversial and is rarely used. The lesion described as such is usually found with concomitant papillary urothelial carcinoma or in followup biopsies of these patients.[2,101,102] Undulating folds of urothelium that lack cytologic atypia and fibrovascular cores characterize papillary hyperplasia (**Figs. 3-42** and **3-43**). Although considered "hyperplastic," papillary hyperplasia is typically surfaced by normal-appearing urothelium only four to seven cells in thickness. Cytologically, the cells in papillary hyperplasia lack atypia and maintain nuclear polarity. There may be increased vascularity in the stroma at the base of the papillary

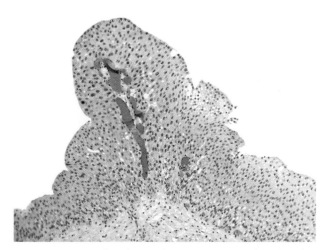

Figure 3-42 Papillary hyperplasia. Microscopic papillary growth without cytologic atypia. This represents early papilloma or papillary hyperplasia.

folds. This lesion is considered by some to be the clonal precursor of papillary urothelial carcinoma based on associated genetic anomalies,[2,103] but critics contend that it actually represents early undiagnosed papillary carcinoma.

Clinical studies of papillary hyperplasia are very limited. Taylor et al. reported 16 cases of "typical" papillary hyperplasia occurring in patients with either a prior or a concurrent low grade papillary urothelial neoplasia.[101] The majority of their patients were men (11 men and 5 women) with a mean age of 67.5 years (range, 40 to 89 years). In a subsequent study, Swierczynski and Epstein reported 15 cases of papillary urothelial hyperplasia with varying degrees of atypia, ranging from dysplasia to flat carcinoma in situ (atypical papillary urothelial hyperplasia).[104] Most of the patients in Swierczynski and Epstein's study developed high grade urothelial neoplasms. This is in contrast to low grade tumors occurring in patients with papillary hyperplasia without atypia previously reported by Taylor et al. Taken together, these clinicopathologic studies suggest that papillary hyperplasia may be a precursor of low grade papillary neoplasms, and that atypical papillary hyperplasia may progress to carcinoma in situ and high grade papillary cancer.

The primary differential diagnoses of papillary hyperplasia include papilloma, low grade papillary carcinoma, and polypoid cystitis.[1,4] In contrast to low grade papillary neoplasms or papilloma, papillary hyperplasia lacks well-defined central fibrovascular cores, arborization, and detached papillary fronds. There may be increased vascularity in the stroma at the base of the papillary folds in papillary hyperplasia. However, these changes do not

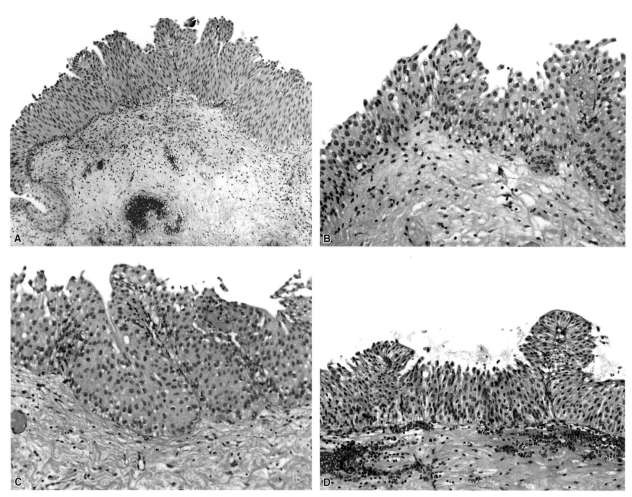

Figure 3-43   Papillary hyperplasia (A to D).

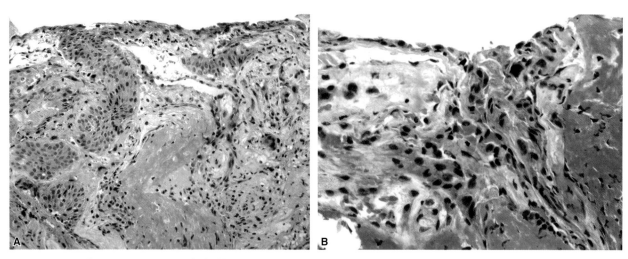

Figure 3-44   Pseudocarcinomatous epithelial hyperplasia (A and B).

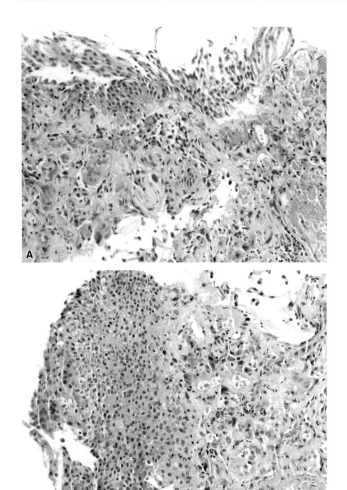

extend upward into the papilla. In diffuse papillomatosis, the mucosa is more extensively involved by small delicate papillary processes, creating a velvety cystoscopic appearance (see also **Chapter 5**). Papillary hyperplasia also lacks the broad-based stalks and inflammation seen in polypoid cystitis. Some cases of polypoid cystitis have thin finger-like papillae. However, papillary urothelial hyperplasia is not accompanied by the abundant chronic inflammation that is seen in polypoid cystitis.

Inflammatory "papillary hyperplasia" of the bladder may be confused with cancer at cystoscopy; we contend that the best term for this finding is "papillary cystitis" (see also **Chapter 2**). Microscopically, there is characteristic granulation tissue with varying amounts of acute and chronic inflammation and, occasionally, denuded papillae. Cases of this type are referred to in older literature as "cystitis granulosa."

Pseudocarcinomatous Epithelial Hyperplasia

Recently, a lesion named "pseudocarcinomatous epithelial proliferation" (hyperplasia), a rare form of florid von Brunn nests first described in association with radiation therapy or chemotherapy, has been reported as unassociated with either.[37,105] It is characterized histologically by pseudoinfiltrative nests of epithelium, sometimes with squamous metaplasia, which are adjacent to ectatic blood vessels that often contain fibrin thrombi (**Figs. 3-44** and **3-45**). These nests, especially because of their irregular shape, can resemble invasive carcinoma.

Figure 3-45   Pseudocarcinomatous epithelial hyperplasia (A and B).

REFERENCES

1. Young RH. Non-neoplastic disorders of the urinary bladder. In: Bostwick DG, Cheng L, eds. Urologic Surgical Pathology, 2nd ed. Philadelphia: Elsevier/Mosby, 2008; 215–58.

2. Wiener DP, Koss LG, Sablay B, Freed SZ. The prevalence and significance of Brunn's nests, cystitis cystica and squamous metaplasia in normal bladders. *J Urol* 1979;122:317–21.

3. Young RH, Wick MR. Transitional cell carcinoma of the urinary bladder with pseudosarcomatous stroma. *Am J Clin Pathol* 1988;90:216–9.

4. Cheng L, Bostwick DG. Overdiagnosis of bladder carcinoma. *Anal Quant Cytol Histol* 2008;30:261–4.

5. Volmar KE, Chan TY, De Marzo AM, Epstein JI. Florid von Brunn nests mimicking urothelial carcinoma: a morphologic and immunohistochemical comparison to the nested variant of urothelial carcinoma. *Am J Surg Pathol* 2003;27:1243–52.

6. Lopez-Beltran A, Luque RJ, Moreno A, Bollito E, Carmona E, Montironi R. The pagetoid variant of bladder urothelial carcinoma in situ. A clinicopathological study of 11 cases. *Virchows Arch* 2002;441:148–53.

7. Lopez-Beltran A, Luque RJ, Oliveira PS, Aydin NE, Mazerolles C, Montironi R. Urothelial carcinoma of the bladder, lipid cell variant (UCBLCV). Immunohistochemical and clinico-pathologic findings in seven cases (abstract). *Mod Pathol* 2002;15:171A.

8. Williamson SR, Montironi R, Lopez-Beltran A, MacLennan GT, Davidson DD, Cheng L. Diagnosis, evaluation and treatment of carcinoma in situ of the urinary bladder: the state of the art. *Crit Rev Oncol Hematol* 2010;76:112–26.

9. Ito N, Hirose M, Shirai T, Tsuda H, Nakanishi K, Fukushima S. Lesions of the urinary bladder epithelium in 125 autopsy cases. *Acta Pathol Jpn* 1981;31:545–57.

10. Singh I, Ansari MS. Cystitis cystica glandularis masquerading as a bladder tumor. *Int Urol Nephrol* 2001;33:635–6.

11. Montironi R, Lopez-Beltran A, Scarpelli M, Mazzucchelli R, Cheng L. Morphological classification and definition of benign, preneoplastic and non-invasive neoplastic lesions of the urinary bladder. *Histopathology* 2008;53:621–33.

12. Williamson SR, Lopez-Beltran A, Montironi R, Cheng L. Glandular lesions of the urinary bladder:clinical significance and differential diagnosis. *Histopathology* 2011;58:811–34.

13. Jost SP, Dixon JS, Gosling JA. Ultrastructural observations on cystitis cystica in human bladder urothelium. *Br J Urol* 1993;71:28–33.

14. Parker C. Cystitis cystica and glandularis: a study of 40 cases. *Proc R Soc Med* 1970;63:239–42.

15. Defoor W, Minevich E, Sheldon C. Unusual bladder masses in children. *Urology* 2002;60:911.

16. Tong RS, Larner T, Finlay M, Agarwal D, Costello AJ. Pelvic lipomatosis associated with proliferative cystitis occurring in two brothers. *Urology* 2002;59:602.

17. Granados EA, Algaba F, Vicente Rodriguez J. Cystitis glandularis. *Arch Esp Urol* 1999;52:119–22.

18. Delnay KM, Stonehill WH, Goldman H, Jukkola AF, Dmochowski RR. Bladder histological changes associated with chronic indwelling urinary catheter. *J Urol* 1999;161:1106–8; discussion 1108–9.

19. Sung MT, Lopez-Beltran A, Eble JN, MacLennan GT, Tan PH, Montironi R, Jones TD, Ulbright TM, Blair JE, Cheng L. Divergent pathway of intestinal metaplasia and cystitis glandularis of the urinary bladder. *Mod Pathol* 2006;19:1395–401.

20. Ward AM. Glandular neoplasia within the urinary tract. The aetiology of adenocarcinoma of the urothelium with a review of the literature. I. Introduction: the origin of glandular epithelium in the renal pelvis, ureter and bladder. *Virchows Arch A Pathol Pathol Anat* 1971;352:296–311.

21. Wells M, Anderson K. Mucin histochemistry of cystitis glandularis and primary adenocarcinoma of the urinary bladder. *Arch Pathol Lab Med* 1985;109:59–61.

22. Corica FA, Husmann DA, Churchill BM, Young RH, Pacelli A, Lopez-Beltran A, Bostwick DG. Intestinal metaplasia is not a strong risk factor for bladder cancer: study of 53 cases with long-term followup. *Urology* 1997;50:427–31.

23. Bell TE, Wendel RG. Cystitis glandularis: Benign or malignant? *J Urol* 1968;100:462–5.

24. Susmano D, Rubenstein AB, Dakin AR, Lloyd FA. Cystitis glandularis and adenocarcinoma of the bladder. *J Urol* 1971;105:671–4.

25. Belman AB. The clinical significant of cystitis cystica in girls: results of a prospective study. *J Urol* 1978;119:661–3.

26. Bullock PS, Thoni DE, Murphy WM. The significance of colonic mucosa (intestinal metaplasia) involving the urinary tract. *Cancer* 1987;59:2086–90.

27. Theuring F. Cystitis glandularis of the intestinal type (= intestinal metaplasia) in the urinary bladder mucosa with functionally significant pseudotumor formation. *Pathologe* 1992;13:235–40.

28. Willemen P, Van Poppel H, Baert L. Ectopic colonic epithelium of the bladder complicated by development of an adenocarcinoma. *Acta Urol Belg* 1992;60:147–9.

29. Davies G, Castro JE. Cystitis glandularis. *Urology* 1977;10:128–9.

30. Davis EL, Goldstein AM, Morrow JW. Unusual bladder mucosal metaplasia in a case of chronic prostatitis and cystitis. *J Urol* 1974;111:767–9.

31. Lin JI, Yong HS, Tseng CH, Marsidi PS, Choy C, Pilloff B. Diffuse cystitis glandularis. Associated with adenocarcinomatous change. *Urology* 1980;15:411–5.

32. Gordon A. Intestinal metaplasia of the urinary tract epithelium. *J Pathol Bacteriol* 1963;85:441–4.

33. Mostofi FK. Potentialities of bladder epithelium. *J Urol* 1954;71:705–14.

34. Young RH, Bostwick DG. Florid cystitis glandularis of intestinal type with mucin extravasation: a mimic of

adenocarcinoma. *Am J Surg Pathol* 1996;20:1462–8.

35. Morton MJ, Zhang S, Lopez-Beltran A, MacLennan GT, Eble JN, Montironi R, Sung MT, Tan PH, Zheng S, Zhou H, Cheng L. Telomere shortening and chromosomal abnormalities in intestinal metaplasia of the urinary bladder. *Clin Cancer Res* 2007;13:6232–6.

36. Smith AK, Hansel DE, Jones JS. Role of cystitis cystica et glandularis and intestinal metaplasia in development of bladder carcinoma. *Urology* 2008;71:915–8.

37. Young RH. Tumor-like lesions of the urinary bladder. *Mod Pathol* 2009;22 Suppl 2:S37–52.

38. Heyns CF, De Kock ML, Kirsten PH, van Velden DJ. Pelvic lipomatosis associated with cystitis glandularis and adenocarcinoma of the bladder. *J Urol* 1991;145:364–6.

39. Jacobs LB, Brooks JD, Epstein JI. Differentiation of colonic metaplasia from adenocarcinoma of urinary bladder. *Hum Pathol* 1997;28:1152–7.

40. Sauty L, Ravery V, Toublanc M, Boccon-Gibod L. Florid glandular cystitis: study of 3 cases and review of the literature. *Prog Urol* 1998;8:561–4.

41. Quilter TN. Embryoma of the urinary bladder. *J Urol* 1956;76:392–5.

42. Kaufman JM, Fam B, Jacobs SC, Gabilondo F, Yalla S, Kane JP, Rossier AB. Bladder cancer and squamous metaplasia in spinal cord injury patients. *J Urol* 1977;118:967–71.

43. Montgomerie JZ, Holshuh HJ, Keyser AJ, Bennett CJ, Schick DG. 28 K in squamous metaplasia of the bladder in patients with spinal cord injury. *Paraplegia* 1993;31:105–10.

44. Stonehill WH, Dmochowski RR, Patterson AL, Cox CE. Risk factors for bladder tumors in spinal cord injury patients. *J Urol* 1996;155:1248–50.

45. Widran J, Sanchez R, Gruhn J. Squamous metaplasia of the bladder: a study of 450 patients. *J Urol* 1974;112:479–82.

46. Ozbey I, Aksoy Y, Polat O, Bicgi O, Demirel A. Squamous metaplasia of the bladder: findings in 14 patients and review of the literature. *Int Urol Nephrol* 1999;31:457–61.

47. Khan MS, Thornhill JA, Gaffney E, Loftus B, Butler MR. Keratinising squamous metaplasia of the bladder: natural history and rationalization of management based on review of 54 years experience. *Eur Urol* 2002;42:469–74.

48. Morgan RJ, Cameron KM. Vesical leukoplakia. *Br J Urol* 1980;52:96–100.

49. Locke JR, Hill DE, Walzer Y. Incidence of squamous cell carcinoma in patients with long-term catheter drainage. *J Urol* 1985;133:1034–5.

50. O'Flynn JD, Mullaney J. Vesical leukoplakia progressing to carcinoma. *Br J Urol* 1974;46:31–7.

51. Reece RW, Koontz WW Jr. Leukoplakia of the urinary tract: a review. *J Urol* 1975;114:165–71.

52. Walts AE, Sacks SA. Squamous metaplasia and invasive epidermoid carcinoma of bladder. *Urology* 1977;9:317–20.

53. Benson RC Jr, Swanson SK, Farrow GM. Relationship of leukoplakia to urothelial malignancy. *J Urol* 1984;131:507–11.

54. Khafagy MM, el-Bolkainy MN, Mansour MA. Carcinoma of the bilharzial urinary bladder. A study of the associated mucosal lesions in 86 cases. *Cancer* 1972;30:150–9.

55. Long ED, Shepherd RT. The incidence and significance of vaginal metaplasia of the bladder trigone in adult women. *Br J Urol* 1983;55:189–94.

56. Tyler DE. Stratified squamous epithelium in the vesical trigone and urethra: findings correlated with the menstrual cycle and age. *Am J Anat* 1962;111:319–35.

57. Bhagavan BS, Tiamson EM, Wenk RE, Berger BW, Hamamoto G, Eggleston JC. Nephrogenic adenoma of the urinary bladder and urethra. *Hum Pathol* 1981;12:907–16.

58. Ford TF, Watson GM, Cameron KM. Adenomatous metaplasia (nephrogenic adenoma) of urothelium. An analysis of 70 cases. *Br J Urol* 1985;57:427–33.

59. Friedman NB, Kuhlenbeck H. Adenomatoid tumors of the bladder reproducing renal structures (nephrogenic adenomas). *J Urol* 1950;64:657–70.

60. Molland EA, Trott PA, Paris AM, Blandy JP. Nephrogenic adenoma: a form of adenomatous metaplasia of the bladder. A clinical and electron microscopical study. *Br J Urol* 1976;48:453–62.

61. Oliva E, Young RH. Nephrogenic adenoma of the urinary tract: a review of the microscopic appearance of 80 cases with emphasis on unusual features. *Mod Pathol* 1995;8:722–30.

62. Fournier G, Menut P, Moal MC, Hardy E, Volant A, Mangin P. Nephrogenic adenoma of the bladder in renal transplant recipients: A report of 9 cases with assessment of deoxyribonucleic acid ploidy and long-term followup. *J Urol* 1996;156:41–4.

63. Pycha A, Mian C, Reiter WJ, Brossner C, Haitel A, Wiener H, Maier U, Marberger M. Nephrogenic adenoma in renal transplant recipients: A truly benign lesion? *Urology* 1998;52:756–61.

64. Mazal PR, Schaufler R, Altenhuber-Muller R, Haitel A, Watschinger B, Kratzik C, Krupitza G, Regele H, Meisl FT, Zechner O, Kerjaschki D, Susani M. Derivation of nephrogenic adenomas from renal tubular cells in kidney-transplant recipients. *N Engl J Med* 2002;347:653–9.

65. Young RH, Scully R. Clear cell adenocarcinoma of the bladder and urethra: a report of three cases and review of the literature. *Am J Surg Pathol* 1985;9:816–26.

66. Heidenreich A, Zirbes TK, Wolter S, Engelmann UH. Nephrogenic adenoma: a rare bladder tumor in children. *Eur Urol* 1999;36:348–53.

67. Porcaro AB, D'Amico A, Ficarra V, Balzarro M, Righetti R, Martignoni G, Cavalleri S, Malossini G. Nephrogenic adenoma of the urinary bladder: our experience and review of the literature. *Urol Int* 2001;66:152–5.

68. Davis TA. Hamartoma of the urinary bladder. *Northwest Med* 1949;48:182–5.

69. Muto G, Comi L, Baldini D. Nephrogenic adenoma of the bladder associated with urinary tuberculosis. Case report. *Minerva Urol Nefrol* 1993;45:77–81.

70. O'Shea PA, Callaghan JF, Lawlor JB, Reddy VC. "Nephrogenic adenoma": an unusual metaplastic change of urothelium. *J Urol* 1981;125:249–52.

71. Pierre-Louis ML, Kovi J, Jackson A, Ucci A, Pinn-Wiggins VW. Nephrogenic adenoma: a light and electron microscopic and immunohistochemical study. *J Natl Med Assoc* 1985;77:201–5.

72. Devine P, Ucci AA, Krain H, Gavris VE, Bhagavan BS, Heaney JA, Alroy J. Nephrogenic adenoma and embryonic kidney tubules share PNA receptor sites. *Am J Surg Pathol* 1984;81:728–32.

73. Emmett JL, McDonald JD. Proliferation of glands of the urinary bladder simulating malignant neoplasm. *J Urol* 1942;48:257–61.

74. McIntire TL, Soloway MS, Murphy WM. Nephrogenic adenoma. *Urology* 1987;29:237–41.

75. Cheng L, Leibovich BC, Cheville JC, Ramnani DM, Sebo TJ, Nehra A, Malek RS, Zincke H, Bostwick DG. Squamous papilloma of the urinary tract is unrelated to condyloma acuminata. *Cancer* 2000;88:1679–86.

76. Hung SY, Tseng HH, Chung HM. Nephrogenic adenoma associated with cytomegalovirus infection of the ureter in a renal transplant patient: presentation as ureteral obstruction. *Transpl Int* 2001;14:111–4.

77. Raghavaiah NV, Noe HN, Parham DM, Murphy WM. Nephrogenic adenoma of urinary bladder associated with malakoplakia. *Urology* 1980;15:190–3.

78. Wiener HG, Remkes GW, Birner P, Pycha A, Schatzl G, Susani M, Breitenecker G. DNA profiles and numeric histogram classifiers in nephrogenic adenoma. *Cancer* 2002;96:117–22.

79. Aldenborg F, Peeker R, Fall M, Olofsson A, Enerback L. Metaplastic transformation of urinary bladder epithelium: effect on mast cell recruitment, distribution, and phenotype expression. *Am J Pathol* 1998;153:149–57.

80. Young RH. Pseudoneoplastic lesions of the urinary bladder and urethra: a selective review with emphasis on recent information. *Semin Diagn Pathol* 1997;14:133–46.

81. Young RH, Oliva E, Garcia JA, Bhan AK, Clement PB. Urethral caruncle with atypical stromal cells simulating lymphoma or sarcoma—a distinctive pseudoneoplastic lesion of females. A report of six cases. *Am J Surg Pathol* 1996;20:1190–5.

82. Cheng L, Lopez-Beltran A, MacLennan GT, Montironi R, Bostwick DG. Neoplasms of the urinary bladder. In: Bostwick DG, Cheng L, eds. Urologic Surgical Pathology, 2nd ed. Philadelphia: Elsevier/Mosby, 2008;259–352.

83. Cheng L, Cheville JC, Sebo TJ, Eble JN, Bostwick DG. Atypical nephrogenic metaplasia of the urinary tract: A precursor lesion? *Cancer* 2000;88:853–61.

84. Sung MT, Zhang S, MacLennan GT, Lopez-Beltran A, Montironi R, Wang M, Tan PH, Cheng L. Histogenesis of clear cell adenocarcinoma in the urinary tract: evidence of urothelial origin. *Clin Cancer Res* 2008;14:1947–55.

85. Tong GX, Weeden EM, Hamele-Bena D, Huan Y, Unger P, Memeo L, O'Toole K. Expression of PAX8 in nephrogenic adenoma and clear cell adenocarcinoma of the lower urinary tract: Evidence of related histogenesis? *Am J Surg Pathol* 2008;32:1380–7.

86. Young RH, Scully RE. Nephrogenic adenoma. A report of 15 cases, review of the literature, and comparison with clear cell adenocarcinoma of the urinary tract. *Am J Surg Pathol* 1986;10:268–75.

87. Malpica A, Ro JY, Troncoso P, Ordonez NG, Amin MB, Ayala AG. Nephrogenic adenoma of the prostatic urethra involving the prostate gland: a clinicopathologic and immunohistochemical study of eight cases. *Hum Pathol* 1994;25:390–5.

88. Schultz RE, Bloch MJ, Tomaszewski JE, Brooks JS, Hanno PM. Mesonephric adenocarcinoma of the bladder. *J Urol* 1984;132:263–5.

89. Alsanjari N, Lynch MJ, Fisher C, Parkinson MC. Vesical clear cell adenocarcinoma. V. Nephrogenic adenoma: a diagnostic problem. *Histopathology* 1995;27:43–9.

90. Gilcrease MZ, Delgado R, Vuitch F, Albores-Saavedra J. Clear cell adenocarcinoma and nephrogenic adenoma of the urethra and urinary bladder: a histopathologic and immunohistochemical comparison. *Hum Pathol* 1998;29:1451–6.

91. Skinnider BF, Oliva E, Young RH, Amin MB. Expression of alpha-methylacyl-CoA racemase (P504S) in nephrogenic adenoma: a significant immunohistochemical pitfall compounding the differential diagnosis with prostatic adenocarcinoma. *Am J Surg Pathol* 2004;28:701–5.

92. Gupta A, Wang HL, Policarpio-Nicolas ML, Tretiakova MS, Papavero V, Pins MR, Jiang Z, Humphrey PA, Cheng L, Yang XJ. Expression of alpha-methylacyl-coenzyme A racemase in nephrogenic adenoma. *Am J Surg Pathol* 2004;28:1224–9.

93. Hansel DE, Nadasdy T, Epstein JI. Fibromyxoid nephrogenic adenoma: a newly recognized variant mimicking mucinous adenocarcinoma. *Am J Surg Pathol* 2007;31:1231–7.

94. Huang Q, Chu PG, Lau SK, Weiss LM. Urothelial carcinoma of the urinary bladder with a component of acinar/tubular type differentiation simulating prostatic adenocarcinoma. *Hum Pathol* 2004;35:769–73.

95. Ayala AG, Ro JY. Premalignant lesions of the urothelium and transitional cell tumors. *Contem Issues in Surg Pathol of the Urinary Bladder* 1989;13:65–101.

96. Koss LG. Tumors of the Urinary Bladder, Fascicle 11. Washington, DC: Armed Forces Institute of Pathology, 1975.

97. Obermann EC, Junker K, Stoehr R, Dietmaier W, Zaak D, Schubert J, Hofstaedter F, Knuechel R, Hartmann A. Frequent genetic alterations in flat urothelial hyperplasias and concomitant papillary bladder cancer as detected by CGH, LOH, and FISH analyses. *J Pathol* 2003;199:50–7.

98. Hartmann A, Moser K, Kriegmair M, Hofstetter A, Hofstaedter F, Knuechel R. Frequent genetic alterations in simple urothelial hyperplasias of the bladder in patients with papillary urothelial carcinoma. *Am J Pathol* 1999;154:721–7.

99. Lopez-Beltran A, Cheng L, Andersson L, Brausi M, de Matteis A, Montironi R, Sesterhenn I, van det Kwast KT, Mazerolles C. Preneoplastic non-papillary lesions and conditions of the urinary bladder: an update based on the Ancona International Consultation. *Virchows Arch* 2002;440:3–11.

100. Majewski T, Lee S, Jeong J, Yoon DS, Kram A, Kim MS, Tuziak T, Bondaruk J, Lee S, Park WS, Tang KS, Chung W, et al. Understanding the development of human bladder cancer by using a whole-organ genomic mapping strategy. *Lab Invest* 2008;88:694–721.

101. Taylor DC, Bhagavan BS, Larsen MP, Cox JA, Epstein JI. Papillary urothelial hyperplasia. A precursor to papillary neoplasms. *Am J Surg Pathol* 1996;20:1481–8.

102. Hodges KB, Lopez-Beltran A, Davidson DD, Montironi R, Cheng L. Urothelial dysplasia and other flat lesions of the urinary bladder: clinicopathologic and molecular features. *Hum Pathol* 2010;41:155–62.

103. Chow NH, Cairns P, Eisenberger CF, Schoenberg MP, Taylor DC, Epstein JI, Sidransky D. Papillary urothelial hyperplasia is a clonal precursor to papillary transitional cell bladder cancer. *Int J Cancer* 2000;89:514–8.

104. Swierczynski SL, Epstein JI. Prognostic significance of atypical papillary urothelial hyperplasia. *Hum Pathol* 2002;33:512–7.

105. Lane Z, Epstein JI. Pseudocarcinomatous epithelial hyperplasia in the bladder unassociated with prior irradiation or chemotherapy. *Am J Surg Pathol* 2008;32:92–7.

Chapter 4

Polyps and Other Nonneoplastic Benign Conditions

Bladder Pathology, First Edition. Liang Cheng, Antonio Lopez-Beltran, David G. Bostwick.
© 2012 Wiley-Blackwell. Published 2012 by John Wiley & Sons, Inc.

Polyps and Polypoid Lesions of the Bladder

Fibroepithelial Polyp

This rare lesion arises most frequently in children with a mean age of 8.9 years,[1] and there is a strong male predilection.[1,2] It involves the renal pelvis ureteropelvic junction, the upper one-third of the ureter, the posterior urethra, and the bladder neck,[3,4] where it may appear as a large polypoid mass.[5–7] The origin may be congenital (sometimes referred to as congenital posterior urethral polyp)[8,9] or possibly acquired.[3] Patients are asymptomatic or present with hematuria, urgency, dysuria, flank pain, and hesitancy.[1–12] The radiologic and/or endoscopic differential diagnosis may include malignancy, especially if the lesion is large and appears to represent a mesenchymal process.[10]

The biologic behavior of fibroepithelial polyp is uniformly benign, although one study identified translocation of chromosomes 4 and 6 in a single case, raising the question of whether such lesions represent a benign neoplasm or whether a constitutional abnormality was present in this particular case.[12]

Histologically, it is similar to fibroepithelial polyps seen elsewhere, appearing as a solitary polyp with a broad stalk containing a fibrous or edematous core usually devoid of significant inflammation or edema masses (**Figs. 4-1** to **4-3**). The epithelial lining is flat, or hyperplastic in some cases. The fibrovascular cores contain blood vessels and a few clusters of chronic inflammatory cells; areas of ulceration or erosion may be present. Rarely, there may be atypical stromal myofibroblasts or stromal xanthoma cells.[13] Three patterns are identified: (1) papillary growth with a core of fibrous connective tissue punctuated by numerous minute round vessels; (2) papillary growth with secondary elongated delicate finger-like projections (secondary branching), and (3) polypoid growth with broad leaf-like or club-shaped papillae with nonintestinal-type cystitis glandularis of the stalk.[3,6] One case was associated with Beckwith–Wiedemann syndrome.[4] Another unusual case arose in a diverticular abscess draining into the vagina.[14] Most cases in the lower urinary tract are treated successfully by transurethral resection; giant fibroepithelial polyps may be removed successfully by ureterocystoscopy; more extensive resection is rarely required.[6]

Benign atypical stromal cells similar to those in giant cell cystitis are sometimes present in fibroepithelial polyps, referred to as pseudosarcomatous stroma, and may be mistaken for sarcoma (**Figure 4-4**).[15] Such cells are often large, multinucleated, and contain smudged featureless chromatin; mitotic figures are invariably lacking.

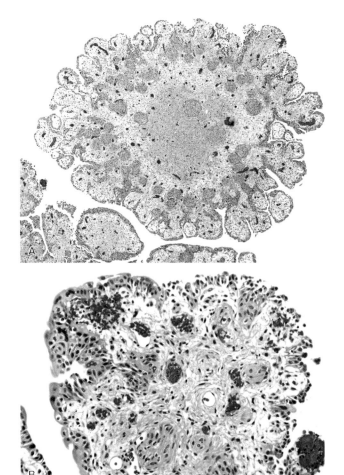

Figure 4-1   Fibroepithelial polyp (A and B).

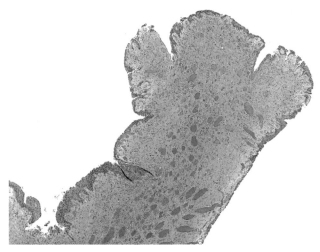

Figure 4-2   Fibroepithelial polyp, with a flat atrophic urothelial surface lining.

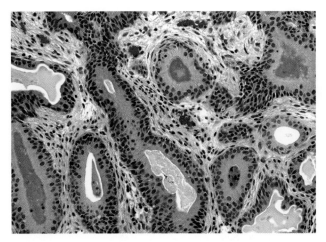

Figure 4-3 Fibroepithelial polyp with a fibrotic stroma.

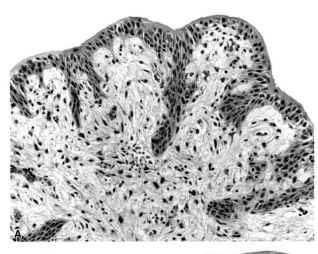

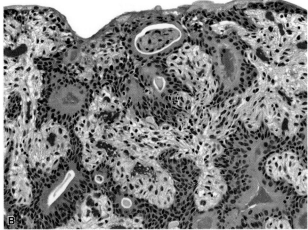

Figure 4-4 Pseudosarcomatous stroma in fibroepithelial polyps (A and B).

It is critical to separate fibroepithelial polyp from urothelial carcinoma. Fortunately, these lesions usually affect different patient populations, have different locations in the urinary tract, and differ radiographically.[16] Distinguishing fibroepithelial polyp from urothelial papilloma may be challenging; however, the complex, interanastomosing, and budding papillary architecture of papilloma is not characteristic of fibroepithelial polyp. Fibroepithelial polyp differs from polypoid cystitis in that it is a solitary polypoid growth, usually with a more fibrous than inflammatory stroma. Although the differential diagnosis also includes botryoides-type rhabdomyosarcoma, which may present as a polypoid mass in the region of the bladder neck and prostatic urethra, fibroepithelial polyp lacks the features of the latter, which include cytologic atypia, mitotic activity, necrosis, and cambium layer formation.

Ectopic Prostatic Tissue

Papillary, polypoid, and sessile masses of benign prostatic epithelium are rarely found in the male bladder and resembling similar findings in the urethra.[17–21] These lesions probably represent persistent embryologic remnants. A variety of terms have been used to describe them, including ectopic prostatic tissue, benign polyps with prostate-type epithelium, villous polyps, papilloma, papillary adenoma, urethral adenoma, glandular polyps, and prostatic caruncle.[17,22]

Ectopic prostatic tissue is more common at the trigone, arising in men between 30 and 84 years of age.[35,40] The average age is 60 years.[17] Hematuria is the usual presenting symptom. Ectopic prostatic tissue consists of acini lined by columnar epithelium that displays prostate-specific antigen (PSA), prostatic-specific acid phosphatase (PSAP), and prostein (P501S) immunoreactivity (**Figs. 4-5** and **4-6**). High molecular weight cytokeratin (CK; 34βE12) positivity is seen in basal cells.[23] Rarely, the acini of ectopic prostatic tissue are partially covered by urothelium. Associated inflammation is uncommon. Rare cases may yield atypical cells on urine cytology.

The main differential diagnosis in the bladder includes cystitis cystica/glandularis due to the presence of glandular structures in a subepithelial location. The key to distinguishing the two is recognition of the undulating architectural appearance of the ectopic prostatic glands and appreciation of the presence of a dual cell layer (columnar epithelial cells and basal cells) in ectopic prostatic glands, histologic features that are not seen in cystitis cystica/glandularis. The presence of corpora amylacea can be very helpful in the distinction. It was reported previously that ectopic prostatic tissue invariably occurs in association with cystitis cystica/glandularis and hence represents a metaplastic process.[1,10,33]

In the largest series of ectopic prostate tissue presented in the urinary tract, Halat et al. showed cystitis

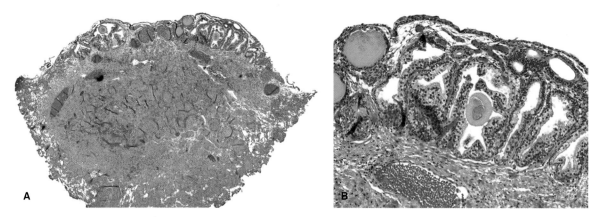

Figure 4-5   Ectopic prostate (A and B).

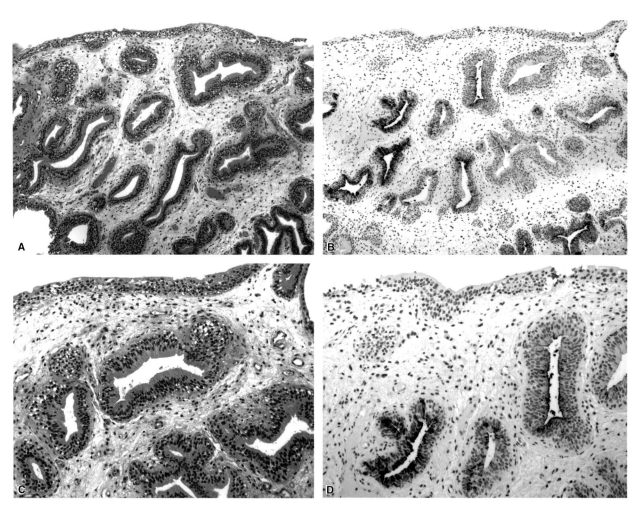

Figure 4-6   Ectopic prostate (A to D). Prostate-specific antigen immunostaining is positive (B and D).

cystica/glandularis in only 25% of the specimens.[17] None of these cases showed any other form of metaplasia, such as intestinal or squamous metaplasia, which often occur in association with chronic irritation.[17] In all cases, the prostatic glandular tissue was in a submucosal location, with no apparent communication with the surface urothelium or the cystitis cystica urothelium.

Immunohistochemistry is helpful in difficult cases. PSA and PSAP are relatively specific and sensitive markers for tissue of prostatic origin; however, both have been reported to be positive in periurethral glands in males[24,25] and females.[25] It is therefore recommended that they should be used in conjunction with other markers for prostatic tissue, such as P501S, which is a transmembrane protein that is prostate specific and so far has been detected only in prostate tissue in males.[26,27] CD10, a putative marker of tissue of mesonephric origin, is another useful biomarker. CD10 is usually positive in epithelial and basal cells of normal and hyperplastic prostatic acini, but is negative in prostatic adenocarcinoma. The pattern of CD10 immunostaining is consistently apically luminal in the epithelial cells.[28] If these stains are inconclusive, basal cell markers such as p63 and high molecular weight cytokeratins, or a PIN4 cocktail to demonstrate the presence of populations of both basal cells and secretory epithelial cells are used.

Polypoid Hamartoma

Hamartoma of the bladder usually arises in children between the ages of 4 and 15 years, often in association with hamartomatous polyps of the gastrointestinal tract.[29–31] It consists of a mixture of tissues resembling von Brunn nests, cystitis cystica, and cystitis glandularis. The stroma may be muscular, fibrous (**Fig. 4-7**), or edematous.[32] The intestinal form of cystitis glandularis may be present, and some authors consider this an unusual and florid variant of cystitis glandularis. A unique case of urachal polypoid hamartoma was reported in a 45-year-old woman.[33]

Papillary–Polypoid Cystitis

See **Chapter 2** for further discussion.

Nephrogenic Adenoma

See **Chapter 3** for further discussion.

Papilloma

See **Chapter 5** for further discussion.

Villous Adenoma

See **Chapter 5** for further discussion.

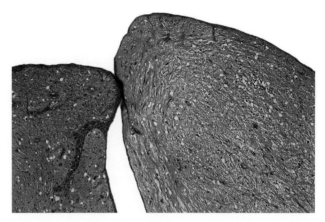

Figure 4-7   Polypoid hamartoma.

Condyloma Acuminata

See **Chapter 14** for further discussion.

Squamous Papilloma

See **Chapters 5** and **14** for further discussion.

Inverted Papilloma

See **Chapters 5** and **17** for further discussion.

Miscellaneous Nonneoplastic Benign Conditions

Diverticulosis

Diverticula are saccular evaginations of the urinary bladder (**Figs. 4-8** and **4-9**). They are most common in men (90% of cases), and occur in ages ranging from 21 to 90 years. Patients usually have bladder outlet obstruction at the bladder base.[34] Bladder diverticula vary from a few millimeters to several centimeters in diameter, and about one-half are multiple. At surgery, most are inflamed, with thinning of the sac wall, fibrosis, and loss of muscle fibers in the wall (**Fig. 4-10**). Neutrophils often infiltrate the lamina propria, and focal squamous or glandular metaplasia of the mucosa may be present. Calculi may also be present. Neoplasms are more common in diverticula than in the normal bladder, and a variety of mesenchymal and epithelial benign and malignant tumors may coexist.[34,35] The survival rate with diverticular carcinoma is poor. Diverticular cancer is more likely to be high grade urothelial carcinoma, squamous cell carcinoma, carcinosarcoma, or sarcoma than typical bladder cancer.

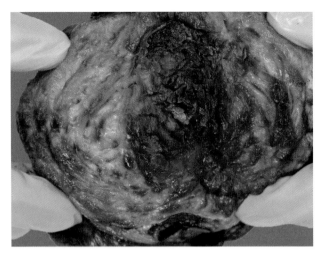

Figure 4-8   Diverticulosis of the bladder.

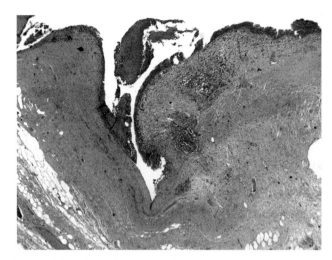

Figure 4-10   Chronic diverticulitis.

Endocervicosis

The term "endocervicosis" refers to an uncommon glandular tumor-like condition occurring in the bladder of women between 31 and 44 years of age. All lesions reported were diagnostically challenging, and some were misinterpreted as adenocarcinoma. Symptoms include suprapubic pain, dysuria, frequency, and hematuria.[36]

Macroscopically, endocervicosis typically arises in the posterior wall and posterior dome of the bladder. Microscopically, there is extensive involvement of the wall by irregular benign-appearing or mildly atypical endocervical-type glands, some that are typically cystically dilated (Figs. 4-11 and 4-12). Although the stroma surrounding the glands may demonstrate a constellation of patterns, including normal smooth muscle, an acutely and chronically inflamed fibrous cuff, endometrial-type stroma, or elastosis, a desmoplastic response is not present and may help in the discrimination from adenocarcinoma.[36–38]

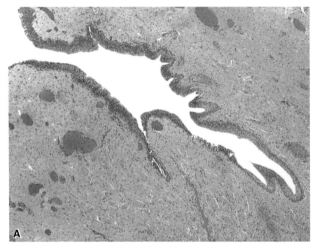

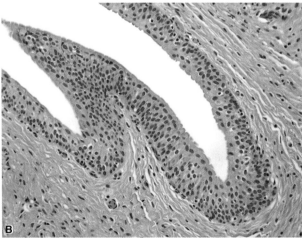

Figure 4-9   Diverticulosis (A and B).

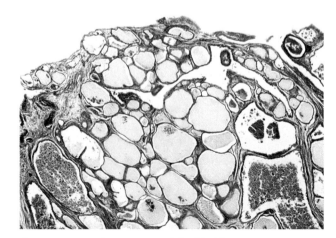

Figure 4-11   Endocervicosis of the bladder.

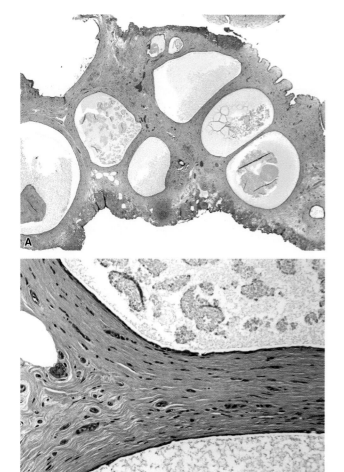

Figure 4-12 Endocervicosis of the bladder (A and B).

Clement and Young concluded that these lesions were müllerian and presented examples of endocervicosis as the mucinous counterpart of endometriosis.[37]

Differentiation from intestinal metaplasia (cystitis glandularis of the intestinal type) may be challenging; however, the architectural pattern of deep muscular involvement in endocervicosis is a contrasting feature to the superficial location of cystitis glandularis. Intestinal metaplasia appears to be composed more uniformly of goblet-type cells with genuine intestinal differentiation, as evidenced by staining with intestinal markers. Urachal remnants, which may also demonstrate a columnar lining, are typically identified incidentally, as opposed to the symptomatic mass lesion of endocervicosis. However, asymptomatic, incidentally identified endocervicosis has been reported.[39]

As these lesions carry a challenging differential diagnosis, careful workup should include exclusion of a primary endocervical adenocarcinoma or well-differentiated adenocarcinoma of the bladder.[40] The absence of a primary cervical lesion by clinical history may be helpful, especially if the cervix has been, at least in part, submitted to pathologic examination, combined with the absence of cytologic atypia and mitosis in bladder endocervicosis. Although some cervical adenocarcinoma is associated with a bland histologic appearance, so-called minimal deviation adenocarcinoma, generally, focal atypia may be appreciated.[41] Primary well-differentiated bladder adenocarcinoma without at least focal significant identifiable atypia has not been reported.

Immunohistochemical markers also appear to confirm the benign and endocervical origin of these lesions. In a case report, HBME-1, a marker typically described as positive in the endocervical epithelium, demonstrated strong positivity in the reported bladder endocervicosis lesion in comparison to control samples of endocervical tissue (sparsely positive) and urothelium (negative).[38] Estrogen receptor (ER) and progesterone receptor (PR) exhibited a similar strong pattern of staining in the bladder lesion compared with control endocervix (heterogeneous staining). DF3, a marker of apomucin MUC1, was strongly positive in both lesional tissue and controls. These authors also found a low proliferative index with Ki67/MIB1, supporting the benign nature of the lesion.[38]

Endometriosis

The bladder is the most common organ (68% to 85%) in the urinary tract to harbor foci of ectopic endometrial tissue (**Fig. 4-13**).[41–45] Most cases occur in women during the reproductive years (25 to 40 years of age), and many occur following pelvic surgery. Endometriosis of the bladder has rarely been reported in men.[46,47] Cystoscopically, the involved areas may be ulcerated, resulting in hematuria. If the implants are deep within the muscularis propria, they

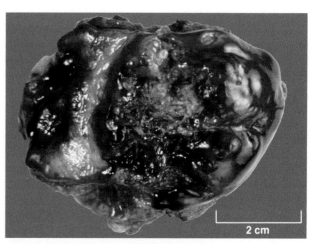

Figure 4-13 Endometriosis of the bladder. Disabling diffuse endometriosis in a young woman that required cystectomy.

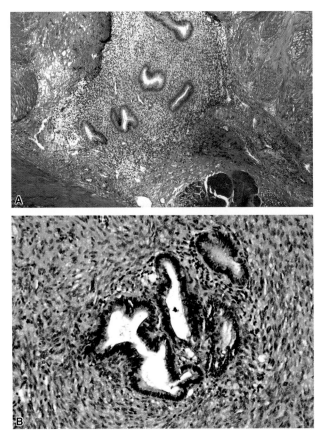

Figure 4-14   Endometriosis of the bladder (A and B).

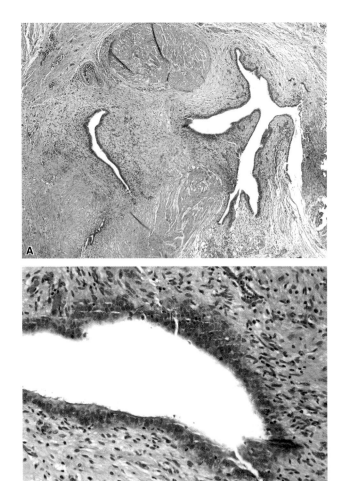

Figure 4-15   Endometriosis of the bladder (A and B).

may elicit a prominent fibrous response, resulting in a mass lesion with wall distortion. The pathogenetic mechanism by which endometriosis occurs is not entirely clear. Proposed pathways include reflux through the fallopian tube, direct extension of adenomyosis, lymphatic/hematogenous "metastasis," metaplasia, embryologic remnants, immunologic disorder, postsurgical implantation, or a combination of the above.[44,45,48–50]

Histopathologic diagnosis is typically based on the presence of both endometrial glands and stroma (**Figs. 4-14** to **4-16**). In some cases, these features may be obscured, leading to significant differential diagnostic difficulties.[41–45,51] The glands observed in these lesions typically resemble those of an inactive or proliferative pattern endometrium, although occasionally a secretory pattern is seen. The stromal component at least focally resembles normal endometrial stroma, although it may be quite inconspicuous and confined to a limited zone surrounding the glandular component. Similarly, the stromal component may be obscured by infiltrating histiocytes, either with foamy or hemosiderin-laden cytoplasm. Endometriosis, in general, may produce a fibrotic reaction composed of small, stellate fibroblasts or extensive smooth muscle

metaplasia, creating a mass-like lesion. Involvement of native smooth muscle, however, is more common.

Awareness of a variety of histologic findings in cases of endometriosis is also important to avoid misdiagnosis. Although, overall, the process is uncommon in the urinary tract, endometriosis, in general, sometimes demonstrates abundant extracellular mucin, postmenopausal changes, or treatment-related changes.[42] Features that may cause confusion with a glandular malignancy include cytologic atypia (mild to moderate), which is seen with relatively high frequency in endometriosis and, less commonly, an Arias–Stella type of reaction similar to that seen in native endometrial specimens associated with pregnancy. Notably, endometrial hyperplasia may be present and is probably similar in significance to native uterine lesions.[45,51] Along these lines, malignancy may sometimes arise in endometriosis. This does occur in the urinary tract, although infrequently, and virtually all types of endometrial-type adenocarcinoma may rarely be seen. Such a diagnosis is typically based on evidence of

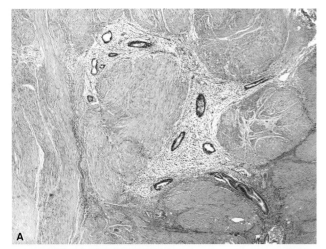

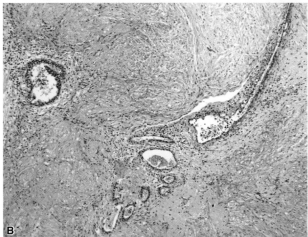

Figure 4-16 Endometriosis of the bladder (A and B).

concurrent readily identifiable endometriosis, absence of alternate primary tumor, and morphology compatible with endometrial origin.

Immunohistochemistry may be helpful in demonstrating the ectopic nature of this tissue type, especially in the case of small biopsy specimens. Positivity with CD10, similar to normal or neoplastic endometrium, may be a useful diagnostic feature, although nonspecific to endometrial tissue.[45,52] In cases of ureteral endometriosis, Al-Khawaja and colleagues identified significant positivity for ER, PR, CK7, and CA125 in the epithelial component, with CD10 expression in the stromal component, suggesting that these markers may be helpful for resolving the differential diagnosis.[45]

The pathogenesis of vesical endometriosis is uncertain. The main theories can be categorized as embryonic, migratory, and immunologic. Embryonic theories suggest that endometriosis may result from metaplastic changes of wolffian, müllerian, and occasionally peritoneal (coelomic-derived) structures. On the other hand, migratory theories

propose that retrograde menstruation, lymphovascular metastasis, and direct extension are different ways for the endometrial cells to transplant into ectopic sites. Immunologic theories suggest that suboptimal immune response may result in ectopic endometrial implantation.

Treatment of endometriosis is either medical or surgical, depending on the patient's age, symptoms, degree of obstruction, and the desire to preserve reproductive function. Hormonal therapy is best suited for patients of childbearing age who wish to retain reproductive capability. Therapy involves the use of any of the following agents: danazol, gonadotropin-releasing hormone agonist, medroxyprogesterone, estrogen–progestin combinations, or progestin alone. These drugs inhibit ovulation and reduce stimulation of endometriotic tissue, but their effects on fibrosis and scarring are minimal. Surgical treatment is also a feasible option.

Endosalpingiosis

Collectively referred to as müllerianosis, components of endometriosis, endocervicosis, and endosalpingiosis may sometimes be seen in varying combinations in the bladder.[41] In such cases, the epithelium of a tubal-type component may be lined by low cuboidal, partially ciliated cells, intermingled with intercalated cells and peg cells, similar to endosalpingiosis seen elsewhere. Differentiation from atrophic endometriosis (without significant endometrial stroma) may be achieved and is frequently based on a relative abundance or lack of a ciliated cell constituent. Like other müllerian lesions, a tumoral mass composed of one or more glandular types may be present. Curative treatment includes partial cystectomy and transurethral resection of the bladder.[53–55]

Müllerianosis

In cases in which endosalpingiosis is associated with endocervicosis, endometriosis, or both, the term "müllerianosis" has been proposed (**Fig. 4-17**).[56]

Pigmented Lesions

Melanosis of the bladder (lipofuscinosis vesicalis)
Excess lipofuscin deposition is a normal process of aging, but is rarely found in the bladder, with only a handful of cases having been reported (**Figs. 4-18 and 4-19**).[57–61] The cystoscopic or macroscopic appearance of multifocal dark pigmented spots or patches may create concern for melanoma, and coexistent melanosis and melanoma may occur.[62] Melanocytes are apparently not present in the normal urothelium; however, S100 immunoreactive dendritic cells are present in inflamed urothelium, urothelial carcinoma, and cystitis follicularis.[63] Adriamycin toxicity may be associated with vesical melanosis.[64]

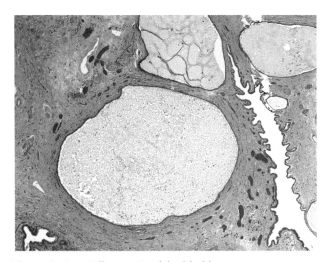

Figure 4-17   Müllerianosis of the bladder.

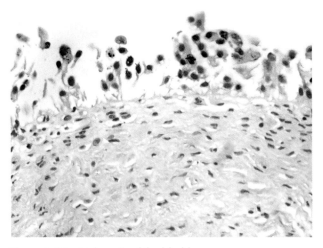

Figure 4-18   Melanosis of the bladder.

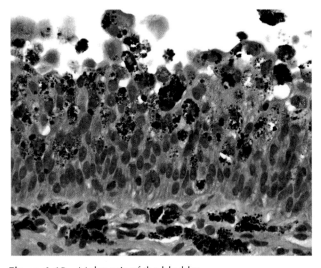

Figure 4-19   Melanosis of the bladder.

Metabolic Deposits

Amyloidosis

Amyloidosis is a disorder in which abnormal proteinaceous deposits occupy the parenchyma, interstitium, and blood vessel walls in multiple organs.[65] The condition is classified as primary or secondary. Many patients present with primary amyloidosis, which includes monoclonal IgG abnormalities of serum, urine, or both, as well as amyloid deposits in the skin, tongue, heart, gastrointestinal tract, and carpal ligaments. Secondary amyloidosis is more common and accompanies chronic inflammation or an infectious process such as rheumatoid arthritis, osteomyelitis, tuberculosis, syphilis, bronchiectasia, or ankylosing spondylitis. Amyloidosis is considered a generic term that refers to the deposition of various proteins that share a β-pleated sheet x-rayed diffraction pattern. Different clinical types of amyloidosis are now more specifically associated with identifiable proteins usually derived from circulating serum precursors. The abnormal protein of the amyloid fibril in patients with nonhereditary primary systemic amyloidosis, or those with plasma cell dyscrasia, is either an intact immunoglobulin light chain (L) or a fragment of its variable region (hence, amyloid L or AL). In localized amyloidosis of the genitourinary tract, the amyloid fibrils appear to have kappa and lambda determinants, indicating immunocytic derivation. The abnormal protein associated with secondary amyloidosis is not immunoglobulin derived but appears to follow cleavage in the liver of the serum protein known as SAA, with the formation of amyloid A (AA). Anti-AA monoclonal antibodies may be used to identify this type of amyloid. AA also constitutes the abnormal protein in patients with hereditary amyloidosis (familial Mediterranean fever). Other types of inherited amyloidosis (autosomal dominant) are associated with other β-pleated proteins, such as the variant of normal thyroxine-binding prealbumin, in the amyloidotic polyneuropathies, cardiomyopathies, or nephropathies. Fibrillar protein deposition of monomers and dimers of β_2 microglobulin occurs in patients on long-term dialysis, and this fibrillar protein has the same staining properties as those of amyloid. Most, but not all, cases of vesical amyloid are not associated with a systemic disorder and present with localized tumefactions in the bladder.

Primary vesical amyloidosis occurs with equal frequency in men and women, and typically causes gross painless hematuria. Men appear to be affected at a younger age than women. This disorder may be associated with suprapubic pain, frequency, nocturia, dysuria, recurrent urinary tract infection, and ureteral obstruction. Primary vesical amyloidosis may clinically mimic interstitial cystitis. At cystoscopy, primary amyloidotic lesions are usually localized, appearing as hemorrhagic ulcers, erythematous and inflammatory excrescences, yellow tumefactions (ulcerated or necrotic), smooth round masses that are occasionally calcified, or as polyps.[66] Localized deposits frequently resemble infiltrating neoplasms.

Microscopically, there is eosinophilic, acellular, amorphous material in primary amyloidosis that thickens and distorts arteries and veins in the suburothelial stroma and inner layers of the muscularis propria (Fig. 4-20). Connective tissue in these layers also becomes involved. There is usually no inflammatory response, although a lymphoplasmacytic and giant cell reaction may occasionally occur. Smooth muscle amyloid deposition apparently begins at the periphery of muscle bundles and progresses centrally.[65]

Vesical amyloidosis associated with systemic disorders is similar to the primary type. The secondary type is uncommon and, rather than forming a localized mass, presents with diffuse erythema and petechiae or focal necrosis. There is more prominent vascular than stromal involvement, presumably accounting for the propensity for massive spontaneous hemorrhage or torrential bleeding after biopsy.[67]

A distinctive subtype of AA amyloidosis shows massive vascular infiltration with protein AA fibrils. Amyloid stained by hematoxylin and eosin may be difficult to distinguish from hyalinized collagen, which usually is found in hyalinized blood vessel walls and some papillae of urothelial carcinomas. Amyloid may be missed if there are few deposits and the pathologist is not considering this possibility. Unlike collagen, amyloid is not birefringent in polarized light. Its tinctorial qualities do not distinguish between primary and secondary types. However, β-pleated protein fibrils are metachromatic (red) with crystal or methyl violet; they fluoresce after thioflavin T staining, and appear bright apple green following staining with alkaline Congo red and use of polarized light. Monoclonal antibodies may be used to further analyze these deposits.

Tamm–Horsfall Protein Deposit (Tamm–Horsfall Pseudotumor)

Tamm–Horsfall protein (THP) is a high molecular weight glycoprotein synthesized exclusively by the ascending loop of Henle and the distal tubule of normal kidney. Under pathologic conditions, THP may accumulate in the renal parenchyma, perirenal soft tissue, or renal hilar lymph nodes. Deposits of THP have been described in the bladder and ureter, and are more frequent in men (male-to-female ratio, 8 : 1) between the ages of 45 and 78 years (mean, 68 years). Two morphologic patterns of presentation have been described.[68] The most common presents with THP appearing as large waxy pale or weakly eosinophilic masses (Fig. 4-21). In such cases, THP was strongly positive by periodic acid–Schiff, pale on Masson trichrome stain, and ultrastructurally composed of nonbranching 4-nm-wide fibrils arranged in a parallel fashion. In the second pattern, THP appears as inconspicuous flecks of interconnecting strands of eosinophilic material obscured by a large amount of adjacent fibrinous exudate or necrotic tissue. In these cases, Masson trichrome and periodic acid–Schiff stains are not always helpful in making the diagnosis. Immunohistochemical studies using anti-THP antibody allow identification of even small amounts of THP. Also, staining is helpful in differentiating THP from amyloidosis or hyalinized collagen. Typically, the areas where THP is deposited invariably show necrosis, inflammation, fibrinous exudate, ulcer, or crystalline material. THP is frequently seen in bladder tissue, and probably represents an incidental finding of morphologic interest but no clinical significance.[68] Recently, we observed two tumors of the renal pelvis that were associated with THP deposits, including an inflammatory myofibroblastic tumor and an invasive urothelial carcinoma.

Calcium oxalate crystal deposit may rarely be seen in patients with bladder stone (Fig. 4-22).

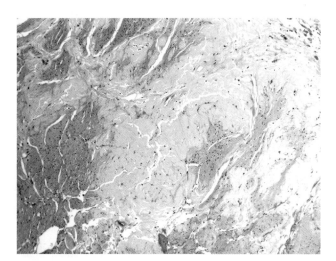

Figure 4-20   Amyloid deposit in the bladder.

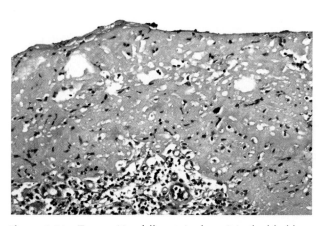

Figure 4-21   Tamm–Horsfall protein deposit in the bladder.

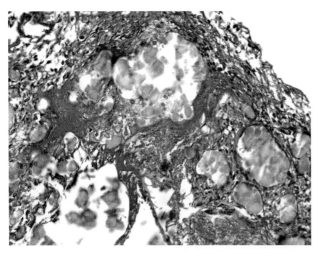

Figure 4-22 Calcium oxalate crystal deposit in the bladder.

Other Rare Benign Lesions

Submucosal Calcification and Ossification

Massive calcification rarely occurs in the bladder, similar to its counterpart in the renal pelvis (**Fig. 4-23**).[69] Patients often have a long history of chronic cystitis, frequently with nephrogenic metaplasia or urachal carcinoma.[70] A case of massive submucosal bone metaplasia was reported in association with encrusted cystitis.[71]

Hemorrhage and Rupture

Subepithelial hemorrhage, similar to the Antopol–Goldman lesion of the renal pelvis, rarely occurs in bladder masses (**Fig. 4-24**). [72-74] The lesion, termed "subepithelial pelvic hematoma," closely mimics cancer clinically. Pseudoneoplastic healing reactions may occur following traumatic bladder rupture. Spontaneous rupture of the urinary bladder

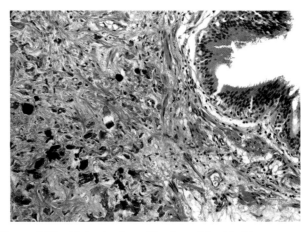

Figure 4-23 Heterotopic ossification of the bladder.

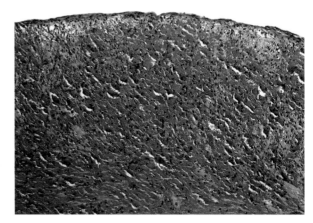

Figure 4-24 Subepithelial pelvic hematoma of the renal pelvis. It mimics cancer clinically.

is a late complication of radiotherapy.[75] A unique case of prolapse of the fallopian tube into the bladder was misinterpreted as carcinoma.[76]

REFERENCES

1. Gleason PE, Kramer SA. Genitourinary polyps in children. *Urology* 1994;44:106–9.
2. Demircan M, Ceran C, Karaman A, Uguralp S, Mizrak B. Urethral polyps in children: a review of the literature and report of two cases. *Int J Urol* 2006;13:841–3.
3. Tsuzuki T, Epstein JI. Fibroepithelial polyp of the lower urinary tract in adults. *Am J Surg Pathol* 2005;29:460–6.
4. Wolgel CD, Parris AC, Mitty HA, Schapira HE. Fibroepithelial polyp of renal pelvis. *Urology* 1982;19:436–9.
5. Barzilai M, Shinawi M, Ish-Shalom N, Mecz Y, Peled N, Lurie A. A fibroepithelial urethral polyp protruding into the base of the bladder: sonographic diagnosis. *Urol Int* 1996;57:129–31.
6. Al-Ahmadie H, Gomez AM, Trane N, Bove KE. Giant botryoid fibroepithelial polyp of bladder with myofibroblastic stroma and cystitis cystica et glandularis. *Pediatr Dev Pathol* 2003;6:179–81.
7. Zachariou AG, Manoliadis IN, Kalogianni PA, Karagiannis GK, Georgantzis DJ. A rare case of bladder fibroepithelial polyp in childhood. *Arch Ital Urol Androl* 2005;77:118–20.
8. Tayib AM, Al-Maghrabi JA, Mosli HA. Urethral polyp verumontanum. *Saudi Med J* 2004;25:1115–6.

9. Fathi K, Azmy A, Howatson A, Carachi R. Congenital posterior urethral polyps in childhood. A case report. *Eur J Pediatr Surg* 2004;14:215–7.

10. Natsheh A, Prat O, Shenfeld OZ, Reinus C, Chertin B. Fibroepithelial polyp of the bladder neck in children. *Pediatr Surg Int* 2008;24:613–5.

11. Kumar A, Das SK, Trivedi S, Dwivedi US, Singh PB. Genito-urinary polyps: summary of the 10-year experiences of a single institute. *Int Urol Nephrol* 2008;40:901–7.

12. Isaac J, Snow B, Lowichik A. Fibroepithelial polyp of the prostatic urethra in an adolescent. *J Pediatr Surg* 2006;41:e29–31.

13. Elson EC, McLaughlin AP 3rd. Xanthomatous ureteral polyp. *Urology* 1974;4:214–6.

14. Lore CE, Mobley J, Zaslau S. Fibroepithelial polyp of the ureter presenting incidentally in a patient with a diverticular abscess. *W V Med J* 2004;100:70–1.

15. Young RH. Fibroepithelial polyp of the bladder with atypical stromal cells. *Arch Pathol Lab Med* 1986;110:241–2.

16. Williams TR, Wagner BJ, Corse WR, Vestevich JC. Fibroepithelial polyps of the urinary tract. *Abdom Imaging* 2002;27:217–21.

17. Halat S, Eble JN, Grignon DG, Lacy S, Montironi R, MacLennan GT, Lopez-Beltran A, Tan PH, Baldridge LA, Cheng L. Ectopic prostatic tissue: histogenesis and histopathologic characteristics. *Histopathology* 2011;58:750–8.

18. Remick DG Jr, Kumar NB. Benign polyps with prostatic-type epithelium of the urethra and the urinary bladder. A suggestion of histogenesis based on histologic and immunohistochemical studies. *Am J Surg Pathol* 1984;8:833–9.

19. Morey AF, Kreder KJ, Wikert GA, Cooper G, Dresner ML. Ectopic prostate tissue at the bladder dome. *J Urol* 1989;141:942–3.

20. Hansen BJ, Christensen SW, Eldrup J. Prostatic-type polyp in the bladder. A case report. *APMIS* 1989;97:664–6.

21. Dogra PN, Ansari MS, Khaitan A, Safaya R, Rifat. Ectopic prostate: an unusual bladder tumor. *Int Urol Nephrol* 2002;34:525–6.

22. Hara S, Horie A. Prostatic caruncle: a urethral papillary tumor derived from prolapse of the prostatic duct. *J Urol* 1977;117:303–5.

23. Yajima I, Ogawa H, Yamaguchi K, Akimoto M. Ectopic prostatic tissue in the bladder. *Hinyokika Kiyo* 1993;39:761–4.

24. Elgamal AA, Van de Voorde W, Van Poppel H, Lauweryns J, Baert L. Immunohistochemical localization of prostate-specific markers within the accessory male sex glands of Cowper, Littre, and Morgagni. *Urology* 1994;44:84–90.

25. Frazier HA, Humphrey PA, Burchette JL, Paulson DF. Immunoreactive prostatic specific antigen in male periurethral glands. *J Urol* 1992;147:246–8.

26. Chuang AY, Demarzo AM, Veltri RW, Sharma RB, Bieberich CJ, Epstein JI. Immunohistochemical differentiation of high grade prostate carcinoma from urothelial carcinoma. *Am J Surg Pathol* 2007;31:1246–55.

27. Hammerich KH, Ayala GE, Wheeler TM. Application of immunohistochemistry to the genitourinary system (prostate, urinary bladder, testis, and kidney). *Arch Pathol Lab Med* 2008;132:432–40.

28. Tawfic S, Niehans GA, Manivel JC. The pattern of CD10 expression in selected pathologic entities of the prostate gland. *Hum Pathol* 2003;34:450–6.

29. Keating MA, Young RH, Lillehei CW, Retik AB. Hamartoma of the bladder in a 4-year-old girl with hamartomatous polyps of the gastrointestinal tract. *J Urol* 1987;138:366–9.

30. Ota T, Kawai K, Hattori K, Uchida K, Akaza H, Harada M. Hamartoma of the urinary bladder. *Int J Urol* 1999;6:211–4.

31. Brancatelli G, Midiri M, Sparacia G, Martino R, Rizzo G, Lagalla R. Hamartoma of the urinary bladder: case report and review of the literature. *Eur Radiol* 1999;9:42–4.

32. McCallion WA, Herron BM, Keane PF. Bladder hamartoma. *Br J Urol* 1993;72:382–3.

33. Park C, Kim H, Lee YB, Song JM, Ro JY. Hamartoma of the urachal remnant. *Arch Pathol Lab Med* 1989;113:1393–5.

34. Peterson LJ, Paulson DF, Glenn JF. The histopathology of vesical diverticula. *J Urol* 1973;110:62–4.

35. Rajan N, Makhuli ZN, Humphrey DM, Batra AK. Metastatic umbilical transitional cell carcinoma from a bladder diverticulum. *J Urol* 1996;155:1700.

36. Nazeer T, Ro JY, Tornos C, Ordonez NG, Ayala AG. Endocervical type glands in urinary bladder: a clinicopathologic study of six cases. *Hum Pathol* 1996;27:816–20.

37. Clement PB, Young RH. Endocervicosis of the urinary bladder. A report of six cases of a benign müllerian lesion that may mimic adenocarcinoma. *Am J Surg Pathol* 1992;16:533–42.

38. Julie C, Boye K, Desgrippes A, Regnier A, Staroz F, Fontaine E, Franc B. Endocervicosis of the urinary bladder. Immunohistochemical comparative study between a new case and normal uterine endocervices. *Pathol Res Pract* 2002;198:115–20.

39. Preusser S, Diener PA, Schmid HP, Leippold T. Submucosal endocervicosis of the bladder: an ectopic, glandular structure of müllerian origin. *Scand J Urol Nephrol* 2008;42:88–90.

40. Cheng L, Bostwick DG. Overdiagnosis of bladder carcinoma. *Anal Quant Cytol Histol* 2008;30:261–4.

41. Young RH. Tumor-like lesions of the urinary bladder. *Mod Pathol* 2009;22 Suppl 2:S37–52.

42. Young RH. Non-neoplastic disorders of the urinary bladder. In: Bostwick DG, Cheng L, eds. Urologic Surgical Pathology, 2nd ed. Philadelphia: Elsevier/Mosby, 2008; 215–58.

43. Williamson SR, Lopez-Beltran A, Montironi R, Cheng L. Glandular lesions of the urinary bladder: clinical significance and differential diagnosis. *Histopathology* 2011;58:811–34.

44. Vercellini P, Meschia M, De Giorgi O, Panazza S, Cortesi I, Crosignani PG. Bladder detrusor endometriosis: clinical and pathogenetic implications. *J Urol* 1996;155:84–6.

45. Al-Khawaja M, Tan PH, MacLennan GT, Lopez-Beltran A, Montironi R, Cheng L. Ureteral endometriosis: clinicopathological and immunohistochemical study of 7 cases. *Hum Pathol* 2008;39:954–9.

46. Schrodt GR, Alcorn MO, Ibanez J. Endometriosis of the male urinary system: a case report. *J Urol* 1980;124:722–3.

47. Arap Neto W, Lopes RN, Cury M, Montelatto NI, Arap S. Vesical endometriosis. *Urology* 1984;24:271–4.

48. al-Izzi MS, Horton LW, Kelleher J, Fawcett D. Malignant transformation in endometriosis of the urinary bladder. *Histopathology* 1989;14:191–8.

49. Vara AR, Ruzics EP, Moussabeck O, Martin DC. Endometrioid adenosarcoma of the bladder arising from endometriosis. *J Urol* 1990;143:813–5.

50. Comiter CV. Endometriosis of the urinary tract. *Urol Clin North Am* 2002;29:625–35.

51. Clement PB. The pathology of endometriosis: a survey of the many faces of a common disease emphasizing diagnostic pitfalls and unusual and newly appreciated aspects. *Adv Anat Pathol* 2007;14:241–60.

52. McCluggage WG, Oliva E, Herrington CS, McBride H, Young RH. CD10 and calretinin staining of endocervical glandular lesions, endocervical stroma and endometrioid adenocarcinomas of the uterine corpus: CD10 positivity is characteristic of, but not specific for, mesonephric lesions and is not specific for endometrial stroma. *Histopathology* 2003;43:144–50.

53. Seman EI, Stewart CJ. Endocervicosis of the urinary bladder. *Aust N Z J Obstet Gynaecol* 1994;34:496–7.

54. Bladamura S, Palma PD, Meneghini A. Paramesonephric remnants with prominent mucinous secretion, so-called endocervicosis of the urinary bladder. *J Urol Pathol* 1995;3:165–72.

55. Parivar F, Bolton DM, Stoller ML. Endocervicosis of the bladder. *J Urol* 1995;153:1218–9.

56. Young RH, Clement PB. Müllerianosis of the urinary bladder. *Mod Pathol* 1996;9:731–7.

57. Sanborn SL, MacLennan G, Cooney MM, Zhou M, Ponsky LE. High grade transitional cell carcinoma and melanosis of urinary bladder: case report and review of the literature. *Urology* 2009;73:928 e13–5.

58. Gupta SR, Seidl E, Oberpenning F. An unusual and rare case of urinary bladder melanosis. *J Endourol* 2010;24:525–6.

59. Alroy J, Ucci AA, Heaney JA, Mitcheson HD, Gavris VE, Woods W. Multifocal pigmentation of prostatic and bladder urothelium. *J Urol* 1986;136:96–7.

60. Herrera GA, Turbat-Herrera EA, Lockard VG. Unusual pigmented vesical lesion in a middle-aged woman. *Ultrastruct Pathol* 1990;14:529–35.

61. Henderson DW. Unusual pigmented vesical lesion in a middle-aged woman. *Ultrastruct Pathol* 1991;15:311.

62. Kerley SW, Blute ML, Keeney GL. Multifocal malignant melanoma arising in vesicovaginal melanosis. *Arch Pathol Lab Med* 1991;115:950–2.

63. Anichkov NM, Nikonov AA. Primary malignant melanomas of the bladder. *J Urol* 1982;128:813–5.

64. Rothberg H, Place CH, Shteir O. Adriamycin (NSC–123127) toxicity: unusual melanotic reaction. *Cancer Chemother Rep* 1974;58:749–51.

65. Fujihara S, Glenner GG. Primary localized amyloidosis of the genitourinary tract: immunohistochemical study on eleven cases. *Lab Invest* 1981;44:55–60.

66. Malek RS, Greene LF, Farrow GM. Amyloidosis of the urinary bladder. *Br J Urol* 1971;43:189–200.

67. Hinsch R, Thompson L, Conrad R. Secondary amyloidosis of the urinary bladder: a rare cause of massive haematuria. *Aust N Z J Surg* 1996;66:127.

68. Truong LD, Ostrowski ML, Wheeler TM. Tamm-Horsfall protein in bladder tissue. Morphologic spectrum and clinical significance. *Am J Surg Pathol* 1994;18:615–22.

69. Firstater M, Farkas A. Submucosal renal pelvic calcification simulating a pelvic stone. *J Urol* 1981;126:802–3.

70. Lopez-Beltran A, Nogales F, Donne CH, Sayag JL. Adenocarcinoma of the urachus showing extensive calcification and stromal osseous metaplasia. *Urol Int* 1994;53:110–3.

71. Collings CW, Welebir F. Osteoma of the bladder. *J Urol* 1941;46:494–6.

72. Iczkowski KA, Sweat SD, Bostwick DG. Subepithelial pelvic hematoma of the kidney clinically mimicking cancer: report of six cases and review of the literature. *Urology* 1999;53:276–9.

73. Antopol W, Goldman L. Subepithelial hemorrhage of renal pelvis simulating neoplasm. *Urol Cutaneous Rev* 1948;52:189–95.

74. Levitt S, Waisman J, deKernion J. Subepithelial hematoma of the renal pelvis (Antopol-Goldman lesion): a case report and review of the literature. *J Urol* 1984;131:939–41.

75. Addar MH, Stuart GC, Nation JG, Shumsky AG. Spontaneous rupture of the urinary bladder: a late complication of radiotherapy—case report and review of the literature. *Gynecol Oncol* 1996;62:314–6.

76. Anastasiades KD, Majmudar B. Prolapse of fallopian tube into urinary bladder, mimicking bladder carcinoma. *Arch Pathol Lab Med* 1983;107:613–4.

Chapter 5

Benign Epithelial Tumors

Papilloma of the Urinary Bladder

Urothelial Papilloma

The diagnosis of urothelial papilloma of the urinary bladder has been controversial.[1–8] Much of the difficulty in diagnosis and acceptance of this lesion is based on varying diagnostic criteria. Some authors believe that papilloma should include the World Health Organization (WHO) grade 1 urothelial carcinoma,[9] but we, and most others, do not follow this suggestion.[1,10–12] If one employs restrictive diagnostic criteria as recommended by the WHO (1973)[13] and the International Society of Urologic Pathologists (ISUP; 1998),[14] as we do, then this lesion is uncommon, representing no more than 1% of papillary urothelial tumors.[13,15] The posterior or lateral walls close to the ureteric orifices and the urethra are the most common locations. The male-to-female ratio is 1.9:1.[11,16] Urothelial papilloma usually arises as a de novo or primary neoplasm, but may occasionally occur in patients with a known clinical history of bladder cancer as a secondary papilloma.[12]

The restrictive criteria for papilloma as defined by the WHO[13] include a small, usually solitary papillary lesion with one or more delicate fibrovascular cores lined by cytologically and architecturally normal urothelium (lacking hyperplastic changes) without mitotic figures (see also **Chapter 9**) (**Figs. 5-1** to **5-6**).[13] The papillary architecture varies from simple and small to complex and anastomosing, with primary and secondary budding. The fibrovascular cores contain loose delicate fibrous connective tissue that may be edematous or, uncommonly, contain dilated lymphatics, foamy macrophages, or chronic lymphoid inflammation. Cells maintain normal polarity. Mild cytologic atypia of the superficial cells, including vacuolization, multinucleation, eosinophilic syncytial metaplasia, moderate cytologic atypia, mucinous metaplasia, or apocrine-like metaplasia, does not exclude the diagnosis of papilloma, particularly when accompanied by an inflammatory infiltrate (**Fig. 5-7**).[11,12,14–18]

Papilloma by itself does not have the capacity to invade or metastasize.[19] The clinical course in most patients is benign, with a very low recurrence rate (7.0% to 8.8%).[12,17] Cheng and his colleagues reported the largest series (52 patients) of urothelial papillomas using modern diagnostic criteria.[11] With up to a 58-year followup (mean, 9.8 years), only four patients (7.6%) developed recurrence. One other patient developed papillary urothelial neoplasm of low malignant potential (PUNLMP) (Ta WHO grade 1 papillary urothelial carcinoma) six years after the initial diagnosis of papilloma. None of these patients developed dysplasia, carcinoma in situ, or invasive urothelial carcinoma or died

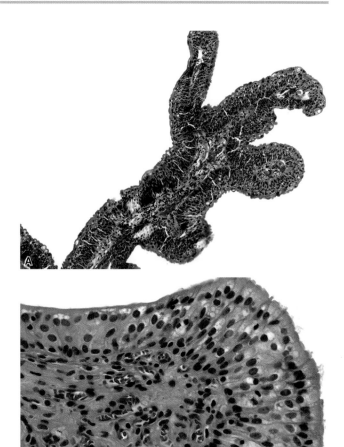

Figure 5-1 Urothelial papilloma. (A) A single delicate elongate 1.1-cm-long papillary growth is present in the posterior wall of the bladder of a 51-year-old woman. (B) The urothelium is of normal thickness, with no cytologic atypia and an intact superficial cell layer.

of bladder cancer.[11] Recurrence may be predicted in the majority of cases with basal cell layer cytokeratin (CK) 5 immunostaining or loss of CK20 immunoreactivity.[20,21] It is likely that some of these recurrences result from underdiagnosed grade 1 or low grade carcinoma that was interpreted as papilloma, owing to small or limited tissue samples. Thus, papilloma is currently considered neoplastic, based on the potential for recurrence and the occasional association with subsequent progression to a higher grade (low grade carcinoma). In one study, urothelial papilloma accounted for 25% of papillary neoplasms of the bladder, considerably higher than other reported series, calling into question the apparently liberal diagnostic criteria for papilloma in that report. As might be expected, 3.3% of patients

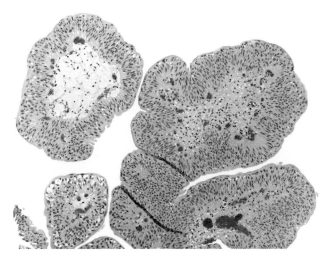

Figure 5-2   Urothelial papilloma. Solitary 1.5-cm-diameter papillary growth found in the bladder of a 45-year-old man. The urothelium is focally thickened due to tangential sectioning, but in most areas is of normal thickness (less than seven layers).

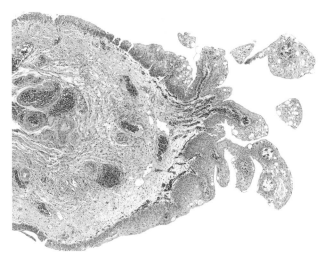

Figure 5-3   Urothelial papilloma.

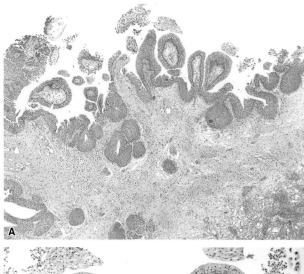

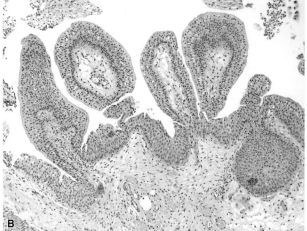

Figure 5-4   Urothelial papilloma (A and B).

developed higher grade lesions, and 4.4% died of urothelial carcinoma.[19] In another study that probably overdiagnosed papilloma, additional papillary tumors arose in up to 73% of 100 patients followed for a minimum of 15 years; invasive carcinoma developed in up to 10% of patients.[22,23] Aggressive behavior was reported in a patient with urothelial papilloma who was on immunosuppressive therapy secondary to a renal transplant.[12] Urothelial papilloma usually occurred in patients with a mean age at diagnosis of 57 years (range, 22 to 89 years).[11]

Urothelial papilloma is diploid and has a low proliferation rate as measured by an immunohistochemical study with Ki67/MIB1 (mean 2.8%), similar to PUNLMP (mean, 2.9%) and lower than the Ki67/MIB1 labeling index in low grade carcinoma (mean, 4.6%).[24] CK20 expression was identical to that in normal urothelium, present only in the superficial (umbrella) cells.[21] No expression of p53 was observed in papilloma. Fibroblast growth factor receptor 3 (*FGFR3*) mutations are present in 75% of cases of urothelial papillomas, similar to that of PUNLMP and low grade carcinoma.[25]

The histopathologic features that are useful to distinguish urothelial papilloma from noninvasive grade 1 urothelial carcinoma or PUNLMP are listed in Table 5-1 (see Chapter 9 for further discussion) (Fig. 5-8). The key difference is the number of cell layers covering the papillae. The number of cell layers in urothealial papilloma is usually between three and seven; however, in grade 1 urothelial carcinoma, it usually exceeds seven layers. Urothelial papilloma should also be distinguished from nephrogenic adenoma with a papillary growth pattern. Nephrogenic adenoma is covered by a single cell layer (Fig. 5-9) and stains positively for PAX2 and PAX8. Ductal adenocarcinoma of the prostate should also be considered in the differential

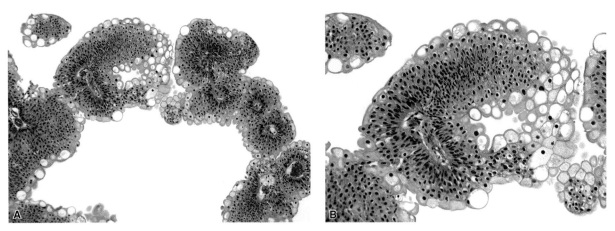

Figure 5-5   Urothelial papilloma (A and B). Note the prominent superficial cells.

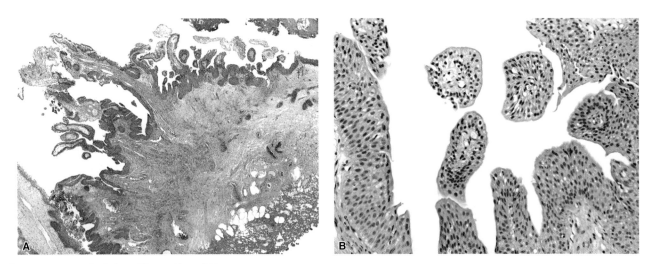

Figure 5-6   Urothelial papilloma (A and B).

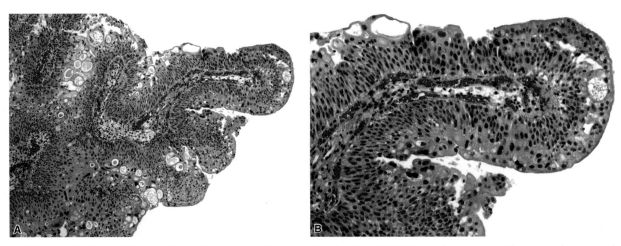

Figure 5-7   Urothelial papilloma with nuclear atypia of the superficial cells. (A) A 2.0-cm-diameter papillary growth removed from the left bladder wall of a 47-year-old man. (B) Cytologic atypia is present but restricted to the superficial cells.

Table 5-1   Urothelial Papilloma Versus Modified Grade 1 Urothelial Carcinoma (Low Grade[a])

	Architecture at Low Power (×10)	Number of Epithelial Layers	Superficial (Umbrella) Cells	Nuclear Enlargement	Nuclear Hyperchromasia	Mitosis
Papilloma	Epithelium, orderly arrangement	5–7 or less	Present/small[b]	No[c]	Absent	Absent
Modified grade 1 (PUNLMP)	Slight distortion but overall orderly	7 or more	Present/variable size	Minimal	Minimal	Absent to rare, basally located

[a]Formerly, papillary urothelial neoplasm of low malignant potential (PUNLMP). See **Chapter 9** for further discussion on grading of bladder cancer.
[b]In rare instances, superficial cells may be conspicuous and enlarged.
[c]Some nuclear enlargement of superficial cells may be present.

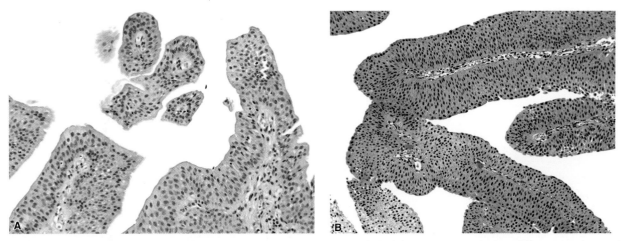

Figure 5-8   Urothelial papilloma (A) and grade I noninvasive papillary urothelial carcinoma (B). The key difference is the number of cell layers covering the papillae. Both are lined by normal-appearing urothelium; however, the thickness of cell layers in urothelial papilloma is usually between three and seven.

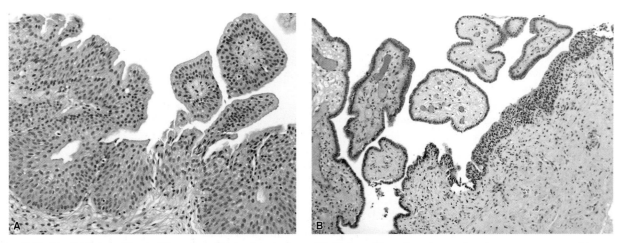

Figure 5-9   Urothelial papilloma (A) and nephrogenic adenoma (B). The papillae of nephrogenic adenoma are covered by a single cell layer.

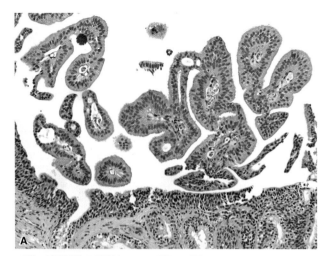

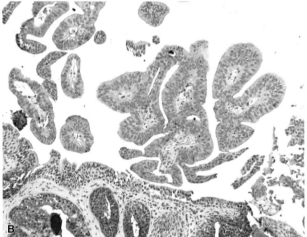

Figure 5-10 Prostatic adenocarcinoma, ductal type (A and B). Ductal adenocarcinoma of the prostate may also mimic urothelial papilloma. Immunostaining for prostate-specific antigen confirms the diagnosis (B).

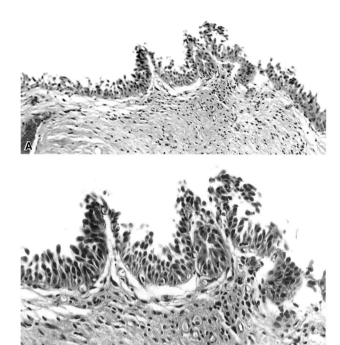

Figure 5-11 Diffuse papillomatosis. (A) Multiple minute papillary excrescences identified in the posterior wall of the bladder of a 46-year-old man. (B) The urothelium is invariably less than seven cells in thickness, with no cytologic atypia.

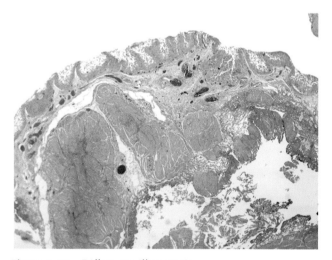

Figure 5-12 Diffuse papillomatosis.

diagnosis. Immunostaining for prostate-specific antigen is positive in ductal prostatic adenocarcinoma (Fig. 5-10).

Diffuse Papillomatosis

This rare lesion is characterized by replacement of most or all of the bladder mucosa by delicate papillary processes, creating a "velvety" cystoscopic appearance.[26] The papillae are covered by urothelium that is indistinguishable from normal mucosa or may have slight cytologic changes. Histologically, there is a proliferation of small papillae covered by cells with conspicuous eosinophilic cytoplasm, minimal or no architectural distortion, little or mild nuclear atypia, and no mitotic figures (Figs. 5-11 to 5-13). These lesions are occasionally focal,[15] and may be seen in the followup biopsies of patients with a known clinical history of bladder papillary tumors. The malignant potential of this lesion is uncertain.

Inverted Papilloma

Inverted papilloma, diagnosed according to strictly defined criteria, is a benign urothelial neoplasm not related to urothelial carcinoma.[27] Hematuria or obstructive symptoms are a common presentation, and less than 1% of cases recur.[27]

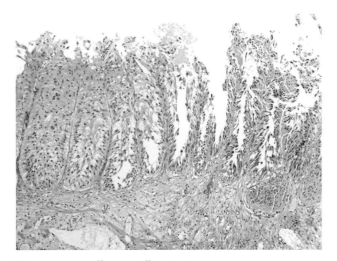

Figure 5-13   Diffuse papillomatosis.

Inverted papilloma applies to a benign urothelial tumor
that has an inverted growth pattern with normal to minimal
cytologic atypia of the cells.[27–32] Most cases are solitary
nodular or sessile lesions, smaller than 3 cm, and arise in
the bladder trigone but can also be found along the urinary
tract. Microscopically, inverted papilloma has a smooth surface covered by normal urothelium, and endophytic cords
of urothelial cells invaginating extensively from the surface
urothelium into the subjacent lamina propria but not into
the muscularis propria wall (**Figs. 5-14** to **5-16**). Trabecular and glandular patterns have been described. Foci of
nonkeratinizing squamous metaplasia and neuroendocrine
differentiation have been reported. Focal minor cytological
atypia may be present, but mitotic figures are not seen or
are very rare.

Recent studies indicate that inverted papilloma is a
monoclonal process; however, the low incidence of loss of
heterozygosity supports the view that inverted papilloma
in urinary bladder is a benign neoplasm with molecular
genetic abnormalities different from those of urothelial
carcinoma.[28,33]

See **Chapter 17** for further discussion.

Squamous Papilloma

Squamous cell papilloma is a rare benign neoplasm;
presumably the squamous counterpart of urothelial
papilloma.[1,34] It is unrelated to human papillomavirus
(HPV) infection. It occurs in elderly women and follows
a benign clinical course with infrequent recurrence. Histologically, it is composed of papillary cores with overlying
benign squamous epithelium (**Figs. 5-17** and **5-18**). It is
diploid, with no or minimal p53 nuclear accumulation, and

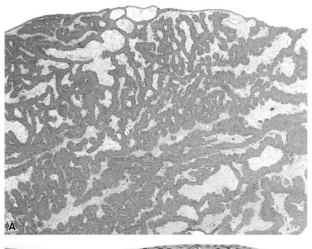
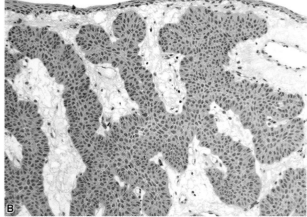

Figure 5-14   Inverted papilloma (A and B).

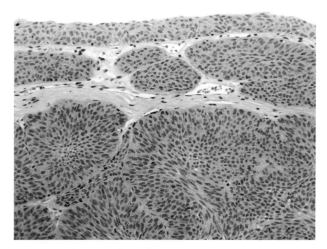

Figure 5-15   Inverted papilloma.

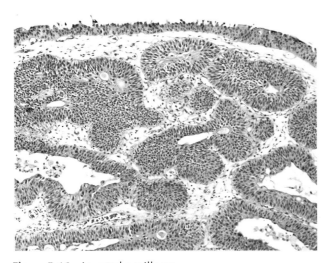

Figure 5-16   Inverted papilloma.

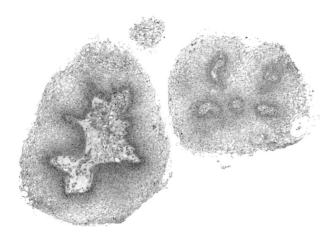

Figure 5-17   Squamous papilloma of the bladder.

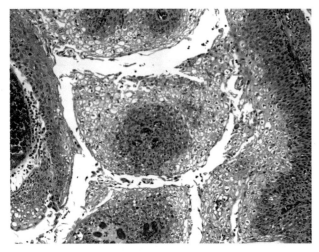

Figure 5-18   Squamous papilloma of the bladder.

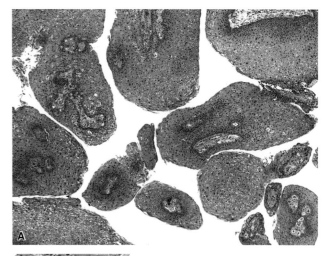

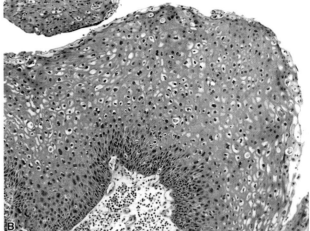

Figure 5-19   Condyloma acuminata of the bladder (A and B).

is HPV negative.[34] Some lesions demonstrate immunohistochemical expression of epidermal growth factor receptor (EGFR) protein.[35]

In the bladder or urethra, squamous papilloma has to be differentiated from condyloma acuminata (**Fig. 5-19**), an aneuploid lesion positive for HPV with increased p53 and p16 nuclear accumulation. It should also be differentiated from papillary cystitis, a common reactive lesion in which the urothelium is occasionally replaced by metaplastic squamous epithelium. The uncommon verrucous type of squamous cell carcinoma rarely enters into the differential diagnosis.[18,34]

See **Chapter 14** for further discussion.

Villous Adenoma and Tubulovillous Adenoma

There are only a modest number of documented cases of villous adenoma, tubulovillous adenoma, and pure tubular adenoma of the bladder, and these are histologically identical to their counterparts in the colon.[36] As seen in the literature, the terminology of this lesion is somewhat variable, with similar lesions termed "tubulovillous adenoma," "villous tumor," "villous metaplasia of intestinal type with dysplasia," "papillary adenocarcinoma in situ," and others.[36–43] This lesion is more common in the urachus.[44] Patients usually present with hematuria and/or irritative symptoms.[36,45] Tumors appear cystoscopically as exophytic papillary masses. Villous adenoma of the urinary bladder is more common in men than in women (3:1 ratio), presenting in patients between 52 and 79 years of age (mean age, 65 years)[36,39,46] and occurring most frequently in the bladder dome and trigone.

Light microscopic examination shows morphologic similarity to its colonic counterpart. The tumor is composed of pointed or blunt finger-like processes lined by pseudostratified columnar epithelium (**Figs. 5-20** to **5-22**). Papillary

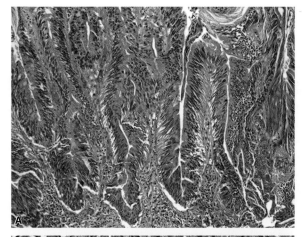

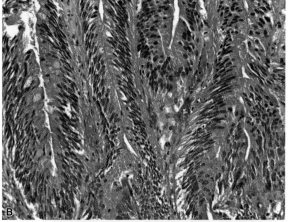

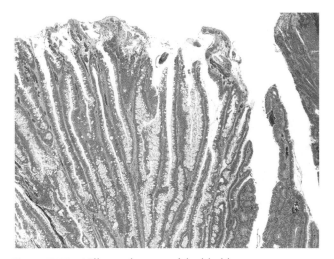

Figure 5-20   Villous adenoma of the bladder.

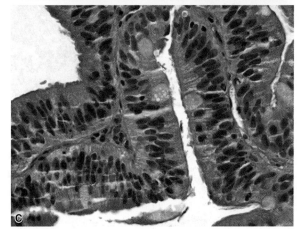

Figure 5-22   Tubulovillous adenoma of the bladder (A and B).

fronds are covered by columnar mucus-secreting epithelium with goblet cells. The epithelial cells display nuclear stratification, nuclear crowding, nuclear hyperchromasia, and occasional prominent nucleoli and mitotic figures. Neuroendocrine cells may be present.[36]

A confounding histologic feature is the uncommon finding of lakes of extravasated mucin in the stroma, raising the possibility of invasion.[47] However, acellular

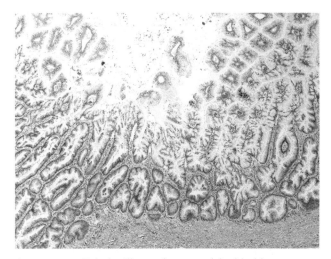

Figure 5-21   Tubulovillous adenoma of the bladder.

pools of mucin are not considered definitive evidence of malignancy at this site. Some cases are associated with invasive urothelial carcinoma of the bladder or adenocarcinoma.[36,39,41,48]

The differential diagnosis of villous adenoma includes florid intestinal-type cystitis glandularis (polypoid cystitis glandularis), well-differentiated adenocarcinoma, adenocarcinoma in situ, papillary urothelial carcinoma with glandular differentiation, ectopic prostate tissue with cytologic abnormalities, and the recently described villous-like papillary urothelial carcinoma.[49,50] Adenocarcinoma with villous architecture occurs rarely in the urinary bladder, usually with severe anaplasia of the pseudostratified epithelium and invasion of the underlying stroma. Villous adenoma may coexist with adenocarcinoma in situ and invasive adenocarcinoma; therefore, the entire specimen should be submitted for pathologic examination to exclude the presence of invasive tumor.

Differentiation of villous adenoma with coexistent adenocarcinoma in the urinary tract from secondary involvement by colonic cancer may be impossible on morphologic grounds alone.[36,51] Because of limited sampling, the biopsy specimen may show only changes of villous adenoma. The difficulty in orienting fragments of tissue removed by transurethral resection is another confounding factor. Accordingly, a diagnosis of villous adenoma of the urinary tract should be made only after adequate tissue sampling and exclusion of secondary involvement from a primary site. Similarly, secondary involvement from other primary sites, such as the prostate gland and the female genital tract, should be considered in the differential diagnosis. Prostate-specific membrane antigen is less specific than prostate-specific antigen for establishing prostatic origin, and may be positive in villous adenoma.[52] Young and Johnston reported a case of serous adenocarcinoma of the uterus mimicking primary bladder adenocarcinoma.[53] The papillary and glandular patterns of growth closely resemble those of primary neoplasm of the bladder. Cancer involving the bladder secondarily tends to invade deeply into the muscularis propria and may be preceded by symptoms related to the primary cancer. Relevant clinical history is important in establishing accurate diagnosis. Noninvasive urothelial carcinoma with glandular differentiation typically lacks the villous finger-like projection seen in villous adenoma.[54]

The immunohistochemical profile of these lesions is remarkable for positivity with CK20 (100% of cases), CK7 (56%), and carcinoembryonic antigen (89%), suggesting limited utility in the differentiation of primary villous adenoma from secondary involvement of colonic adenocarcinoma.[36] Acid mucin has been demonstrated in 78% of cases with Alcian blue/periodic acid–Schiff stain. Das1, a marker found on colonic epithelium and primary adenocarcinomas of the bladder and urachus, is expressed in 80% of cases of villous adenoma.[39] Normal and neoplastic urothelium do not express the mAbDas1 epitope.

Patients with isolated villous adenoma have an excellent prognosis. Transurethral resection of the bladder is the treatment of choice, resulting in no reported recurrences. Recurrent or invasive adenocarcinoma did not develop in any patient with isolated villous adenoma during a mean followup of 9.9 years.[36] However, rare patients with coexistent adenocarcinoma may experience recurrence or distant metastasis.[39,55]

Villous and tubulovillous adenomas of the bladder are rare. Secondary involvement by ductal adenocarcinoma of the prostate should always be considered in the differential diagnosis (**Fig. 5-23**).

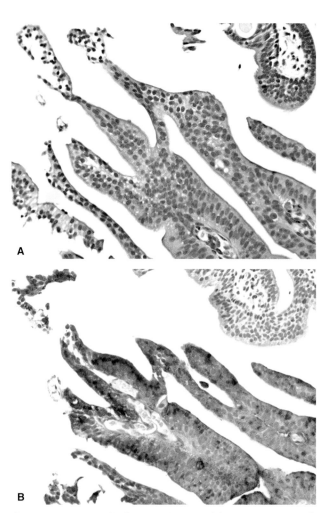

Figure 5-23 Ductal adenocarcinoma of the prostate (A) with positive prostate-specific antigen immunostaining (B). Involvement of the bladder by prostatic adenocarcinoma is far more common than villous adenoma of the bladder. It should always be in the differential consideration.

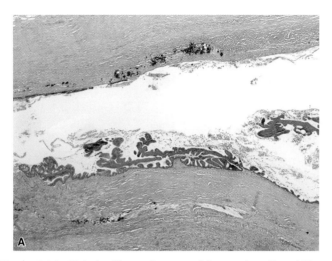
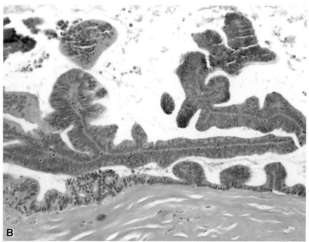

Figure 5-24   Tubulovillous adenoma of the urachus (A and B).

Urachal Adenoma

Urachal adenoma is rare (see also **Chapter 24**).[15,36–43,45,46,48,56–59] It occurs most often in the lower one-third of the urachus and involves the bladder wall.[57] Macroscopically, adenoma is cystic and may be multilocular, varying in size from 1 to 8 cm in diameter. The cysts are often filled with mucus, and mucinuria is a characteristic finding.[56] Microscopically, the epithelium consists of tall columnar cells and goblet cells, often with a striking resemblance to colonic glandular epithelium (**Fig. 5-24**). The epithelium may be papillary or flat, sometimes admixed with urothelium. The distinction between multilocular urachal cysts and adenoma may be difficult in some cases, particularly when the lesion is not complex, and the surface epithelium is simple. Invasion may be difficult to evaluate in superficial specimens, and repeat biopsy or transurethral resection may be of value.

REFERENCES

1. Cheng L, Lopez-Beltran A, MacLennan GT, Montironi R, Bostwick DG. Neoplasms of the urinary bladder. In: Bostwick DG, Cheng L, eds. Urologic Surgical Pathology, 2nd ed. Philadelphia: Elsevier/Mosby, 2008; 259–352.
2. Bostwick DG, Mikuz G. Urothelial papillary (exophytic) neoplasms. *Virchows Arch* 2002;441:109–16.
3. Lerman R, Hutter R, Whitmore J,WF. Papilloma of the urinary bladder. *Cancer* 1970;25:333–42.
4. Nichols JA, Marshall BF. Treatment of histologically benign papilloma of the urinary bladder by local excision and fulguration. *Cancer* 1956;9:566–71.
5. Bostwick DG, Ramnani D, Cheng L. Diagnosis and grading of bladder cancer and associated lesions. *Urol Clin North Am* 1999;26:493–507.
6. Cheng L, Bostwick DG. World Health Organization and International Society of Urological Pathology classification and two-number grading system of bladder tumors: reply. *Cancer* 2000;88:1513–6.
7. Jones TD, Cheng L. Papillary urothelial neoplasm of low malignant potential: evolving terminology and concepts. *J Urol* 2006;175:1995–2003.
8. Maclennan GT, Kirkali Z, Cheng L. Histologic grading of noninvasive papillary urothelial neoplasms. *Eur Urol* 2007;51:889–98.
9. Murphy WM, Beckwith JB, Farrow GM. Tumors of the kidney, bladder, and related urinary structures. In: Rosai J, ed. Atlas of Tumor Pathology, 3rd ed., Fascicle 11. Washington, DC: Armed Forces Institute of Pathology, 1994;202–48.
10. Epstein JI, Amin MB, Reuter VR, Mostofi FK. The World Health Organization/International Society of Urological Pathology consensus classification of urothelial (transitional cell) neoplasms of the urinary bladder. Bladder Consensus Conference Committee. *Am J Surg Pathol* 1998;22:1435–48.
11. Cheng L, Darson M, Cheville JC, Neumann RM, Zincke H, Nehra A, Bostwick DG. Urothelial papilloma of the bladder. Clinical and biologic implications. *Cancer* 1999;86:2098–101.
12. McKenney JK, Amin MB, Young RH. Urothelial (transitional cell) papilloma of the urinary bladder: a clinicopathologic study of 26 cases. *Mod Pathol* 2003;16:623–9.

13. Mostofi FK, Sobin LH, Torloni H. Histological Typing of Urinary Bladder Tumours, Vol. 10. Geneva: World Health Organization, 1973.

14. Epstein JL, Amin MB, Reuter VR, Mostofi FK. The Bladder Consensus Conference Committee. The World Health Organization/International Society of Urologic Pathology consensus classification of urothelial (transitional cell) neoplasms of the urinary bladder. *Am J Surg Pathol* 1998;22:1435–38.

15. Eble JN, Young RH. Benign and low grade papillary lesions of the urinary bladder: a review of the papilloma-papillary carcinoma controversy and a report of five typical papillomas. *Sem Diagn Pathol* 1989;6:351–71.

16. Busch C, Johansson SL. Urothelial Papilloma. In: Eble JN Sauter G, Epstein JI, Sesterhenn I, eds. World Health Organization Classification of Tumors. Pathology and Gentics of Tumors of the Urinary System and Male Genital Organs. Lyon, France: IARCC Press, 2003.

17. Magi-Galluzzi C, Epstein JI. Urothelial papilloma of the bladder: a review of 34 de novo cases. *Am J Surg Pathol* 2004;28:1615–20.

18. Cheng L, Bostwick DG. Overdiagnosis of bladder carcinoma. *Anal Quant Cytol Histol* 2008;30:261–4.

19. Jordan AM, Weingarten J, Murphy WM. Transitional cell neoplasms of the urinary bladder. Can biologic potential be predicted from histologic grading? *Cancer* 1987;60:2766–74.

20. Celis JE, Celis P, Palsdottir H, Ostergaard M, Gromov P, Primdahl H, Orntoft TF, Wolf H, Celis A, Gromova I. Proteomic strategies to reveal tumor heterogeneity among urothelial papillomas. *Mol Cell Proteomics* 2002;1:269–79.

21. Harnden P, Mahmood N, Southgate J. Expression of cytokeratin 20 redefines urothelial papillomas of the bladder. *Lancet* 1999;353:974–7.

22. Greene L, Hanash K, Farrow G. Benign papilloma or papillary carcinoma of the bladder. *J Urol* 1973;110:205–7.

23. Prout GJ Jr, Barton BA, Griffin PP, Friedell GH. Treated history of noninvasive grade 1 transitional cell carcinoma. The National Bladder Cancer Group. *J Urol*. 1992;148:1413–9.

24. Cina SJ, Lancaster-Weiss KJ, Lecksell K, Epstein JI. Correlation of Ki–67 and p53 with the new World Health Organization/International Society of Urological Pathology Classification System for Urothelial Neoplasia. *Arch Pathol Lab Med* 2001;125:646–51.

25. van Rhijn BW, Montironi R, Zwarthoff EC, Jobsis AC, van der Kwast TH. Frequent FGFR3 mutations in urothelial papilloma. *J Pathol* 2002;198:245–51.

26. Mostofi FK. Pathological aspects and spread of carcinoma of the bladder. *JAMA* 1968;206:1764–9.

27. Sung MT, Maclennan GT, Lopez-Beltran A, Montironi R, Cheng L. Natural history of urothelial inverted papilloma. *Cancer* 2006;107:2622–7.

28. Jones TD, Zhang S, Lopez-Beltran A, Eble JN, Sung MT, MacLennan GT, Montironi R, Tan PH, Zheng S, Baldridge LA, Cheng L. Urothelial carcinoma with an inverted growth pattern can be distinguished from inverted papilloma by fluorescence in-situ hybridization, immunohistochemistry, and morphologic analysis. *Am J Surg Pathol* 2007;31:1861–7.

29. Hodges KB, Lopez-Beltran A, Maclennan GT, Montironi R, Cheng L. Urothelial lesions with inverted growth patterns: histogenesis, molecular genetic findings, differential diagnosis and clinical management. *BJU Int* 2011;107:532–7.

30. Montironi R, Lopez-Beltran A, Scarpelli M, Mazzucchelli R, Cheng L. Morphological classification and definition of benign, preneoplastic and non-invasive neoplastic lesions of the urinary bladder. *Histopathology* 2008;53:621–33.

31. Montironi R, Mazzucchelli R, Scarpelli M, Lopez-Beltran A, Cheng L. Morphological diagnosis of urothelial neoplasms. *J Clin Pathol* 2008;61:3–10.

32. Montironi R, Cheng L, Lopez-Beltran A, Scarpelli M, Mazzucchelli R, Mikuz G, Kirkali Z, Montorsi F. Inverted (endophytic) noninvasive lesions and neoplasms of the urothelium: The Cinderella group has yet to be fully exploited. *Eur Urol* 2011;59:225–30.

33. Sung MT, Eble JN, Wang M, Tan PH, Lopez-Beltran A, Cheng L. Inverted papilloma of the urinary bladder: a molecular genetic appraisal. *Mod Pathol* 2006;19:1289–94.

34. Cheng L, Leibovich BC, Cheville JC, Ramnani DM, Sebo TJ, Nehra A, Malek RS, Zincke H, Bostwick DG. Squamous papilloma of the urinary tract is unrelated to condyloma acuminata. *Cancer* 2000;88:1679–86.

35. Guo CC, Fine SW, Epstein JI. Noninvasive squamous lesions in the urinary bladder: a clinicopathologic analysis of 29 cases. *Am J Surg Pathol* 2006;30:883–91.

36. Cheng L, Montironi R, Bostwick DG. Villous adenoma of the urinary tract: a report of 23 cases, including 8 with coexistent adenocarcinoma. *Am J Surg Pathol* 1999;23:764–71.

37. Miller DC, Gang DL, Gavris V, Alroy J, Ucci AA, Parkhurst EC. Villous adenoma of the urinary bladder: A morphologic or biologic entity? *Am J Clin Pathol* 1983;79:728–31.

38. Trotter SE, Philp B, Luck R, Ali M, Fisher C. Villous adenoma of the bladder. *Histopathology* 1994;24:491–3.

39. Seibel JL, Prasad S, Weiss RE, Bancila E, Epstein JI. Villous adenoma of the urinary tract: a lesion frequently associated with malignancy. *Hum Pathol* 2002;33:236–41.

40. Adegboyega PA, Adesokan A. Tubulovillous adenoma of the urinary bladder. *Mod Pathol* 1999;12:735–8.

41. Val-Bernal JF, Mayorga M, Garijo MF. Villous adenoma of the urinary tract: a lesion frequently associated with malignancy. *Hum Pathol* 2002;33:1150.

42. Tamboli P, Ro JY. Villous adenoma of urinary tract: a common tumor in an uncommon location. *Adv Anat Pathol* 2000;7:79–84.

43. Rubin J, Khanna OP, Damjanov I. Adenomatous polyp of the bladder: a rare cause of hematuria in young men. *J Urol* 1981;126:549–50.

44. Mazzucchelli R, Scarpelli M, Montironi R. Mucinous adenocarcinoma with superficial stromal invasion and villous adenoma of urachal remnants: a case report. *J Clin Pathol* 2003;56:465–7.

45. Husain AS, Papas P, Khatib G. Villous adenoma of the urinary bladder presenting as gross hematuria. *J Urol Pathol*. 1996;4:299–306.

46. Billis A, Lima AC, Queiroz LS, Cia EM, Oliveira ER, Pinto W Jr. Adenoma of bladder in siblings with renal dysplasia. *Urology* 1980;16:299–302.

47. Grignon DJ, Sakr W. Inflammatory and other conditions that can mimic carcinoma in the urinary bladder. *Pathol Annu* 1995;30 (Pt 1):95–122.

48. West D, Orihuela E, Pow-sang M, et al. Villous adenoma-like lesions associated with invasive transitional cell carcinoma of the bladder. *J Urol Pathol* 1995;3:263–68.

49. Williamson SR, Lopez-Beltran A, Montironi R, Cheng L. Glandular lesions of the urinary bladder: clinical significance and differential diagnosis. *Histopathology* 2011;58:811–34.

50. Lopez-Beltran A, Jimenez RE, Montironi R, Patriarca C, Blanca A, Menendez C, Algaba F, Cheng L. Flat urothelial carcinoma in situ of the bladder with glandular differentiation. *Hum Pathol* 2011;42:1653–9.

51. Silver SA, Epstein JI. Adenocarcinoma of the colon simulating primary urinary bladder neoplasia. A report of nine cases. *Am J Surg Pathol* 1993;17:171–8.

52. Lane Z, Hansel DE, Epstein JI. Immunohistochemical expression of prostatic antigens in adenocarcinoma and villous adenoma of the urinary bladder. *Am J Surg Pathol* 2008;32:1322–6.

53. Young RH, Johnston WH. Serous adenocarcinoma of the uterus metastatic to the urinary bladder mimicking primary bladder neoplasia. A report of a case. *Am J Surg Pathol* 1990;14:877–80.

54. Miller JS, Epstein JI. Noninvasive urothelial carcinoma of the bladder with glandular differentiation: report of 24 cases. *Am J Surg Pathol* 2009;33:1241–8.

55. Powell I, Cartwright H, Jano F. Villous adenoma and adenocarcinoma of female urethra. *Urology* 1981;18:612–4.

56. Eble JN, Hull MT, Rowland RG, Hostetter M. Villous adenoma of the urachus with mucusuria: a light and electron microscopic study. *J Urol* 1986;135:1240–4.

57. Hamm FC. Benign cytadenoma of the bladder probably of urachal origen. *J Urol* 1940;44:227–30.

58. Copp HL, Wong IY, Krishnan C, Malhotra S, Kennedy WA. Clinical presentation and urachal remnant pathology: implications for treatment. *J Urol* 2009;182:1921–4.

59. Ashley RA, Inman BA, Routh JC, Rohlinger AL, Husmann DA, Kramer SA. Urachal anomalies: a longitudinal study of urachal remnants in children and adults. *J Urol* 2007;178:1615–8.

Chapter 6

Flat Urothelial Lesions with Atypia and Urothelial Dysplasia

Bladder Pathology, First Edition. Liang Cheng, Antonio Lopez-Beltran, David G. Bostwick.
© 2012 Wiley-Blackwell. Published 2012 by John Wiley & Sons, Inc.

The classification of nonpapillary (flat) intraepithelial lesions and conditions of the urothelium has evolved over the years and was recently redefined at the *International Consultation on the Diagnosis of Noninvasive Urothelial Neoplasms* held in Ancona, Italy in 2001 (**Table 6-1**).[1] This classification includes epithelial abnormalities (reactive urothelial atypia and flat urothelial hyperplasia), presumed preneoplastic lesions and conditions (keratinizing squamous and glandular metaplasia, and malignancy-associated cellular changes), and preneoplastic (dysplasia) and neoplastic noninvasive [carcinoma in situ (CIS)] lesions.[1-10] Each of these lesions is defined with strict morphological criteria in order to provide more accurate information to urologists in managing patients. Flat urothelial lesions with atypia include reactive urothelial atypia, atypia of unknown significance, and urothelial dysplasia and urothelial CIS. Reactive urothelial atypia is a benign condition. The term "atypia of unknown significance" should be avoided in surgical pathology reporting (other than in cytology). We recommend use of the terms "dysplasia" and "CIS" to describe flat lesions with atypia that have biologic potential to progress to invasive disease.[1,5,6,8-11] Grading and subclassification of dysplasia are not recommended.

Reactive Urothelial Atypia

Urothelial abnormalities whose architectural and cytologic changes are of lesser degree than those of dysplasia have often been termed "atypia,"[1,11] a term that is, by its very nature, nonspecific. The intra- and interobserver variation in recognition and interpretation of "urothelial atypia" is substantial. Nevertheless, the term "atypia" is still in use at many institutions.

Table 6-1 Classification of Flat Urothelial Lesions of the Urinary Bladder Based on the Ancona International Consultation

Flat urothelial hyperplasia

Reactive urothelial atypia

Presumed preneoplastic lesions and conditions
  Keratinizing squamous metaplasia
  Intestinal metaplasia
  Malignancy associated cellular changes

Preneoplastic lesions
  Dysplasia

Neoplastic noninvasive lesion
  Urothelial carcinoma in situ

Source: Modified from Ref. 1.

Reactive urothelial atypia is characterized by mild nuclear abnormalities occurring in acutely or chronically inflamed urothelium (**Figs. 6-1** and **6-2**). Most patients with reactive atypia have a history of cystitis, infection, stones, instrumentation, or prior treatments (**Fig. 6-3**) and present with hematuria and/or irritative symptoms, including frequency, urgency, and dysuria. Under cystoscopic evaluation, the urothelium appears abnormally erythematous or inflamed.[4]

Microscopically, the urothelium may be normal or slightly thickened, but it still maintains orderly maturation from basal to superficial cells (**Table 6-2**). Frequently, the cells are enlarged and have abundant cytoplasm. Nuclei are uniformly enlarged, vesicular, and may have prominent nucleoli. Overall nuclear polarity is maintained. There may be frequent mitoses involving the lower layers of the urothelium (**Figs. 6-4** and **6-5**). The cells are often larger than normal, with more abundant cytoplasm than that of normal urothelial cells. These features occasionally impart a squamoid appearance. The lamina propria is typically inflamed, and inflammatory cells often extend into the mucosa. In the absence of nuclear hyperchromasia, pleomorphism, or coarse chromatin pattern, reactive atypia should not be considered dysplastic. One caveat is that reactive atypia may coexist with dysplasia or CIS. Cytokeratin (CK)20, CD44, and p53 immunohistochemical stains may be particularly useful from a differential diagnosis perspective (see "Urothelial Dysplasia" section) (**Table 6-3**).[8,12,13]

Clinical studies of patients with reactive atypia are limited. Cheng et al. studied 25 patients with reactive atypia and a mean followup of 3.7 years and found that none of the patients developed dysplasia, CIS, or urothelial carcinoma (**Table 6-4**).[4] Reactive urothelial atypia is not a premalignant lesion and is currently placed under benign urothelial abnormalities.[1,2]

Atypia of Unknown Significance

"Atypia of unknown significance" is a descriptive term used when there is uncertainty whether the changes are reactive or preneoplastic in nature.[14] It has been proposed as a diagnosis to encompass lesions with nuclear abnormalities similar to those of reactive changes (fewer than those of dysplasia), but out of proportion to the degree of inflammation. Patients with atypia of unknown significance usually present with hematuria or irritative symptoms.[4] In contrast to reactive atypia, patients with atypia of unknown significance often have a previous diagnosis of urothelial dysplasia or have undergone various types of treatment, such as intravesical chemotherapy or radiotherapy.[1,8,15]

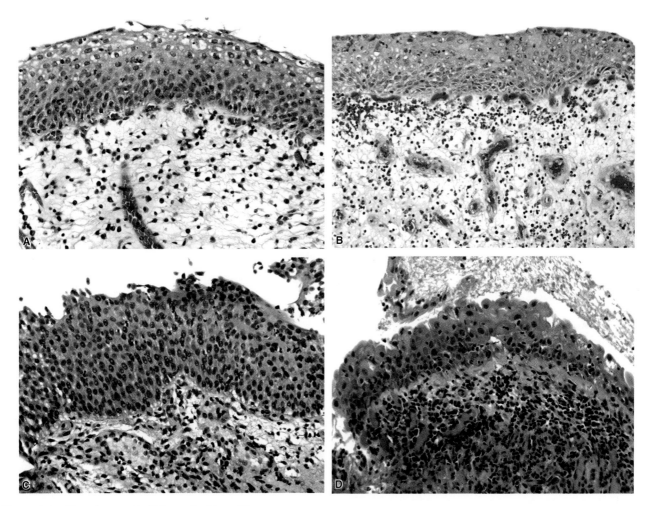

Figure 6-1   Reactive urothelial atypia (A to D).

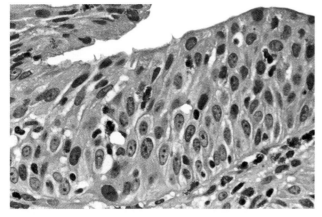

Figure 6-2   Reactive urothelial atypia. There is some thickening and loss of polarity and crowding of the mucosal cells, but they are relatively uniform in size and show maturation at the surface.

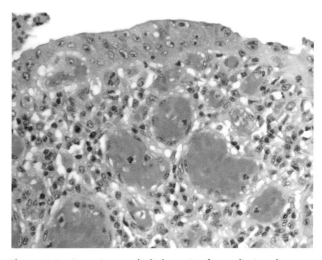

Figure 6-3   Reactive urothelial atypia after radiation therapy.

Table 6-2 Morphologic Features of Flat Urothelial Lesions

	Normal Urothelium	Flat (Simple) Urothelial Hyperplasia	Reactive Urothelial Atypia	Atypia of Unknown Significance	Urothelial Dysplasia
Architecture					
Cell layers	4–7	10 or more	Normal to mildly thickened	Normal to mildly thickened	Usually normal, but may be increased or decreased
Organization of cells	Maturation from basal to superficial cell layer	Normal	Normal	Normal	Lack of maturation in basal and intermediate cell layers (not full thickness)
Cytology					
Nuclear size	Small	Normal	May be mildly enlarged	May be mildly enlarged	Variable
Nuclear shape	Round to oval	Normal	Normal	Normal	Variable
Nuclear chromatin	Smooth	Normal	Vesicular	Vesicular	Coarse
Nucleoli	Absent	Absent	Prominent	Prominent	Inconspicuous
Mitoses	Absent	Absent	Present in lower layers	Present in lower layers	Variable
Umbrella cells	Present	Present	Present	Present	Present

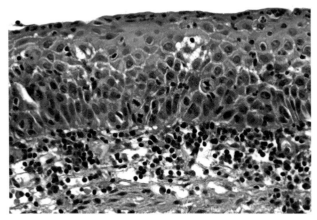

Figure 6-4   Reactive urothelial atypia. Note the mitotic figures in the lower portion of the urothelium.

Microscopically, one sees inflammation of the lamina propria and variable degrees of nuclear atypia (Fig. 6-6). The severity of nuclear atypia, however, is disproportionate to the extent of inflammation. Atypia of unknown significance may be difficult to distinguish from dysplasia. This distinction is critical because of important therapeutic and prognostic implications. In difficult cases, discriminatory immunohistochemical staining may be helpful.[8,13,16–18]

Overall, CK20 and CD44 appear to be the most useful objective markers for distinguishing atypia of unknown significance from dysplasia (Table 6-3). As mentioned earlier, CK20 expression is normally limited to the superficial umbrella cells. In contrast, CK20 expression in the deeper mucosal layers is characteristic of atypia of unknown significance.[17] Reactive urothelium typically shows staining with CD44 in a diffuse membranous full-thickness pattern or with patchy basal and intermediate cell expression. This is in contrast to the absence of CD44 staining in dysplasia. It is important to note that these staining patterns are not absolute. Therefore, caution must be exercised when interpreting them, and correlation with morphology is critical.

Atypia of unknown significance is not associated with adverse outcomes and may reasonably be combined diagnostically with reactive changes. Currently, there is no evidence supporting premalignant potential of atypia of unknown significance. Of the 35 patients with atypia of unknown significance and a mean followup of 3.7 years, Cheng et al. found that none progressed to dysplasia, CIS, or urothelial carcinoma (Table 6-4).[4] Because the diagnosis of atypia of unknown significance appears to be of little value clinically, use of this term is strongly discouraged.[1,4,8]

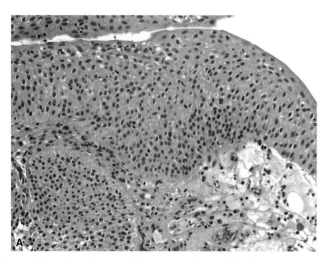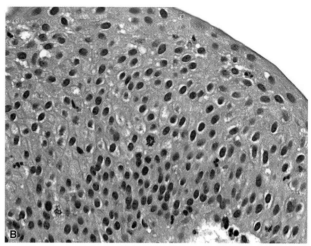

Figure 6-5   Reactive urothelial atypia (A and B). Despite mucosal thickening and the presence of mitotic figures, this lesion is still within the spectrum of reactive changes. The cells are relatively uniform in size and show maturation at the surface. Note the presence of intraepithelial neutrophils.

Table 6-3   Immunohistochemical Features of Flat Urothelial Lesions

	Normal Urothelium	Flat (Simple) Urothelial Hyperplasia	Reactive Urothelial Atypia	Atypia of Unknown Significance	Urothelial Dysplasia
Markers					
CK20	Limited to umbrella cells	Limited to umbrella cells	Limited to umbrella cells	Limited to umbrella cells	Deep layers
CD44	Limited to basal cells	Limited to basal cells	Increased reactivity in all cell layers	Increased reactivity in all cell layers	Absent
p53	Absent	Absent	Absent	Absent	Positive

Table 6-4   Clinical Findings of Patients with Reactive Atypia, Atypia of Unknown Significance, and Dysplasia of the Urinary Bladder

Characteristics	Reactive Atypia ($n = 25$)	Atypia of Unknown Significance ($n = 35$)	Dysplasia ($n = 26$)
Mean age (range), years	66 (39–88)	64 (24–80)	69 (50–85)
Male-to-female ratio	4 : 1	2 : 1	4 : 1
Major symptoms	Hematuria or irritative symptoms	Hematuria or irritative symptoms	Hematuria or irritative symptoms
Major cystoscopic findings	Erythematous/inflamed or suspicious for tumor	Erythematous/inflamed or suspicious for tumor	Erythematous/inflamed or suspicious for tumor
Mean followup (range), years	3.6 (0.1–9.9)	3.7 (0.2–11.4)	3.9 (0.1–13.4)
Clinical outcome	No adverse outcome[a]	No adverse outcome[a]	15% developed biopsy-proven cancer progression

Source: Modified from Ref. 4; with permission.
[a]None developed dysplasia, carcinoma in situ, or urothelial carcinoma.

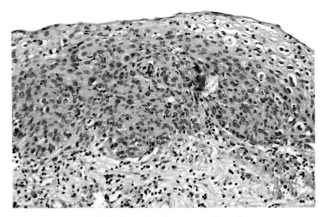

Figure 6-6 Urothelial atypia, favor reactive changes. Although considered dysplastic by multiple observers, this focus has many features of partial involvement by immature squamous metaplasia. Some investigators may consider this "atypia of unknown significance," although we discourage the use of "atypia of unknown significance" in surgical specimens. The diagnostic term "atypia of unknown significance" is used more appropriately in cytology specimens.

Urothelial Dysplasia

The difficulty in standardizing nomenclature for urothelial cytologic abnormalities is compounded by the lack of reproducibility in classification and grading. (Table 6-5).[1,4,9,11,19-32] Some investigators have categorized urothelial dysplasia into mild, moderate, and severe dysplasia in the past. CIS and high grade dysplasia are considered synonymous by most but not all investigators,[33] as there are no apparent distinguishing histologic features, and there is a relatively high level of agreement for these lesions. However, separation of epithelial changes with fewer cytologic and architectural abnormalities than CIS, such as intermediate (moderate)- and low grade dysplasia is difficult, and the morphologic continuum does not provide any absolute features that allow unequivocal separation. Some authors propose categories of reactive atypia and dysplasia, culminating in the final preinvasive stage of CIS; others suggest a two- or four-tiered system. One group lumped all neoplastic epithelial lesions into the category of CIS, apparently in response to the clinical and biologic uncertainty of these changes, whereas others graded CIS as 1, 2, or 3. Some authors preferred the terms "low grade intraurothelial neoplasia" and "high grade intraurothelial neoplasia" to dysplasia and CIS, respectively. The histologic criteria for distinguishing severe dysplasia from CIS are unreliable. It is also difficult to distinguish mild dysplasia from moderate dysplasia. Recognizing these limitations, it is recommended that severe dysplasia and CIS be combined into a single

category.[14] It is also recommended that dysplasia not be further subclassified into mild or moderate dysplasia.

Urothelial dysplasia is defined as abnormal urothelium with cytologic and architectural changes that do not meet all the criteria for an unequivocal diagnosis of urothelial CIS (Figs. 6-7 to 6-12).[3] Dysplasia represents an early morphologic manifestation of progressive alterations between normal urothelium and CIS. The thickness of dysplastic urothelium is usually normal, but it may be increased or decreased. Superficial umbrella cells are usually present, and most of the cytologic changes are restricted to the intermediate and basal cells (i.e., less than full-thickness atypia as frequently seen in CIS). The overall appearance is that of the urothelium in low grade papillary urothelial carcinoma.[3,4,12]

The cytologic abnormalities in urothelial dysplasia include nuclear and nucleolar enlargement, nuclear hyperchromasia and coarse chromatin, variation in nuclear shape, nuclear membrane irregularity, and notching of the chromatinic rim. However, there is no significant nuclear pleomorphism as seen in CIS. Nucleoli are usually small and inconspicuous, but may occasionally be enlarged. Loss of nuclear polarity is one of the earliest changes observed in neoplasia.[34] Loss of nuclear polarity in urothelial dysplasia is evidenced by crowding and nuclei with the long axis parallel to the basement membrane. Normal cytoplasmic clearing may be lost. Mitotic figures are usually absent; if present, usually only the basal layers, are involved. CK20 and p53 immunostains typically highlight the dysplastic cells (Table 6-3).

The lamina propria is usually normal, in contrast to atypia of unknown significance and urothelial CIS (see also Chapter 7), although it may contain scattered inflammatory cells and demonstrate increased neovascularity. The transition from normal urothelium to dysplasia is usually subtle, and dysplastic urothelial cells may show pagetoid spread in normal urothelium.

The main differential consideration for urothelial dysplasia is with reactive atypia and urothelial CIS (see also Chapter 7). Distinction may be particularly challenging in patients previously treated for CIS. Nuclear and architectural features are the primary criteria for distinguishing dysplasia from reactive atypia and urothelial CIS. Immunohistochemical stains such as CK20, CD44, p53, and Ki67 may be helpful (Table 6-3).[8,13,16-18] As mentioned earlier, CK20 expression is restricted to the umbrella cells in normal urothelium. In dysplasia, aberrant CK20 expression is seen in the deeper layers of the urothelium (Figs. 6-13 and 6-14). Increased reactivity of CD44 in all layers of the urothelium is more commonly seen in reactive atypia than in dysplasia. p53 immunostaining can also be helpful by highlighting dysplastic cells (Fig. 6-15). A conservative approach with repeat cystoscopy and biopsy after the inflammation has resolved is recommended in equivocal cases.

Table 6-5   Terminology for Flat (Nonpapillary) Intraepithelial Lesions of the Urothelium[a]

Koss et al.[23]	Nagy et al.[24]	Mostofi and Sesterhenn[25]	Murphy[59]	CIS Workshop[26]	Koss et al.[27]	Reuter and Melamed[28]	Amin et al.[29]	Grignon[30]	WHO/ISUP[31]	WHO[32]	Cheng et al.[4]	Ancona Proposal[1]	Current Proposal
Simple hyperplasia	Atypia (NOS)	—	—	—	—	—	Urothelial atypia, reactive	—	Reactive atypia	Reactive atypia	Reactive atypia	Reactive atypia[b]	Reactive atypia
Atypical hyperplasia	Mild dysplasia	CIS, grade 1	Dysplasia	Slight dysplasia (IUN1)	IUN1	CIS, low grade	Urothelial atypia, unknown significance	Low grade dysplasia	Atypia of unknown significance	Atypia of unknown significance		Presumed preneoplastic lesions[c]	
	Moderate dysplasia	CIS, grade 2	—	Moderate dysplasia (IUN2)	IUN2	CIS, moderate grade	Urothelial dysplasia, low grade	Moderate dysplasia	Dysplasia	Dysplasia	Dysplasia	Low grade IUN (dysplasia)[d]	Dysplasia
CIS	Severe dysplasia	CIS, grade 3	CIS	Severe dysplasia (IUN3)	IUN3	CIS, high grade	High grade dysplasia/CIS	High grade dysplasia/CIS	CIS	CIS	CIS	High grade IUN (CIS)[e]	CIS

Source: Modified from Ref. 4; with permission.

[a] CIS, carcinoma in situ; IUN, intraurothelial neoplasia; NOS, not otherwise specified.
[b] Including cases previously called "atypia of unknown significance," "mild dysplasia," "flat urothelial hyperplasia," and "CIS grade 1."
[c] Including keratinizing squamous metaplasia, glandular metaplasia, and malignancy-associated cellular changes.
[d] Mild dysplasia, moderate dysplasia, atypical hyperplasia, CIS grade 2, and dysplasia in other classifications.
[e] Urothelial CIS in other classifications, including severe dysplasia.

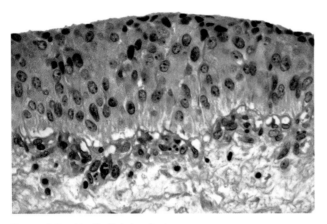

Figure 6-7   Urothelial dysplasia.

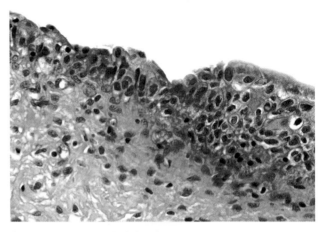

Figure 6-10   Urothelial dysplasia.

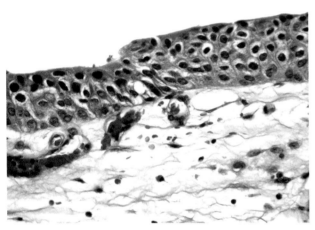

Figure 6-8   Urothelial dysplasia. Despite cytologic changes, including enlargement and hyperchromasia, the urothelium maintains cellular polarity and maturation. Multiple observers felt that this focus was dysplastic and not reactive, due largely to the lack of coexistent inflammation.

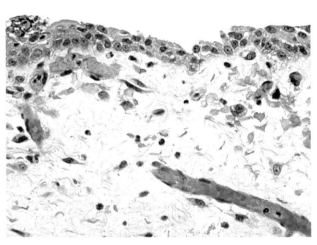

Figure 6-11   Urothelial dysplasia. The changes seen here are considered to fall just short of the threshold for urothelial carcinoma in situ.

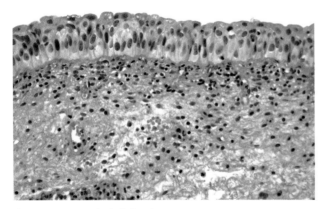

Figure 6-9   Urothelial dysplasia.

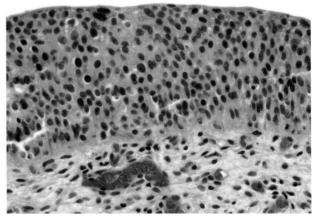

Figure 6-12   Urothelial dysplasia. The thickened urothelium is populated by dysplastic cells that are variable in size and shape.

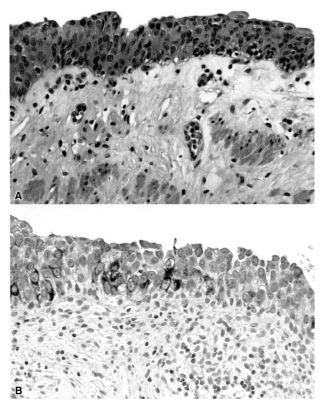

Figure 6-13 Urothelial dysplasia (A and B) with aberrant cytokeratin 20 expression (B).

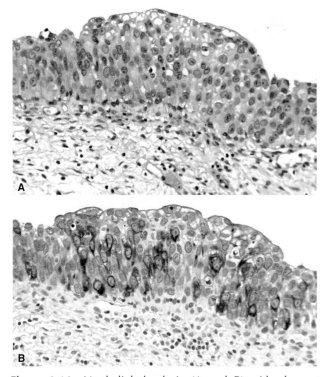

Figure 6-14 Urothelial dysplasia (A and B) with aberrant cytokeratin 20 expression (B).

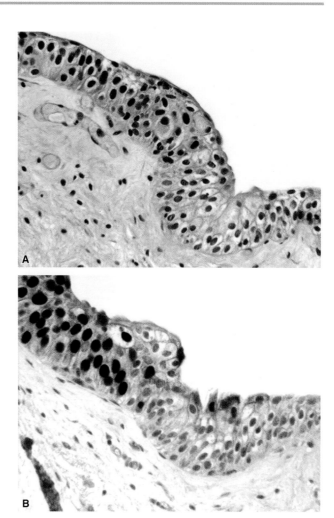

Figure 6-15 Urothelial dysplasia (A and B). p53 stain highlights dysplastic cells (B). (From Ref. 7; with permission.)

Another important differential diagnosis is the chemotherapy-related treatment effect. Systemic cyclophosphamide treatment may produce large binucleate or multinucleate cells with enlarged bizarre nuclei. Because cyclophosphamide causes arrest of the cell cycle, there is both cellular and nuclear enlargement. Nucleoli in these cells may be single or double, with angulated edges (see also **Chapters 2** and **24**). Awareness of the clinical history is critical to avoid misdiagnosis.

Clinically, dysplasia occurs in two distinct clinical settings: (1) de novo (primary or isolated) and (2) in patients with concurrent or previous urothelial neoplasms (secondary, concurrent). The true incidence of de novo dysplasia in the general population is unknown due to lack of large-scale screening studies and an inability to identify most cases cystoscopically. In an autopsy series of 313 cases, Shirai et al.[35] found dysplasia in 6.8% of males and 5.7% of females. Clinical followup information on patients with de novo dysplasia is limited as well.[3,4,36,37] Cheng et al. studied 26 patients with primary dysplasia.[4]

Table 6-6   Progression of Primary Urothelial Dysplasia of the Bladder[a]

	Patient Age	Gender	Clinical Presentation	Endoscopic Findings	Cytology	Location of Dysplasia	Interval from the Diagnosis to Progression (years)	Diagnosis[b]	Location of Cancer
1	71	F	Irritative symptoms	Erythematous	Positive	Posterior wall	1.0	Noninvasive papillary UC	Trigone
2	71	M	Incidental	Erythematous	Negative	Dome	1.4	Urothelial CIS	Posterior wall
3	74	M	Hematuria	Erythematous	Not done	Vesical neck	1.2	Urothelial CIS; noninvasive papillary UC	Trigone osterior wall
4	79	M	Incidental	Erythematous	Negative	Posterior wall	0.6	Urothelial CIS	Posterior wall
5	78	M	Irritative symptoms	Suspicious for neoplasm	Not done	Posterior wall	8.0	Invasive UC (stage T1)	Dome
6	54	M	Irritative symptoms	Suspicious for neoplasm	Not done	Right lateral wall	2.2	Urothelial CIS; invasive UC (stage T2)	Unspecified
7	48	F	Incidental	Suspicious for neoplasm	Negative	Base	3.0	Invasive UC (stage T1)	Posterior wall

Source: Modified from Ref. 3; with permission.
[a]Seven of 36 cases of de novo urothelial dysplasia progressed during a mean followup of 8.2 years.
[b]Diagnosis of cancer recurrence/progression; CIS, carcinoma in situ; UC, urothelial carcinoma.

Table 6-7   Clinical Outcomes of Patients with Atypical Urothelial Proliferations of the Urinary Bladder

1998 WHO/ISUP Classification	Clinical Significance
Reactive atypia	None developed dysplasia, carcinoma in situ, or urothelial carcinoma[4]
Atypia of unknown significance	None developed dysplasia, carcinoma in situ, or urothelial carcinoma[4]
Dysplasia	14–19% developed biopsy-proven progression[4,60]
Carcinoma in situ	74% 15-year cancer-specific surival[60]

Source: Modified from Ref. 4; with permission.

During a mean followup of 3.9 years, 15% developed biopsy-proven cancer, including CIS and high grade invasive carcinoma. In another study from a different patient cohort, Cheng et al. identified 36 patients with isolated urothelial dysplasia.[3] The patients ranged in age from 25 to 79 years (mean, 60 years), and the male-to-female ratio was 2.6 : 1. Patients presented with urinary tract obstructive symptoms (11/36), hematuria (10/36), both (3/36), and incidental findings (1/36). Dysplasia had a predilection for the posterior wall. Seven patients (19%) developed biopsy-proven progression, including 11% with CIS and 8% with invasive cancer (mean followup, 8.2 years) (Table 6-6). Mean time to progression was 2.5 years (range, 0.5 to 8 years). These data indicate

that isolated urothelial dysplasia was a significant risk factor for urothelial carcinoma (Table 6-7). Close clinical followup and regular cystoscopic examinations are recommended for patients with a diagnosis of de novo urothelial dysplasia.

Dysplasia in the mucosa adjacent to papillary urothelial carcinoma (secondary dysplasia) is associated with an increased risk of recurrence and progression.[26,38–41] In one study, 87% of patients with concomitant (secondary) dysplasia developed recurrence, whereas only 26% of those without dysplasia recurred.[39] Secondary dysplasia is more common than primary dysplasia and has a higher rate of progression to carcinoma than that of de novo dysplasia, with estimates ranging from 30% to 36%.[3]

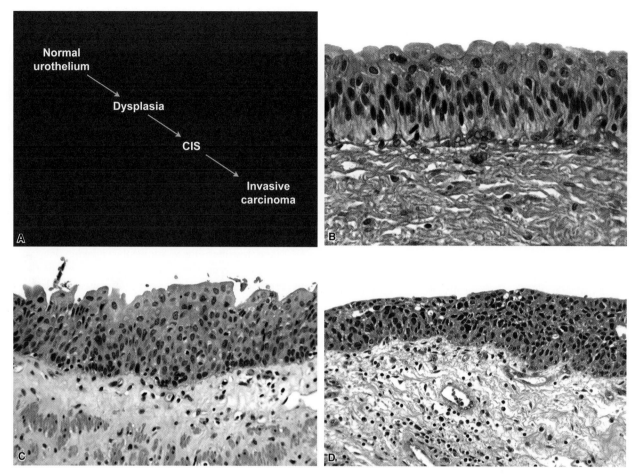

Figure 6-16   Continuum from normal urothelium through dysplasia to carcinoma in situ (CIS), according to the disease-continuum concept. (A) Progression scheme; (B) normal urothelium; (C) urothelial dysplasia; (D) CIS.

Molecular Alterations in Flat Lesions

Urothelial carcinogenesis is thought to proceed through two distinct genetic pathways.[1,7,42–44] These two genetic pathways are associated with marked differences in genetic instability and correspond to the morphologically entities low grade noninvasive lesions and its precursors, on the one hand, and CIS and invasive carcinoma, on the other. The low grade pathway involves inactivation of cyclin-dependent kinase inhibitors, including p15, p16 (9p21), and p21WAF/CIP1 in genetically stable premalignant and low grade tumors. In contrast, 17p13 (TP53)-mediated abnormalities occur in genetically unstable CIS (high grade intraurothelial neoplasia) and invasive carcinoma (Fig. 6-16).

Studies of blood group isoantigen expression, nuclear morphometry, DNA ploidy, and molecular genetic alterations indicate that the findings in dysplasia are intermediate between benign urothelium and CIS, as expected. Numerous deletions and genetic abnormalities occur in CIS,

reflecting generalized genetic instability, whereas premalignant flat lesions and dysplasia show a low rate of gene deletions. DNA aneuploidy occurs in less than 50% of cases of dysplasia and low grade lesions, whereas CIS demonstrates DNA aneuploidy in more than 90% of cases. Genetic alterations can also be found in histologically normal urothelium in bladder cancer patients, a change of uncertain significance.[1,44–49]

Chromosome 9 abnormalities and mutations in the fibroblast growth factor receptor 3 gene (FGFR3) are common in low grade papillary tumors and its precursors. TP53 mutations, on the other hand, are frequent in CIS.[7,50–55] The small fraction of cases of dysplasia which harbor TP53 mutations suggests that dysplasia is a precursor of CIS in some cases. The timing of chromosome 9 and p53 gene alterations during urothelial tumorigenesis may explain differences in the premalignant potential of flat lesions. Alterations in chromosome 9 may occur early in dysplasia, while p53 mutations occur in CIS. The p53 gene product functions in cell cycle regulation at the G1/S checkpoint[42] and mutations in the *TP53* gene prevent cell cycle arrest, leading to generalized genetic instability and possibly further genetic alterations. Inactivation of the *p53* gene in CIS may therefore explain the propensity of these lesions to progress to invasive carcinoma.

Recent studies using whole-organ mapping support the concepts of malignancy-associated cellular changes (MACC) and field effect in urothelial carcinogenesis.[7,8,50,56,57] Majewski et al.[50] identified a complex of genetic alterations involving chromosome regions 3q22–q24, 5q22–q31, 9q21–q22, 10q26, 13q14, and 17p13 ("forerunner genes") occurring prior to identifiable phenotypic changes in bladders. They identified three waves of genetic "hits" involving morphologically normal mucosa and regions of evident dysplasia. It was proposed that the first wave involves allelic loss of *RB1* (retinoblastoma gene) on 3q, resulting in plaque-like clonal expansion of morphologically normal urothelium in large patches.[50] The second wave is associated with clonal expansion of cells showing the first morphologically

detectable features of dysplasia. The third wave of genetic alterations occurs when the fully transformed phenotype of CIS is apparent. Similarly, Lopez-Beltran et al. recently demonstrated MACC with loss of heterozygosity (LOH) at 9q32–33 *DBC1* (deleted in bladder cancer 1) in normal urothelium from patients with low grade papillary urothelial tumors.[58] The most striking observation in their study was the association between *DBC1* locus in normal urothelium with tumor recurrence and progression.[58] Of the 38 low grade Ta papillary urothelial carcinomas and associated samples of 11 normal urothelium specimens, which were informative in their 9q32–33 LOH study, 12 (31.6%) showed tumor recurrence, and five (13.1%) showed tumor stage progression when there was deletion of *DBC1*.

Taken together, these molecular genetic data suggest that dysplasia represents a genetically unstable preneoplastic process, which places some patients with flat lesions at increased risk for the development of CIS and invasive urothelial carcinoma.

REFERENCES

1. Lopez-Beltran A, Cheng L, Andersson L, Brausi M, de Matteis A, Montironi R, Sesterhenn I, van det Kwast KT, Mazerolles C. Preneoplastic non-papillary lesions and conditions of the urinary bladder: an update based on the Ancona International Consultation. *Virchows Arch* 2002;440:3–11.
2. Bostwick DG, Cheng L, eds. Urologic Surgical Pathology, 2nd ed. Philadelphia: Elsevier/Mosby, 2008.
3. Cheng L, Cheville JC, Neumann RM, Bostwick DG. Natural history of urothelial dysplasia of the bladder. *Am J Surg Pathol* 1999;23:443–7.
4. Cheng L, Cheville JC, Neumann RM, Bostwick DG. Flat intraepithelial lesions of the urinary bladder. *Cancer* 2000;88:625–31.
5. Cheng L, Montironi R, Davidson DD, Lopez-Beltran A. Staging and reporting of urothelial carcinoma of the urinary bladder. *Mod Pathol* 2009;22 (Suppl 2):S70–95.
6. Bostwick DG, Ramnani D, Cheng L. Diagnosis and grading of bladder cancer and associated lesions. *Urol Clin North Am* 1999;26:493–507.
7. Cheng L, Davidson DD, Maclennan GT, Williamson SR, Zhang S, Koch MO, Montironi R, Lopez-Beltran A. The origins of urothelial carcinoma. *Expert Rev Anticancer Ther* 2010;10:865–80.
8. Hodges KB, Lopez-Beltran A, Davidson DD, Montironi R, Cheng L. Urothelial dysplasia and other flat lesions of the urinary bladder: clinicopathologic and molecular features. *Hum Pathol* 2010;41: 155–62.
9. Montironi R, Lopez-Beltran A, Scarpelli M, Mazzucchelli R, Cheng L. 2004 World Health Organization classification of the noninvasive urothelial neoplasms: inherent problems and clinical reflections. *Eur Urol* 2009;Suppl 8:453–7.
10. Montironi R, Mazzucchelli R, Scarpelli M, Lopez-Beltran A, Cheng L. Morphological diagnosis of urothelial neoplasms. *J Clin Pathol* 2008;61:3–10.
11. Cheng L, Lopez-Beltran A, MacLennan GT, Montironi R, Bostwick DG. Neoplasms of the urinary bladder. In: Bostwick DG, Cheng L, eds. Urologic Surgical Pathology, 2nd ed. Philadelphia: Elsevier/Mosby, 2008;259–352.
12. Montironi R, Lopez-Beltran A, Scarpelli M, Mazzucchelli R, Cheng L. Morphological classification and definition of benign, preneoplastic and non-invasive neoplastic lesions of the urinary bladder. *Histopathology* 2008;53:621–33.
13. McKenney JK, Desai S, Cohen C, Amin MB. Discriminatory immunohistochemical staining of urothelial carcinoma in situ and non-neoplastic urothelium: an analysis of cytokeratin 20, p53, and CD44 antigens. *Am J Surg Pathol* 2001;25:1074–8.
14. Epstein JL, Amin MB, Reuter VR, Mostofi FK. The bladder consensus conference committee. The World Health Organization/International Society of Urologic Pathology consensus classification of urothelial (transitional cell) neoplasms of the urinary bladder. *Am J Surg Pathol* 1998;22:1435–8.
15. Lopez-Beltran A, Luque RJ, Mazzucchelli R, Scarpelli M, Montironi R. Changes produced in the urothelium by traditional and newer therapeutic procedures for bladder cancer. *J Clin Pathol* 2002;55:641–7.

16. Harnden P, Eardley I, Joyce AD, Southgate J. Cytokeratin 20 as an objective marker of urothelial dysplasia. *Br J Urol* 1996;78:870–5.

17. Kunju LP, Lee CT, Montie J, Shah RB. Utility of cytokeratin 20 and Ki–67 as markers of urothelial dysplasia. *Pathol Int* 2005;55:248–54.

18. Sun W, Herrera GA. E-cadherin expression in urothelial carcinoma in situ, superficial papillary transitional cell carcinoma, and invasive transitional cell carcinoma. *Hum Pathol* 2002;33:996–1000.

19. Bostwick DG. Natural history of early bladder cancer. *J Cell Biochem* 1992;161 (Supp l):31–8.

20. Jones TD, Cheng L. Papillary urothelial neoplasm of low malignant potential: evolving terminology and concepts. *J Urol* 2006;175:1995–2003.

21. Maclennan GT, Kirkali Z, Cheng L. Histologic grading of noninvasive papillary urothelial neoplasms. *Eur Urol* 2007;51:889–98.

22. Grignon DJ. The current classification of urothelial neoplasms. *Mod Pathol* 2009;22 (Suppl 2):S60–90.

23. Koss LG. Tumors of the Urinary Bladder, Fascicle 11. Washington, DC: Armed Forces Institute of Pathology, 1975.

24. Nagy G, Frable W, Murphy W. Classificiation of premalignant urothelial abnormalities: a delphi study of the national bladder cancer collaborative group A. *Pathol Annul* 1982;17:219–33.

25. Mostofi FK, Sesterhenn IA. Pathology of epithelial tumors and carcinoma in situ of the bladder. *Prog Clin Biol Res* 1984;162A:55–74.

26. Friedell G, Soloway M, Hilgar A, Farrow G. Summary of workshop on carcinoma in situ of the bladder. *J Urol* 1986;136:1047–8.

27. Koss LG, Woyke S, Olszewski W. Aspiration biopsy. Cytologic Interpretation and Histologic Bases, 2nd ed. New York: Igaku Shoin, 1992.

28. Reuter VE, Melamed MR. Diagnostic Surgical Pathology. In: Sternberg SS, ed. Diagnostic Surgical Pathology. New York: Raven Press, 1989;1355–92.

29. Amin MB, Murphy WM, Reuter VE, Ro JY, Ayala AG, Weiss MA, Eble JN, Young RH. A symposium on controversies in the pathology of transitional cell carcinomas of the urinary bladder. Part I. *Anat Pathol* 1996;1:1–39.

30. Grignon DJ. Neoplasms of the urinary bladder. In: Bostwick DG, Eble JN, eds. Urologic Surgical Pathology. St. Louis: Mosby-Year Book, Inc, 1997;214–305.

31. Epstein JI, Amin MB, Reuter VR, Mostofi FK. The World Health Organization/International Society of Urological Pathology consensus classification of urothelial (transitional cell) neoplasms of the urinary bladder. Bladder Consensus Conference Committee. *Am J Surg Pathol* 1998;22:1435–48.

32. Mostofi FK, Davis CJ, Sesterhenn IA. WHO Histologic Typing of Urinary Bladder Tumors. Berlin: Springer, 1999.

33. Adsay NV, Sakr WA, Grignon DJ. Flat-type transitional cell carcinoma in situ. *Pathol Case Rev* 1997;2:115–21.

34. Chandramouly G, Abad PC, Knowles DW, Lelievre SA. The control of tissue architecture over nuclear organization is crucial for epithelial cell fate. *J Cell Sci* 2007;120:1596–1606.

35. Shirai T, Fukushima S, Hirose M, Ohshima M, Ito N. Epithelail lesions of the urinary bladder in 313 autopsy cases. *Jpn J Cancer Res* 1987;78:1073–80.

36. Zuk R, Rogers H, Martin J, Baithun S. Clinicopathological importance of primary dsyplasia of bladder. *J Clin Pathol* 1988;41:1277–80.

37. Baithun S, Rogers H, martin J, Zuk R, Blandy J. Primary dysplasia of bladder. *Lancet* 1988;1(8583):483.

38. Smith G, Elton RA, Beynon LL, Newsam JE, Chisholm GD, Hargreave TB. Prognostic significance of biopsy results of normal-looking mucosa in cases of superficial bladder cancer. *Br J Urol* 1983;55:665–9.

39. Wolf H, Hojgaard K. Urothelial dysplasia concomitant with bladder tumours as a determinant factor for future new occurrences. *Lancet* 1983;2:134–6.

40. Heney NM. Natural history of superficial bladder cancer: prognostic features and long-term disease course. *Urol Clin North Am* 1992;19:429–33.

41. Kiemeney LA, Witjes JA, Heijbroek RP, Debruyne FM, Verbeek AL. Dysplasia in normal-looking urothelium increases the risk of tumour progression in primary superficial bladder cancer. *Eur J Cancer* 1994;30A:1621–5.

42. Spruck CH 3rd, Ohneseit PF, Gonzalez-Zulueta M, Esrig D, Miyao N, Tsai YC, Lerner SP, Schmutte C, Yang AS, Cote R, et al. Two molecular pathways to transitional cell carcinoma of the bladder. *Cancer Res* 1994;54:784–8.

43. Wu XR. Urothelial tumorigenesis: a tale of divergent pathways. *Nat Rev Cancer* 2005;5:713–25.

44. Cheng L, Zhang S, Maclennan GT, Williamson SR, Lopez-Beltran A, Montironi R. Bladder cancer: translating molecular genetic insights into clinical practice. *Hum Pathol* 2011;42:455–81.

45. Baithun SI, Naase M, Blanes A, Diaz-Cano SJ. Molecular and kinetic features of transitional cell carcinomas of the bladder: biological and clinical implications. *Virchows Arch* 2001;438:289–97.

46. Baud E, Catilina P, Boiteux J-P, Bignon Y-J. Human bladder cancers and normal bladder mucosa present the same hot spot of heterozygous chromosome–9 deletion. *Int J Cancer* 1998;77:821–4.

47. Hart KC, Robertson SC, Kanemitsu MY, Meyer AN, Tynan JA, Donoghue DJ. Transformation and stat activation by derivatives of FGFR1, FGFR3, and FGFR4. *Oncogene* 2000;19:3309–20.

48. Jebar AH, Hurst CD, Tomlinson DC, Johnston C, Taylor CF, Knowles MA. FGFR3 and Ras gene mutations are mutually exclusive genetic events in urothelial cell carcinoma. *Oncogene* 2005;24:5218–25.

49. Muto S, Horie S, Takahashi S, Tomita K, Kitamura T. Genetic and epigenetic alterations in normal bladder epithelium in patients with metachronous bladder cancer. *Cancer Res* 2000;60:4021–5.

50. Majewski T, Lee S, Jeong J, Yoon DS, Kram A, Kim MS, Tuziak T, Bondaruk J, Lee S, Park WS, Tang KS, Chung W, et al. Understanding the development of human bladder cancer by using a whole-organ genomic mapping strategy. *Lab Invest* 2008;88:694–721.

51. Hartmann A, Rosner U, Schlake G, Dietmaier W, Zaak D, Hofstaedter F, Knuechel R. Clonality and genetic divergence in multifocal low grade superficial urothelial carcinoma as determined by chromosome 9 and p53 deletion analysis. *Lab Invest* 2000;80:709–18.

52. Hartmann A, Schlake G, Zaak D, Hungerhuber E, Hofstetter A, Hofstaedter F, Knuechel R. Occurrence of chromosome 9 and p53 alterations in multifocal dysplasia and carcinoma in situ of human urinary bladder. *Cancer Res* 2002;62:809–18.

53. Hartmann A, Moser K, Kriegmair M, Hofstetter A, Hofstaedter F, Knuechel R. Frequent genetic alterations in simple urothelial hyperplasias of the bladder in patients with papillary urothelial carcinoma. *Am J Pathol* 1999;154:721–7.

54. Steidl C, Simon R, Burger H, Brinkschmidt C, Hertle L, Bocker W, Terpe HJ. Patterns of chromosomal aberrations in urinary bladder tumours and adjacent urothelium. *J Pathol* 2002;198:115–20.

55. Williamson SR, Montironi R, Lopez-Beltran A, MacLennan GT, Davidson DD, Cheng L. Diagnosis, evaluation and treatment of carcinoma in situ of the urinary bladder: the state of the art. *Crit Rev Oncol Hematol* 2010;76:112–26.

56. Lee S, Jeong J, Majewski T, Scherer SE, Kim MS, Tuziak T, Tang KS, Baggerly K, Grossman HB, Zhou JH, Shen L, Bondaruk J, et al. Forerunner *genes* contiguous to RB1 contribute to the development of in situ neoplasia. *Proc Natl Acad Sci U S A* 2007;104:13732–7.

57. Tuziak T, Jeong J, Majewski T, Kim MS, Steinberg J, Wang Z, Yoon DS, Kuang TC, Baggerly K, Johnston D, Czerniak B. High-resolution whole-organ mapping with SNPs and its significance to early events of carcinogenesis. *Lab Invest* 2005;85:689–701.

58. Lopez-Beltran A, Alvarez-Kindelan J, Luque RJ, Blanca A, Quintero A, Montironi R, Cheng L, Gonzalez-Campora R, Requena MJ. Loss of heterozygosity at 9q32–33 (DBC1 locus) in primary non-invasive papillary urothelial neoplasm of low malignant potential and low grade urothelial carcinoma of the bladder and their associated normal urothelium. *J Pathol* 2008;215:263–72.

59. Murphy WM, ed. Atlas of Bladder Carcinoma. Chicago: American Society of Clinical Pathologists Press, 1986.

60. Cheng L, Cheville JC, Neumann RM, Leibovich BC, Egan KS, Spotts BE, Bostwick DG. Survival of patients with carcinoma in situ of the urinary bladder. *Cancer* 1999;85:2469–74.

Chapter 7

Urothelial Carcinoma in Situ

Bladder Pathology, First Edition. Liang Cheng, Antonio Lopez-Beltran, David G. Bostwick.
© 2012 Wiley-Blackwell. Published 2012 by John Wiley & Sons, Inc.

Definition, Terminology, and Historical Perspective

Carcinoma in situ (CIS) of the urinary bladder, also referred to as "urothelial carcinoma in situ" or "high grade intraurothelial neoplasia," is defined by the replacement of part or all of the normal epithelium by cells that have microscopic—and now molecular—features of carcinoma, yet are confined to the epithelium (**Fig. 7-1**).[1-5] The number of cell layers in CIS may be increased, normal, or decreased. CIS is therefore a "flat" lesion, designated Tis according to the tumor, lymph node, and metastasis (TNM) pathologic staging. In contrast, noninvasive papillary urothelial carcinomas are considered Ta lesions. In many cases, an in situ carcinoma component is adjacent to or associated with invasive carcinoma. In such cases, the CIS is referred to as secondary. In the less common clinical scenario, invasive carcinoma is absent and CIS is associated with a lower grade intraurothelial lesion (dysplasia). These cases are referred to as primary CIS.

Although other types of carcinoma in situ, such as adenocarcinoma in situ and squamous cell CIS, have been described in the urinary bladder, they are somewhat controversial and far less common than urothelial CIS. Most investigators typically use the term "urothelial carcinoma in situ" and "carcinoma in situ" interchangeably. Urothelial CIS was traditionally referred to as transitional cell CIS, based on the premise that the urothelium has features intermediate or transitional between stratified squamous epithelium and pseudostratified columnar epithelium. In recent years, the term "urothelium" has been used increasingly to describe this specialized epithelium.

In 1952, Melicow[2,6,7] recognized the significance of examining the grossly normal bladder mucosa between exophytic tumors, in an attempt to explain the high recurrence rate of bladder cancer, even after extensive organ-preserving surgical treatment. Later that year, Melicow and Hollowell[2,6,7] described CIS of the urinary system, referring to lesions "... whose gross features are inconspicuous and seemingly benign but whose microscopic picture is that of malignancy." This concise

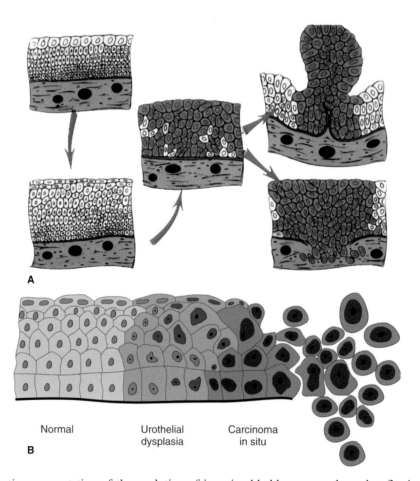

A

B

| Normal | Urothelial dysplasia | Carcinoma in situ |

Figure 7-1 Diagrammatic representation of the evolution of invasive bladder cancer through a flat in situ phase (A and B). Formation of a papillary neoplasm may also occur.

description remains accurate today. Melamed et al.[6–8] first described the natural history of urothelial CIS and found that nine of 25 patients (36%) developed invasive carcinoma within five years after the initial diagnosis.

Nomenclature for CIS has historically been somewhat confusing. In Melicow's original papers, the terms "Bowen disease" and "intraurothelial cancer" are used somewhat interchangeably with CIS. Over the years, precancerous bladder lesions have been referred to by a variety of names, including dysplasia (mild, moderate, or severe), intraepithelial neoplasia (low or high grade), intraurothelial neoplasia (grade 1 or 2), atypical hyperplasia, and marked atypia (see **Chapter 6** for additional discussion).[6–8] Urothelial carcinoma in situ and high grade intraurothelial neoplasia are indistinguishable and have been used interchangeably. To avoid miscommunication, we recommend use of the terminology "urothelial carcinoma in situ" in the reporting.[3,9–15]

CIS exists in two settings: de novo or isolated CIS and secondary CIS associated with papillary urothelial carcinoma (see the discussion below). De novo or isolated CIS (often referred to as primary CIS) is less common, and accounts for approximately 10% of all CIS and 1% to 3% of bladder neoplasms.[16,17]

Clinical Features

CIS usually occurs in elderly men and presents most frequently at 60 to 70 years of age. Clinical presentation often closely mimics that of interstitial cystitis. Symptoms typically include gross and microscopic hematuria, irritative symptoms (dysuria, pain, and/or frequency), nocturia, and sterile pyuria.[18–27]

Approximately 25% of patients are asymptomatic.[1–3,11,28] In Cheng et al.'s study of 138 patients with CIS, 41% had macroscopic hematuria at presentation, 44% had microscopic hematuria, 49% had irritative symptoms, and 26% were identified incidentally, reinforcing these clinical parameters.[1] Irritative symptoms may be particularly prominent when CIS is primary and diffusely present.

Cystoscopically, detection and accurate assessment of flat lesions is difficult. In most cases, CIS appears as erythematous velvety or granular patches (**Figs. 7-2 to 7-4**), although it may be visually undetectable.[3,29,30] Characteristic lesions are sometimes described as a "red velvety patch," although this finding is nonspecific.

CIS is frequently multifocal. Two or more separate locations are involved by CIS in 50% of cases, with a predilection for the trigone, lateral wall, and dome of the bladder. Additional sites of multifocal involvement include distal ureters, prostatic urethra (20% to 67% of cases), prostatic ducts or acini (up to 40%), renal pelvis, and proximal ureters.[3] Mapping studies of cystectomy specimens show

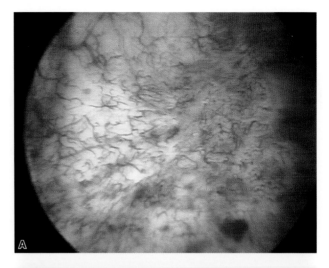
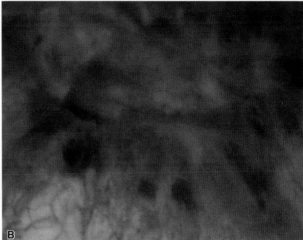
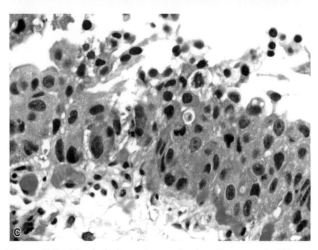

Figure 7-2 Urothelial carcinoma in situ. Cystoscopic (A), gross (B), and microscopic (C) appearance. Note the prominent vascular proliferations immediately below the basement membrane of urothelium (C).

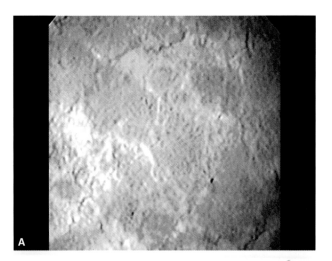

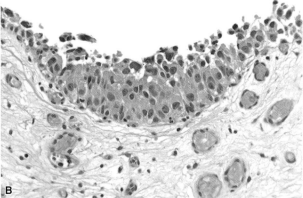

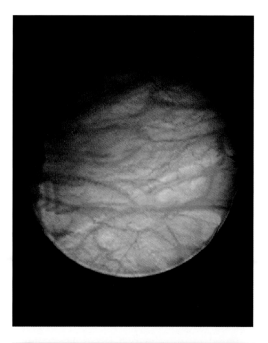

Figure 7-3 Urothelial carcinoma in situ. Cystoscopic (A) and microscopic (B) appearance. At cystoscopy, the mucosa appears slightly raised (whitish area), focally reddish, and bleeds easily (A). (Photo courtesy of Dr. Koch.)

extensive CIS, with involvement of the prostatic urethra and of the ureter in as many as 67% and 57% of cases, respectively.[31–34]

Urothelial CIS has a high likelihood of progressing to invasive carcinoma if untreated, occurring in up to 83% of cases.[1,3,11,35–43] Cystectomy reveals foci of microinvasion in 34% of bladders with CIS, and muscle-invasive cancer in 9%.[44] In a recent large series of 243 CIS patients treated with radical cystectomy from eight centers in the United States, Canada, and Europe, Tilki and colleagues found that 36% of patients had cancer upstaged, including 11% of patients with extravesical (pT3 or higher) extension and 5.8% of patients with lymph node metastasis.[43] The five-year cancer-specific survival was 85%.[43] In Cheng et al.'s study, the mean interval between a diagnosis of CIS and the detection of cancer progression is five years.[1] The actuarial progression-free survival, cancer-specific survival, and all-cause survival rates are 63%, 79%, and 55%, respectively, at 10 years and 59%, 74%, and 40%, respectively, at 15 years (Fig. 7-5).[1]

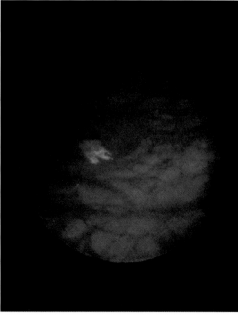

Figure 7-4 Urothelial CIS visualized by standard white-light cystoscopy (top) and fluorescence cystoscopy (bottom). Sharp (red) appearance of CIS lesion under fluorescence cystoscopy (bottom). These CIS lesions as shown may be difficult to detect using standard white-light cystoscopy (top). Hexaminolevulinate causes photoactive porphyrins to accumulate preferentially in rapidly proliferating tumor cells. These porphyrins emit red fluorescence when exposed to blue light. (Photo courtesy of Dr. Montironi.)

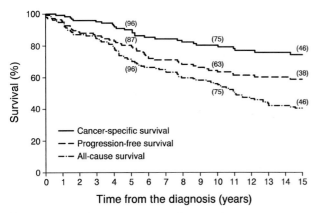

Figure 7-5 Kaplan–Meier survival curves for 138 patients with primary urothelial carcinoma in situ of the bladder. No patients had invasive urothelial carcinoma at the time of diagnosis. The numbers in parentheses represent the number of patients under observation at 5, 10, and 15 years. Progression was defined as development of invasive carcinoma, distant metastasis, or death from bladder cancer. (From Ref. 1; with permission.)

Urothelial CIS is often associated with invasive carcinoma elsewhere in the bladder (referred to as secondary or concomitant CIS). The frequency of CIS increases with the grade and stage of the associated urothelial neoplasm. Up to 24% of random biopsies from patients with Ta and T1 carcinoma show epithelial abnormalities that include dysplasia and CIS.

Patients with lower stage and higher grade tumors more commonly had CIS, and patients with involvement of the prostatic urethra by tumor were also more likely to have CIS.[45] Patients with coexisting invasive urothelial carcinoma have a higher risk of cancer progression and cancer-specific death than that of patients with primary CIS.[2,11]

Special Considerations

Primary Versus Secondary Carcinoma in Situ

Definitions of primary and secondary CIS vary somewhat in the pathologic and urologic literature. Takenaka et al.[16] separated lesions into the following categories: (1) primary CIS, occurring without associated previous urothelial tumor; (2) concomitant CIS, occurring in conjunction with a newly diagnosed bladder tumor; and (3) secondary CIS, diagnosed during followup of a known bladder tumor, with or without a concomitant tumor at the time of CIS diagnosis. This convention was used by some other authors, and may be gaining in usage.[15,46–49]

In many cases, however, the terminology is less clearly defined, so "primary" and "secondary" refer presumptively to the presence or absence of any current or past tumor. Admittedly, this is perhaps the most important distinction, since it appears to make little clinical difference whether CIS is related to a synchronous or metachronous primary tumor. Other synonyms are sometimes used, including "isolated," "solitary," and "concurrent" CIS, but the meaning of these is even less clearly defined than that of the terms above.[15,46–49]

Primary (de novo or isolated) CIS is uncommon, accounting for less than 10% of cases of CIS and 1% to 3% of bladder tumors.[47–51] It occurs in the absence of other urothelial tumors, almost exclusively in men over 50 years of age. Primary CIS has a lower risk of progression (28% vs. 59%) and death (7% vs. 45%) than that of secondary CIS.[49] However, a recent study of 476 CIS patients indicated that patients with primary CIS have a worse prognosis than that of patients with primary CIS.[42] Cancer progression rate was 43% for patients with primary CIS compared to 32% for those with secondary CIS.[42] Factors predictive of high risk of progression include multifocality, coexistent bladder neoplasm, prostatic urethral involvement, and recurrence after treatment.

Prostatic Ducts and Prostatic Urethra Involvement

Patel and colleagues examined 308 patients who underwent radical cystoprostatectomy with whole-mount processing of the prostate component.[52] Of the 121 (39%) patients with prostatic urothelial carcinoma, 59 (49%) had dysplasia/CIS of the prostatic urethra and 20 (17%) had involvement of the prostatic ducts. The remaining patients had involvement by invasive urothelial carcinoma. Risk factors for overall prostatic involvement included a bladder tumor location in the trigone and associated bladder CIS by both univariate and multivariate analyses. Presence of bladder CIS was the sole risk factor associated specifically with nonstromal involvement (CIS/dysplasia of ducts/urethra).[52] Similar to the tumor cell mobility seen in the bladder, the malignant cells may spread in a pagetoid fashion through the prostatic epithelium or undermine the epithelium of the prostatic ducts/acini, resulting in a layer of malignant cells sandwiched between the basal cell layer and the epithelial layer.

In the newly revised 2010 TNM staging system,[4,9] subepithelial invasion of prostatic urethra will not constitute T4a staging status. T4a tumor is defined by prostatic stromal invasion directly from the bladder cancer.

Histopathology and Diagnostic Criteria

CIS is defined as a flat noninvasive neoplastic mucosal change of the urothelium with substantial cytologic and architectural abnormalities that lack papillary changes.

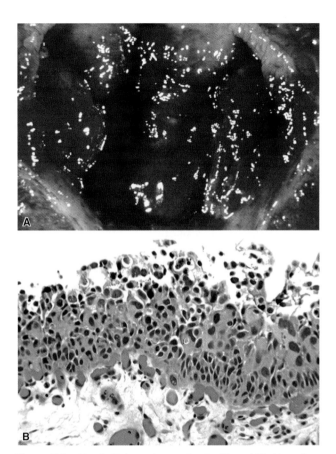

Figure 7-6   Urothelial carcinoma in situ (A and B). Note the velvety appearance of the carcinoma in situ.

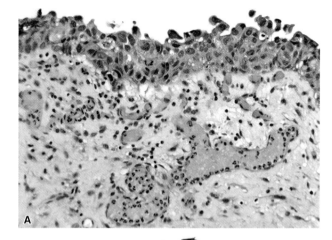

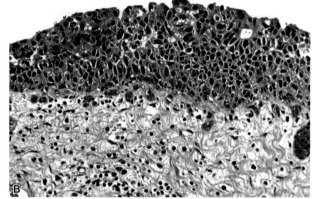

Figure 7-7   Urothelial carcinoma in situ (A and B). Note the full-thickness involvement of the urothelium by the carcinoma in situ.

Grossly, the mucosa may range from unremarkable to erythematous velvety, granular patches, edematous, or eroded (Fig. 7-6); lesions may be found both near an invasive tumor and at a distance from it. The diagnosis of CIS requires the presence of severe cytologic atypia (nuclear anaplasia); full-thickness change is not essential, although it is usually present (Fig. 7-7). The cells of CIS may form a layer that is only one cell layer thick, of normal thickness (up to seven cells), or the thickness of hyperplasia (greater than seven cells) (Fig. 7-8).

Prominent disorganization of cells is characteristic, with loss of polarity and cohesiveness. Superficial (umbrella) cells may be present except in areas of full-thickness abnormality. The tumor cells tend to be large and pleomorphic, with moderate to abundant cytoplasm, although they are sometimes small with a high nuclear-to-cytoplasmic ratio. The chromatin tends to be coarse and clumped. Morphometrically, the cells display increased nuclear area, nuclear perimeter, and maximum nuclear diameter. Nucleoli are usually large and prominent in at least some of the cells, and may be multiple. Mitotic figures are often seen in the uppermost urothelium, and may be atypical (Fig. 7-9). The

adjacent mucosa often contains lesser degrees of cytologic abnormality.

The small cell pattern of CIS is usually associated with an increased number of cell layers. In such cases, the cytoplasm is scant and nuclei are enlarged and hyperchromatic, with coarse unevenly distributed chromatin; scattered prominent nucleoli are distorted and angulated. Mitotic figures are frequently present, often with abnormal forms. The cells are randomly oriented and disorganized, often with striking cellular dyscohesion that, in some cases, results in few or no recognizable epithelial cells on the surface, a condition referred to as denuding cystitis.[53] Careful search of all residual mucosa is important in biopsies that have little or no mucosa in order to exclude the denuding cystitis of CIS.

CIS is often associated with focal discontinuity of the basement membrane. Tissue edema, vascular ectasia, and proliferation of small capillaries are frequently observed in the lamina propria. There may be intense chronic inflammation in the superficial lamina propria in some cases, and vascular ectasia and proliferation of small capillaries is frequent. In denuded areas, residual CIS may

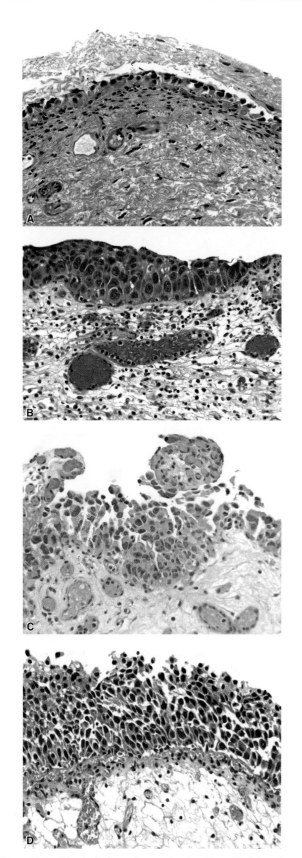

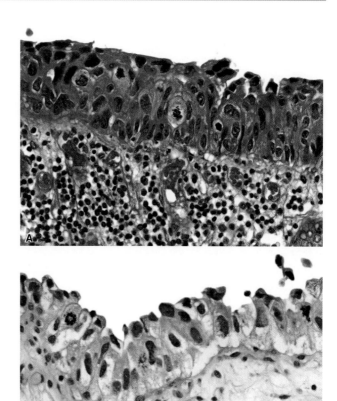

Figure 7-9 Urothelial carcinoma in situ (A and B). Note the atypical mitotic figures.

involve von Brunn nests (**Fig. 7-10**). Rarely, CIS exhibits pagetoid growth, characterized by large single cells or small clusters of cells within otherwise normal urothelium, in squamous metaplasia, or within prostatic ducts.[48,54–56] Individual cells showing pagetoid spread have enlarged nuclei with coarse chromatin, single or multiple nucleoli, and abundant pale to eosinophilic cytoplasm that is mucin negative. A careful search should be made for subepithelial invasion (microinvasion), often appearing as single cells or small nests of cells with retraction artifact. Microinvasion may be masked by chronic inflammation, denuded mucosa, or stromal fibrosis.

Variants of Urothelial Carcinoma in Situ

To avoid misdiagnosis, it is useful to recognize the histopathologic variants of urothelial CIS, such as large cell CIS, pagetoid CIS, and small cell CIS.[3,15] Nevertheless, these variants connote no known prognostic differences. Morphologic grading has historically been applied to

Figure 7-8 Urothelial carcinoma in situ (A to D). Note the variable layers of carcinoma in situ.

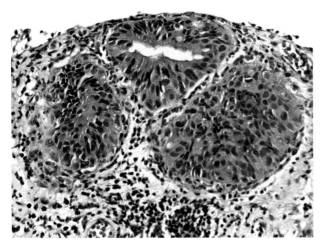

Figure 7-10 Urothelial carcinoma in situ involves von Brunn nests. The overlying urothelium is denuded.

Table 7-1   Variants of Urothelial Carcinoma in Situ (CIS)

Large cell CIS
Small cell CIS
Denuding and "clinging pattern" CIS
Pagetoid and undermining (lepedic) CIS
CIS with squamous differentiation
CIS with glandular differentiation
CIS with micropapillary growth
CIS with microinvasion

CIS, but the current World Health Organization and International Society of Urologic Pathology (WHO/ISUP) classification system recognizes only two grades of atypia, defined as dysplasia and CIS. Each of these grades has been shown to have clinical prognostic importance.

A number of morphologic variants and growth patterns of CIS have been recognized over the years (**Table 7-1**). Although it is not necessary to mention these specific growth patterns or morphologic variants in the surgical pathology report, awareness of the histologic diversity of CIS may aid in the diagnosis of this therapeutically and biologically important lesion.[15,57] These lesions may be associated with microinvasion, sometimes clinically unsuspected and histologically subtle.[57]

Large Cell Carcinoma in Situ

Large cell CIS constitutes the most common morphologic form of this entity. Cytologic findings include nuclear pleomorphism, variably abundant cytoplasm, and anaplastic nuclear features (**Fig. 7-11**). In rare cases, large cell CIS may have minor nuclear pleomorphism but still exhibit architectural disarray. Rare cases of large cell CIS with pleomorphic giant cells have been reported as "giant cell" CIS (**Fig. 7-12**).

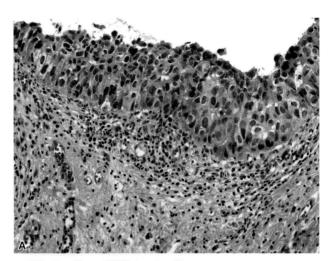

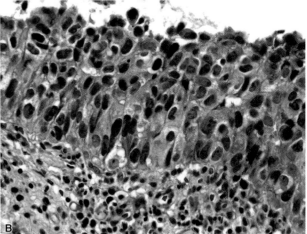

Figure 7-11 Urothelial carcinoma in situ (A and B), large cell variant. Carcinoma in situ involving a thickened urothelium.

Small Cell Carcinoma in Situ

The small cell pattern refers to the size of the cells, may or may not coexist with small cell carcinoma, and is unrelated to neuroendocrine differentiation of CIS. In such cases, the pleomorphism is usually minimal; the cytoplasm is scant; and nuclei are enlarged and hyperchromatic, with coarse, unevenly distributed chromatin (**Figs. 7-13 and 7-14**). The scattered prominent nucleoli are distorted and angulated. Recognition of the small cell pattern of CIS is important to avoid misdiagnosis of basal cell hyperplasia, which has been observed in patients treated with bacillus Calmette–Guérin (BCG). These show a small cell pattern but lack nuclear atypia or loss of polarity.

Denuding and "Clinging Pattern" Carcinoma in Situ

In some cases, the neoplastic urothelial cells are strikingly discohesive and undergo extensive exfoliation, with the result that biopsies may show only a few residual

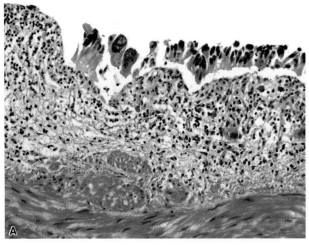

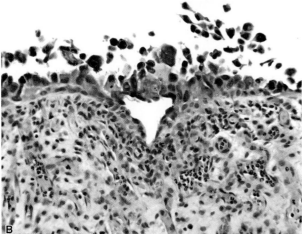

Figure 7-12 Urothelial carcinoma in situ (CIS) with pleomorphic giant cells ("giant cell" CIS) (A and B). Bizarre hyperchromatic cells of CIS separating from the basement membrane; note the underlying chronic cystitis (A).

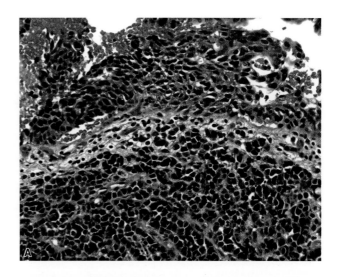

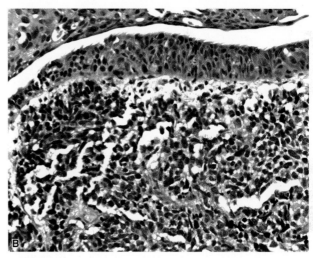

Figure 7-13 Urothelial carcinoma in situ (A and B), small cell variant.

carcinoma cells on the surface ("clinging CIS") or no recognizable epithelial cells on the surface (denuding cystitis) (**Figs. 7-15** and **7-16**).[58] In the clinging pattern of CIS, there is a patchy, usually single layer of atypical cells (**Figs. 7-17** and **7-18**). In mucosal biopsies entirely lacking surface epithelium, CIS may be present only in von Brunn nests. A careful search for CIS in deeper sections or in other submitted biopsy fragments is important, and a recommendation for evaluation of urine cytology for carcinoma cells is warranted.

Pagetoid and Undermining (Lepidic) Carcinoma in Situ

Another pattern of CIS, also referred to as cancerization of the urothelium, shows either pagetoid spread (clusters or isolated single cells) (**Figs. 7-19** and **7-20**) or undermining or overriding of the normal urothelium (lepidic growth)

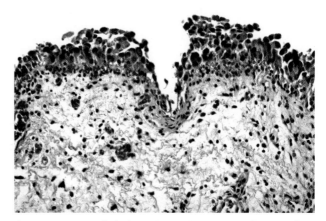

Figure 7-14 Urothelial carcinoma in situ (A and B), small cell variant.

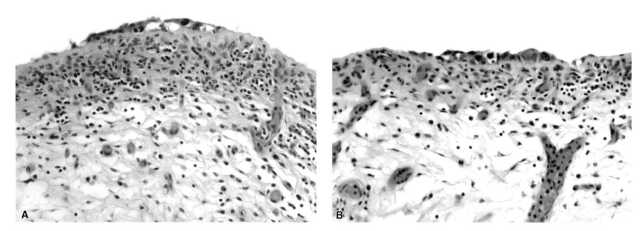

Figure 7-15   Urothelial carcinoma in situ (A and B), denuding variant.

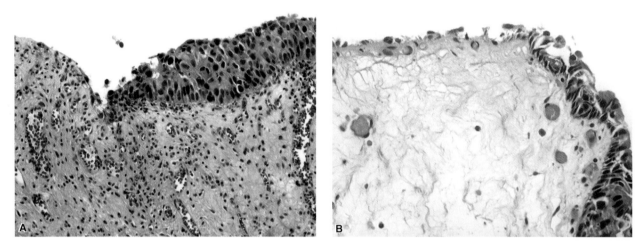

Figure 7-16   Urothelial carcinoma in situ (A and B). Partially denuded urothelium; the remainder is lined by cells with marked cytologic abnormalities.

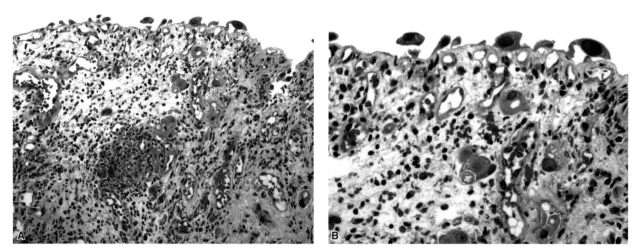

Figure 7-17   Urothelial carcinoma in situ (A and B), denuding and clinging variant. Note the single cell invasion of the lamina propria by carcinoma in situ.

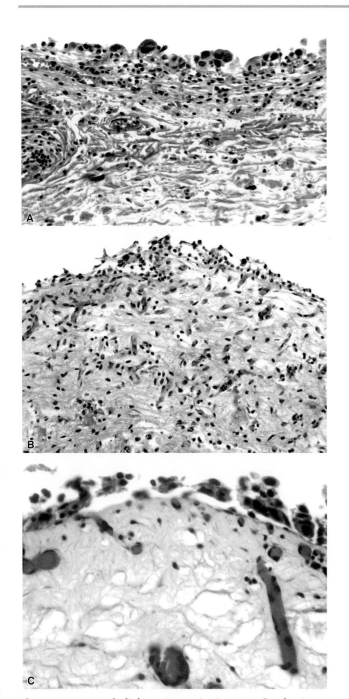

Figure 7-18 Urothelial carcinoma in situ (A to C), clinging variant.

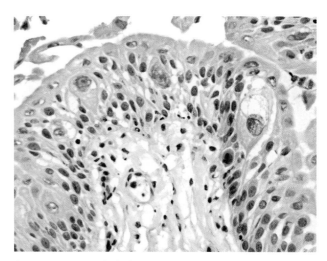

Figure 7-19 Urothelial carcinoma in situ, pagetoid spread.

(**Figs. 7-21** and **7-22**).[15,57] CIS exhibiting pagetoid growth is characterized by large single cells or small clusters of cells within otherwise normal urothelium of ureter, urethra, prostatic ducts, or in areas of squamous metaplasia. Individual cells showing pagetoid spread have enlarged nuclei with coarse chromatin; frequently, the cytoplasm is clear.

Pagetoid growth patterns can be found in up to 15% of CIS cases.[15] Most patients are male and their ages range from 31 to 78 years (mean, 64 years).[15,57] Pagetoid CIS is usually a focal lesion and is easily overlooked. It occurs in a clinical and histological setting of conventional CIS with coexisting invasive urothelial carcinoma; such patients essentially have the same progression and survival rates as patients without pagetoid changes. In cases with extensive urothelial denudation, pagetoid CIS may be focally present in adjacent, otherwise normal-looking urothelium, thus alerting the surgical pathologist to search for additional CIS elsewhere in the bladder.

Since primary extramammary Paget disease of the external genitalia and of the anal canal may extend to the bladder, and conversely, some cases of pagetoid CIS of the bladder may extend to the urethra, ureter, and external genitalia, differentiating between these two entities represents an important diagnostic and therapeutic challenge. A panel of immunostains, including cytokeratin (CK) 7, CK20, and thrombomodulin, may assist in differentiating pagetoid urothelial CIS from extramammary Paget disease, which is known to be CK7 positive and CK20 negative.[15,57]

Carcinoma in Situ with Squamous or Glandular Differentiation

Rare cases of CIS may exhibit squamous differentiation characterized by intercellular bridges (**Fig. 7-23**). CIS with squamous features is most often observed in association with urothelial carcinoma, showing extensive squamous differentiation elsewhere in the bladder.

A much less frequently encountered pattern is CIS with morphological and immunohistochemical (IHC) evidence of glandular differentiation (**Fig. 7-24**). Some authors refer to this as adenocarcinoma in situ; such lesions may show papillary, cribriform, or flat morphology. CIS involving cystitis glandularis (**Fig. 7-25**), cystitis cystica (**Fig. 7-26**), or von Brunn nests (**Figs. 7-27** and **7-28**) may be difficult

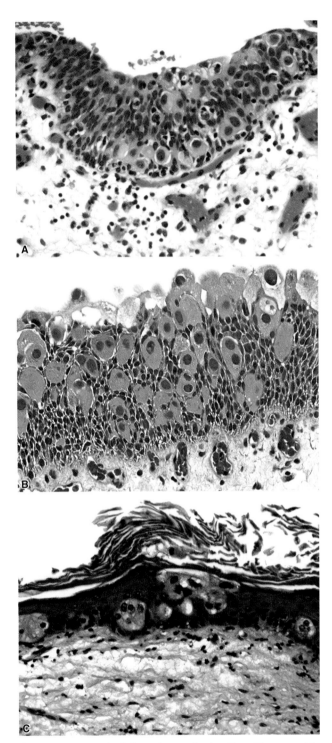

Figure 7-20 Urothelial carcinoma in situ (A to C), pagetoid spread.

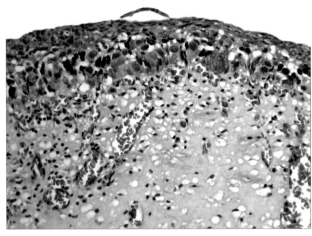

Figure 7-21 Urothelial carcinoma in situ with lepidic growth.

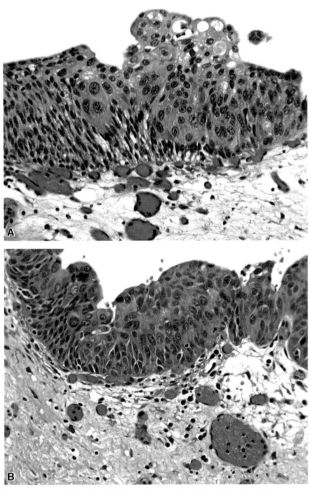

Figure 7-22 Urothelial carcinoma in situ with lepidic growth (A and B).

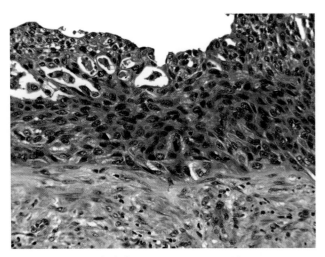

Figure 7-23 Urothelial carcinoma in situ with squamous differentiation.

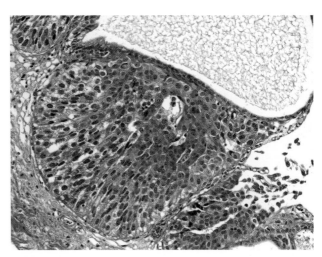

Figure 7-26 Urothelial carcinoma in situ involving cystitis cystica.

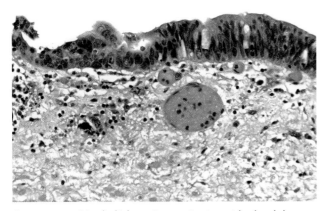

Figure 7-24 Urothelial carcinoma in situ with glandular differentiation. Note the presence of goblet cells.

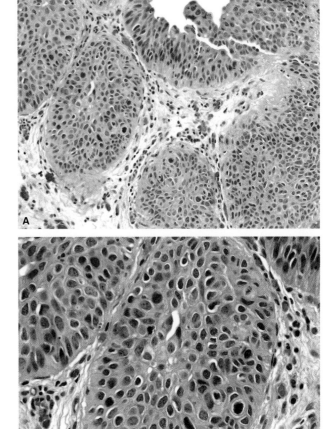

Figure 7-27 Urothelial carcinoma in situ involving von Brunn nests (A and B).

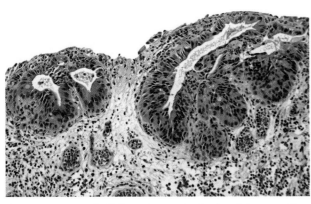

Figure 7-25 Urothelial carcinoma in situ involving cystitis glandularis.

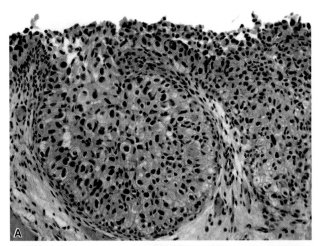

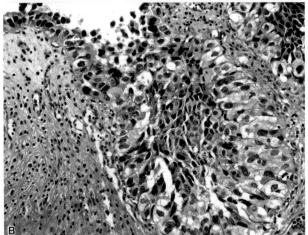

Figure 7-28 Urothelial carcinoma in situ involving von Brunn nests (A and B).

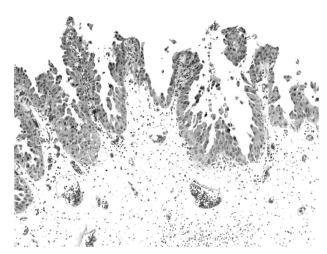

Figure 7-29 Urothelial carcinoma in situ, micropapillary variant.

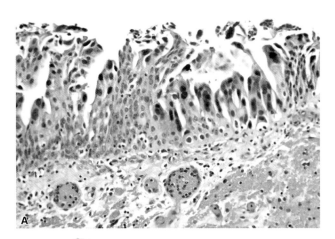

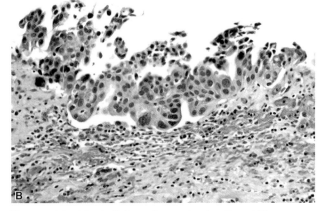

Figure 7-30 Urothelial carcinoma in situ (A and B), micropapillary variant.

to distinguish from adenocarcinoma in situ in the absence of concurrent invasive adenocarcinoma.

We consider urothelial carcinoma in situ with glandular differentiation a rare variant of urothelial carcinoma in situ.[59] Some of the lesions have been reported as adenocarcinoma in situ of the bladder[60] or, more recently, as noninvasive urothelial carcinoma of the bladder with glandular differentiation.[61,62] None of the reported cases was associated with pure invasive adenocarcinoma or villous adenoma, or developed these lesions on followup.[59–62] Therefore, their status as a precursor for adenocarcinoma is questionable.

Carcinoma in Situ with Micropapillary Growth

Rarely, CIS may present with micropapillary growth. It does not necessarily indicate the presence of micropapillary variant of urothelial carcinoma (**Figs. 7-29** and **7-30**).

Carcinoma in Situ with Microinvasion

CIS with microinvasion was initially defined by Farrow and Utz as invasion into the lamina propria to a depth of 5 mm or less from the basement membrane.[44] In the original study by Farrow et al., cystectomy specimens with urothelial CIS were totally embedded.[25,26] Of the 70 cases studied, 24 contained microinvasion, and two patients died of cancer. A recent consensus conference suggested that cases with more than 20 cells measured from the stromal epithelial interface should be classified as fully invasive.[15] Microinvasion appears as a direct extension in cords (tentacular), single cells, or single cells and clusters of cells (**Figs. 7-31** and **7-32**).[15,57,63,64] The clusters of cells may have a retraction artifact that mimics vascular invasion. Stromal response may be present, but in most cases is absent. In cases with a prominent stromal inflammatory response, the invasive neoplastic cells may be interspersed among lymphocytes, making them inconspicuous. In these circumstances, IHC staining with antibodies against cytokeratins (such as AE1/AE3) exposes the

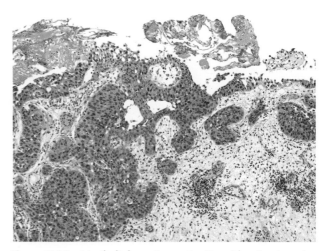

Figure 7-32 Urothelial carcinoma in situ with microinvasion and tentacular growth. It may be difficult to distinguish carcinoma in situ involving cystitis glandularis and von Brunn nests from true invasion. This tumor has finger-like projections in a desmoplastic stroma. Note the irregular-sized nests and loss of smooth contour of those nests.

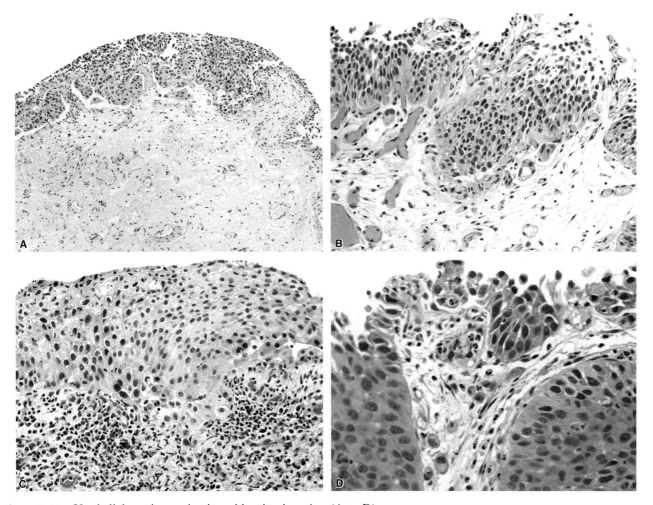

Figure 7-31 Urothelial carcinoma in situ with microinvasion (A to D).

Table 7-2 Major Differential Diagnosis of Urothelial Carcinoma in Situ

	Reactive Atypia	Hyperplasia	Dysplasia	Carcinoma in Situ
Cell layers	Variable	>7 cells	Variable	Variable
Polarization	Slightly abnormal	Normal	Slightly abnormal	Abnormal
Cytoplasm	Vacuolated	Homogeneous	Homogeneous	Homogeneous
Nuclear-to-cytoplasmic ratio	Normal or slightly increased	Normal or slightly increased	Slightly increased	Increased
Nuclei				
Anisonucleosis	Normal	Normal	Mild	Moderate to severe
Borders	Regular/smooth	Regular/smooth	Notches/creases	Pleomorphic
Chromatin	Fine/dusty	Fine	Slight hyperchromasia	Coarse/hyperchromatic
Chromatin distribution	Even	Even	Even	Uneven
Nucleoli	Large	Small/absent	Small/absent	Large/prominent
Mitotic figures	Variable	Absent	Variable to rare	Often
Denudation	Variable	No	No	Variable
Stromal microvascular proliferation	Variable	Variable	Less prominent	Prominent in some cases
Cytokeratin 20	Surface	Surface	Surface and deeper layers	Surface and deeper layers

invading cells. It is important to keep in mind that bladder lamina propria myofibroblasts can immunoreact with cytokeratin antibodies.

Differential Diagnosis

The main differential diagnoses include reactive atypia, flat urothelial hyperplasia, dysplasia, and therapy-induced changes (Table 7-2; see Chapters 2, 3, 6, and 24 for further discussion). Flat urothelial hyperplasia is characterized by an increase in the number of cell layers (usually, more than seven) without the hyperchromasia, nuclear membrane irregularities, or architectural disarray of carcinoma or CIS. There may be slight nuclear enlargement, but the nuclei of hyperplastic epithelium are of approximately uniform size. Flat urothelial hyperplasia is frequently seen in conjunction with low grade papillary urothelial tumors, as well as inflammatory disorders and lithiasis.[15,65]

Lesions classified as urothelial dysplasia are frequently observed in a context of known cancer diagnosis (secondary dysplasia) or in conjunction with a noninvasive papillary neoplasm. Nevertheless, dysplasia is also sometimes identified de novo (primary dysplasia) and has the potential to progress to neoplasia (see Chapter 6 for further discussion). Urothelial dysplasia includes a spectrum of cytologic and architectural abnormalities that do appear preneoplastic but are insufficient for the diagnosis of CIS.[23] There is nuclear enlargement and nucleolar prominence, nuclear membrane irregularity, and nuclear hyperchromasia. There may be nuclear crowding and architectural disturbance, including loss of polarity, but altogether to a lesser degree than those of unequivocal CIS. The cytologic abnormalities in urothelial dysplasia, characterized by cellular crowding, loss of orderly maturation, and loss of cellular polarity, are usually not present in the full thickness of the urothelium, although full-thickness involvement of abnormal cells is not required for the diagnosis of CIS.

In reactive atypia, nuclear abnormalities are less than those of dysplasia or CIS, and these changes occur in conjunction with mucosal inflammation.[3,15] Thus, the nuclear aberrations of reactive atypia can reasonably be attributed to urothelial repair or regeneration. These cells have enlarged vesicular nuclei, prominent nucleoli, and abundant cytoplasm, and their presence can often be correlated with a clinical setting of previous manipulation or irritation.

Therapy-related atypia may follow many of the therapeutic modalities currently used for bladder carcinoma, and drugs used for other cancers can cause therapy-related changes that confound the diagnosis of flat urothelial lesions like CIS.[15,66,67] Such cases may have markedly abnormal cytologic and histologic features in nonneoplastic urothelium. Thiotepa (triethylenethiophosphoramide) and mitomycin C, for example, may induce cell exfoliation and mucosal denudation, similar to denuding cystitis. After intravesical administration of these agents, umbrella cells become large, vacuolated, and multinucleated; prominent small nucleoli may be apparent within these enlarged nuclei. These findings may persist for weeks or months after discontinuation of treatment.

Several agents are given systemically to treat neoplastic and nonneoplastic disorders. Among these agents, cyclophosphamide is known to have severe effects on the bladder mucosa (Figs. 7-33 and 7-34; see also Chapter 24). Systematic cyclophosphamide treatment may induce reactivation of polyomavirus infection, causing marked nuclear atypia in the surface urothelium. In rare cases, polyomavirus (BK virus) infection mimics carcinoma in situ in immunocompromised patients.

Radiation therapy, similarly, causes urothelial cell enlargement, multinucleation, and vacuolization, with a normal nuclear-to-cytoplasmic ratio (Fig. 7-35).[57] Hemorrhage, fibrin deposition, and multinucleated stromal cells may create a tumor-like appearance in long-standing cases. There may even be nodules of squamoid epithelium pushing into the lamina propria without true infiltrative growth.[66,68]

Awareness of the therapy-induced changes noted above may assist the pathologist in avoiding a misdiagnosis of CIS. Unfortunately, the information needed is often not provided by the clinician when the diagnostic specimens are submitted for pathologic evaluation.

Diagnostic and Predictive Biomarkers

IHC staining may be useful in differentiating CIS from reactive changes in difficult biopsy cases (see Chapters 6 and 26 for further discussion). Normal urothelium typically exhibits CK20 staining in only the umbrella cell layer and p53 staining primarily in the basal layer.[11,27,57,69-71] A pattern of CK20 and p53 positivity throughout the neoplastic urothelium combined with negative staining for CD44 favors a diagnosis of CIS (Fig. 7-36).[57] The combination of triple staining with CK20, p53, and CD44 may be used to confirm cases of strongly favored CIS, primary CIS, or the less common patterns of undermining and pagetoid CIS (Fig. 7-37). In the reactive setting, the urothelium is often strongly positive for CD44 and lacks extensive staining for CK20 and p53. Mallofré and colleagues[72] reported similar findings utilizing CK20 and p53 immunostaining, and proposed Ki67 as a third "positive marker" in the neoplastic urothelium of CIS.

p53 is sometimes called "the guardian of the genome." p53 is a cell cycle control protein that acts at the transition of G1 to S-phase, preventing cells with DNA damage from progressing, either by inducing apoptosis or by delaying the S-phase until DNA repair is accomplished. Deletions and mutations of p53 are implicated in a variety of tumors, so it is not surprising that high grade lesions, including CIS, are also associated with p53 abnormalities.[5,73] Ick and colleagues[74] demonstrated that following BCG therapy, cases of recurrent CIS with persistent p53 staining have an ominous prognosis, with 75% progressing to muscle-invasive disease over 2 to 6 months. Using a PCR technique, Ecke and colleagues found *TP53* mutation to be an independent prognostic factor for poor progression-free survival in noninvasive bladder cancer. These authors suggest

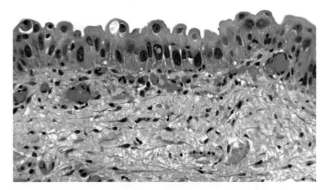

Figure 7-33 Cyclophophamide (cytoxan)-induced urothelial atypia, mimicking carcinoma in situ.

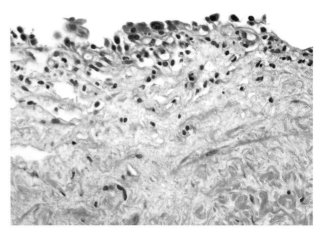

Figure 7-34 Cyclophophamide (cytoxan)-induced urothelial atypia, mimicking carcinoma in situ.

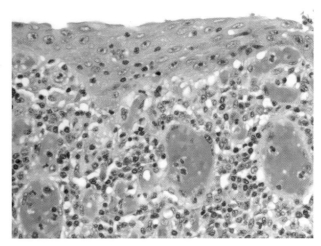

Figure 7-35 Radiation-induced urothelial atypia, mimicking carcinoma in situ.

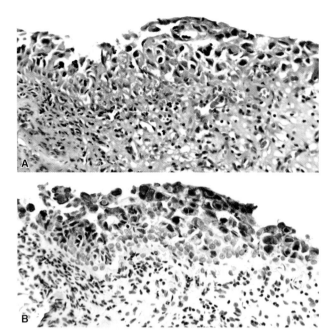

Figure 7-36   Urothelial carcinoma in situ (A and B). Aberrant expression of cytokeratin 20 (B). In normal urothelium, cytokeratin 20 expression is limited to superficial cells.

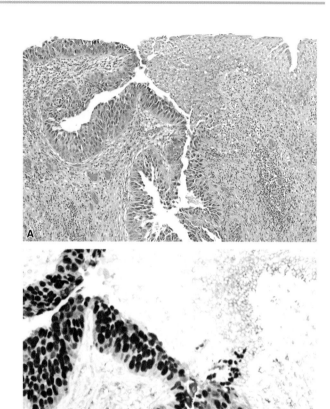

Figure 7-37   Urothelial carcinoma in situ (A and B). URO-3 triple stain (B): CD44 (blue) is cytoplasmic, p53 (brown) is nuclear, and cytokeratin 20 (red) is cytoplasmic.

that *TP53* mutation analysis may be useful for determining treatment options for patients with high grade lesions.[75] Although several authors have found similar adverse risk from p53 abnormalities, other studies have found negative results, leaving the overall predictive capacity of p53 somewhat controversial.[76,77]

Shariat et al. found that p21 positivity by IHC was associated with bladder cancer recurrence and progression in patients with CIS and without muscle-invasive disease. Furthermore positive p21 and p53 staining was associated with increased risk of recurrence, progression, and mortality. Negative staining for both was associated with the best outcome. In cases where p53 was positive and p21 was negative, the difference in outcome compared to double-negative patients was minimal and not statistically significant. This observation led the authors to propose an abrogating effect of normal p21 on the adverse effect of abnormal p53.[78]

Loss of E-cadherin IHC staining in CIS seems, in some studies, to correlate with increased likelihood of recurrence, progression, and bladder cancer–specific death. This suggests a role for E-cadherin annulment in tumor cells surmounting cell–cell adhesion to develop invasion.[79] Sun and Herrera found that E-cadherin is strongly expressed in CIS and that loss occurs only with invasion. Moreover, the loss of E-cadherin staining appeared to be in direct proportion to the depth of the invasion.[80]

Prognosis

Primary Carcinoma in Situ

Although urothelial CIS is by definition a noninvasive lesion, it is, as discussed above, a precancerous lesion, with 20% to 83% of cases progressing to invasive carcinoma (**Fig. 7-38**).[45] There are relatively few studies of primary CIS (without concurrent or prior papillary tumor). In Cheng et al.'s 1999 study of 80 patients with primary CIS (mean followup 11 years), it was found that progression-free survival, cancer-specific survival, and all-cause survival were 54%, 72%, and 36%, respectively, at 15 years.[1] Similarly, in a study of 62 patients with CIS, Utz et al. found that 60% of those with CIS developed invasive carcinoma and 39% died of bladder carcinoma over a period of five years.[38] In Melamed's early study, patients with CIS progressed to invasion over a median period of 26 to 33 months.[8] Short-term outcome appears favorable after cystectomy. Only six patients

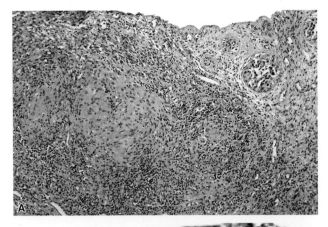

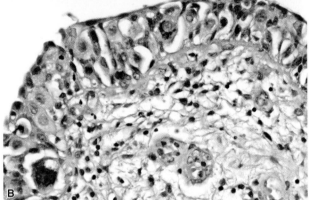

Figure 7-38 Recurrent urothelial carcinoma in situ. (A) There is prominent granulomatous inflammation resulting from BCG therapy, but the carcinoma in situ (B) is resistant.

(12%) developed metastatic disease among 52 patients with CIS only at cystectomy during a mean followup of 37 months.[17]

Carcinoma in Situ with Noninvasive Bladder Carcinoma

Cheng and colleagues found no significant difference in outcome between patients with isolated CIS and those with noninvasive papillary urothelial carcinoma (concurrent or prior) in addition to CIS.[1] This finding supports the hypothesis that CIS is a high grade lesion and the more worrisome of the two components. Examining the opposite relationship, a study by Shariat et al. demonstrated that concomitant CIS conferred a significant increase in risk of disease recurrence after cystectomy in patients with nonmuscle-invasive bladder cancer (<pT2 stage) in univariate analysis.[45] Similarly, bladder cancer-specific survival also decreased in the same population for patients with CIS (57%) compared to those without CIS (87.7%; $P = 0.0198$).[45]

Carcinoma in Situ with Invasive Bladder Carcinoma

In patients with organ confined, muscle-invasive bladder carcinoma (pT2), the increased risk of disease recurrence was maintained for patients with CIS in Shariat et al.'s study. However, the difference in bladder cancer-specific survival did not reach statistical significance between the groups with and without coexisting CIS. For patients with pT3 stage tumors or higher (nonorgan confined), the study found no significant difference in recurrence or survival related to concurrent CIS, suggesting that the invasive component has the greater impact on the overall prognosis.[45]

Multicentricity

In the 1999 Cheng et al. study, there was no significant difference between patients with three or more CIS foci and those with only a single focus identified (Fig. 7-39).[1] However, Takenaka and colleagues found that patients with "extensive" CIS had a lower progression-free survival than that of patients with "limited" CIS.[16] The distinction between extensive and limited disease was made on the basis of three or more positive biopsy sites out of six, although the number of sites biopsied was not uniform in this study. Other studies have found no significant differences between extensive and limited disease, similar to the Cheng et al. study. However, the discrepancy between results is interesting and warrants further investigation. An objective and formal system to determine the extent of disease would probably prove helpful for overall assessment of prognosis.[81,82]

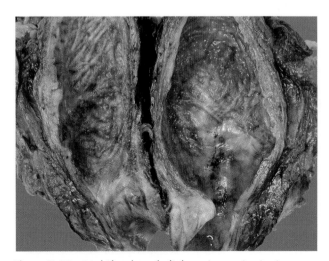

Figure 7-39 Multifocal urothelial carcinoma in situ in a gross specimen.

Upper Urinary Tract and Urethral Carcinoma in Situ Involvement

CIS is an established risk factor for recurrence in the upper urinary tract (UUT) in patients treated for superficial (Ta, Tis, and T1) bladder cancer. In patients treated with radical cystectomy for invasive urothelial carcinoma, however, there is controversy as to whether the CIS risk burden for UUT neoplasia persists.[83] In a series by Solsona et al., UUT recurrence after radical cystectomy was significantly higher in patients with CIS than those with muscle-invasive urothelial carcinoma.[84] However, other studies have found no association between the presence of bladder CIS and UUT recurrence.[83,85,86] These conflicting findings may be related to the longer overall survival of patients with CIS only, since these patients had a longer life span during which an upper UUT cancer might develop.[83] Similarly, some authors have suggested that primary bladder CIS may impart less risk of UUT neoplasia than secondary bladder CIS, whereas others have found no significant difference.[81,87]

Although intraoperative frozen section analysis is frequently performed to assess the ureteral margins at the time of cystectomy, the literature suggests that routine performance is unnecessary. UUT recurrence indeed appears higher in patients with involved margins, but concomitant ureteral CIS is uncommon. Postcystectomy ureteral CIS is infrequently associated with local morbidity, and significance of the implications for clinical outcome are not clear.[31,88,89]

In 1997, Tobisu et al. examined 52 patients who underwent radical cystoprostatectomy with simultaneous en bloc urethrectomy for bladder cancer.[90] This included 21 patients with diffuse primary CIS (with or without microscopic invasion). Of them, four (19%) had abnormalities of the anterior urethra, three with CIS in the bulbar urethra extending from the prostatic and membranous urethra, and one with severe dysplasia. Of the 10 patients with diffuse CIS in addition to nodular/papillary tumor, one had invasive urothelial carcinoma involving the corpus spongiosum of the penile urethra. These authors conclude that diffuse bladder CIS extending to the prostatic urethra is a risk factor for synchronous anterior urethra involvement.[90]

Molecular Characteristics

Noninvasive papillary tumors and CIS represent distinct entities with different frequencies of progression to invasive cancer (Fig. 7-40).[2,91,92] It is, therefore, fitting that they differ at the genetic level. In general, loss of heterozygosity (LOH) of chromosome 9 is reported more frequently in papillary tumors than in CIS, while the reverse is true for I gene mutation.[93,94] However, Hartmann et al. found that many cases of CIS (86%) had significant chromosome 9 abnormalities, calling this relationship into question. These investigators found that cases of moderate dysplasia were slightly less likely to exhibit chromosome 9 deletions (75%) than CIS or high grade dysplasia, supporting the notion that dysplasia is a precursor to CIS. In addition, they found by LOH studies and fluorescent in situ hybridization (FISH) that deletions of 17p13.1 at the *TP53* locus were present in 84% of CIS cases and 53% of dysplasia cases,

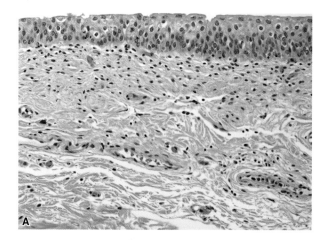

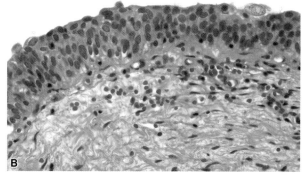

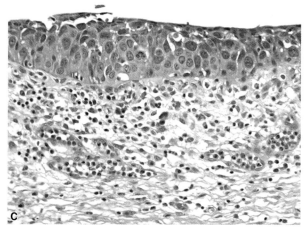

Figure 7-40 Morphologic progression from urothelial dysplasia to urothelial carcinoma in situ. (A) Normal urothelium; (B) urothelial dysplasia; (C) urothelial carcinoma in situ.

reinforcing the association between *TP53* abnormalities and high grade lesions.[95]

Hopman et al. propose that molecular differences exist between primary CIS (termed "isolated") and secondary CIS (associated with a papillary tumor). In their study, chromosome 9 deletions were not present in cases of primary CIS and were frequently present in secondary CIS. This finding supports the hypothesis that *TP53* mutations precede chromosome 9 aberrations in the progression from CIS to invasive cancer.[96] In contrast, the Hartmann study did not identify differences between primary and secondary CIS, perhaps due to the limited total number of cases, a majority of which included concurrent papillary tumors.[95] Zieger et al. have recently elucidated this issue further. They demonstrated gains of chromosome 5p only in CIS, whereas fibroblast growth factor receptor 3 (*FGFR3*) mutations were identified only in papillary tumors. These findings suggest that noninvasive papillary- and CIS-type tumors originate along different pathways, merging in some cases with disease progression, as CIS eventually develops in some patients with papillary tumors. (see **Chapters 6, 29**, and **34** for further discussion). This proposed mechanistic pathway is also compatible with the findings of overlap between chromosome 9 and *TP53* abnormalities in CIS by some investigators.[97]

Dyrskjøt and colleagues recently identified a multigene molecular classifier for CIS using microarray analysis, comparing CIS lesions to normal urothelium, papillary tumors with and without associated CIS, and invasive tumors.[98] Interestingly, the group found that in CIS cases with associated papillary tumors, the CIS lesions demonstrated similar expression patterns to both the concurrent papillary tumors and the adjacent normal urothelium. This pattern of similar molecular findings, even in adjacent normal urothelium, would support the "field effect" theory of bladder carcinogenesis. In papillary lesions without concurrent CIS, the expression profile was notably different between these primary papillary tumors and the usual CIS profile.[98] Contrary to the common hypothesis that invasive tumors typically arise from CIS-type lesions, however, the group found a distinct characteristic profile for invasive carcinoma. In a large-scale validation, a 68-gene signature had 80% sensitivity (36 of 45 samples) and 68% specificity (71 of 105) for CIS.[98,99] Together, these findings suggest that such molecular techniques may provide an accurate prediction of CIS presence even when CIS itself is not seen in the tissue biopsy

CIS typically does not express normal A, B, and O (H) blood group isoantigens.[100] Conversely, carcinoembryonic antigen, usually absent in normal urothelium, is frequently found in the cells of CIS. DNA ploidy studies by flow cytometry and image analysis reveal a high frequency of aneuploidy.[101–103]

REFERENCES

1. Cheng L, Cheville JC, Leibovich BC, Weaver AL, Egan KS, Spotts BE, Neumann RM, Bostwick DG. Survival of patients with carcinoma in situ of the urinary bladder. *Cancer* 1999;85:2469–74.

2. Cheng L, Davidson DD, Maclennan GT, Williamson SR, Zhang S, Koch MO, Montironi R, Lopez-Beltran A. The origins of urothelial carcinoma. *Expert Rev Anticancer Ther* 2010;10:865–80.

3. Cheng L, Lopez-Beltran A, MacLennan GT, Montironi R, Bostwick DG. Neoplasms of the urinary bladder. In: Bostwick DG, Cheng L, eds. Urologic Surgical Pathology, 2nd ed. Philadelphia: Elsevier/Mosby, 2008;259–352.

4. Edge SB, Byrd DR, Compton CC, Fritz AG, Greene FL, Trotti A. American Joint Committee on Cancer Staging Manual, 7th ed. New York: Springer, 2010.

5. Cheng L, Zhang S, Maclennan GT, Williamson SR, Lopez-Beltran A, Montironi R. Bladder cancer: translating molecular genetic insights into clinical practice. *Hum Pathol* 2011;42:455–81.

6. Melicow M. Histological study of vesical urothelium intervening between gross neoplasms in total cytectomy. *J Urol* 1952;68:261–79.

7. Melicow M, Hollowell J. Intra-urothelial cancer: carcinoma in situ, Nowens's disease of the urinary system: discussion of thirty cases. *J Urol* 1952;68:763–72.

8. Melamed M, Voutsa N, Grabstald H. Natural history and clinical behavior of in situ carcinoma of the human urinary bladder. *Cancer* 1964;17:1533–45.

9. Cheng L, Montironi R, Davidson DD, Lopez-Beltran A. Staging and reporting of urothelial carcinoma of the urinary bladder. *Mod Pathol* 2009;22 (Suppl 2):S70–95.

10. Bostwick DG, Ramnani D, Cheng L. Diagnosis and grading of bladder cancer and associated lesions. *Urol Clin North Am* 1999;26:493–507.

11. Williamson SR, Montironi R, Lopez-Beltran A, MacLennan GT, Davidson DD, Cheng L. Diagnosis, evaluation and treatment of carcinoma in situ of the urinary bladder: the state of the art. *Crit Rev Oncol Hematol* 2010;76:112–26.

12. Hodges KB, Lopez-Beltran A, Davidson DD, Montironi R, Cheng L. Urothelial dysplasia and other flat lesions of the urinary bladder: clinicopathologic and molecular features. *Hum Pathol* 2010;41:155–62.

13. Montironi R, Lopez-Beltran A, Scarpelli M, Mazzucchelli R, Cheng L. 2004 World Health Organization classification of the noninvasive urothelial neoplasms: Inherent problems and clinical reflections. *Eur Urol* 2009;Suppl 8:453–57.

14. Montironi R, Mazzucchelli R, Scarpelli M, Lopez-Beltran A, Cheng L. Morphological diagnosis of urothelial neoplasms. *J Clin Pathol* 2008;61:3–10.

15. Lopez-Beltran A, Cheng L, Andersson L, Brausi M, de Matteis A, Montironi R, Sesterhenn I, van det Kwast KT, Mazerolles C. Preneoplastic non-papillary lesions and conditions of the urinary bladder: an update based on the Ancona International Consultation. *Virchows Arch* 2002;440:3–11.

16. Takenaka A, Yamada Y, Miyake H, Hara I, Fujisawa M. Clinical outcomes of bacillus Calmette-Guérin instillation therapy for carcinoma in situ of urinary bladder. *Int J Urol* 2008;15:309–13.

17. Hassan JM, Cookson MS, Smith JA Jr, Johnson DL, Chang SS. Outcomes in patients with pathological carcinoma in situ only disease at radical cystectomy. *J Urol* 2004;172:882–4.

18. Althausen A, Prout G, Daly J. Non-invasive papillary carcinoma of the bladder associated with carcinoma in situ. *J Urol* 1976;116:575–80.

19. Altaffer LF 3rd, Wilkerson SY, Jordan GH, Lynch DF. Malignant inverted papilloma and carcinoma in situ of the bladder. *J Urol* 1982;128:816–8.

20. Brawn PN. The origin of invasive carcinoma of the bladder. *Cancer* 1982;50:515–9.

21. Prout G, Griffin P, Daly J, Heney N. carcinoma in situ of the urinary bladder with and without association vesical neoplasms. *Cancer* 1983;52:524–32.

22. Vicente J, Laguna MP, Duarte D, Algaba F, Chechile G. Carcinoma in situ as a prognostic factor for G3pT1 bladder tumours. *Br J Urol* 1991;68:380–2.

23. Cheng L, Cheville JC, Neumann RM, Bostwick DG. Natural history of urothelial dysplasia of the bladder. *Am J Surg Pathol* 1999;23:443–7.

24. Farrow GM, Barlebo H, Enjoji M, Chisholm G, Friedell GH, Jackse G, Kakizoe T, Koss LG, Kotake T, Vanlensieck W. Transitional cell carcinoma in situ. *Prog Clin Biol Res* 1986;221:85–96.

25. Farrow G, Utz D, Rife C. Morphological and clinical observations of patients with early bladder cancer treated with total cystectomy. *Cancer Res* 1976;36:2495–501.

26. Farrow G, Utz D, Rife C, Greene L. Clinical observations on sixty-nine cases of in situ carcinoma of the urinary bladder. *Cancer Res* 1977;37:2794–8.

27. Hodges KB, Lopez-Beltran A, Davidson DD, Montironi R, Cheng L. Urothelial dysplasia and other flat lesions of the urinary bladder: clinicopathologic and molecular features. *Hum Pathol* 2010;41:155–62.

28. Hudson MA, Herr HW. Carcinoma in situ of the bladder. *J Uro* 1995;153:564–72.

29. Zincke H, Utz D, Farrow G. Review of Mayo Clinic experience with carcinoma in situ. *Urology* 1985;26:39–46.

30. Wolf H, Melsen F, Pedersen SE, Nielsen KT. Natural history of carcinoma in situ of the urinary bladder. *Scand J Urol Nephrol Suppl* 1994;157:147–51.

31. Batista J, Palou J, Iglesias J, Sanchotene E, Da Luz P, Algaba F, Villavicencio H. Significance of urethral carcinoma in situ in speciments of cystectomy. *Eur Urol* 1994;25:313–5.

32. Khan AU, Farrow GM, Zincke H, Utz DC, Greene LF. Primary carcinoma in situ of the ureter and renal pelvis. *J Urol* 1979;121:681–3.

33. Koss LG, Tiamson EM, Robbins MA. Mapping cancerous and precancerous bladder changes. A study of the urothelium in ten surgically removed bladders. *JAMA* 1974;227:281–6.

34. Mahadevia PS, Koss LG, Tar IJ. Prostatic involvement in bladder cancer. Prostate mapping in 20 cystoprostatectomy specimens. *Cancer* 1986;58:2096–102.

35. Daly JJ. Carcinoma-in-situ of the urothelium. *Urol Clin North Am* 1976;3:87–105.

36. Utz D, Hanash K, Farrow G. The plight of the patient with carcinoma in situ of the bladder. *J Urol* 1970;103:160–4.

37. Utz D, Farrow G. Management of carcinoma in situ of the bladder: the case for surgical management. *Urol Clin North Am* 1980;7:533–41.

38. Utz D, Farrow G. Carinoma in situ of the urinary tract. *Urol Clin North Am* 1984;11:735–40.

39. Dean PJ, Murphy WM. Carcinoma in situ and dysplasia of the bladder urothelium. *World J Urol* 1987;5:103–7.

40. Hudson MA, Herr HW. Carcinoma in situ of the bladder. *J Urol* 1995;153:564–72.

41. Chade DC, Shariat SF, Godoy G, Savage CJ, Cronin AM, Bochner BH, Donat SM, Herr HW, Dalbagni G. Clinical outcomes of primary bladder carcinoma in situ in a contemporary series. *J Urol* 2010;184:74–80.

42. Chade DC, Shariat SF, Adamy A, Bochner BH, Donat SM, Herr HW, Dalbagni G. Clinical outcome of primary versus secondary bladder carcinoma in situ. *J Urol* 2010;184:464–9.

43. Tilki D, Reich O, Svatek RS, Karakiewicz PI, Kassouf W, Novara G, Ficarra V, Chade DC, Fritsche HM, Gerwens N, Izawa JI, Lerner SP, Schoenberg M, Stief CG, Skinner E, Lotan Y, Sagalowsky AI, Shariat SF. Characteristics and outcomes of patients with clinical carcinoma in situ only treated with radical cystectomy: an international study of 243 patients. *J Urol* 2010;183:1757–63.

44. Farrow GM, Utz DC. Observation on microinvasive transitional cell carcinoma of the urinary bladder. *Clin Oncol* 1982;1:609–15.

45. Shariat SF, Palapattu GS, Karakiewicz PI, Rogers CG, Vazina A, Bastian PJ, Schoenberg MP, Lerner SP, Sagalowsky AI, Lotan Y. Concomitant carcinoma in situ is a feature of aggressive disease in patients with organ-confined TCC at radical cystectomy. *Eur Urol* 2007;51:152–60.

46. Bostwick DG, Ramnani DM, Cheng L. Diagnosis and grading of bladder cancer and associated lesions. *Urol Clin North Am* 1999;26:493–507.

47. Cheng L, Cheville JC, Neumann RM, Leibovich BC, Egan KS, Spotts BE, Bostwick DG. Survival of patients with carcinoma in situ of the urinary bladder. *Cancer* 1999;85:2469–74.

48. Farrow G. Pathology of carcinoma in situ of the urinary bladder and related lesions. *J Cell Biochem* 1992;161:39–43.

49. Orozco R, Martin A, Murphy W. Carcinoma in situ of the urinary bladder: clues to host involvement in human carcinogenesis. *Cancer* 1994;74:115–22.

50. Cifuentes Delatte L, Oliva H, Navarro V. Intraepithelial carcinoma of the bladder. *Urol Int* 1970;25:169–86.

51. Okaneya T, Ikado S, Ogawa A. [The progress pattern of carcinoma in situ of the urinary bladder]. *Nippon Hinyokika Gakkai Zasshi* 1991;82:1227–32.

52. Patel SG, Cookson MS, Barocas DA, Clark PE, Smith JAJ, Chang SS. Risk factors for urothelial carcinoma of the prostate in patients undergoing radical cystoprostatectomy for bladder cancer. *BJU Int* 2009;104:934–7.

53. Elliott GB, Moloney PJ, Anderson GH. "Denuding cystitis" and in situ urothelial carcinoma. *Arch Pathol* 1973;96:91–4.

54. Begin LR, Deschenes J, Mitmaker B. Pagetoid carcinomatous involvement of the penile urethra in association with high grade transitional cell carcinoma of the urinary bladder. *Arch Pathol Lab Med* 1991;115:632–5.

55. Orozco R, Vander Zwaag R, Murphy W. The pagetoid variant of urothelial carcinoma in situ. *Hum Pathol* 1993;24:1199–1202.

56. Jendresen M, Kvist E, Beck B. Paget's disease in a squamous metaplasia of the urinary bladder. The first published case of a disease which is usually found in the epidermis. *Scand J Urol Nephrol* 1994;28:327–9.

57. McKenney JK, Gomez JA, Desai S, Lee MW, Amin MB. Morphologic expressions of urothelial carcinoma in situ: a detailed evaluation of its histologic patterns with emphasis on carcinoma in situ with microinvasion. *Am J Surg Pathol* 2001;25:356–62.

58. Owens CL, Epstein JI. Significance of denuded urothelium in papillary urothelial lesions. *Am J Surg Pathol* 2007;31:298–303.

59. Lopez-Beltran A, Jimenez RE, Montironi R, Patriarca C, Blanca A, Menendez C, Algaba F, Cheng L. Flat urothelial carcinoma in situ of the bladder with glandular differentiation. *Hum Pathol* 2011;42:1653–9.

60. Chan TY, Epstein JI. In situ adenocarcinoma of the bladder. *Am J Surg Pathol* 2001;25:892–9.

61. Miller JS, Epstein JI. Noninvasive urothelial carcinoma of the bladder with glandular differentiation: report of 24 cases. *Am J Surg Pathol* 2009;33:1241–8.

62. Lim M, Adsay NV, Grignon D, Osunkoya AO. Urothelial carcinoma with villoglandular differentiation: a study of 14 cases. *Mod Pathol* 2009;22:1280–6.

63. Lopez-Beltran A, Cheng L. Stage pT1 bladder carcinoma: diagnostic criteria, pitfalls and prognostic significance. *Pathology* 2003;35:484–91.

64. Benson RC Jr, Farrow GM, Kinsey JH, Cortese DA, Zincke H, Utz DC. Detection and localization of In situ carcinoma of the bladder with hematoporphyrin derivative. *Mayo Clin Proc* 1982;57:548–55.

65. van Oers JM, Adam C, Denzinger S, Stoehr R, Bertz S, Zaak D, Stief C, Hofstaedter F, Zwarthoff EC, van der Kwast TH, Knuechel R, Hartmann A. Chromosome 9 deletions are more frequent than FGFR3 mutations in flat urothelial hyperplasias of the bladder. *Int J Cancer* 2006;119:1212–5.

66. Chan TY, Epstein JI. Radiation or chemotherapy cystitis with "pseudocarcinomatous" features. *Am J Surg Pathol* 2004;28:909–13.

67. Lopez-Beltran A. Bladder treatment. Immunotherapy and chemotherapy. *Urol Clin North Am* 1999;26:535–54.

68. Lopez-Beltran A, Luque RJ, Mazzucchelli R, Scarpelli M, Montironi R. Changes produced in the urothelium by traditional and newer therapeutic procedures for bladder cancer. *J Clin Pathol* 2002;55:641–7.

69. Hodges KB, Lopez-Beltran A, Emerson RE, Montironi R, Cheng L. Clinical utility of immunohistochemistry in the diagnoses of urinary bladder neoplasia. *Appl Immunohistochem Mol Morphol* 2010;18:401–10.

70. Emerson RE, Cheng L. Immunohistochemical markers in the evaluation of tumors of the urinary bladder: a review. *Anal Quant Cytol Histol* 2005;27:301–16.

71. Harnden P, Eardley I, Joyce AD, Southgate J. Cytokeratin 20 as an objective marker of urothelial dysplasia. *Br J Urol* 1996;78:870–5.

72. Mallofré C, Castillo M, Morente V, Sole M. Immunohistochemical expression of CK20, p53, and Ki–67 as objective markers of urothelial dysplasia. *Mod Pathol* 2003;16:187–91.

73. Schrier BP, Vriesema JL, Witjes JA, Kiemeney LA, Schalken JA. The predictive value of p53, p27(Kip1), and alpha-catenin for progression in superficial bladder carcinoma. *Eur Urol* 2006;50:76–82.

74. Ick K, Schultz M, Stout P, Fan K. Significance of p53 overexpression in urinary bladder transitional cell carcinoma in situ before and after bacillus Calmette-Guérin treatment. *Urology* 1997;49:541–6; discussion 546–7.

75. Ecke TH, Sachs MD, Lenk SV, Loening SA, Schlechte HH. TP53 gene mutations as an independent marker for urinary bladder cancer progression. *Int J Mol Med* 2008;21:655–61.

76. Salinas-Sanchez AS, Lorenzo-Romero JG, Gimenez-Bachs JM, Sanchez-Sanchez F, Donate-Moreno MJ, Rubio-Del-Campo A, Hernandez-Millan IR, Segura-Martin M, Atienzar-Tobarra M, Escribano-Martinez J. Implications of p53 gene mutations on patient survival in transitional cell carcinoma of the bladder: a long-term study. *Urol Oncol* 2008;26:620–6.

77. Gonzalez S, Aubert S, Kerdraon O, Haddad O, Fantoni JC, Biserte J, Leroy X. Prognostic value of combined p53 and survivin in pT1G3 urothelial carcinoma of the bladder. *Am J Clin Pathol* 2008;129:232–7.

78. Shariat SF, Kim J, Raptidis G, Ayala GE, Lerner SP. Association of p53 and p21 expression with clinical outcome in patients with carcinoma in situ of the urinary bladder. *Urology* 2003;61:1140–5.

79. Shariat SF, Pahlavan S, Baseman AG, Brown RM, Green AE, Wheeler TM, Lerner SP. E-cadherin expression predicts clinical outcome in carcinoma in situ of the urinary bladder. *Urology* 2001;57:60–5.

80. Sun W, Herrera GA. E-cadherin expression in urothelial carcinoma in situ, superficial papillary transitional cell carcinoma, and invasive transitional cell carcinoma. *Hum Pathol* 2002;33:996–1000.

81. Van Gils-Gielen R, Witjes W, Caris C, Debruyne F, Witjes J, Oosterhof G. Risk factors in carcinoma in situ of the urinary bladder. *Urol* 1995;45:581–6.

82. Terakawa T, Miyake H, Muramaki M, Takenaka A, Hara I, Fujisawa M. Risk factors for intravesical recurrence after surgical management of transitional cell carcinoma of the upper urinary tract. *Urology* 2008;71:123–7.

83. Sanderson KM, Cai J, Miranda G, Skinner DG, Stein JP. Upper tract urothelial recurrence following radical cystectomy for transitional cell carcinoma of the bladder: an analysis of 1,069 patients with 10-year followup. *J Urol* 2007;177:2088–94.

84. Solsona E, Iborra I, Ricos J, Dumont R, Casanova J, Calabuig C. Upper urinary tract involvement in patients with bladder carcinoma in situ (Tis): its impact on management. *Urol* 1997;49:347–52.

85. Kenworthy P, Tanguay S, Dinney CP. The risk of upper tract recurrence following cystectomy in patients with transitional cell carcinoma involving the distal ureter. *J Urol* 1996;155:501–3.

86. Balaji KC, McGuire M, Grotas J, Grimaldi G, Russo P. Upper tract recurrences following radical cystectomy: an analysis of prognostic factors, recurrence pattern and stage at presentation. *J Urol* 1999;162:1603–6.

87. Talic RF, Hargreave TB, Bishop MC, Kirk D, Prescott S. Intravesical Evans bacille Calmette-Guérin for carcinoma in situ of the urinary bladder. Scottish Urological Oncology Group. *Br J Urol* 1994;73:645–8.

88. Raj GV, Tal R, Vickers A, Bochner BH, Serio A, Donat SM, Herr H, Olgac S, Dalbagni G. Significance of intraoperative ureteral evaluation at radical cystectomy for urothelial cancer. *Cancer* 2006;107:2167–72.

89. Silver D, Stroumbakis N, Russo P, Fair W, Herr H. Ureteral carcinoma in situ at radical cystectomy: Does the margin matter? *J Urol* 1997;158:768–71.

90. Tobisu K, Kanai Y, Sakamoto M, Fujimoto H, Doi N, Horie S, Kakizoe T. Involvement of the anterior urethra in male patients with transitional cell-carcinoma of the bladder undergoing radical cystectomy with simultaneous urethrectomy. *Jpn J Clin Oncol* 1997;27:406–9.

91. Cheng L, Zhang D. Molecular Genetic Pathology. New York: Humana Press/Springer, 2008.

92. Cheng L, Zhang S, Maclennan GT, Williamson SR, Lopez-Beltran A, Montironi R. Bladder cancer: translating molecular genetic insights into clinical practice. *Hum Pathol* 2011;42:455–81.

93. Spruck CH 3rd, Ohneseit PF, Gonzalez-Zulueta M, Esrig D, Miyao N, Tsai YC, Lerner SP, Schmutte C, Yang AS, Cote R, et al. Two molecular pathways to transitional cell carcinoma of the bladder. *Cancer Res* 1994;54:784–8.

94. Cheng L, Zhang S, Davidson DD, MacLennan GT, Koch MO, Montironi R, Lopez-Beltran A. Molecular determinants of tumor recurrence in the urinary bladder. *Future Oncol* 2009;5:843–57.

95. Hartmann A, Schlake G, Zaak D, Hungerhuber E, Hofstetter A, Hofstaedter F, Knuechel R. Occurrence of chromosome 9 and p53 alterations in multifocal dysplasia and carcinoma in situ of human urinary bladder. *Cancer Res* 2002;62:809–18.

96. Hopman AH, Kamps MA, Speel EJ, Schapers RF, Sauter G, Ramaekers FC. Identification of chromosome 9 alterations and p53 accumulation in isolated carcinoma in situ of the urinary bladder versus carcinoma in situ associated with carcinoma. *Am J Pathol* 2002;161:1119–25.

97. Zieger K, Marcussen N, Borre M, Orntoft TF, Dyrskjot L. Consistent genomic alterations in carcinoma in situ of the urinary bladder confirm the presence of two major pathways in bladder cancer development. *Int J Cancer* 2009;125:2095–103.

98. Dyrskjøt L, Kruhoffer M, Thykjaer T, Marcussen N, Jensen JL, Moller K, Orntoft TF. Gene expression in the urinary bladder: a common carcinoma in situ gene expression signature exists disregarding histopathological classification. *Cancer Res* 2004;64:4040–8.

99. Dyrskjøt L, Zieger K, Real FX, Malats N, Carrato A, Hurst C, Kotwal S, Knowles M, Malmstrom PU, de la Torre M, Wester K, Allory Y, et al. Gene expression signatures predict outcome in non-muscle-invasive bladder carcinoma: a multicenter validation study. *Clin Cancer Res* 2007;13:3545–51.

100. Coon JS, McCall A, Miller AW 3rd, Farrow GM, Weinstein RS. Expression of blood-group-related antigens in carcinoma in situ of the urinary bladder. *Cancer* 1985;56:797–804.

101. Norming U, Tribukait B, Gustafson H, Nyman C, Wang N, Wijkstrom H. Deoxyribonucleic acid profile and tumor progression in primary carcinoma in situ of the bladder: a study of 63 patients with grade 3 lesions. *J Urol* 1992;147:11–5.

102. Norming U, Tribukait B, Nyman CR, Nilsson B, Wang N. Prognostic significance of mucosal aneuploidy in stage Ta/T1 grade 3 carcinoma of the bladder. *J Urol* 1992;148:1420–7.

103. Tyrkus M, Powell I, Fakr W. Cytogenetic studies of carcinoma in situ of the bladder: prognostic implications. *J Urol* 1992;148:44–6.

Chapter 8

Bladder Cancer: General Features

Bladder Pathology, First Edition. Liang Cheng, Antonio Lopez-Beltran, David G. Bostwick.
© 2012 Wiley-Blackwell. Published 2012 by John Wiley & Sons, Inc.

Epidemiology and Risk Factors

Worldwide, bladder cancer is the seventh most common cancer.[1] An average of 386,300 new cases of urinary bladder cancer are diagnosed worldwide every year, accounting for 150,200 deaths.[1–6] In the United States, Canada, and the European Union, the urinary bladder is estimated to be the fourth leading site of new cancer diagnoses in men, following prostatic, pulmonary, and colorectal cancers.[1,2] Bladder cancer is morphologically heterogeneous; more than 90% of bladder cancer cases are urothelial (transitional cell) carcinoma, whereas primary squamous cell carcinoma, adenocarcinoma, small cell carcinoma, and other tumors are less common.[5,7–10]

Bladder cancer presents mainly as nonmuscle invasive disease, which has a high recurrence of 50% to 70% with low progression rate in 15% to 25% of the patients (**Fig. 8-1**). The high recurrence rate and low aggressiveness of these tumors have resulted in close followup of patients. In the United States, the Medicare expenditure on patients with bladder cancer was higher than that of other cancers. Such high costs are due, in part, to the high propensity for recurrence and progression of bladder tumor. Early detection and identification of precursor lesions may reduce costs and may eventually lead to decreased morbidity and mortality.[5,10]

There are significant variations in incidence, morbidity, and mortality rates of bladder cancer in different countries and ethnic groups.[5,10–15] The bladder cancer incidence is nearly twice as high in Caucasians than in African-Americans and has been increasing steadily for decades, but in some countries a decline has been observed recently. The mortality rate for bladder cancer is higher in female and African-American patients than in male and Caucasian patients. The higher mortality risk in African-American males and females is limited primarily to late-stage bladder cancer.[16] Mallin and colleagues recently analyzed a large cohort of bladder cancer patients diagnosed in 1993 to 2007 from the National Cancer Database.[16] There were 310,257 Caucasian male, 102,345 Caucasian female, 13,313 African-American male, and 7439 African-American female patients. The male-to-female ratio was 3:1. African-American and female patients had a higher proportion of muscle-invasive tumors than those of Caucasian and male patients, and African-American patients had a larger proportion of higher grade tumors. Notably, African-American patients, especially African-American females, had higher stage and higher grade cancer throughout the 15-year study period (1993–1997).[16] Five-year relative survival for all stages did not differ significantly between 1993 to 1997 and 1998 to 2002 in any race or gender group. Five-year survival rates were 58% for African-American female, 72% for

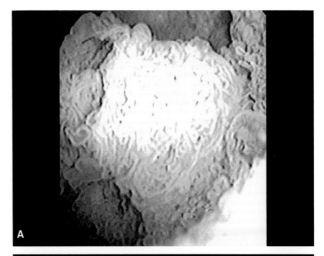

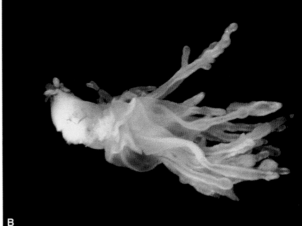

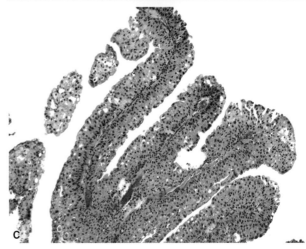

Figure 8-1 Early-stage bladder cancer (pTa). Cystoscopic (A), gross (B), and microscopic (C) appearance of papillary noninvasive urothelial carcinoma. (Photo courtesy of Dr. Koch.)

African-American male, 78% for Caucasian female, and 84% for Caucasian male patients during the 1998–2002 period.[16]

Bladder cancer in the United States occurs two to five times more frequently in men than in women. This has been attributed to different smoking habits and more prevalent occupational exposure in men than in women.[4,11–14,17,18] Although bladder cancer is more common in men, the incidence of bladder cancer in women is increasing.

Multiple risk factors have been linked to bladder cancer.[12,13,19] Exogenous factors such as tobacco smoking, occupational risk, and lifestyle exposure to carcinogens all play important roles. Smokers have two to four times the risk of urothelial cancer as that of the general population, and heavy smokers have five times the risk. Nevertheless, the specific urothelial carcinogens associated with smoking are still unknown. It is estimated that 20 years of smoking is needed for the development of bladder cancer, and the probability of this event is directly correlated with the lifetime number of cigarettes consumed. The relative risk of active smokers developing bladder cancer compared to never-smokers is 3 : 1, and for previous smokers it is 1.9 : 1. Although the exact mechanism by which tobacco causes bladder cancer is not known, many known carcinogens in cigarette smoke, such as acrolein, 4-aminobiphenyl, arylamine, and oxygen free radicals, have been implicated. Furthermore, increased duration, intensity of tobacco consumption, and degree of inhalation contribute significantly to cancer development.

The beneficial effects of smoking cessation, on the other hand, include an almost immediate decline in the risk of bladder cancer. Continued smokers have a poorer recurrence-free survival rate than that of those who quit at the time of diagnosis. Occupational exposure to aniline dyes and aromatic amines, such as 2-naphthylamine and benzidine, are the second most prevalent risk factors for bladder cancer. Benzidine, the most carcinogenic aromatic amine, is used in dye production and as a hardener in the rubber industry. The degree of carcinogenesis due to occupational exposure varies with the degree of industrialization, but in heavily industrialized nations, occupational exposure may account for up to one-fourth of all urothelial cancers. The latency period between exposure and tumor development is usually prolonged. Occupational bladder cancer has also been observed in gas workers, painters, and hairdressers. Nutrition may also play a role. Vitamin A supplementation apparently reduces the risk of bladder cancer, while fried food and fat ingestion cause a risk increase. A high fluid intake reduced the risk of bladder cancer in one study, but this remains controversial. Epidemiologic studies in Taiwan and Chile have shown an increased risk for urothelial cancer in people whose drinking water has a high arsenic content. Other water contaminants with putative toxic effects on urothelium are also being investigated actively.[12]

Additional factors implicated in the development and progression of bladder cancer include analgesic use; urinary tract infections, whether bacterial, parasitic, fungal, or viral; urinary lithiasis; pelvic radiation; and chemotherapeutic agents such as cyclophosphamide. Although caffeine ingestion has been implicated as a risk factor for bladder cancer, risk estimates for this association decrease after controlling for concomitant tobacco use. Similarly, saccharin-containing artificial sweeteners induce bladder neoplasia in rats, but human epidemiological studies have failed to establish this relationship. There is a relationship between the parasite *Bilharzia* (schistosomiasis) and squamous cell cancer in the bladder, more frequently seen in the Middle East, where the waterborne flatworms are endemic. A variety of other infectious conditions, including urinary tract infection, gonorrhea, syphilis, other bacteria, human papillomavirus, human immunodeficiency virus, herpes simplex virus, and BK, virus have been studied as potential risk factors for bladder carcinoma.[20]

In a meta-analysis of 30 epidemiologic studies, Zeegers et al.[13] found that alcohol consumption in men, when adjusted for cigarette smoking, confers a small increased risk compared to no alcohol consumption. This result, however, was not statistically significant. The same relationship in women was not demonstrated. Similarly, coffee consumption is heavily confounded by a frequent association with tobacco smoking, yet has been shown by some investigators to confer a slightly increased risk.

Analgesic use has also been implicated in bladder carcinogenesis, particularly with regard to phenacetin-containing compounds. This observation has raised concern over the use of acetaminophen (its metabolite) and nonsteroidal antiinflammatory drugs (NSAIDs). Conversely, some studies have found that NSAIDs, including acetaminophen, may be associated with decreased risk.

Malignancy developing in patients receiving bladder augmentation is a growing concern, and increasing reports have recognized this surgical procedure as a potential risk factor for subsequent cancer initiation and progression (see **Chapter 21** for further discussion).[21,22]

Genetic Predisposition and Syndromic Associations

Bladder cancer has been linked to certain familial cancer syndromes, such as hereditary nonpolyposis colorectal cancer (HNPCC) syndrome.[23] HNPCC syndrome is related to mutation of mismatch repair genes, including *MLH1, MSH2, MSH6*, and *PMS2*. In the background of defective DNA mismatch repair via such mechanisms, microsatellite regions may accumulate errors more rapidly than normal as a part of tumor carcinogenesis. The HNPCC patients are predisposed to certain types of extracolonic tumors, including endometrial, ovarian, small bowel, stomach, hepatobiliary, skin, brain, and urinary tract sites. Upper tract urothelial neoplasms reportedly occur at a higher incidence and at a slightly younger median age of onset (56 years).[24] However, evidence of increased risk of urothelial neoplasia in the bladder of these patients is less compelling.[24,25] Currently there is no evidence of increased risk of urothelial neoplasia in pediatric patients with HNPCC syndrome, as noted by Wild et al. in their study of urothelial neoplasms in patients under age 20 years.[26] In the same patient group, no familial bladder cancer history was identified.[27]

Bladder cancer has been reported in patients with hereditary retinoblastoma, in whom its occurrence has been attributed to radiation and/or cyclophosphamide therapy. However, even in the absence of such treatment, increased mortality from bladder cancer in comparison to the general population has been noted, suggesting that it may indeed be a component of the hereditary retinoblastoma spectrum.[25]

Bladder cancer is sometimes a component of Costello syndrome, a rare autosomal dominant disorder in which patients are at risk for various malignancies, such as rhabdomyosarcoma, neuroblastoma, and urinary bladder urothelial carcinoma (UC).[25,28] These patients have been reported to develop papillary UC during childhood,[28,29] sometimes with recurrence, suggesting that hematuria or other urinary tract symptoms in patients with Costello syndrome should prompt consideration of a bladder tumor workup.[29]

Clinical Features and Natural History of Bladder Cancer

Approximately three-fourths of patients with bladder cancer present with painless intermittent hematuria.[11–14,30,31] It is estimated that approximately 20% of patients being evaluated for gross hematuria will subsequently be diagnosed with bladder cancer. Similarly, of patients presenting with microscopic hematuria, up to CIS 10% will be diagnosed with bladder cancer. Total gross hematuria without pain is the typical sign for suspicion of bladder cancer. Varkarakis et al. studied 95 patients with gross painless hematuria and found 13% with bladder cancer.[32] In a similar study of 1000 patients with gross painless hematuria by Lee and Davis, 15% of the patients had bladder cancer.[33] Careful characterization of hematuria as initial, terminal, and total hematuria is important in identifying the location of bleeding. Therefore, with these high incidences of bladder cancer in patients with gross hematuria, examination by flexible cystoscopy seems to be necessary. However, hematuria is

quite often intermittent, so that a negative result on one or two specimens has little meaning in ruling out the presence of bladder cancer.

Similarly, of patients presenting with microscopic hematuria, up to 10% will be diagnosed with bladder cancer. Microscopic hematuria in patients with bladder cancer tends to be unpredictable and inconsistent; therefore, a single negative urinalysis does not exclude the possibility of cancer. Mohr et al. reported that asymptomatic microhematuria occurred in 13% of the general population, and, of those patients, only 0.4% had urothelial neoplasia.[34] On the other hand, Golin and Howard found that 6.5% had bladder cancer among 246 patients with asymptomatic microscopic hematuria who were referred to a urology clinic.[35] Extrapolating the clinical importance of macroscopic hematuria to microscopic hematuria has not been rewarding, so the usefulness of testing for microhematuria is now in doubt.[36] Testing for microhematuria is considered not helpful in evaluating men with lower urinary tract symptoms. Therefore, the clinical significance of asymptomatic microscopic hematuria is uncertain.

Although the vast majority of bladder cancers are diagnosed as a result of evaluating patients for hematuria, one-fourth of patients with bladder cancer will present with irritative voiding symptoms, including urgency, frequency, and dysuria, symptoms often mistakenly attributed to urinary tract infection.[7,10,37]

The initial evaluation and management for patients with suspected bladder cancer involves cystoscopic evaluation of the bladder, transurethral resection (TUR) of visible tumor, and assessment of the appearance of the uninvolved bladder and prostatic urethra, which may be indicated when visible abnormalities of the prostatic urothelium exist (Figs. 8-2 to 8-5). Small lesions and flat lesions worrisome for carcinoma in situ (CIS) can be sampled with cold-cup biopsy forceps, while larger lesions should be completely resected. In addition, during TUR, attempts should be made to obtain muscularis propria. The presence of smooth muscle in the pathologic specimen is an important indicator for an adequately performed resection.[38] It is clear that up to 4% patients with early-stage bladder cancer are at risk for synchronous and metachronous upper urinary tract tumors.[39] Patients with a history of CIS, tumors adjacent to the ureteral orifices, or those with persistently unexplained positive cytologies might be at increased risk of an upper urinary tract tumor or prostatic urethral tumor involvement.

Nearly 80% of patients who initially present with bladder urothelial carcinoma have tumors confined to the mucosa or submucosa—so-called superficial "nonmuscle invasive" bladder cancers, more appropriately reported as stage Ta/T1 urothelial tumors.[13,18,40–42] "Superficial" bladder tumors represent a heterogeneous group of cancers that include those that are (1) papillary in nature and limited to the mucosa (stage Ta), and (2) those that are

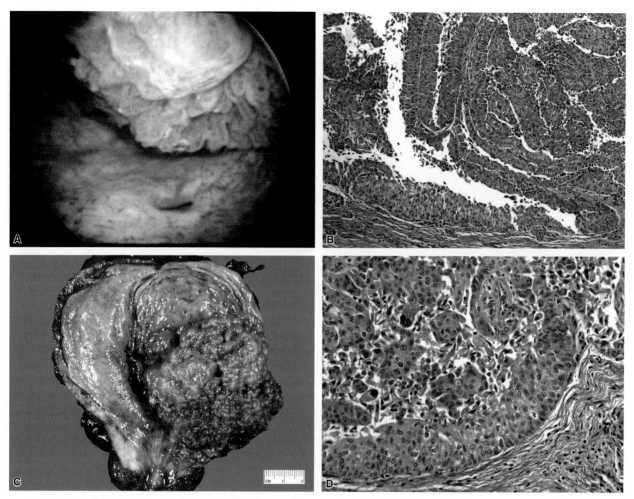

Figure 8-2 Papillary urothelial carcinoma of the bladder. Cystoscopic (A), gross (C), and microscopic B and D appearance. The bladder is partially filled with a velvety mass. (Photo courtesy of Dr. Koch.)

invasive into the lamina propria or submucosa when the muscularis mucosae is present (stage T1). Flat urothelial CIS (Tis) has been included historically as part of the group of superficial bladder cancer patients. The rest of bladder cancer patients present initially with bladder tumors invading the muscularis propria of the bladder or beyond (stages T2 to T4) (**Figs. 8-6** to **8-8**).[7,38,43–47] However, the recent consensus is not to group these diseases under the umbrella term "superficial bladder cancer."[48] The term "superficial" should be abandoned.[49]

The natural history of bladder cancer is difficult to predict, due to biologic heterogeneity; features that characterize early-stage (stage Ta or T1) bladder cancer are disease recurrence and progression. The risks for both recurrence and tumor progression are related to multiple histopathologic factors, including grade, depth of invasion, multiplicity, tumor size, tumor morphology, presence or absence of vascular or lymphatic invasion, and presence or absence of CIS and some molecular features (**Table 8-1**).[50] Although these conventional measures

provide some degree of prognostic information, they fail to clearly evaluate each individual tumor's malignant potential. These shortcomings with traditional clinical and histopathologic features have therefore lead to significant efforts to better define a tumor's true biological potential on a molecular level.[5,51,52]

Nearly 60% to 90% of patients with early-stage bladder cancer will have a tumor recurrence if treated by TUR alone; 25% of cancers that recur will ultimately progress to invasive cancers.[5,6,53–55] Eighty percent of urothelial bladder cancer patients suffer from recurrence within one to two years of initial treatment. Despite radical cystectomy and systemic therapy, 50% of patients with invasive tumors die from metastasis.[44,46,56,57]

A retrospective analysis of 176 patients from Sweden with early-stage urothelial carcinoma, who were followed until death or for at least 20 years (with no adjuvant therapy), provides some insight into the importance and natural history of this disease when left untreated.[58] An overall recurrence rate of 80% was reported, with 22% of patients

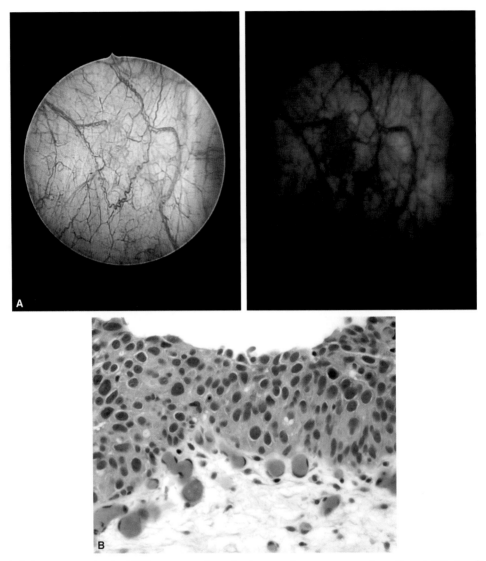

Figure 8-3 Urothelial carcinoma in situ (CIS), cystoscopic and microscopic appearance. A urothelial CIS visualized by standard white light cystoscopy (A, left) and fluorescence cystoscopy (A, right). Prominent microvascular proliferation immediately below the basement of the urothelium has been replaced by CIS cells (B). (Photo courtesy of Dr. Montironi.)

dying from the disease if followed long enough: 11% of patients with Ta disease and 30% of patients with T1 disease. In this study, death was related directly to tumor grade, number of tumors, and volume of recurrences.[58]

Urinary bladder cancer is a heterogeneous disease with diverse morphologic and clinical manifestations.[43,59] Three major risks for patients after initial management of tumor include recurrence, progression into higher grade and higher stage tumors, and metastasis. These risks are well known for each stage of the disease, but are not sufficiently quantifiable to prospectively assess risk for individuals. Clinical and pathological parameters are widely used to predict clinical outcome, but these parameters have limited utility for predicting tumor recurrence. Reliable parameters for tumor recurrence risk would be valuable when advising patients

about surveillance measures and aggressiveness of therapy (see **Chapters 29, 32, 33,** and **34** for further discussion).

Morphologic Characteristics of Invasive Urothelial Carcinoma

Infiltrating (or invasive) urothelial carcinoma is defined as a urothelial tumor that invades beyond the basement membrane. Infiltrative carcinomas grossly span a range of morphology, including papillary, polypoid, nodular, solid, ulcerative, or transmural diffuse. They may be solitary or multifocal. The histology of infiltrating urothelial carcinomas is variable and includes stage pT1–T4

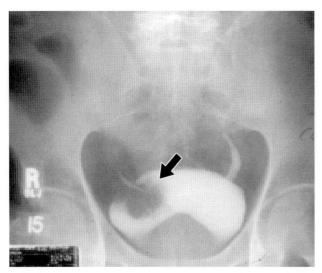

Figure 8-4 Urothelial carcinoma of the bladder. Radiographically, urothelial carcinomas are visualized as filling defects. (Photo courtesy of Dr. Koch.)

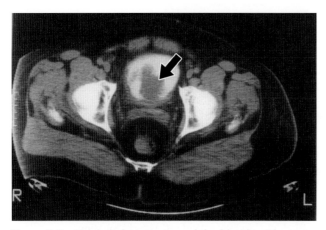

Figure 8-5 Urothelial carcinoma of the bladder. The arrow indicates the tumor. With superficial tumors, there is usually little deformity to the bladder wall, and on CT scan, the thickness of the bladder wall is thin. (Photo courtesy of Dr. Koch.)

tumors (**Fig. 8-9**; see **Chapters 9, 10**, and **11** for further discussion).[38] Infiltrating urothelial carcinomas are graded as low or high grade according to the new 2004 WHO classification, depending on the degree of nuclear anaplasia and architectural abnormalities.[3]

Invasive urothelial carcinoma may present as polypoid, sessile, ulcerated, or infiltrative tumor, in which the neoplastic cells invade the bladder wall as nests, cords, trabeculae, small clusters, or single cells that are often separated by a desmoplastic stroma (**Figs. 8-10** to **8-14**). The tumor sometimes grows in a more diffuse, sheet-like pattern, but even in these cases, focal nests and clusters are generally present. The cells show moderate to abundant amphophilic or eosinophilic cytoplasm and

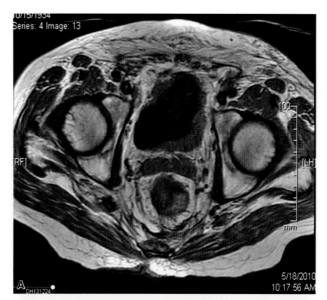

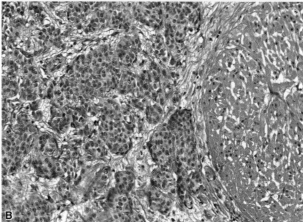

Figure 8-6 Invasive urothelial carcinoma. Magnetic resonance imaging shows an invasive cancer (A). Tumor invades the muscularis propria wall (B). (Photo courtesy of Dr. Koch.)

large hyperchromatic nuclei. In larger nests, palisading nuclei may be seen at the edges of the nests. The nucleus is typically pleomorphic and often has irregular contours with angular profiles. Nuclear grooves may be identified in some cells. Nucleoli are highly variable in number and appearance; with some cells containing single or multiple small nucleoli and others having large eosinophilic nucleoli. Foci of marked pleomorphism may be seen, with bizarre and multinuclear tumor cells. Mitotic figures are common, with numerous abnormal forms.

Urothelial carcinoma has a propensity for divergent differentiation, with the most common being squamous (**Fig. 8-15**), followed by glandular differentiation.[8] Tumor heterogeneity is also common, with different histologic grades in the same tumor (**Fig. 8-16**).[59] Virtually, the entire spectrum of bladder cancer variants may be seen

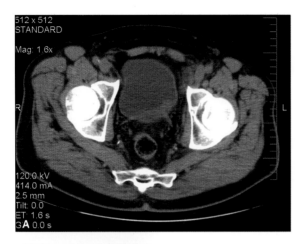

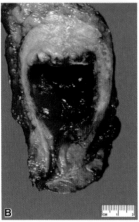

Figure 8-7 Invasive urothelial carcinoma with a thickened bladder wall (A and B). (Photo courtesy of Dr. Koch.)

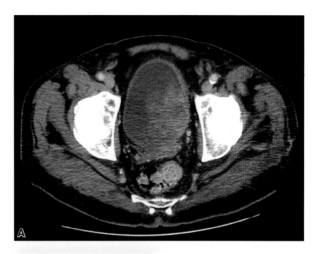

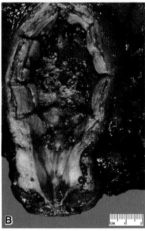

Figure 8-8 Bulky invasive urothelial carcinoma with a thickened bladder wall. (A and B). (Photo courtesy of Dr. Koch.)

in variable proportions accompanying otherwise typical urothelial carcinoma. It has been proposed that sarcomatoid carcinoma represents the final common pathway of urothelial carcinoma differentiation (see **Chapters 16 and 34** for further discussion).[60] The clinical outcome of some of these variants differs from typical urothelial carcinoma; therefore, recognition of these variants is important. Pathologic features of the most common variants of urothelial carcinoma are discussed in **Chapter 12**.

Urothelial Carcinoma in Young Adults

Various studies have used differing age criteria for "young" patients; however, in patients 20 to 40 years of age, urothelial carcinoma generally remains less common than in patients over 40 years of age. Most studies have found urothelial tumors to be somewhat more common in this age group than in true pediatric patients (under 20 years).[22,61,62] Similarly, the male predilection is maintained

Table 8-1 Factors Predictive of Recurrence and Progression in Bladder Carcinoma Without Muscle Invasion

Number of Tumors
Solitary
2–7
>8
Cancer size
<3 cm in greatest dimension
>3 cm in greatest dimension
Prior recurrence rate
<1 recurrence/year
>1 recurrence/year
Pathologic stage
Ta
T1
Coexistent carcinoma in situ
Histologic grade (WHO 1973)
Grade 1
Grade 2
Grade 3

Source: Modified from Ref. 50.

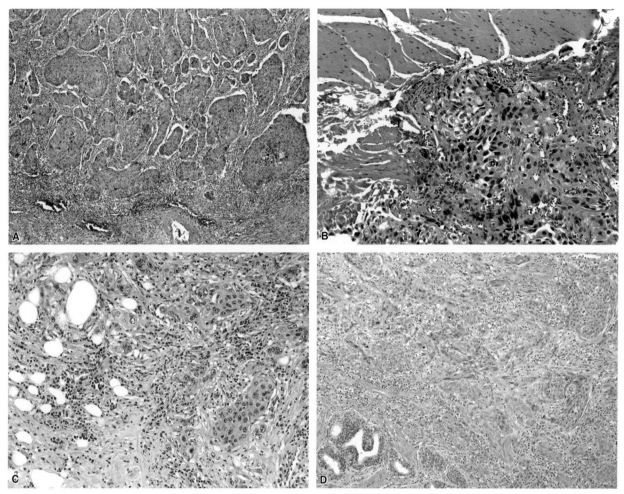

Figure 8-9   Different stages of bladder cancer. (A) Tumor invades the lamina propria (pT1). (B) Tumor invades the muscularis propria (pT2). (C) Tumor with extravesical fat invasion (pT3). (D) Urothelial carcinoma invades the prosate (pT4).

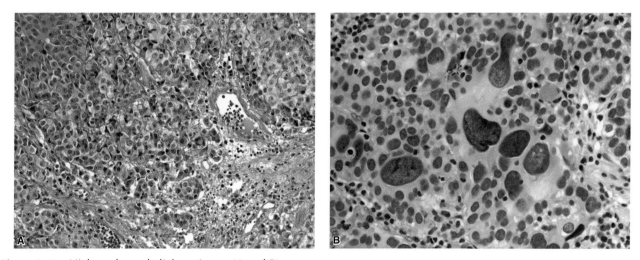

Figure 8-10   High grade urothelial carcinoma (A and B).

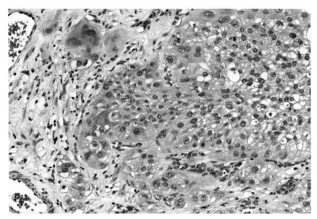

Figure 8-11 Early-stage (pT1) urothelial carcinoma. Note the presence of small nests and individual single cells invading the lamina propria.

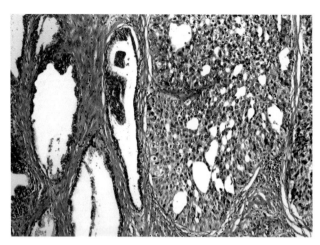

Figure 8-14 Urothelial carcionoma invading the prostate.

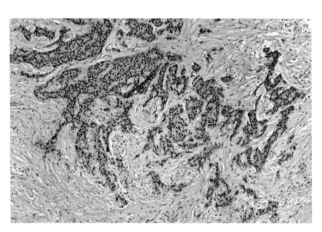

Figure 8-12 Invasive urothelial carcinoma. Tentacular pattern of stromal invasion with desmoplasia.

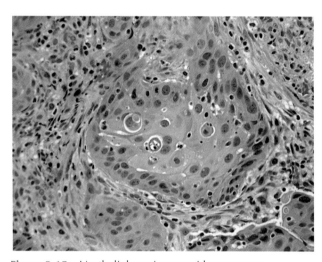

Figure 8-15 Urothelial carcinoma with squamous differentiation.

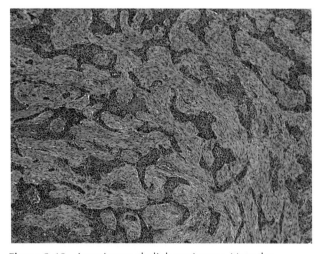

Figure 8-13 Invasive urothelial carcinoma. Note the prominent desmoplasia.

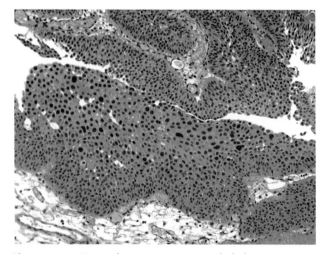

Figure 8-16 Tumor heterogeneity in urothelial carcinoma. Mixed histologic grades are seen in the same tumor.

in this age group,[61,62] although the male predominance may be somewhat less marked in young patients.[63] When patients are stratified by decade of life, tumors occurring in patients during the third and fourth decades of life exhibit more indolent tumor behavior than do those that arise in older individuals.

Yossepowitch and Dalbagni studied 74 patients aged 40 years or younger, finding that the clinical presentation and disease outcome were similar to those of older patients, with a comparable male-to-female ratio, stage distribution, and disease-free progression/recurrence rates in the Ta, Tis, and T1 categories.[64] In particular, young patients who underwent radical cystectomy were prone to an aggressive clinical course and poor outcome, with a higher rate of distant metastasis. However, the authors noted that all but one of 14 patients below age 30 years presented with stage Ta disease and were disease-free at the last followup.[64] In contrast, Migaldi and colleagues[63] reported 58 patients ranging from 20 to 45 years of age who developed urothelial neoplasms: histologically superficial urothelial carcinoma (86%), muscle-invasive urothelial carcinoma (2%), and urothelial (10%). The authors contrasted the group of 50 superficial tumors (pTa and pT1) with a second group of 90 superficial tumors occurring in patients over 55 years of age. Interestingly, when limiting the analysis to these stage restrictions (pTa and pT1), patient populations revealed a significantly better outcome in young patients, with statistically significant decreases in tumor grade and recurrence for the under-45 population. Similarly, pTa tumors were more common in the "young" group.[63] Of note, the male predilection was greater for older patients (7 : 1) than for younger patients (2 : 1),[63] in contrast to the findings of Yossepowitch and Dalbagni.[64]

Some authors have found that the indolent biologic behavior of urothelial neoplasms arising in patients aged less than 19 years is not seen with young adult patients (ages 20 to 30), whose urothelial neoplasms exhibit a poorer prognosis, more similar to that of typical urothelial carcinoma patients.[61,64] In a study including 15 patients in the third decade of life, 40% developed recurrence and two patients with grade 2/3 tumors progressed to invasive carcinoma. One patient died of metastatic cancer, while the other was alive with tumor recurrence.[61] Similarly, in a study of patients under age 30, recurrences developed in 11 patients, although those above and below age 20 were not analyzed separately.[62] Thus, differences in the biologic behavior of pediatric and young adult tumors may at least partially account for these increased incidences of tumor recurrence.

The study by Migaldi et al. found by univariate analysis that high Ki67 and low cyclin D1 immunohistochemical expressions were associated with an increased risk of recurrence in the young adult group (ages 20 to 45), while reduced p27^{Kip1} expression and p53 overexpression were not. In contrast, reduced p27^{Kip1} expression did correlate with increased risk of recurrence in the elderly patient group (greater than 55 years of age), suggesting that distinct molecular pathways may be involved in the development and progression of these tumors.[63]

Prognosis of Invasive Urothelial Cancer

The prognosis for patients with invasive urothelial carcinoma is poor, with five-year survival of less than 50%, despite therapy.[5,37,44,46,65,66] Numerous pathologic factors have been shown in select cohorts of patients with bladder cancer to correlate with recurrence, progression, and survival. The immune response to the tumor as measured by immunohistochemical staining for lymphocytes and antigen-presenting dendritic cells is useful in predicting recurrence.[67] The number of papillary tumors also predicts recurrence but does not appear to be a significant determinant of invasive cancer.[68]

Patients with a single focus of papillary cancer develop recurrence after transurethral resection in 45% of cases; however, patients who develop a second tumor have an 84% risk of developing a third tumor. Tumors larger than 5 cm in diameter also increase the risk of muscle invasion.[69,70] Tumor recurrence more than four years after resection of the primary tumor is an ominous sign.[58,71] It is an important goal to exclude dysplasia or CIS in the adjacent mucosa or elsewhere in the bladder, as this is a significant factor predictive of recurrence and invasion.[72–74]

The presence of lymphovascular invasion is predictive of poor outcome, and this finding should be included in the pathology report according to the Cancer Committee of the College of American Pathologists.[65,75] Identification of lymphovascular invasion may be difficult, and can be confused with artifactual clefting around nests of invasive carcinoma, including perineural invasion.[65,75] The incidence of lymphovascular invasion is variable, reportedly as high as 7% of cases. Immunohistochemical studies directed against endothelial cells that employ *Ulex europeus* lectin, factor VIII, CD31, or CD34 may be of value in identifying lymphovascular invasion, although less than 40% of cases with lymphovascular invasion by routine examination can be confirmed immunohistochemically.[76] Invasion is an important predictor of patient outcome, regardless of tumor grade.[65,77]

Prostatic involvement by urothelial carcinoma is common.[38,78,79] In patients with muscle-invasive bladder cancer, the prostate is involved in up to 50% of cases, and the frequency is even higher in those who have multifocal CIS of the bladder. Prostatic involvement is classified into three groups: (1) carcinoma confined to the prostatic urethral lining, (2) carcinoma extending into ducts and acini but confined by the basement membrane, and (3) carcinoma that invades the prostatic stroma.[80] Metastases are most likely with prostatic stromal invasion.[78] The presence of prostatic urethral CIS indicates a high risk for urethral recurrence after radical surgery.[78,79,81] Prostatic stromal invasion is a strong predictor of poor patient survival (see **Chapter 11** for further discussion).[78,82]

Field Cancerization and Tumor Multicentricity

The morbidity and high cost of care for urothelial carcinoma result from its proclivity for multifocality and frequent recurrence, requiring expensive surveillance and multiple endoscopic and/or intravesical treatments. Development of multifocal tumors in the same patient, either synchronous or metachronous, is a common characteristic of urothelial malignancy (**Figs. 8-17** and **8-18**).[6,68,83–90] Multiple coexisting tumors have often arisen before clinical symptoms are apparent. The separate tumors may or may not share a similar histology. Two theories have been proposed to explain the frequency of urothelial tumor multifocality. One theory, the monoclonal theory, suggests that the multiple tumors arise from a single transformed cell that proliferates and spreads throughout the urothelium either by intraluminal implantation or by intraepithelial migration. The second theory, the field effect theory, explains tumor multifocality as a development secondary to field cancerization effect. Chemical carcinogens cause independent transforming genetic alterations at different sites in the urothelial lining, leading to multiple genetically unrelated tumors.

The issue of monoclonal versus oligoclonal origin of multifocal urothelial carcinomas is clinically important for understanding patterns of early tumor development when planning treatment and surgical strategies.[5,6,23,51,83,89–94] The cause of multifocality also influences test design for genetic detection of recurrent or residual tumor cells in posttreatment urine samples. There is currently no consensus concerning which theory is most important in the development of multifocal urothelial carcinoma.[95–106] Many studies have suggested a monoclonal origin for multifocal urothelial carcinoma, but other studies have shown an independent origin for some multicentric urothelial tumors using similar methods.[83,97,100,104,105,107–113] A recent study suggests that both field cancerization and monoclonal tumor spread may coexist in the same patient.[83] Molecular evidence supporting an oligoclonal origin for multifocal urothelial carcinomas in the majority of cases was found, consistent with the field cancerization theory for multicentric urothelial carcinogenesis. This finding is clinically important to understanding early

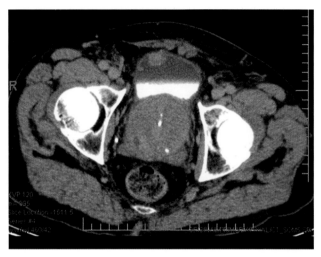

Figure 8-17 Multifocality of bladder cancer. CT scan shows a large prostate and two superficial urothelial tumors on the anterior bladder wall. (Photo courtesy of Dr. Koch.)

tumor development, and spread must be considered in the development of appropriate treatment and surgical strategies and when molecular diagnostic techniques are utilized in the detection of recurrent or residual disease.

Field cancerization, which is an important cause of multicentric squamous cell carcinomas of the head and neck, postulates that multifocal urothelial carcinomas arise in the same way.[5] In the field cancerization process, simultaneous or sequential tumors result from numerous independent mutational events at different sites in the urothelial tract. These independent transformations are a consequence of external cancer-causing influences. In support of the field effect theory is the frequent finding of genetic instability in normal-appearing bladder mucosa in patients with bladder cancer in the adjacent urothelium.[114,115] Premalignant changes such as dysplasia or CIS often are found in urothelial mucosa away from an invasive bladder cancer.

Many genetic comparisons and mapping of atypia in cystectomy specimens have emphasized the role of oligoclonality and field cancerization in the development of multifocal urothelial tumors, especially in early-stage disease. Since the monoclonal and oligoclonal theories explaining urothelial tumor multifocality are not mutually exclusive, various theories have been proposed to combine the two mechanisms. It has been suggested that oligoclonality is more common in early lesions, with progression to higher stages, leading to the overgrowth of one clone and pseudomonoclonality.[105,116] Thus, early or preneoplastic lesions may arise independently with a specific clone undergoing malignant transformation, which subsequently spreads through the urothelium by either an intraluminal or an intraepithelial dissemination.

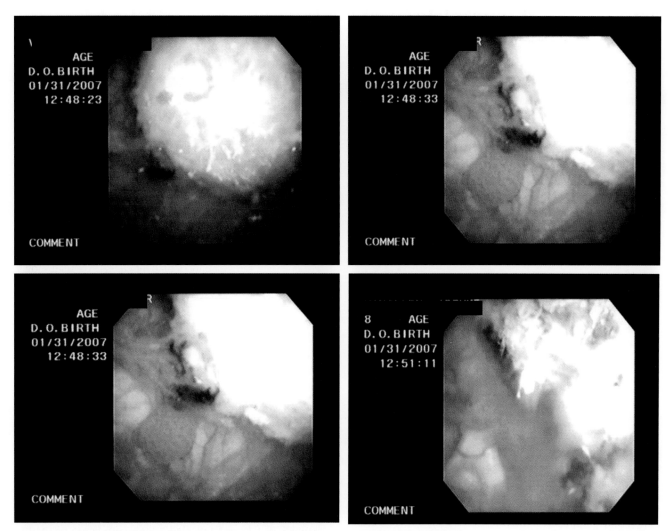

Figure 8-18 Multifocality of bladder cancer. Cystoscopic examination revealing multiple early-stage bladder cancer from the same patient. (Photo courtesy of Dr. Koch.)

Whereas tumor multifocality seems to be an oligoclonal phenomenon in the majority of cases, there is undeniable support for the monoclonal hypothesis in some cases.[83]

The Origin of Bladder Cancer

Current carcinogenesis models suggests that malignancy represents clonal expansion of one or a few cancer stem cells (CSCs) in the fields affected.[5,6,23,51,117,118] CSCs comprise 1% to 4% of the viable cell population in a malignant tumor. These cells proliferate through asymmetric differentiation and can diversify into heterogeneous cancer cell lineages. Asymmetric differentiation means that following cell division, one daughter cell retains the capacity to divide again, and the other daughter cell possesses genetic plasticity, allowing phenotypic variation in the offspring. When tumors arise from CSCs or progenitor cells, a specific set of genomic, epigenomic, and/or microenvironmental niche alterations is essential for continued clonal expansion. Therefore, each CSC and its progeny possesses a unique set of genetic, epigenetic, and phenotypic features. Urothelial CSCs may harbor either fibroblast growth factor receptor 3 (FGFR3) mutation or TP53 mutations. Although pure populations of bladder CSCs have not yet been isolated, many investigators have reported putative populations of stem cell-like cells in bladder cancer. Bladder CSCs in urothelial carcinoma can be identified by their properties of colony formation, self-renewal, high proliferation rate, and expression of stem cell-related genes.[119-121] Genetic alterations of stromal somatic cells assist CSCs in the niche to promote cancer development and progression. CSCs gain growth advantage and develop into an expanding clonal patch with genetically altered daughter cells. The subsequent clonal explanation gradually displaces the normal epithelium to form a field. The process is driven by the enhanced proliferative capacity of a genetically altered clonal unit. Urothelial carcinomas arise from CSCs that are distributed in the primary tumor and also in the shared field, and which appear to be the source of tumor recurrences, tumor progression, and tumor metastasis.[23,38,51,91,92,94,122,123]

Chan et al. used the expression of protein markers to isolate and characterize a tumor-initiating cell (TIC) subpopulation in primary human bladder cancer. The cells of this subpopulation exhibited enhanced ability to induce xenograft tumors in vivo that recapitulated the heterogeneity of the original tumor.[124] These investigators analyzed over 300 bladder cancer specimens and found heterogeneity among activated oncogenic pathways in TIC (e.g., 80% Gli1, 45% Stat3, 10% Bmi-1, and 5% β-catenin) and a unique bladder TIC gene signature was identified by gene chip analysis.[124] It is suggested that variations in the clinical behavior of different urothelial carcinomas, even within clinical and pathological staging groups, results from this heterogeneity of activated oncogenic pathways and T-IC gene signatures.[124]

CSC and field carcinogenesis theories explain urothelial carcinoma clonality and multifocality, and provide a rationale for novel therapeutic strategies.[23,38,125] Understanding the mechanisms of CSC/field carcinogenesis may lead to the identification of novel molecular markers that could be critically important in tumor identification and classification, and also in the development of targeted therapeutic regimens aimed not only at treatment of established cancer but in prevention of metastases as well.

Molecular Genetics

Traditional morphological analysis is of limited utility for identifying cases in which cancer recurrence and progression will occur. However, molecular and genetic analyses offer new perspectives on the prediction of clinical outcome (see also **Chapters 29 to 34**). Recent studies have suggested that urothelial carcinogenesis occurs as a "field effect" that can involve any number of sites in the bladder mucosa.[6] Accumulating evidence supports the notion that resident urothelial stem cells in the affected field are transformed into CSCs by acquiring genetic alterations that lead to tumor formation through clonal expansion. Both initial and recurrent tumors are derived from CSCs in the affected field via two distinct molecular pathways. These provide a genetic framework for understanding urothelial carcinogenesis, tumor recurrence, and progression: the *FGFR3*- and *TP53*-associated pathways. These two pathways are characterized by different genomic, epigenetic, and gene expression alterations. Their outcomes correlate with the markedly different clinical and pathologic features of both relatively indolent low grade cancers and the aggressive high grade cancers. As such, these molecular findings are potentially useful for counseling patients and for assessing the risk of recurrence and progression. The molecular changes may additionally prove useful for developing preventive and therapeutic strategies for bladder cancer.

Bladder cancer, in particular, shows a loss of heterozygosity (LOH) on chromosome 9, with the most common site of loss at 9p21. The most common genetic alterations of bladder tumors are gains of 1q, 8p/q, and 20q and losses of 8p, 11p, 9p, and 9q.[5,6,23,57,60,83,89,91,97,113,122,123,126–149] Invasive bladder cancer commonly shows losses of 2q, 5q, 8p, 9p, 9q, 10q, 11p, 18q, and Y (see **Chapters 29, 32, 33, and 34** for further discussion). Gains include 1q, 5p, 8q, and 17q. LOH in bladder cancer can be detected by cytogenetics, restriction fragment length polymorphisms, and microsatellite polymorphism analysis.[23]

Some chromosomal deletions are common in urothelial carcinoma, and the most common is loss of chromosome 9p, present in more than 50% of T1 and T2 cancers.[97,113,145] Both 9p and 9q probably harbor tumor suppressor genes involved in the initiation of bladder carcinogenesis[150] and recurrence.[151] The total number of alterations is higher in pT1 tumors than in pTa tumors.[152]

Chromosome 9p21 deletion is frequently observed in early stages of urothelial carcinogenesis. Hyperplastic urothelium and adjacent papillary urothelial carcinoma have both been found to share chromosome 9 deletions, which is a very interesting observation in the tumorigenesis of these neoplasms.[5,113,148] LOH and fluorescence in situ hybridization (FISH) were compared in microdissected samples of CIS and revealed a high correlation of the two methods, with 86% and 75% chromosome 9 deletion rates, respectively; for dysplasia, the rates were 84% and 53%, respectively.[113]

Low grade papillary tumors are diploid or near-diploid and have been found to express *P16* inactivation and missense mutations of *FGFR3* (see **Chapters 9, 29, 33, and 34** for further discussion). Low grade tumors also show altered expression of cytokeratin 20, CD44, p53, and p63.[3] Ultimately, deletions of chromosome 9 and mutations of *FGFR3* are the most commonly found alterations in these tumors.[153]

High grade papillary tumors are aneuploid (which includes CIS and invasive tumors) and show alterations in *TP53* and *P16*.[126–128,146,154] In fact, mutations of *FGFR3* and *TP53* may show an inverse relationship, as *FGFR3* mutations are found in lower stage and lower grade tumors, whereas *TP53* mutations are found more commonly in invasive and more aggressive tumors.[155–158] High grade tumors show overexpression of p53, HER2, or EGFR, and loss of p21 (CDKN1A/Waf1) or p27(CDKN1B/Kip1) (especially in invasive cancers).[3] Furthermore, other common genetic areas of LOH include 14q (70%), 8p (65%), 13q (56%), 11p (54%), and 4q (52%) in CIS.

pT1 tumors have an average of 6.5 to 9.8 chromosomal imbalances, whereas low grade pTa tumors have an average of 2.3 to 3.7 chromosomal imbalances.[137,152] In more aggressive forms of bladder carcinoma, gains and amplifications of genes, rather than deletions, predominate.[137,152,159] Amplifications on the long arm of chromosome 3 have been found to decrease p63 expression, which is thereby associated with loss of tumor differentiation and increased depth of tumor invasion, although studies suggest that p63 alterations are not useful as prognostic indicators in patients' survival rates.[159,160]

LOH of 15q has been reported to be present in 40% of urothelial tumors.[141] LOH of 11p has been reported to be found in approximately 40% of bladder tumors, but it is more commonly associated with higher stage and higher grade tumors.[142,143] A loss at 13q14 indicates a loss at *RB1*, and a loss of 17p indicates a loss at *TP53*.[161–163]

LOH of chromosomes 11p and 17p13 (the *TP53* locus) usually occurred in high grade invasive cancer,[113,164] whereas allelic loss of chromosome 3 was seen in only 26% of high stage urothelial cancers.[165] Loss of the Y chromosome was common in urothelial carcinoma and was associated with advanced stage, coexistent CIS, and poor prognosis.[166] LOH on chromosome 2q revealed a candidate tumor suppressor gene, *LRP1B*, that was more frequent in high grade cancer.[167] LOH of the short arm of chromosome 3 was not present in superficial papillary cancer, whereas it is present in 54% of cases of muscle-invasive cancer. LOH has also been observed on chromosomes 4p, 4q, 5q, 8p, and 10q.[168] Loss of 14q is common in invasive bladder cancer and suggests that there are potential tumor suppressor loci on 14q12 and 14q32.1–32.2.[169] LOH of chromosome 18q was associated with muscle-invasive bladder cancer.[170] LOH at the DEL-27 locus on 5p13–12 predicted progression in bladder cancer.[171] In contrast, LOH of 8p 22 *N*-acetyltransferase 2, a polymorphic enzyme that metabolizes aromatic amines, was not associated with cancer progression in bladder cancer.[172] FISH revealed that polysomy of chromosomes 1 and 8 were linked to muscle invasion but not recurrence.[151] LOH of *D11S490* or *D17S928* predicted recurrence in superficial cancer.[172]

Genome-wide single-nucleotide polymorphism assays revealed that homozygous *TP53* mutations were more often associated with high LOH than with low LOH.[173] The *GSTM1* null genotype was associated with bladder cancer.[174] Tissue microarray screening revealed amplification of three putative target genes on chromosome region 12q13–q15, including *MDM2, CDK4,* and *GLI*.[175]

Other genetic alterations, such as aberrant DNA methylations and microRNA deregulations, have also been investigated extensively in bladder cancer (see **Chapters 29, 30, 31, 32, 33,** and **34** for further discussion).

Molecular Therapies Targeting Molecular Pathways

Traditional therapies such as surgery, radiation, and chemotherapy have limited success in the treatment of advanced bladder cancer.[176] Over the last decade, great strides have been made in identifying the molecular pathways in urothelial carcinogenesis.[5,6,23,51,57,60,122,130,134,148] Molecular alterations such as *FGFR3* and *TP53* abnormalities have been found to be associated with tumor grade, recurrence, clinical phenotype, and prognosis (see also **Chapters 29** to **34**). These molecular pathways lead to aberrant cell cycle control, apoptosis, self-sufficient replication, enhanced angiogenesis, insensitivity to antigrowth signals, and varying tumor phenotypes.[177] In recent years, there has been substantial interest in developing novel therapeutic agents targeted against the molecular pathways that are deregulated in tumor cells. Identification of these molecular alterations provides the possibility for finding novel therapeutic agents that can specifically target these alterations, eliminating tumor cells while having little impact on normal tissues.[6,178–183]

Epidermal growth factor receptor (*EGFR*) is expressed in 31% to 48% of urothelial carcinomas and among the best-studied receptors in urothelial carcinomas, having been associated with increased probability of progression and death.[184,185] Among the functions of this pathway are mediation of cell differentiation, proliferation, migration, angiogenesis, and apoptosis. The most thoroughly evolved treatment strategies targeted against the *EGFR* pathway include cetuximab and trastuzumab, monoclonal antibodies that block the extracellular ligand-binding domain, as well as gefitinib, erlotinib, and lapatinib, inhibitors of the intracellular tyrosine kinase domain.[6,186,187] A number of other monoclonal antibodies have been produced against *EGFR*,[188] and treatment of experimental animal tumors with anti-*EGFR* has demonstrated marked reduction in tumor growth, reduced vascular endothelial growth factor (*VEGF*) production, and prevention of metastases to the lungs and lymph nodes that were observed in control mice.[6,60,189,190]

Similarly, *VEGF*, an important factor regulating angiogenesis, has been correlated with increasing disease stage and tumor invasion into muscle.[191,192] For this reason, it has also been considered as a potential therapeutic target. Blocking signaling through the *VEGF* pathway has demonstrated a significant antiangiogenic effect via inhibition of endothelial proliferation. Novel therapeutics inhibiting *VEGF* signaling include sunitinib, sorafenib, pazopanib, aflibercept, and bevacizumab.[193] Of note, tumors treated with cisplatin, sunitinib, and a combination of the two agents exhibited reduced Ki67 expression compared to untreated lesions. The two agents, used in combination, also demonstrated a statistically significant difference compared to cisplatin alone.[194]

Gain of function mutations in *FGFR3* have been identified in 65% of papillary and in 20% of muscle-invasive bladder carcinomas.[195] *RAS* is a factor downstream of the *FGFR3* pathway, and its mutations have been associated with low grade bladder tumors, similar to *FGFR3* itself.[196,197] Anti-FGFR3 monoclonal antibody, R3Mab, binds selectively to *FGFR3* and blocks the *FGFR3*-dependent tumor proliferation.[198] With regard to the other major molecular pathway in urothelial carcinogenesis, the cell cycle is controlled primarily by the *TP53* and *Rb* pathways. *TP53* is also involved in several other important cellular processes related to cancer development, progression, and response to treatment, including angiogenesis, apoptosis, and DNA repair.[199–201] Viral transfer of *TP53* to human bladder cancer patients in preliminary studies has been proposed as a safe and potentially feasible emerging treatment, warranting further investigation.[202]

Additionally, hypermethylation of the promoter of tumor suppressor genes is one of the major mechanisms in carcinogenesis. Demethylation agents such as zebularine, 5-Aza-Cdr, and 5-Aza-CR reverse the hypermethylated CpG sites and functionally activate the hypermethylation-silenced tumor suppressor genes (see also **Chapter 34**).[203,204]

REFERENCES

1. Jemal A, Bray F, Center MM, Ferlay J, Ward E, Forman D. Global cancer statistics. *CA Cancer J Clin* 2011;61:69–90.
2. Siegel R, Ward E. Brawley O. Jemal A, Cancer statistics, 2011: The impact of eliminating socioeconomic and racial disparities on premature cancer death, *CA Cancer J Clin* 2011;61:212–36.
3. Eble JN, Sauter G, Epstein JI, Sesterhenn IA. eds. World Health Organization Classification of Tumours: Pathology and Genetics of Tumours of the Urinary System and Male Genital Organs. Lyon, France: IARC Press, 2004.
4. Kaufman DS, Shipley WU, Feldman AS. Bladder cancer. *Lancet* 2009;374:239–49.
5. Cheng L, Davidson DD, Maclennan GT, Williamson SR, Zhang S, Koch MO, Montironi R, Lopez-Beltran A. The origins of urothelial carcinoma. *Expert Rev Anticancer Ther* 2010;10:865–80.
6. Cheng L, Zhang S, Maclennan GT, Williamson SR, Lopez-Beltran A, Montironi R. Bladder cancer: translating molecular genetic insights into clinical practice. *Hum Pathol* 2011;42:455–81.
7. Cheng L, Lopez-Beltran A, MacLennan GT, Montironi R, Bostwick DG. Neoplasms of the urinary bladder. In: Bostwick DG, Cheng L, eds. Urologic Surgical Pathology, 2nd ed. Philadelphia: Elsevier/Mosby, 2008;259–352.
8. Lopez-Beltran A, Cheng L. Histologic variants of urothelial carcinoma: differential diagnosis and clinical implications. *Hum Pathol* 2006;37:1371–88.
9. Bostwick DG, Ramnani D, Cheng L. Diagnosis and grading of bladder cancer and associated lesions. *Urol Clin North Am* 1999;26:493–507.
10. Lopez-Beltran A. Bladder cancer: clinical and pathological profile. *Scand J Urol Nephrol Suppl* 2008;95–109.
11. Hartge P, Harvey EB, Linehan WM, Silverman DT, Sullivan JW, Hoover RN, Fraumeni JF. Unexplained excess risk of bladder cancer in men. *J Natl Cancer Inst* 1990;82:1636–40.
12. Kirkali Z, Chan T, Manoharan M, Algaba F, Busch C, Cheng L, Kiemeney L, Kriegmair M, Montironi R, Murphy WM, Sesterhenn IA, Tachibana M, Weider J. Bladder cancer: epidemiology, staging and grading, and diagnosis. *Urology* 2005;66:4–34.
13. Zeegers MP, Kellen E, Buntinx F, van den Brandt PA. The association between smoking, beverage consumption, diet and bladder cancer: a systematic literature review. *World J Urol* 2004;21:392–401.
14. Cohen SM, Shirai T, Steineck G. Epidemiology and etiology of premalignant and malignant urothelial changes. *Scand J Urol Nephrol Suppl* 2000;S205:105–15.
15. Ferlay J, Bray F, Pisani P, Parkin DM. GLOBOCAN 2000: Cancer Incidence, Mortality and Prevalence Worldwide. France: Lyon,IARC Press, 2001.
16. Mallin K, David KA, Carroll PR, Milowsky MI, Nanus DM. Transitional cell carcinoma of the bladder: racial and gender disparities in survival (1993 to 2002), stage and grade (1993 to 2007). *J Urol*;185:1631–6.
17. Dinney CP, McConkey DJ, Millikan RE, Wu X, Bar-Eli M, Adam L, Kamat AM, Siefker-Radtke AO, Tuziak T, Sabichi AL, Grossman HB, Benedict WF, Czerniak B. Focus on bladder cancer. *Cancer Cell* 2004;6:111–6.
18. Johansson SL, Cohen SM. Epidemiology and etiology of bladder cancer. *Semin Surg Oncol* 1997;13:291–8.
19. Cheng L, MacLennan GT, Lopez-Beltran A. Histologic grading of urothelial carcinoma: A reappraisal. *Hum Pathol* 2012 (in press).

20. Escudero AL, Luque RJ, Quintero A, Alvarez-Kindelan J, Requena MJ, Montironi R, Lopez-Beltran A. Association of human herpesvirus type 6 DNA with human bladder cancer. *Cancer Lett* 2005;230:20–4.

21. Sung MT, Zhang S, Lopez-Beltran A, Montironi R, Wang M, Davidson DD, Koch MO, Cain MP, Rink RC, Cheng L. Urothelial carcinoma following augmentation cystoplasty: an aggressive variant with distinct clinicopathological characteristics and molecular genetic alterations. *Histopathology* 2009;55:161–73.

22. Williamson SR, Lopez-Beltran A, Maclennan GT, Montironi R, Cheng L. Unique clinicopathologic and molecular characteristics of urinary bladder tumors in children and young adults. *Urol Oncol* 2012 (in press).

23. Cheng L, Zhang D. Molecular Genetic Pathology. New York: Humana Press/Springer, 2008.

24. Roupret M, Hupertan V, Yates DR, Comperat E, Catto JW, Meuth M, Lackmichi A, Ricci S, Lacave R, Gattegno B, Richard F, Hamdy FC, Cussenot O. A comparison of the performance of microsatellite and methylation urine analysis for predicting the recurrence of urothelial cell carcinoma, and definition of a set of markers by Bayesian network analysis. *BJU Int* 2008;101: 1448–53.

25. Mueller CM, Caporaso N, Greene MH. Familial and genetic risk of transitional cell carcinoma of the urinary tract. *Urol Oncol* 2008;26:451–64.

26. Wild PJ, Giedl J, Stoehr R, Junker K, Boehm S, van Oers JM, Zwarthoff EC, Blaszyk H, Fine SW, Humphrey PA, Dehner LP, Amin MB, Epstein JI, Hartmann A. Genomic aberrations are rare in urothelial neoplasms of patients 19 years or younger. *J Pathol* 2007;211:18–25.

27. Fine SW, Humphrey PA, Dehner LP, Amin MB, Epstein JI. Urothelial neoplasms in patients 20 years or younger: a clinicopathological analysis using the World Health Organization 2004 bladder consensus classification. *J Urol* 2005;174:1976–80.

28. Franceschini P, Licata D, Di Cara G, Guala A, Bianchi M, Ingrosso G, Franceschini D. Bladder carcinoma in Costello syndrome: report on a patient born to consanguineous parents and review. *Am J Med Genet* 1999;86:174–9.

29. Urakami S, Igawa M, Shiina H, Shigeno K, Kikuno N, Yoshino T. Recurrent transitional cell carcinoma in a child with the Costello syndrome. *J Urol* 2002;168:1133–4.

30. Esrig D, Freeman JA, Stein JP, Skinner DG. Early cystectomy for clinical stage T1 transitional cell carcinoma of the bladder. *Semin Urol Oncol* 1997;15:154–60.

31. Jemal A, Siegel R, Ward E, Hao Y, Xu J, Thun MJ. Cancer statistics, 2009. *CA Cancer J Clin* 2009;59:225–49.

32. Varkarakis MJ, Gaeta J, Moore RH, Murphy GP. Superficial bladder tumor. Aspects of clinical progression. *Urology* 1974;4: 414–20.

33. Lee LW, Davis E Jr. Gross urinary hemorrhage: a symptom, not a disease. *J Am Med Assoc* 1953;153:782–4.

34. Mohr DN, Offord KP, Owen RA, Melton LJ 3rd. Asymptomatic microhematuria and urologic disease. A population-based study. *JAMA* 1986;256:224–9.

35. Golin AL, Howard RS. Asymptomatic microscopic hematuria. *J Urol* 1980;124:389–91.

36. Malmstrom PU. Time to abandon testing for microscopic haematuria in adults? *BMJ* 2003;326:813–5.

37. Droller MJ. Bladder cancer: State-of-the-art care. *CA Cancer J Clin* 1998;48:269–84.

38. Cheng L, Montironi R, Davidson DD, Lopez-Beltran A. Staging and reporting of urothelial carcinoma of the urinary bladder. *Mod Pathol* 2009;22 (Suppl 2):S70–95.

39. Hoglund M. On the origin of syn- and metachronous urothelial carcinomas. *Eur Urol* 2007;51:1185–93; discussion 93.

40. Melamed M, Voutsa N, Grabstald H. Natural history and clinical behavior of in situ carcinoma of the human urinary bladder. *Cancer* 1964;17:1533–45.

41. Melicow M. Histological study of vesical urothelium intervening between gross neoplasms in total cytectomy. *J Urol* 1952;68:261–79.

42. Lopez-Beltran A, Cheng L, Andersson L, Brausi M, de Matteis A, Montironi R, Sesterhenn I, van det Kwast KT, Mazerolles C. Preneoplastic non-papillary lesions and conditions of the urinary bladder: an update based on the Ancona International Consultation. *Virchows Arch* 2002;440:3–11.

43. Cheng L, Neumann RM, Weaver AL, Cheville JC, Leibovich BC, Ramnani DM, Scherer BG, Nehra A, Zincke H, Bostwick DG. Grading and staging of bladder carcinoma in transurethral resection specimens. Correlation with 105 matched cystectomy specimens. *Am J Clin Pathol* 2000;113:275–9.

44. Cheng L, Neumann RM, Weaver AL, Spotts BE, Bostwick DG. Predicting cancer progression in patients with stage T1 bladder carcinoma. *J Clin Oncol* 1999;17:3182–7.

45. Cheng L, Weaver AL, Bostwick DG. Predicting extravesical extension of bladder carcinoma: a novel method based on micrometer measurement of the depth of invasion in transurethral resection specimens. *Urology* 2000;55:668–72.

46. Cheng L, Weaver AL, Leibovich BC, Ramnani DM, Neumann RM, Scherer BG, Nehra A, Zincke H, Bostwick DG. Predicting the survival of bladder carcinoma patients treated with radical cystectomy. *Cancer* 2000;88:2326–32.

47. Cheng L, Weaver AL, Neumann RM, Scherer BG, Bostwick DG. Substaging of T1 bladder carcinoma based on the depth of invasion as measured by micrometer. A new proposal. *Cancer* 1999;86:1035–43.

48. Epstein JI, Amin MB, Reuter VR, Mostofi FK. The World Health Organization/International Society of Urological Pathology consensus classification of urothelial (transitional cell) neoplasms of the urinary bladder. Bladder Consensus Conference Committee. *Am J Surg Pathol* 1998;22:1435–48.

49. Soloway MS. It is time to abandon the "superficial" in bladder cancer. *Eur Urol* 2007;52:1564–5.

50. van Rhijn BW, Burger M, Lotan Y, Solsona E, Stief CG, Sylvester RJ, Witjes JA, Zlotta AR. Recurrence and progression of disease in non-muscle-invasive bladder cancer:

from epidemiology to treatment strategy. *Eur Urol* 2009;56:430–42.

51. Cheng L, Zhang S, Davidson DD, MacLennan GT, Koch MO, Montironi R, Lopez-Beltran A. Molecular determinants of tumor recurrence in the urinary bladder. *Future Oncol* 2009;5:843–57.

52. Lopez-Beltran A, Jimenez RE, Montironi R, Patriarca C, Blanca A, Menendez C, Algaba F, Cheng L. Flat urothelial carcinoma in situ of the bladder with glandular differentiation. *Hum Pathol* 2011;42:1653–9.

53. Bostwick DG, Cheng L, eds. Urologic Surgical Pathology, 2nd ed. Philadelphia: Elsevier/Mosby, 2008.

54. Raghavan D, Shipley WU, Garnick MB, Russell PJ, Richie JP. Biology and management of bladder cancer. *N Engl J Med* 1990;322:1129–38.

55. Grossman HB, Soloway M, Messing E, Katz G, Stein B, Kassabian V, Shen Y. Surveillance for recurrent bladder cancer using a point-of-care proteomic assay. *JAMA* 2006;295:299–305.

56. Black PC, Brown GA, Dinney CP. Molecular markers of urothelial cancer and their use in the monitoring of superficial urothelial cancer. *J Clin Oncol* 2006;24:5528–35.

57. Wu XR. Urothelial tumorigenesis: a tale of divergent pathways. *Nat Rev Cancer* 2005;5:713–25.

58. Holmang S, Hedelin H, Anderstrom C, Johansson SL. The relationship among multiple recurrences, progression and prognosis of patients with stages Ta and T1 transitional cell cancer of the bladder followed for at least 20 years. *J Urol* 1995;153:1823–7.

59. Cheng L, Neumann RM, Nehra A, Spotts BE, Weaver AL, Bostwick DG. Cancer heterogeneity and its biologic implications in the grading of urothelial carcinoma. *Cancer* 2000;88:1663–70.

60. Cheng L, Zhang S, Alexander R, MacLennan GT, Hodges KB, Harrison BT, Lopez-Beltran A, Montironi R. Sarcomatoid carcinoma of the urinary bladder: the final common pathway of urothelial carcinoma dedifferentiation. *Am J Surg Pathol* 2011;35:e34–46.

61. Madgar I, Goldwasser B, Nativ O, Hanani Y, Jonas P. Long-term followup of patients less than 30 years old with transitional cell carcinoma of bladder. *J Urol* 1988;139:933–4.

62. McCarthy JP, Gavrell GJ, LeBlanc GA. Transitional cell carcinoma of bladder in patients under thirty years of age. *Urology* 1979;13:487–9.

63. Migaldi M, Rossi G, Maiorana A, Sartori G, Ferrari P, De Gaetani C, Cittadini A, Trentini GP, Sgambato A. Superficial papillary urothelial carcinomas in young and elderly patients: a comparative study. *BJU Int* 2004;94:311–6.

64. Yossepowitch O, Dalbagni G. Transitional cell carcinoma of the bladder in young adults: presentation, natural history and outcome. *J Urol* 2002;168:61–6.

65. Lopez JI, Angulo JC. The prognostic significance of vascular invasion in stage T1 bladder cancer. *Histopathology* 1995;27:27–33.

66. Lopez-Beltran A, Cheng L, Mazzucchelli R, Bianconi M, Blanca A, Scarpelli M, Montironi R. Morphological and molecular profiles and pathways in bladder neoplasms. *Anticancer Res* 2008;28:2893–900.

67. Lopez-Beltran A, Morales C, Reymundo C, Toro M. T-zone histiocytes and recurrence of papillary urothelial bladder carcinoma. *Urol Int* 1989;44:205–9.

68. Lutzeyer W, Rubben H, Dahm H. Prognostic parameters in superficial bladder cancer: an analysis of 315 cases. *J Urol* 1982;127:250–52.

69. Heney NM, Ahmed S, Flanagan MJ, Frable W, Corder MP, Hafermann MD, Hawkins IR. Superficial bladder cancer: progression and recurrence. *J Urol* 1983;130:1083–6.

70. Reading J, Hall RR, Parmar MK. The application of a prognostic factor analysis for Ta.T1 bladder cancer in routine urological practice. *Br J Urol* 1995;75:604–7.

71. Morris SB, Gordon EM, Shearer RJ, Woodhouse CR. Superficial bladder cancer: For how long should a tumour-free patient have check cystoscopies? *Br J Urol* 1995;75:193–6.

72. Coloby PJ, Kakizoe T, Tobisu K, Sakamoto M. Urethral involvement in

female bladder cancer patients: mapping of 47 consecutive cysto-urethrectomy specimens. *J Urol* 1994;152:1438–42.

73. Kiemeney LA, Witjes JA, Heijbroek RP, Debruyne FM, Verbeek AL. Dysplasia in normal-looking urothelium increases the risk of tumour progression in primary superficial bladder cancer. *Eur J Cancer* 1994;30A:1621–5.

74. Thrasher JB, Frazier HA, Robertson JE, Dodge RK, Paulson DF. Clinical variables which serve as predictors of cancer-specific survival among patients treated by radical cystectomy for transitional cell carcinoma of the bladder and prostate. *Cancer* 1994;73:1708–15.

75. Hammond EH, Henson DE. Practice protocol for the examination of specimens removed from patients with carcinoma of the urinary bladder, ureter, renal pelvis, and urethra. *Arch Pathol Lab Med* 1996;120:1103–10.

76. Deen S, Ball RY. Basement membrane and extracellular interstitial matrix components in bladder neoplasia—evidence of angiogenesis. *Histopathology* 1994;25:475–81.

77. Jaeger TM, Weidner N, Chew K, Moore DH, Kerschmann RL, Waldman FM, Carroll PR. Tumor angiogenesis correlates with lymph node metastases in invasive bladder cancer. *J Urol* 1995;154:69–71.

78. Solsona E, Iborra I, Ricos JV, Monros JL, Casanova JL, Almenar S. The prostate involvement as prognostic factor in patients with superficial bladder tumors. *J Urol* 1995;154:1710–3.

79. Sakamoto N, Tsuneyoshi M, Naito S, Kumazawa J. An adequate sampling of the prostate to identify prostatic involvement by urothelial carcinoma in bladder cancer patients. *J Urol* 1993;149:318–21.

80. Hardeman SW, Soloway MS. Transitional cell carcinoma of the prostate: diagnosis, staging, and management. *World J Urol* 1998;6:170–4.

81. Tobisu K, Tanaka Y, Mizutani T, Kakizoe T. Transitional cell carcinoma of the urethra in men following cystectomy for bladder

cancer: multivariate analysis for risk factors. *J Urol* 1991;146:1551–3; discussion 1553–4.

82. Cheville JC, Dundore PA, Bostwick DG, Lieber MM, Batts KP, Sebo TJ, Farrow GM. Transitional cell carcinoma of the prostate: clinicopathologic study of 50 cases. *Cancer* 1998;82:703–7.

83. Jones TD, Wang M, Eble JN, MacLennan GT, Lopez-Beltran A, Zhang S, Cocco A, Cheng L. Molecular evidence supporting field effect in urothelial carcinogenesis. *Clin Cancer Res* 2005;11:6512–9.

84. Koss LG, Tiamson EM, Robbins MA. Mapping cancerous and precancerous bladder changes. A study of the urothelium in ten surgically removed bladders. *JAMA* 1974;227:281–6.

85. Weinstein RS. Origin and dissemination of human urinary bladder carcinoma. *Semin Oncol* 1979;6:149–56.

86. Kiemeney LA, Witjes JA, Heijbroek RP, Verbeek AL, Debruyne FM. Predictability of recurrent and progressive disease in individual patients with primary superficial bladder cancer. *J Urol* 1993;150:60–4.

87. Mazzucchelli R, Barbisan F, Stramazzotti D, Montironi R, Lopez-Beltran A, Scarpelli M. Chromosomal abnormalities in macroscopically normal urothelium in patients with bladder pT1 and pT2a urothelial carcinoma: a fluorescence in situ hybridization study and correlation with histologic features. *Anal Quant Cytol Histol* 2005;27:143–51.

88. Cheng L, Cheville JC, Neumann RM, Bostwick DG. Flat intraepithelial lesions of the urinary bladder. *Cancer* 2000;88:625–31.

89. Cheng L, MacLennan GT, Pan CX, Jones TD, Moore CR, Zhang S, Gu J, Patel NB, Kao C, Gardner TA. Allelic loss of the active X chromosome during bladder carcinogenesis. *Arch Pathol Lab Med* 2004;128:187–90.

90. Davidson DD, Cheng L. Field cancerization in the urothelium of the bladder. *Anal Quant Cytol Histol* 2006;28:337–8.

91. Jones TD, Carr MD, Eble JN, Wang M, Lopez-Beltran A, Cheng L. Clonal origin of lymph node metastases in bladder carcinoma. *Cancer* 2005;104:1901–10.

92. Cheng L, Gu J, Ulbright TM, MacLennan GT, Sweeney CJ, Zhang S, Sanchez K, Koch MO, Eble JN. Precise microdissection of human bladder carcinomas reveals divergent tumor subclones in the same tumor. *Cancer* 2002;94:104–10.

93. Cheng L, Cheville JC, Neumann RM, Bostwick DG. Natural history of urothelial dysplasia of the bladder. *Am J Surg Pathol* 1999;23:443–7.

94. Paterson RF, Ulbright TM, MacLennan GT, Zhang S, Pan CX, Sweeney CJ, Moore CR, Foster RS, Koch MO, Eble JN, Cheng L. Molecular genetic alterations in the laser-capture-microdissected stroma adjacent to bladder carcinoma. *Cancer* 2003;98:1830–6.

95. Sidransky EA, Frost P, von Eschenbach A, Oyasu R, Preisinger AC, Vogelstein B. Clonal origin of bladder cancer. *N Engl J Med* 1992;326:737–40.

96. Habuchi T, Takahashi R, Yamada H, Kakehi Y, Sugiyama T, Yoshida O. Metachronous multifocal development of urothelial cancers by intraluminal seeding. *Lancet* 1993;342:1087–8.

97. Miyao N, Tsai YC, Lerner SP, Olumi AF, Spruck CHI, Goñzalez-Zulueta M, Nichols PW, Skinner DG, Jones PA. Role of chromosome 9 in human bladder cancer. *Cancer Res* 1993;53:4066–70.

98. Xu X, Stower MJ, Reid IN, Garner RC, Burns PA. Molecular screening of multifocal transitional cell carcinoma of the bladder using p53 mutations as biomarkers. *Clin Cancer Res* 1996;2:1795–800.

99. Chern HD, Becich MJ, Persad RA, Romkes M, Smith P, Collins C, Li YH, Branch RA. Clonal analysis of human recurrent superficial bladder cancer by immunohistochemistry of p53 and retinoblastoma proteins. *J Urol* 1996;156:1846–9.

100. Takahashi T, Kakehi Y, Mitsumori K, Akao T, Terachi T, Kato T, Ogawa O, Habuchi T. Distinct microsatellite alterations in upper urinary tract tumors and subsequent bladder tumors. *J Urol* 2001;165:672–7.

101. Takahashi T, Habuchi T, Kakehi Y, Mitsumori K, Akao T, Terachi T, Yoshida O. Clonal and chronological genetic analysis of multifocal cancers of the bladder and upper urinary tract. *Cancer Res* 1998;58:5835–41.

102. Li M, Cannizzaro LA. Identical clonal origin of synchronous and metachronous low grade, noninvasive papillary transitional cell carcinomas of the urinary tract. *Hum Pathol* 1999;30:1197–1200.

103. Fadl-Elmula I, Gorunova L, Mandahl N, Elfving P, Lundgren R, Mitelman F, Heim S. Cytogenetic monoclonality in multifocal uroepithelial carcinomas: evidence of intraluminal tumour seeding. *Br J Cancer* 1999;81:6–12.

104. Hartmann A, Rosner U, Schlake G, Dietmaier W, Zaak D, Hofstaedter F, Knuechel R. Clonality and genetic divergence in multifocal low grade superficial urothelial carcinoma as determined by chromosome 9 and p53 deletion analysis. *Lab Invest* 2000;80:709–18.

105. Hafner C, Knuechel R, Zanardo L, Dietmaier W, Blaszyk H, Cheville J, Hofstaedter F, Hartmann A. Evidence for oligoclonality and tumor spread by intraluminal seeding in multifocal urothelial carcinomas of the upper and lower urinary tract. *Oncogene* 2001;20:4910–5.

106. Simon R, Eltze E, Schafer KL, Burger H, Semjonow A, Hertle L, Dockhorn-Dworniczak B, Terpe HJ, Bocker W. Cytogenetic analysis of multifocal bladder cancer supports a monoclonal origin and intraepithelial spread of tumor cells. *Cancer Res* 2001;61:355–62.

107. Goto K, Konomoto T, Hayashi K, Kinukawa N, Naito S, Kumazawa J, Tsuneyoshi M. p53 mutations in multiple urothelial carcinomas: a molecular analysis of the development of multiple carcinomas. *Mod Pathol* 1997;10:428–37.

108. Spruck CH 3rd, Ohneseit PF, Gonzalez-Zulueta M, Esrig D, Miyao N, Tsai YC, Lerner SP, Schmutte C, Yang AS, Cote R, et al. Two molecular pathways to transitional cell carcinoma of the bladder. *Cancer Res* 1994;54:784–8.

109. Petersen I, Ohgaki H, Ludeke BI, Kleihues P. p53 mutations in phenacetin-associated human urothelial carcinomas. *Carcinogenesis* 1993;14:2119–22.

110. Hartmann A, Moser K, Kriegmair M, Hofstetter A, Hofstaedter F, Knuechel R. Frequent genetic alterations in simple urothelial hyperplasias of the bladder in patients with papillary urothelial carcinoma. *Am J Pathol* 1999;154:721–7.

111. Yoshimura I, Kudoh J, Saito S, Tazaki H, Shimizu N. p53 gene mutation in recurrent superficial bladder cancer. *J Urol* 1995;153:1711–5.

112. Stoehr R, Hartmann A, Hiendlmeyer E, Murle K, Wieland W, Knuechel R. Oligoclonality of early lesions of the urothelium as determined by microdissection-supported genetic analysis. *Pathobiology* 2000;68:165–72.

113. Hartmann A, Schlake G, Zaak D, Hungerhuber E, Hofstetter A, Hofstaedter F, Knuechel R. Occurrence of chromosome 9 and p53 alterations in multifocal dysplasia and carcinoma in situ of human urinary bladder. *Cancer Res* 2002;62:809–18.

114. Cianciulli AM, Leonardo C, Guadagni F, Marzano R, Iori F, De Nunzio C, Franco G, Merola R, Laurenti C. Genetic instability in superficial bladder cancer and adjacent mucosa: an interphase cytogenetic study. *Hum Pathol* 2003;34:214–21.

115. Junker K, Boerner D, Schulze W, Utting M, Schubert J, Werner W. Analysis of genetic alterations in normal bladder urothelium. *Urology* 2003;62:1134–8.

116. Hafner C, Knuechel R, Stoehr R, Hartmann A. Clonality of multifocal urothelial carcinomas: 10 years of molecular genetic studies. *Int J Cancer* 2002;101:1–6.

117. Cheng L, Alexander RE, Zhang S, Pan CX, MacLennan GT, Lopez-Beltran A, Montironi R. Clinical and therapeutic implications of cancer stem cell biology. *Exp Rev Anticancer Ther* 2011;11:1131–43.

118. Cheng L, Zhang S, Davidson DD, Montironi R, Lopez-Beltran A. Implications of cancer stem cells for cancer therapy. In: Bagley R, G, Teicher BA, eds. Cancer Drug Discovery and Development: Stem Cells and Cancer. New York: Humana Press/Springer, 2009;252–62.

119. Yang YM, Chang JW. Bladder cancer initiating cells (BCICs) are among EMA-CD44v6+ subset: novel methods for isolating undetermined cancer stem (initiating) cells. *Cancer Invest* 2008;26:725–33.

120. Ben-Porath I, Thomson MW, Carey VJ, Ge R, Bell GW, Regev A, Weinberg RA. An embryonic stem cell-like gene expression signature in poorly differentiated aggressive human tumors. *Nat Genet* 2008;40:499–507.

121. Sanchez-Carbayo M, Socci ND, Lozano J, Saint F, Cordon-Cardo C. Defining molecular profiles of poor outcome in patients with invasive bladder cancer using oligonucleotide microarrays. *J Clin Oncol* 2006;24:778–89.

122. Sung MT, Wang M, MacLennan GT, Eble JN, Tan PH, Lopez-Beltran A, Montironi R, Harris JJ, Kuhar M, Cheng L. Histogenesis of sarcomatoid urothelial carcinoma of the urinary bladder: evidence for a common clonal origin with divergent differentiation. *J Pathol* 2007;211:420–30.

123. Cheng L, Jones TD, McCarthy RP, Eble JN, Wang M, MacLennan GT, Lopez-Beltran A, Yang XJ, Koch MO, Zhang S, Pan CX, Baldridge LA. Molecular genetic evidence for a common clonal origin of urinary bladder small cell carcinoma and coexisting urothelial carcinoma. *Am J Pathol* 2005;166:1533–9.

124. Chan KS, Espinosa I, Chao M, Wong D, Ailles L, Diehn M, Gill H, Presti J Jr, Chang HY, van de Rijn M, Shortliffe L, Weissman IL. Identification, molecular characterization, clinical prognosis, and therapeutic targeting of human bladder tumor-initiating cells. *Proc Natl Acad Sci U S A* 2009;106:14016–21.

125. Braakhuis BJ, Tabor MP, Kummer JA, Leemans CR, Brakenhoff RH. A genetic explanation of Slaughter's concept of field cancerization: evidence and clinical implications. *Cancer Res* 2003;63:1727–30.

126. Dalbagni G, Presti J, Reuter V, Fair WR, Cordon-Cardo C. Genetic alterations in bladder cancer. *Lancet* 1993;342:469–71.

127. Knowles MA, Elder PA, Williamson M, Cairns JP, Shaw ME, Law MG. Allelotype of human bladder cancer. *Cancer Res* 1994;54:531–8.

128. Rosin MP, Cairns P, Epstein JI, Schoenberg MP, Sidransky D. Partial allelotype of carcinoma in situ of the human bladder. *Cancer Res* 1995;15:5213–6.

129. Cheng L, MacLennan GT, Zhang S, Wang M, Pan CX, Koch MO. Laser capture microdissection analysis reveals frequent allelic losses in papillary urothelial neoplasm of low malignant potential of the urinary bladder. *Cancer* 2004;101:183–8.

130. Sung MT, Lopez-Beltran A, Eble JN, MacLennan GT, Tan PH, Montironi R, Jones TD, Ulbright TM, Blair JE, Cheng L. Divergent pathway of intestinal metaplasia and cystitis glandularis of the urinary bladder. *Mod Pathol* 2006;19:1395–401.

131. Sung MT, Maclennan GT, Lopez-Beltran A, Zhang S, Montironi R, Cheng L. Primary mediastinal seminoma: a comprehensive assessment integrated with histology, immunohistochemistry, and fluorescence in situ hybridization for chromosome 12p abnormalities in 23 cases. *Am J Surg Pathol* 2008;32:146–55.

132. Jones TD, Zhang S, Lopez-Beltran A, Eble JN, Sung MT, MacLennan GT, Montironi R, Tan PH, Zheng S, Baldridge LA, Cheng L. Urothelial carcinoma with an inverted growth pattern can be distinguished from inverted papilloma by fluorescence in-situ hybridization, immunohistochemistry, and morphologic analysis. *Am J Surg Pathol* 2007;31:1861–7.

133. Cheng L, Bostwick DG, Li G, Zhang S, Vortmeyer AO, Zhuang Z. Conserved genetic findings in metastatic bladder cancer: a possible utility of allelic loss of chromosomes 9p21 and 17p13 in diagnosis. *Arch Pathol Lab Med* 2001;125:1197–9.

134. Sung MT, Eble JN, Wang M, Tan PH, Lopez-Beltran A, Cheng L. Inverted papilloma of the urinary bladder: a molecular genetic appraisal. *Mod Pathol* 2006;19:1289–94.

135. Houskova L, Zemanova Z, Babjuk M, Melichercikova J, Pesl M, Michalova K. Molecular cytogenetic characterization and diagnostics of bladder cancer. *Neoplasma* 2007;54:511–6.

136. Prat E, Bernues M, Caballin MR, Egozcue J, Gelabert A, Miro R. Detection of chromosomal imbalances in papillary bladder tumors by comparative genomic hybridization. *Urology* 2001;57:986–92.

137. Simon R, Burger H, Brinkschmidt C, Bocker W, Hertle L, Terpe HJ. Chromosomal aberrations associated with invasion in papillary superficial bladder cancer. *J Pathol* 1998;185:345–51.

138. Richter J, Wagner U, Schraml P, Maurer R, Alund G, Knonagel H, Moch H, Mihatsch MJ, Gasser TC, Sauter G. Chromosomal imbalances are associated with a high risk of progression in early invasive (pT1) urinary bladder cancer. *Cancer Res* 1999;59:5687–91.

139. Simon R, Burger H, Semjonow A, Hertle L, Terpe HJ, Bocker W. Patterns of chromosomal imbalances in muscle invasive bladder cancer. *Int J Oncol* 2000;17:1025–9.

140. Bruch J, Wohr G, Hautmann R, Mattfeldt T, Bruderlein S, Moller P, Sauter S, Hameister H, Vogel W, Paiss T. Chromosomal changes during progression of transitional cell carcinoma of the bladder and delineation of the amplified interval on chromosome arm 8q. *Genes Chromosomes Cancer* 1998;23:167–74.

141. Natrajan R, Louhelainen J, Williams S, Laye J, Knowles MA. High-resolution deletion mapping of 15q13.2-q21.1 in transitional cell carcinoma of the bladder. *Cancer Res* 2003;63:7657–62.

142. Shaw ME, Knowles MA. Deletion mapping of chromosome 11 in carcinoma of the bladder. *Genes Chromosomes Cancer* 1995;13:1–8.

143. Tsai YC, Nichols PW, Hiti AL, Williams Z, Skinner DG, Jones PA. Allelic losses of chromosomes 9, 11, and 17 in human bladder cancer. *Cancer Res* 1990;50:44–7.

144. Sandberg AA, Berger CS. Review of chromosome studies in urological tumors. II. Cytogenetics and molecular genetics of bladder cancer. *J Urol* 1994;151:545–60.

145. Seripa D, Parrella P, Gallucci M, Gravina C, Papa S, Fortunato P, Alcini A, Flammia G, Lazzari M, Fazio VM. Sensitive detection of transitional cell carcinoma of the bladder by microsatellite analysis of cells exfoliated in urine. *Int J Cancer* 2001;95:364–9.

146. Cairns P, Shaw ME, Knowles MA. Initiation of bladder cancer may involve deletion of a tumor suppressor gene on chromosome 9. *Oncogene* 1993;8:1083–5.

147. Linnenbach AJ, Pressler LB, Seng BA, Kimmel BS, Tomaszewski JE, Malkowicz SB. Characterization of chromosome 9 deletions in transitional cell carcinoma by microsatellite assay. *Hum Mol Genet* 1993;2:1407–11.

148. Lacy S, Lopez-Beltran A, MacLennan GT, Foster SR, Montironi R, Cheng L. Molecular pathogenesis of urothelial carcinoma: the clinical utility of emerging new biomarkers and future molecular classification of bladder cancer. *Anal Quan Cytol Histol* 2009;31:5–16.

149. Hartmann A, Zanardo L, Bocker-Edmonston T, Blaszyk H, Dietmaier W, Stoehr R, Cheville JC, Junker K, Wieland W, Knuechel R, Rueschoff J, Hofstaedter F, Fishel R. Frequent microsatellite instability in sporadic tumors of the upper urinary tract. *Cancer Res* 2002;62:6796–802.

150. Simoneau AR, Spruck CH 3rd, Gonzalez-Zulueta M, Gonzalgo ML, Chan MF, Tsai YC, Dean M, Steven K, Horn T, Jones PA. Evidence for two tumor suppressor loci associated with proximal chromosome 9p to q and distal chromosome 9q in bladder cancer and the initial screening for GAS1 and PTC mutations. *Cancer Res* 1996;56:5039–43.

151. Edwards J, Duncan P, Going JJ, Watters AD, Grigor KM, Bartlett JM. Identification of loci associated with putative recurrence genes in transitional cell carcinoma of the urinary bladder. *J Pathol* 2002;196:380–5.

152. Richter J, Jiang F, Gorog JP, Sartorius G, Egenter C, Gasser TC, Moch H, Mihatsch MJ, Sauter G. Marked genetic differences between stage pTa and stage pT1 papillary bladder cancer detected by comparative genomic hybridization. *Cancer Res* 1997;57:2860–4.

153. Fadl-Elmula I, Gorunova L, Mandahl N, Elfving P, Lundgren R, Mitelman F, Heim S. Karyotypic characterization of urinary bladder transitional cell carcinomas. *Genes Chromosomes Cancer* 2000;29:256–65.

154. Ruppert JM, Tokino K, Sidransky D. Evidence for two bladder cancer suppressor loci on human chromosome 9. *Cancer Res* 1993;53:5093–5.

155. Bakkar AA, Wallerand H, Radvanyi F, Lahaye JB, Pissard S, Lecerf L, Kouyoumdjian JC, Abbou CC, Pairon JC, Jaurand MC, Thiery JP, Chopin DK, de Medina SG. FGFR3 and TP53 gene mutations define two distinct pathways in urothelial cell carcinoma of the bladder. *Cancer Res* 2003;63:8108–12.

156. van Rhijn BW, van der Kwast TH, Vis AN, Kirkels WJ, Boeve ER, Jobsis AC, Zwarthoff EC. FGFR3 and p53 characterize alternative genetic pathways in the pathogenesis of urothelial cell carcinoma. *Cancer Res* 2004;64:1911–4.

157. Lamy A, Gobet F, Laurent M, Blanchard F, Varin C, Moulin C, Andreou A, Frebourg T, Pfister C. Molecular profiling of bladder tumors based on the detection of FGFR3 and TP53 mutations. *J Urol* 2006;176:2686–9.

158. Mhawech-Fauceglia P, Cheney RT, Fischer G, Beck A, Herrmann FR. FGFR3 and p53 protein expressions in patients with pTa and pT1 urothelial bladder cancer. *Eur J Surg Oncol* 2006;32:231–7.

159. Richter J, Beffa L, Wagner U, Schraml P, Gasser TC, Moch H, Mihatsch MJ, Sauter G. Patterns of chromosomal imbalances in advanced urinary bladder cancer detected by comparative genomic hybridization. *Am J Pathol* 1998;153:1615–21.

160. Koga F, Kawakami S, Fujii Y, Saito K, Ohtsuka Y, Iwai A, Ando N, Takizawa T, Kageyama Y, Kihara K. Impaired p63 expression associates with poor prognosis and uroplakin III

expression in invasive urothelial carcinoma of the bladder. *Clin Cancer Res* 2003;9:5501–7.

161. Helpap B, Schmitz-Drager BJ, Hamilton PW, Muzzonigro G, Galosi AB, Kurth KH, Lubaroff D, Waters DJ, Droller MJ. Molecular pathology of non-invasive urothelial carcinomas (part I). *Virchows Arch* 2003;442:309–16.

162. Chatterjee SJ, Datar R, Youssefzadeh D, George B, Goebell PJ, Stein JP, Young L, Shi SR, Gee C, Groshen S, Skinner DG, Cote RJ. Combined effects of p53, p21, and pRb expression in the progression of bladder transitional cell carcinoma. *J Clin Oncol* 2004;22:1007–13.

163. Malats N, Bustos A, Nascimento CM, Fernandez F, Rivas M, Puente D, Kogevinas M, Real FX. P53 as a prognostic marker for bladder cancer: a meta-analysis and review. *Lancet Oncol* 2005;6:678–86.

164. Olumi AF, Tsai YC, Nichols PW, Skinner DG, Cain DR, Bender LL, Jones PA. Allelic loss of chromosome 17p distinguishes high grade from low grade transitional cell carcinomas of the bladder. *Cancer Res* 1990;50:7081–3.

165. Li M, Zhang ZF, Reuter VE, Cordon-Cardo C. Chromosome 3 allelic losses and microsatellite alterations in transitional cell carcinoma of the urinary bladder. *Am J Pathol* 1996;149:229–35.

166. Sidransky D, Messing E. Molecular genetics and biochemical mechanisms in bladder cancer. Oncogenes, tumor suppressor genes, and growth factors. *Urol Clin North Am* 1992;19:629–39.

167. Langbein S, Szakacs O, Wilhelm M, Sukosd F, Weber S, Jauch A, Lopez Beltran A, Alken P, Kalble T, Kovacs G. Alteration of the LRP1B gene region is associated with high grade of urothelial cancer. *Lab Invest* 2002;82:639–43.

168. Cappellen D, Gil Diez de Medina S, Chopin D, Thiery JP, Radvanyi F. Frequent loss of heterozygosity on chromosome 10q in muscle-invasive transitional cell carcinomas of the bladder. *Oncogene* 1997;14:3059–66.

169. Chang F, Syrjanen S, Syrjanen K. Implications of the p53 tumor-suppressor gene in clinical oncology. *J Clin Oncol* 1995;13:1009–22.

170. Brewster SF, Gingell JC, Browne S, Brown KW. Loss of heterozygosity on chromosome 18q is associated with muscle-invasive transitional cell carcinoma of the bladder. *Br J Cancer* 1994;70:697–700.

171. Bohm M, Kirch H, Otto T, Rubben H, Wieland I. Deletion analysis at the DEL–27, APC and MTS1 loci in bladder cancer: LOH at the DEL–27 locus on 5p13–12 is a prognostic marker of tumor progression. *Int J Cancer* 1997;74:291–5.

172. Edwards J, Duncan P, Going JJ, Grigor KM, Watters AD, Bartlett JM. Loss of heterozygosity on chromosomes 11 and 17 are markers of recurrence in TCC of the bladder. *Br J Cancer* 2001;85:1894–9.

173. Celis JE, Celis P, Palsdottir H, Ostergaard M, Gromov P, Primdahl H, Orntoft TF, Wolf H, Celis A, Gromova I. Proteomic strategies to reveal tumor heterogeneity among urothelial papillomas. *Mol Cell Proteomics* 2002;1:269–79.

174. Lee YL, Shih MC, Wu WJ, Chou YH, Huang CH. Clinical and urographic presentation of transitional cell carcinoma of the ureter in a blackfoot disease endemic area in southern Taiwan. *Kaohsiung J Med Sci* 2002;18:443–9.

175. Simon R, Struckmann K, Schraml P, Wagner U, Forster T, Moch H, Fijan A, Bruderer J, Wilber K, Mihatsch MJ, Gasser T, Sauter G. Amplification pattern of 12q13-q15 genes (MDM2, CDK4, GLI) in urinary bladder cancer. *Oncogene* 2002;21:2476–83.

176. Jacobs BL, Lee CT, Montie JE. Bladder cancer in 2010: How far have we come? *CA Cancer J Clin* 2010;60:244–72.

177. Hanahan D, Weinberg RA. The hallmarks of cancer. *Cell* 2000;100:57–70.

178. Wallerand H, Bernhard JC, Culine S, Ballanger P, Robert G, Reiter RE, Ferriere JM, Ravaud A. Targeted therapies in non-muscle-invasive bladder cancer according to the signaling pathways. *Urol Oncol* 2011;29:4–11.

179. Iyer G, Milowsky MI, Bajorin DF. Novel strategies for treating relapsed/refractory urothelial carcinoma. *Expert Rev Anticancer Ther* 2010;10:1917–32.

180. Pan CX, Zhang H, Lara PN, Cheng L. Small-cell carcinoma of the urinary bladder: diagnosis and management. *Expert Rev Anticancer Ther* 2006;6:1707–13.

181. Black PC, Agarwal PK, Dinney CP. Targeted therapies in bladder cancer—an update. *Urol Oncol* 2007;25:433–8.

182. Chen M, Cassidy A, Gu J, Delclos GL, Zhen F, Yang H, Hildebrandt M, Lin J, Ye Y, Chamberlain RM, Dinney CP, Wu X. Genetic variations in PI3K-AKT-mTOR pathway and bladder cancer risk. *Carcinogenesis* 2009.

183. Pant-Purohit M, Lopez-Beltran A, Montironi R, MacLennan GT, Cheng L. Small cell carcinoma of the urinary bladder. *Histol Histopathol* 2010;25:217–21.

184. Chow NH, Chan SH, Tzai TS, Ho CL, Liu HS. Expression profiles of ErbB family receptors and prognosis in primary transitional cell carcinoma of the urinary bladder. *Clin Cancer Res* 2001;7:1957–62.

185. Turkeri LN, Erton ML, Cevik I, Akdas A. Impact of the expression of epidermal growth factor, transforming growth factor alpha, and epidermal growth factor receptor on the prognosis of superficial bladder cancer. *Urology* 1998;51:645–9.

186. Dominguez-Escrig JL, Kelly JD, Neal DE, King SM, Davies BR. Evaluation of the therapeutic potential of the epidermal growth factor receptor tyrosine kinase inhibitor gefitinib in preclinical models of bladder cancer. *Clin Cancer Res* 2004;10:4874–84.

187. Nutt JE, Lazarowicz HP, Mellon JK, Lunec J. Gefitinib ('Iressa', ZD1839) inhibits the growth response of bladder tumour cell lines to epidermal growth factor and induces TIMP2. *Br J Cancer* 2004;90:1679–85.

188. Prewett M, Rockwell P, Rockwell RF, Giorgio NA, Mendelsohn J, Scher HI, Goldstein NI. The biologic effects of C225, a chimeric monoclonal antibody to the EGFR, on human prostate carcinoma. *J Immunother Emphasis Tumor Immunol* 1996;19:419–27.

189. Mendelsohn J. Targeting the epidermal growth factor receptor for cancer therapy. *J Clin Oncol* 2002;20:1S–13S.

190. Cheng L, Zhang S, Alexander R, Yao Y, Maclennan GT, Pan CX, Huang J, Wang M, Montironi R, Lopez-Beltran A. The landscape of EGFR pathways and personalized management of non-small-cell lung cancer. *Future Oncol* 2011;7:519–41.

191. Birkhahn M, Mitra AP, Williams AJ, Lam G, Ye W, Datar RH, Balic M, Groshen S, Steven KE, Cote RJ. Predicting recurrence and progression of noninvasive papillary bladder cancer at initial presentation based on quantitative gene expression profiles. *Eur Urol* 2009;57:12–20.

192. Xia G, Kumar SR, Hawes D, Cai J, Hassanieh L, Groshen S, Zhu S, Masood R, Quinn DI, Broek D, Stein JP, Gill PS. Expression and significance of vascular endothelial growth factor receptor 2 in bladder cancer. *J Urol* 2006;175:1245–52.

193. Youssef RF, Mitra AP, Bartsch G Jr, Jones PA, Skinner DG, Cote RJ. Molecular targets and targeted therapies in bladder cancer management. *World J Urol* 2009;27:9–20.

194. Sonpavde G, Jian W, Liu H, Wu MF, Shen SS, Lerner SP. Sunitinib malate is active against human urothelial carcinoma and enhances the activity of cisplatin in a preclinical model. *Urol Oncol* 2009;27:391–9.

195. Knowles MA. Novel therapeutic targets in bladder cancer: mutation and expression of FGF receptors. *Future Oncol* 2008;4:71–83.

196. Fitzgerald JM, Ramchurren N, Rieger K, Levesque P, Silverman M, Libertino JA, Summerhayes IC. Identification of H-ras mutations in urine sediments complements cytology in the detection of bladder tumors. *J Natl Cancer Inst* 1995;87:129–33.

197. Boulalas I, Zaravinos A, Karyotis I, Delakas D, Spandidos DA. Activation of RAS family genes in urothelial carcinoma. *J Urol* 2009;181:2312–9.

198. Qing J, Du X, Chen Y, Chan P, Li H, Wu P, Marsters S, Stawicki S, Tien J, Totpal K, Ross S, Stinson S, Dornan D, French D, Wang QR, Stephan JP, Wu Y, Wiesmann C, Ashkenazi A. Antibody-based targeting of FGFR3 in bladder carcinoma and t(4;14)-positive multiple myeloma in mice. *J Clin Invest* 2009;119:1216–29.

199. Shariat SF, Chade DC, Karakiewicz PI, Ashfaq R, Isbarn H, Fradet Y, Bastian PJ, Nielsen ME, Capitanio U, Jeldres C, Montorsi F, Lerner SP, Sagalowsky AI, Cote RJ, Lotan Y. Combination of multiple molecular markers can improve prognostication in patients with locally advanced and lymph node positive bladder cancer. *J Urol* 2010;183:68–75.

200. Shariat SF, Youssef RF, Gupta A, Chade DC, Karakiewicz PI, Isbarn H, Jeldres C, Sagalowsky AI, Ashfaq R, Lotan Y. Association of angiogenesis related markers with bladder cancer outcomes and other molecular markers. *J Urol* 2010;183:1744–50.

201. Bentley J, L'Hote C, Platt F, Hurst CD, Lowery J, Taylor C, Sak SC, Harnden P, Knowles MA, Kiltie AE. Papillary and muscle invasive bladder tumors with distinct genomic stability profiles have different DNA repair fidelity and KU DNA-binding activities. *Genes Chromosomes Cancer* 2009;48:310–21.

202. Kuball J, Wen SF, Leissner J, Atkins D, Meinhardt P, Quijano E, Engler H, Hutchins B, Maneval DC, Grace MJ, Fritz MA, Storkel S, Thuroff JW, Huber C, Schuler M. Successful adenovirus-mediated wild-type p53 gene transfer in patients with bladder cancer by intravesical vector instillation. *J Clin Oncol* 2002;20:957–65.

203. Cheng JC, Matsen CB, Gonzales FA, Ye W, Greer S, Marquez VE, Jones PA, Selker EU. Inhibition of DNA methylation and reactivation of silenced genes by zebularine. *J Natl Cancer Inst* 2003;95:399–409.

204. Cote RJ, Laird PW, Datar RH. Promoter hypermethylation: a new therapeutic target emerges in urothelial cancer. *J Clin Oncol* 2005;23:2879–81.

Chapter 9

Grading of Bladder Cancer

Bladder Pathology, First Edition. Liang Cheng, Antonio Lopez-Beltran, David G. Bostwick.
© 2012 Wiley-Blackwell. Published 2012 by John Wiley & Sons, Inc.

Pathologic Classification and Grading of Urothelial Carcinoma: An Overview

Urothelial carcinoma of the bladder is the second most common malignancy of the genitourinary system, after prostate cancer.[1,2] It represents a diverse group of diseases with various morphologic and biologic manifestations (**Fig. 9-1**). Two predominant diagnostic categories are assigned based on the presence or absence of stromal invasion: noninvasive papillary urothelial carcinoma and invasive urothelial carcinoma. The majority of bladder cancer patients have a relatively indolent, low grade tumor confined to the superficial mucosa. Despite the relatively indolent nature of these tumors, the recurrence rate may be as high as 70%, thus necessitating long-term followup.[3,4] In addition, about one-third of recurrent tumors eventually progress to a higher grade or stage. The most important predictors of progression are histologic grade, multiplicity of tumors, early recurrence, and tumor size. The presence of dysplasia or carcinoma in situ (CIS) in the adjacent urothelium is an especially ominous feature (see **Chapters 6 and 7**).[3-13]

The topic of classification and grading for noninvasive papillary neoplasia has been debated and should be considered unsettled.[14-17] The 1973 World Health Organization (WHO) classification is preferred by some authors because it allows comparison of results between different clinical centers. It is a robust, clinically proven, widely used, time tested, and reasonably reproducible method for pathologic reporting of bladder tumors, and therefore is still recommended. The 1998 WHO/International Society of Urological Pathology (ISUP) classification of bladder tumors was controversial, mainly because it had no validation, reproducibility, and translation studies.[16,18-32] In particular, there is poor interobserver agreement for papillary urothelial neoplasm of low malignant potential (PUNLMP) and low grade urothelial carcinoma, two new categories in the 2004 system.[15-17,33,34] Use of both the 1973 and 2004 WHO classifications (former 1998 ISUP/WHO) have been recommended.[5,15,17,19,35] In this chapter we also propose a new grading scheme based on cumulative data, combining the features of the 1973 and 2004 WHO grading systems (**Fig. 9-2; Table 9-1**).

Because of the subjective nature of histologic grading, some have questioned whether better descriptive morphology and criteria would be the best approach for grading urothelial neoplasia.[36] Incorporation of biomarker expression and molecular findings into the grading process may be a more objective and quantitative measure of clinical outcome. The fibroblast growth factor receptor 3 (*FGFR3*) mutations are usually present in low grade papillary carcinomas, whereas high grade urothelial carcinomas are characterized by *TP53* mutation. *TP53* mutations are almost

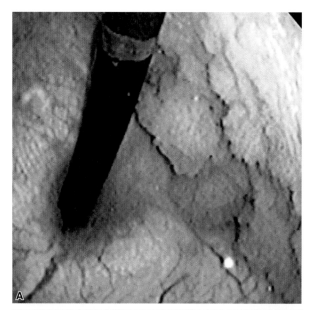

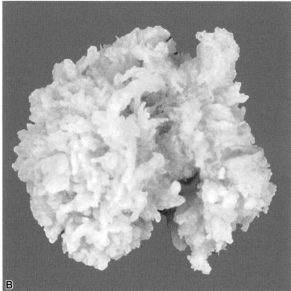

Figure 9-1 Noninvasive papillary urothelial carcinoma. Note the broad-based tumor cystoscopically (A) and macroscopically (B). (Photo courtesy of Dr. Koch.)

always mutually exclusive of *FGFR3* mutations, a fact that could potentially be exploited as a tool for the molecular grading of bladder cancer (see also **Chapters 29 to 34**).[4,6,37]

Histologic Grading According to the 1973 WHO Classification

Histologic grading is one of the most important prognostic factors in bladder cancer. The first widely accepted

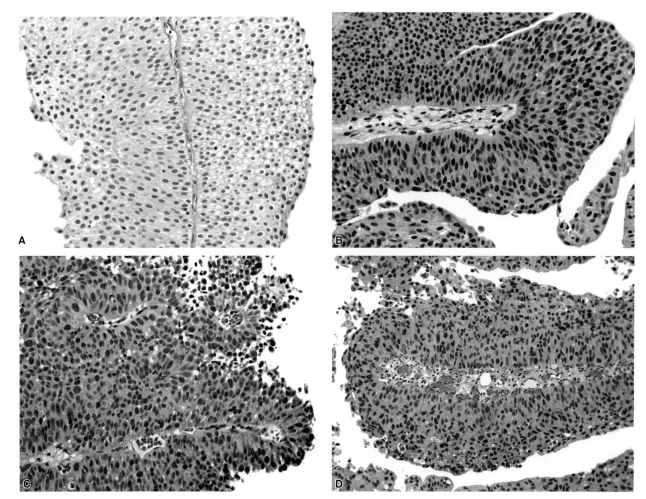

Figure 9-2 Newly proposed grading system (grades 1 to 4). (A) Grade 1 urothelial carcinoma (low grade); (B) grade 2 urothelial carcinoma (low grade); (C) grade 3 urothelial carcinoma (high grade); (D) grade 4 urothelial carcinoma (high grade) (discussed later in this chapter).

Table 9-1   Grading of Urothelial Carcinoma of the Urinary Bladder[a]

1973 WHO	1998 WHO/ISUP	1999 WHO	2004 WHO	Current Proposal
Papilloma	Papilloma	Papilloma	Papilloma	Papilloma
Grade 1	PUNLMP	PUNLMP	PUNLMP	Grade 1 (low grade)
Grade 2	Low grade	Grade 1 Grade 2	Low grade	Grade 2 (low grade) Grade 3 (high grade)
Grade 3	High grade	Grade 3	High grade	Grade 4 (high grade)

[a]All the grading schemes have substantial inter- and intraobserver variabilities. There is no exact correlation between different grading systems. WHO, World Health Organization; IUSP, International Society of Urological Pathology; PUNLMP, papillary urothelial neoplasm of low malignant potential.

grading system for papillary urothelial neoplasms was the WHO (1973) classification system, which divided urothelial tumors into four categories: papilloma, grade 1 carcinoma, grade 2 carcinoma, and grade 3 carcinoma.[38] Histologic grading is based on the degree of cellular anaplasia, with grade 1 tumors having the least degree of anaplasia compatible with a diagnosis of malignancy, and grade 3 tumors having the most severe degree of anaplasia.[38] Morphologic criteria for grading were quite detailed in the original 1973 WHO classification. Anaplasia was defined by the authors of the 1973 WHO classification as increased cellularity, nuclear crowding, disturbed cellular polarity, failure of differentiation from the base to the surface, nuclear polymorphism, irregular cell size, variation in nuclear shape and chromatin pattern, displaced or abnormal mitotic figures, and giant cells.[38]

Urothelial Papilloma

Urothelial papilloma is a benign exophytic neoplasm composed of a delicate fibrovascular core covered by normal-appearing urothelium (**Fig. 9-3**; see also **Chapter 5**).[22] The superficial cells are often prominent. Mitoses are absent or, if present, located in the basal cell layer. The stroma may show edema and inflammatory cells.[22] Papillomas are diploid with low proliferation, uncommon p53 expression, and frequent *FGFR3* (75%) mutation. Cytokeratin (CK) 20 expression is limited to the superficial (umbrella) cells as in normal urothelium. The incidence is below 1% of all bladder tumors and the male-to-female ratio is 1.9 : 1. Hematuria is common. Most papillomas are single and occur in younger patients (mean age, 46 years), close to the ureteric orifices. Urothelial papillomas may recur but do not progress.

Grade 1 Urothelial Carcinoma

Grade 1 papillary urothelial carcinoma consists of an orderly arrangement of normal urothelial cells lining delicate papillae with minimal architectural abnormality and minimal nuclear atypia (**Figs. 9-4** to **9-6**). Nuclear grooves are usually present. There may be some complexity and fusion of the papillae, but this is usually not prominent. The urothelium is often thickened to more than seven cell layers. There is normal maturation and cohesiveness, with an intact superficial cell layer. The nuclei tend to be uniform in shape and spacing, although there may be some enlargement and elongation. The chromatin texture is finely granular, without nucleolar enlargement. Mitotic figures are rare and basally located. Grade 1 tumor should be distinguished from urothelial papilloma, which is a benign lesion without invasive potential or risk of progression (see also **Chapter 5**).

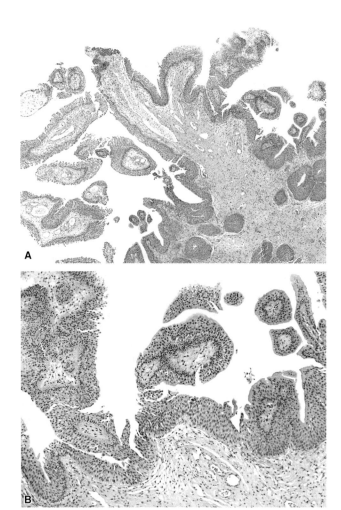

Figure 9-3   Urothelial papilloma (A and B).

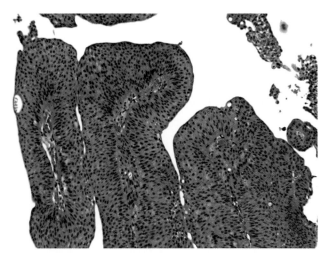

Figure 9-4   Grade 1 urothelial carcinoma, 1973 WHO classification.

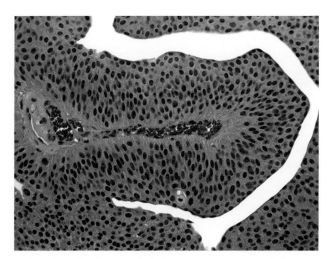

Figure 9-5 Grade 1 urothelial carcinoma, 1973 WHO classification.

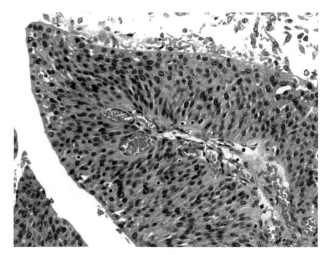

Figure 9-6 Grade 1 urothelial carcinoma, 1973 WHO classification.

Grade 1 urothelial carcinoma appears to have a predilection for the ureteric orifices. In one study, 69% of grade 1 urothelial carcinomas were centered near a ureteric orifice but the remainder was seen in all other portions of the bladder. Patients with grade 1 urothelial carcinoma are at increased risk of local recurrence, progression, and dying of bladder cancer. Significant morbidity and mortality are associated with grade 1 urothelial carcinoma of the bladder if patients are followed for a sufficient interval.[39-52] With 20 years of followup, Holmang et al.[41] found that 14% of patients with noninvasive grade 1 urothelial carcinoma (pTa G1) died of bladder cancer. In a recent review of 152 patients with stage Ta grade 1 urothelial carcinoma, Leblanc et al. found that 83 patients (55%) had tumor recurrence, including 37% with cancer progression.[43] Patients who remained tumor-free for one year still had

a 43% chance of late recurrence. In Greene et al.'s study of 100 patients with grade 1 urothelial carcinoma, 10 patients (10%) died of bladder cancer after more than 15 years; of 73 patients who had recurrences, 22% were of higher grade than the original tumor.[53] The mean interval from diagnosis to development of invasive cancer was eight years. Jordan et al. studied 91 patients with grade 1 papillary urothelial tumors and found that 40% of them had recurrence. Twenty percent of patients with recurrences developed high grade (grade 3) cancer, and four patients (4%) died of bladder cancer.[51] Long-term followup is recommended for patients with grade 1 papillary urothelial carcinoma.

Grade 2 Urothelial Carcinoma

Grade 2 urothelial carcinoma represents a broad group of tumors encompassing a spectrum of cytologic atypia and some variability in the relative proportion of cells with atypical features. Grade 2 urothelial carcinomas retain some of the overall maturation of grade 1 carcinoma, but also display at least focal moderate variation in polarity, nuclear appearance, and chromatin texture apparent at low magnification (**Figs. 9-7** to **9-9**). Cytologic abnormalities are invariably present in grade 2 urothelial carcinoma, with moderate nuclear crowding, moderate loss of cell polarity, moderate nuclear hyperchromasia, moderate anisonucleosis, and mild nucleolar enlargement. Mitotic figures are usually limited to the lower one-half of the urothelium, but may focally rise higher. Superficial cells are usually present, and the urothelial cells are predominantly cohesive, although variation in cohesion may be present. Some tumors may be extremely orderly, reminiscent of grade 1 urothelial carcinoma, with only a small focus of obvious disorder or

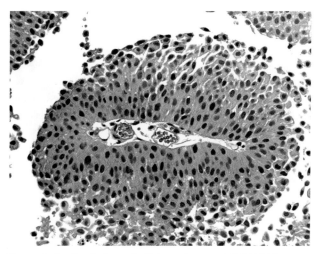

Figure 9-7 Grade 2 urothelial carcinoma, 1973 WHO classification.

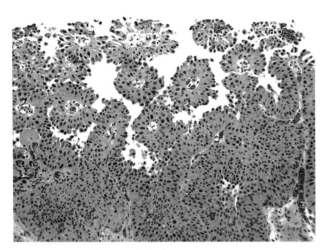

Figure 9-8 Grade 2 urothelial carcinoma, 1973 WHO classification.

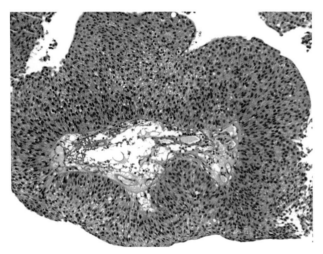

Figure 9-9 Grade 2 urothelial carcinoma, 1973 WHO classification.

atypia. These are considered grade 2 urothelial cancer, recognizing that tumor grade is based on the highest level of abnormality present.

The prognosis for patients with grade 2 urothelial carcinoma is significantly worse than for those with lower grade papillary cancer.[18,54,55] Recurrence risk for patients with noninvasive grade 2 urothelial carcinoma is 45% to 67%.[18,54,55] Invasion occurs in up to 20% and cancer-specific death is expected in 13% to 20% following surgical treatment. Patients with grade 2 urothelial carcinoma and lamina propria invasion are at even greater risk, with recurrences in 67% to 80% of cases, the development of muscle invasive cancer in 21% to 49%, and cancer-specific death in 17% to 51% of those treated surgically.[18,54,55] Some authors consider both nuclear pleomorphism and mitotic count as criteria for subdividing

grade 2 urothelial carcinoma (grades 2A and 2B), and they have been successful in identifying groups of cancers with different outcomes.[14,56–59] However, subclassification of grade 2 urothelial carcinoma is not recommended, due to significant interobserver variability.

Grade 3 Urothelial Carcinoma

Grade 3 urothelial carcinoma displays the most extreme nuclear abnormality of any papillary urothelial cancer, similar to changes observed in urothelial CIS (**Figs. 9-10** to **9-12**; see also **Chapter 7**). The obvious urothelial disorder and loss of polarity is present at scanning magnification. The superficial cell layer is partially or completely absent, and grade 3 urothelial carcinoma is accompanied by prominent cellular discohesion. There

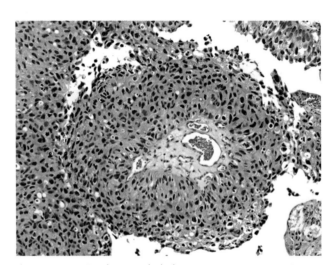

Figure 9-10 Grade 3 urothelial carcinoma, 1973 WHO classification.

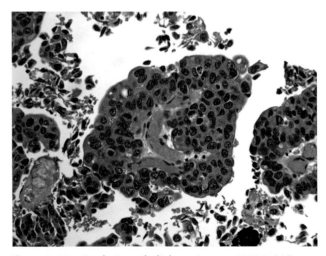

Figure 9-11 Grade 3 urothelial carcinoma, 1973 WHO classification.

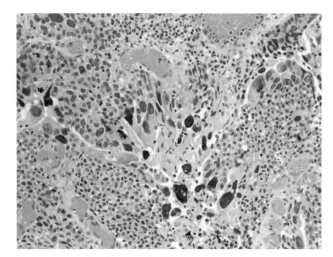

Figure 9-12 Grade 3 urothelial carcinoma, 1973 WHO classification.

is obvious loss of normal architecture and cell polarity, and frequent atypical mitotic figures. Cellular anaplasia, characteristic of grade 3 urothelial carcinoma, is defined as increased cellularity, nuclear crowding, random cellular polarity, absence of normal mucosal differentiation, nuclear pleomorphism, irregularity in cell size, variation in nuclear shape, capricious chromatin pattern, increased frequency of mitotic figures, and occasional neoplastic giant cells.[38] Recurrence risk for patients with noninvasive grade 3 urothelial carcinoma is 65% to 85%, with invasion occurring in 20% to 52% and cancer-specific death in up to 35% following surgical treatment.[54,60] Of surgically treated patients with grade 3 urothelial carcinoma and lamina propria invasion, 46% to 71% develop recurrences, 24% to 48% develop muscle invasive cancer, and 25% to 71% suffer cancer-specific death, emphasizing a need for aggressive treatment of these patients.[18,19,55]

Histologic Grading According to the 1998 ISUP/2004 WHO Classification

The first widely accepted grading system for papillary urothelial neoplasms was the 1973 WHO classification system.[38] In 1998, a revised system of classifying noninvasive papillary urothelial neoplasms of the urinary bladder was proposed.[21] This system was subsequently formally adopted by the WHO. In 2004, a classification system for noninvasive papillary urothelial neoplasms, identical to the 1998 WHO/ISUP classification system, was adopted in Pathology and Genetics of Tumours of the Urinary System and Male Genital Organs, one of the WHO "Blue Books" for the classification of tumors.[61] This new system separates noninvasive papillary urothelial neoplasms into four

categories: papilloma, PUNLMP, low grade carcinoma, and high grade carcinoma. The recommendations in this book reflect the views of a Working Group of urologic pathologists assembled at an Editorial and Consensus Conference held in Lyon, France, in December 2002. Their findings and recommendations were stated to be a work in progress.[61]

Urothelial Papilloma

The diagnostic criteria and terminology are identical to those of the 1973 WHO classification.[22,38] (See the previous section and **Chapter 5** for further discussion.)

Papillary Urothelial Neoplasm of Low Malignant Potential

PUNLMP is a low grade urothelial tumor with a papillary architecture and a purported low incidence of recurrence and progression.[15,16,19,62–65] This lesion is defined histologically by the 2004 WHO classification system as a papillary urothelial tumor that resembles the exophytic urothelial papilloma, but with increased cellular proliferation exceeding the thickness of normal urothelium (**Fig. 9-13**). All such tumors would be grade 1 urothelial carcinomas by the 1973 WHO grading system. Cytologic atypia is minimal or absent and architectural abnormalities are slight with preserved polarity. Mitotic figures are infrequent and usually limited to the basal layer. Clinically, these tumors show a male predominance (3 : 1) and occur at a mean age of 65 years.[66] They are most commonly identified during investigation of gross or microscopic hematuria. Cystoscopically, these lesions are typically 1 to 2 cm in greatest dimension, and located on the lateral wall of the bladder or near the ureteric orifices.[66] They have been described as having a "seaweed in the ocean" appearance.

See the following section for further discussion.

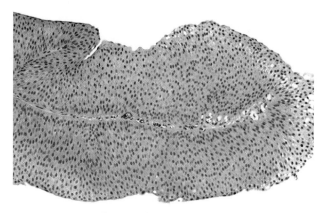

Figure 9-13 Papillary urothelial neoplasm of low malignant potential, 2004 WHO classification.

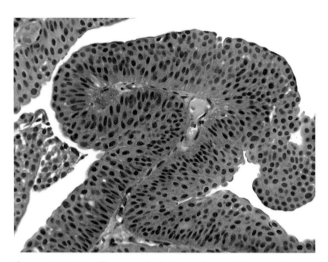

Figure 9-14   Papillary urothelial neoplasm of low malignant potential, 2004 WHO classification.

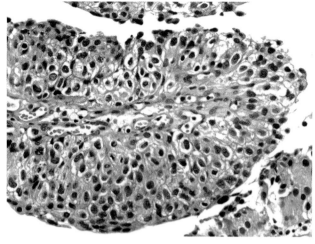

Figure 9-15   High grade urothelial carcinoma, 2004 WHO classification.

Low Grade Urothelial Carcinoma

Low grade papillary urothelial carcinoma shows fronds with recognizable variation in architecture and cytology (**Fig. 9-14**).[19,61] The tumor consists of slender papillae with frequent branching and variation in nuclear polarity. The nuclei show enlargement and irregularity with vesicular chromatin, and nucleoli are often present. Mitotic figures may occur at any level in low grade papillary urothelial carcinoma. Such cases would have been considered grade 1 or grade 2 in the 1973 WHO classification schema. Altered expression of CK20, CD44, p53, and p63 is frequent. Some tumors are diploid, but aneuploidy is the rule. *FGFR3* mutations are seen with about the same frequency as in PUNLMP.[19,61] The male-to-female ratio is 2.9 : 1 and the mean age is 70 years (range, 28 to 90 years). Most patients present with hematuria and have a single tumor in the posterior or lateral bladder wall. However, 22% of patients with low grade papillary urothelial carcinoma have two or more tumors. Tumor recurrence, stage progression, and tumor related mortality are 50%, 10%, 13%, and 5%, respectively. In another series of 215 patients with low grade noninvasive papillary urothelial carcinoma, 17 patients (8%) had grade or stage progression, and one patient (0.5%) died of bladder cancer.[67] Grade and stage progression occurred in 18% and 7% of patients, respectively, in another study.[68]

High Grade Urothelial Carcinoma

In high grade papillary urothelial carcinoma, the cells lining the papillary fronds show obviously disordered arrangement with cytologic atypia (**Figs. 9-15** and **9-16**). All tumors classified as grade 3 in the 1973 WHO schema, as well as some tumors assigned grade 2 in

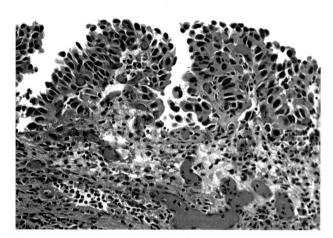

Figure 9-16   High grade urothelial carcinoma, 2004 WHO classification.

that classification, would be considered high grade carcinoma in the 2004 WHO classification. The papillae are frequently fused. Both architectural and cytologic abnormalities are recognizable at scanning power.[19] The nuclei are pleomorphic with prominent nucleoli and altered polarity. Mitotic figures are frequent. The thickness of the urothelium varies considerably. CIS is frequently evident in the adjacent mucosa. Changes in CK20, p53, and p63 expressions, as well as aneuploidy, are more frequent than in low grade lesions. Molecular alterations in these tumors include overexpression of p53, HER2, or EGFR, and loss of p21Waf1 or p27Kip1 as seen with invasive cancers. Genetically, high grade noninvasive lesions (pTa G3) resemble invasive tumors.[19,61] A comparative genomic hybridization study showed deletions at 2q, 5q, 10q, and 18q as well as gains at 5p and 20q.[69] Hematuria is common and the endoscopic appearance varies from papillary to nodular or solid. There may be single or multiple tumors. Stage progression and death due to disease are observed in as many as 65% of patients.[19,61]

Histologic Grading According to the 1999 WHO Classification

The 1999 WHO blue book introduced a new grading scheme.[70] This new classification retained the three-tiered numbering system (grade 1, grade 2, and grade 3 carcinomas). However, tumors formerly classified as 1973 WHO grade 1 tumors were subdivided into PUNLMP and grade 1 tumors (Table 9-1). In the 1999 WHO classification, which differed from both the 1998 WHO/ISUP and 1973 WHO classifications, papillary tumors of the urinary bladder were subclassified as papilloma, PUNLMP, and grade 1, grade 2, and grade 3 papillary urothelial carcinomas. The definition of papilloma remains the same in all new grading systems, and is defined as a papillary tumor with a delicate fibrovascular stroma lined by cytologically and architecturally normal urothelium without increased cellularity or mitotic figures.[71]

Should We Abandon PUNLMP?

The greatest source of controversy with the WHO (2004)/ISUP classification system centers on the diagnosis of the PUNLMP.[14,18,55,72–75] Some authors consider PUNLMP to be an essentially benign tumor with a negligible progression rate. However, others feel that PUNLMP terminology increases the complexity of histologic grading and does not accurately reflect biological potential. Since PUNLMP is a low grade papillary urothelial tumor with a relatively high incidence of recurrence and a low but similar progression rate to that of low grade urothelial carcinoma, some investigators believe they should be considered grade 1 urothelial carcinomas as in the 1973 WHO grading system.

What Constitutes a Carcinoma?

A great deal of the confusion and controversy regarding the proper histologic grading of bladder tumors stems from the fact that the term "carcinoma" is used routinely to describe noninvasive neoplasms in this organ. Nonetheless, the term "carcinoma" or "adenocarcinoma" has also been used to describe tumors without evidence of invasion in other organ systems. Another criticism of the 1973 WHO classification of urothelial tumors is that very low grade noninvasive

tumors with a low probability of progressing are labeled as "carcinomas," thus subjecting patients with these tumors to psychosocial stigmata as well as financial and insurance consequences that follow a diagnosis of cancer. Indeed, the creation of the diagnostic category of PUNLMP was designed, in part, to free patients with this diagnosis from these burdens. However, as detailed above, PUNLMP has a reported recurrence rate of up to 60% and a progression rate of up to 8%.[25,27,28,72,76] Thus, a diagnosis of PUNLMP carries with it a real and significant potential for an adverse clinical outcome similar to low grade noninvasive urothelial carcinomas, as defined by the WHO (2004)/ISUP classification system.

In the study by Cheng et al.,[77] the mean interval from initial diagnosis of PUNLMP to development of an invasive carcinoma was 13.3 years (range, 10 to 14 years). Therefore, claims that PUNLMP is benign should be viewed within the context of length of followup. On the other hand, some noninvasive papillary urothelial carcinomas (both low and high grade) may never recur or progress after removal. Why, then, do these tumors warrant a designation as "carcinoma" in the WHO (2004)/ISUP classification when many behave as an indolent tumor? A greater understanding of urothelial tumor genetics and of clinical diagnostic applications may eventually discern which genetic derangements are responsible for aggressive biological behavior. This molecular prognostic detail would allow pathologists to sort out which noninvasive tumors should be called "carcinoma." However, until that time, it seems prudent to treat PUNLMP as a low grade noninvasive carcinoma and follow these patients closely. In the study by Samaratunga et al.,[76] a statistically significant difference in progression rates was seen for PUNLMP (8%) and low grade noninvasive urothelial carcinoma (13%). However, based on high reported rates of interobserver variability when diagnosing PUNLMP (see below), it may not be necessary or clinically justified to create a distinct diagnostic category for these low grade urothelial tumors. Accumulated data suggest that PUNLMP should be treated in a manner similar to low grade noninvasive carcinoma. Indeed, there is no consensus recommendation regarding the clinical management of patients with PUNLMP. It is understood by urologists that 1973 WHO grade 1 noninvasive tumors have an excellent prognosis. However, followup of patients at regular intervals is warranted. The length of clinical followup and frequency of surveillance cystoscopy should be determined by the clinical behavior of these low grade neoplasms over time rather than by the histologic grade alone.[78] Tumors with early recurrence, rapid growth, or evidence of progression should have frequent cystoscopy. What, then, is the purpose in creating a diagnostic category without a distinct clinical management?

Recurrence and Progression of PUNLMPs

Several studies have shown the WHO (2004)/ISUP classification to differentiate noninvasive papillary urothelial tumors into prognostic groups.[27,79] When applied to transurethral resection of bladder tumor specimens, this system also predicted the pathologic stage of the corresponding cystectomy.[80] However, the published recurrence and progression rates are conflicting, and some studies have shown the prognostic value of the WHO (2004)/ISUP system to be limited.[27,72] In a series of 112 patients diagnosed with PUNLMP, with up to 35 years of followup (median, greater than 12 years), tumor recurrence was observed in 29% of patients.[77] Seventy-five percent of patients with tumor recurrence had a higher tumor grade (i.e., low grade or high grade urothelial carcinomas according to the WHO (2004)/ISUP classification). The stage progression rate was 4%.[77] This study was criticized by some authors because the project was initiated before the appearance of the WHO/ISUP 1998 publication.[76] However, the WHO/ISUP 1998 manuscript was circulated among the consensus meeting participants prior to its publication. In another study, Samaratunga et al. found that PUNLMP and low grade urothelial carcinoma had progression rates of 8% and 13%, respectively.[76] Recurrence and progression rates were 18% and 2% for PUNLMP in a recent study.[81]

Similar recurrence and stage progression results were subsequently found in additional studies. The tumor recurrence rate after the diagnosis of PUNLMP was reported to be 35% in the study by Holmang et al.[82] and 47% in the study by Pich et al.[83] Holmang et al. concluded that PUNLMP and low grade carcinoma have similar risks of progression compared to high grade carcinoma.[82] In a study of 53 PUNLMP tumors with a mean followup period of 11.7 years, Fujii et al. report a recurrence rate of 60%, with 34% progressing to low grade carcinoma and 8% progressing to invasive carcinoma (stage T1).[28] In a study of 322 patients with a mean followup period of 6.6 years, Oosterhuis et al.[72] found no difference with regard to tumor recurrence or disease progression between patients with PUNLMP and patients with low grade urothelial carcinoma. They concluded that there are insufficient data to justify a different clinical approach or the introduction of a new pathologic category. Samaratunga et al.[76] studied 134 patients with noninvasive papillary urothelial tumors from Johns Hopkins Hospital and found that both the 1973 WHO and WHO (2004)/ISUP grading systems were predictive of patient outcome ($P = 0.003$ and $P = 0.002$, respectively). However, their reported progression rate to invasive disease for patients with PUNLMP was the highest in any published study.[15,16] With a median followup of 56 months, the 1973 WHO grade 1 tumors were found to have a progression rate

of 11%, whereas the WHO (2004)/ISUP PUNLMP tumors were found to have a progression rate of 8%.[76] These data indicate that patients with PUNLMP do not have a benign neoplasm, but instead have significant risk of tumor recurrence and disease progression. Long-term clinical followup is recommended for these patients.

Interobserver Variability

Grading systems always involve a degree of subjectivity, which affects the interobserver reproducibility. The subjective nature of bladder tumor grading was highlighted by Coblentz et al., who found 18% of bladder specimens with a referring diagnosis of urothelial carcinoma had significant discrepancies from the review pathologist with regard to the diagnosis, stage, grade, or tumor histologic type.[30] Because the reproducibility of grading systems is usually tested within small groups of pathologists who have previously worked or trained together, an international system often has even greater variation than the rates reported for interobserver discrepancy for institutional grading systems. One of the main goals of the WHO (2004)/ISUP classification was to create a reproducible classification system where the histologic criteria for each diagnostic category were explained in detail. Noninvasive papillary urothelial neoplasms, formerly classified as urothelial carcinomas grades 1, 2, and 3 in the 1973 WHO system, are now classified according to a new three-tiered system with new terminology. Despite the detailed histologic criteria provided by the WHO (2004)/ISUP system for grading, intra- and interobserver variability is not significantly different when either this system or the 1973 WHO classification is used. In fact, Mikuz demonstrated that interobserver agreement was higher using the 1973 WHO classification than when using either the WHO (2004)/ISUP or 1999 WHO systems.[31]

Yorukoglu et al. assessed the intra- and interobserver reproducibility of both the WHO (2004)/ISUP and 1973 WHO systems by allowing six urologic pathologists to independently review 30 slides of noninvasive papillary urothelial tumors in a study set. They found that the newer classification does not increase the reproducibility.[32] While a moderate and substantial intra- and interobserver reproducibility was seen with both systems, there was no statistical difference ($P > 0.05$) between the reproducibility achieved with either system.[32] There was disagreement for PUNLMP in 52% of cases, and reproducibility was lower for low grade tumors in both the WHO (2004)/ISUP and 1973 WHO systems.[32] Similar results were seen by Murphy et al.,[33] who found a 50% discrepancy among pathologists when distinguishing PUNLMP from low grade papillary urothelial carcinoma even after a period of structured pathologist education.

In a recent study, Bol et al. found that agreement among three experienced pathologists on the diagnosis of PUNLMP was 0%.[74] Using the 1999 WHO classification system, the distribution of papilloma, PUNLMP, grades 1, 2, and 3 urothelial carcinoma was 0.8%, 0%, 50.8%, 25.4%, and 23% after second review by three different pathologists.[74] Oyasu[73] believed that the new term "PUNLMP" should not be used in the bladder classification considering that bladder cancer is a disease of field change and that progression to a high grade cancer is a common event among patients who are constantly exposed to carcinogens.[8,73]

The WHO (2004)/ISUP classification replaced a three-tiered grading system (1973 WHO) with another three-tiered system. It is thus understandable that reproducibility is not significantly different. A two-tiered grading system may improve the reproducibility, as demonstrated by Lipponen et al. using morphometry.[84] Two-tiered grading systems have been proposed by Murphy and other investigators. However, none of these systems have gained acceptance among pathologists and urologists. Perhaps subjective grading systems need an intermediate category for cases that are not clearly either high or low grade.

Does PUNLMP Exist in the Upper Urinary Tract?

Approximately 5% of urothelial tumors occur in the upper urinary tract.[85] The classifications of urothelial tumors of the renal pelvis and ureter have traditionally been similar or identical to that of the urinary bladder. The WHO (2004)/ISUP classification system states that the grading system for urothelial tumors of the upper urinary tract is identical to that employed for bladder tumors and states that PUNLMPs may arise from upper urinary tract urothelium.[75] A 9.3% frequency of 1973 WHO grade 1 urothelial carcinomas has been reported in the upper urinary tract,[86] which would suggest that at least some of these lesions would be classified as PUNLMP tumors according to the WHO (2004)/ISUP classification. However, in several large series, PUNLMP tumors do not appear to exist in the upper urinary tract.[87,88] In a study of 102 renal pelvic urothelial neoplasms, Genega et al. did not identify a single PUNLMP.[87] Similarly, Olgac et al. examined 130 urothelial tumors of the renal pelvis and also did not identify a single PUNLMP.[88] The vast majority of urothelial tumors occurring in the upper urinary tract were found to be carcinomas, most of which were high grade.[87,88] The rarity of PUNLMP tumors in the upper urinary tract suggests either that upper urinary tract urothelium is intrinsically different in some way from that of the bladder or that these tumors do not typically cause symptoms that lead to clinical investigation of the upper urinary tract. Alternatively, the high degree of interobserver variability and subjectivity that has been seen in the grading of low grade urothelial tumors may account for their reported absence in the upper tract. It may also

be that these lesions come to clinical attention only after a progression in grade or stage, which implies that low grade tumors, if they exist in the upper urinary tract, have the capacity for aggressive biological behavior. It is also possible, although it has not been studied, that PUNLMP tumors of the upper tract progress more commonly and at a faster rate than similar tumors occurring in the urinary bladder. Regardless of the reason why PUNLMP tumors are so rare (or do not exist) in the upper urinary tract, it appears that they have little clinical or pathologic relevance when applied to this region of the urothelial tract.

PUNLMPs and Urinary Cytopathology

The impact of the WHO (2004)/ISUP classification and the effect of PUNLMP diagnoses on urinary cytopathology have been studied. It was proposed that the diagnostic sensitivity of urine cytology for low grade urothelial neoplasms would improve with the advent of the WHO (2004)/ISUP classification system. The authors of the WHO (2004)/ISUP classification hypothesized that PUNLMP tumors would be difficult to diagnose by urinary cytopathology because of their minimal cytologic atypia, while the majority of WHO (2004)/ISUP low grade carcinomas could be diagnosed by this method.[21] Whisnant et al. studied 86 transurethral surgical biopsies, representing the spectrum of urothelial papillary lesions, and the corresponding urine cytology specimens and reported no significant difference in the distribution of cytologic diagnoses for PUNLMP and low grade papillary urothelial cases $(P>0.05)$.[89] Curry and Wojcik[90] examined 100 bladder biopsies and corresponding voided urine specimens and found that the cytologic detection of low grade urothelial carcinomas was much lower than expected. The sensitivity of urinary cytology for low grade lesions did not improve and there was no difference in the diagnostic accuracy of urinary cytology when the WHO (2004)/ISUP grading system was applied to the corresponding biopsy.[90] The identification of *FGFR3* gene mutations in urine sediment DNA samples may complement standard cytology for low grade bladder tumor screening.[91] Inability to differentiate PUNLMP from low grade carcinoma by urinary cytopathology may be another reason for possible elimination of PUNLMP terminology in future classification systems.

Genetics of PUNLMPs

Development of urothelial carcinoma involves a series of successive oncogenic alterations. The early events are probably caused by molecular changes in tumor suppressor genes, as evidenced by the frequent finding of loss of heterozygosity (LOH) at loci on multiple chromosomes in these tumors. In a study of 26 cases of PUNLMP, 21 tumors (81%) showed allelic loss from at least one of five chromosome loci examined by LOH analysis.[29] In addition, concurrent allelic loss of multiple chromosome loci involved in urothelial carcinoma was often observed in PUNLMP. The incidence and chromosomal location of LOH in PUNLMP tumors is comparable to that found in urothelial carcinoma. Additional studies are needed to determine whether the genetic changes observed in PUNLMP affect the biological behavior of these neoplasms, the risk of progression and recurrence, or the responsiveness of these tumors to therapy.

PUNLMP Treatment and Followup

Because of the high incidence of cancer recurrence (up to 60%[28]) and progression (up to 8%[28,76]) from PUNLMP, most urologists treat and followup patients with this diagnosis in a manner identical to patients with a diagnosis of low grade noninvasive carcinoma. Patients with PUNLMP and noninvasive low grade carcinoma are typically treated by transurethral resection and subsequently monitored by regular cystoscopy. Frequent followup cystoscopies are expensive.[92] Soloway et al. showed that small, recurrent low grade urothelial tumors are slow growing and may be observed rather than subjecting patients to repeated transurethral resections.[93] Studies of the recurrence and progression rates of PUNLMP tumors recommend long-term clinical followup for patients with these lesions.[27,28,72,76,77] Treatment protocol for PUNLMP tumors did not differ from the standard treatment for low grade noninvasive urothelial carcinomas. Thus, a diagnosis of PUNLMP is no different from one of noninvasive low grade papillary carcinoma in terms of clinical management.

As a result of the risks and expenses of frequent followup cystoscopies, a variety of less invasive and expensive alternatives have been investigated. The low grade nature of PUNLMP, however, makes detection of recurrence difficult without cystoscopy and biopsy. As mentioned above, urine cytology has been used for followup. This technique, however, is more effective for monitoring recurrence of high grade lesions. Immunocytochemical analysis of exfoliated urothelial cells for overexpression of Lewis X antigen and p53 protein has been investigated as an aid to urine cytologic examination; however, both antibodies suffer from a lack of specificity. Flow cytometry and image analysis of exfoliated tumor cells have similarly been found to be insensitive techniques for low grade lesions, as DNA aneuploidy is more characteristic of higher grade neoplasms. Urine assays for soluble elements associated with urothelial neoplasia, such as bladder tumor antigen, nuclear matrix proteins, fibrin/fibrinogen degradation products, telomerase, and hyaluronic acid/hyaluronidase have also been used to monitor patients for recurrent tumors. Fluorescence in situ hybridization (FISH) has also been performed on urine cytology specimens with promising results

for stratifying patients with superficial bladder cancer into low and high risk groups for tumor recurrence or progression. Additional studies are needed to determine whether these techniques are useful in monitoring patients with low grade neoplasms, such as PUNLMP. Lotan and Roehrborn have proposed a modified followup protocol incorporating a urine-based tumor marker alternating with cystoscopy or cytology. A prospective randomized trial is needed to validate this approach.[94] As of now, flexible cystoscopy is still the mainstay of surveillance for patients with a history of low grade noninvasive papillary tumors of the bladder.

A recent study by Mariappan and Smith[95] examined 115 patients with 1973 WHO grade 1, stage Ta disease over a period of 19.4 years. They found tumor status at 3 months to be the strongest prognostic factor for recurrence. Of patients without recurrence after five years of followup, 98.3% remained tumor-free for 20 years. Thus, they conclude that patients who are free of recurrence after five years can be safely discharged without additional cystoscopic examinations.[95] Holmang and Johansson found that 68% of patients who are tumor-free at the first followup cystoscopy remain tumor-free during a followup period of five years.[96] Others recommend urological followup, including cystoscopy, for at least 10 years in patients who remain recurrence-free.[28] Additional studies are necessary to confirm the findings of Mariappan and Smith or Holmang and Johansson. Such studies may determine an optimal surveillance schedule for patients with low grade noninvasive urothelial tumors, including PUNLMP. Clinical studies to determine an optimal length and frequency of followup in these patients would be especially important given the reported mean interval from initial diagnosis of PUNLMP to development of invasive carcinoma was 13 years.[77] Thompson et al. have shown that superficial, low grade urothelial tumors can become muscle-invasive despite careful surveillance and a long dormant period.[97] The general frequency and cause of this phenomenon are unknown.

Because a uniform grading system will allow for valid comparison of treatment results among different centers, the advent of the WHO (2004)/ISUP classification is a welcome first step toward standardization of treatment and followup regimens. Since PUNLMP terminology does not change clinical management of low grade noninvasive tumors from the 1973 WHO scheme, its terminology is confusing to urologists, pathologists, and oncologists, in light of its reported high recurrence and progression rates, substantial interobserver variability, and overlap with both benign papilloma and noninvasive low grade papillary carcinoma. Additionally, treatment and followup regimens for patients with PUNLMP do not typically differ from those prescribed for low grade, noninvasive urothelial carcinoma, further minimizing the clinical need for the PUNLMP distinction to be made.

We propose to abandon the terminology "papillary urothelial neoplasm of low malignant potential (PUNLMP)" in bladder tumor classification (see further discussion below).

Histologic Grading of Urothelial Carcinoma: Current Proposal

The histopathologic grade of urothelial tumors is one of the best predictors of biological behavior. The criteria for pathologic grading of noninvasive papillary urothelial neoplasms have been a source of controversy for many decades.[98] Numerous classification schemes have been proposed, but the most widely accepted and used is the 1973 WHO classification.[38] The major criticism of this classification scheme is vague and poorly defined morphologic criteria for grading these neoplasms. Because no clearly defined cutoff points between the different grades were defined in the 1973 WHO classification system, there is considerable debate among pathologists concerning the proper assignment of grade in noninvasive urothelial tumors, especially those falling into the grade 1 and grade 2 categories. This has resulted in a lumping of cases into the grade 2 category with a wide range of reported incidences for grade 2 carcinomas, ranging from 13% to 69%.[18] There is inevitably a degree of heterogeneity within the grades when comparing studies using the 1973 WHO classification.

In 1998, the WHO/ISUP proposed a new consensus classification system (WHO/ISUP 1998) intended to provide better morphologic criteria for grading, to achieve better standardization, and to avoid using the term "carcinoma" for tumors with a very low probability of progressing or recurring.[21] The diagnostic category of PUNLMP was created to achieve these goals. In 1999, within a 12-month period from publication of the WHO/ISUP 1998 system, the WHO again changed their preferred classification system (1999 WHO) to closely mirror the three-tiered 1973 WHO grading system, preserving PUNLMP as the lowest risk category. Considering the discussion above on the biologic behavior and the molecular characteristics of PUNLMP, it seems evident that PUNLMP is an indolent variety of what we generally regard as "carcinoma." A diagnosis of PUNLMP implies a real and significant potential for an adverse clinical outcome that does not differ greatly from that of 2004 WHO low grade noninvasive urothelial carcinomas. In a series of 504 patients with noninvasive urothelial tumors, Schned and his colleagues found no clear advantage of the 2004 WHO grading system over the 1973 WHO grading system.[99] With a mean followup of 7.2 years (range, 3 to 11 years), five-year survival for PUNLMP (94%) was essentially identical to that of low grade urothelial carcinoma (93%) (**Fig. 9-17**).[99]

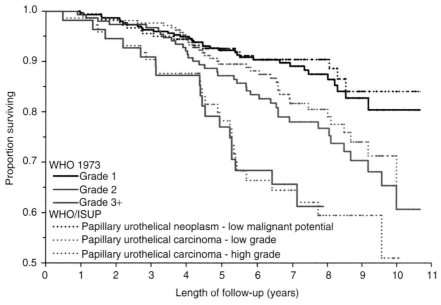

Figure 9-17 Kaplan—Meier survival probability curves in 504 bladder cancer patients: comparison of WHO (1973) and WHO/ISUP classification schemes. Solid lines illustrate survival curves for categories of WHO (1973) classification. Dashed lines illustrate survival curves for categories of WHO/ISUP classification. Note that the survival curve of LGPUC, a category comprised of subsets of grade 1 and grade 2 tumors in the WHO classification, falls as expected between survival curves of grade 1 and grade 2 tumors. Followup was defined as the date of diagnosis until the death of the patient or the date of the last followup. (From Ref. 99; with permission.)

Speculations about the psychosocial burdens of a carcinoma diagnosis are unproven. It is difficult to accept the rationale behind retaining three categories of noninvasive papillary urothelial tumors in the new 2004 WHO system, yet giving them new and unfamiliar names. What benefit is there to calling two categories carcinoma while being ambivalent about the third category (PUNLMP), which, by many criteria, qualifies as a "carcinoma"?

In the current proposal, noninvasive papillary urothelial tumors are separated into five categories: papilloma, grade 1 urothelial carcinoma (low grade), grade 2 urothelial carcinoma (low grade), grade 3 urothelial carcinoma (high grade), and grade 4 urothelial carcinoma (high grade) (Tables 9-1 to 9-3; Figs. 9-18 to 9-20). PUNLMP is classified as "grade 1 urothelial carcinoma (low grade)."

Urothelial Papilloma

The diagnostic criteria and terminology are identical to those defined in the 1973 and 2004 WHO classification (Figs. 9-21 and 9-22).[38] See Chapter 5 for further discussion.[22]

Grade 1 Urothelial Carcinoma (Low Grade)

The diagnostic criteria are identical to those defined in the 1998 WHO/ISUP and 2004 WHO classification for PUNLMP.[20,21] We propose to change the terminology of PUNLMP to "grade 1 urothelial carcinoma (low grade)"(Figs. 9-23 to 9-25; see also the section "Should We Abandon PUNLMP?"). The key difference between papilloma and grade 1 urothelial carcinoma (low grade) is the number of epithelial layers covering the papillae (Fig. 9-26; Tables 9-2 and 9-3).[66]

Grade 2 Urothelial Carcinoma (Low Grade)

The diagnostic criteria are identical to those defined in the 1998 WHO/ISUP and 2004 WHO classification for low grade urothelial carcinomas.[20,21] These tumors are characterized by an overall orderly appearance but with areas of variation in architectural and cytologic features recognizable at scanning power (Figs. 9-27 to 9-31). They are differentiated from grade 1 urothelial carcinoma (low grade) by the presence of easily recognizable cytologic atypia, including variation of polarity and nuclear size, shape, and chromatin texture. Mitotic figures are infrequent and may be seen at any level of the urothelium.

Grade 3 Urothelial Carcinoma (High Grade)

We feel that the spectrum of high grade urothelial carcinomas under the 2004 WHO classification scheme are quite broad, and there is a need to separate these tumors for further investigation. The grade 3 urothelial carcinomas (high grade) display an intermediate degree of architectural and cytologic abnormality between grade 2 urothelial carcinomas (low grade) and grade 4 urothelial carcinomas (high grade) (Figs. 9-32 to 9-35). Architectural disorder in these tumors is obvious, with branching and bridging of papillary projections. Nevertheless, a certain degree of polarity and nuclear uniformity is still discernible. Severe anaplasia is not seen in these tumors. Most grade 3 urothelial carcinomas (high grade) would be classified as grade 2 urothelial carcinoma using the 1973 WHO classification scheme.[38]

Grade 4 Urothelial Carcinoma (High Grade)

The diagnostic criteria are the same as in the 1973 and 1999 WHO classification for grade 3 urothelial carcinomas.[38,70] These tumors present an overall impression of complete architectural disorder with absence of polarity, loss of superficial umbrella cells, and marked variation of all nuclear parameters (Figs. 9-36 to 9-38). Numerous irregularly distributed mitotic figures are frequently noted (Figs. 9-39 and 9-40).[38,70] Cases with nuclear anaplasia are also considered grade 4 urothelial carcinoma in the current proposal (Figs. 9-40 to 9-42). These cases are typically associated with stromal invasion and advanced-stage bladder cancer.

Grading of Invasive Bladder Carcinoma

Invasive tumors are invariably high grade (grade 3/4 in current classification) (Fig. 9-43). Some cases also exhibit marked anaplasia with focal giant cell formation (Figs. 9-40 to 9-42), although low grade (grade 2) urothelial carcinoma may also display invasive behavior (Fig. 9-44). Some invasive urothelial carcinomas exhibit vascular invasion (see Chapters 10, 11, and 25 for further discussion). The most important morphology-based prognostic factors for advanced bladder cancer are tumor stage and lymph node status. In an attempt to identify new parameters to assess bladder cancer prognosis, Jimenez et al.[100] recently introduced a new morphologic classification of invasive bladder tumors distinguishing three patterns of growth (nodular, trabecular, and infiltrative) (Figs. 9-45 to 9-47). Tumors with an infiltrative growth pattern are associated with a worse prognosis than tumors displaying a nodular or trabecular growth pattern.

Tumor Heterogeneity

The WHO (2004)/ISUP system provides clearly defined histologic criteria for each diagnostic category, but urothelial

Table 9-2 Diagnostic Criteria for the Newly Proposed Grading System of Urothelial Carcinoma of the Bladder

Characteristics	Grade 1[a] (Low Grade)	Grade 2 (Low Grade)	Grade 3 (High Grade)	Grade 4 (High Grade)
Increased cell layers (>7)	Yes	Variable	Variable	Variable
Superficial umbrella cells	Present	Often present	Often absent	Usually absent
Polarity/overall architecture	Normal	Mildly distorted	Moderately distorted	Severely distorted
Clear cytoplasm	May be present	May be present	Usually absent	Absent
Nuclear size	Normal or slightly increased	Mildly increased	Moderately increased	Markedly increased
Nuclear pleomorphism	Uniform, slightly elongated to oval	Mild, round to oval with slight variation in shape and contour	Moderate	Marked
Nuclear polarization	Normal to slightly abnormal	Abnormal	Abnormal	Absent
Nuclear hyperchromasia	Slight or minimal	Mild	Moderate	Severe
Nuclear grooves	Present	Present	Absent	Absent
Nucleoli	Absent or inconspicuous	Inconspicuous	Enlarged, often prominent	Multiple prominent nucleoli
Mitotic figures	None/rare, basal location	May be present, at any level	Often present	Prominent and frequent, atypical forms
Stromal invasion	Rare	Uncommon	May be present	Often present

[a]These tumors are classified as PUNLMP, "papillary urothelial neoplasm of low malignant potential," in the 2004 WHO classification system. (From Ref. 2; with permission.)

Table 9-3 Differential Diagnosis of Urothelial Papilloma and Grade 1 (Low Grade) Urothelial Carcinoma[a]

	Urothelial Papilloma	Grade 1 (low grade) Urothelial Carcinoma
Age	Younger	Older
Gender (male-to-female ratio)	2:1	3:1
Size	Small, usually <2 cm	Typically larger than papilloma
Microscopic findings		
Well-formed papillae	Present	Present, rarely fused
Thickness of urothelium	≤7 layers	>7 layers
Superficial umbrella cells	Present	Usually present
Cytology	Minimal or absent	Mild
Nuclear enlargement	Rare or none	None or slightly enlarged
Nuclear hyperchromasia	Rare or none	Slight or minimal
Chromatin	Fine	Fine, slightly granular
Nucleolar enlargement	Absent	Absent or inconspicuous
Nuclear pleomorphism	Absent	Absent
Mitotic figures	None	Rare or basal location
Stromal invasion	Absent	Rare

[a]Grade 1 (low grade) urothelial carcinoma in the newly proposed grading system corresponds to those previously classified "papillary urothelial neoplasm of low malignant potential" (PUNLMP) in the 2004 WHO classification system.

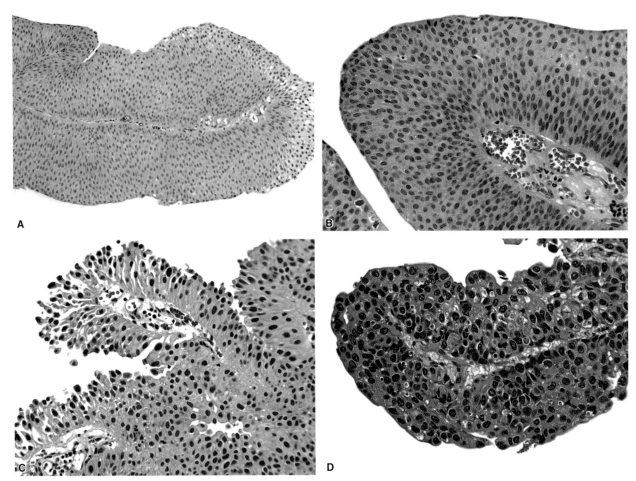

Figure 9-18 Histologic grading of urothelial carcinoma, new proposal. (A) Grade 1 urothelial carcinoma (low grade); (B) grade 2 urothelial carcinoma (low grade); (C) grade 3 urothelial carcinoma (high grade); (D) grade 4 urothelial carcinoma (high grade).

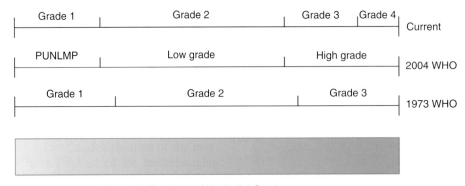

Histologic Spectrum of Urothelial Carcinoma

Figure 9-19 Comparison of the 1973 and 2004 WHO classification with the current proposal for grading of urothelial carcinoma. The 1973 WHO grade 1 carcinomas are reassigned, some to the PUNLMP category and some to the low grade carcinoma category. Similarly, 1973 WHO grade 2 carcinomas are reassigned, some to the low grade carcinoma category, and others to the high grade carcinoma category. All 1973 WHO tumors are assigned to the high grade carcinoma category. In the current proposal, PUNLMP and low grade tumors have been reassigned as grade 1 and grade 2 tumors. The high grade tumors (WHO 2004) have been further divided into grade 3 and grade 4 tumors in the new proposal. (From Ref. 2; with permission.)

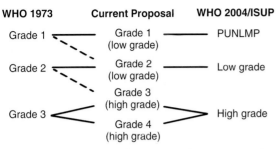

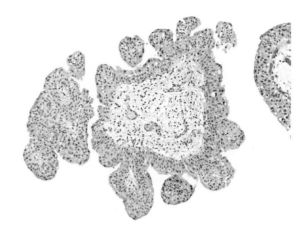

Figure 9-22   Urothelial papilloma.

Figure 9-20   Comparison of various grading systems. The 1973 WHO grade 1 carcinomas are reassigned, some to the PUNLMP category, and some to the low grade carcinoma category. Similarly, 1973 WHO grade 2 carcinomas are reassigned, some to the low grade carcinoma category and others to the high grade carcinoma category. All 1973 WHO tumors are assigned to the high grade carcinoma category. In the current proposal, PUNLMP has been reassigned as grade 1 tumor; 2004 low grade urothelial carcinoma has been reassigned as grade 2 urothelial carcinoma; and 2004 high grade urothelial carcinoma has been divided into grade 3 and grade 4 urothelial carcinomas. Grade 4 urothelial carcinomas are more commonly associated with invasion. (From Ref. 2; with permission.)

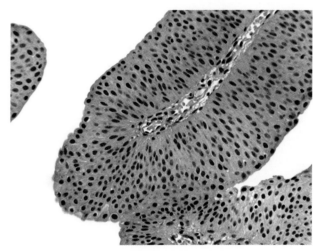

Figure 9-23   Grade 1 urothelial carcinoma (low grade), current proposal.

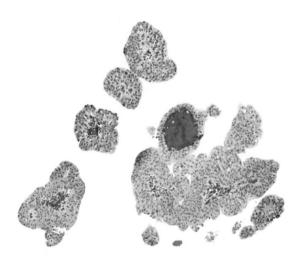

Figure 9-21   Urothelial papilloma.

neoplasms frequently demonstrate features of more than one grade (**Figs. 9-47** and **9-48**). The grading of papillary urothelial tumors is typically based on the worst grade present. However, cancer heterogeneity could have a significant impact on patient outcome. Cheng et al.[79] examined 164 patients with stage Ta urothelial tumors and found that approximately one-third of tumors had areas consistent with more than one histologic grade. They graded both the primary and secondary patterns of tumor growth by the WHO (2004)/ISUP criteria with PUNLMP, low grade carcinoma, and high grade carcinoma patterns, receiving

scores of 1, 2, and 3, respectively. Each tumor was then evaluated by a combined scoring system on a scale of 2 to 6. With a median followup of 9.2 years, the prognosis of patients with a combined score of 6 (the entire tumor consisting of high grade carcinoma) was considerably worse than those with a combined score of 5 (a tumor consisting of low grade and high grade carcinoma) (26% 10-year progression-free survival versus 68% 10-year progression free survival, $P = 0.02$) (**Figs. 9-49** and **9-50**).[79] The significant survival difference (42%) between score 5 and score 6 groups may suffice to warrant different management strategies in appropriate settings. Subsequent studies have confirmed that combined scoring systems may be useful in the grading of bladder tumors.[101] Grading should take cancer heterogeneity into consideration because prognostic accuracy was increased when both the primary and secondary grades were applied.[79]

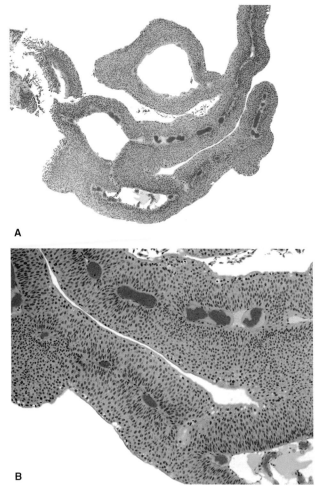

A

B

Figure 9-24 Grade 1 urothelial carcinoma (low grade), current proposal (A and B).

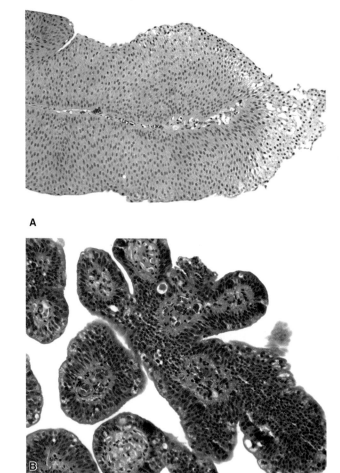

A

B

Figure 9-26 Comparison of grade 1 urothelial carcinoma (low grade) (A) and urothelial papilloma (B). The key difference is the lesser number of cell layers covering the papillae in papilloma.

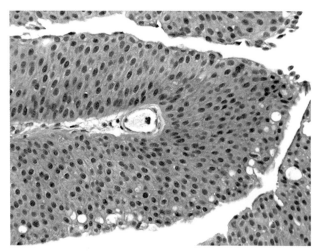

Figure 9-25 Grade 1 urothelial carcinoma (low grade), current proposal.

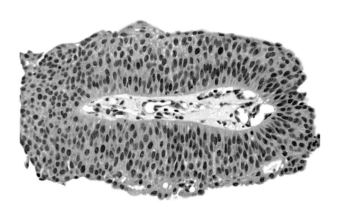

Figure 9-27 Grade 2 urothelial carcinoma (low grade), current proposal.

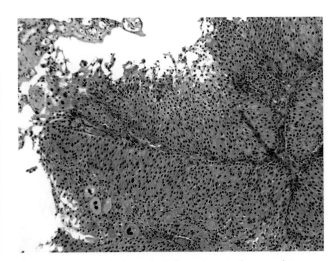

Figure 9-28   Grade 2 urothelial carcinoma (low grade), current proposal.

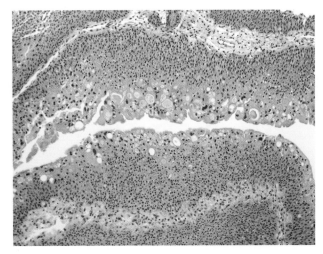

Figure 9-31   Grade 2 urothelial carcinoma (low grade), current proposal. Note the "bull's-eye" features in the superficial umbrella cells.

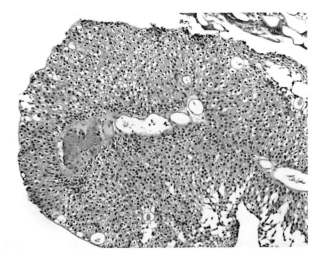

Figure 9-29   Grade 2 urothelial carcinoma (low grade), current proposal.

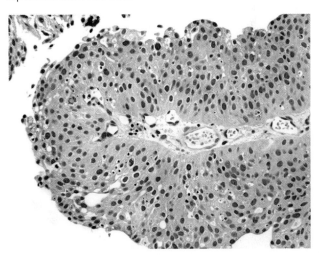

Figure 9-32   Grade 3 urothelial carcinoma (high grade), current proposal.

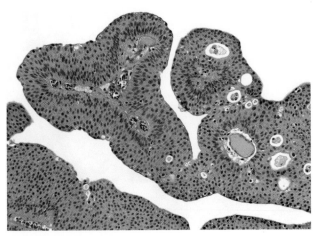

Figure 9-30   Grade 2 urothelial carcinoma (low grade), current proposal. Note the intracytoplasmic lumina.

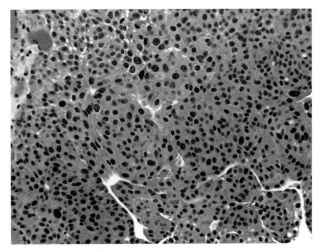

Figure 9-33   Grade 3 urothelial carcinoma (high grade), current proposal.

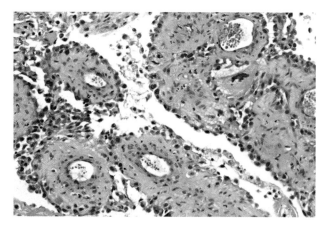

Figure 9-34 Grade 3 urothelial carcinoma (high grade), current proposal. Note the hyalinized fibrovascular core.

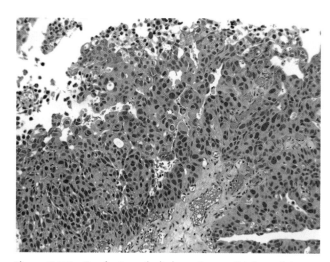

Figure 9-37 Grade 4 urothelial carcinoma (high grade), current proposal.

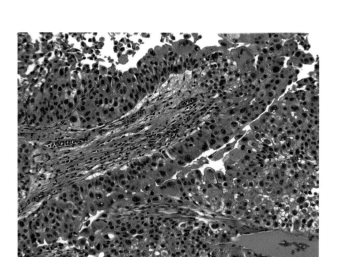

Figure 9-35 Grade 3 urothelial carcinoma (high grade), current proposal. Note the cytoplasmic eosinophilia.

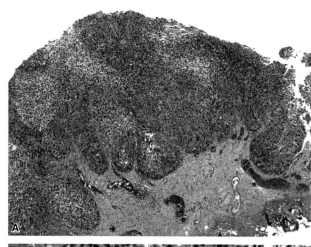

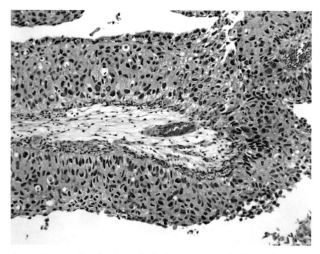

Figure 9-36 Grade 4 urothelial carcinoma (high grade), current proposal.

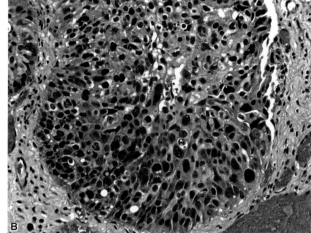

Figure 9-38 Grade 4 urothelial carcinoma (high grade), current proposal (A and B).

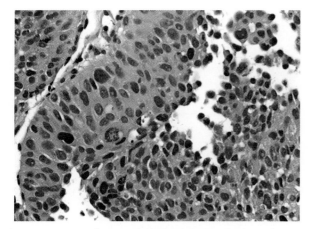

Figure 9-39 Grade 4 urothelial carcinoma (high grade), current proposal. Note the atypical mitotic figures.

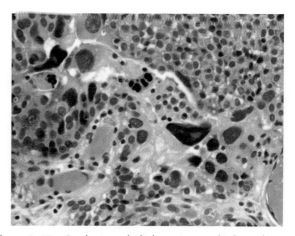

Figure 9-42 Grade 4 urothelial carcinoma (high grade), current proposal. Note the nuclear anaplasia.

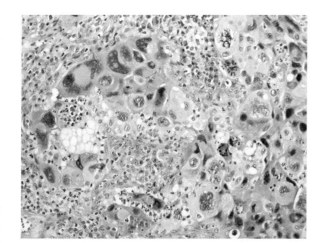

Figure 9-40 Grade 4 urothelial carcinoma (high grade), current proposal. Note the atypical mitotic figures and nuclear anaplasia.

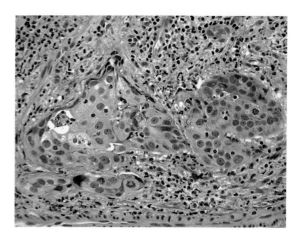

Figure 9-43 Invasive grade 4 urothelial carcinoma (high grade), current proposal. Note the atypical mitotic figures.

Neither the WHO (2004)/ISUP system nor the 1973 WHO system takes tumor heterogeneity into account; however, the 1973 WHO system does allow a greater amount of diagnostic flexibility in that tumors are frequently classified as grade 1/2 or grade 2/3. This added flexibility may actually give a more accurate representation of the tumor histology than attempting to force a lesion into a single diagnostic category. Future investigation is needed to fully address the impact of tumor heterogeneity on clinical outcome.

Molecular Grading

Several molecular classifications have been reported in the literature, and current genetic data support two major pathways, corresponding to two morphologically defined entities (see **Chapters 29** to **34** for further discussion).[4,6] The

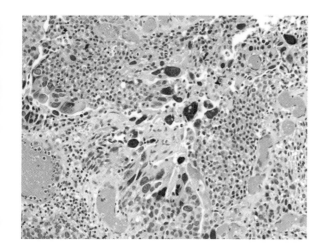

Figure 9-41 Grade 4 urothelial carcinoma (high grade), current proposal. Note the nuclear anaplasia.

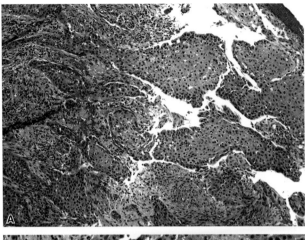

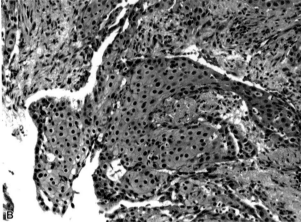

Figure 9-44   Invasive urothelial carcinoma, grade 2 (low grade), current proposal (A and B).

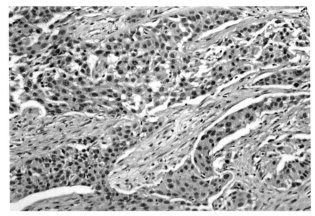

Figure 9-46   Invasive urothelial carcinoma, trabecular growth pattern.

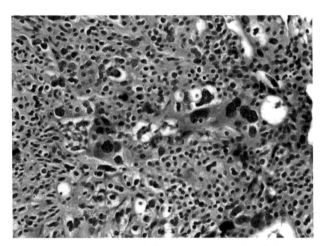

Figure 9-47   Invasive urothelial carcinoma with solid growth pattern. Note the various degrees of differentiation in the same field.

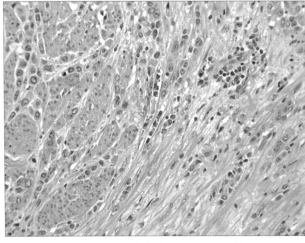

Figure 9-45   Invasive urothelial carcinoma, infiltrative growth pattern.

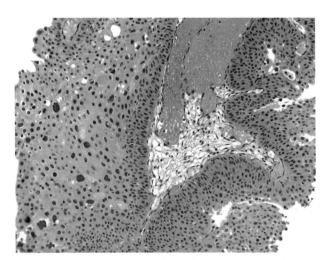

Figure 9-48   Heterogeneity of histologic grade. Note the various degrees of differentiation in the same field.

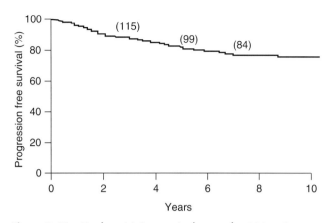

Figure 9-49 Kaplan–Meier survival curve for 164 patients with noninvasive papillary urothelial carcinoma of the bladder (classified as Ta). None of the patients had previous or coexistent urothelial carcinoma in situ or invasive carcinoma. Progression was defined as the development of invasive carcinoma, distant metastasis, or death from bladder cancer. Numbers in parentheses represent numbers of patients under observation at three, five, and seven years. (From Ref. 79; with permission.)

genetically stable category includes low grade (grade 1 and some grade 2, 1973 WHO schema) noninvasive papillary tumors.[16,18,19,22–32] The genetically unstable category contains high grade (some grade 2 and all grade 3, 1973 WHO schema) noninvasive CIS, and invasively growing carcinomas (stages T1 to T4). Noninvasive low grade bladder neoplasms have few genomic alterations and should be viewed as genetically stable.

The natural history of urothelial neoplasia shows that bladder cancer is actually two diseases. The first is low grade papillary noninvasive urothelial tumors (PUNLMP and low grade) previously classified as grade 1. These are characterized by genetic stability with common chromosome 9 alterations and *(FGFR3)* mutations.[31,32] These tumors have a high propensity to recur but rarely invade or metastasize. The second type of bladder cancer is the high grade lesion that originates as urothelial dysplasia and begins as CIS or high grade noninvasive papillary carcinoma (grade 3 and some grade 2, 1973 WHO schema). They have common alterations at the *TP53* and *RB* tumor suppressor genes. Both types of neoplasm can develop in the same patient, either simultaneously or sequentially.

The morphological grades of bladder cancer are influenced by molecular events involved in carcinogenesis. The morphological criteria used for bladder cancer grading have been updated continuously over the past few decades. The current bladder cancer classification of urothelial neoplasms was based on an attempt to reconcile molecular genetic and pathologic findings. Most of the WHO 2004 categories have

been validated successfully by expression and genome profiling and by identification of distinctive genetic alterations.

Mutations in the *FGFR3* and *TP53* genes define two independent and distinct pathways in superficial papillary and invasive or flat urothelial carcinomas.[4,6,102,103] Tumors characterized by these two pathways have markedly different biological behaviors and clinical outcomes. Activating point mutations of the *FGFR3* gene have been demonstrated in a number of malignancies, including urothelial carcinomas,[104] and in a variety of skeletal anomalies. Several studies have examined the importance of these *FGFR3* gene mutations in urothelial carcinomas.[102,104] *FGFR3* mutations are seen most commonly in noninvasive papillary tumors (stage Ta), including papillomas, PUNLMPs, and low grade carcinomas. This mutation is associated with a favorable disease course.[102] High grade and high stage urothelial neoplasms and flat CIS rarely show these mutations but have frequent inactivating mutations of *TP53* or *RB*. Thus, molecular analysis of bladder tumors for *FGFR3* mutations may eventually serve as a means for predicting clinical outcome. van Rhijn et al. found *FGFR3* mutation status to be a stronger predictor of decreased recurrence than stage and grade ($P = 0.008$).[105] Their results suggest that the frequency of followup cystoscopies could be reduced for patients with tumors harboring *FGFR3* gene mutations.

In the grading study of Lamy et al., *FGFR3* mutations were detected in 54% of grade 1 and 85% of grade 2 but in only 20% of grade 3 tumors. *TP53* mutations were found in 26% of grade 1/2 tumors but in 44% of grade 3 tumors.[106] The data suggest that pathologic grading alone may not predict tumor behavior accurately.

In a prospective study, Burger et al. analyzed Ki67 expression and *FGFR3* status in urothelial carcinomas from 221 patients. Pathologic grading was performed according to the WHO classification systems of 1973 and 2004, and molecular grading was done using *FGFR3* mutation status and Ki67 expression levels. Grade 1 tumors showed a 65% incidence of *FGFR3* mutation and a 6% incidence of a high Ki67 index; grade 2 tumors showed a 67% incidence of *FGFR3* mutation, and 35% had a high Ki67 index. Only 9% of grade 3 tumors showed *FGFR3* mutation, and 16% had high Ki67 indices. In multivariate analyses, either the 1973 or 2004 WHO grading system was a statistically significant and independent predictor of progression.[107]

Molecular grading may discriminate high risk cases from low risk cases in patients with similar pathological grades (**Figs. 9-51** and **9-52**).[3,4,6,108] Combining morphological and molecular grading markers may allow better risk stratification for patients with bladder cancer. In a study of *FGFR3* mutation status and three molecular markers (Ki67, p53, and P27[Kip1]) on 286 patients with primary urothelial carcinoma, van Rhijn et al. determined

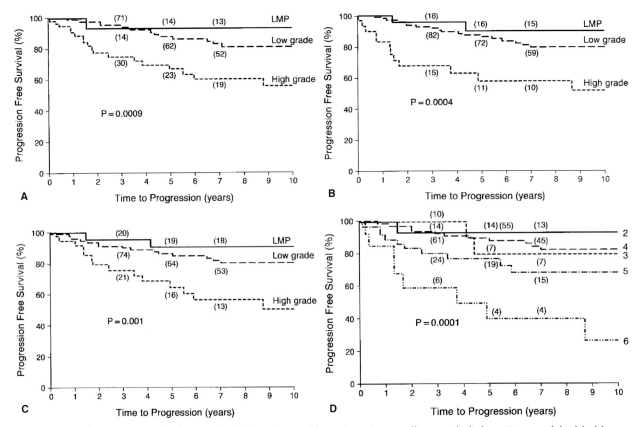

Figure 9-50   Kaplan–Meier survival curves for 164 patients with noninvasive papillary urothelial carcinoma of the bladder (classified as Ta) according to (A) worst grade, (B) primary grade, (C) secondary grade, and (D) combined primary and secondary grades. Histologic grading was performed according to the newly proposed World Health Organization and International Society of Urological Pathology (WHO/ISUP) grading system.1 The primary (most common) and secondary (second most common) grades were evaluated for each tumor, and combined scores were derived from the summation of primary and secondary grades. Scores of 1, 2, and 3 were assigned to papillary urothelial neoplasms of low malignant potential (PUNLMP), low grade urothelial carcinomas, and high grade urothelial carcinomas, respectively. Numbers in parentheses represent numbers of patients under observation at three, five, and seven years. (From Ref. 79; with permission.)

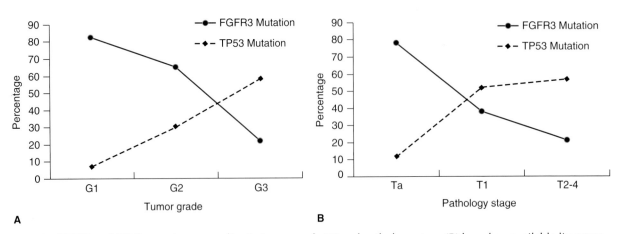

Figure 9-51   *FGFR3* and *TP53* mutations according to tumor grade (A) and pathology stage (B) based on available literature. (From Ref. 4; with permission.)

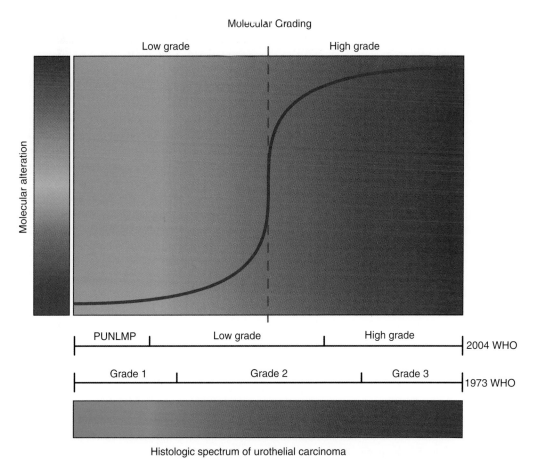

Molecular Grading

Low grade   High grade

Molecular alteration

PUNLMP | Low grade | High grade | 2004 WHO

Grade 1 | Grade 2 | Grade 3 | 1973 WHO

Histologic spectrum of urothelial carcinoma

Figure 9-52 Molecular grading of urothelial carcinomas. The grading of urothelial carcinomas encompasses a continuous spectrum, both molecularly and morphologically. Histological grading according to the severity of atypia is shown on the horizontal bar with progression from green to red; molecular grading reflects the severity of molecular alterations, and is shown in the vertical bar, gradient from blue to red. The blue curve represents the probability of significant molecular alterations in tumors exhibiting morphologic features commensurate with their degree of architectural and cytologic atypia (grade) at each point along the grading spectrum. The blue curve, as it proceeds from green to red zones, may more precisely define tumor behavior. (From Ref. 4; with permission.)

the reproducibility of pathologic grade and molecular variables. *FGFR3* mutations were detected in 88% of grade 1 urothelial carcinomas, in contrast to 16% of grade 3 tumors. Conversely, aberrant expression patterns of Ki67, p53, and P27[Kip1] were seen in 5%, 2%, and 3% of grade 1 tumors and in 85%, 60%, and 56% of grade 3 tumors, respectively. Three molecular grades (mG) could be identified: mG1 had *FGFR3* mutation, normal expression, and portended a favorable prognosis. The intermediate grade, mG2, has either mutated *FGFR3* or elevated Ki67 and was associated with an outcome intermediate between mG1 and mG3 tumors; and mG3 tumors with wild type *FGFR3* and high expression of Ki67 were associated with a poor clinical outcome.[109] The molecular variables were more reproducible than the pathologic grade (85% to 100% agreement between determinations versus 47% to 61% for different morphological grading). Molecular

grading provides a new, simple, and highly reproducible tool for clinical decision making in bladder cancer patients.

Differential gene expression profiles may also be used to stratify tumor grade.[108] Microarray data show clear distinctions between low grade and high grade tumors in bladder washing samples in a study of patients with low grade and high grade urothelial carcinomas.[110] Catto et al. studied the profiles of 322 miRNAs in 78 normal or malignant urothelial samples and found that miRNA alterations occurred in a tumor phenotype-specific manner.[111] High grade urothelial carcinomas were characterized by miRNA upregulation, including miRNA-21, which suppresses p53 function. Low grade urothelial carcinomas, on the other hand, were characterized by downregulation of miRNA-99a and miRNA-100, which lead to upregulation of *FGFR3* even before its mutation.[111]

A retrospective study was performed to evaluate differences in chromosomal aberrations in recurrent urothelial carcinomas. The number of chromosomal aberrations differed significantly between tumor grades, regardless of whether grading was done using 1973 or 2004 WHO grading parameters.[112] The most frequent gains of chromosomal material were found on 19p, 7q, 16, 19q, 8q, 12q, and 20 and the most frequent losses of chromosomal material were detected on 9, 13q, 5q, 8p, 11p, and 18q. Chromosomal aberrations correlated well with either grading system. High grade tumors showed aberrations usually associated with higher grade chromosomal alteration panels (1p+, 16p+, −2 and −5q) and poor clinical outcome. Polysomy of chromosome 17 by FISH was not seen in grade 1 tumors, but was seen in 8/29 grade 2 tumors and 29/29 grade 3 tumors.[113]

Distinct molecular pathways for superficial papillary urothelial carcinoma and flat invasive urothelial carcinoma are well established. Molecular markers efficiently distinguish low grade bladder tumors from high grade tumors.[3,102] Low grade (grade 1 to grade 2) tumors possess few molecular alterations apart from deletions involving chromosome 9 and activating mutations of the *FGFR3*. However, loss of 11p and inactivation of *TP53* is more commonly seen in tumors of higher grade.[102]

Some studies have examined CK20 expression in urothelial tumors and urothelial dysplasia. CK20 immunohistochemistry has been suggested to be a useful adjunct to hematoxylin and eosin in the diagnosis of urothelial dysplasia and for predicting malignant potential in low grade urothelial tumors.[114] Alsheikh et al. investigated CK20 expression in 49 stage Ta papillary tumors of the bladder (20 PUNLMPs and 29 low grade carcinomas) and found a lower recurrence rate among tumors with normal CK20 expression versus those with an abnormal pattern of CK20 expression.[92] However, a significant number of PUNLMPs with a normal CK20 expression pattern (20%) recurred.[92] Thus, CK20 immunohistochemistry is an unreliable method for identifying tumors with a sufficiently low likelihood of recurrence to change the recommended clinical management.

Several studies have demonstrated a positive correlation between immunohistochemical expression of p53 or mutations of the *TP53* gene and tumor grade and stage. Similarly, expression of Ki67, a marker of proliferative activity, has been shown to correlate with the growth rate of urothelial carcinomas, with tumor grade, and with tumor stage. Yin and Leong analyzed 84 noninvasive papillary urothelial tumors with immunostains for CK20, Ki67, and p53. They found that each of the biomarkers and the probability of tumor recurrence was significantly different between the WHO (2004)/ISUP system and the 1973 WHO system.[115] By contrast, Karakok et al. found no significant association between p53 expression and grade when the WHO (2004)/ISUP criteria were applied.[116]

The value of many additional biomarkers and molecular findings for grading urothelial neoplasms have been studied. High molecular weight cytokeratin (34βE12) immunohistochemistry to assess basal cell status, p21/WAF expression, combined CK20 and CD44 expression patterns, pRb expression, proliferating cell nuclear antigen (PCNA) expression, DNA content and ploidy, cellular apoptosis information, and karyotyping have all been examined as potential aids in the grading of bladder tumors with both promising and discouraging results. Additionally, nuclear morphometry, assessment of mitotic indices, cytometry, and image analysis have been applied to the grading of these tumors. Despite these studies, classical descriptive morphology remains essential to the assessment of tumor grade and probability of recurrence and progression.

Recent studies using single-strand conformation polymorphism analysis, DNA sequencing, and full genome expression analysis have identified specific molecular markers and a 45-gene molecular signature present in superficial bladder tumors. These newer methods may facilitate molecular grading of urothelial carcinoma and may make it possible to identify patients with a high risk of disease progression at an early stage.[117] It is not possible to distinguish which noninvasive papillary tumors of the bladder will recur or progress based solely on tumor histology. Therefore, if patients with tumors that will not recur or progress could be selected, overtreatment of these individuals may be averted. Other tumors with many adverse markers may behave in an aggressive manner despite being treated according to standard protocols. It is possible that molecular and immunohistochemical adjuncts may help in predicting biologic behavior. These may eventually be included in a grading scheme once their clinical usefulness and reproducibility are well established. However, until that time, diagnosis and grading based on tumor morphology will continue to be used.

Future Prospectives

The clinical behaviors of noninvasive papillary urothelial carcinoma are related directly to the degree of architectural, cytological, and molecular alterations of the neoplastic cells confined within the urothelium. The WHO (2004)/ISUP classification is a positive first step toward the standardization of urothelial tumor grading. The creation of "papillary urothelial neoplasm of low malignant potential" has been the most contentious aspect of the WHO (2004)/ISUP classification of papillary bladder tumors. Studies have shown that this terminology may not reflect its true biological behavior and that interobserver variability in making this diagnosis is very high, despite detailed histologic criteria. Additionally, urine cytology in the context of the WHO (2004)/ISUP classification does not appear to effectively discriminate PUNLMP from low grade carcinoma. For practical purposes, patients with PUNLMP should be managed as patients with low grade noninvasive urothelial carcinoma are managed. Many issues have been raised regarding the use of either the 1973 or 2004 WHO grading system. We propose a four-tier grading system (grades 1 to 4) to replace existing grading systems. We believe that this proposed grading system incorporates the strengths of both the 1973 and 2004 grading systems. The new grading system is simple to use and to apply in daily practice. The use of both numerical (grades 1 to 4) and categorical schemes (low vs. high grade) in a single grading system will allow better stratification for research purposes and facilitate clinical decision making. There are many categorical management decisions regarding noninvasive papillary urothelial tumors, such as when to administer intravesical antitumor agents, how often to repeat cystoscopic surveillance, and whether to fulgurate or biopsy small tumors. It is anticipated that the identification of high grade and low grade papillary tumors will help make such clinical decisions.

Full genome searches for prognostic and predictive molecular gene expression signatures as cancer markers have shown significant promise. GeneChip technology and proteomic techniques may help to stratify patients into prognostic groups in the future. Several new biomarkers and molecular tests have shown promise in objectively differentiating patients at risk for adverse clinical outcome. It may eventually be useful to include these markers in future grading schemes when their clinical utility is better established. Recent advances in the molecular grading of these tumors may eventually supplant traditional morphologic classification, allowing a more precise and objective assessment of the tumors' biological potential.

REFERENCES

1. Siegel R, Ward E, Brawley O, Jemal A. Cancer statistics, 2011: The impact of eliminating socioeconomic and racial disparities on premature cancer death CA. *Cancer J Clin* 2011;61:212–36.
2. Cheng L, MacLennan GT, Lopez-Beltran A. Histologic grading of urothelial carcinoma: A reapraisal. *Hum Pathol* 2012 (in press).
3. Cheng L, Zhang S, Davidson DD, MacLennan GT, Koch MO, Montironi R, Lopez-Beltran A. Molecular determinants of tumor recurrence in the urinary bladder. *Future Oncol* 2009;5:843–57.
4. Cheng L, Zhang S, Maclennan GT, Williamson SR, Lopez-Beltran A, Montironi R. Bladder cancer: translating molecular genetic insights into clinical practice. *Hum Pathol* 2011;42:455–81.
5. Cheng L, Lopez-Beltran A, MacLennan GT, Montironi R, Bostwick DG. Neoplasms of the urinary bladder. In: Bostwick DG, Cheng L, eds. Urologic Surgical Pathology, 2nd ed. Philadelphia: Elsevier/Mosby, 2008:259–352.
6. Cheng L, Davidson DD, Maclennan GT, Williamson SR, Zhang S, Koch MO, Montironi R, Lopez-Beltran A. The origins of urothelial carcinoma. *Expert Rev Anticancer Ther* 2010;10:865–80.
7. Cheng L, Cheville JC, Leibovich BC, Weaver AL, Egan KS, Spotts BE, Neumann RM, Bostwick DG. Survival of patients with carcinoma in situ of the urinary bladder. *Cancer* 1999;85:2469–74.
8. Cheng L, Cheville JC, Neumann RM, Bostwick DG. Natural history of urothelial dysplasia of the bladder. *Am J Surg Pathol* 1999;23:443–7.
9. Cheng L, Cheville JC, Neumann RM, Bostwick DG. Flat intraepithelial lesions of the urinary bladder. *Cancer* 2000;88:625–31.
10. Cheng L, Neumann RM, Scherer BG, Weaver AL, Nehra A, Zincke H, Bostwick DG. Tumor size predicts the survival of patients with pathologic stage T2 bladder carcinoma: a critical evaluation of the depth of muscle invasion. *Cancer* 1999;85:2638–47.
11. Cheng L, Neumann RM, Weaver AL, Spotts BE, Bostwick DG. Predicting cancer progression in patients with stage T1 bladder carcinoma. *J Clin Oncol* 1999;17:3182–7.
12. van Rhijn BW, Burger M, Lotan Y, Solsona E, Stief CG, Sylvester RJ, Witjes JA, Zlotta AR. Recurrence and progression of disease in non-muscle-invasive bladder cancer: from epidemiology to treatment strategy. *Eur Urol* 2009;56:430–42.
13. Montironi R, Lopez-Beltran A, Scarpelli M, Mazzucchelli R, Cheng L. Morphological classification and definition of benign, preneoplastic and non-invasive neoplastic lesions of the urinary bladder. *Histopathology* 2008;53:621–33.
14. Cheng L, Bostwick DG. World Health Organization and International Society of Urological Pathology classification and two-number grading system of bladder tumors: reply. *Cancer* 2000;88:1513–6.
15. Maclennan GT, Kirkali Z, Cheng L. Histologic grading of noninvasive papillary urothelial neoplasms. *Eur Urol* 2007;51:889–98.
16. Jones TD, Cheng L. Papillary urothelial neoplasm of low malignant potential: evolving terminology and concepts. *J Urol* 2006;175:1995–2003.
17. Montironi R, Lopez-Beltran A, Scarpelli M, Mazzucchelli R, Cheng L. 2004 World Health Organization classification of the noninvasive urothelial neoplasms: inherent problems and clinical reflections. *Eur Urol* 2009;Suppl 8:453–7.
18. Bostwick DG, Mikuz G. Urothelial papillary (exophytic) neoplasms. *Virchows Arch* 2002;441:109–16.

19. Lopez-Beltran A, Montironi R. Non-invasive urothelial neoplasms: according to the most recent WHO classification. *Eur Urol* 2004;46:170–6.

20. Eble JN, Sauter G, Epstein JI, Sesterhenn IA, eds. WHO Classification of Tumours: Pathology and Genetics. Tumours of the Urinary and Male Reproductive System. Lyon, France: IARC Press, 2004.

21. Epstein JI, Amin MB, Reuter VR, Mostofi FK. The World Health Organization/International Society of Urological Pathology consensus classification of urothelial (transitional cell) neoplasms of the urinary bladder. Bladder Consensus Conference Committee. *Am J Surg Pathol* 1998;22:1435–48.

22. Cheng L, Darson M, Cheville JC, Neumann RM, Zincke H, Nehra A, Bostwick DG. Urothelial papilloma of the bladder. Clinical and biologic implications. *Cancer* 1999;86:2098–101.

23. Pich A, Chiusa L, Formiconi A, Galliano D, Bortolin P, Comino A, Navone R. Proliferative activity is the most significant predictor of recurrence in noninvasive papillary urothelial neoplasms of low malignant potential and grade 1 papillary carcinomas of the bladder *Cancer* 2002;95:784–90.

24. Oosterhuis JSR, Janssen-Heijnen ML, Pauwels RP, Newling DW, ten Kate F. Histological grading of papillary urothelial carcinoma of the bladder: prognostic value of the 1998 WHO/ISUP classification system and comparison with conventional grading systems. *J Clin Pathol*. 2002;55:900–5.

25. Pich A, Chiusa L, Formiconi A, Galliano D, Bortolin P, Navone R. Biologic differences between noninvasive papillary urothelial neoplasms of low malignant potential and low grade (grade 1) papillary carcinomas of the bladder. *Am J Surg Pathol* 2001;25:1528–33.

26. Samaratunga H, Makarov DV, Epstein JI. Comparison of WHO/ISUP and WHO classification of noninvasive papillary urothelial neoplasms for risk of progression. *Urology* 2002;60:315–9.

27. Holmang S, Hedelin H, Anderstrom C, Holmberg E, Busch C, Johansson SL. Recurrence and progression in low grade papillary urothelial tumors. *J Urol* 1999;162:702–7.

28. Fujii Y, Kawakami S, Koga F, Nemoto T, Kihara K. Long-term outcome of bladder papillary urothelial neoplasms of low malignant potential. *BJU Int* 2003;92:559–62.

29. Cheng L, MacLennan GT, Zhang S, Wang M, Pan CX, Koch MO. Laser capture microdissection analysis reveals frequent allelic losses in papillary urothelial neoplasm of low malignant potential of the urinary bladder. *Cancer* 2004;101:183–8.

30. Coblentz TR, Mills SE, Theodorescu D. Impact of second opinion pathology in the definitive management of patients with bladder carcinoma. *Cancer* 2001;91:1284–90.

31. Mikuz G. The reliability and reproducibility of the different classifications of bladder cancer. In: Hauptmann S, Dietel M, Sorbino-Simoes M. Surgical pathology update 2001 Berlin: ABW-Wissenschaftsverlag, 2001:114–5.

32. Yorukoglu K, Tuna B, Dikicioglu E, Duzcan E, Isisag A, Sen S, Mungan U, Kirkali Z. Reproducibility of the 1998 World Health Organization/International Society of Urologic Pathology classification of papillary urothelial neoplasms of the urinary bladder. *Virchows Arch* 2003;443:734–40.

33. Murphy WM, Takezawa K, Maruniak NA. Interobserver discrepancy using the 1998 World Health Organization/International Society of Urologic Pathology classification of urothelial neoplasms: practical choices for patient care. *J Urol* 2002;168:968–72.

34. Bol MG, Baak JP, Buhr-Wildhagen S, Kruse AJ, Kjellevold KH, Janssen EA, Mestad O, Ogreid P. Reproducibility and prognostic variability of grade and lamina propria invasion in stages Ta, T1 urothelial carcinoma of the bladder. *J Urol* 2003;169:1291–4.

35. Cheng L, Montironi R, Davidson DD, Lopez-Beltran A. Staging and reporting of urothelial carcinoma of the urinary bladder. *Mod Pathol* 2009;22 (Suppl 2):S70–95.

36. Harnden P, Southgate J. Revised classification of urothelial neoplasms. *Am J Surg Pathol* 2000;24:160–2.

37. Wu XR. Urothelial tumorigenesis: a tale of divergent pathways. *Nat Rev Cancer* 2005;5:713–25.

38. Mostofi FK, Sobin LH, Torloni H. Histological Typing of Urinary Bladder Tumours, Vol. 10. Geneva: World Health Organization, 1973.

39. Malmstrom PU, Bush C, Norlen BJ. Recurrence, progression, and survival in bladder cancer. A retrospective analysis of 232 patients with greater than or equal to 5-year followup. *Scand J Urol Nephrol* 1987;21:185–95.

40. Prout Jr, Barton BA, Griffin PP, Friedell GH. Treated history of noninvasive grade 1 transitional cell carcinoma. The National Bladder Cancer Group. *J Urol*. 1992;148:1413–9.

41. Holmang S, Hedelin H, Anderstrom C, Johansson SL. The relationship among multiple recurrences, progression and prognosis of patients with stages Ta and T1 transitional cell cancer of the bladder followed for at least 20 years. *J Urol* 1995;153:1823–7.

42. England HR, Paris AM, Blandy JP. The correlation of T1 bladder tumour history with prognosis and followup requirements. *Br J Urol* 1981;53:593–7.

43. Leblanc B, Duclos AJ, Benard F, Cote J, Valiquette L, Paquin JM, Mauffette F, Faucher R, Perreault JP. Long-term followup of initial Ta grade 1 transitional cell carcinoma of the bladder. *J Urol* 1999;162:1946–60.

44. Pocock RD, Ponder BA, O'Sullivan JP, Ibrahim SK, Easton DF, Shearer RJ. Prognostic factors in non-infiltrating carcinoma of the bladder: a preliminary report. *Br J Urol* 1982;54:711–5.

45. Gilbert HA, Logan JL, Kagan AR, Friedman HA, Cove JK, Fox M, Muldoon TM, Lonni YW, Rowe JH, Cooper JF, Nussbaum H, Chan P, Rao A, Starr A. The natural history of papillary transitional cell carcinoma of the bladder and its

treatment in any unselected population on the basis of histologic grading. *J Urol* 1978;119:488–92.

46. Heney NM, Ahmed S, Flanagan MJ, Frable W, Corder MP, Hafermann MD, Hawkins IR. Superficial bladder cancer: progression and recurrence. *J Urol* 1983;130:1083–6.

47. Fitzpatrick JM, West AB, Butler MR, Lane V, O'Flynn JD. Superficial bladder tumors (stage pTa, grades 1 and 2): the importance of recurrence pattern following initial resection. *J Urol* 1986;135:920–2.

48. Prout G, Bassil B, Griffin P. The treated histories of patients with Ta grade 1 transitional-cell carcinoma of the bladder. *Arch Surg* 1986;121:1463–8.

49. Hemstreet GP 3rd, Rollins S, Jones P, Rao JY, Hurst RE, Bonner RB, Hewett T, Smith BG. Identification of a high risk subgroup of grade 1 transitional cell carcinoma using image analysis based deoxyribonucleic acid ploidy analysis of tumor tissue. *J Urol* 1991;146:1525–9.

50. Mufti GR, Virdi JS, Singh M. "Solitary" Ta-T1 G1 bladder tumour—history and long-term prognosis. *Eur Urol* 1990;18:101–6.

51. Jordan AM, Weingarten J, Murphy WM. Transitional cell neoplasms of the urinary bladder. Can biologic potential be predicted from histologic grading? *Cancer* 1987;60:2766–74.

52. Fitzpatrick JM. Superficial bladder carcinoma. *World J Urol* 1993;11:142–7.

53. Greene L, Hanash K, Farrow G. Benign papilloma or papillary carcinoma of the bladder. *J Urol* 1973;110:205–07.

54. Bostwick DG. Natural history of early bladder cancer. *J Cell Biochem* 1992;161 (Suppl):31–8.

55. Bostwick DG, Ramnani D, Cheng L. Diagnosis and grading of bladder cancer and associated lesions. *Urol Clin North Am* 1999;26:493–507.

56. Pauwels RP, Schapers RF, Smeets AW, Debruyne FM, Geraedts JP. Grading in superficial bladder cancer: morphological criteria. *Br J Urol* 1988;61:129–34.

57. Schapers RF, Pauwels RP, Wijnen JT, Arends JW, Thunnissen FB, Coebergh JW, Smeets AW, Bosman

FT. A simplified grading method of transitional cell carcinoma of the urinary bladder: reproducibility, clinical significance and comparison with other prognostic parameters. *Br J Urol* 1994;73:625–31.

58. Carbin B, Ekman P, Gustafson H, Christensen NJ, Sandstedt B, Silfversward C. Grading of human urothelial carcinoma based on nuclear atypia and mitotic frequency. I. Histological description. *J Urol* 1991;145:968–71.

59. Lipponen PK, Eskelinen MJ, Kiviranta J, Pesonen E. Prognosis of transitional cell bladder cancer: a multivariate prognostic score for improved prediction. *J Urol* 1991;146:1535–40.

60. Bostwick DG, Lopez-Beltran A. Bladder Biopsy Interpretation. Washington DC: United Pathologists Press, 1999.

61. Eble JN, Sauter G, Epstein JI, Sesterhenn IA, eds. World Health Organization Classification of Tumours: Pathology and Genetics of Tumours of the Urinary System and Male Genital Organs. Lyon, France: IARC Press, 2004.

62. Alsheikh A, Mohamedali Z, Jones E, Masterson J, Gilks CB. Comparison of the WHO/ISUP classification and cytokeratin 20 expression in predicting the behavior of low grade papillary urothelial tumors. World/Health Organization/Internattional Society of Urologic Pathology. *Mod Pathol* 2001;14:267–72.

63. Alvarez KJ, Lopez-Beltran A, Anglada CF, Moreno AP, Carazo CJL, Regueiro LJC, Leva VM, Prieto CR, Requena TMJ. Clinico-pathologic differences between bladder neoplasm with low malignant potential and low grade carcinoma. *Actas Urol Esp* 2001;25:645–50.

64. Montironi R, Lopez-Beltran A. The 2004 WHO Classification of Bladder Tumors: a summary and commentary. *Int J Surg Pathol* 2005;13:143–53.

65. Montironi R, Lopez-Beltran A, Mazzucchelli R, Bostwick DG. Classification and grading of the non-invasive urothelial neoplasms: recent advances and controversies. *J Clin Pathol* 2003;56:91–5.

66. Cheng L, Neumann RM, Bostwick DG. Papillary urothelial neoplasms of low malignant potential. Clinical and biologic implications. *Cancer* 1999;86:2102–8.

67. Herr HW, Donat SM, Reuter VE. Management of low grade papillary bladder tumors. *J Urol* 2007;178:1201–5; discussion 1205.

68. Miyamoto H, Brimo F, Schultz L, Ye H, Miller JS, Fajardo DA, Lee TK, Epstein JI, Netto GJ. Low grade papillary urothelial carcinoma of the urinary bladder: a clinicopathologic analysis of a post-World Health Organization/International Society of Urological Pathology classification cohort from a single academic center. *Arch Pathol Lab Med* 2010;134:1160–3.

69. Habuchi T, Ogawa O, Kakehi Y, Ogura K, Koshiba M, Hamazaki S, Takahashi R, Sugiyama T, Yoshida O. Accumulated allelic losses in the development of invasive urothelial cancer. *Int J Cancer* 1993;53:5093–5.

70. Mostofi FK, Davis CJ, Sesterhenn IA. WHO Histologic Typing of Urinary Bladder Tumors. Berlin: Springer, 1999.

71. Cheng L, Darson M, Cheville JC, Neumann RM, Zincke Z, Nehra A, Bostwick DG. Urothelial papilloma of the bladder: clinical and biologic implications. *Cancer* 1999;86:2098–101.

72. Oosterhuis JW, Schapers RF, Janssen-Heijnen ML, Pauwels RP, Newling DW, ten Kate F. Histological grading of papillary urothelial carcinoma of the bladder: prognostic value of the 1998 WHO/ISUP classification system and comparison with conventional grading systems. *J Clin Pathol* 2002;55:900–5.

73. Oyasu R. World Health Organization and International Society of Urological Pathology Classification and two-number grading system of bladder tumors. *Cancer* 2000;88:1509–12.

74. Bol MG, Baak JP, Buhr-Wildhagen S, Kruse AJ, Kjellevold KH, Janssen EA, Mestad O, Øgreid P. Reproducibility and prognostic variability of grade and lamina propria invasion in stages Ta, T1

urothelial carcinoma of the bladder. *J Urol* 2003;169:1291–4.

75. Eble JN, Sauter G, Epstein JI, Sesterhenn IAE. World Health Organization Classification of Tumours: Pathology and Genetics of Tumours of the Urinary System and Male Genital Organs. Lyon, France: IARC Press, 2004.

76. Samaratunga H, Makarov DV, Epstein JI. Comparison of WHO/ISUP and WHO classification of noninvasive papillary urothelial neoplasms for risk of progression. *Urology* 2002;60:315–9.

77. Cheng L, Neumann RM, Bostwick DG. Papillary urothelial neoplasms of low malignant potentia: clinical and biological implications. *Cancer* 1999;86:2102–8.

78. Haukaas S, Daehlin L, Maartmann-Moe H, Ulvik NM. The long-term outcome in patients with superficial transitional cell carcinoma of the bladder: a single-institutional experience. *BJU Int* 1999;83:957–63.

79. Cheng L, Neumann RM, Nehra A, Spotts BE, Weaver AL, Bostwick DG. Cancer heterogeneity and its biologic implications in the grading of urothelial carcinoma. *Cancer* 2000;88:1663–70.

80. Cheng L, Neumann RM, Weaver AL, Cheville JC, Leibovich BC, Ramnani DM, Scherer BG, Nehra A, Zincke H, Bostwick DG. Grading and staging of bladder carcinoma in transurethral resection specimens. Correlation with 105 matched cystectomy specimens. *Am J Clin Pathol* 2000;113:275–9.

81. Pan CC, Chang YH, Chen KK, Yu HJ, Sun CH, Ho DM. Prognostic significance of the 2004 WHO/ISUP classification for prediction of recurrence, progression, and cancer-specific mortality of non-muscle-invasive urothelial tumors of the urinary bladder: a clinicopathologic study of 1,515 cases. *Am J Clin Pathol* 2010;133:788–95.

82. Holmang S, Andius P, Hedelin H, Wester K, Busch C, Johansson SL. Stage progression in Ta papillary urothelial tumors: relationship to grade, immunohistochemical expression of tumor markers, mitotic frequency and DNA ploidy. *J Urol* 2001;165:1124–8; discussion 1128–30.

83. Pich A, Chiusa L, Formiconi A, Galliano D, Bortolin P, Comino A, Navone R. Proliferative activity is the most significant predictor of recurrence in noninvasive papillary urothelial neoplasms of low malignant potential and grade 1 papillary carcinomas of the bladder. *Cancer* 2002;95:784–90.

84. Lipponen P, Simpanen H, Pesonen E, Eskelinen M, Sotarauta M, Collan Y. Potential of morphometry in grading transitional cell carcinoma of the urinary bladder. *Path Res Pract* 1989;185:617–20.

85. Genega EM, Porter CR. Urothelial neoplasms of the kidney and ureter. An epidemiologic, pathologic, and clinical review. *Am J Clin Pathol* 2002;117 (Suppl):S36–48.

86. Hall MC, Womack S, Sagalowsky AI, Carmody T, Erickstad MD, Roehrborn CG. Prognostic factors, recurrence, and survival in transitional cell carcinoma of the upper urinary tract: a 30-year experience in 252 patients. *Urology* 1998;52:594–601.

87. Genega EM, Kapali M, Torres-Quinones M, Huang WC, Knauss JS, Wang LP, Raghunath PN, Kozlowski C, Malkowicz SB, Tomaszewski JE. Impact of the 1998 World Health Organization/International Society of Urological Pathology classification system for urothelial neoplasms of the kidney. *Mod Pathol* 2005;18:11–18.

88. Olgac S, Mazumdar M, Dalbagni G, Reuter VE. Urothelial carcinoma of the renal pelvis: a clinicopathologic study of 130 cases. *Am J Surg Pathol* 2004;28:1545–52.

89. Whisnant RE, Bastacky SI, Ohori NP. Cytologic diagnosis of low grade papillary urothelial neoplasms (low malignant potential and low grade carcinoma) in the context of the 1998 WHO/ISUP classification. *Diagn Cytopathol* 2003;28:186–90.

90. Curry JL, Wojcik EM. The effects of the current World Health Organization/International Society of Urologic Pathologists bladder neoplasm classification system on urine cytology results. *Cancer* 2002;96:140–5.

91. Rieger-Christ KM, Mourtzinos A, Lee PJ, Zagha RM, Cain J, Silverman M, Libertino JA, Summerhayes IC. Identification of fibroblast growth factor receptor 3 mutations in urine sediment DNA samples complements cytology in bladder tumor detection. *Cancer* 2003;98:737–44.

92. Alsheikh A, Mohamedali Z, Jones E, Masterson J, Gilks CB. Comparison of the WHO/ISUP classification and cytokeratin 20 expression in predicting the behavior of low grade papillary urothelial tumors. World/Health Organization/Internattional Society of Urologic Pathology. *Mod Pathol* 2001;14:261–72.

93. Soloway MS, Bruck DS, Kim SS. Expectant management of small, recurrent, noninvasive papillary bladder tumors. *J Urol* 2003;170:438–41.

94. Lotan Y, Roehrborn CG. Cost-effectiveness of a modified care protocol substituting bladder tumor markers for cystoscopy for the followup of patients with transitional cell carcinoma of the bladder: a decision analytical approach. *J Urol* 2002;167:75–9.

95. Mariappan P, Smith G. A surveillance schedule for G1Ta bladder cancer allowing efficient use of check cystoscopy and safe discharge at 5 years based on a 25-year prospective database. *J Urol* 2005;173:1108–11.

96. Holmang S, Johansson SL. Stage Ta-T1 bladder cancer: the relationship between findings at first followup cystoscopy and subsequent recurrence and progression. *J Urol* 2002;167:1634–7.

97. Thompson RA Jr, Campbell EW Jr, Kramer HC, Jacobs SC, Naslund MJ. Late invasive recurrence despite long-term surveillance for superficial bladder cancer. *J Urol* 1993;149:1010–11.

98. Eble JN, Young RH. Benign and low grade papillary lesions of the urinary bladder: A review of the papilloma-papillary carcinoma controversy, and a report of five typical papillomas. *Semin Diag Pathol* 1989;6:351–71.

99. Schned AR, Andrew AS, Marsit CJ, Zens MS, Kelsey KT, Karagas MR. Survival following the diagnosis of noninvasive bladder cancer: WHO/International Society of Urological Pathology versus WHO classification systems. *J Urol* 2007;178:1196–1200.

100. Jimenez RE, Gheiler E, Oskanian P, Tiguert R, Sakr W, Wood DP Jr, Pontes JE, Grignon DJ. Grading the invasive component of urothelial carcinoma of the bladder and its relationship with progression-free survival. *Am J Surg Pathol* 2000;24:980–7.

101. Bircan S, Candir O, Serel TA. Comparison of WHO 1973, WHO/ISUP 1998, WHO 1999 grade and combined scoring systems in evaluation of bladder carcinoma. *Urol Int* 2004;73:201–8.

102. van Rhijn BW, van der Kwast TH, Vis AN, Kirkels WJ, Boeve ER, Jobsis AC, Zwarthoff EC. FGFR3 and P53 characterize alternative genetic pathways in the pathogenesis of urothelial cell carcinoma. *Cancer Res* 2004;64:1911–4.

103. Bakkar AA, Wallerand H, Radvanyi F, Lahaye JB, Pissard S, Lecerf L, Kouyoumdjian JC, Abbou CC, Pairon JC, Jaurand MC, Thiery JP, Chopin DK, de Medina SG. FGFR3 and TP53 gene mutations define two distinct pathways in urothelial cell carcinoma of the bladder. *Cancer Res* 2003;63:8108–12.

104. Gomez-Roman JJ, Saenz P, Molina M, Cuevas Gonzalez J, Escuredo K, Santa Cruz S, Junquera C, Simon L, Martinez A, Gutierrez Banos JL, Lopez-Brea M, Esparza C, Val-Bernal JF. Fibroblast growth factor receptor 3 is overexpressed in urinary tract carcinomas and modulates the neoplastic cell growth. *Clin Cancer Res* 2005;11:459–65.

105. van Rhijn BW, Lurkin I, Radvanyi F, Kirkels WJ, van der Kwast TH, Zwarthoff EC. The fibroblast growth factor receptor 3 (FGFR3) mutation is a strong indicator of superficial bladder cancer with low recurrence rate. *Cancer Res* 2001;61:1265–8.

106. Lamy A, Gobet F, Laurent M, Blanchard F, Varin C, Moulin C, Andreou A, Frebourg T, Pfister C. Molecular profiling of bladder tumors based on the detection of FGFR3 and TP53 mutations. *J Urol* 2006;176:2686–9.

107. Burger M, van der Aa MN, van Oers JM, Brinkmann A, van der Kwast TH, Steyerberg EC, Stoehr R, Kirkels WJ, Denzinger S, Wild PJ, Wieland WF, Hofstaedter F, Hartmann A, Zwarthoff EC. Prediction of progression of non-muscle-invasive bladder cancer by WHO 1973 and 2004 grading and by FGFR3 mutation status: a prospective study. *Eur Urol* 2008;54:835–43.

108. Lauss M, Ringner M, Hoglund M. Prediction of stage, grade, and survival in bladder cancer using genome-wide expression data: a validation study. *Clin Cancer Res* 2010;16:4421–33.

109. van Rhijn BW, Vis AN, van der Kwast TH, Kirkels WJ, Radvanyi F, Ooms EC, Chopin DK, Boeve ER, Jobsis AC, Zwarthoff EC. Molecular grading of urothelial cell carcinoma with fibroblast growth factor receptor 3 and MIB-1 is superior to pathologic grade for the prediction of clinical outcome. *J Clin Oncol* 2003;21:1912–21.

110. Mengual L, Burset M, Ars E, Lozano JJ, Villavicencio H, Ribal MJ, Alcaraz A. DNA microarray expression profiling of bladder cancer allows identification of noninvasive diagnostic markers. *J Urol* 2009;182:741–8.

111. Catto JW, Miah S, Owen HC, Bryant H, Myers K, Dudziec E, Larre S, Milo M, Rehman I, Rosario DJ, Di Martino E, Knowles MA, Meuth M, Harris AL, Hamdy FC. Distinct microRNA alterations characterize high- and low grade bladder cancer. *Cancer Res* 2009;69:8472–81.

112. Brunner A, Schonhuber G, Waldner M, Schaefer G, Mikuz G, Verdorfer I. Chromosomal aberrations in urothelial carcinoma of the bladder and the World Health Organization 2004 grading system. *Anal Quant Cytol Histol* 2008;30:297–305.

113. Simonetti S, Russo R, Ciancia G, Altieri V, De Rosa G, Insabato L. Role of polysomy 17 in transitional cell carcinoma of the bladder: immunohistochemical study of HER2/neu expression and fish analysis of c-erbB–2 gene and chromosome 17. *Int J Surg Pathol* 2009;17:198–205.

114. Harnden P, Mahmond N, Southgate J. Expression of cytokeratin 20 defines urothelial papillomas of the bladder. *Lancet* 1999;353:974–7.

115. Yin H, Leong AS. Histologic grading of noninvasive papillary urothelial tumors: validation of the 1998 WHO/ISUP system by immunophenotyping and followup. *Am J Clin Pathol* 2004;121:679–87.

116. Karakok M, Aydin A, Bakir K, Ucak R, Korkmaz C. AgNOR/p53 expression compared with different grades in bladder carcinoma. *Int Urol Nephrol* 2001;33:353–5.

117. Dyrskjot L, Zieger K, Kruhoffer M, Thykjaer T, Jensen JL, Primdahl H, Aziz N, Marcussen N, Moller K, Orntoft TF. A molecular signature in superficial bladder carcinoma predicts clinical outcome. *Clin Cancer Res* 2005;11:4029–36.

Chapter 10

Stage pT1 Urothelial Carcinoma

Bladder Pathology, First Edition. Liang Cheng, Antonio Lopez-Beltran, David G. Bostwick.
© 2012 Wiley-Blackwell. Published 2012 by John Wiley & Sons, Inc.

The 2010 tumor, lymph node, and metastasis (TNM) staging system defines pT1 tumors of the bladder as those invading the lamina propria but not the muscularis propria (**Figs. 10-1** and **10-2**).[1] The recognition of lamina propria invasion by urothelial carcinoma is one of the most challenging fields in surgical pathology, and the pathologist should follow strict criteria in its assessment (**Table 10-1**).[2,3] Clinical management of pT1 bladder cancer has been reviewed extensively by Soloway.[4] Patients with primary T1 urothelial carcinoma may have a higher risk of cancer progression than do those patients who initially present with Ta or CIS cancers.[5] However, an earlier study indicated that patients with primary stage T1 bladder cancers had a higher progression rate than that of those with nonprimary pT1 cancer.[6]

Table 10-1   Histologic Features Useful for the Diagnosis of Stromal Invasion

Histologic grade
  Invasive cells are usually higher nuclear grade

Invading epithelium
  Irregularly shaped nests
  Single cell infiltration
  Irregular or absent basement membrane
  Tentacular finger-like projections
  Paradoxical differentiation
  Angiolymphatic invasion

Stromal response
  Desmoplasia or fibrotic stroma
  Retraction artifact
  Inflammation
  Myxoid stroma
  Pseudosarcomatous stroma

Diagnosis of Lamina Propria Invasion (pT1 Urothelial Carcinoma)

Histologic Grade

Most invasive urothelial carcinomas are high grade tumors (**Figs. 10-3** and **10-4**). While invasion is not necessarily an unexpected finding in low grade tumors (**Fig. 10-5**), it is much more commonly encountered in high grade lesions, reaching 96% in some series.[2,3] In addition, the histologic grade of transurethral resection (TUR) specimens correlates closely with the pathologic stage at cystectomy.[7]

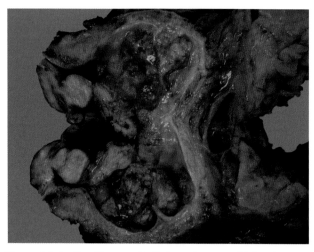

Figure 10-1   Papillary urothelial carcinoma with lamina propria invasion (pT1 cancer).

Stroma–Epithelial Interface

Tangentially sectioned, densely packed noninvasive papillary tumors exhibit a stroma–epithelial interface that is smooth and regular. In instances of true invasion, one is likely to see variably sized and irregularly shaped nests or individual tumor cells insinuating through the stroma (**Figs. 10-6** to **10-10**). When the specimen includes tangential sections through noninvasive tumor or when urothelial carcinoma involves von Brunn nests, the basement membrane preserves a regular contour, whereas it is frequently absent or disrupted in cases of true invasion. The smoothness of the stroma–epithelial interface may be assessed using hematoxylin and eosin (H&E) stains. In some cases, however, additional findings may be helpful; for example, there is a parallel array of thin-walled vessels that evenly line the basement membrane of noninvasive nests. These are absent in patients with invasive tumors.

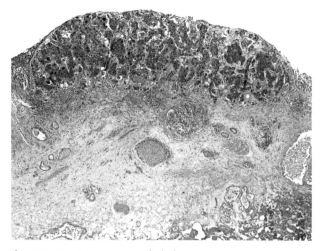

Figure 10-2   Stage pT1 urothelial carcinoma.

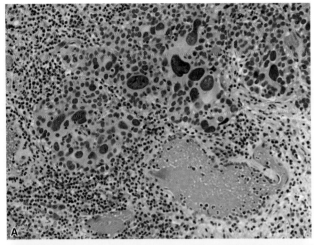

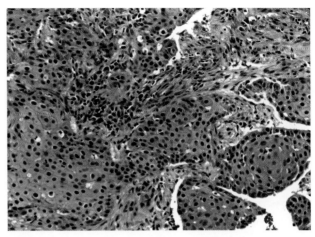

Figure 10-5 Grade 2 (low grade) invasive urothelial carcinoma.

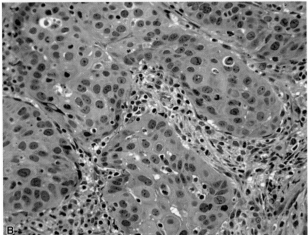

Figure 10-3 Stage pT1 urothelial carcinoma (A and B). The majority of pT1 urothelial carcinomas are high grade (grade 3–4 in the new classification; see **Chapter 9** for further discussion).

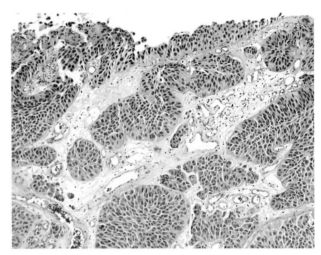

Figure 10-6 Stage pT1 urothelial carcinoma. Note the variable-sized tumor nests.

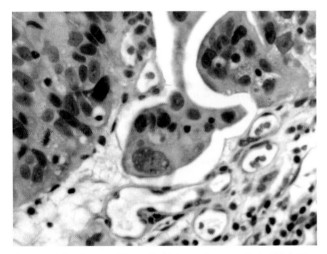

Figure 10-4 Stage pT1 urothelial carcinoma. Note the high nuclear grade of the tumor cells and retraction artifact, which is relatively common in early invasive bladder carcinoma.

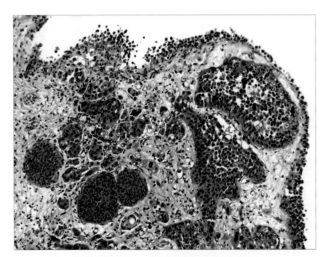

Figure 10-7 Stage pT1 urothelial carcinoma. Note the variable-sized tumor nests and infiltrating individual tumor cells.

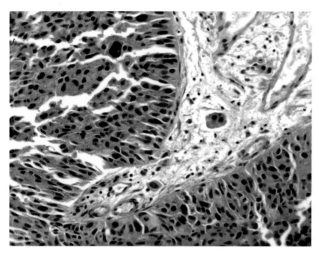

Figure 10-8 Stage pT1 urothelial carcinoma. Note the infiltrating single tumor cell and retraction artifact.

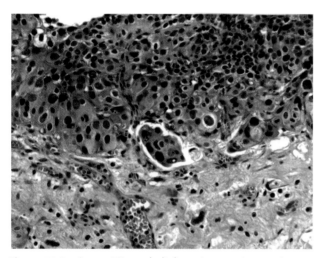

Figure 10-9 Stage pT1 urothelial carcinoma. A retraction artifact is one of most helpful features in identifying early stromal invasion.

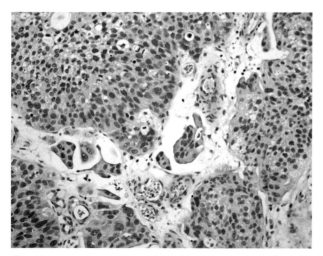

Figure 10-10 Stage pT1 urothelial carcinoma. Note the retraction artifact.

Invading Epithelium

The invasive front of the neoplasm may show one of several features. Most commonly, tumors invade the underlying stroma as single cells or irregularly shaped nests of tumor cells (**Figs. 10-11** and **10-12**). Sometimes, tentacular or finger-like extensions can be seen arising from the base of the papillary tumor (**Fig. 10-13**). Frequently, the invading nests appear cytologically different from cells at the base of the noninvasive component. Invasive tumor cells often have more abundant cytoplasm and a higher degree of nuclear pleomorphism. In some cases, particularly in microinvasive disease, the invasive tumor cells may acquire abundant eosinophilic cytoplasm. At low to medium power magnification, these microinvasive cells seem to be more differentiated than the overlying noninvasive disease, a feature known as paradoxical differentiation (**Figs. 10-14** to **10-16**).

Stromal Response

The stromal response to invading carcinoma is not always uniformly present in invasive urothelial carcinoma, and the diagnosis of invasion may rely on identification of the typical characteristics of the invading epithelium. The stromal reaction in the lamina propria associated with invasive tumor may be inflammatory (**Figs. 10-17** to **10-19**), myxoid (**Figs. 10-20** and **10-21**), or fibrous (**Figs. 10-22** and **10-23**). Assessment of differences in the stromal growth pattern provides an important diagnostic clue.[8] Although the majority of bladder tumors with unquestionable lamina propria invasion exhibit some sort of stromal reaction, microinvasive disease usually does not, making its identification even more difficult. In some cases, retraction artifact around superficially invasive individual tumor cells may mimic angiolymphatic invasion. This finding is often focal and

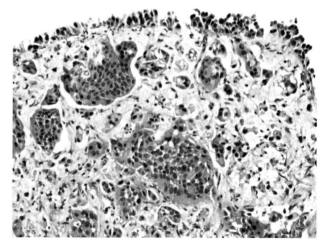

Figure 10-11 Stage pT1 urothelial carcinoma. Note the single cells and irregularly shaped tumor nests.

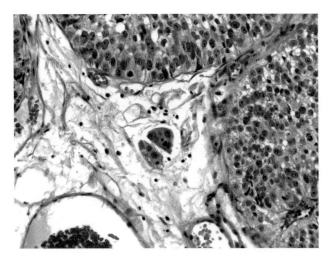

Figure 10-12 Stage pT1 urothelial carcinoma. Note the retraction artifact.

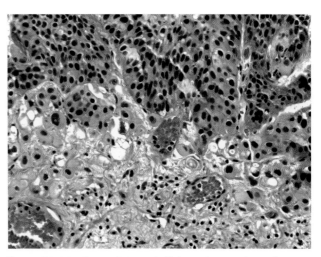

Figure 10-14 Stage pT1 urothelial carcinoma. Note the paradoxical differentiation.

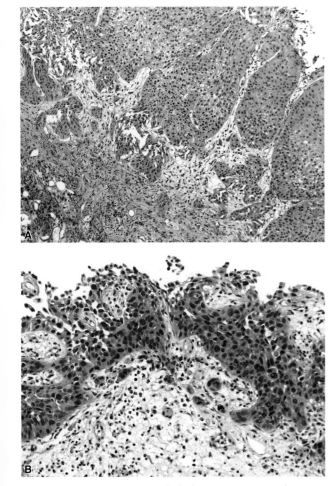

Figure 10-13 Stage pT1 urothelial carcinoma (A and B). Note the tentacular or finger-like projects of an early invasive urothelial carcinoma.

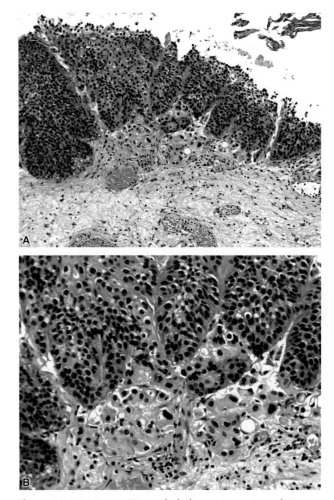

Figure 10-15 Stage pT1 urothelial carcinoma (A and B). Note the paradoxical differentiation.

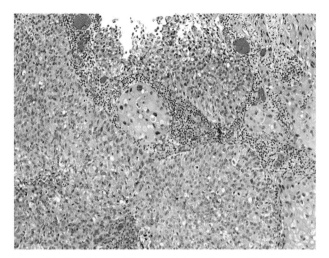

Figure 10-16 Stage pT1 urothelial carcinoma. Note the paradoxical differentiation.

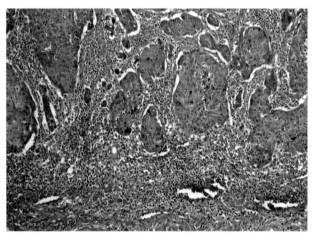

Figure 10-17 Stage pT1 urothelial carcinoma with inflammatory stroma.

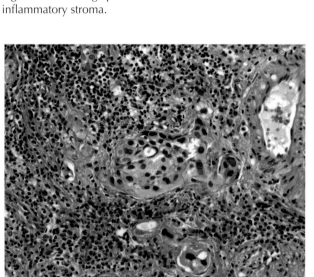

Figure 10-18 Stage pT1 urothelial carcinoma with inflammatory stroma.

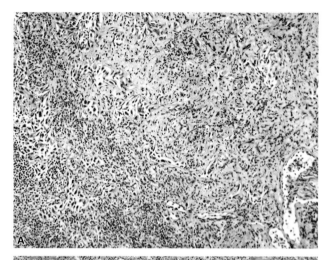

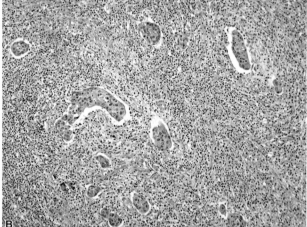

Figure 10-19 Stage pT1 urothelial carcinoma with inflammatory stroma (A and B).

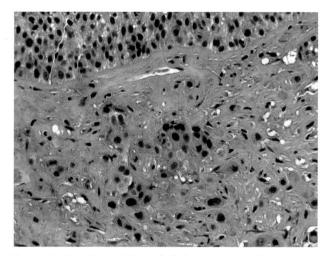

Figure 10-20 Stage pT1 urothelial carcinoma with myxoid stroma.

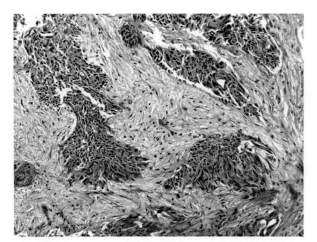

Figure 10-21 Stage pT1 urothelial carcinoma with myxoid stroma.

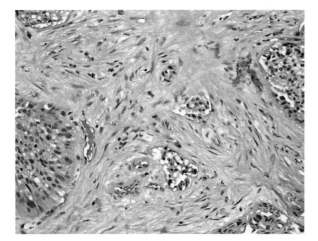

Figure 10-22 Stage pT1 urothelial carcinoma with fibrotic stroma.

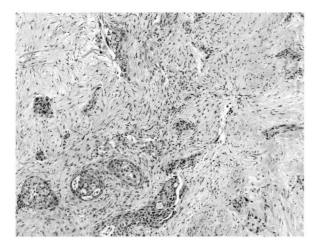

Figure 10-23 Stage pT1 urothelial carcinoma with fibrotic stroma.

may itself be one of the early signs of invasion into the lamina propria.

Lamina propria invasion may elicit a brisk inflammatory response. Numerous inflammatory cells in the lamina propria often obscure the interface between epithelium and stroma. This makes a small nest or single cell invasion difficult to recognize. Cytokeratin immunostaining is useful in difficult cases (**Figs. 10-24** and **10-25**).

Invasive urothelial carcinoma may have a cellular stroma with spindled fibroblasts and variable collagenization, or a hypocellular stroma with myxoid background (**Figs. 10-26** and **10-27**). Rarely, the tumor induces an exuberant proliferation of fibroblasts, which may display alarming cellular atypia similar to giant cell cystitis. This feature, although a helpful clue to invasion, should not be mistaken for the spindle cell component of sarcomatoid urothelial carcinoma. Immunostains for cytokeratin are helpful in difficult cases although some myofibroblasts may also be positive for keratin.[9] The proliferating stroma is usually nonexpansile, being limited to areas around the neoplasm, and is composed of cells that have a degenerate or smudged appearance.

Unusual Histologic Patterns of Lamina Propria Invasion

Carcinoma in Situ with Microinvasion (CISmic)

Invasion may be seen in urothelial CIS (**Figs. 10-28** and **10-29**). A recent proposal based on the Ancona International Consultation, has suggested a cutoff for CISmic of no more than 20 invading cells, measured from the stroma–epithelial interface.[10] It is useful to recognize a number of morphologic patterns of CISmic, including single cell invasion, clustered invasive cells with retraction artifact, and tentacular extension.[2]

Papillary Urothelial Carcinoma with Microinvasion

Microinvasion of papillary urothelial carcinoma is defined in a manner similar to CISmic and its presence should be noted in the report (**Figs. 10-30** to **10-32**).[10] The extent of microinvasion may also be quantified accurately using a micrometer.[11–13]

Papillary Urothelial Carcinoma with Invasion into the "Stalk"

It is uncommon for papillary urothelial carcinoma to invade the stalk of a papilla (**Fig. 10-33**). Appreciation of this pattern requires optimal orientation of the entire papillary tumor, which may not always be the case, especially in the TUR specimens.

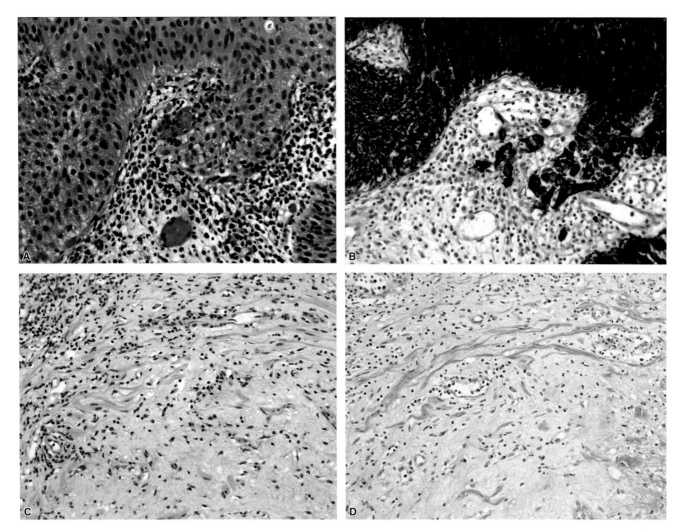

Figure 10-24 Stage pT1 urothelial carcinoma. (A) Prominent inflammation at the stroma–epithelial interface may obscure isolated cells or small nests of invasive carcinoma. (B) Immmunostaining with anticytokeratin antibodies highlights the tumor cells. (C and D) Myofibroblasts and smooth muscle cells may show positive cytokeratin immunoreactivity. The intensity of staining, however, is weak and the nuclei are small with indistinct smudged chromatin. (From Ref. 3; with permission.)

Variants of Invasive Urothelial Carcinoma with Deceptively Bland Cytology

Deceptively bland patterns of invasive urothelial carcinoma may make recognition of pT1 disease extremely difficult in small biopsies (see also **Chapter 12**).[2,14] For example, microcystic variant of urothelial carcinoma may mimic cystitis cystica and cystitis glandularis (**Fig. 10-34**). The nested variant of urothelial carcinoma may be confused with von Brunn nest hyperplasia, particularly in limited superficial biopsies (**Figs. 10-35** and **10-36**).[2,15] Attention should be paid to general features useful in assessing invasion, such as cytological atypia, infiltrative architecture, desmoplasia, and architectural complexity, and pathologists should be aware that these signs may be subtle in superficial biopsies.

Invasion in Urothelial Carcinoma with Inverted Growth

A more difficult pattern of invasion is seen in large papillary tumors with prominent endophytic growth (**Figs. 10-37** and **10-38**). These carcinomas often invade the lamina propria with a pushing border, much akin to cutaneous and mucosal verrucous carcinoma. Applying strict morphologic criteria for the diagnosis of stromal invasion should minimize diagnostic discrepancies among pathologists (see **Chapter 17** for further discussion).

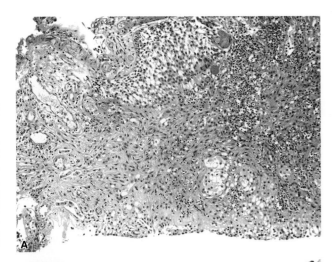

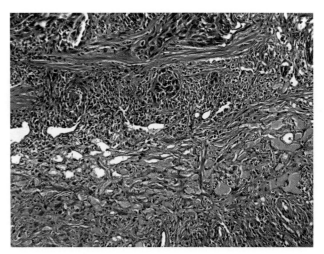

Figure 10-27 Invasive urothelial carcinoma with pseudosarcomatous and myxoid stroma.

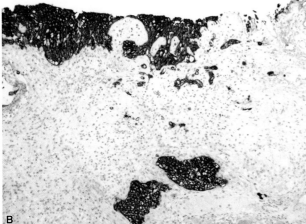

Figure 10-25 Stage pT1 urothelial carcinoma (A and B). The inflammatory response may obscure the interface between the epithelium and the stroma. Cytokeratin staining highlights infiltrative tumor cells (B).

Table 10-2 Unusual Histologic Patterns of Lamina Propria Invasion

Carcinoma in situ with microinvasion
Papillary urothelial carcinoma with microinvasion
Papillary urothelial carcinoma with invasion into the "stalk"
Variants of invasive urothelial carcinoma with deceptively bland cytology
Invasion in urothelial carcinoma with inverted growth

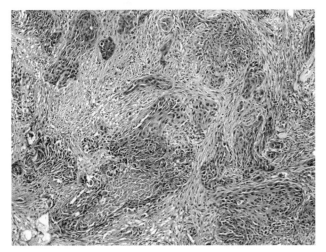

Figure 10-26 Invasive urothelial carcinoma with pseudosarcomatous stroma.

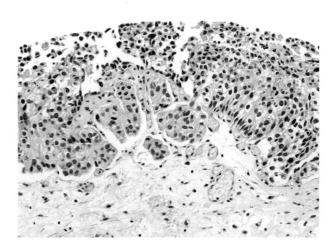

Figure 10-28 Carcinoma in situ with microinvasion.

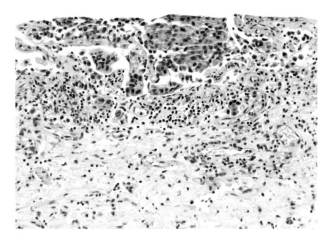

Figure 10-29   Carcinoma in situ with microinvasion.

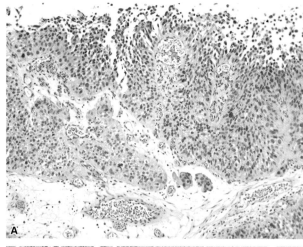

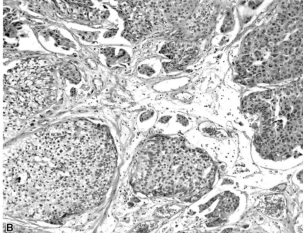

Figure 10-31   Papillary urothelial carcinoma with early invasion (A and B).

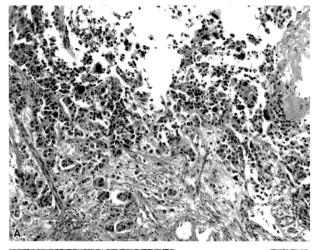

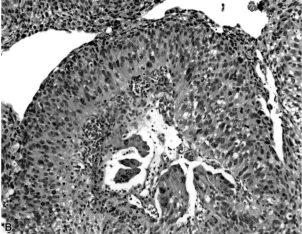

Figure 10-30   Papillary urothelial carcinoma with early invasion (A and B).

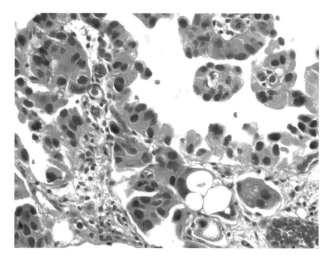

Figure 10-32   Papillary urothelial carcinoma with early invasion.

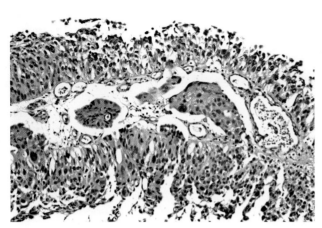

Figure 10-33 Papillary urothelial carcinoma with invasion into the stalk.

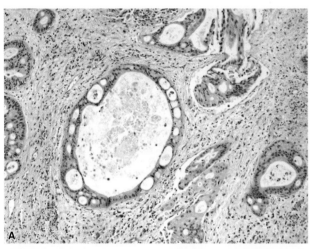

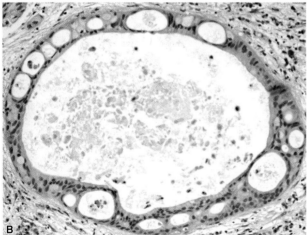

Figure 10-34 Microcystic variant of urothelial carcinoma (A and B).

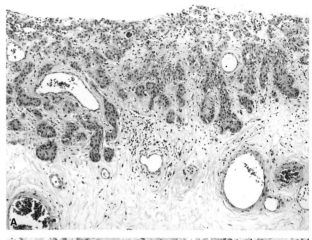

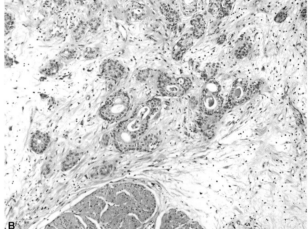

Figure 10-35 Nested variant of urothelial carcinoma (A and B).

Pitfalls in the Diagnosis of Stage pT1 Urothelial Carcinoma

Tangential Sectioning and Poor Orientation

TUR specimens are excised in a piecemeal fashion. The specimens resulting from this procedure are often fragmented with frequent disruption of the tumor architecture, and thus may be difficult to orient. Furthermore, due to their complex architecture, papillary tumors are inevitably tangentially sectioned in multiple planes, resulting in the presence of isolated nests of noninvasive tumor cells within connective tissue. Smooth, round, and regular contours favor tangential sectioning, whereas irregular, jagged nests with a haphazard arrangement favor stromal invasion.

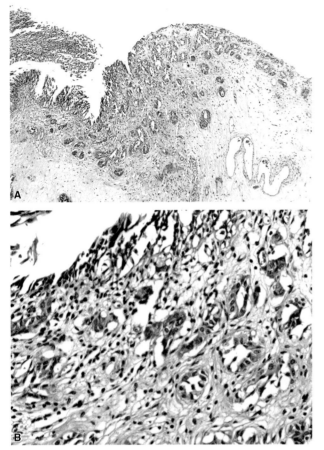

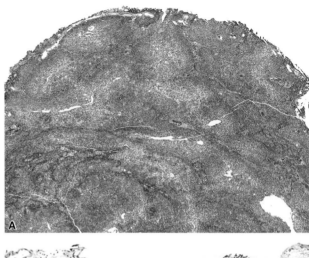

Figure 10-36 Nested variant of urothelial carcinoma (A and B).

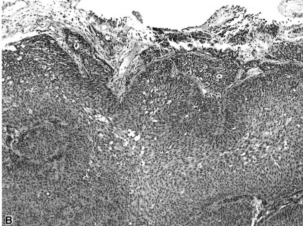

Figure 10-37 Inverted variant of urothelial carcinoma (A and B).

Thermal Injury

Thermal injury or cautery artifact produces severely distorted morphology in TUR specimens (**Figs. 10-39 to 10-41**) and is a frequent source of difficulty for the pathologist.[16,17] Unfortunately, pathologists have no control over this problem, although deeper levels may occasionally display better preserved areas. Some cases may also benefit from the use of immunohistochemistry with anticytokeratin antibodies.[17] When this proves unhelpful, an inability to render a definitive diagnosis due to thermal effect should be stated clearly in the report.

Obscuring Inflammation

Papillary tumors may show variable and often brisk inflammation at the tumor–stroma interface (**Figs. 10-42 and 10-43**). This may obscure isolated cells or small nests of invasive tumor. Diagnosis of invasion in some of these cases can be facilitated by immunohistochemical study with anticytokeratin antibodies.

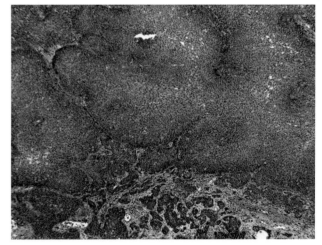

Figure 10-38 Inverted variant of urothelial carcinoma with invasion.

Table 10-3   Pitfalls in the Diagnosis of Stage pT1 Urothelial Carcinoma

Tangential sectioning and poor orientation

Thermal injury

Obscuring inflammation

Urothelial carcinoma in situ involving von Brunn nests

Urothelial carcinoma with endophytic or broad-front growth pattern

Pseudoinvasive nests of benign proliferative urothelial lesions

Muscle invasion indeterminate for the type of muscle (muscularis propria versus muscularis mucosae)

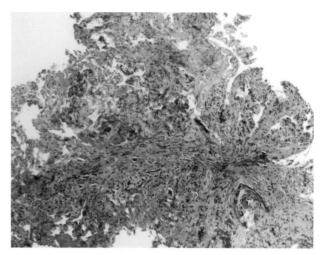

Figure 10-40   Thermal artifact in transurethral resection. The specimen is uninterpretable.

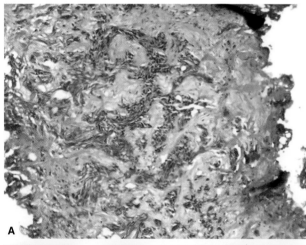

A

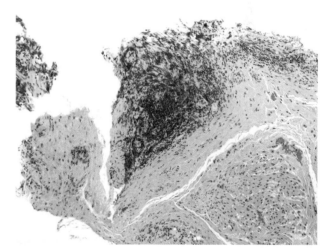

Figure 10-41   Thermal artifact in transurethral resection.

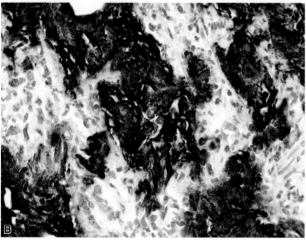

B

Figure 10-39   Transurethral resection with associated thermal artifact showing crushed tumor nests infiltrating the lamina propria (A). Immunostaining for cytokeratin AE1/AE3 highlights the epithelial nature of the invading nests (B).

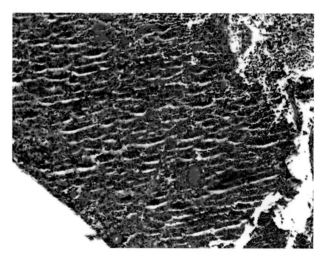

Figure 10-42   Obscuring inflammation in transurethral resection.

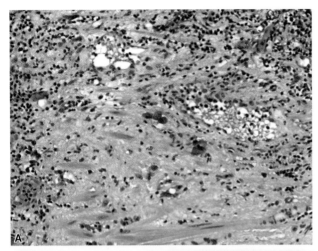

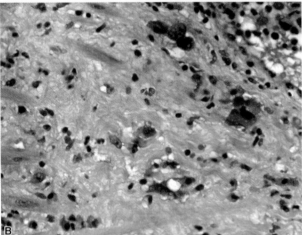

Figure 10-43 Bizarre stromal cells in an inflamed stroma (A and B). These atypical stromal cells may mimic infiltrating tumor cells. Cytokeratin immunostaining is helpful in difficult cases. These stromal cells were negative for cytokeratin staining (not shown).

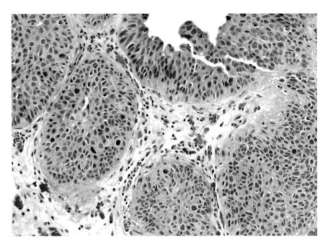

Figure 10-44 Urothelial carcinoma in situ involving von Brunn nests. The smooth contours are retained. No invasion is seen.

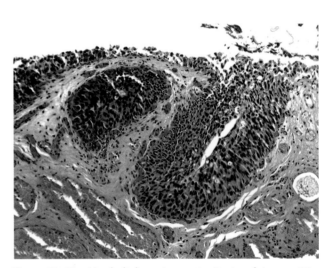

Figure 10-45 Urothelial carcinoma in situ involving cystitis glandularis and von Brunn nests. No invasion is seen.

Carcinoma in Situ Involving von Brunn Nests

Tumor cells involving von Brunn nests may also mimic lamina propria invasion (**Figs. 10-44** and **10-45**). This is especially problematic when von Brunn nests are prominent or when they have been distorted by inflammatory or cautery artifact (see **Chapter 7** for further discussion).

Urothelial Carcinoma with Endophytic or Broad-Front Growth Pattern

Strict diagnostic criteria for stromal invasion should apply in cases of urothelial carcinoma with endophytic or broad-front growth pattern. Admission of an inability to identify invasion definitively is appropriate in difficult cases with suboptimal tissue preservation or orientation.

Pseudoinvasive Nests of Benign Proliferative Urothelial Lesions

In rare cases, benign proliferative urothelial lesions such as florid von Brunn nest proliferations, florid cystitis glandularis, inverted papilloma, and nephrogenic metaplasia manifest as pseudoinvasive nests of urothelium within the lamina propria (**Figs. 10-46** and **10-47**).[18,19] The problem is often compounded by lack of orientation and by cautery artifact. Pseudocarcinomatous epithelial hyperplasia, typically associated with radiation and chemotherapy, should also occur in other settings. The presence of a prominent inflammatory background should alert the pathologists to the possibility of dealing with those cancer mimickers (**Figs. 10-48** and **10-49**; see **Chapters 3** and **24** for further discussion).

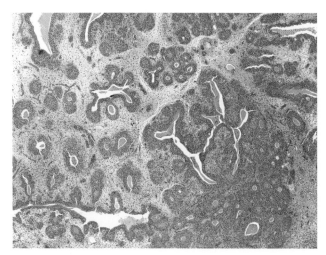

Figure 10-46   Florid von Brunn nest proliferations and cystitis glandularis.

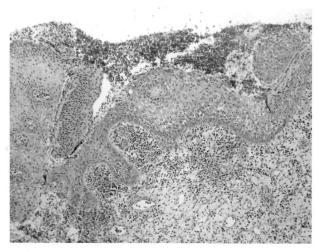

Figure 10-48   Pseudocarcinomatous epithelial hyperplasia.

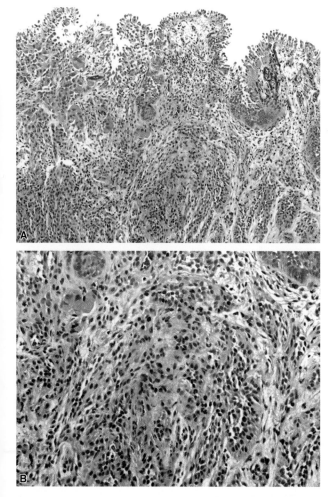

Figure 10-47   Florid von Brunn nest proliferations (A and B).

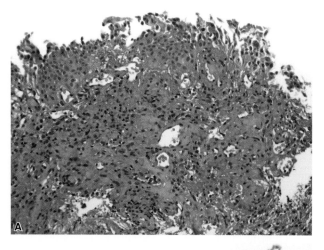

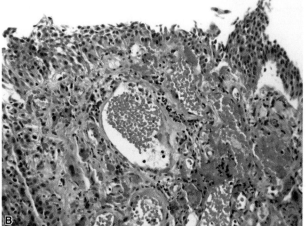

Figure 10-49   Pseudocarcinomatous epithelial hyperplasia (A and B).

Muscle Invasion Indeterminate for the Type of Muscle

In some cases, invasive tumor is juxtaposed to muscle fibers, but due to obscuring factors (i.e., inflammation, tangential sectioning, cautery artifact, desmoplastic response, or poor orientation), it may be difficult to determine whether the muscle fibers are from the muscularis mucosae or muscularis propria (detrusor muscle) (**Figs. 10-50 to 10-53**). Muscularis mucosae is often present in the lamina propria and consists of thin and wavy fascicles of smooth muscle, which are frequently associated with large-caliber blood vessels (also see **Chapter 1**).[2,7,20] Occasionally, muscularis mucosae bundles undergo hypertrophy that renders distinction from muscularis propria difficult. Smoothelin is a recently identified biomarker that facilitates distinguishing muscularis mucosae from muscularis propria. Muscularis propria typically displays intense and strong smoothelin staining, in contrast to muscularis mucosae, which has weak or negative smoothelin staining.[21–23]

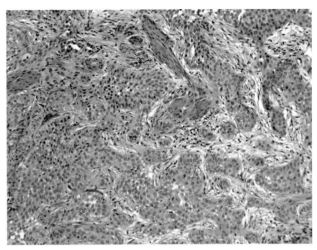

Figure 10-50 Muscularis mucosae invasion by urothelial carcinoma.

Substaging of Urothelial Carcinoma

The recurrence and progression rates for pT1 tumors are highly variable.[2,3,11,12,24,25] This is partly due to intrinsic difficulty in assessing the presence and extent of invasion. There is need for an accurate, easy-to-use, reproducible substaging system to stratify pT1 patients into different prognostic groups. Several studies have explored the utility of evaluating the spatial relationship of invasive tumor to the muscularis mucosae for subclassification of pT1 tumor.[2,26–32] Others have divided cases between those tumors that involve the stromal core of the papillae and those that invade the lamina propria. A novel approach to substaging pT1 tumors based on the micrometric measurement of invasion was recently proposed by Cheng et al.[11,33]

In most instances, the subepithelial connective tissue of the bladder is divided by a thin layer of smooth muscle fibers, referred to as muscularis mucosae (**Fig. 10-54**). The subepithelial layer is thus subdivided into lamina propria, superficial to the muscle fibers, and a submucosal layer, located between the muscularis mucosae and muscularis propria. The importance of identification of the muscularis mucosae has been emphasized for the substaging of pT1 disease.[26–32] Microscopically, muscularis mucosae fibers are usually thin and often discontinuous. There are wispy and wavy fascicles of smooth muscle, which are frequently associated with large-caliber blood vessels, and surrounded by loose fibroconnective tissue.[34,35] The muscularis mucosae is present in 94% of cystectomy specimens and in up to 83% of specimens from biopsies or TUR.[11,26–31,34–37]

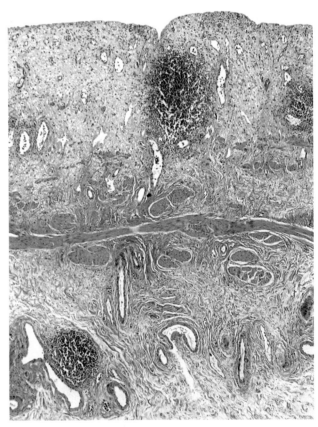

Figure 10-51 Muscularis mucosae can become hypertrophic and difficult to distinguish from muscularis propria in small biopsy specimens without appropriate orientation.

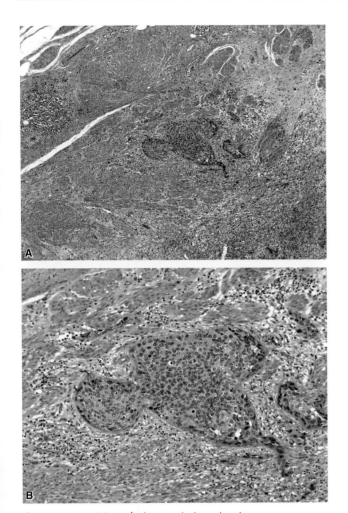

Figure 10-52   Muscularis propria invasion in a cystectomy specimen. Tumor invades into the outer layer of the muscularis propria wall (pT2b) (A). Muscle fibers are often fragmented and discontiguous (B). In a limited biopsy specimen, it is difficult to distinguish muscularis mucosae from muscularis propria (detrusor muscle) invasion.

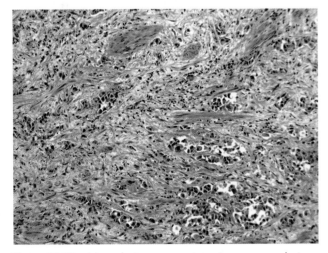

Figure 10-53   Muscularis mucosae invasion or muscularis propria invasion?

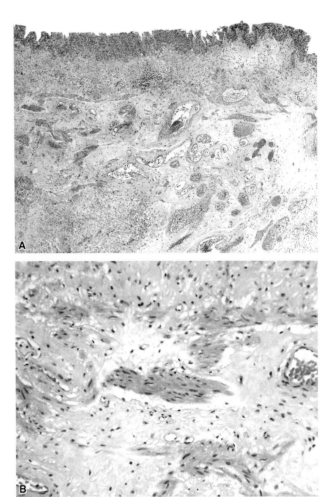

Figure 10-54   Muscularis mucosae of the bladder (A and B).

Younes et al. found a 75% five-year all-cause survival for tumors invading above or into the muscularis mucosae, compared to an 11% survival for those tumors invading below the muscularis mucosae.[31] In this study, the five-year survival of patients with pT1c disease (i.e., invasion beyond the muscularis mucosae) was similar to those with pT2 disease (14% vs. 20%, respectively).[31] Similarly, Hasui et al.,[27] Angulo et al.,[26] and Holmang et al.[29] were able to determine different progression rates, five-year all-cause survival, and cancer-specific survival, respectively, for those tumors with invasion above and below the muscularis mucosae. Hermann et al.[28] found that tumors with invasion beyond the muscularis mucosae had a less favorable prognosis than those with invasion in the tumor stalk or above the muscularis mucosae and, in a multivariate analysis, depth of invasion was the only significant parameter that predicted outcome. The main problem with this method of substaging pT1 urothelial carcinomas is that the muscularis mucosae, as noted above, is not a consistent histologic finding in bladder tumor resection specimens. Most of the authors mentioned above have at least partially overcome this problem by using the large blood vessels in the submucosa as a substitute anatomic landmark when muscularis mucosae bundles are not present (**Fig. 10-55**).[30] For example, Angulo et al. were able to identify muscularis mucosae in 39% of their cases and utilized the blood vessel landmark in 26%.[26] Thus, in 35% of their cases, substaging could not be performed. Platz et al. identified muscularis mucosae in only 33% of their cases.[30] Furthermore, when they used the vascular surrogate anatomic landmark in the remainder of the cases, they did not find any prognostic significance in substaging pT1 disease.[30] In a recent study,[38] Kondylis et al. found no difference in recurrence and progression rates between patients with T1a and T1b cancer using muscularis mucosae invasion for substaging, with a median followup of 71 months. Cancer progression rates were 78% and 71% for T1a and T1b cancer, respectively.[38] Furthermore, significant topographical variation of muscularis mucosae in different regions of the bladder has recently been documented.[39] These practical problems have prompted recent questioning as to whether substaging pT1 disease based on the muscularis mucosae is the best system and, as a consequence, whether substaging of pT1 tumors based on muscularis mucosae invasion should not be advocated.[40]

Cheng et al. proposed a novel system of substaging pT1 tumors based on the micrometric measurement of the depth of invasion of tumor into the subepithelial connective tissue (**Figs. 10-56 and 10-57**).[11,33] They studied a series of 55 patients with stage pT1 urothelial carcinomas diagnosed on TUR specimens and eventually treated by cystectomy.[33] By using an ocular micrometer to measure the depth of invasion from the mucosal basement membrane, they found a significant correlation between depth of invasion in the TUR specimen and final pathologic stage at cystectomy. A depth of invasion of 1.5 mm predicted an advanced stage of disease at cystectomy with a sensitivity of 81%, a specificity of 83%, and positive and negative predictive values of 95% and 56%, respectively. They applied the same criteria to a group of 83 consecutive patients diagnosed with pT1 bladder cancer and found a five-year progression-free survival of 67% in patients with a depth of tumor invasion greater than 1.5 mm, compared to 93% for those tumors with a depth of invasion below 1.5 mm (**Figs. 10-56 and 10-57**).[11]

Substaging of pT1 bladder tumors may benefit from cytokeratin immunohistochemistry. Mhawech et al.[41] found this to be useful in difficult cases where specimen orientation and tissue artifact created a hindrance to accurate diagnosis. Total agreement between hematoxylin and eosin (H&E) and immunohistochemistry was reached in 76 of 93 cases (82%). Immunohistochemistry downstaged seven cases, upstaged four cases, and failed to subclassify pT1 tumors in only 5% of cases studied.[41]

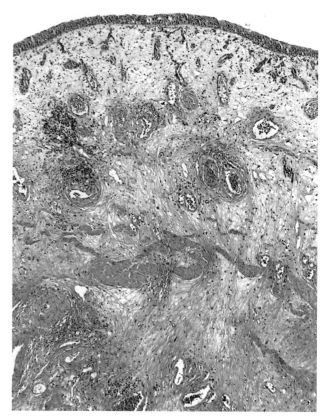

Figure 10-55 Muscuaris mucosae of the bladder. Muscularis mucosae are commonly associated with thick-walled vessels. However, thick-walled vessels should not be used as a substitute for muscularis mucosae. Some thick-walled vessels are located close to the superficial lamina propria.

The collective data indicate the level of invasion, whether assessed by the relation of the tumor to the muscularis mucosae or by direct micrometric measurement, and identify a subset of patients with pT1 bladder cancer who have a more adverse prognosis. It would be advisable to express some assessment of the depth of lamina propria invasion in a pathology report. It seems appropriate to use 1.5 mm as the cutoff in evaluating the depth of invasion in pT1 urothelial carcinomas.

Lymphovascular Invasion in pT1 Urothelial Carcinoma

The incidence of lymphovascular invasion is variable and has been reported to range from 5% to 28% of stage pT1 urothelial carcinoma (**Figs. 10-58 to 10-60**).[2,42–44] Lymphovascular invasion is more frequent in larger (>5 cm) high grade tumors without papillary configuration

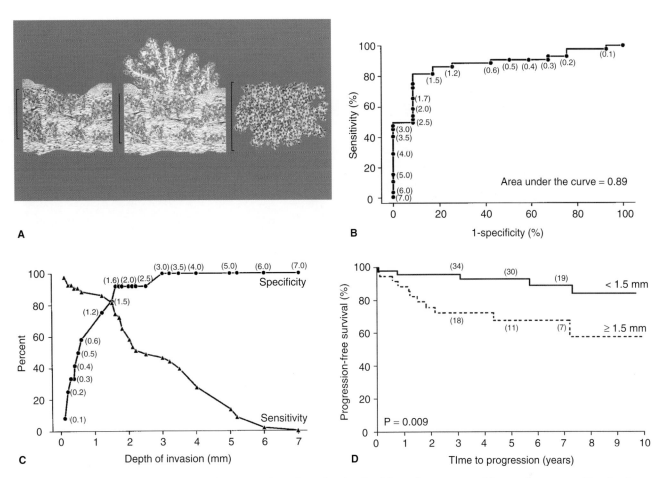

Figure 10-56 Substaging of pT1 bladder cancer based on the depth of invasion measured by a micrometer. Depth of invasion in pT1 urothelial carcinoma is a powerful predictor of clinical outcome. (A) The depth of stromal invasion in the transurethral resection or biopsy specimens is measured from the basement membrane of the bladder mucosae to the deepest invasive cancer cells using an ocular micrometer, whether the lesion is flat (AI) or papillary (AII). When tissue fragments contain cancer without adjacent basement membrane or when the specimen is not oriented, the depth of invasion is the shortest dimension of an intact tumor fragment to avoid overestimation of the depth of invasion (AIII). (B) Receiver operating characteristic (ROC) analysis of invasion depth as a predictor of advanced stage ($\geq$T2) bladder carcinoma. The area under the ROC curve was 0.89. (C) Sensitivity and specificity of invasion depth as a predictor for advanced stage ($\geq$T2) bladder carcinoma. The optimal depth of invasion for maximizing both sensitivity and specificity in predicting advanced stage bladder carcinoma is 1.5 mm. (D) Cancer progression-free survival curves comparing invasion depths < 1.5 mm and $\geq$ 1.5 mm in transurethral resection specimens. Progression consisted of muscle-invasive or more advanced stage carcinoma, of distant metastasis, or of death from bladder cancer. (From Refs. 3,11,13, and 33; with permission.)

and is associated with poor prognosis. In a study of 170 patients with pT1 urothelial carcinoma, five-year survival for pT1 cases without vascular invasion was 81% versus 44% for those with vascular invasion.[44] Lymphovascular invasion appeared to be an independent predictor of poor outcome regardless of tumor grade. Therefore, the presence of lymphovascular invasion should be included in the pathology report (see also **Chapter 27**).[3]

The identification of vascular/lymphatic invasion can be difficult and confused with artifactual clefting around nests of invasive carcinoma on conventional H&E evaluation. In suspicious cases, immunostaining using antibodies against CD31 or CD34 may be helpful. However, the problem of differentiating lymphovascular invasion versus artifactual space entrapment by tumor cells may not be resolved in selected cases, and it is appropriate to report these cases as indeterminate for lymphovascular invasion.

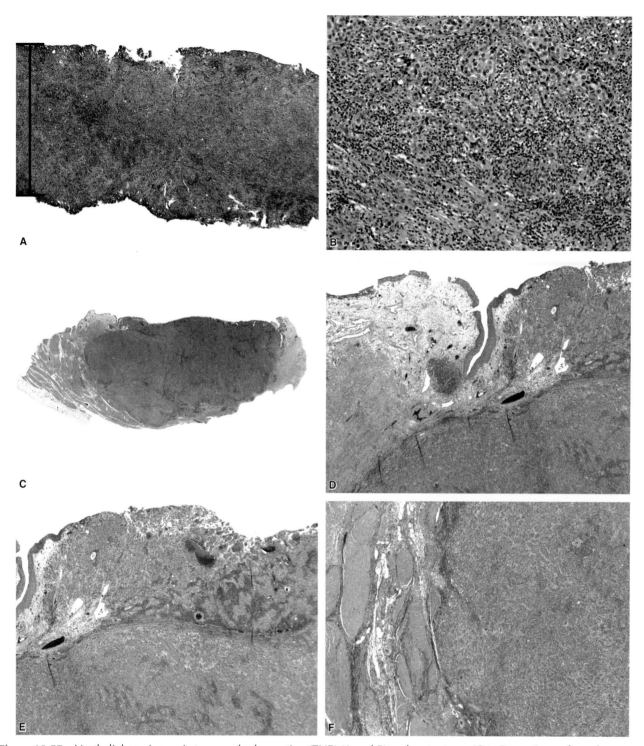

Figure 10-57 Urothelial carcinoma in transurethral resection (TUR) (A and B) and cystectomy (C to F) specimens from the same patient. Muscularis propria is not present in the transurethral resection specimen (A and B). The depth of invasion is 5.1 mm in the TUR specimens. Based on the depth of invasion, the patient underwent a cystectomy, which revealed a pT3N2 cancer. It should be noted that it is not always possible to demonstrate muscularis propria invasion in TUR or biopsy specimens when the tumor presents as expansile or pushing growth.

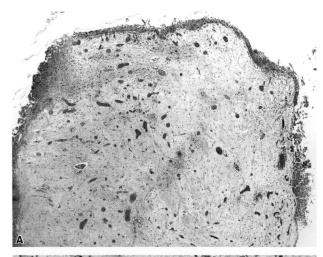

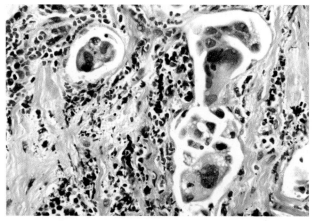

Figure 10-59 Lymphovascular invasion in pT1 bladder cancer.

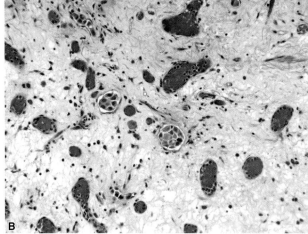

Figure 10-58 Lymphovascular invasion in pT1 bladder cancer.

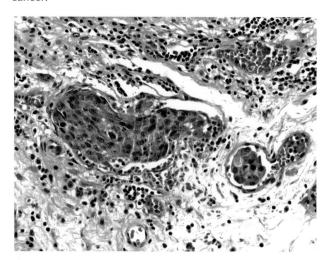

Figure 10-60 Lymphovascular invasion in pT1 bladder cancer.

REFERENCES

1. Edge SB, Byrd DR, Compton CC, Fritz AG, Greene FL, Trotti A. American Joint Committee on Cancer Staging Manual, 7th ed. New York: Springer, 2010.
2. Lopez-Beltran A, Cheng L. Stage pT1 bladder carcinoma: diagnostic criteria, pitfalls and prognostic significance. *Pathology* 2003;35:484–91.
3. Cheng L, Montironi R, Davidson DD, Lopez-Beltran A. Staging and reporting of urothelial carcinoma of the urinary bladder. *Mod Pathol* 2009;22(Suppl 2):S70–95.
4. Soloway MS, Sofer M, Vaidya A. Contemporary management of stage T1 transitional cell carcinoma of the bladder. *J Urol* 2002;167:1573–83.
5. Alkhateeb SS, Van Rhijn BW, Finelli A, van der Kwast T, Evans A, Hanna S, Vajpeyi R, Fleshner NE, Jewett MA, Zlotta AR. Nonprimary pT1 nonmuscle invasive bladder cancer treated with bacillus Calmette-Guérin is associated with higher risk of progression compared to primary T1 tumors. *J Urol* 2010;184:81–6.
6. Kwak C, Ku JH, Park JY, Lee E, Lee SE, Lee C. Initial tumor stage and grade as a predictive factor for recurrence in patients with stage T1 grade 3 bladder cancer. *J Urol* 2004;171:149–52.
7. Cheng L, Neumann RM, Weaver AL, Cheville JC, Leibovich BC, Ramnani DM, Scherer BG, Nehra A, Zincke H, Bostwick DG. Grading and staging of bladder carcinoma in transurethral resection specimens. Correlation with 105 matched cystectomy specimens. *Am J Clin Pathol* 2000;113:275–9.
8. Jimenez RE, Keany TE, Hardy HT, Amin MB. pT1 Urothelial carcinoma of the bladder: criteria for diagnosis, pitfalls, and clionical implications. *Adv Anat Pathol* 2000;7:13–25.

9. Tamas EF, Epstein JI. Detection of residual tumor cells in bladder biopsy specimens: pitfalls in the interpretation of cytokeratin stains. *Am J Surg Pathol* 2007;31:390–7.

10. Lopez-Beltran A, Cheng L, Andersson L, Brausi M, de Matteis A, Montironi R, Sesterhenn I, van det Kwast KT, Mazerolles C. Preneoplastic non-papillary lesions and conditions of the urinary bladder: an update based on the Ancona International Consultation. *Virchows Arch* 2002;440:3–11.

11. Cheng L, Neumann RM, Weaver AL, Spotts BE, Bostwick DG. Predicting cancer progression in patients with stage T1 bladder carcinoma. *J Clin Oncol* 1999;17:3182–7.

12. Cheng L, Bostwick DG. Progression of T1 bladder tumors: better staging or better biology. *Cancer* 1999;86:910–2.

13. Cheng L, Weaver AL, Bostwick DG. Predicting extravesical extension of bladder carcinoma: a novel method based on micrometer measurement of the depth of invasion in transurethral resection specimens. *Urology* 2000;55:668–72.

14. Eble JN, Young RH. Carcinoma of the urinary bladder: a review of its diverse morphology. *Semin Diagn Pathol* 1997;14:98–108.

15. Drew PA, Furman J, Civantos F, Murphy WM. The nested variant of transitional cell carcinoma: an aggressive neoplasm with innocuous histology. *Mod Pathol* 1996;9:989–94.

16. Lopez-Beltran A. Bladder treatment. Immunotherapy and chemotherapy. *Urol Clin North Am* 1999;26:535–54.

17. Lopez-Beltran A, Luque RJ, Mazzucchelli R, Scarpelli M, Montironi R. Changes produced in the urothelium by traditional and newer therapeutic procedures for bladder cancer. *J Clin Pathol* 2002;55:641–7.

18. Young RH. Non-neoplastic disorders of the urinary bladder. In: Bostwick DG, Cheng L, eds. Urologic Surgical Pathology, 2nd ed. Philadelphia: Elsevier/Mosby, 2008;215–58.

19. Young RH. Tumor-like lesions of the urinary bladder. *Mod Pathol* 2009;22Suppl 2:S37–52.

20. Lopez-Beltran A, Sauter G, Gasser T, Hartmann A, Schmitz-Dräger BJ, Helpap B, Ayala AG, Tamboli P, Knowles MA, Sidransky D, Cordon-Cardo C, Jones PA, Cairns P, Simon R, Amin MB. Urothelial tumors: infiltrating urothelial carcinoma. In: Eble JN, Sauter G, Epstein JI, Sesterhenn I, eds. World Health Organization Classification of Tumors. Pathology and Gentics of Tumors of the Urinary System and Male Genital Organs Lyon, France: IARC Press, 2004.

21. Paner GP, Shen SS, Lapetino S, Venkataraman G, Barkan GA, Quek ML, Ro JY, Amin MB. Diagnostic utility of antibody to smoothelin in the distinction of muscularis propria from muscularis mucosae of the urinary bladder: a potential ancillary tool in the pathologic staging of invasive urothelial carcinoma. *Am J Surg Pathol* 2009;33:91–8.

22. Council L, Hameed O. Differential expression of immunohistochemical markers in bladder smooth muscle and myofibroblasts, and the potential utility of desmin, smoothelin, and vimentin in staging of bladder carcinoma. *Mod Pathol* 2009;22:639–50.

23. Miyamoto H, Sharma RB, Illei PB, Epstein JI. Pitfalls in the use of smoothelin to identify muscularis propria invasion by urothelial carcinoma. *Am J Surg Pathol* 2010;34:418–22.

24. Nieder AM, Brausi M, Lamm D, O'Donnell M, Tomita K, Woo H, Jewett MA. Management of stage T1 tumors of the bladder: International Consensus Panel. *Urology* 2005;66:108–25.

25. Quintero A, Alvarez-Kindelan J, Luque RJ, Gonzalez-Campora R, Requena MJ, Montironi R, Lopez-Beltran A. Ki–67 MIB1 labelling index and the prognosis of primary TaT1 urothelial cell carcinoma of the bladder. *J Clin Pathol* 2006;59:83–8.

26. Angulo JC, Lopez JI, Grignon DJ, Sanchez-Chapado M. Muscularis mucosae differentiates two populations with different prognosis in stage T1 bladder cancer. *Urology* 1995;45:47–53.

27. Hasui Y, Osada Y, Kitada S, Nishi S. Significance of invasion to the muscularis mucosae on the progression of superficial bladder cancer. *Urology* 1994;43:782–6.

28. Hermann GG, Horn T, Steven K. The influence of the level of lamina propria invasion and the prevalence of p53 nuclear accumulation on survival in stage T1 transitional cell bladder cancer. *J Urol* 1998;159:91–4.

29. Holmang S, Hedelin H, Anderstrom C, Holmberg E, Johansson SL. The importance of the depth of invasion in stage T1 bladder carcinoma: a prospective cohort study. *J Urol* 1997;157:800–4.

30. Platz CE, Cohen MB, Jones MP, Olson DB, Lynch CF. Is microstaging of early invasive cancer of the urinary bladder possible or useful? *Mod Pathol* 1996;11:1035–9.

31. Younes M, Sussman J, True LD. The usefulness of the level of the muscularis mucosae in the staging of invasive transitional cell carcinoma of the urinary bladder. *Cancer* 1990;66:543–8.

32. Sozen S, Akbal C, Sokmensuer C, Ekici S, Ozen H. Microstaging of pT1 transitional cell carcinoma of the bladder: Does it really differentiate two populations with different prognoses? *Urol Int* 2002;69:200–6.

33. Cheng L, Weaver AL, Neumann RM, Scherer BG, Bostwick DG. Substaging of T1 bladder carcinoma based on the depth of invasion as measured by micrometer. A new proposal. *Cancer* 1999;86:1035–43.

34. Dixon JS, Gosling JA. Histology and fine structure of the muscularis mucosae of the human urinary bladder. *J Anat* 1983;136:265–71.

35. Ro JY, Ayala AG, el-Naggar A. Muscularis mucosae of urinary bladder. Importance for staging and treatment. *Am J Surg Pathol* 1987;11:668–73.

36. Keep JC, Piehl M, Miller A, Oyasu R. Invasive carcinomas of the urinary bladder. Evaluation of tunica muscularis mucosae involvement. *Am J Clin Pathol* 1989;91:575–9.

37. Engel P, Anagnostaki L, Braendstrup O. The muscularis mucosae of the human urinary bladder. *Scand J Urol Nephrol* 1992;26:249–52.

38. Kondylis FI, Demirci S, Ladaga L, Kolm P, Schellhammer PF. Outcomes after intravesical bacillus Calmette-Guérin are not affected by

substaging of high grade T1 transitional cell carcinoma. *J Urol* 2000;163:1120–3.

39. Paner GP, Ro JY, Wojcik EM, Venkataraman G, Datta MW, Amin MB. Further characterization of the muscle layers and lamina propria of the urinary bladder by systematic histologic mapping: implications for pathologic staging of invasive urothelial carcinoma. *Am J Surg Pathol* 2007;31:1420–9.

40. Epstein JI, Amin MB, Reuter VR, Mostofi FK. The World Health Organization/International Society of Urological Pathology consensus classification of urothelial (transitional cell) neoplasms of the urinary bladder. Bladder Consensus Conference Committee. *Am J Surg Pathol* 1998;22:1435–48.

41. Mhawech P, Iselin C, Pelte MF. Value of immunohistochemistry in staging T1 urothelial bladder carcinoma. *Eur Urol* 2002;42:459–63.

42. Cho KS, Seo HK, Joung JY, Park WS, Ro JY, Han KS, Chung J, Lee KH. Lymphovascular invasion in transurethral resection specimens as predictor of progression and metastasis in patients with newly diagnosed T1 bladder urothelial cancer. *J Urol* 2009;182:2625–30.

43. Andius P, Johansson SL, Holmang S. Prognostic factors in stage T1 bladder cancer: tumor pattern (solid or papillary) and vascular invasion more important than depth of invasion. *Urology* 2007;70:758–62.

44. Lopez JI, Angulo JC. The prognostic significance of vascular invasion in stage T1 bladder cancer. *Histopathology* 1995;27:27–33.

Chapter 11

Staging of Bladder Cancer

The pathologic stage is the most important determinant of prognosis and treatment for bladder cancer.[1-8] An ideal staging system should accurately reflect the natural history of cancer at this site, describe the total cancer burden, assess the extent of spread at the time of diagnosis (**Figs. 11-1 to 11-3**), and stratify patients into prognostic groups for treatment planning. Adoption of a uniform staging system permits comparison of therapeutic interventions between different institutions. The 2010 revision of the American Joint Committee on Cancer/International Union Against Cancer/Union Internationale Contre le Cancer (AJCC/UICC) tumor, lymph node, and metastasis (TNM) system is recommended (**Tables 11-1 and 11-2**).[9]

Stage pT0 Carcinoma

Stage pT0 tumor is a condition in which there is no evidence of residual carcinoma in the cystectomy specimen after an initial cancer diagnosis in the biopsy or transurethral resection (TUR) specimen. The incidence of stage pT0 bladder carcinoma is approximately 5% to 10%.[7,10-15] The clinical outcome among patients with stage pT0 bladder cancer is variable. In a large series of 120 patients with pT0 carcinomas, the five-year recurrence-free, cancer-specific, and overall survivals were 84%, 88%, and 84%, respectively.[11] Multivariate analysis showed that lymphovascular invasion and carcinoma in situ (CIS) in the TUR specimens were independent predictors of adverse clinical outcome.[11] The five-year overall survival for patients with lymphovascular invasion was 70%, compared to 89% for those patients without

lymphovascular invasion.[11] The incidence of lymph node metastasis among pT0 patients is 3% to 8%.[10,13,15]

More recently, Tilki and his colleagues reported the largest series of pT0 bladder cancer from the records of 4430 patients treated with radical cystectomy for bladder urothelial carcinoma without neoadjuvant chemotherapy at 12 centers in the United States, Canada, and Europe.[15] The incidence of pT0 bladder cancer was 5.1%. Overall, 17 patients (7.5%) had regional lymph node metastasis. During a median followup of 48 months, 15 patients (6.6%) died of bladder cancer. Five-year recurrence-free and cancer-specific survival estimates were 90% (95% confidence interval, 85.3–93.1) and 93%. Lymph node metastasis and female gender were independent predictors of recurrence-free and cancer-specific survival in multivariate analysis.[15]

Stage pTa Carcinoma

pTa carcinoma is defined by the 2010 TNM staging system as noninvasive papillary carcinoma (**Fig. 11-4**).[9] It should be distinguished from pT1 cancer by the absence of lamina propria invasion. Recognition of diagnostic pitfalls associated with lamina propria, submucosa, or muscularis propria invasion is critical for evaluation of bladder tumor specimens.[16]

Historically, the term "superficial bladder cancer" has been used to describe tumors that have not invaded the muscularis propria. This designation includes noninvasive papillary urothelial carcinoma (pTa), CIS (pTis), and tumor invading the lamina propria (pT1).

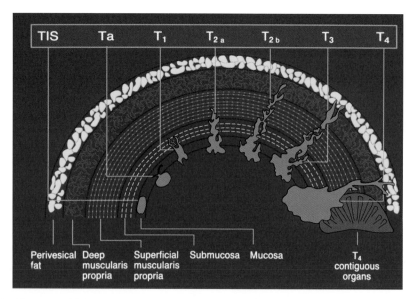

Figure 11-1 Schematic diagram of bladder carcinoma staging according to the 2002 TNM (tumor, lymph node, and metastasis) staging system. The staging system is based on the depth of invasion.

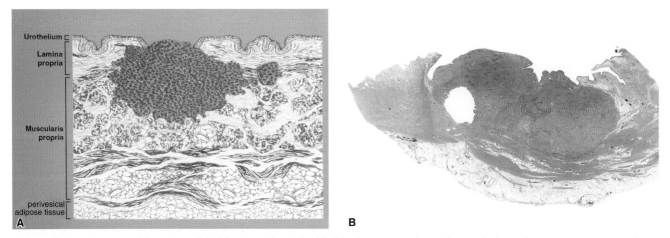

Figure 11-2   Anatomy of the urinary bladder (A and B). The bladder is organized into the urothelium, lamina propria, muscularis propria, and perivesical adipose tissue. Adipose tissue can be present in the lamina propria or muscularis propria layer. Current staging system for bladder cancer is based on the depth of invasion. A tumor invading into muscular propria (detrusor muscle) is illustrated. (From Ref. 57; with permission.)

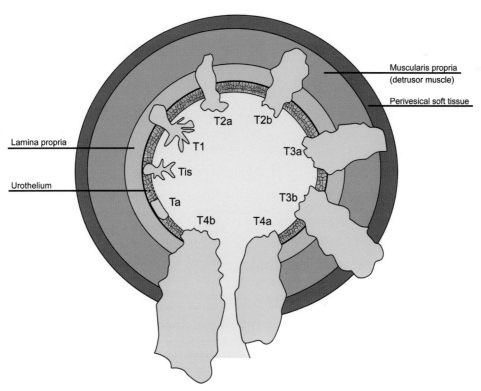

Figure 11-3   Schematic diagram of bladder carcinoma staging according to the 2002 TNM (tumor, lymph node, and metastasis) staging system.

Table 11-1 TNM Classification of Bladder Carcinoma (2010 Revision)

Primary tumor (T)

TX	Primary tumor cannot be assessed
T0	No evidence of primary tumor
Ta	Noninvasive papillary carcinoma
Tis	Carcinoma in situ
T1	Tumor invades subepithelial connective tissue (lamina propria)
T2	Tumor invades muscularis propria bladder wall
	T2a Tumor invades superficial muscularis propria (inner half)
	T2b Tumor invades deep muscularis propria (outer half)
T3	Tumor invades perivesical tissue
	T3a Microscopically
	T3b Macroscopically (extravesical mass)
T4	Tumor invades any of the following: prostate, uterus, vagina, pelvic wall, and abdominal wall
T4a	Tumor invades prostatic stroma, uterus, vagina
T4b	Tumor invades pelvic or abdominal wall

Regional lymph nodes (N)

NX	Regional lymph nodes cannot be assessed
N0	No regional lymph node metastasis
N1	Single regional lymph node metastasis in the true pelvis (hypogastric, obturator, external iliac, or presacral lymph node)
N2	Multiple regional lymph node metastasis in the true pelvis
N3	Lymph node metastasis to the common iliac lymph node

Distant metastasis (M)

M0	No distant metastasis
M1	Distant metastasis

Table 11-2 TNM Stage Groupings

Stage 0a	Ta	N0	M0
Stage 0is	Tis	N0	M0
Stage I	T1	N0	M0
Stage II	T2a	N0	M0
	T2b	N0	M0
Stage III	T3a	N0	M0
	T3b	N0	M0
	T4a	N0	M0
Stage IV	T4b	N0	M0
	Any T	N1, 2, 3	M0
	Any T	Any N	M1

[a]M0 is defined as "no distant metastasis."

This terminology is still in use by many practicing urologists. However, it is now recommended that the term "superficial" be eliminated entirely from bladder tumor nomenclature.[17,18]

Histologic grading is one of the most important prognostic factors for pTa bladder tumors (see also **Chapter 9**).[19–22]

Stage pT1 Carcinoma

See **Chapters 10** and **25** for further discussion.

Stage pT2 Carcinoma

Stage pT2 carcinoma is defined by tumor invasion into muscularis propria (**Figs. 11-5** to **11-12**). The 2010 TNM staging system subclassifies pT2 carcinoma into two categories: cancer invading less than one-half of the depth of muscular propria (pT2a) and cancer invading greater than one-half of the muscle wall.[9] The clinical utility of pT2 tumor substaging has been questioned.[23]

Current subclassification of T2 carcinomas is based on the work by Jewett in 1952.[24] In a study of 18 patients with muscle-invasive carcinoma, from five T2a (B1) cases and 13 T2b (B2) urothelial carcinomas, the author found that 80% of T2a bladder carcinoma patients survived, whereas only 8% of those with stage T2b survived.[24] Data that have accumulated in the 47 years since this original publication do not lend solid support to the subdivision of T2 by depth of muscularis propria invasion (**Table 11-3**).[7,24–58] However, a recent multi-institutional study indicated that substaging of pT2 bladder cancer may be of value in stratifying different risk groups.[59]

Based on the Mayo Clinic data, Cheng et al. found no survival difference between pT2a and pT2b cancer during a mean followup of 8.3 years.[57] Ten-year cancer-specific survival rates were 82% and 81%, respectively, for patients with pT2a and pT2b bladder cancer.[57] In contrast, tumor

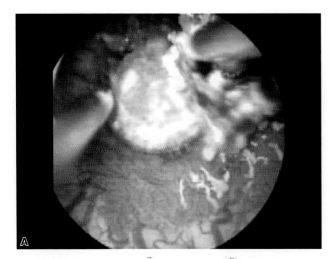

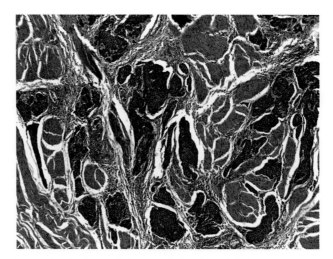

Figure 11-6   Muscularis propria invasion (pT2).

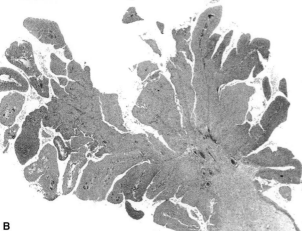

Figure 11-4   Low grade noninvasive papillary urothelial carcinoma.

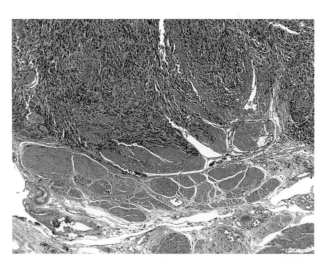

Figure 11-7   pT2b bladder cancer. Tumor invades into the outer one-half of the muscularis propria wall. Substaging of T2 can be done only in cystectomy specimen.

size (the largest tumor dimension) was predictive of distant metastasis-free and cancer-specific survival in patients with muscularis propria invasion.[57] Ten-year cancer-specific survival rates were 94% and 73%, respectively, for patients with tumors < 3 cm and patients with tumors ≥ 3 cm in greatest dimension (**Fig 11-13**).[57] In a recent study of 311 patients with pT2 bladder cancer, Yu et al. found no significant difference in clinical outcome between pT2a and pT2b cancers after controlling for lymph node status.[53] Ten-year recurrence-free survival rates were 84% and 72%, respectively, for pT2a and pT2b lymph node-negative bladder cancers. Among lymph node-positive bladder cancer patients, 10-year recurrence-free survival was 50% for pT2a carcinoma and 48% for pT2b carcinoma.[53]

In 1978, Jewett concluded: "It seems probable that our arbitrary dividing line drawn 30 years ago at the halfway

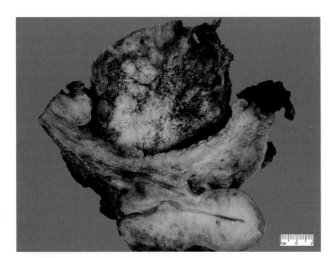

Figure 11-5   Stage T2 bladder cancer. Bulky tumor mass protruding into the luminal space of the bladder.

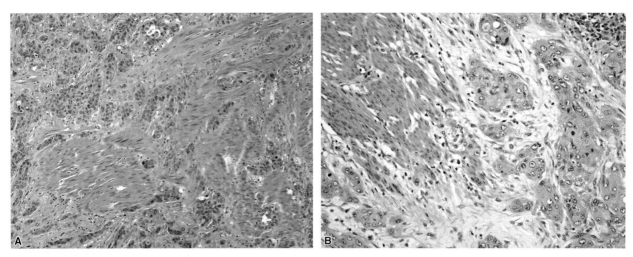

Figure 11-8 Muscularis propria invasion (pT2) (A and B).

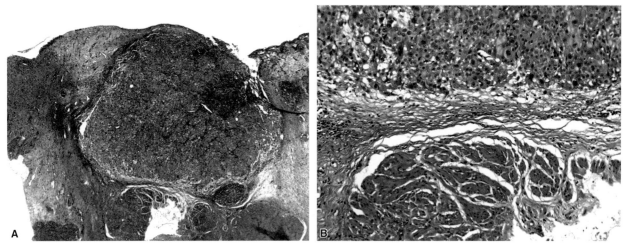

Figure 11-9 pT2b bladder cancer. Tumor invades into the outer one-half of the muscularis propria wall and presents as expansile growth (A). Tumor does not infiltrate through muscularis propria (B). It would be difficult to document muscularis propria invasion in biopsy specimens.

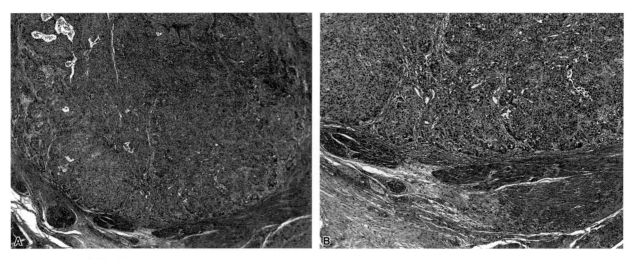

Figure 11-10 pT2b bladder cancer with expansile growth (A and B).

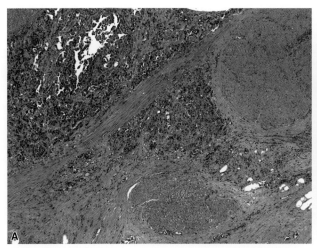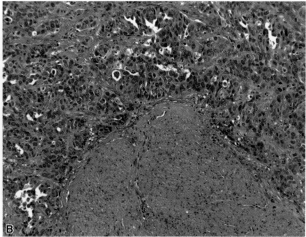

Figure 11-11 pT2b bladder cancer (A and B). Tumor is surrounding the muscularis propria. Note the desmoplastic stroma.

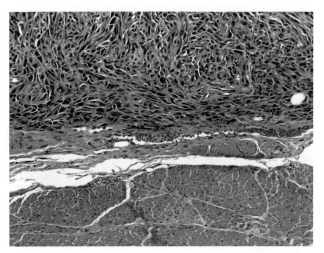

Figure 11-12 pT2 bladder cancer. Another case illustrating the expansile growth of tumor without directly infiltrating through the muscularis propria. It is not always feasible to document muscularis propria invasion in TUR or biopsy specimens. We recommend the depth of invasion measured by a micrometer be reported for invasive urothelial carcinoma (see the discussion in **Chapter 10**).

level to separate B1 (pT2a) from B2 (pT2b) tumors was too superficial."[60] Substaging of T2 bladder carcinoma based on the level of muscularis propria invasion is of limited value for stratifying patients into prognostic groups and should be eliminated from future TNM classification. Tumor size may be a more pertinent parameter for the subclassification of T2 bladder cancer.[57]

Stage pT3 Carcinoma

Stage pT3 bladder carcinoma is defined by tumor invasion into perivesical soft tissue (**Figs. 11-14** to **11-18**). The

presence of intramural adipose tissue is well documented in the bladder (**Fig. 11-19**).[61,62] The appearance of fat invasion in a biopsy or TUR specimen, therefore, does not necessarily indicate invasive pT3 carcinoma. As a consequence, it is not feasible to document pT3 cancer in biopsy or TUR specimens.

The subdivision of pT3 tumors into pT3a (tumors with microscopic extravesical extension) and pT3b (tumors with gross extravesical extension) is controversial. Quek et al. examined 236 patients with pT3 bladder carcinoma.[63] With a median followup of 8.9 years, there was no difference in recurrence or survival rates between patients with pT3a and pT3b tumors. Lymph node metastasis and surgical margin status were the only factors to significantly affect patient prognosis in this study.[63] A more recent study, however, has found that macroscopic perivesical fat invasion on gross examination (pT3b) is associated with increased risk of cancer recurrence and cancer death.[64] In a multi-institutional study of 808 patients with pT3 bladder cancer, subclassification of pT3 cancer as microscopic (pT3a) versus macroscopic perivesical fat extension was not a significant predictor of recurrence and cancer-specific survival.[65] Only age, soft tissue surgical margin status, lymphovascular invasion, and lymph node metastasis were independent predictors of patient outcome. However, pT3 subclassification was a significant predictor in a subset analysis among node-negative patients, excluding patients with lymph node metastasis.[65] The presence or absence of macroscopic perivesical fat invasion, therefore, should be reported.

Currently, there is no reliable method to predict extravesical extension (pT3) from TUR or biopsy specimens. The presence of fat invasion in TUR or biopsy specimens does not constitute a pT3 cancer. Cheng and his colleagues analyzed 90 bladder cancer patients diagnosed with invasive bladder cancer at TUR.[66] The depth of invasion were measured from the TUR specimens by ocular micrometer. All patients were treated by radical cystectomy. Median

Table 11-3   Comparison of Clinical Outcome Between pT2a and pT2b Bladder Carcinomas

Reference	Year	Number of Cases (T2a and T2b)	Five-year Survival (%)	
			T2a	T2b
Jewett[24]	1952	18	80	8
Bowles and Cordonnier[32]	1963	40	52	50
Cox et al.[33]	1968	75	45	40
Sorensen et al.[46]	1969	38	7	0
Pomerase[40]	1972	46	15	29
Utz et al.[47]	1975	73	47	40
Cordonnier[37]	1974	76	52	40
Richie et al.[42]	1975	58	40	40
Pearse et al.[50]	1978	26	64	50
Prout et al.[41]	1976	112	31	31
Boileau et al.[34]	1980	67	38	52
Bredael et al.[36]	1980	61	54	48
Mathur et al.[38]	1981	18	86	64
Skinner et al.[55]	1982	33	53	39
Bcahrs et al.[35]	1984	61	42	35
Montie et al.[51]	1984	27	62	63
Pagano et al.[52]	1991	95	63	50
Roehrborn et al.[44]	1991	145	65	61
Wishnow et al.[49]	1992	35	75	78
Pollack et al.[39]	1995	140	78	77
Cuesta et al.[56]	1997	50	73	67
Cheng et al.[59]	1999	64	62	56
Dalbagni et al.[7]	2001	58	62	58
Girgin et al.[54]	2005	75	84	66
Yu et al.[53]	2006	242[a]	87	75
		69[b]	50	50
Tokgoz et al.[58]	2007	57	44	43

[a]Lymph node-negative patients.
[b]Lymph node-positive patients.

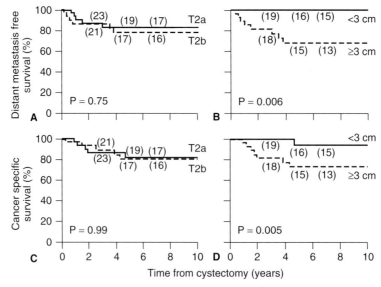

Figure 11-13   Substaging of pT2 urothelial carcinoma. Distant metastasis-free (A and B) and cancer-specific (C and D) survivals for patients with pT2 urothelial carcinoma. Tumor size (B and D) was more clinically relevant than the pT2 substaging (pT2a vs. pT2b) (A and C). (From Ref. 57; with permission.)

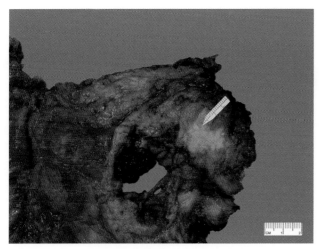

Figure 11-14   pT3b bladder cancer. Tumor grossly invades perivesical soft tissue (arrow).

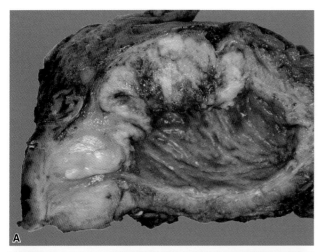

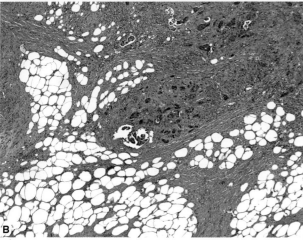

Figure 11-15   pT3b bladder cancer. Tumor invades perivesical adipose tissue (A and B).

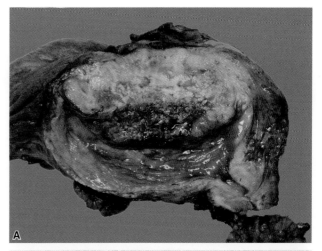

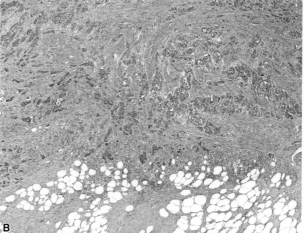

Figure 11-16   pT3b bladder cancer. Tumor invades perivesical adipose tissue (A and B).

interval from TUR to cystectomy was 44 days. Extravesical extension (≥ T3) at cystectomy was present in 39 patients (43%). The authors found that the depth of invasion was associated with final pathologic stage (Spearman correlation $r = 0.58$, $P < 0.001$).[66] The overall accuracy of the depth of invasion for the prediction of extravesical extension, measured by the area under the receiver operating characteristic (ROC) curve, was 0.81 (standard error, 0.045) (Figs. 11-20 and 11-21). The mean depth of invasion among patients with extravesical extension at cystectomy was 4.0 mm, compared to 2.2 mm for those without extravesical extension. Based on a 4.0-mm cutoff point, the sensitivity, specificity, positive predictive value, and negative predictive value for extravesical extension were 54%, 90%, 81%, and 72%, respectively (Table 11-4). Among patients with a depth of invasion greater than 4 mm in biopsies, 100% had advanced-stage (≥pT2) bladder cancer; 81% had pT3 or pT4 bladder cancer. The authors concluded that patients with bladder cancer depth of invasion above 4 mm in the

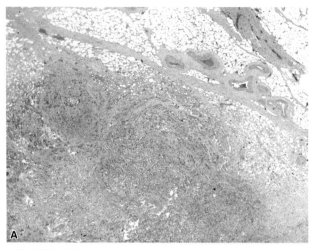

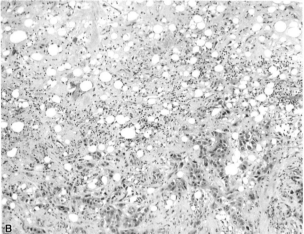

Figure 11-17   pT3 bladder cancer. Tumor invades perivesical adipose tissue (A and B).

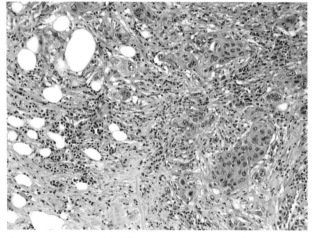

Figure 11-18   pT3 bladder cancer. Tumor invades perivesical soft tissue.

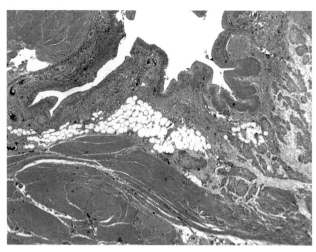

Figure 11-19   pT2 bladder cancer. Note the presence of adipose tissue in the lamina propria. Fat invasion into TUR or biopsy specimens does not indicate pT3 cancer.

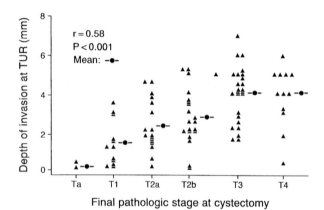

Figure 11-20   The depth of invasion in the transurethral resection specimens is associated with the final pathologic stage at cystectomy (Spearman correlation, $r = 0.58, P < 0.001$). The mean depth of invasion among patients with extravesical extension ($\geq$ T3) at cystectomy was 4.0 mm, compared to 2.2 mm for those without extravesical extension. Among patients with depth of invasion > 4 mm in biopsies, 100% had advanced-stage ($\geq$ pT2) bladder cancer; 81% had pT3 or pT4 bladder cancer. (From Ref. 66; with permission.)

TUR specimens, measured by micrometer, are likely to have extravesical extension, and more aggressive treatment should be considered.[66]

Stage pT4 Carcinoma

Stage pT4 bladder cancer is defined by tumor invasion into an adjacent organ, including uterus, vagina, prostatic

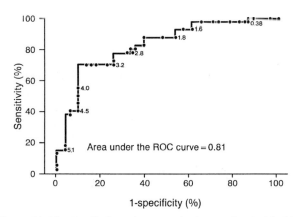

Figure 11-21   Prediction of extravesical extension in bladder cancer patients. Receiver operating characteristic analysis of the depth of invasion as a predictor of extravesical extension. The numbers (mm) represent the depth of invasion measured by a micrometer from transurethral resection specimens. (From Ref. 66; with permission.)

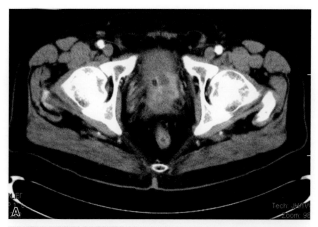

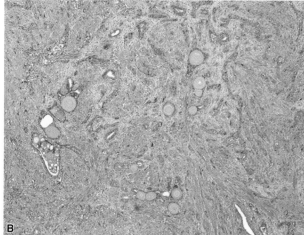

Figure 11-22   pT4 bladder cancer. Tumor invades the prostate. CT scan (A) and microscopic appearance (B). (Photo courtesy of Dr. Koch.)

stroma, pelvic wall, or abdominal wall (**Figs. 11-22** to **11-24**). In the 2010 AJCC/UICC bladder cancer TNM staging guidelines, pT4a includes invasion of prostate, uterus, or vagina and pT4b indicates pelvic or abdominal wall invasion. The major modification of 2010 TNM staging is the clarification of pT4 cancer. In men, T4 cancer is defined as prostatic stromal invasion directly from bladder cancer (**Figs. 11-25** to **11-28**). Subepithelial invasion of prostatic urethra does not constitute T4 cancer.

The designation of prostate invasion by bladder carcinoma as stage pT4 cancer has been debated.[67] Donat et al. identified three pathways for prostatic stromal invasion by urothelial carcinoma.[68] These include extravesical, intraurethral, and bladder neck invasion.[68] However, the prognostic significance of stromal invasion through these different pathways is uncertain. Esrig et al. studied 143 bladder cancers with prostatic involvement, dividing them into two groups. Group I penetrated the full thickness of bladder wall to involve the prostate, and group II involved the prostate by extension from the prostatic urethra.[69] Five-year overall survival rates were 21% and 55% for

groups I and II, respectively. Among group II patients, the presence of prostatic stromal invasion was associated with a worse prognosis than for patients in whom urothelial cancer was confined to the urethral mucosa only.[69] Similarly, Pagano et al. found that five-year survival was only 7% among group I patients, compared to 46% among group II patients.[70] In group II, all patients with urethral mucosal

Table 11-4   **Prediction of Extravesical Extension by the Depth of Invasion Measured by Micrometer in Transurethral Resection of Bladder Specimens**[a]

Depth of Invasion (mm)	Cystectomy (Number of Patients)						
	Ta	T1	T2a	T2b	T3	T4	Totals
≤4.0	2	12	15	17	11	7	64
>4.0	0	0	2	3	15	6	26
Totals	2	12	17	20	26	13	90

Source: Ref. 66, with permission.
[a]Using 4.0 mm as a cutoff point, the sensitivity, specificity, positive predictive value, and negative predictive value for the prediction of extravesical extension (≥T3) at cystectomy were 54%, 90%, 81%, and 72%, respectively. Among patients with depth of invasion >4 mm in biopsies, 100% had advanced-stage (≥pT2) bladder cancer; 81% had pT3 or pT4 bladder cancer.

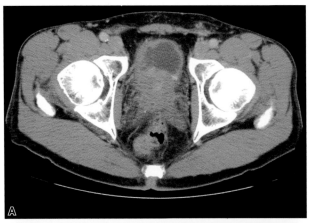

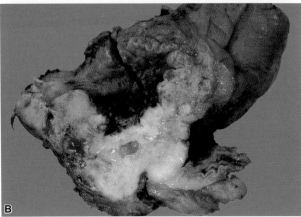

Figure 11-23 pT4 bladder cancer. Tumor invades the prostate and rectum. CT scan (A) and gross appearance (B). (Photo courtesy of Dr. Koch.)

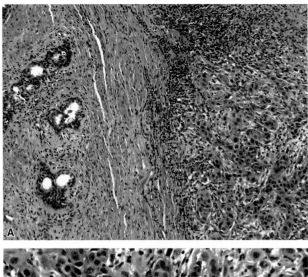

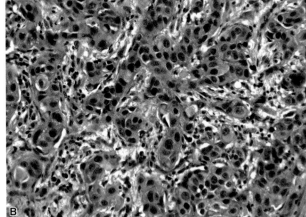

Figure 11-25 pT4 bladder cancer. Tumor invades the prostate (A and B).

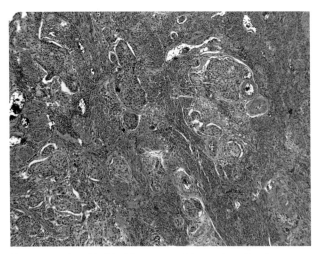

Figure 11-24 pT4 bladder cancer. Tumor invades the myometrium of the uterus.

involvement only were alive and free of cancer after five years, compared to 40% to 50% survival among patients with prostatic stromal invasion.[70] In a detailed mapping study of 214 radical cystoprostatectomy specimens with prostatic involvement by urothelial carcinoma, 26% of invasive bladder carcinomas resulted from direct infiltration of the prostate from the bladder. In the remaining 74% of cases, the prostate was invaded by urothelial carcinoma extending from the prostatic urethra.[71] More recently, Montironi et al. reported a detailed histopathologic analysis of 248 consecutive prostates from cystoprostatectomies for muscle-invasive bladder carcinoma using the whole-mount technique.[72] Involvement by bladder cancer was present in 38% of the prostates. Incidental prostate cancer was also seen in 50% of the specimens, but 81% of these prostate cancers were clinically insignificant.[72] These findings emphasize the importance of thorough sampling and histologic evaluation of the prostate for cystoprostatectomy specimens removed for bladder carcinoma.

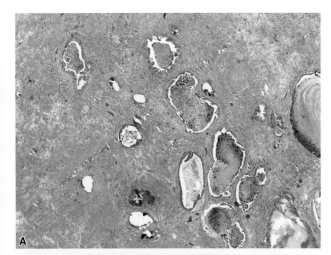

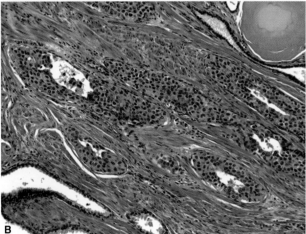

Figure 11-26 pT4 bladder cancer. Tumor invades the prostate (A and B).

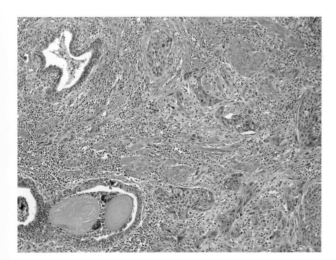

Figure 11-27 pT4 bladder cancer. Tumor invades the prostate.

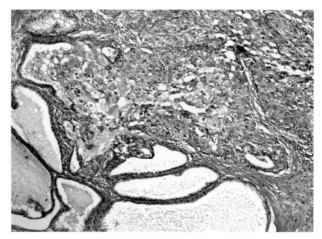

Figure 11-28 pT4 bladder cancer. Tumor invades the prostate.

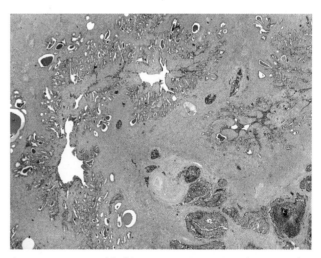

Figure 11-29 pT4 bladder cancer. Tumor invades seminal vesicles of the prostate. These tumors tend to be more aggressive than those invading prostatic parenchyma only.

Direct perivesical tumor extension involving the seminal vesicles was associated with poor prognosis, similar to that of pT4b bladder cancer (**Fig. 11-29**).[73,74] Five-year overall survival for these patients was only 10%, similar to pT4b cancer (7%). The five-year overall survival for patients with prostatic stromal involvement was 38%.[73] However, the prognostic significance of seminal vesicle invasion via intraepithelial extension from the prostate is less certain and should be reported separately.[75]

The prognostic significance of different prostatic involvement patterns is uncertain. The prostatic urethra may be involved by urothelial carcinoma, with or without stromal invasion. CIS involving the prostatic urethra should not be designated as pT4a cancer. Similarly, prostatic ducts and acini may be involved by urothelial carcinoma without stromal invasion. Prostatic stromal invasion is usually associated with poor clinical outcome and should be stated clearly. Seminal vesicle involvement by direct perivesical tumor extension is a poor prognostic indicator.[73,74]

On a larger population-based analysis of 2043 pT4 bladder cancer patients from 17 Surveillance, Epidemiology and End Results (SEER) registries diagnosed between 1988 and 2006, Liberman and his colleagues found that cancer-specific mortality was 2.3-fold higher in pT4b versus pT3 ($P < 0.001$), 1.1-fold higher in pT4a versus pT3 ($P = 0.002$), and 2.0-fold higher in pT4a versus pT4b patients.[76] Among node-negative patients, pT4b patients had a 2.3-fold higher rate of cancer-specific mortality than pT3 patients ($P < 0.001$) and pT4b patients had a 2.1-fold higher rate of cancer-specific mortality than pT4a patients ($P < 0.001$). Interestingly, the cancer-specific mortality was the same for pT4a and pT3 patients ($P = 0.1$). These findings support clinical utility of stratifications of pT4 bladder cancer patents.[76]

Lymphovascular and Perineural Invasion

See **Chapter 25** for further discussion (**Figs. 11-30** and **11-31**).

Nodal Classification (N Staging)

The 2010 TNM staging system categorizes nodal status based on the number of positive lymph nodes and location of positive nodes (**Figs. 11-32** to **11-35**; **Table 11-1**).[9] N1 is defined as a single positive node in primary drainage

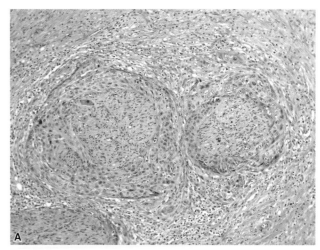
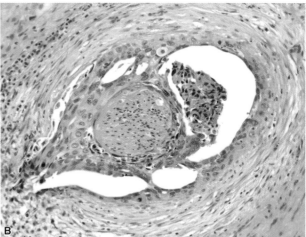

Figure 11-31   Perineural invasion (A and B).

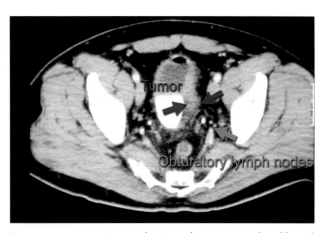

Figure 11-32   Imaging evaluation of tumor spread and lymph node metastasis. This bladder wall thickening is evident on CT scans as well. CT scans are poorly predictive of local extension of tumor. CT scans or MRI scans of the pelvis are obtained to rule out spread to the pelvic lymph nodes. The most common sites of spread are the obturator lymph nodes located posterior to the external iliac artery and vein. (Photo courtesy of Dr. Koch.)

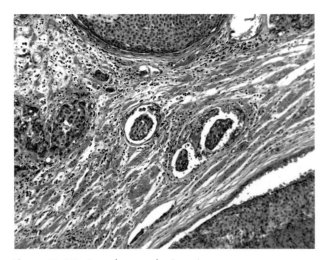

Figure 11-30   Lymphovascular invasion.

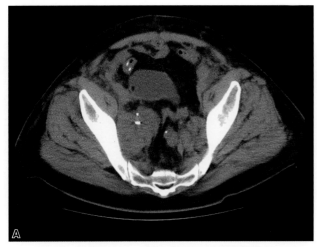

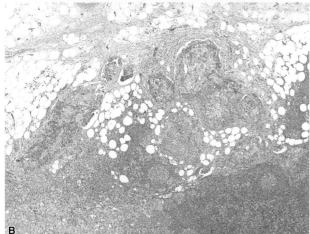

Figure 11-33   Lymph node metastasis. CT scan showed extensive pelvic lymphadenopathy in a bladder cancer patient (A). Lymph node dissection was performed and microscopic examination revealed near-replacement of lymph node by bladder cancer. Note the extranodal extension of lymph node metastasis (B). (Photo courtesy of Dr. Koch.)

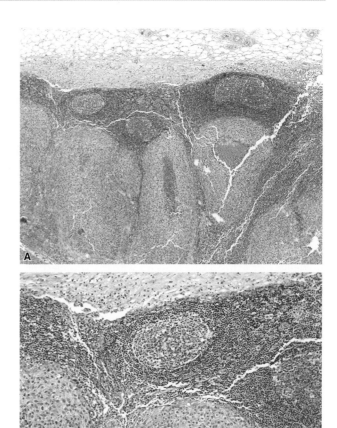

Figure 11-34   Lymph node metastasis (A and B).

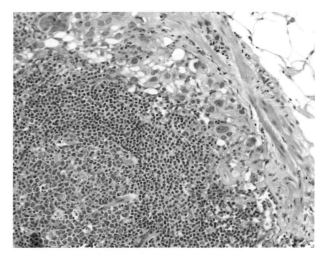

Figure 11-35   Lymph node metastasis. Note the subcapsular location of the micrometastasis.

regions; N2 is defined as multiple positive nodes in primary drainage regions; N3 is defined as common iliac node involvement. The previous N subclassification,[77] based on the size of the metastasis using 2 cm and 5 cm as thresholds, has been abandoned.

Recent studies have emphasized the importance of lymph node density for nodal staging.[78-82] Lymph node density is defined by the ratio of positive lymph nodes to the total number of lymph nodes sampled. In an analysis of 248 patients with positive nodal metastasis, Kassouf et al. found that lymph node density was an independent predictor of cancer survival.[79] The five-year cancer-specific survival for patients with lymph node density > 20% was 15%, compared to 55% five-year cancer-specific survival among patients with lymph node density ≤ 20%.[79]

However, the minimum number of lymph nodes in the specimen for optimal lymph node density estimation is yet to be established. Moreover, the best cutoff for lymph node density has not been determined in a systematic way. In a multivariate analysis of 101 lymph node-positive bladder carcinomas, using 20% as the cutoff, lymph node density was not a significant predictor of survival.[83] In another series of 154 node-positive patients, only the number of positive nodes was an independent predictor of survival.[84] Each level of increase by one positive node increased the risk of cancer death by 20%.[84]

Additional factors, such as the largest dimension of metastasis, extranodal extension, and anatomic location of positive nodes, may also be important. Fleischmann et al. found that extranodal extension was the strongest predictor of clinical outcome.[83] The incidence of extranodal extension in 101 patients with pelvic node metastases was 58%.[83] During a median followup of 21 months, patients with extranodal extension had significantly worse recurrence-free survival (median, 12 months) and overall (median, 16 months) survival than those without extranodal extension (median, 60 months for both recurrence-free survival and overall survival).[85]

Occult lymph node metastasis may be present but undetectable by routine hematoxylin and eosin examinations. The detection of lymph node micrometastasis by molecular methods is a promising technique in overcoming this limitation. The reverse transcriptase–polymerase chain reaction (RT-PCR) assay for uroplakin II was more sensitive than cytokeratin 20 for detecting occult lymph node metastasis.[86] Of 66 pelvic lymph node samples without histologic evidence of metastasis, uroplakin II was detected in six (10%), whereas cytokeratin 20 was not detected in any samples.[86] In the analysis by Seraj et al., the incidence of positive RT-PCR for uroplakin II mRNA was 25% of 27 patients with histologically negative lymph nodes.[87] Copp et al. found positive uroplakin II RNA transcripts in 33% of pelvic lymphadenectomy specimens without morphologic evidence of lymph node metastasis.[88] The investigators found that only 5% of histologically and RT-PCR node-negative patients had cancer recurrence, whereas 91% of histologically and RT-PCR node-positive patients recurred after a mean followup of 6 months.[88] Using the quantitative real-time RT-PCR approach, Marin-Aguilera et al. found positive RT-PCR results in 21% of histologically negative lymph nodes.[89] However, there was no survival difference between RT–PCR-positive and RT–PCR-negative groups during a median followup of 35 months.[89] The use of cytokeratin immunohistochemistry for detection of occult metastasis appeared to be of no practical value.[90]

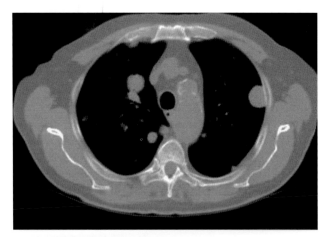

Figure 11-36 Distant metastasis. CT scan shows lung metastasis from bladder cancer. (Photo courtesy of Dr. Koch.)

Distant Metastasis

The presence of distant metastasis is designated as M1. The common sites of distant metastasis include liver, lung, bone, adrenal, and gastrointestinal tract (**Figs. 11-36** to **11-41**).[1,22] Bone metastasis often presents as alytic lesion in the spine. Metastasis to the ovary, skin, and soft tissue has also been documented.

TNM Descriptors

Pathologic staging depends on pathologic documentation of the anatomic extent of cancer, whether or not the primary tumor has been removed completely. It is mandatory that TNM staging information is included in the final pathology report (see **Chapter 25** for further discussion). By AJCC/UICC convention, the designation "T" refers to a primary tumor that has not been treated previously. The symbol "p" refers to the pathologic classification of the TNM, as opposed to the clinical classification, and is based on gross and microscopic examination (**Table 11-5**). pT indicates a resection of the primary tumor or biopsy adequate to evaluate the highest pT category, pN indicates removal of nodes adequate to validate lymph node metastasis, and pM implies microscopic examination of distant lesions. Clinical classification (cTNM) is usually carried out by the physician before treatment during initial evaluation of the patient or when pathologic classification is not possible. The suffix "is" may be added to any T to indicate the presence of associated carcinoma in situ.

For identification of special cases of TNM or pTNM classification, the "m" suffix and "y" and "r" prefixes are used (**Table 11-5**). The suffix "m" should be added to the

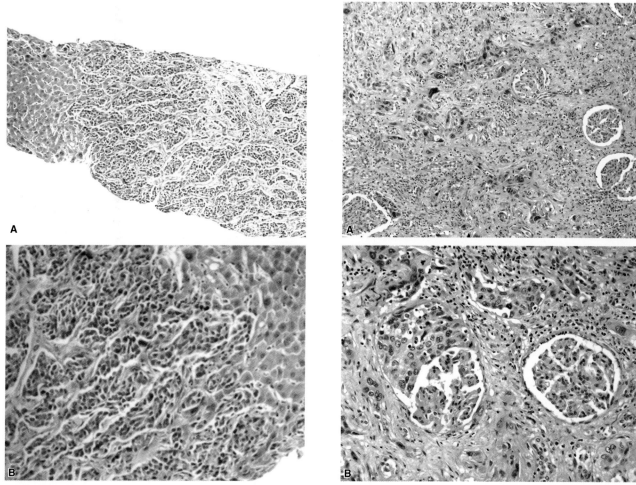

Figure 11-37 Distant metastasis (liver) from primary bladder cancer (A and B).

Figure 11-39 Distant metastasis (kidney) from primary bladder cancer (A and B).

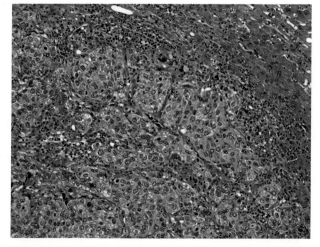

Figure 11-38 Distant metastasis (liver) from primary bladder cancer.

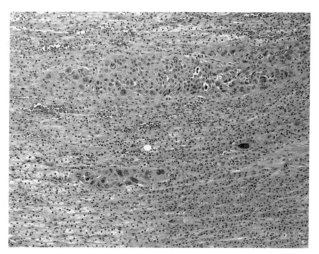

Figure 11-40 Distant metastasis (adrenal) from primary bladder cancer.

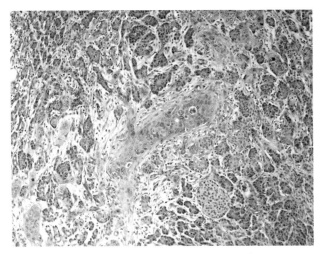

Figure 11-41 Distant metastasis (pancreas) from primary bladder cancer.

Table 11-5 Selected TNM Descriptors

Primary tumor (T)	
c	Stage given by clinical examination of a patient; the "c" prefix is implicit in the absence of the "p" prefix
p	Stage given by pathologic examination of a surgical specimen
m	Indicates multiple primary tumors
r	Recurrent tumor after a documented disease-free interval
y	Stage assessed after neoadjuvant therapy (posttreatment)

R Classification	
RX	Presence of residual tumor cannot be assessed
R0	No residual tumor
R1	Microscopic residual tumor
R2	Macroscopic residual tumor

appropriate T category to indicate the presence of multiple primary tumors in a single site and is recorded in parentheses: pT(m)NM. The "y" prefix indicates those cases in which classification is performed during or following initial multimodality therapy (i.e., neoadjuvant chemotherapy, radiation therapy, or both chemotherapy and radiation therapy). In such instances, the cTNM or pTNM category is qualified by a "y" prefix. The ycTNM or ypTNM categorizes the extent of tumor actually present at the time of pathologic examination. Recurrent tumor,

when staged after a documented disease-free interval, is identified by the "r" prefix: rTNM.

Additional descriptors may be used when residual tumor (r) is used. Tumor remaining in a patient after therapy with curative intent (e.g., surgical resection for cure) is categorized by a system known as R classification (Table 11-5). For the surgeon, the R classification may be useful to indicate the known or assumed status of the completeness of a surgical excision.

REFERENCES

1. Cheng L, Montironi R, Davidson DD, Lopez-Beltran A. Staging and reporting of urothelial carcinoma of the urinary bladder. *Mod Pathol* 2009;22(Suppl 2):S70–95.
2. Droller MJ. Bladder cancer: State-of-the-art care. *CA Cancer J Clin* 1998;48:269–84.
3. Cheng L, Neumann RM, Nehra A, Spotts BE, Weaver AL, Bostwick DG. Cancer heterogeneity and its biologic implications in the grading of urothelial carcinoma. *Cancer* 2000;88:1663–70.
4. Cheng L, Neumann RM, Weaver AL, Cheville JC, Leibovich BC, Ramnani DM, Scherer BG, Nehra A, Zincke H, Bostwick DG. Grading and staging of bladder carcinoma in transurethral resection specimens. Correlation with 105 matched cystectomy specimens. *Am J Clin Pathol* 2000;113:275–9.
5. Cheng L, Weaver AL, Leibovich BC, Ramnani DM, Neumann RM, Scherer BG, Nehra A, Zincke H, Bostwick DG. Predicting the survival of bladder carcinoma patients treated with radical cystectomy. *Cancer* 2000;88:2326–32.
6. Stein JP, Lieskovsky G, Cote R, Groshen S, Feng AC, Boyd S, Skinner E, Bochner B, Thangathurai D, Mikhail M, Raghavan D, Skinner DG. Radical cystectomy in the treatment of invasive bladder cancer: long-term results in 1,054 patients. *J Clin Oncol* 2001;19:666–75.
7. Dalbagni G, Genega E, Hashibe M, Zhang ZF, Russo P, Herr H, Reuter V. Cystectomy for bladder cancer: a contemporary series. *J Urol* 2001;165:1111–6.
8. Shariat SF, Karakiewicz PI, Palapattu GS, Lotan Y, Rogers CG, Amiel GE, Vazina A, Gupta A, Bastian PJ, Sagalowsky AI, Schoenberg MP, Lerner SP. Outcomes of radical cystectomy for transitional cell carcinoma of the bladder: a contemporary series from the Bladder Cancer Research Consortium. *J Urol* 2006;176:2414–22.
9. Edge S, B, Byrd DR, Compton CC, Fritz AG, Greene FL, Trotti A. American Joint Committee on Cancer Staging Manual, 7th ed. New York: Springer, 2010.
10. Palapattu GS, Shariat SF, Karakiewicz PI, Bastian PJ, Rogers CG, Amiel G, Lotan Y, Vazina A, Gupta A, Sagalowsky AI, Lerner SP, Schoenberg MP. Cancer specific outcomes in patients with pT0 disease following radical cystectomy. *J Urol* 2006;175:1645–9.

11. Kassouf W, Spiess PE, Brown GA, Munsell MF, Grossman HB, Siefker-Radtke A, Dinney CP, Kamat AM. P0 stage at radical cystectomy for bladder cancer is associated with improved outcome independent of traditional clinical risk factors. *Eur Urol* 2007;52:769–74.

12. Thrasher JB, Frazier HA, Robertson JE, Paulson DF. Does of stage pT0 cystectomy specimen confer a survival advantage in patients with minimally invasive bladder cancer? *J Urol* 1994;152:393–6.

13. Volkmer BG, Kuefer R, Bartsch G Jr, Straub M, de Petriconi R, Gschwend JE, Hautmann RE. Effect of a pT0 cystectomy specimen without neoadjuvant therapy on survival. *Cancer* 2005;104:2384–91.

14. Yiou R, Patard JJ, Benhard H, Abbou CC, Chopin DK. Outcome of radical cystectomy for bladder cancer according to the disease type at presentation. *BJU Int* 2002;89:374–8.

15. Tilki D, Svatek RS, Novara G, Seitz M, Godoy G, Karakiewicz PI, Kassouf W, Fradet Y, Fritsche HM, Sonpavde G, Izawa JI, Ficarra V, et al. Stage pT0 at radical cystectomy confers improved survival: an international study of 4,430 patients. *J Urol* 2010;184:888–94.

16. Lopez-Beltran A, Cheng L. Stage pT1 bladder carcinoma: diagnostic criteria, pitfalls and prognostic significance. *Pathology* 2003;35:484–91.

17. Soloway MS. It is time to abandon the "superficial" in bladder cancer. *Eur Urol* 2007;52:1564–5.

18. Nieder AM, Soloway MS. Eliminate the term "superficial" bladder cancer. *J Urol* 2006;175:417–8.

19. Maclennan GT, Kirkali Z, Cheng L. Histologic grading of noninvasive papillary urothelial neoplasms. *Eur Urol* 2007;51:889–98.

20. Montironi R, Lopez-Beltran A, Scarpelli M, Mazzucchelli R, Cheng L. 2004 World Health Organization classification of the noninvasive urothelial neoplasms: Inherent problems and clinical reflections. *Eur Urol* 2009;Suppl 8:453–7.

21. Bostwick DG, Ramnani D, Cheng L. Diagnosis and grading of bladder cancer and associated lesions. *Urol Clin North Am* 1999;26:493–507.

22. Cheng L, Lopez-Beltran A, MacLennan GT, Montironi R, Bostwick DG. Neoplasms of the urinary bladder. In: Bostwick DG, Cheng L, eds. Urologic Surgical Pathology, 2nd ed. Philadelphia: Elsevier/Mosby, 2008:259–352.

23. Cheng L, Neumann RM, Weaver AL, Spotts BE, Bostwick DG. Predicting cancer progression in patients with stage T1 bladder carcinoma. *J Clin Oncol* 1999;17:3182–7.

24. Jewett HJ. Carcinoma of the bladder: Influence of depth of infiltration on the 5-year results following complete extirpation of the primary growth. *J Urol* 1952;67:672–80.

25. Bayraktar Z, Gurbuz G, Tasci AI, Sevin G. Staging error in the bladder tumor: the correlation between stage of TUR and cystectomy. *Int J Urol Nephrol* 2002;33:627–9.

26. Herr HW. Staging invasive bladder tumors. *J Surg Oncol* 1992;51:217–20.

27. Herr HW. A propsed simplified staging system of invasive bladder tumors. *Urol Int* 1993;50:17–20.

28. Hall RR, Prout GR. Staging of bladder cancer: Is the tumor, node, metastasis system adequate? *Semin Oncol* 1990;17:517–23.

29. Skinner DG. Current state of classification and staging of bladder cancer. *Cancer Res* 1977;37:2838–42.

30. Skinner DG. Current perspectives in the management of high grade invasive bladder cancer. *Cancer* 1980;45:1866–74.

31. Cummings KB, Barone JG, Ward WS. Diagnosis and staging of bladder cancer. *Urol Clin North Am* 1992;19:455–65.

32. Bowles WT, Cordonnier JJ. Total cystectomy for carcinoma of the bladder. *J Urol* 1963;90:731–5.

33. Cox CE, Cass AS, Boyce WH. Bladder cancer: a 26-year review. *Trans Am Assoc Genitourin Surg* 1968;60:22–30.

34. Boileau MA, Johnson DE, Chan RC, Gonzales MO. Bladder carcinoma. Results with preoperative radiation therapy and radical cystectomy. *Urology* 1980;16:569.

35. Beahrs JR, Fleming TR, Zincke H. Risk of local urethral recurrence after radical cystectomy for bladder cancer. *J Urol* 1984;131:264–66.

36. Bredael JJ, Croker BP, Glenn JF. The curability of invasive bladder cancer treated by radical cystectomy. *Eur Urol* 1980;6:206–10.

37. Cordonnier JJ. Simple cystectomy in the management of bladder carcinoma. *Arch Surg* 1974;108:190–91.

38. Mathur VK, Krahn HP, Ramsey EW. Total cystectomy for bladder cancer. *J Urol* 1981;125:784–6.

39. Pollack A, Zagars GK, Cole CJ, Dinney CPN, Swanson DA, Grossman HB. The relationship of local control to distant metastasis in muscle invasive bladder cancer. *J Urol* 1995;154:2059–64.

40. Pomerance A. Pathology and prognosis following total cystectomy for carcinoma of bladder. *Br J Urol* 1972;44:451–8.

41. Prout GR Jr. The surgical management of bladder carcinoma. *Urol Clin North Am* 1976;3:149–75.

42. Richie JP, Skinner DG, Kaufman JJ. Radical cystectomy for carcinoma of the bladder: 16 years of experience. *J Urol* 1975;113:186–9.

43. Richie JP, Skinner DG, Kaufman JJ. Carcinoma of the bladder: treatment by radical cystectomy. *J Surg Res* 1975;18:271–5.

44. Roehrborn CG, Sagalowsky AI, Peters PC. Long-term patient survival after cystectomy for regional metastatic transitional cell carcinoma of the bladder. *J Urol* 1991;146:36–9.

45. Skinner DG. Management of invasive bladder cancer: a meticulous pelvic node dissection can make a difference. *J Urol* 1982;128:34–6.

46. Sorensen BL, Ohlsen AS, Barlebo H. Carcinoma of the urinary bladder. Clinical staging and histologic grading in relation to survival. *Scand J Urol Nephrol* 1969;3:189–92.

47. Utz DC, Schmitz SE, Fugelso PD, Farrow GM. A clinicopathologic evaluation of partial cystectomy for carcinoma of the urinary bladder. *Cancer* 1975;32:1075–7.

48. Whitemore WF. Management of invasive bladder Nnoplasms. *Semin Urol* 1983;1:34–41.

49. Wishnow KI, Levinson AK, Johnson DE, Tenney DM, Grignon DJ, Ro JY, Ayala AJ, Logothetis CJ, Babaian RJ, von Eschenbach AC. Stage B (P 2/3A/N0) transitional cell carcinoma of bladder highly curable by radical cystectomy. *Urology* 1992;39:12–16.

50. Pearse HD, Reed RR, Hodges CV. Radical cystectomy for bladder cancer. *J Urol* 1978;119:216–18.

51. Montie JE, Straffon RA, Stewart BH. Radical cystectomy without radiation therapy for carcinoma of the bladder. *J Urol* 1984;131:477–82.

52. Pagano F, Bassi P, Galetti TP, Meneghini A, Milani C, Artibani W, A G. Results of contemporary radical cystectomy for invasive bladder cancer: a clinicopathological study with an emphasis on the inadequacy of the tumor, nodes and metastases classification. *J Urol* 1991;145:45–50.

53. Yu RJ, Stein JP, Cai J, Miranda G, Groshen S, Skinner DG. Superficial (pT2a) and deep (pT2b) muscle invasion in pathological staging of bladder cancer following radical cystectomy. *J Urol* 2006;176:493–9.

54. Girgin C, Sezer A, Delibas M, Sahin O, Oder M, Dincel C. Impact of the level of muscle invasion in organ-confined bladder cancer. *Urol Int* 2007;78:145–9.

55. Skinner DG, Tift JP, Kaufman JJ. High dose, short course preoperative radiation therapy and immediate single stage radical cystectomy with pelvic node dissection in the management of bladder cancer. *J Urol* 1982;127:671–4.

56. Cuesta JA, Chapado MS, Cid MG, Corral NF, Pontes EJ, Grignon DJ. Survival of patiens with stage T2-T3a baldder cancer treated by radical cystectomy. *Arch Esp De Urol* 1997;50:17–25.

57. Cheng L, Neumann RM, Scherer BG, Weaver AL, Nehra A, Zincke H, Bostwick DG. Tumor size predicts the survival of patients with pathologic stage T2 bladder carcinoma: a critical evaluation of the depth of muscle invasion. *Cancer* 1999;85:2638–47.

58. Tokgoz H, Turkolmez K, Resorlu B, Kose K, Tulunay O, Beduk Y. Pathological staging of muscle invasive bladder cancer. Is substaging of pT2 tumors really necessary? *Int Braz J Urol* 2007;33:777–83.

59. Tilki D, Reich O, Karakiewicz PI, Novara G, Kassouf W, Ergun S, Fradet Y, Ficarra V, Sonpavde G, Stief CG, Skinner E, Svatek RS, Lotan Y, Sagalowsky AI, Shariat SF. Validation of the AJCC TNM substaging of pT2 bladder cancer: deep muscle invasion is associated with significantly worse outcome. *Eur Urol* 2010;58:112–7.

60. Jewett HJ. Editorial: Comments on the staging of invasive bladder cancer two B's or not to B's: That is the question. *J Urol* 1978;119:39.

61. Bochner BH, Nichols PW, Skinner DG. Overstaging of transitional cell carcinoma: clinical significance of lamina propria fat within the urinary bladder. *Urology* 1995;45:528–31.

62. Philip AT, Amin MB, Tamboli P, Lee TJ, Hill CE, Ro JY. Intravesical adipose tissue: a quantitative study of its presence and location with implications for therapy and prognosis. *Am J Surg Pathol* 2000;24:1286–90.

63. Quek ML, Stein JP, Clark PE, Daneshmand S, Miranda G, Cai J, Groshen S, Cote RJ, Lieskovsky G, Quinn DI, Skinner DG. Microscopic and gross extravesical extension in pathological staging of bladder cancer. *J Urol* 2004;171:640–5.

64. Bastian PJ, Hutterer GC, Shariat SF, Rogers CG, Palapattu GS, Lotan Y, Vazina A, Amiel GE, Gupta A, Sagalowsky AI, Lerner SP, Schoenberg MP, Karakiewicz PI, Bladder Cancer Research Consortium. Macroscopic, but not microscopic, perivesical fat invasion at radical cystectomy is an adverse predictor of recurrence and survival. *BJU Int* 2008;101:450–4.

65. Tilki D, Svatek RS, Karakiewicz PI, Novara G, Seitz M, Sonpavde G, Gupta A, Kassouf W, Fradet Y, Ficarra V, Skinner E, Lotan Y, Sagalowsky AI, Stief CG, Reich O, Shariat SF. pT3 Substaging is a prognostic indicator for lymph node negative urothelial carcinoma of the bladder. *J Urol* 2010;184:470–4.

66. Cheng L, Weaver AL, Bostwick DG. Predicting extravesical extension of bladder carcinoma: a novel method based on micrometer measurement of the depth of invasion in transurethral resection specimens. *Urology* 2000;55:668–72.

67. Palou J, Baniel J, Klotz L, Wood D, Cookson M, Lerner S, Horie S, Schoenberg M, Angulo J, Bassi P. Urothelial carcinoma of the prostate. *Urology* 2007;1 (Suppl):50–61.

68. Donat SM, Genega EM, Herr HW, Reuter VE. Mechanisms of prostatic stromal invasion in patients with bladder cancer: clinical significance. *J Urol* 2001;165:1117–20.

69. Esrig D, Freeman JA, Elmajian DA, Stein JP, Chen SC, Groshen S, Simoneau A, Skinner EC, Lieskovsky G, Boyd SD, Cote RJ, Skinner DG. Transitional cell carcinoma involving the prostate with a proposed staging classification for stromal invasion. *J Urol* 1996;156:1071–6.

70. Pagano F, Bassi P, Ferrante GL, Piazza N, Abatangelo G, Pappagallo GL, Garbeglio A. Is stage pT4a (D1) reliable in assessing transitional cell carcinoma involvement of the prostate in patients with a concurrent bladder cancer? A necessary distinction for contiguous or noncontiguous involvement. *J Urol* 996;155:244–7.

71. Shen SS, Lerner SP, Muezzinoglu B, Truong LD, Amiel G, Wheeler TM. Prostatic involvement by transitional cell carcinoma in patients with bladder cancer and its prognostic significance. *Hum Pathol* 2006;37:726–34.

72. Montironi R, Cheng L, Mazzucchelli R, Scarpelli M, Kirkali Z, Montorsi F, Lopez-Beltran A. Critical evaluation of the prostate from cystoprostatectomies for bladder cancer: insights from a complete sampling with the whole mount technique. *Eur Urol* 2009;55:1305–9.

73. Daneshmand S, Stein JP, Lesser T, Quek ML, Nichols PW, Miranda G, Cai J, Groshen S, Skinner EC, Skinner DG. Prognosis of seminal vesicle involvement by transitional cell carcinoma of the bladder. *J Urol* 2004;2004:81–4.

74. Volkmer BG, Küfer R, Maier S, Bartsch G, Bach D, Hautmann R, Gschwend JE. Outcome in patients with seminal vesicle invasion after radical cystectomy. *J Urol* 2003;169:1299–1302.

75. Murphy WM, Crissman JD, Johansson SL, Ayala AG. Recommendations for the reporting of urinary bladder specimens that contain bladder neoplasms. *Mod Pathol* 1996;9:796–8.

76. Liberman D, Alasker A, Sun M, Ismail S, Lughezzani G, Jeldres C, Budaus L, Thuret R, Shariat SF, Widmer H, Perrotte P, Graefen M, Montorsi F, Karakiewicz PI. Radical cystectomy for patients with pT4 urothelial carcinoma in a large population-based study. *BJU Int* 2011;107:905–11.

77. Greene FL, Page DL, Fleming ID, Fritz AG, Balch CM, Haller DG, Morrow M. American Joint Committee on Cancer Staging Manual, 6th ed. New York: Springer, 2002.

78. Herr HW. Superiority of ratio based lymph node staging for bladder cancer. *J Urol* 2003;169:943–5.

79. Kassouf W, Agarwal PK, Herr HW, Munsell MF, Spiess PE, Brown GA, Pisters L, Grossman HB, Dinney CP, Kamat AM. Lymph node density is superior to TNM nodal status in predicting disease-specific survival after radical cystectomy for bladder cancer: analysis of pooled data from MDACC and MSKCC. *J Clin Oncol* 2008;26:121–6.

80. Stein JP, Cai J, Groshen S, Skinner DG. Risk factors for patients with pelvic lymph node metastases following radical cystectomy with en bloc pelvic lymphadenectomy: concept of lymph node density. *J Urol* 2003;170:35–41.

81. Kassouf W, Leibovici D, Munsell MF, Dinney CP, Grossman HB, Kamat AM. Evaluation of the relevance of lymph node density in a contemporary series of patients undergoing radical cystectomy. *J Urol* 2006;176:53–7.

82. May M, Herrmann E, Bolenz C, Tiemann A, Brookman-May S, Fritsche HM, Burger M, Buchner A, Gratzke C, Wulfing C, Trojan L, Ellinger J, et al. Lymph node density affects cancer-specific survival in patients with lymph node-positive urothelial bladder cancer following radical cystectomy. *Eur Urol* 2011;59:712–8.

83. Fleischmann A, Thalmann GN, Markwalder R, Studer UE. Extracapsular extension of pelvic lymph node metastases from urothelial carcinoma of the bladder is an independent prognostic factor. *J Clin Oncol* 2005;23:2358–65.

84. Frank I, Cheville JC, Blute ML, Lohse CM, Nehra A, Weaver AL, Karnes RJ, Zincke H. Transitional cell carcinoma of the urinary bladder with regional lymph node involvement treated by cystectomy: clinicopathologic features associated with outcome. *Cancer* 2003;97:2425–31.

85. Fleischmann A, Thalmann GN, Markwalder R, Studer UE. Prognostic implications of extracapsular extension of pelvic lymph node metastases in urothelial carcinoma of the bladder. *Am J Surg Pathol* 2005;29:89–95.

86. Wu X, Kakehi Y, Zeng Y, Taoka R, Tsunemori H, Inui M. Uroplakin II as a promising marker for molecular diagnosis of nodal metastases from bladder cancer: comparison with cytokeratin 20. *J Urol* 2005;174:2138–43.

87. Seraj MJ, Thomas AR, Chin JL, Theodorescu D. Molecular determination of perivesical and lymph node metastasis after radical cystectomy for urothelial carcinoma of the bladder. *Clin Cancer Res* 2001;7:1516–22.

88. Copp HL, Chin JL, Conaway M, Theodorescu D. Prospective evaluation of the prognostic relevance of molecular staging for urothelial carcinoma. *Cancer* 2006;107:60–6.

89. Marin-Aguilera M, Mengual L, Burset M, Oliver A, Ars E, Ribal MJ, Colomer D, Mellado B, Villavicencio H, Algaba F, Alcaraz A. Molecular lymph node staging in bladder urothelial carcinoma: impact on survival. *Eur Urol* 2008;54:1363–72.

90. Yang XJ, Lecksell K, Epstein JI. Can immunohistochemistry enhance the detection of micrometastases in pelvic lymph nodes from patients with high grade urothelial carcinoma of the bladder? *Am J Clin Pathol* 1999;112:649–53.

Histologic Variants of Urothelial Carcinoma

David G. Bostwick.

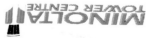

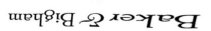

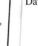

For use in the Pinnacle Restaurant on Apr. 17th at

MINOLTA
TOWER CENTRE

or

Domestic Beer, House Wine, House Mixed Drink

Host Bar Ticket

Baker & Bigham

Urothelial carcinoma has a tremendous morphologic plasticity. A remarkably wide diversity of histologic patterns, some that mimic other malignancies, may be seen in the same tumor. Some variants of urothelial carcinoma appear to represent unique morphologic characteristics of the same disease process; thus, no distinction in clinical behavior has been identified. However, in other variants, tumors behave more aggressively than the histologic features would otherwise suggest, making their correct diagnosis critical (Tables 12-1 and 12-2). Divergent differentiation may be appreciated in 25% of urothelial carcinoma, and overall, its presence appears to carry a worse prognosis. Therefore, recognition of these and other forms is important to avoid misdiagnosis or confusion with other benign-appearing lesions.

Urothelial Carcinoma with Squamous Differentiation

Urothelial carcinoma with mixed differentiation includes urothelial carcinoma with squamous (Figs. 12-1 to 12-3) and/or glandular differentiation. The exact biological significance of mixed differentiation in urothelial carcinoma has not come to a definite conclusion in the literature. Some investigators report that urothelial carcinomas harboring squamous or glandular differentiation have a less favorable response to therapy than does pure urothelial carcinoma.[1] In a mapping study of 38 bladder carcinomas, Jozwicki et al. found that those urothelial carcinomas with more than 80% of conventional urothelial differentiation seemed to have a more favorable clinical course.[2] However, in a larger study comprising 448 bladder carcinomas, the presence of mixed differentiation failed to predict disease-specific survival by either univariate or multivariate analysis.[3] To further define the prognostic significance of these mixed differentiations, squamous and glandular differentiation should be reported separately.

Squamous differentiation, defined by the presence of intercellular bridges or keratinization, occurs in approximately 20% of urothelial carcinomas of the bladder,[1] but its frequency increases up to 40% in high grade and advanced-stage bladder cancers with a similar incidence in renal pelvis carcinomas. In general, urothelial carcinoma with a squamous or glandular component has a less favorable response to therapy than that of pure urothelial carcinoma.[4-7]

In a study of patients with metastatic carcinoma, 46% with a mixed component of squamous differentiation (squamous cell carcinoma) experienced disease progression despite intense chemotherapy, while less than 30% of patients with pure urothelial histology progressed.[4]

Table 12-1 Histologic Variants of Urothelial Carcinoma

Urothelial carcinoma with squamous differentiation
Urothelial carcinoma with glandular differentiation
   Urothelial carcinoma with villoglandular differentiation

Urothelial carcinoma, nested variant
Urothelial carcinoma, micropapillary variant
Urothelial carcinoma, microcystic variant
Urothelial carcinoma, inverted variant
Urothelial carcinoma, lipid cell variant
Urothelial carcinoma, plasmacytoid variant
Lymphoepithelioma-like carcinoma
Urothelial carcinoma, clear cell (glycogen-rich) variant
Sarcomatoid carcinoma
Large cell undifferentiated carcinoma
Osteoclast-rich undifferentiated carcinoma
Pleomorphic giant cell carcinoma

Other morphological variations in bladder cancer
   Urothelial carcinoma with chordoid features
   Urothelial carcinoma with small tubules/acini
   Urothelial carcinoma with syncytiotrophoblastic giant cells
   Urothelial carcinoma with discohesive growth pattern
   Urothelial carcinoma with rhabdoid features

Urothelial carcinoma with multiple histologic patterns
   Urothelial carcinoma with small cell carcinoma component

Urothelial carcinoma with tumor-associated stromal reactions
   Urothelial carcinoma with pseudosarcomatous stromal reaction
   Urothelial carcinoma with osseous and chondroid metaplasia
   Urothelial carcinoma with osteoclast-type giant cell reaction
   Urothelial carcinoma with prominent lymphoid reaction

Low grade urothelial carcinoma with focal squamous differentiation also has a higher recurrence rate.

The proportion of the squamous component may vary considerably, with some cases having urothelial carcinoma in situ (CIS) as the only urothelial component. The morphologic patterns of keratinizing and nonkeratinizing squamous differentiation include (1) wide nests and cords showing dyskeratosis, intercellular bridges, and corneous pearls; (2) small foci frequently overlooked under conventional evaluation showing intercellular bridges but not dyskeratosis or corneous pearls; (3) additional features suggestive of koilocytosis; (4) occasional but focally prominent intracytoplasmic lumina in nests of squamous differentiation; and (5) rare cases with rather clear cells forming nests of

Table 12-2 Pathologic Variants of Urothelial Bladder Carcinoma According to Their Suggested Clinical Significance

Pathologic Variants of Invasive Bladder Cancer and Their Potential Pitfalls	Main Lesions and Tumors in Differential Diagnosis
Urothelial carcinoma with deceptively benign features	
Urothelial carcinoma, nested variant	von Brunn nest and hyperplasia
Urothelial carcinoma, inverted variant	Inverted papilloma
Urothelial carcinoma, microcystic variant	Cystitis cystica et glandularis, endocervicosis
Urothelial carcinoma with small tubules	Nephrogenetic metaplasia, von Brunn nests, cystitis glandularis, prostatic adenocarcinoma
Differential diagnosis with metastases to the bladder	
Urothelial carcinoma, micropapillary variant	Serous carcinoma of the ovary; micropapillary carcinomas from other sites
Urothelial carcinoma, plasmacytoid variant	Plasmacytoma
Urothelial carcinoma, clear cell (glycogen-rich) variant	Clear cell carcinomas from kidney, and others
Large cell undifferentiated carcinoma	Metastasis from other sites such as lung
Complex therapeutic approach	
Urothelial carcinoma, lymphoepithelioma-like variant	Chemotherapy, metastases from other sites
Small cell carcinoma	Chemotherapy, metastases from lung
Misdiagnosis as choriocarcinoma either primary/secondary	
Urothelial carcinoma with syncytiotrophoblastic giant cells	Choriocarcinoma either primary or secondary
Misdiagnosis as myofibroblastic proliferation	
Sarcomatoid carcinoma	Inflammatory myofibroblastic tumor; urothelial carcinoma with pseudocarcinomatous stromal reaction
Misdiagnosis as squamous cell carcinoma or adenocarcinoma either primary or secondary	
Urothelial carcinoma with squamous and/or glandular differentiation	Squamous cell carcinoma, adenocarcinoma
Misdiagnosis as other tumor types	
Urothelial carcinoma, lipid-cell variant	Sarcomatoid carcinoma with heterologous component
Urothelial carcinoma with pseudosarcomatous stroma	Sarcomatoid carcinoma
Urothelial carcinoma with stromal osseous or cartilaginous metaplasia	Carcinosarcoma/sarcomatoid carcinoma heterologous type
Urothelial carcinoma with osteoclast-type giant cells	Reactive granulomatous lesion
Urothelial carcinoma with prominent lymphoid infiltrate	Lymphoma
Urothelial carcinomas with discohesive growth	Signet ring cell adenocarcinoma, lobular carcinoma of breast

variable size well demarcated from concomitant urothelial carcinoma.[6] Basaloid or clear cell-type squamous differentiation can be observed rarely. Mac387, cytokeratin (CK) 14, L1 antigen, and caveolin-1 have been reported as immunohistochemical markers of squamous differentiation.[8-10]

Urothelial carcinoma with squamous differentiation should be distinguished from pure squamous cell carcinoma. In the urinary bladder, the term "squamous cell carcinoma" should be reserved for tumors with an exclusive squamous cell component. Tumors with any identifiable urothelial element should be classified as urothelial carcinoma with squamous differentiation, and an estimate of the percentage of the squamous component should be provided.[1,11-16]

Urothelial Carcinoma with Glandular Differentiation

Glandular differentiation is less common than squamous differentiation and may be present in about 6% to 18% of urothelial carcinomas of the bladder depending on histologic grade.[1,3,6,17,18] Glandular differentiation is more frequently identified in high grade urothelial carcinoma and associated with poor prognosis.[1,3,4] Of 91 patients with metastatic carcinoma, there was cancer progression despite intense chemotherapy in 83% with admixed adenocarcinoma, but in less than 30% with pure urothelial carcinoma.[4]

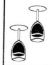

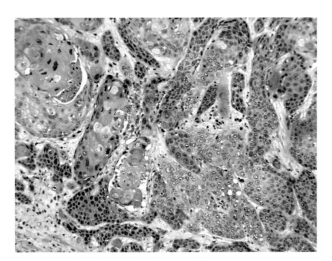

Figure 12-1 Urothelial carcinoma with squamous differentiation.

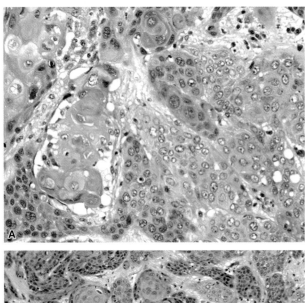

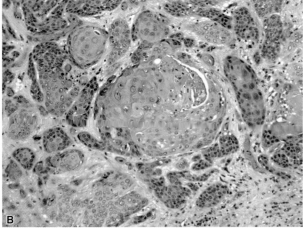

Figure 12-2 Urothelial carcinoma with squamous differentiation (A and B).

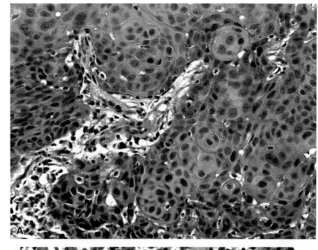

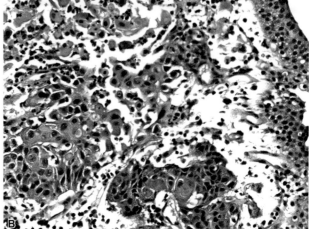

Figure 12-3 Urothelial carcinoma with squamous differentiation (A and B).

Glandular differentiation is defined as the presence of true glandular spaces within the tumor. These may be tubular or enteric glands with mucin secretion (Figs. 12-4 to 12-6). However, individual cells containing cytoplasmic mucin are present in a significant number of typical urothelial carcinomas and are not considered to represent true glandular differentiation. A colloid–mucinous pattern characterized by nests of cells floating in extracellular mucin, occasionally with signet ring cells, may be present. Cytoplasmic mucin-containing cells are present in 14% to 63% of typical urothelial carcinoma and are not considered to represent glandular differentiation.[19,20] In rare cases, the glandular component has the morphology of hepatoid or clear cell adenocarcinoma. Glandular differentiation may occasionally occur in low grade noninvasive papillary carcinoma.[18]

Urothelial carcinoma following augmentation cystoplasty often shows glandular differentiation; however, its prognosis is much worse for urothelial carcinomas with

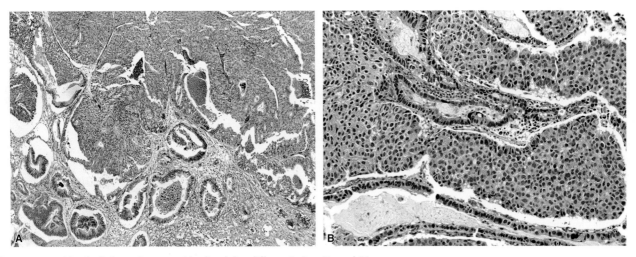

Figure 12-4 Urothelial carcinoma with glandular differentiation (A and B).

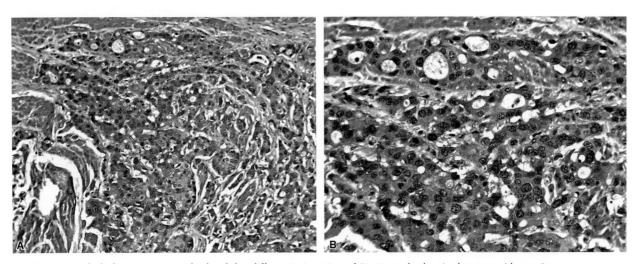

Figure 12-5 Urothelial carcinoma with glandular differentiation (A and B). Note the luminal space with mucin.

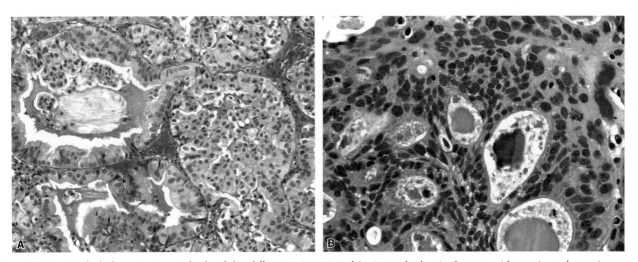

Figure 12-6 Urothelial carcinoma with glandular differentiation (A and B). Note the luminal space with mucin and proteinaceous secretions.

mixed differentiation arising in other settings.[21] Wasco et al. have reported a three-year disease-specific survival rate in urothelial carcinoma with mixed differentiation of 69%.[3] This is more favorable than in the report by Sung et al., who reported that all patients receiving augmentation cystoplasty series who developed carcinoma died of widespread metastases within months.[21] The dramatic discrepancy in biological behavior indicates that urothelial carcinoma following augmentation cystoplasty is a distinct variant rather than a conventional urothelial carcinoma with mixed differentiation (see **Chapter 21** for further discussion).

The differential diagnosis includes villous adenoma, CIS with glandular differentiation, and adenocarcinoma of the bladder (see also **Chapters 5** and **13**). The diagnosis of adenocarcinoma of the bladder is reserved for pure tumors. The expression of MUC5AC apomucin may be useful as an immunohistochemical marker of the usual forms of glandular differentiation in urothelial tumors.[19] A particularly important exercise is the differential diagnosis of glandular tumors that can occur primarily and secondarily in the bladder. Immunostaining is helpful in these settings. Urothelial carcinoma with glandular differentiation can be distinguished from colonic adenocarcinoma since the former is CK7 positive, CK20 positive, and villin negative, whereas the latter is CK20 positive, villin positive, and CK7 negative. Lack of CDX2 and villin immunoreactivity suggests a bladder primary adenocarcinoma (see also **Chapters 13** and **23**). In general, primary adenocarcinoma of the urinary bladder is uncommon. Uroplakin, thrombomodulin, p63, CK7, CK20, and high molecular weight cytokeratins are useful in confirming urothelial origin. Metastasis from other sites should be ruled out. Thyroid transcription factor 1 is helpful in the differential diagnosis of lung adenocarcinoma.

Urothelial Carcinoma with Villoglandular Differentiation

Recently, Lim et al. identified 14 cases of papillary urothelial carcinoma with villoglandular differentiation, containing both components of glandular differentiation and villous architecture similar to villous adenoma (**Figs. 12-7** to **12-9**).[22] Patients had a mean age of 70 years with a male-to-female ratio of 5:1. By definition, these cases included a component of invasive urothelial carcinoma or urothelial CIS, a significant feature in discriminating such tumors from villous adenoma. In contrast, in the 1999 study of villous adenoma by Cheng and colleagues, a subset of tumors were associated with concurrent bladder adenocarcinoma but not urothelial carcinoma.[23]

Microscopically, these tumors are composed superficially of finger-like, villous processes with the epithelial

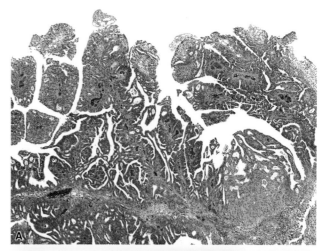
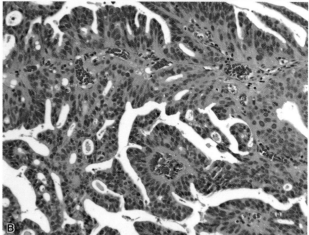

Figure 12-7 Urothelial carcinoma with villoglandular differentiation (A and B).

lining containing true glandular lumina, some with cribriform morphology. These tumors are intermixed with other components, including typical urothelial carcinoma with or without glandular differentiation, micropapillary and plasmacytoid variant, and small cell carcinoma. Concurrent cystitis cystica and glandularis was present for 21% of cases.[22] Key differential diagnosis is ductal prostatic adenocarcinoma involving the bladder (**Fig. 12-10**).

Clinical outcome data are limited. Based on the frequent presence of divergent differentiation and the clinical behavior of the tumors studied, this variant is probably aggressive.

Urothelial Carcinoma, Nested Variant

This rare pattern of urothelial carcinoma was first described as a tumor with a "deceptively benign" appearance that

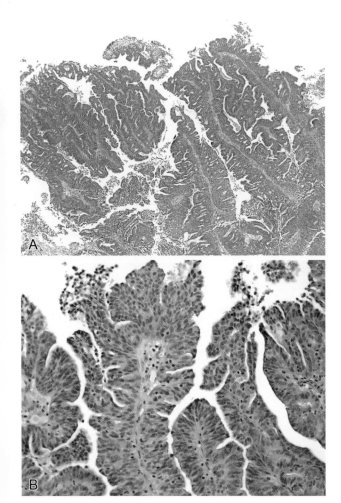

Figure 12-8 Urothelial carcinoma with villoglandular differentiation (A and B).

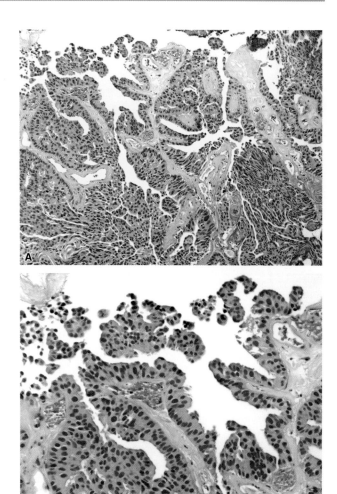

Figure 12-9 Urothelial carcinoma with villoglandular differentiation (A and B).

closely resembles von Brunn nests infiltrating the lamina propria.[24] The tumor is highly aggressive and should always be considered high grade carcinoma (**Figs. 12-11** to **12-13**).[24-30] It has a male predominance, and many patients (70%) die 4 to 40 months after diagnosis, despite therapy.[24,26]

This variant contains a variable proportion of infiltrating cell nests (**Figs. 12-14** to **12-18**). Some nests have small tubular lumens. Nuclei generally show little or no atypia, but invariably the tumor contains foci of unequivocal cancer with cells exhibiting enlarged nucleoli and coarse nuclear chromatin. This feature is most apparent in the deeper aspects of the cancer. The differential diagnosis of nested urothelial carcinoma therefore includes prominent von Brunn nests, cystitis cystica, cystitis glandularis, or inverted papilloma. Useful features in recognizing this lesion as malignant include the tendency for increasing cellular anaplasia in the deeper aspects of the lesion, its infiltrative nature, disorderly proliferation of discrete, small

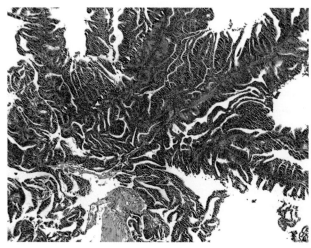

Figure 12-10 Ductal prostatic adenocarcinoma mimicking urothelial carcinoma with villoglandular differentiation. Prostate-specific antigen (PSA) staining is strongly positive (not shown).

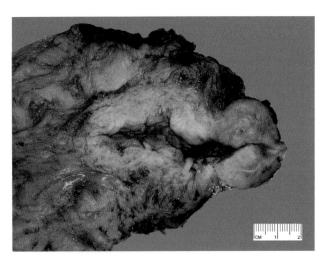

Figure 12-11 Nested variant urothelial carcinoma (gross appearance). Tumor also invades the prostate (pT4a cancer).

variably sized nests/tubules, and the frequent presence of muscle invasion (**Fig. 12-19**).[24,28,31] A focal myxoid or desmoplastic stroma may be present (**Fig. 12-20**); however, in many cases, minimal stromal response is present, further compounding this challenging diagnosis.

Nested urothelial carcinoma, seen either in pure form or with a component of usual urothelial carcinoma, has a poor outcome. In a study of 30 urothelial carcinoma cases with pure or predominant nested morphology, the patients' ages ranged from 41 to 83 years (mean, 63 years) with a male-to-female ratio of 2.3:1.[29] The nested pattern comprised 50% to 100% of the tumors studied, with some cases including typical/usual urothelial carcinoma or urothelial CIS concurrently. The architectural patterns of nested carcinoma components ranged from a predominantly disorderly proliferation of discrete, small, variably sized nests (90%) to focal areas demonstrating confluent nests (40%), cord-like growth (37%), and cystitis cystica-like areas (33%) to tubular growth pattern (13%). The deep tumor stroma interface was invariably (100%) jagged and infiltrative. Despite overall bland cytology, tumor nests demonstrated focal random cytologic atypia (90%) and focal high grade cytologic atypia centered within the base of the tumor (40%). The tumor stroma ranged from having minimal stromal response to being focally desmoplastic and myxoid. A component of usual urothelial carcinoma was present in 63% of cases. These authors found the nested pattern to represent a highly unfavorable feature, with muscle invasion, extravesical disease, and metastasis occurring more commonly than typical urothelial carcinoma.[29] When compared with pure high grade urothelial carcinoma, nested urothelial carcinoma was associated with muscle invasion at transurethral resection (31% vs. 70%), extravesical disease at cystectomy (33% vs. 83%), and metastatic disease (19% vs. 67%).[29] Followup was available on 29 patients (97%) with a median

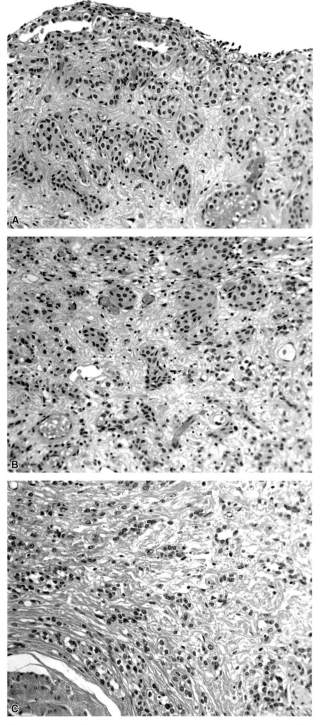

Figure 12-12 Urothelial carcinoma, nested variant (A to C). The tumor is in contact with the overlying urothelium (A). The deceptively benign appearance of cells in the superficial nests belies the malignant nature of this process (B and C).

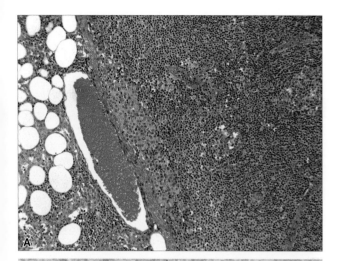

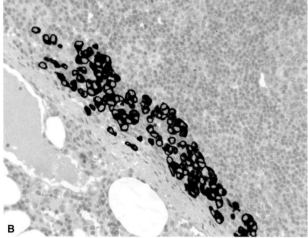

Figure 12-13   Lymph node metastasis (A and B) from the same case as **Fig. 12-12**. Cytokeratin AE1/AE3 staining highlights the tumor cells (B).

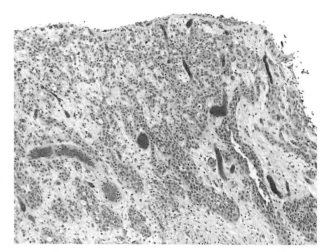

Figure 12-15   Urothelial carcinoma, nested variant.

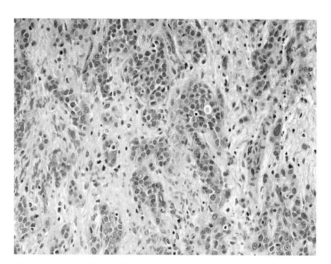

Figure 12-16   Urothelial carcinoma, nested variant.

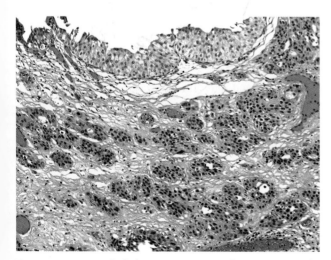

Figure 12-14   Urothelial carcinoma, nested variant. Note the separation of intact urothelium and cancer.

of 12 months (range, 1 to 31 months); three (10%) died of disease, 16 (55%) were alive with persistent or recurrent disease, and 10 (34%) were alive without disease. Response to neoadjuvant chemotherapy was observed in two (13%) of 15 patients.

The immunohistochemical features of the nested variant are similar to those of high grade urothelial carcinoma, with frequent loss of p27 and a high Ki67 (MIB1) labeling index.[25] Tumor cells are positive for high molecular weight cytokeratin (92%), CK7 (93%), and p63 (92%) with high frequency, and variable CK20 (68%).[29]

The differential diagnosis of the nested variant of urothelial carcinoma includes prominent von Brunn nests, cystitis cystica and glandularis, inverted papilloma, nephrogenic adenoma, paraganglionic tissue, paraganglioma, and urothelial carcinoma with nested-like features (**Table 12-3**).[31,32] In the differential diagnosis between

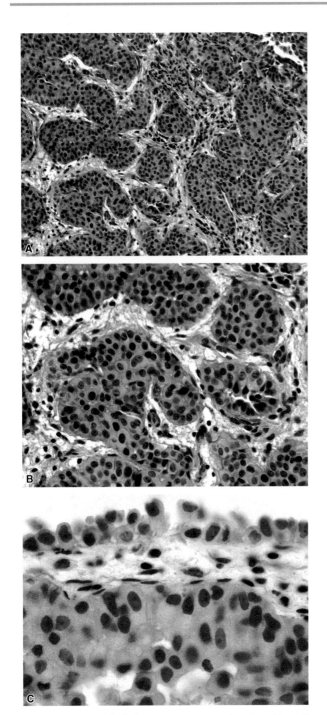

Figure 12-17   Urothelial carcinoma, nested variant (A to C).

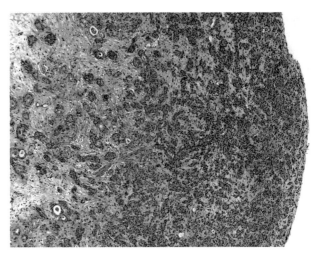

Figure 12-18   Urothelial carcinoma, nested variant.

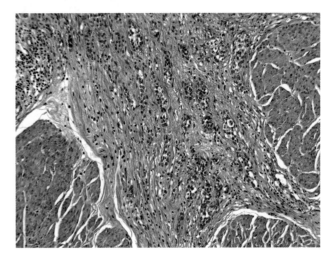

Figure 12-19   Urothelial carcinoma, nested variant. Tumor invades the muscularis propria.

florid von Brunn nests and the nested variant, CK20 IHC evaluation does not appear to be useful, but significantly greater Ki67 and p53 expression are seen in nested variant urothelial carcinoma compared to florid von Brunn nests. Ki67 expression in more than 7% of tumor cells and p53 expression in more than 3% of tumor cells is seen only in carcinoma.[33] The presence of deep invasion is most useful in distinguishing carcinoma from benign proliferations, and nuclear atypia is also of value. Closely packed and irregularly distributed small tumor cell nests favor carcinoma. Inverted papilloma lacks a nested architecture. Nephrogenic adenoma typically has a mixed pattern, including tubular, papillary, and other components, and only rarely has deep muscle invasion in the urethra. The nested variant of carcinoma may mimic paraganglioma, but the prominent vascular network of paraganglioma that surrounds individual nests is different than in carcinoma.[8,34,35]

Urothelial Carcinoma, Micropapillary Variant

Micropapillary carcinoma should be considered a distinct variant of urothelial carcinoma with a poor prognosis.[1,36–38]

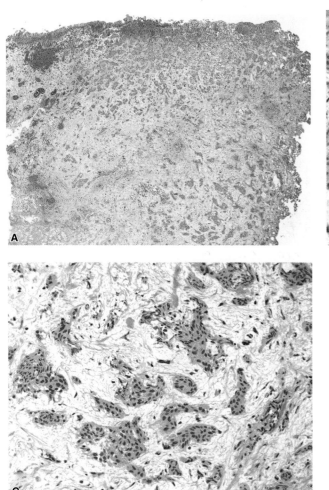

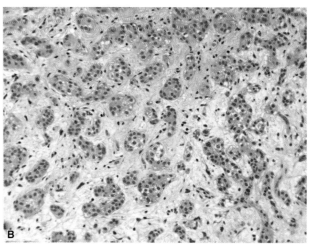

Figure 12-20 Urothelial carcinoma, nested variant (A to C). Note the myxoid stroma.

Table 12-3   Key Features in the Differential Diagnosis of the Nested Variant of Urothelial Carcinoma

	Lumen Formation	Marked Cytologic Atypia in Deeper Portion	Infiltrative Base	Muscle Invasion	Immunohistochemistry
Nested variant	Yes, variable	Yes, frequent	Yes, frequent	Yes, frequent	Low p27^{Kip1}, high proliferation
Florid von Brunn nests	Yes, variable	No	No	No	Variable
Nephrogenic metaplasia	Yes, frequent associated papillary component	No	Yes, frequent	Yes, rare	PAX2 and PAX8 +
Cystitis cystica, cystitis glandularis	Yes	No	No	No	Variable
Paraganglionic tissue and paraganglioma	No, associated prominent vascular network	No	No	Yes	Neuroendocrine markers +

There is a male predominance with a male-to-female ratio of 5 : 1. The patients' ages range from the fifth to the ninth decade, with a mean age of 66 years. The most common presenting symptom is hematuria.

The micropapillary component is found in association with noninvasive papillary urothelial carcinoma, consisting of slender delicate filiform processes or small papillary clusters of tumor cells with prominent retraction artifact (clefts); when present in invasive carcinoma, it is composed of infiltrating tight clusters of micropapillary aggregates that are often within lacunae (Figs. 12-21 to 12-25). It is important to keep in mind that retraction artifact, or prominent clefts can also be present in an otherwise conventional urothelial carcinoma; therefore, the diagnosis of micropapillary carcinoma might need the presence of additional features. Vascular/lymphatic invasion is common, and most cases show invasion of the muscularis propria or deeper, often with metastases. Psammoma bodies are infrequent, unlike ovarian papillary serous carcinoma. The presence of a surface micropapillary component in bladder biopsy specimens with cancer is an unfavorable prognostic feature (Figs. 12-26 and 12-27), and deeper biopsies may be useful to determine the level of muscle invasion.

Twenty-five percent of cases show glandular differentiation, leading some authors to consider it as a variant of adenocarcinoma.[39] Micropapillary carcinoma is likely to express CA-125, supporting the hypothesis that this phenotype is a form of glandular differentiation.[40] Lopez-Beltran et al. recently reported 13 cases of invasive micropapillary carcinoma.[41] The micropapillary component varied from 50% to 100% of the tumor specimen; in 10 cases, the micropapillary component comprised greater than 70% of the tumor, with five cases showing pure micropapillary carcinoma. The architectural pattern of the tumor varied from solid expansile nests with slender papillae within tissue retraction spaces to pseudoglandular growth with prominent ring-like structures (two cases, 15%), and invasive micropapillary carcinoma with squamous differentiation (two cases, 15%); a streaking solid architectural pattern of micropapillary carcinoma was additionally present in two cases (15%). The individual tumor cells had abundant eosinophilic cytoplasm and nuclei with prominent nucleoli and irregular distribution of chromatin, and frequent mitotic figures. Most neoplastic cells had nuclei of low to intermediate nuclear grade with occasional nuclear pleomorphism. Eight mixed cases had concurrent conventional high grade urothelial carcinoma with squamous or glandular differentiation in three and one cases, respectively. All patients had advanced stage cancer (>pT2); and eight (62%) had lymph node metastases.[41] During a mean followup of 10 months, 11 patients (85%) had died of bladder cancer. The mean interval from diagnosis to cancer death was 6.2 months.

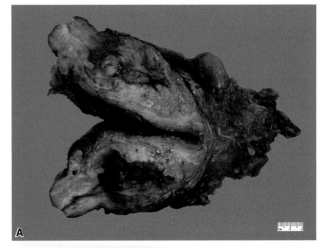
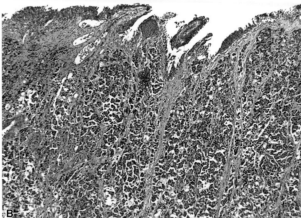
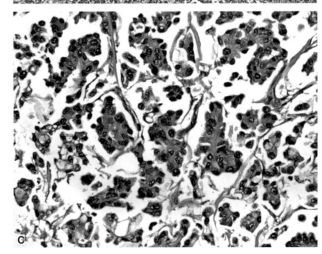

Figure 12-21   Urothelial carcinoma, micropapillary variant. Gross (A) and microscopic appearance (B and C).

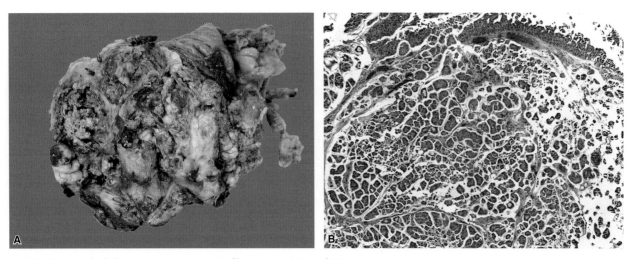

Figure 12-22   Urothelial carcinoma, micropapillary variant (A and B).

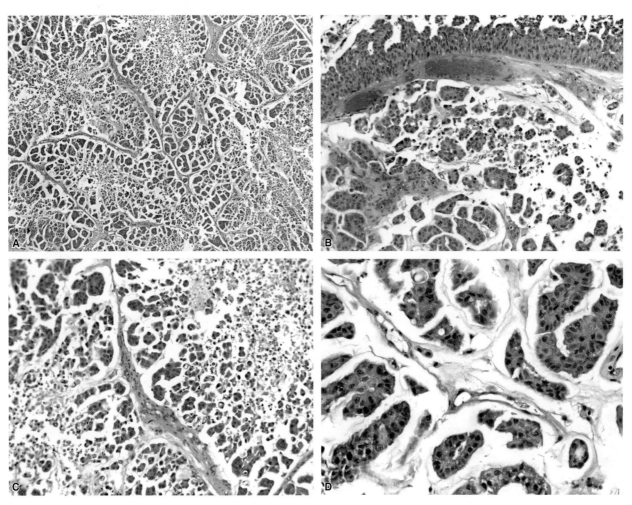

Figure 12-23   Urothelial carcinoma, micropapillary variant (A to D).

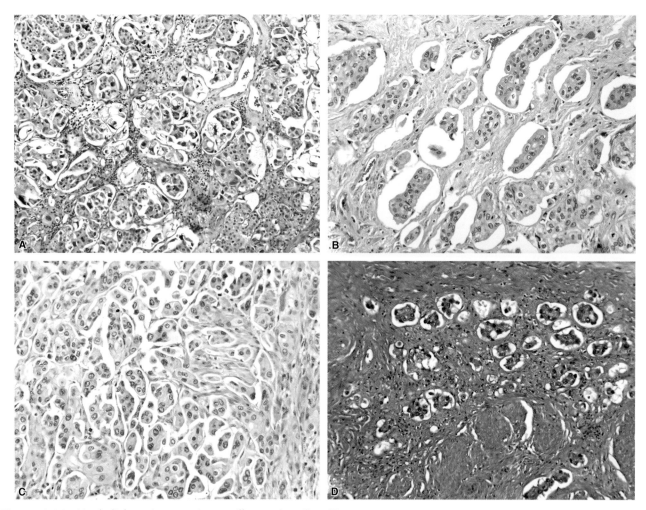

Figure 12-24   Urothelial carcinoma, micropapillary variant (A to D).

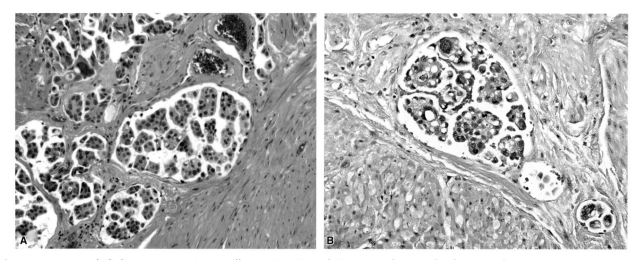

Figure 12-25   Urothelial carcinoma, micropapillary variant (A and B). Tumor also invades the muscularis propria.

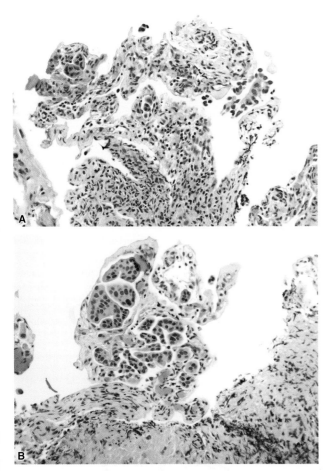

Figure 12-26 Urothelial carcinoma, micropapillary variant (A and B). Note the surface involvement.

Immunohistochemical studies disclosed immunoreactivity of the micropapillary carcinoma for epithelial membrane antigen (EMA), both CK7 and CK20, and LeuM1 (CD15) in all 20 cases studied.[39] Samaratunga and Khoo confirmed these observations and noted that immunohistochemical staining was positive for CK7, CK20, EMA, carcinoembryonic antigen (CEA), and high molecular weight cytokeratin 34bE12 in micropapillary carcinoma and conventional urothelial carcinoma (Fig. 12-28).[40] In this series, CA125 staining was seen in only 43% of the micropapillary carcinomas. In another recent series, micropapillary and associated conventional urothelial carcinoma were positive for MUC1 and MUC2, CK7, phosphatase and tensin homolog (PTEN), p53, uroplakin, CA125, CK20, high molecular weight cytokeratin 34βE12, and p16.[41] MUC5A, MUC6, and CDX2 were negative in all micropapillary cases.[41]

In the micropapillary pattern of invasive carcinoma, the expression of MUC1 is largely limited to the basal surface of the cells facing the stroma, in contrast to the conventional carcinomas in which MUC1 is largely apical, intracytoplasmic, or intercellular.[42] The MUC1 expression was

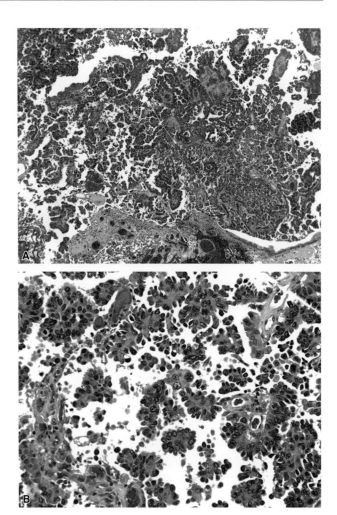

Figure 12-27 Urothelial carcinoma, micropapillary variant (A and B). Note the surface involement.

predominantly in the aspect of the cell clusters facing the stroma, accentuating the outlines of the micropapillary units by forming a distinct band on the surface.[42] This observation provides support for the hypothesis that the reversal of cell polarity is an important factor in the pathogenesis of invasive micropapillary carcinoma. Because MUC1 is known to be involved in lumen formation and has an inhibitory effect on cell–stroma interaction, it may play an important role in the detachment of cells from the stroma, easing the spread of neoplastic cells.

Differential considerations include serous ovarian carcinoma in women or mesothelioma in both sexes.[43] Carcinomas with micropapillary histology have also been reported in the lung, breast, pancreas, and salivary glands. Clinical correlation is usually required, but the possibility of a bladder primary may be suggested if there is no obvious primary tumor at another anatomic site. Identification of an admixed urothelial carcinoma of more typical morphology or immunohistochemical support (CK7, CK20, and uroplakin III positivity) would be helpful.[44]

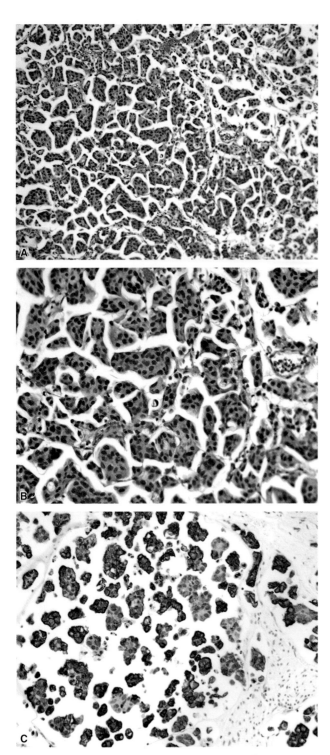

Figure 12-28 Urothelial carcinoma, micropapillary variant (A to C). Cytokeratin 7 staining is strongly positive.

Micropapillary carcinoma is considered a highly malignant variant histologic subtype of urothelial carcinoma that closely resembles papillary serous carcinoma of the ovary.[45] A series by Kamat et al. is remarkable for the high proportion of nonmuscle invasive disease compared with other variant histologies; 44% had pT1 disease.[46] These authors suggested that intravesical therapy should not be given. Patients are likely to progress while receiving bacillus Calmette–Guérin (BCG) or intravesical chemotherapy, and will have a worse outcome after subsequent cystectomy. In patients who underwent cystectomy after failed intravesical therapy, the median survival was 62 months. In those who underwent primary cystectomy, the median survival had not yet been reached after up to 15 years of followup.[46] Samaratunga and Khoo found that the prognosis is related to the proportion and location of the micropapillary component.[40] Cases with a moderate or extensive micropapillary component are at high risk for having an advanced stage at presentation. Cases with less than 10% micropapillary component and a surface micropapillary component have a high chance of detection at an early stage.

Urothelial Carcinoma, Microcystic Variant

The rare microcystic variant of urothelial carcinoma is characterized by the formation of microcysts, macrocysts, or tubular structures ranging in size from microscopic to 2 cm in diameter (**Figs. 12-29** and **12-30**).[47–49] The cysts and tubules may be empty or contain necrotic debris or mucin that stains with periodic acid–Schiff stain after diastase digestion. This morphologic variant has also been reported in association with renal pelvic carcinoma.

This variant of cancer may be confused with benign proliferations such as florid polypoid cystitis cystica and glandularis and nephrogenic metaplasia[48,50] and thus represents a potential pitfall. Helpful diagnostic features may include the characteristic variation in cyst size as well as the infiltrative growth pattern throughout the bladder wall. In comparison, cystitis cystica/glandularis may exhibit a similar tubular proliferation, without extension into the bladder wall. The microcystic variant should be separated from the nested variant of urothelial carcinoma and from urothelial carcinoma with small tubules.[27,50] A case of urothelial carcinoma of the urinary bladder with microcystic component simulating prostatic adenocarcinoma Gleason pattern 3 has been reported recently.[51] Immunohistochemical studies showed that the acinar/tubular component of the tumor was negative for prostate-specific antigen (PSA) and prostate-specific acid phosphatase (PSAP), but positive for CK7,

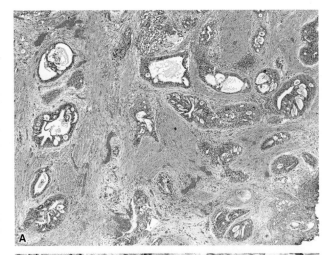

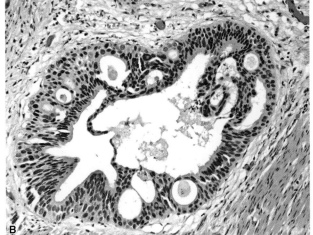

Figure 12-29 Urothelial carcinoma, microcystic variant (A and B).

CK20, high molecular weight cytokeratin (34βE12), and thrombomodulin.

Urothelial Carcinoma, Inverted Variant (Urothelial Carcinoma with Inverted Growth)

Recent interest in urothelial carcinoma with inverted growth arose because they can be misdiagnosed as a benign inverted papilloma (**Figs. 12-31** and **12-32**).[52] Inverted variant of urothelial carcinoma can show variable cytological and architectural abnormalities, but invariably has a higher mitotic count and cell proliferation, as seen by Ki67, high p53 accumulation, aberrant CK20 expression, and frequent polysomies at chromosome 3, 7, and 17, and loss of 9p21.[53] This profile has been very useful in the differential diagnosis with inverted papilloma.

See **Chapter 17** for further discussion.

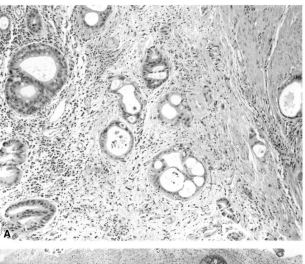

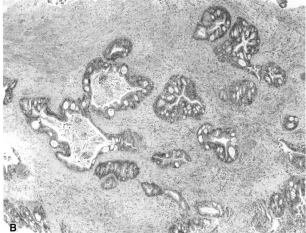

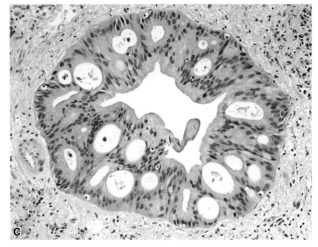

Figure 12-30 Urothelial carcinoma, microcystic variant (A to C).

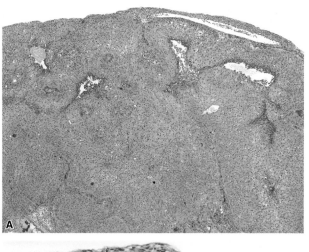

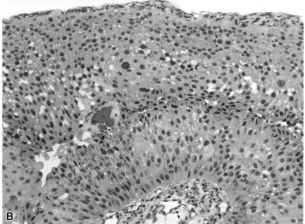

Figure 12-31 Urothelial carcinoma, inverted variant (A and B). Note the cytologic atypia.

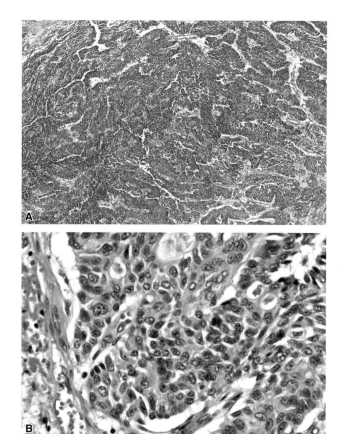

Figure 12-32 Urothelial carcinoma, inverted variant (A and B). Note the cytologic atypia.

Urothelial Carcinoma, Lipid Cell Variant

The lipid cell variant is a rare neoplasm defined by the World Health Organization (WHO) as a type of urothelial carcinoma that exhibits transition to cells resembling signet ring lipoblasts (**Figs. 12-33** and **12-34**). It frequently presents with gross hematuria.[54] These tumors are typically associated with advanced-stage high grade urothelial carcinoma, where the prognosis is poor, and is clonally related to the concurrent conventional urothelial carcinoma.

A recent report based on 27 cases showed that the lipid cell component varied from 10% to 50% of the tumor specimen; in 11 cases, the lipid cell component comprised more than 30% of the tumor.[55] Pathologic stage at diagnosis was Ta ($n = 1$), T1 ($n = 2$), T2, (at least $n = 7$), T3a ($n = 4$), T3b ($n = 8$), and T4a ($n = 5$). Sixteen of the patients died of disease within 16 to 58 months (mean, 33 months) and eight patients were alive with disease at 8 to 25 months (mean, 22 months). Three additional patients died of other causes at 6 to 15 months (mean, 10 months).

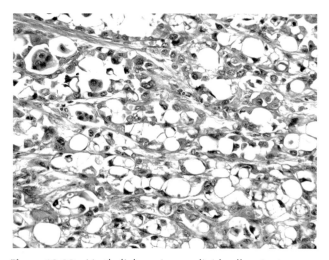

Figure 12-33 Urothelial carcinoma, lipid cell variant.

The architectural pattern of the tumor varied from solid expansile to infiltrative nests. The large epithelial tumor cells had an eccentrically placed nucleus and abundant vacuolated cytoplasm resembling signet ring lipoblasts. Mucin stains were negative in all cases. Typical features of high grade conventional urothelial carcinoma were present

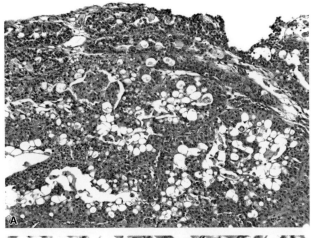

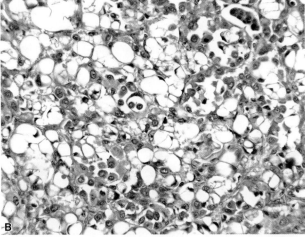

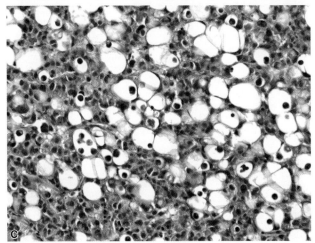

Figure 12-34 Urothelial carcinoma, lipid cell variant (A to C).

in all cases, with micropapillary or plasmacytoid carcinoma in two and one cases, respectively; extensive squamous or glandular differentiation was present in two additional cases. Most neoplastic cells had nuclei of intermediate nuclear grade with occasional nuclear pleomorphism.

Immunohistochemical staining demonstrated that the lipid cell component was positive for cytokeratins 7, 20, CAM5.2, high molecular weight (34βE12) and AE1/AE3, epithelial membrane antigen, and thrombomodulin; vimentin and S100 protein were negative. The loss of heterozygosity (LOH) analysis was performed on eight cases using four polymorphic microsatellite markers (D9S171, D9S177, IFNA, and TP53); LOH (at least in one marker) was present in six cases. The LOH results were the same for lipid variant and conventional urothelial carcinoma. Electron microcopy analysis based on two cases supported lipid content in tumor cells.[55]

In limited samples, lipid cell variant urothelial carcinoma may be misdiagnosed as liposarcoma, sarcomatoid carcinoma (carcinosarcoma) with a liposarcomatous component, or signet ring cell carcinoma. The finding of lipid cells immunoreactive for epithelial markers can be very useful in this setting.

Urothelial Carcinoma, Plasmacytoid Variant

This is a rare aggressive variant of urothelial carcinoma with poor prognosis. These patients typically present with hematuria at an advanced stage (Figs. 12-35 to 12-40).[1,56–65]

Zukerberg et al. described two cases of bladder carcinoma that diffusely permeated the bladder wall and were

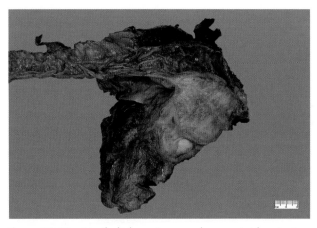

Figure 12-35 Urothelial carcinoma, plasmacytoid variant. Tumor invades the rectum, involving rectal mucosa. It also invades the prostate.

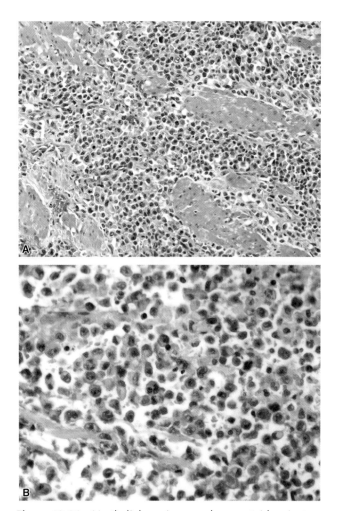

Figure 12-36 Urothelial carcinoma, plasmacytoid variant (A and B).

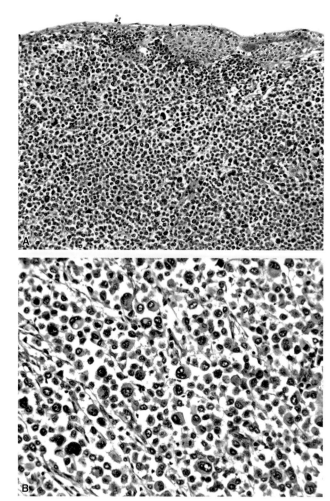

Figure 12-37 Urothelial carcinoma, plasmacytoid variant (A and B).

composed of cells with a monotonous appearance mimicking lymphoma.[66] The tumor cells were medium-sized, with eosinophilic cytoplasm and eccentric nuclei producing a plasmacytoid appearance. Typical urothelial carcinoma was present in one case. The epithelial nature of the malignancy was confirmed by immunoreactivity for cytokeratin and carcinoembryonic antigen and negative staining for lymphoid markers. A similar bladder tumor with prominent plasmacytoid pattern presented as a scalp metastasis mimicking multiple myeloma.[58]

A recent report based on 11 cases showed that the plasmacytoid component varied from 30% to 100% of the tumor specimen; in eight cases, the plasmacytoid component comprised greater than 50% of the tumor, with two cases showing pure plasmacytoid carcinoma.[59] Seven of nine mixed cases had concurrent conventional high grade urothelial carcinoma, and the remaining two cases presented features of nested or micropapillary urothelial carcinoma. All patients had advanced-stage cancer (>pT3), and eight (73%) had

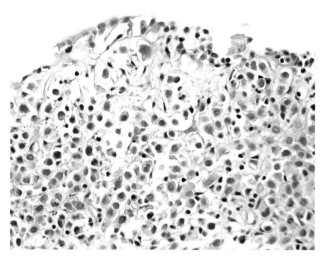

Figure 12-38 Urothelial carcinoma, plasmacytoid variant.

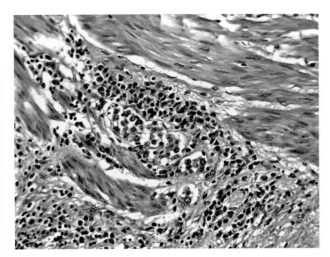

Figure 12-39 Urothelial carcinoma, plasmacytoid variant. Tumor invades the muscularis propria.

lymph node metastasis. On followup, nine of the patients (82%) died of disease within 2 to 11 months, and two patients were alive with disease at 8 and 16 months.

The architectural pattern of the tumor varied from solid expansile nests with discohesive cells to mixed solid and alveolar growth; a streaking discohesive architecture was additionally present in two cases (18%). Rarely, a myxoid pattern was present. Histologically, the individual tumor cells had an eccentrically placed nucleus and abundant eosinophilic cytoplasm reminiscent of plasma cells. Most neoplastic cells had nuclei of low to intermediate nuclear grade with occasional nuclear pleomorphism. Small intracytoplasmic vacuoles were variably present in all cases. Immunohistochemical staining demonstrated that both plasmacytoid and associated conventional urothelial carcinoma were positive for CK7, CK20, AE1/AE3, and EMA; CD138 was positive in three cases (**Fig. 12-41**).

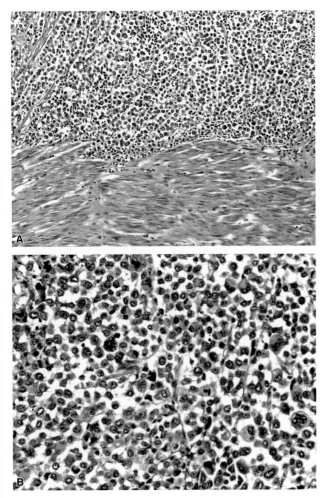

Figure 12-40 Urothelial carcinoma, plasmacytoid variant (A and B). Tumor invades the muscularis propria.

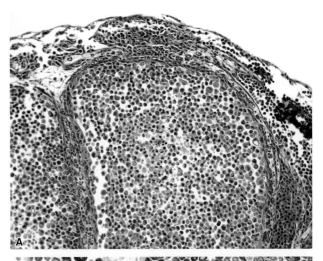

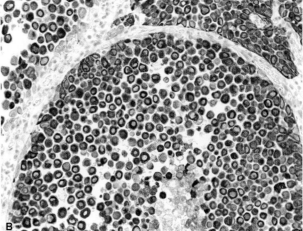

Figure 12-41 Urothelial carcinoma, plasmacytoid variant (A and B). Note the strong and diffuse cytokeratin 20 immunostaining.

Table 12-4   Main Differential Features of Bladder Tumors with Plasmacytoid Cells

	Cytologic Features			Immunohistochemical Features[b]									
	Nuclear Shape	Nucleolus	Cytoplasm[a]	Pan-CK	Vim	CK7	CK20	S100	LCA	HMB45	Syn	CD138	Desmin
Plasmacytoid carcinoma	Round	±	Eosino/ampho	+	−	+	+	−	−	−	−	±	−
Rhabdoid carcinoma	Round	+	Eosino	±	+	±	±	−	−	−	−	−	−
Signet ring cell carcinoma	Indented	±	Ampho/clear	+	−	+	+	−	−	−	−	−	−
Lymphoma/plasmacytoma	Round	±	Eosino/ampho	±	+	−	−	−	+	−	−	+	−
Paraganglioma/ neuroendocrine carcinoma	Round	+	Ampho/clear	±	+	±	−	+	−	−	+	−	−
Melanoma	Round	+	Eosino	±	+	−	−	+	−	+	−	−	−
Rhabdomyosarcoma	Round/fusiform	±	Scant/eosino	±	+	−	−	−	−	−	±	−	+

[a]Ampho, amphophilic; eosino, eosinophilic.
[b]CK, cytokeratin; Vim, vimentin; LCA, leukocyte common antigen; Syn, synaptophysin.

The differential diagnostic considerations include lymphoid reaction, lymphoma, multiple myeloma, urothelial carcinoma with rhabdoid features, signet ring cell adenocarcinoma, paraganglioma, neuroendocrine carcinoma, melanoma, and rhabdomyosarcoma (Table 12-4). Identification of an epithelial component by immunohistochemistry confirms the diagnosis. Immunohistochemistry using CD45 (leukocyte common antigen) or cytokeratins is useful. In limited samples, it may be misdiagnosed as chronic cystitis or plasmacytoma, a pitfall further compounded by CD138 (marker of plasma cells) expression in some cases. Morphologic distinction from other malignant neoplasms with plasmacytoid phenotype is critical for its clinical management (Table 12-4).

Lymphoepithelioma-like Carcinoma

Fewer than 100 cases of carcinoma histologically resembling lymphoepithelioma of the nasopharynx have been described in the urinary bladder (Figs. 12-42 to 12-45).[67–74] This variant is more common in men than in women (male-to-female ratio, 2.8 : 1) and occurs in late adulthood (range, 54 to 84 years; mean, 70 years).[67] Most patients present with hematuria. The tumor is solitary and usually involves the dome, posterior wall, or trigone, often with a sessile growth pattern.

Histologically, it may be pure or mixed with typical urothelial carcinoma. Cases with a typical urothelial carcinoma component have been reported in the ureter and renal pelvis. Glandular and squamous differentiation may be seen. The epithelial component is composed of nests, sheets, and cords of undifferentiated cells with large pleomorphic nuclei and prominent nucleoli. The cytoplasmic borders are poorly defined, imparting a syncytial appearance. The background consists of a prominent polyclonal lymphoid stroma that includes T and B lymphocytes, plasma cells, histiocytes, and occasional neutrophils or eosinophils that frequently invade the epithelial nests. Epstein–Barr virus infection has not been identified in lymphoepithelioma-like carcinoma of the bladder, although it is frequent in cases from the head and neck region. The epithelial cells of this tumor stain with several cytokeratin markers, including AE1/AE3, CK7, and CK8. They are rarely positive for CK20. This tumor has been found to be responsive to chemotherapy when it is encountered in its pure form.[70,73]

Most reported cases in the urinary bladder had a relatively favorable prognosis when pure or in predominant form, but when the lymphoepithelioma-like carcinoma is focally present in an otherwise typical urothelial carcinoma, the neoplasm behaves like conventional urothelial carcinoma of the same grade and stage. Most reported tumors are muscle-invasive carcinomas (pT2 or higher). Some studies have shown that tumors with a predominant lymphoepithelioma-like histology have a more favorable prognosis than those with only a focal component of this histology. In a large series, cases treated with cystectomy had a five-year actuarial survival rate of 59% (62% for pure and 57% for mixed); in comparison the five-year recurrence-free rate of muscle-invasive bladder cancer treated by cystectomy was similar and in the range 65 to 68%.[74]

The major differential diagnostic considerations are poorly differentiated urothelial carcinoma with lymphoid stroma, poorly differentiated squamous cell carcinoma, and lymphoma. The presence of recognizable urothelial or squamous cell carcinoma does not exclude lymphoepithelioma-like carcinoma; rather, the diagnosis is based on finding areas typical of lymphoepithelioma reminiscent of that in the nasopharynx. Differentiation from lymphoma may be difficult, but the presence of a syncytial pattern of large malignant cells with a dense polymorphous lymphoid background is an important clue. Immunohistochemistry reveals cytokeratin immunoreactivity in the malignant cells, confirming their epithelial nature. It is possible to overlook the malignant cells

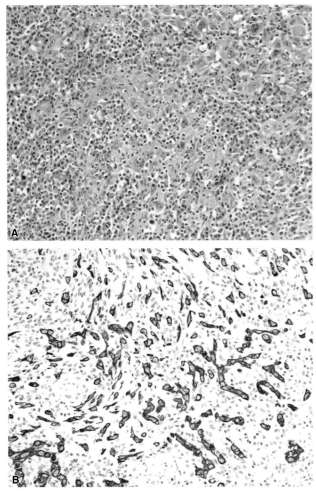

Figure 12-42 Lymphoepithelioma-like carcinoma of the bladder (A and B). Immunostaining for high molecular weight cytokeratin 34βE12 highlights the tumor cells.

in the background of inflamed bladder mucosa and to misdiagnose the condition as florid chronic cystitis. The clinical significance of lymphoepithelioma-like carcinoma rests with the apparent chemosensitivity of this tumor.

Urothelial Carcinoma, Clear Cell (Glycogen-rich) Variant

Up to two-thirds of urothelial carcinoma cases have foci of clear cell change resulting from abundant glycogen. The glycogen-rich clear cell "variant" of urothelial carcinoma, recently described, appears to represent the extreme end of the morphologic spectrum, consisting predominantly or exclusively of cells with abundant clear cytoplasm that stain for CK7 (**Figs. 12-46** and **12-47**).[75–78] Recognition of this pattern avoids confusion with clear cell adenocarcinoma of

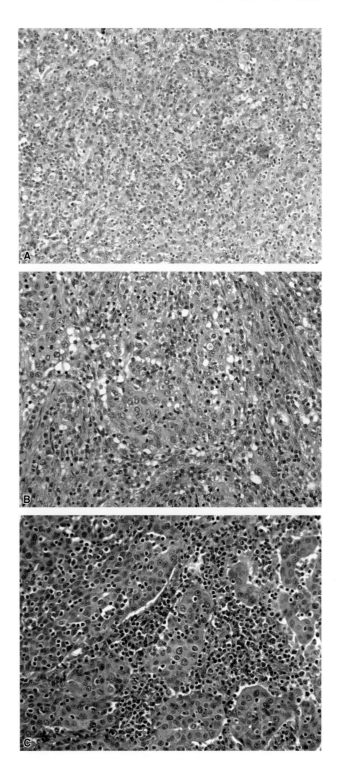

Figure 12-43 Lymphoepithelioma-like carcinoma of the bladder (A to C).

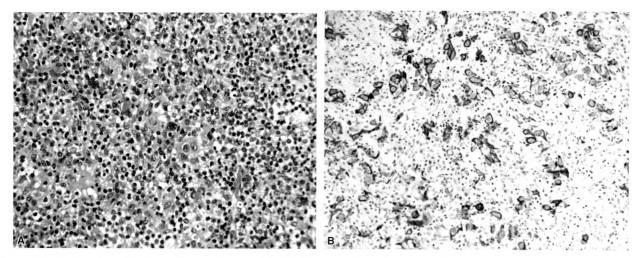

Figure 12-44 Lymphoepithelioma-like carcinoma of the bladder (A and B). The tumor cells are positive for cytokeratin 7 (B).

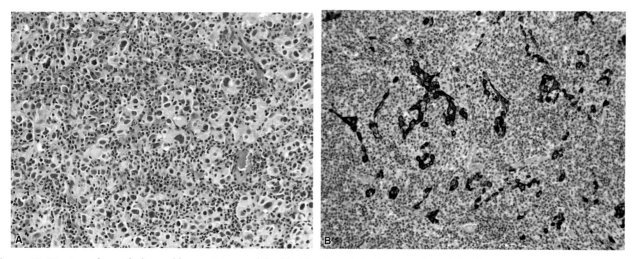

Figure 12-45 Lymphoepithelioma-like carcinoma of the bladder (A and B). Cytokeratin staining is positive (B).

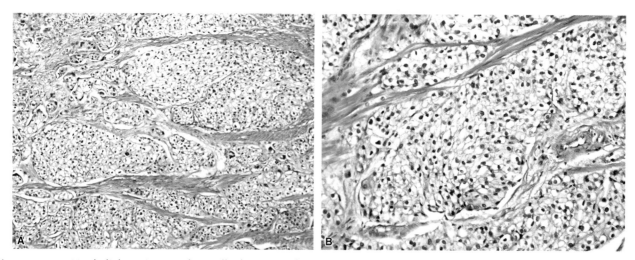

Figure 12-46 Urothelial carcinoma, clear cell (glycogen-rich) variant (A and B).

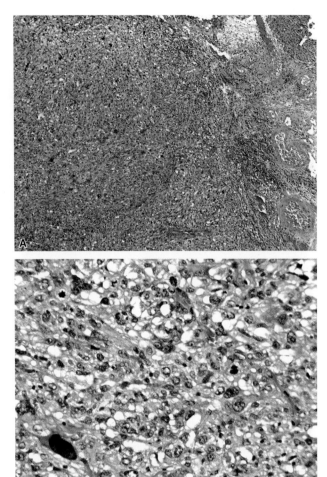

Figure 12-48 Sarcomatoid carcinoma (A and B).

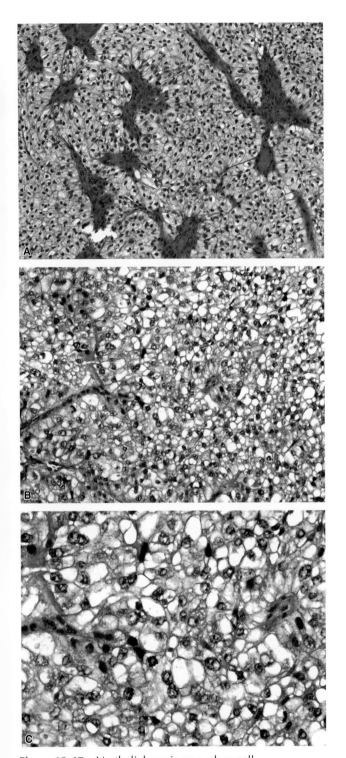

Figure 12-47 Urothelial carcinoma, clear cell (glycogen-rich) variant (A to C). The cytoplasmic vacuoles contain abundant glycogen.

the bladder and metastatic clear cell carcinoma from the kidney or other sites.[79] Also, the recently described variant of bladder paraganglioma may be misdiagnosed as urothelial carcinoma in transurethral resection specimens mainly because of the infiltrative growth pattern and the clear cell appearance of the tumor cells.[80] Paraganglioma cells are characteristically immunoreactive for chromogranin A and S100 protein.[35]

Sarcomatoid Carcinoma

See **Chapter 16** for further discussion (**Fig. 12-48**).

Large Cell Undifferentiated Carcinoma

Large cell undifferentiated carcinoma is more common in the lung but has been described in other organs as a rare and aggressive disease (**Fig. 12-49**). Large cell undifferentiated

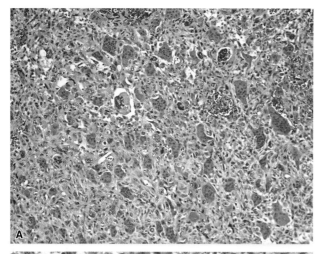

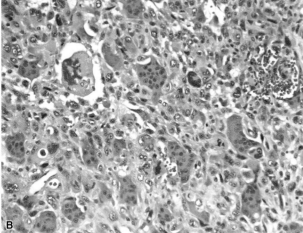

Figure 12-49 Large cell undifferentiated carcinoma (A and B).

carcinoma of the urinary bladder refers to carcinomas that are composed of sheets or isolated undifferentiated cells that do not fit into urothelial, squamous, adenocarcinoma, or any other recognized category of bladder carcinoma. There tumors are rare and if present in a metastatic site, the histology would not suggest a urothelial primary.[81]

A recent report by Lopez-Beltran et al. presented the clinicopathologic features of eight cases of large cell undifferentiated bladder carcinoma.[81] These tumors are characterized by sheets of large polygonal or round cells with moderate to abundant cytoplasm and distinct cell borders. The large cell undifferentiated component varied from 90% to 100% of the tumor specimen, with five cases showing pure tumors. The architectural pattern of the tumor varied from infiltrating tumor to solid expansile nests with focal (< 5%) discohesive growth pattern in two cases.

Immunohistochemical staining demonstrated that large cell undifferentiated cases were positive for AE1/AE3 and CK7. CAM5.2, CK20, thrombomodulin, and uroplakin III were positive in six, three, three, and two

cases, respectively. Other immunohistochemical markers performed in the differential diagnosis context included α-fetoprotein, βhCG, PSA, vimentin, synaptophysin, and chromogranin, and all were negative. Ki67 and p53 labeling indexes ranged from 50% to 90% and 40% to 90%, respectively.

Large cell undifferentiated is an aggressive variant of urothelial carcinoma that presents at an advanced stage with poor prognosis. In a series of eight cases, all patients had advanced-stage cancer (≥ pT3), and seven (88%) had lymph node metastases.[81] Six patients died of disease within 5 to 26 months and two patients were alive with metastases at 6 and 14 months. The prognosis of large cell undifferentiated carcinoma was compared with conventional urothelial carcinoma of similar stages showing survival differences ($P = 0.0004$).[81]

Osteoclast-rich Undifferentiated Carcinoma

Osteoclast-rich "giant cell tumors" or "osteoclastoma-like giant cell tumors" of the pancreas, gallbladder, liver, breast, salivary gland, thyroid, skin, lung, intestines, larynx, and female genital tract have been reported. Fewer than 20 cases of a similar spectrum have been reported in the bladder, most as case reports.[56,82,83] In a series of six cases, four of five patients with followup died of disease, three with documented metastasis.[84] A large majority of patients reported in case reports that have adequate followup also had documented metastatic disease or cancer death.

The tumors are composed of mononuclear cells (frequently positive for epithelial markers), osteoclast-like giant cells (positive CD68, CD51, and CD54), and recognizable usual urothelial neoplasia (CIS, papillary, or invasive carcinoma) in varying proportions (**Figs. 12-50** to **12-52**).[84]

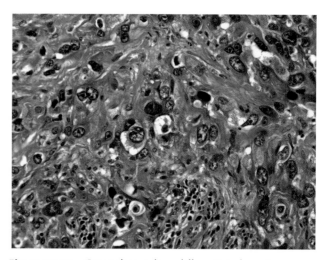

Figure 12-50 Osteoclast-rich undifferentiated carcinoma.

Some areas may be composed entirely of histology similar to giant cell tumors of bone, whereas other areas may show single cells or aggregates of mononuclear cells with a spectrum of atypia, including marked pleomorphism, which are distinct from the nuclei of the osteoclast-like giant cells. These mononuclear cells may stain for pancytokeratin, EMA, CAM5.2, and CK7; and rarely for S100 protein, actin, desmin, and p53.[84] Although these tumors have several histological features of their skeletal counterparts, including areas with blood-filled cysts mimicking aneurysmal bone cyst, it is believed that these tumors represent true undifferentiated carcinomas due to cytokeratin positivity, concurrent presence of high grade urothelial neoplasia, matched p53 positivity in mononuclear cells and urothelial tumor cells, and the poor prognosis of tumors with this histology.[84] These tumors should be distinguished from urothelial carcinoma with syncytiotrophoblastic giant cells and urothelial carcinoma with osteoclast-type giant cell reaction (see the discussion below).

Pleomorphic Giant Cell Carcinoma

Pleomorphic giant cell carcinoma is a rare form of bladder cancer recognized by the current WHO classification of urologic tumors.[54] It is an aggressive variant of urothelial carcinoma associated with poor prognosis that presents at an advanced stage.[85,86]

A recent study based on eight cases showed that the pleomorphic giant cell component varied from 20% to 100% of the tumor specimen; in two cases, the pleomorphic giant cell component comprised more than 50% of the tumor, with one case showing pure pleomorphic giant cell carcinoma.[85] The architectural pattern of the tumor varied from infiltrating pleomorphic tumor with bizarre giant cells to solid expansile nests with discohesive growth pattern; a hypocellular desmoplastic stromal response was present in two cases (25%), with single cells in sclerotic stroma.[85]

Histologically, giant, bizarre, anaplastic cells with frequent typical or atypical mitotic figures were present in all cases (**Figs. 12-53** to **12-55**). Seven mixed cases had concurrent conventional high grade urothelial carcinoma; two cases presented features of micropapillary or lymphoepithelioma-like urothelial carcinoma. Variable-sized intracytoplasmic vacuoles were present in two cases. All patients had advanced-stage cancer (>pT3); and six (75%) had lymph node metastases. Immunohistochemical staining demonstrated that both pleomorphic giant cell carcinoma and associated conventional urothelial carcinoma were positive for CK7, CAM5.2, AE1/AE3, and EMA; p63, thrombomodulin, and uroplakin III were positive in six, three, and two cases, respectively. On followup, five patients died of disease within 6 to 17 months, and two

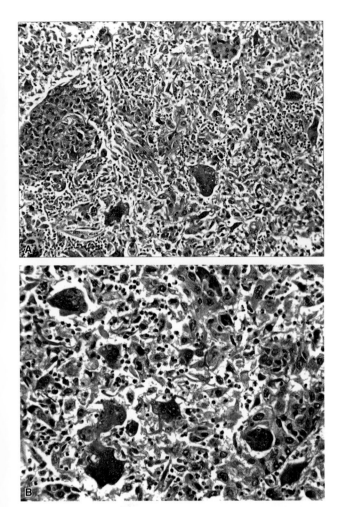

Figure 12-51 Osteoclast-rich undifferentiated carcinoma (A and B).

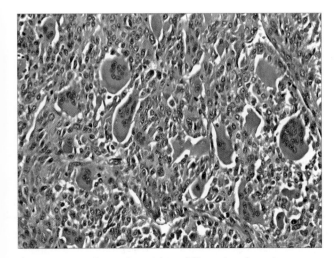

Figure 12-52 Osteoclast-rich undifferentiated carcinoma.

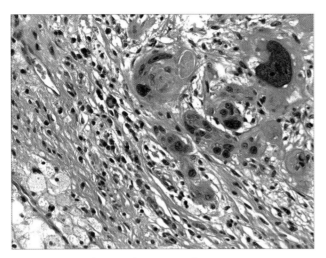

Figure 12-53 Pleomorphic giant cell carcinoma.

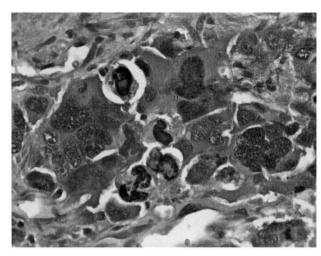

Figure 12-55 Pleomorphic giant cell carcinoma.

patients were alive with metastases at 11 and 19 months. One patient had no evidence of disease at 74 months.

The main differential diagnosis includes giant cell carcinoma in the lung or from other uncommon anatomic locations, and this is currently based on clinical means. The giant cells display cytokeratin and vimentin immunoreactivity. Also, other bladder tumors with giant cells associated with hCG production, osteoclast-type giant cells, and sarcomatoid carcinoma with occasional pleomorphic giant cells should enter the differential diagnosis. In limited samples, pleomorphic giant cell carcinoma may be misdiagnosed as sarcoma, a pitfall of paramount importance for its clinical management.

Other Morphological Variations in Bladder Cancer

Diverse morphologic variations can be seen in urothelial carcinoma. They are usually associated with coexisting high grade urothelial carcinoma.

Urothelial Carcinoma with Chordoid Features

This is a recently described entity with a unique chordoid morphology characterized by prominent cellular cording and associated myxoid stromal matrix, a pattern closely resembling extraskeletal myxoid chondrosarcoma (Figs. 12-56 and 12-57).[87] Urothelial carcinoma with chordoid features has a morphologic pattern of urothelial carcinoma that may potentially mimic a spectrum of primary vesical and nonvesical neoplasms with myxoid or mucinous components. These carcinomas maintain an immunophenotype characteristic of urothelial carcinoma and usually present with high-stage disease.[87]

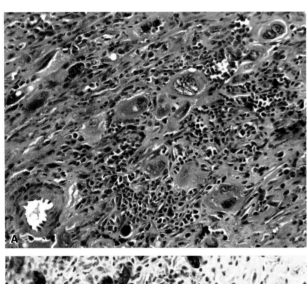

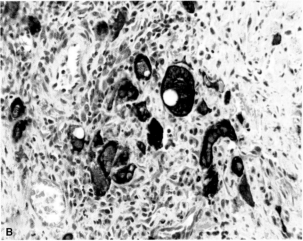

Figure 12-54 Pleomorphic giant cell carcinoma (A and B). Cytokeratin staining is strongly positive (B).

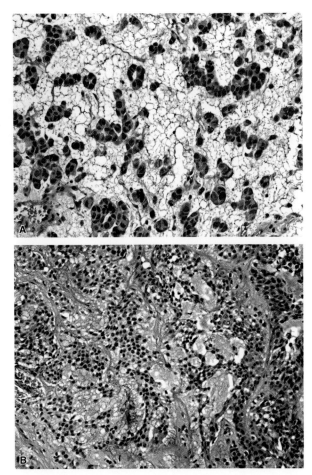

Figure 12-56 Urothelial carcinoma with chordoid features (A and B).

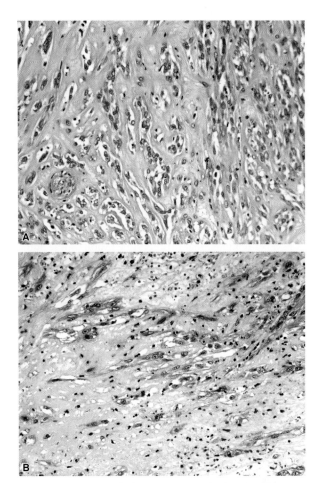

Figure 12-57 Urothelial carcinoma with chordoid features (A and B). (Photo courtesy of Dr. McKenney.)

In Cox's study of 12 cases, the patients' ages ranged from 50 to 85 years (mean, 68 years); there were eight males and four females. The specimens consisted of five cystectomies, six transurethral resections, and one anterior exenteration with right nephroureterectomy. Morphologically, each case had at least focal areas in which acellular myxoid stroma was associated with the carcinoma cells. When well developed, the neoplastic cells had scant eosinophilic cytoplasm and were arranged into cords closely mimicking extraskeletal myxoid chondrosarcoma, chordoma, mixed tumor/myoepithelioma of soft tissue, and yolk sac tumor. The percentage of tumor with a chordoid appearance ranged from 5% to 95% (mean, 39%; median, 25%). No conventional sarcomatous differentiation, no intracytoplasmic mucin, and no glandular formation was present in any case. All 12 cases had foci of typical urothelial carcinoma present at least focally and a gradual transition to the chordoid pattern was commonly seen.[87]

Immunophenotypically, these tumors show strong immunoreactivity for p63 (nuclear) and CK34βE12 (cytoplasmic). Immunostains for CK20, calponin, glial fibrillary acidic protein, oncofetal protein glypican-3, and brachyury and were negative in the seven cases studied, whereas S100 protein had focal staining (< 5%) in one case. The myxoid stromal component was diffusely positive for colloidal iron and Alcian blue; periodic acid–Schiff was negative in all eight cases, whereas mucicarmine was focally positive in only two of eight cases. Most cases were high stage (pT4: five, pT3: four, pT2: two, and pT1: one), and six of eight cases (75%) with nodal sampling had metastatic disease. In one case, the lymph node metastasis had areas with chordoid morphology. Nine of 12 patients had available followup: two were dead of disease (1 and 10 months), four were alive with disease (5 to 8 months) with distant metastasis in three, and three had no evidence of disease at last followup (2 to 120 months).[87]

Urothelial Carcinoma with Small Tubules/Acini

Although a prominent tubular component may accompany a nested carcinoma, some urothelial carcinomas may have an almost exclusive component of small- to medium-sized, round to elongated tubules that may be misdiagnosed as nephrogenic adenoma or cystitis glandularis (**Figs. 12-58** and **12-59**).[27,31,51] Furthermore, the tubules of urothelial carcinoma are lined by attenuated urothelial cells, in contrast to the varying admixture of cuboidal, columnar, and occasionally flattened cells that line the tubules of nephrogenic adenoma. Urothelial carcinoma with small tubules may be widely invasive despite their deceptively bland histology. The biological significance of this pattern is unclear given the rarity of cases, but some of these cases occur in conjunction with the nested pattern and are widely invasive, having an aggressive outcome because of their high stage at presentation. Similar to the nested variant, the chief reason for the awareness of this morphological variant of urothelial carcinoma is not to mistake it in superficial biopsies as a benign glandular proliferative lesion. Some authors believe that urothelial carcinoma with small tubules should be considered within the spectrum of nested carcinoma. The differential diagnosis with an extension of a prostatic carcinoma is often also a consideration but is easily handled by immunohistochemistry (PSA and PSAP are positive in prostate cancer; CK20, high molecular weight cytokeratin, and p63 are positive in more than one-half of urothelial carcinomas).[51]

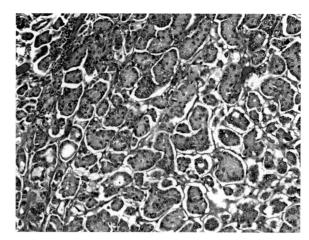

Figure 12-59 Urothelial carcinoma with acini. (Photo courtesy of Dr. Chu.)

Urothelial Carcinoma with Syncytiotrophoblastic Giant Cells

Syncytiotrophoblastic giant cells are present in up to 12% of cases of urothelial carcinoma, producing substantial amounts of immunoreactive β-human chorionic gonadotropin (βhCG) (**Figs. 12-60** to **12-64**).[88-94] The number of βhCG-immunoreactive cells is inversely related to tumor grade.[95,96] Secretion of βhCG into the serum may be associated with a poor response to radiation therapy.[97]

The most important differential diagnostic consideration is choriocarcinoma. Most cases of primary choriocarcinoma

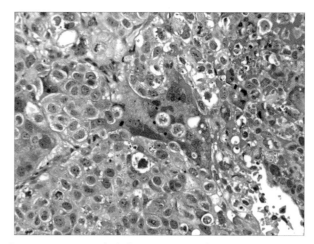

Figure 12-60 Urothelial carcinoma with syncytiotrophoblastic giant cells.

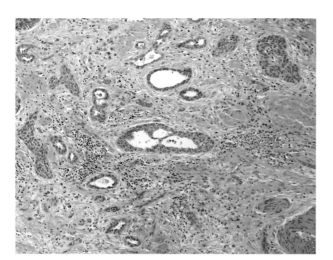

Figure 12-58 Urothelial carcinoma with small tubules.

of the bladder reported previously were actually urothelial carcinoma with syncytiotrophoblasts.[98] Pure choriocarcinoma of the bladder is rare, with fewer than 10 cases reported.[98] Hanna et al. reported a primary choriocarcinoma of the bladder in a 19-year-old man showing a high copy number of the isochromosome 12p that supported germ cell differentiation.[99]

A recent case report[94] showing micropapillary carcinoma with trophoblastic differentiation found that the tumor expressed βhCG and human placental lactogen in trophoblastic areas and CK20 and high molecular weight cytokeratin in all tumor components, suggesting the urothelial origin of the trophoblastic component. Trophoblastic differentiation has also been reported in association with sarcomatoid carcinoma of the bladder (see also **Chapter 16**).

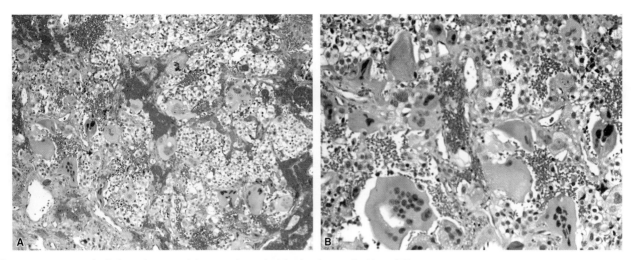

Figure 12-61   Urothelial carcinoma with syncytiotrophoblastic giant cells (A and B).

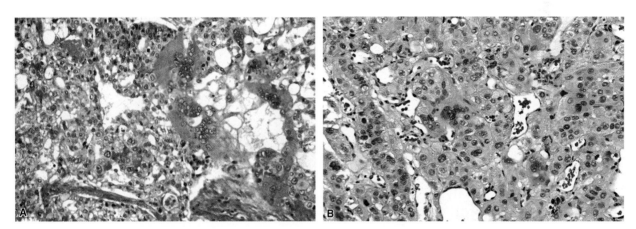

Figure 12-62   Urothelial carcinoma with syncytiotrophoblastic giant cells (A and B).

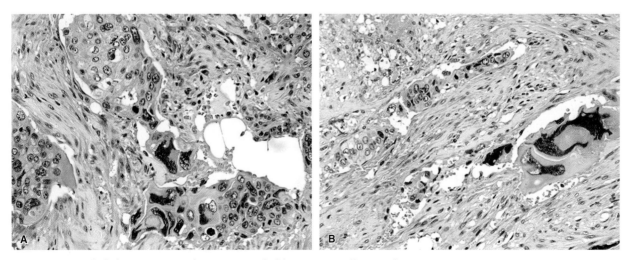

Figure 12-63   Urothelial carcinoma with syncytiotrophoblastic giant cells (A and B).

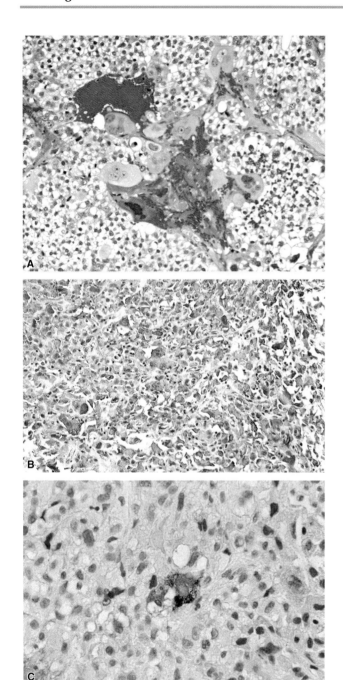

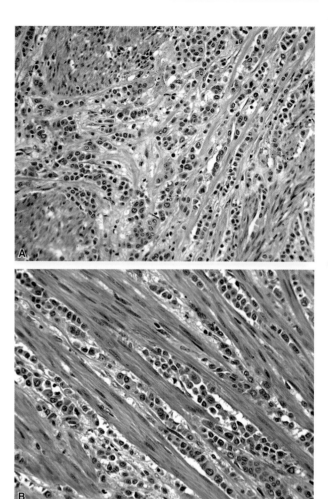

Figure 12-65   Urothelial carcinoma with discohesive growth (A and B).

Figure 12-64   Urothelial carcinoma with syncytiotrophoblastic giant cells (A to C). Cytokeratin AE1/AE3 is strongly positive in urothelial carcinoma (B). Scattered syncytiotrophoblasts are positive for human chorionic gonadotropin immunostaining (C).

Urothelial Carcinoma with Discohesive Growth

Baldwin et al. described a series of 10 cases of urothelial carcinoma with a striking discohesive growth pattern showing morphological features that mimicked infiltrating lobular carcinoma of the breast and diffuse carcinoma of the stomach (**Figs. 12-65** and **12-66**).[100] Eight of the patients were male and two were female. The mean age was 67 years at presentation (range, 52 to 77 years). All the cases showed areas where the tumor was composed of uniform cells with a discohesive, single cell, diffusely infiltrative growth pattern. In some areas, the tumor cells were arranged in linear single cell patterns (Indian-file pattern), and in separate areas, the tumor cells were arranged in solid sheets of discohesive cells. In all of the cases, some tumor cells showed prominent intracytoplasmic vacuoles. In addition to this pattern, four cases showed typical transitional cell carcinoma or CIS. Tumor cells expressed CK20 but not estrogen receptors. This pattern is important to recognize to avoid misdiagnosis of signet ring cell adenocarcinoma and metastatic lobular carcinoma of the breast, especially in small biopsies. Secondary bladder tumors with a characteristic single cell (Indian-file) invading pattern such as lobular carcinoma of the breast or poorly differentiated carcinoma of the stomach are the main differential diagnostic considerations for bladder carcinoma with discohesive growth pattern.

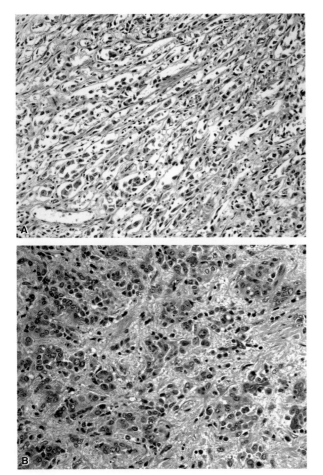

Figure 12-66 Urothelial carcinoma with discohesive growth (A and B).

It is uncertain if urothelial carcinoma with discohesive growth pattern may represent a special variant of plasmacytoid urothelial carcinoma.

Urothelial Carcinoma with Rhabdoid Features

Rarely bladder carcinomas may exhibit rhabdoid features (**Fig. 12-67**).[101] A recent report based on six cases showed that all patients were men, with ages ranging from 53 to 86 years (mean, 66.5 years).[102] Patients initially presented with hematuria or obstructive symptoms. The sites included bladder ($n = 4$) and renal pelvis ($n = 2$). In addition to the rhabdoid component, multiple coexistent histological components were seen, including in situ urothelial carcinoma and high grade papillary urothelial carcinoma ($n = 2$), poorly differentiated carcinoma with small cell features ($n = 1$), sarcomatoid ($n = 2$), and a myxoid component ($n = 2$). All cases in this series had focal or diffuse positive staining with one or more cytokeratin markers (EMA, CAM5.2, AE1/AE3). Of the six patients, two died within 1 month, and a third patient died within 4 months. The

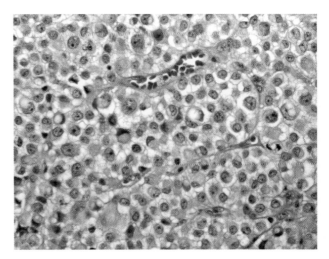

Figure 12-67 Urothelial carcinoma with rhabdoid features.

remaining three patients were alive at 3, 3, and 9 months, respectively, after diagnosis.

Urothelial Carcinoma with Multiple Histologic Patterns

Another important observation when dealing with urothelial carcinoma is that occasionally tumors with divergent (or aberrant) differentiation show multiple histologic patterns within the same tumor, such as sarcomatoid, small cell, micropapillary, squamous, and glandular differentiation, and virtually all variants described above could be present (**Fig. 12-68**).[1] When multiple histologies are encountered,

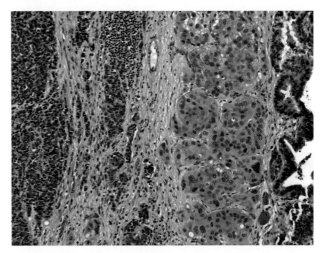

Figure 12-68 Urothelial carcinoma with multiple histologic pattern. Histologic heterogeneity of bladder cancer is relatively common. Different components (small cell carcinoma, urothelial carcinoma, and adenocarcinoma) are seen in the same field.

it is recommended that the relative percentage of each of the different components be provided: for example, invasive high grade urothelial carcinoma (50%), with squamous differentiation (20%), glandular differentiation (10%), and micropapillary variant (10%).

Urothelial Carcinoma with Small Cell Carcinoma Component

When small cell carcinoma is present in association with urothelial carcinoma, even focally, it portends a poor prognosis (**Fig. 12-69**; see **Chapter 15** for further discussion).[103] The pathologist should examine all sections of urothelial carcinoma carefully to exclude this possibility, as small cell carcinoma is an important finding and usually dictates different therapy. Unlike other forms of mixed differentiation that are often considered histologic novelties, small cell carcinoma dominates and should be highlighted in the diagnosis, due to its clinical importance. The pathologists should give the estimated percentage of small cell carcinoma component in the pathology report.

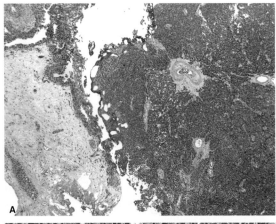
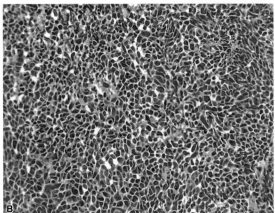

Figure 12-69 Small cell carcinoma of the bladder (A and B). Small cell carcinoma of the bladder is often accompanied by other components, such as conventional urothelial carcinoma (A).

Urothelial Carcinoma with Tumor-associated Stromal Reactions

Urothelial carcinoma may be associated with a variety of stromal reactions that mimic sarcoma or inflammation.

Urothelial Carcinoma with Pseudosarcomatous Stromal Reaction

Urothelial carcinoma and other tumors may have a cellular pseudosarcomatous stroma, which rarely displays sufficient cellularity, cytologic atypia, and spindle cell proliferation, to raise a serious concern for sarcomatoid carcinoma (**Figs. 12-70** to **12-73**).[1,104,105] The stroma is variable in appearance, and may be myxoid or arranged in spindle cell fascicles, usually punctuated by stellate or multinucleated cells.[106] The stromal cells reveal immunohistochemical evidence of fibroblastic and myofibroblastic differentiation, and invariably are cytokeratin negative. Squamous cell carcinoma of the bladder may also have a pseudosarcomatous stroma.[107]

Key differential diagnostic considerations include sarcomatoid carcinoma with prominent myxoid and sclerosing stroma, inflammatory myofibroblastic tumor, and postoperative spindle cell nodule (see also **Chapters 16**, **19**, and **26**). A recent history of urologic surgery is important in making the diagnosis of postoperative spindle cell nodule. The presence of slit-like vessels, the absence of atypical mitotic figures, and the absence of tumor necrosis favor a benign lesion.

Urothelial Carcinoma with Osseous and Chondroid Metaplasia

Osseous metaplasia is present in some cases of urothelial carcinoma and its metastases,[108,109] and this should

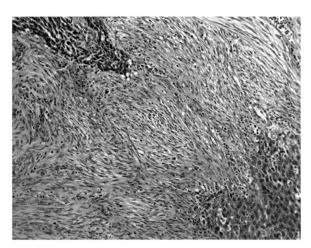

Figure 12-70 Urothelial carcinoma with pseudosarcomatous stromal reaction.

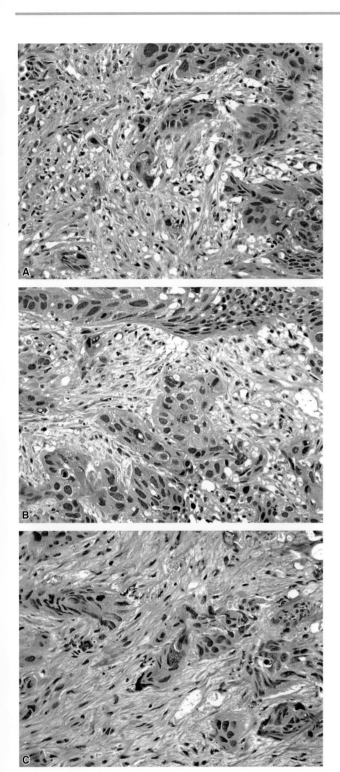

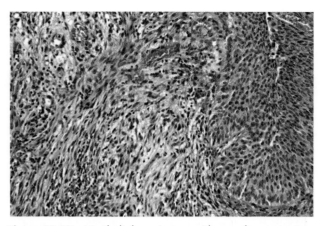

Figure 12-72 Urothelial carcinoma with pseudosarcomatous stromal reaction.

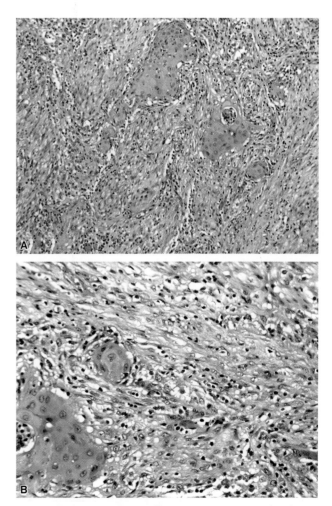

Figure 12-71 Urothelial carcinoma with pseudosarcomatous stromal reaction (A to C).

Figure 12-73 Squamous cell carcinoma associated with pseudosarcomatous stroma.

be differentiated from osteosarcoma. This finding has also been described in metastatic urothelial carcinoma.[109] The metaplastic bone is histologically benign, with a normal lamellar pattern, and is usually adjacent to areas of hemorrhage (**Figs. 12-74** and **12-75**).[110] The cells in the adjacent stroma are cytologically benign.[108]

Urothelial Carcinoma with Osteoclast-type Giant Cell Reaction

Zukerberg and colleagues[66] described the presence of osteoclast-like giant cells in two cases of invasive high grade urothelial carcinoma, both of which had a sarcomatoid spindle cell component. The giant cells had abundant eosinophilic cytoplasm and numerous small, round, regular nuclei, and displayed immunoreactivity for vimentin, CD68, and tartrate-resistant acid phosphatase, but not for epithelial markers—a key feature in differentiating these tumors from osteoclast-rich undifferentiated carcinoma.

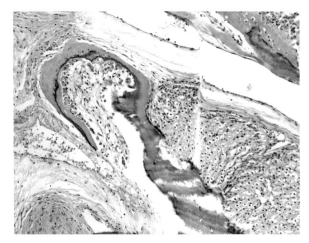

Figure 12-74   Urothelial carcinoma with osseous metaplasia.

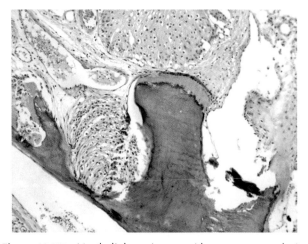

Figure 12-75   Urothelial carcinoma with osseous metaplasia.

Osteoclast-type giant cell reaction may be seen in low grade urothelial carcinoma, suggesting that this might be a nonspecific finding (**Fig. 12-76**). The presence of osteoclast-like giant cells is not related to prognosis, and the giant cells probably reflect a stromal response to the tumor.

Urothelial Carcinoma with Prominent Lymphoid Reaction

An inflammatory cell response in the stroma adjacent to the invasive tumors is relatively common.[66,111–114] This usually takes the form of a lymphocytic infiltrate with a variable admixture of plasma cells (**Figs. 12-77** and **12-78**). Generally, this cellular reaction is mild to moderate, but occasionally may be dense. Sometimes, a neutrophilic response is observed, with or without extensive eosinophilic infiltrate, suggesting that in the absence of cellular response, the carcinoma was likely to be more aggressive in its behavior. The number of eosinophils may be a useful predictive factor for cancer-specific survival.[112] The differential diagnosis with lymphoepithelioma-like carcinoma of the urinary bladder is mandatory in cases with extensive inflammation in the stroma.[67]

Other unusual patterns may also be seen (**Figs. 12-79** to **12-83**). It is critical that prostatic adenocarcinoma be excluded, especially when a solid (and nested) pattern of tumor growth is encountered (**Figs. 12-84** to **12-86**).

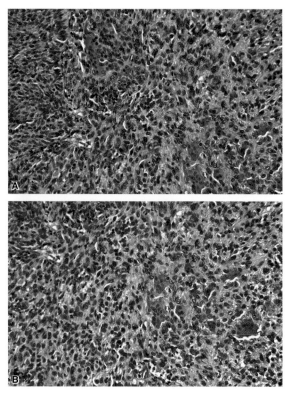

Figure 12-76   Osteoclast type giant cell reaction in association with urothelial carcinoma (A and B).

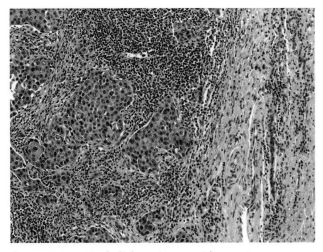

Figure 12-77 Urothelial carcinoma with prominent lymphoid reaction.

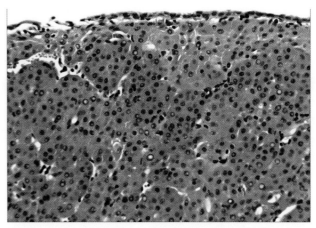

Figure 12-79 Urothelial carcinoma with prominent eosinophilic cytoplasm. Tumor has a nested growth pattern.

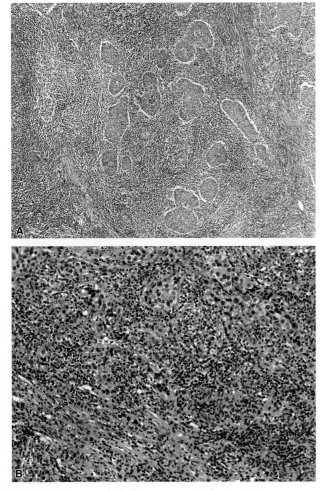

Figure 12-78 Urothelial carcinoma with prominent lymphoid reaction (A and B).

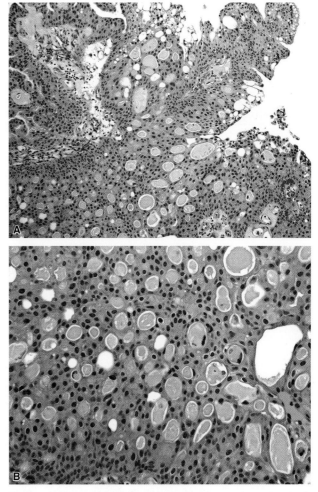

Figure 12-80 Urothelial carcinoma with prominent luminal spaces (A and B). Note the eosinophilic proteinaceous secretions.

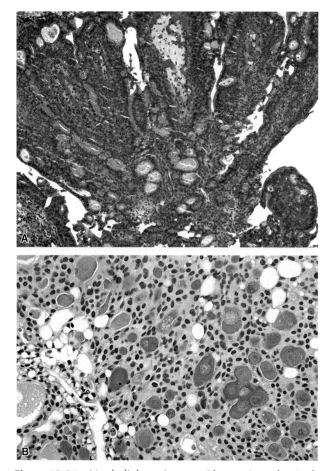

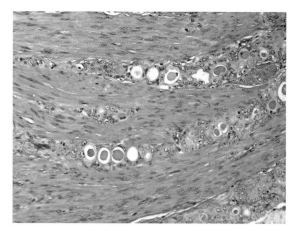

Figure 12-83 Urothelial carcinoma with colloid-like secretions.

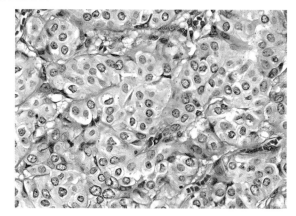

Figure 12-81 Urothelial carcinoma with prominent luminal spaces that are filled with proteinaceous secretions (A and B).

Figure 12-84 Urothelial carcinoma with solid and nested growth pattern.

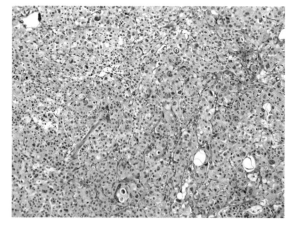

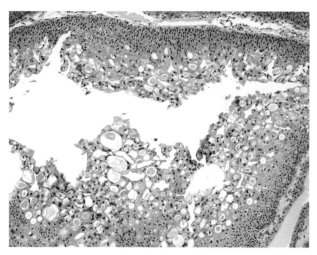

Figure 12-82 Urothelial carcinoma with prominent superficial umbrella cells. Some umbrella cells are atypical and have a bull's-eye appearance.

Figure 12-85 High grade urothelial carcinoma with solid growth. Prostatic carcinoma should be excluded by immunostaining. Prostatic adenocarcinoma is positive for prostatic-specific antigen (PSA), prostate-specific acid phosphatase (PSAP) and P501s (prostein); negative for cytokeratin 20, high molecular weight cytokeratin 34βE12, p63. Urothelial carcinomas are typically positive for high molecular weight cytokeratin 34βE12 and always negative for prostate makers such as PSA, PSAP, and P501S. Cytokeratin 20 is often positive in urothelial carcinoma.

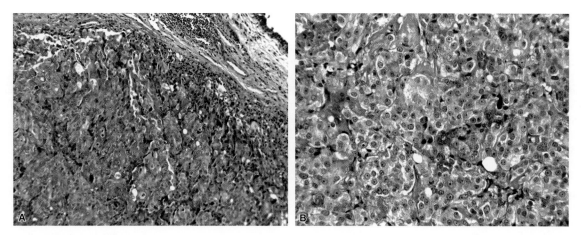

Figure 12-86 Prostatic adenocarcinoma involving the bladder (A and B). Immunostaining for PSA is strongly positive (not shown).

REFERENCES

1. Lopez-Beltran A, Cheng L. Histologic variants of urothelial carcinoma: differential diagnosis and clinical implications. *Hum Pathol* 2006;37:1371–88.
2. Jozwicki W, Domaniewski J, Skok Z, Wolski Z, Domanowska E, Jozwicka G. Usefulness of histologic homogeneity estimation of muscle-invasive urinary bladder cancer in an individual prognosis: a mapping study. *Urology* 2005;66:1122–6.
3. Wasco MJ, Daignault S, Zhang Y, Kunju LP, Kinnaman M, Braun T, Lee CT, Shah RB. Urothelial carcinoma with divergent histologic differentiation (mixed histologic features) predicts the presence of locally advanced bladder cancer when detected at transurethral resection. *Urology* 2007;70:69–74.
4. Ro JY, Staerkel GA, Ayala AG. Cytologic and histologic features of superficial bladder cancer. *Urol Clin North Am* 1992;19:435–53.
5. Akdas A, Turkeri L. The impact of squamous metaplasia in transitional cell carcinoma of the bladder. *Int Urol Nephrol* 1991;23:333–6.
6. Lopez-Beltran A, Martin J, Garcia J, Toro M. Squamous and glandular differentiation in urothelial bladder carcinomas. Histopathology, histochemistry and immunohistochemical expression of carcinoembryonic antigen. *Histol Histopathol* 1988;3:63–8.
7. Ayala AG, Ro JY. Premalignant lesions of urothelium and transitional cell tumors. In: Young RH, ed. Contemporary Issues in Surgical Pathology: Pathology of the Urinary Bladder. New York, NY: Churchill Livingstone, 1989;65–101.
8. Lopez-Beltran A, Luque RJ, Quintero A, Requena MJ, Montironi R. Hepatoid adenocarcinoma of the urinary bladder. *Virchows Arch* 2003;442:381–7.
9. Fong A, Garcia E, Gwynn L, Lisanti MP, Fazzari MJ, Li M. Expression of caveolin-1 and caveolin-2 in urothelial carcinoma of the urinary bladder correlates with tumor grade and squamous differentiation. *Am J Clin Pathol* 2003;120:93–100.
10. Lopez-Beltran A, Requena MJ, Alvarez-Kindelan J, Quintero A, Blanca A, Montironi R. Squamous differentiation in primary urothelial carcinoma of the urinary tract as seen by MAC387 immunohistochemistry. *J Clin Pathol* 2007;60:332–5.
11. Montironi R, Mazzucchelli R, Scarpelli M, Lopez-Beltran A, Cheng L. Morphological diagnosis of urothelial neoplasms. *J Clin Pathol* 2008;61:3–10.
12. Montironi R, Lopez-Beltran A, Scarpelli M, Mazzucchelli R, Cheng L. Morphological classification and definition of benign, preneoplastic and non-invasive neoplastic lesions of the urinary bladder. *Histopathology* 2008;53:621–33.
13. Montironi R, Lopez-Beltran A, Scarpelli M, Mazzucchelli R, Cheng L. 2004 World Health Organization classification of the noninvasive urothelial neoplasms: inherent problems and clinical reflections. *Eur Urol* 2009;Suppl 8:453–7.
14. Montironi R, Lopez-Beltran A, Mazzucchelli R, Bostwick DG. Classification and grading of the non-invasive urothelial neoplasms: recent advances and controversies. *J Clin Pathol* 2003;56:91–5.
15. Cheng L, Lopez-Beltran A, MacLennan GT. Neoplasms of the Urinary Bladder. Philadelphia: Elsevier/Mosby, 2008.
16. Cheng L, Montironi R, Davidson DD, Lopez-Beltran A. Staging and reporting of urothelial carcinoma of the urinary bladder. *Mod Pathol* 2009;22 (Suppl 2):S70–95.
17. Al-Khawaja M, Tan PH, MacLennan GT, Lopez-Beltran A, Montironi R, Cheng L. Ureteral endometriosis: clinicopathological and immunohistochemical study of 7 cases. *Hum Pathol* 2008;39:954–9.

18. Miller JS, Epstein JI. Noninvasive urothelial carcinoma of the bladder with glandular differentiation: report of 24 cases. *Am J Surg Pathol* 2009;33:1241–8.

19. Kunze E, Francksen B, Schulz H. Expression of MUC5AC apomucin in transitional cell carcinomas of the urinary bladder and its possible role in the development of mucus-secreting adenocarcinomas. *Virchows Arch* 2001;439:609–15.

20. Kunze E, Francksen B. Histogenesis of nonurothelial carcinomas of the urinary bladder from pre-existent transitional cell carcinomas. A histopathological and immunohistochemical study. *Urol Res* 2002;30:66–78.

21. Sung MT, Zhang S, Lopez-Beltran A, Montironi R, Wang M, Davidson DD, Koch MO, Cain MP, Rink RC, Cheng L. Urothelial carcinoma following augmentation cystoplasty: an aggressive variant with distinct clinicopathological characteristics and molecular genetic alterations. *Histopathology* 2009;55:161–73.

22. Lim M, Adsay NV, Grignon D, Osunkoya AO. Urothelial carcinoma with villoglandular differentiation: a study of 14 cases. *Mod Pathol* 2009;22:1280–6.

23. Cheng L, Montironi R, Bostwick DG. Villous adenoma of the urinary tract: a report of 23 cases, including 8 with coexistent adenocarcinoma. *Am J Surg Pathol* 1999;23:764–71.

24. Talbert ML, Young RH. Carcinomas of the urinary bladder with deceptively benign-appearing foci. A report of three cases. *Am J Surg Pathol* 1989;13:374–81.

25. Lin O, Cardillo M, Dalbagni G, Linkov I, Hutchinson B, Reuter VE. Nested variant of urothelial carcinoma: a clinicopathologic and immunohistochemical study of 12 cases. *Mod Pathol* 2003;16:1289–98.

26. Drew PA, Furman J, Civantos F, Murphy WM. The nested variant of transitional cell carcinoma: an aggressive neoplasm with innocuous histology. *Mod Pathol* 1996;9:989–94.

27. Young RH, Oliva E. Transitional cell carcinomas of the urinary bladder that may be underdiagnosed. A report of four invasive cases exemplifying the homology between neoplastic and non-neoplastic transitional cell lesions. *Am J Surg Pathol* 1996;20:1448–54.

28. Murphy WM, Deanna DG. The nested variant of transitional cell carcinoma: a neoplasm resembling proliferation of Brunn's nests. *Mod Pathol* 1992;5:240–3.

29. Wasco MJ, Daignault S, Bradley D, Shah RB. Nested variant of urothelial carcinoma: a clinicopathologic and immunohistochemical study of 30 pure and mixed cases. *Hum Pathol* 2010;41:163–71.

30. Holmang S, Johansson SL. The nested variant of transitional cell carcinoma—a rare neoplasm with poor prognosis. *Scand J Urol Nephrol* 2001;35:102–5.

31. Young RH. Tumor-like lesions of the urinary bladder. *Mod Pathol* 2009;22 Suppl 2:S37–52.

32. Patriarca C, Colecchia M, Lopez Beltran A, Sirugo G, Bollito E, di Pasquale M. Nest-like features in bladder, simulating the nested variant of urothelial carcinoma. *Int J Surg Pathol* 2009.

33. Volmar KE, Chan TY, De Marzo AM, Epstein JI. Florid von Brunn nests mimicking urothelial carcinoma: a morphologic and immunohistochemical comparison to the nested variant of urothelial carcinoma. *Am J Surg Pathol* 2003;27:1243–52.

34. Cheng L, Cheville JC, Sebo TJ, Eble JN, Bostwick DG. Atypical nephrogenic metaplasia of the urinary tract: a precursor lesion? *Cancer* 2000;88:853–61.

35. Cheng L, Leibovich B, Cheville J, Ramnani D, Sebo T, Neumann R, Nascimento A, Zincke H, Bostwick D. Paraganglioma of the urinary bladder: Can biologic potential be predicted? *Cancer* 2000;88:844–52.

36. Dominici A, Nesi G, Mondaini N, Amorosi A, Rizzo M. Skin involvement from micropapillary bladder carcinoma as the first clinical manifestation of metastatic disease. *Urol Int* 2001;67:173–4.

37. Hong SP, Park SW, Lee SJ, Chung JP, Song SY, Chung JB, Kang JK, Cho NH. Bile duct wall metastasis from micropapillary variant transitional cell carcinoma of the urinary bladder mimicking primary hilar cholangiocarcinoma. *Gastrointest Endosc* 2002;56:756–60.

38. Amin MB. Histological variants of urothelial carcinoma: diagnostic, therapeutic and prognostic implications. *Mod Pathol* 2009;22 Suppl 2:S96–S118.

39. Johansson SL, Borghede G, Holmang S. Micropapillary bladder carcinoma: a clinicopathological study of 20 cases. *J Urol* 1999;161:1798–1802.

40. Samaratunga H, Khoo K. Micropapillary variant of urothelial carcinoma of the urinary bladder; a clinicopathological and immunohistochemical study. *Histopathology* 2004;45:55–64.

41. Lopez-Beltran A, Montironi R, Blanca A, Cheng L. Invasive micropapillary urothelial carcinoma of the bladder. *Hum Pathol* 2010;41:1159–64.

42. Nassar H, Pansare V, Zhang H, Che M, Sakr W, Ali-Fehmi R, Grignon D, Sarkar F, Cheng J, Adsay V. Pathogenesis of invasive micropapillary carcinoma: role of MUC1 glycoprotein. *Mod Pathol* 2004;19:1045–50.

43. Amin MB, Ro JY, el-Sharkawy T, Lee KM, Troncoso P, Silva EG, Ordonez NG, Ayala AG. Micropapillary variant of transitional cell carcinoma of the urinary bladder. Histologic pattern resembling ovarian papillary serous carcinoma. *Am J Surg Pathol* 1994;18:1224–32.

44. Parker DC, Folpe AL, Bell J, Oliva E, Young RH, Cohen C, Amin MB. Potential utility of uroplakin III, thrombomodulin, high molecular weight cytokeratin, and cytokeratin 20 in noninvasive, invasive, and metastatic urothelial (transitional cell) carcinomas. *Am J Surg Pathol* 2003;27:1–10.

45. Black PC, Brown GA, Dinney CP. The impact of variant histology on the outcome of bladder cancer treated with curative intent. *Urol Oncol* 2009;27:3–7.

46. Kamat AM, Gee JR, Dinney CP, Grossman HB, Swanson DA, Millikan RE, Detry MA, Robinson TL, Pisters LL. The case for early cystectomy in the treatment of

nonmuscle invasive micropapillary bladder carcinoma. *J Urol* 2006;175:881–5.

47. Eble JN, Young RH. Carcinoma of the urinary bladder: a review of its diverse morphology. *Semin Diagn Pathol* 1997;14:98–108.

48. Leroy X, Leteurtre E, De La Taille A, Augusto D, Biserte J, Gosselin B. Microcystic transitional cell carcinoma: a report of 2 cases arising in the renal pelvis. *Arch Pathol Lab Med* 2002;126:859–61.

49. Young RH, Zukerberg LR. Microcystic transitional cell carcinomas of the urinary bladder. A report of four cases. *Am J Clin Pathol* 1991;96:635–9.

50. Williamson SR, Lopez-Beltran A, Montironi R, Cheng L. Glandular lesions of the urinary bladder:clinical significance and differential diagnosis. *Histopathology* 2011;58:811–34.

51. Huang Q, Chu PG, Lau SK, Weiss LM. Urothelial carcinoma of the urinary bladder with a component of acinar/tubular type differentiation simulating prostatic adenocarcinoma. *Hum Pathol* 2004;35:769–73.

52. Cheng L, Bostwick DG. Overdiagnosis of bladder carcinoma. *Anal Quant Cytol Histol* 2008;30:261–4.

53. Jones TD, Zhang S, Lopez-Beltran A, Eble JN, Sung MT, MacLennan GT, Montironi R, Tan PH, Zheng S, Baldridge LA, Cheng L. Urothelial carcinoma with an inverted growth pattern can be distinguished from inverted papilloma by fluorescence in-situ hybridization, immunohistochemistry, and morphologic analysis. *Am J Surg Pathol* 2007;31:1861–7.

54. Eble JN, Sauter G, Epstein JI, Sesterhenn IA, eds. World Health Organization Classification of Tumours: Pathology and Genetics of Tumours of the Urinary System and Male Genital Organs. Lyon, France: IARC Press, 2004.

55. Lopez-Beltran A, Amin MB, Oliveira PS, Montironi R, Algaba F, McKenney JK, de Torres I, Mazerolles C, Wang M, Cheng L. Urothelial carcinoma of the bladder, lipid cell variant: clinicopathologic findings and LOH analysis. *Am J Surg Pathol* 2010;34:371–6.

56. Zukerberg LR, Armin AR, Pisharodi L, Young RH. Transitional cell carcinoma of the urinary bladder with osteoclast-type giant cells: a report of two cases and review of the literature. *Histopathology* 1990;17:407–11.

57. Tamboli P, Amin MB, Mohsin SK, Ben-Dor D, Lopez-Beltran A. Plasmocytoid variant of non-papillary urothelial carcinoma (Abstract). *Mod Pathol* 2000;13:107A.

58. Sahin AA, Myhre M, Ro JY, Sneige N, Dekmezian RH, Ayala AG. Plasmacytoid transitional cell carcinoma. Report of a case with initial presentation mimicking multiple myeloma. *Acta Cytologica* 1991;35:277–80.

59. Lopez-Beltran A, Requena MJ, Montironi R, Blanca A, Cheng L. Plasmacytoid urothelial carcinoma of the bladder. *Hum Pathol* 2009;40:1023–8.

60. Coyne JD, Sim E. Urothelial neoplasia with plasmacytoid morphology. *Histopathology* 2006;48:200–1.

61. Fritsche HM, Burger M, Denzinger S, Legal W, Goebell PJ, Hartmann A. Plasmacytoid urothelial carcinoma of the bladder: histological and clinical features of 5 cases. *J Urol* 2008;180:1923–7.

62. Kohno T, Kitamura M, Akai H, Takaha M, Kawahara K, Oka T. Plasmacytoid urothelial carcinoma of the bladder. *Int J Urol* 2006;13:485–6.

63. Nigwekar P, Tamboli P, Amin MB, Osunkoya AO, Ben-Dor D. Plasmacytoid urothelial carcinoma: detailed analysis of morphology with clinicopathologic correlation in 17 cases. *Am J Surg Pathol* 2009;33:417–24.

64. Ro JY, Shen SS, Lee HI, Hong EK, Lee YH, Cho NH, Jung SJ, Choi YJ, Ayala AG. Plasmacytoid transitional cell carcinoma of urinary bladder: a clinicopathologic study of 9 cases. *Am J Surg Pathol* 2008;32:752–7.

65. Mai KT, Park PC, Yazdi HM, Saltel E, Erdogan S, Stinson WA, Cagiannos I, Morash C. Plasmacytoid urothelial carcinoma of the urinary bladder report of seven new cases. *Eur Urol* 2006;50:1111–4.

66. Zukerberg LR, Harris NL, Young RH. Carcinomas of the urinary

bladder simulating malignant lymphoma. A report of five cases. *Am J Surg Pathol* 1991;15:569–76.

67. Williamson SR, Zhang S, Lopez-Beltran A, Shah RB, Montironi R, Tan PH, Wang M, Baldridge LA, MacLennan GT, Cheng L. Lymphoepithelioma-like carcinoma of the urinary bladder: clinicopathologic, immunohistochemical, and molecular features. *Am J Surg Pathol* 2011;35:474–83.

68. Amin MB, Ro JY, Lee KM, Ordonez NG, Dinney CP, Gulley ML, Ayala AG. Lymphoepithelioma-like carcinoma of the urinary bladder. *Am J Surg Pathol* 1994;18:466–73.

69. Young RH, Eble JN. Unusual forms of carcinoma of the urinary bladder. *Hum Pathol* 1991;22:948–65.

70. Lopez-Beltran A, Luque RJ, Vicioso L, Anglada F, Requena MJ, Quintero A, Montironi R. Lymphoepithelioma-like carcinoma of the urinary bladder: a clinicopathologic study of 13 cases. *Virchows Arch* 2001;438:552–7.

71. Holmang S, Borghede G, Johansson SL. Bladder carcinoma with lymphoepithelioma-like differentiation: a report of 9 cases. *J Urol* 1998;159:779–82.

72. Dinney CP, Ro JY, Babaian RJ, Johnson DE. Lymphoepithelioma of the bladder: a clinicopathological study of 3 cases. *J Urol* 1993;149:840–1.

73. Gulley ML, Amin MB, Nicholls JM, Banks PM, Ayala AG, Srigley JR, Eagan PA, Ro JY. Epstein-Barr virus is detected in undifferentiated nasopharyngeal carcinoma but not in lymphoepithelioma-like carcinoma of the urinary bladder. *Hum Pathol* 1995;26:1207–14.

74. Tamas EF, Nielsen ME, Schoenberg MP, Epstein JI. Lymphoepithelioma-like carcinoma of the urinary tract: a clinicopathological study of 30 pure and mixed cases. *Mod Pathol* 2007;20:828–34.

75. Amin MB, Young RH. Primary carcinomas of the urethra. *Semin Diagn Pathol* 1997;14:147–60.

76. Braslis KG, Jones A, Murphy D. Clear-cell transitional cell carcinoma. *Aust N Z J Surg* 1997;67:906–8.

77. Kotliar SN, Wood CG, Schaeffer AJ, Oyasu R. Transitional cell carcinoma exhibiting clear cell features. A differential diagnosis for clear cell adenocarcinoma of the urinary tract. *Arch Pathol Lab Med* 1995;119:79–81.

78. Oliva E, Amin MB, Jimenez R, Young RH. Clear cell carcinoma of the urinary bladder: a report and comparison of four tumors of müllerian origin and nine of probable urothelial origin with discussion of histogenesis and diagnostic problems. *Am J Surg Pathol* 2002;26:190–7.

79. Bates AW, Baithun SI. The significance of secondary neoplasms of the urinary and male genital tract. *Virchows Arch* 2002;440:640–7.

80. Zhou M, Epstein JI, Young RH. Paraganglioma of the urinary bladder: a lesion that may be misdiagnosed as urothelial carcinoma in transurethral resection specimens. *Am J Surg Pathol* 2004;28:94–100.

81. Lopez-Beltran A, Cheng L, Comperat E, Roupret M, Blanca A, Menendez CL, Montironi R. Large cell undifferentiated carcinoma of the urinary bladder. *Pathology* 2010;42:364–8.

82. Amir G, Rosenmann E. Osteoclast-like giant cell tumour of the urinary bladder. *Histopathology* 1990;17:413–8.

83. Kruger S, Mahnken A, Kausch I, Feller AC. P16 immunoreactivity is an independent predictor of tumor progression in minimally invasive urothelial bladder carcinoma. *Eur Urol* 2005;47:463–7.

84. Baydar D, Amin MB, Epstein JI. Osteoclast-rich undifferentiated carcinomas of the urinary tract. *Mod Pathol* 2006;19:161–71.

85. Lopez-Beltran A, Blanca A, Montironi R, Cheng L, Regueiro JC. Pleomorphic giant cell carcinoma of the urinary bladder. *Hum Pathol* 2009;40:1461–6.

86. Serio G, Zampatti C, Ceppi M. Spindle and giant cell carcinoma of the urinary bladder: a clinicopathological light microscopic and immunohistochemical study. *Br J Urol* 1995;75:167–72.

87. Cox RM, Schneider AG, Sangoi AR, Clingan WJ, Gokden N, McKenney JK. Invasive urothelial carcinoma with chordoid features: a report of 12 distinct cases characterized by prominent myxoid stroma and cordlike epithelial architecture. *Am J Surg Pathol* 2009;33:1213–9.

88. Campo E, Algaba F, Palacin A, Germa R, Sole-Balcells FJ, Cardesa A. Placental proteins in high grade urothelial neoplasms. An immunohistochemical study of human chorionic gonadotropin, human placental lactogen, and pregnancy-specific beta-1-glycoprotein. *Cancer* 1989;63:2497–504.

89. Fowler AL, Hall E, Rees G. Choriocarcinoma arising in transitional cell carcinoma of the bladder. *Br J Urol* 1992;70:333–4.

90. Grammatico D, Grignon DJ, Eberwein P, Shepherd RR, Hearn SA, Walton JC. Transitional cell carcinoma of the renal pelvis with choriocarcinomatous differentiation. Immunohistochemical and immunoelectron microscopic assessment of human chorionic gonadotropin production by transitional cell carcinoma of the urinary bladder. *Cancer* 1993;71:1835–41.

91. Seidal T, Breborowicz J, Malmstrom P. Immunoreactivity to human chorionic gonadotropin in urothelial carcinoma: correlation with tumor grade, stage, and progression. *J Urol Pathol* 1993;1:397–410.

92. Shah VM, Newman J, Crocker J, Chapple CR, Collard MJ, O'Brien JM, Considine J. Ectopic beta-human chorionic gonadotropin production by bladder urothelial neoplasia. *Arch Pathol Lab Med* 1986;110:107–11.

93. Bastacky S, Dhir R, Nangia AK, et al. Choriocarcinomatous differentiation in a high grade urothelial carcinoma of the urinary bladder: case report and litterature review. *J Urol Pathol* 1997;6:223–34.

94. Regalado JJ. Mixed micropapillary and trophoblastic carcinoma of bladder: report of a first case with new immunohistochemical evidence of urothelial origin. *Hum Pathol* 2004;35:382–4.

95. Yamase HT, Wurzel RS, Nieh PT, Gondos B. Immunohistochemical demonstration of human chorionic gonadotropin in tumors of the urinary bladder. *Ann Clin Lab Sci* 1985;15:414–7.

96. Oyasu R, Nan L, Smith P, Kawamata H. Human chorionic gonadotropin β-subunit synthesis by undifferentiated urothelial carcinoma with syncytiotrophoblastic differentiation. *Arch Pathol Lab Med* 1994;118:715–17.

97. Martin JE, Jenkins BJ, Zuk RJ, Oliver RT, Baithun SI. Human chorionic gonadotrophin expression and histological findings as predictors of response to radiotherapy in carcinoma of the bladder. *Virchows Arch A Pathol Anat Histopathol* 1989;414:273–7.

98. Cho JH, Yu E, Kim KH, Lee I. Primary choriocarcinoma of the urinary bladder—a case report. *J Korean Med Sci* 1992;7:369–72.

99. Hanna NH, Ulbright TM, Einhorn LH. Primary choriocarcinoma of the bladder with the detection of isochromosome 12p. *J Urol* 2002;167:1781.

100. Baldwin L, Lee AH, Al-Talib RK, Theaker JM. Transitional cell carcinoma of the bladder mimicking lobular carcinoma of the breast: a discohesive variant of urothelial carcinoma. *Histopathology* 2005;46:50–6.

101. Kumar S, Kumar D, Cowan DF. Transitional cell carcinoma with rhabdoid features. *Am J Surg Pathol* 1992;16:515–21.

102. Parwani AV, Herawi M, Volmar K, Tsay SH, Epstein JI. Urothelial carcinoma with rhabdoid features: report of 6 cases. *Hum Pathol* 2006;37:168–72.

103. Cheng L, Pan C, Yang XJ, Lopez-Beltran A, MacLennan GT, Lin H, Kuzel TM, Papavero V, Tretiakova M, Nigro K, Koch MO, Eble JN. Small cell carcinoma of the urinary bladder: a clinicopathologic analysis of 64 patients. *Cancer* 2004;101:957–62.

104. Bannach G, Grignon D, Shum D. Sarcomatoid transitional cell carcinoma vs pseudosarcomatous stromal reaction in bladder carcinoma: an immunohistolchemical study. *J Urol Pathol* 1993;1:105–13.

105. Mahadevia PS, Alexander JE, Rojas-Corona R, Koss LG. Pseudosarcomatous stromal reaction in primary and metastatic urothelial carcinoma. A source of diagnostic difficulty. *Am J Surg Pathol* 1989;13:782–90.

106. Roth JA. Reactive pseudosarcomatous response in urinary bladder. *Urology* 1980;16:635–7.

107. Kobayashi M, Hashimoto S, Hara Y, Kobayashi Y, Nakamura S, Tokue A, Shimizu H. [Squamous carcinoma with pseudosarcomatous stroma of the renal pelvis and ureter: a case report]. *Hinyokika Kiyo* 1994;40:55–9.

108. Eble JN, Young RH. Stromal osseous metaplasia in carcinoma of the bladder. *J Urol* 1991;145:823–5.

109. Kinouchi T, Hanafusa T, Kuroda M, Usami M, Kotake T. Ossified cystic metastasis of bladder tumor to abdominal wound after partial cystectomy. *J Urol* 1995;153:1049–50.

110. Lam KY. Chondroid and osseous metaplasia in carcinoma of the bladder. *J Urol Pathol* 1995;3:255–62.

111. Sarma KP. The role of lymphoid reaction in bladder cancer. *J Urol* 1970;104:843–9.

112. Flamm J. Tumor-associated tissue inflammatory reaction and eosinophilia in primary superficial bladder cancer. *Urology* 1992;40:180–5.

113. Feeney D, Quesada ET, Sirbasku DM, Kadmon D. Transitional cell carcinoma in a tuberculous kidney: case report and review of the literature. *J Urol* 1994;151:989–91.

114. Lipponen PK, Eskelinen MJ, Jauhiainen K, Harju E, Terho R. Tumour infiltrating lymphocytes as an independent prognostic factor in transitional cell bladder cancer. *Eur J Cancer* 1992;29A:69–75.

Chapter 13

Adenocarcinoma and Its Putative Precursors and Variants

Bladder Pathology, First Edition. Liang Cheng, Antonio Lopez-Beltran, David G. Bostwick.
© 2012 Wiley-Blackwell. Published 2012 by John Wiley & Sons, Inc.

Putative Precursor Lesions

Although some glandular lesions are associated with urinary bladder adenocarcinoma with relative frequency, a definitive pathogenetic mechanism as demonstrated for colorectal adenocarcinoma is difficult to identify in this setting. Intuitively, it seems logical that intestinal differentiation precedes dysplastic changes, which precede primary bladder adenocarcinoma; however, this link is still missing in the bladder.[1-3]

Intestinal Metaplasia

Emerging molecular data suggest that intestinal metaplasia may be implicated in the development of bladder adenocarcinoma (**Fig. 13-1**; see also **Chapter 3**).[4,5] Morton and his colleagues found that intestinal metaplasia harbors genetic alterations typically associated with precursor lesions in other organ sites. There was significant telomere shortening in intestinal metaplasia compared to adjacent normal urothelial cells.[4] A subset of cases with telomere shortening also demonstrated chromosomal abnormalities common to urothelial carcinoma by the UroVysion FISH method.[4] These findings suggest that intestinal metaplasia may indeed be a precursor in the development of adenocarcinoma.[4b]

Villous Adenoma and Tubulovillous Adenoma

Villous adenoma and tubulovillous adenoma are uncommon benign glandular epithelial neoplasms with exophytic growth that are often associated with coexisting adenocarcinoma (**Fig. 13-2**; see also **Chapter 5**).[6] Histologically, these lesions are identical to their colonic counterparts, showing columnar mucinous cells and goblet cells lining delicate fibrovascular stalks with nuclear stratification, crowding, and hyperchromasia. The precursor nature of these lesions has been debated.[7]

Adenocarcinoma in Situ (Carcinoma in Situ with Glandular Differentiation)

This is a controversial entity. Histologically, this lesion overlaps with noninvasive papillary urothelial carcinoma with glandular differentiation (**Fig. 13-3**), villous adenoma, and urothelial carcinoma in situ with glandular differentiation. In practice, it may be impossible to distinguish adenocarcinoma in situ from urothelial carcinoma in situ with glandular differentiation or noninvasive urothelial carcinoma with glandular differentiation.[6,8,9]

Chan and Epstein described the papillary, cribriform, and flat architectural patterns of adenocarcinoma in situ, which demonstrate glandular differentiation with atypical columnar epithelium and apical cytoplasm.[10] In contrast

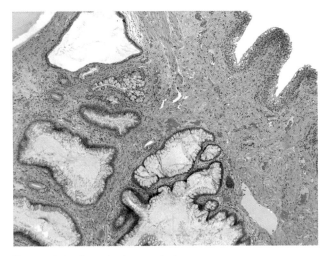

Figure 13-1   Intestinal metaplasia.

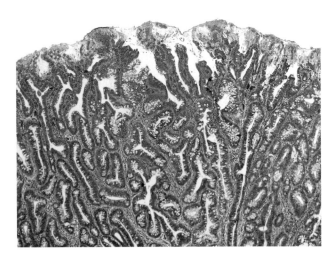

Figure 13-2   Tubullovillous adenoma.

to villous adenoma,[6] adenocarcinoma in situ typically demonstrates a small, focal lesion rather than a significant mass. Similarly, the villous, finger-like projections should be absent, although the papillary form of adenocarcinoma in situ does demonstrate architecture similar to papillary urothelial carcinoma. The flat pattern of adenocarcinoma in situ also resembles typical urothelial carcinoma in situ, although noteworthy glandular differentiation may be appreciated, in contrast to the small, mucin-containing spaces without columnar epithelium, so-called "gland-like lumina," which are present in some cases of urothelial carcinoma in situ.

Adenocarcinoma in situ should also be distinguished from involvement of a von Brunn nest by urothelial carcinoma in situ. The absence of true columnar glandular differentiation may be helpful in resolving this challenge. Due to significant morphologic overlaps, lack of reliable diagnostic criteria, and lack of convincing data linking

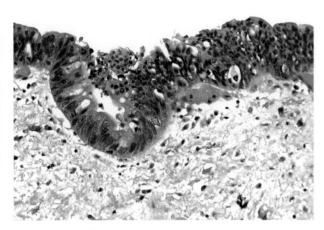

Figure 13-3   Adenocarcinoma in situ.

adenocarcinoma in situ with adenocarcinoma, we recommend replacing "adenocarcinoma in situ" with "carcinoma in situ with glandular differentiation" until additional evidence could link this lesion with adenocarcinoma of the bladder.

Adenocarcinoma

Primary adenocarcinoma of the bladder accounts for 0.5% to 2% of bladder cancers and should be distinguished from adenocarcinoma arising in the urachus (see **Chapter 27** for further discussion).[1,11–13] It occurs at any age, but is most common after the fifth decade of life, with a male predominance. The male-to-female ratio is 2.5 : 1. Patients typically present with hematuria, irritative voiding symptoms, and, rarely, mucinuria. The cancer is often advanced, with metastases in up to 40% of patients at the time of diagnosis.[12] Intestinal metaplasia coexists in up to 67% of patients, and most cancers arising in association with exstrophy are adenocarcinoma.[14] Occasional cases of adenocarcinoma arise within a diverticulum.[15] Other associations with adenocarcinoma include pelvic lipomatosis and *Schistosomiasis haematobium* infection.

Adenocarcinoma may appear as an exophytic, papillary, solid, sessile, ulcerating, or infiltrative mass. The signet ring cell variant frequently shows diffuse thickening of the bladder wall, producing a linitis plastica-like appearance.[16] Cold-cup biopsies of the urothelial mucosa may be unrevealing.

Strict definition includes those tumors derived from urothelium with histopathologic demonstration of only a pure glandular component. In this discussion we exclude any case containing any urothelial carcinoma component, preferring to classify such cases as urothelial carcinoma

Table 13-1   Histologic Patterns of Adenocarcinoma of the Urinary Bladder

Adenocarcinoma, not otherwise specified (NOS)
Adenocarcinoma with colonic (enteric or intestinal type) pattern
Mucinous (colloid) adenocarcinoma
Signet ring cell adenocarcinoma
Adenocarcinoma with hepatoid pattern (hepatoid adenocarcinoma)
Clear cell adenocarcinoma
Adenocarcinoma with mixed patterns

with glandular differentiation (see also **Chapter 12**); this distinction is probably semantic and academic.

There are six main histologic patterns of adenocarcinoma of the bladder (**Table 13-1**). The enteric type closely resembles adenocarcinoma of the colon,[17] while adenocarcinoma without a specific glandular growth pattern may be termed "adenocarcinoma, not otherwise specified (NOS)." Lesions with abundant extracellular mucin containing floating tumor cell clusters are designated mucinous (colloid) type, similar to the counterpart phenomenon in breast and other organs. Tumors are categorized based on the degree of glandular differentiation and nuclear pleomorphism, similar to adenocarcinoma seen elsewhere.

Nonurachal adenocarcinoma is staged using the standard American Joint Committee on Cancer tumor, lymph node, and metastasis (AJCC TNM) staging system.[18] As with other urinary bladder neoplasms, stage is considered the most significant prognostic factor.

Adenocarcinoma, Not Otherwise Specified (NOS)

Adenocarcinoma, NOS, refers to a cancer that does not fit into one of the other categories (**Figs. 13-4** and **13-5**).

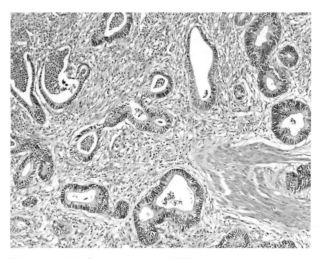

Figure 13-4   Adenocarcinoma, NOS.

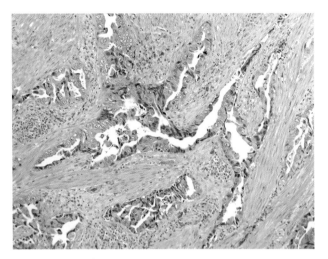

Figure 13-5   Adenocarcinoma, NOS.

Table 13-2   Glandular or Gland-like Lesions Involving the Urinary Bladder

Benign lesions and mimickers with glandular or gland-like
    differentiation
    Cystitis cystica
    Cystitis glandularis (of the usual/typical type)
    Nephrogenic metaplasia
    Urachal remnant
    Endometriosis
    Endocervicosis
    Endosalpingiosis

Putative precursor lesions
    Intestinal metaplasia (cystitis glandularis of the intestinal
        type)
    Villous adenoma
    Urothelial carcinoma in situ with glandular
        differentiation (adenocarcinoma in situ)

Nonurachal bladder adenocarcinoma

Urachal adenocarcinoma

Variants of urothelial carcinoma with glandular or
    gland-like differentiation
    Urothelial carcinoma with glandular differentiation
    Urothelial carcinoma with villoglandular differentiation
    Micropapillary variant urothelial carcinoma
    Microcystic variant urothelial carcinoma
    Urothelial carcinoma with small tubules
    Nested variant urothelial carcinoma
    Lipid (lipoid) cell variant urothelial carcinoma
    Urothelial carcinoma with chordoid features

Remarkably, this and the colonic pattern are the most common forms of adenocarcinoma.

The differential diagnosis of bladder adenocarcinoma is extensive (Tables 13-2 to 13-4). Benign mimics need to be excluded, including florid cystitis cystica and cystitis glandularis with mucin extravasation.[19] These lesions may produce pseudopapillary or polypoid lesions, but the benign cytology of the lining cells and lack of invasion are important distinguishing features. In unusual cases, extracellular mucin is present, and careful evaluation for malignant cells is necessary. Also, it is important to know the location in the bladder of the worrisome tissue, recognizing that cystitis glandularis of intestinal type usually arises in the bladder neck or trigone. Rare cases of florid cystitis glandularis with extensive intestinal metaplasia and mucin extravasation have been reported, and such cases may be difficult to distinguish from adenocarcinoma.[19,20] However, the degree of cytologic and architectural atypicality of adenocarcinoma far exceeds that seen in florid cystitis glandularis. Adenocarcinoma usually exhibits obvious destruction of the lamina propria and, in the colloid variant, clusters of malignant cells are seen floating in pools of mucin, a feature that excludes a diagnosis of extensive intestinal metaplasia with mucin extravasation.

Villous adenoma rarely occurs in the urinary bladder, and shows cytologic and architectural abnormalities of adenomatous epithelium without stromal invasion. Nephrogenic metaplasia must be distinguished from adenocarcinoma, particularly the clear cell pattern (see the discussion below), and this may be difficult in small or distorted superficial biopsies. Endocervicosis is a difficult problem in small biopsy samples, but lacks cytologic atypia of adenocarcinoma.

Differential diagnosis with colonic adenocarcinoma is particularly challenging, as bladder adenocarcinoma may have a similar immunoprofile.[21,22] Positivity for cytokeratin (CK) 7 is variable, while CK20 is positive in most cases of bladder adenocarcinoma.[17] Nuclear transcription factor CDX2 is sometimes used as a marker of intestinal differentiation; however, it has not shown tremendous utility in differentiating primary and secondary adenocarcinoma, as both bladder and colonic primary tumors may be CDX2 positive,[23] as well as intestinal metaplasia of the bladder.[5,21] In fact, tissue microarray studies have demonstrated CDX2 positivity in 2% of urothelial carcinoma.[24] Villin, an actin-binding protein related to the brush border of epithelial cells, exhibited positivity in both colonic adenocarcinoma and enteric-type bladder adenocarcinoma, while urothelial carcinoma with glandular differentiation is negative.[25] Nuclear staining for β-catenin may have some utility, as staining is seen in 81% of colorectal carcinoma involving the bladder, with only membranous or cytoplasmic staining demonstrable in primary bladder adenocarcinoma (Table 13-4).[26]

Direct extension or metastasis from prostatic adenocarcinoma should also be considered in the differential

Table 13-3   Differentiating Histopathologic Characteristics of Cytologically Bland-appearing Glandular and Gland-like Lesions of the Urinary Bladder[a]

von Brunn nests	Solid nests of urothelial cells; extension to a uniform depth in the lamina propria; lobular architecture (especially in the upper urinary tract); lack of muscularis propria involvement
Cystitis cystica	Central cystic degeneration of von Brunn nests without apical glandular differentiation; extension to a uniform depth in the lamina propria; lobular architecture (especially in the upper urinary tract); lack of muscularis propria involvement
Cystitis glandularis	Apical glandular differentiation in von Brunn nests; cuboidal or columnar central lining surrounded by urothelial cells; extension to a uniform depth in the lamina propria; lobular architecture; lack of muscularis propria involvement
Intestinal metaplasia	Glandular proliferation within lamina propria; abundant mucin-producing goblet cells, sometimes Paneth cells; extension to a uniform depth in the lamina propria; lobular architecture; lack of muscularis propria involvement
Microcystic variant UC	Characteristic variation in cyst size, up to 2 cm; infiltrative growth pattern throughout the bladder wall; lumen containing necrotic debris, PAS-diastase positive mucin
UC with small tubules	Predominance of small tubules; extensive invasion of bladder wall; lack of nephrogenic metaplasia features (tubular–papillary architecture, cuboidal epithelium, hobnail cells); negative for PSA, PSAP, and AMACR
Nested variant UC	Infiltrating nests of urothelial cells with a variable proportion of small tubular lumens, resembling von Brunn nests; focal significant atypia present in deeper aspects of infiltrative tumor (enlarged nucleoli and coarse nuclear chromatin); disorderly proliferation; jagged tumor–stroma interface; focal myxoid or desmoplastic stroma; extensive infiltration of bladder wall out of proportion to histologic grade

[a]UC, urothelial carcinoma; AMACR, α-methylacyl-CoA racemase; PSA, prostate-specific antigen; PSAP, prostate-specific acid phosphatase; PAS, periodic acid–Schiff.

Table 13-4   Selected Immunohistochemical Markers in Glandular Lesions of the Urinary Bladder[a]

	Positive	Negative
Cystitis glandularis, usual type	CK7	CDX2, CK20
Intestinal metaplasia (cystitis glandularis, intestinal type)	CDX2, CK20	CK7
Nephrogenic metaplasia	AMACR, PAX2	p63, 34βE12
Endometriosis	CD10 (stromal) CK7, CA-125, ER, PR (epithelial)	
Endocervicosis	HBME-1, ER, PR	
Primary bladder adenocarcinoma	CDX2, CK20, villin CK7 (variable) β-Catenin (cytoplasmic)	PSA, PSAP
Urothelial carcinoma with glandular differentiation	CK7, CK20 34βE12, UP, TM	Villin
Colorectal adenocarcinoma (variable)	CK20, villin β-Catenin (nuclear)	TM, CK7
Prostatic adenocarcinoma	PSA, PSAP, Leu 7 AMACR	UP, TM 34βE12, PAX2

[a]CK, cytokeratin; AMACR, α-methylacyl-CoA racemase (P504S); ER, estrogen receptor; PR, progesterone receptor; PSA, prostate-specific antigen; PSAP, prostatic-specific acid phosphatase; UP, uroplakin III; TM, thrombomodulin; 34βE12, high molecular weight cytokeratin 34βE12.

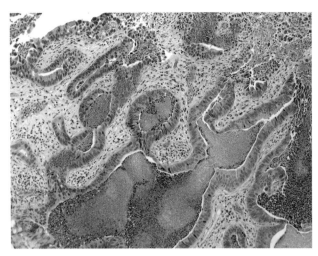

Figure 13-6   Adenocarcinoma, enteric type. Note the central comedonecrosis.

diagnosis. In such cases, basal cell markers such as 34βE12 cytokeratin and p63 (which are negative in prostate cancer), and prostate-specific antigen (PSA) and prostate-specific acid phosphatase (PSAP) immunostaining would help confirm prostatic origin of the tumor (see also **Chapter 23**).

Adenocarcinoma with Colonic (Enteric or Intestinal Type) Pattern

The colonic pattern is composed of pseudostratified columnar cells forming glands, often with central necrosis, typical of colonic adenocarcinoma (**Figs. 13-6** to **13-8**). Paneth cells and argentaffin cells may be present.[27] The distinction from florid cystitis glandularis depends on architectural and cytologic differences between them, but these may be subtle.

Mucinous (Colloid) Adenocarcinoma

The mucinous (colloid) pattern consists of single tumor cells or nests floating in extracellular mucin (**Figs. 13-9** and **13-10**). This pattern is unusual in isolation, and usually coexists with the colonic pattern of adenocarcinoma. Florid cystitis glandularis with mucin extravasation has previously been mistaken for mucinous carcinoma.[19] Complete absence of atypical cells within or at the periphery of the extravasated mucin strongly favors a benign diagnosis, although caution is urged in small or limited samples.[20] Endocervicosis is another benign mimic that rarely has mucin pools, sometimes eliciting an inflammatory response that is very uncommon in adenocarcinoma.

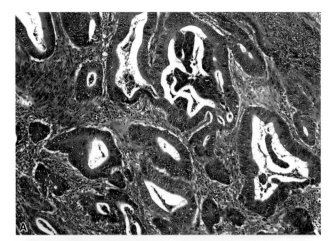

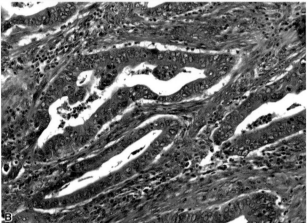

Figure 13-7   Adenocarcinoma, enteric type (A and B).

Signet Ring Cell Carcinoma

The signet ring cell pattern of bladder adenocarcinoma consists of a diffuse infiltrate of distinctive cells involving the bladder wall.[1,16,28-33] The diagnosis requires the presence of at least a focal component of diffuse linitis plastica-like growth and no element of urothelial carcinoma.[16] Microscopic examination reveals diffuse permeation by solitary signet ring cells or nests with single cytoplasmic vacuoles or foamy multivacuolated cytoplasm (**Figs. 13-11** to **13-14**). In some cases, the cytoplasm is pale and eosinophilic, with the nucleus compressed at one end, a pattern referred to as monocytoid. Rare cases are associated with neurogenic bladder.[31]

Signet ring cell carcinoma has an extremely poor prognosis, with less than 13% five-year survival, compared with 33% in cancer with a mixed pattern (urothelial and signet ring cells).[16] Torenbeek and colleagues found that 77% of patients with signet ring cell carcinoma of the bladder died of disease over a mean survival period of 20 months.[32] Radiation therapy and systemic chemotherapy are ineffective in most cases.[30]

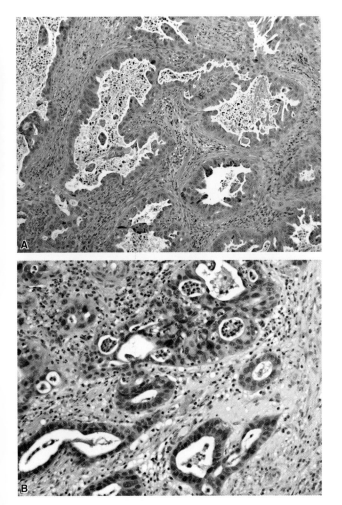

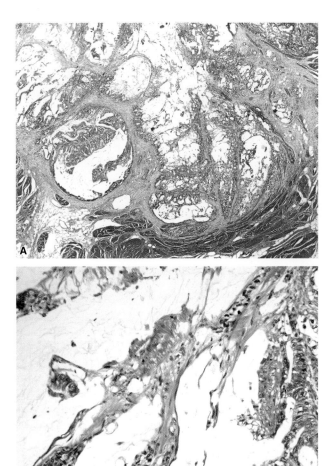

Figure 13-8   Adenocarcinoma, enteric type (A and B).

Figure 13-10   Colloid adenocarcinoma (A and B).

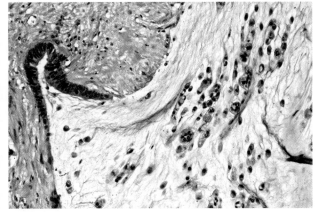

Figure 13-9   Colloid adenocarcinoma. Mucin pool with malignant cells in colloid (mucinous) pattern of adenocarcinoma of the bladder.

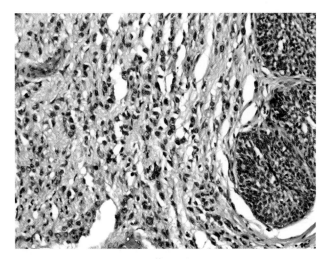

Figure 13-11   Signet ring cell carcinoma.

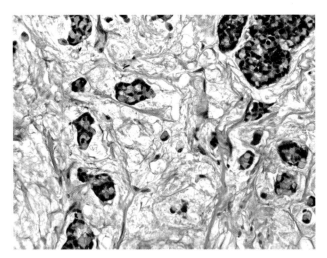

Figure 13-12 Signet ring cell carcinoma with mucin pools.

The signet ring cell variant is exceedingly rare, accounting for an estimated 0.24% of bladder malignancies.[32] However, secondary involvement of the bladder by signet ring cell-type adenocarcinoma, is more common and may be challenging to exclude from the differential diagnosis without thorough clinical information and a adequate tissue specimen. Malignancy of the stomach, colon, breast, pancreas, lung, and prostate demonstrate signet ring cell morphology more commonly than the urinary bladder.[34] Primary bladder signet ring cell-type carcinoma may be composed of diffusely infiltrating single cells or mixed glandular and signet ring components; however, tumors with pure signet ring cell morphology exhibit the worst prognosis. Similar to villous adenoma, cells may have demonstrable acid mucin by mucicarmine, periodic acid–Schiff (PAS), and Alcian blue stains.[16,34] Notably, the lipid cell variant of urothelial carcinoma may exhibit a similar signet ring cell appearance, although true mucin within the vacuole is not readily identifiable by special studies.[35]

Immunohistochemically, Thomas et al. found markers such as CK20, CDX-2, E-cadherin, and β-catenin to have decreased expression in the signet ring cell component compared to areas of colonic-type bladder adenocarcinoma.[33] E-cadherin, in particular, is involved in cell cohesion, and thus, these findings intuitively correspond with the poorly cohesive nature of signet ring cells. In contrast, the study found expression of villin-1 to be preserved in the signet ring cell areas.[33]

Adenocarcinoma with Hepatoid Pattern (Hepatoid Adenocarcinoma)

Adenocarcinoma with hepatoid pattern has been described in the stomach, ovary, pancreas, papilla of Vater, renal pelvis, and, recently, in the bladder (**Figs. 13-15** and **13-16**).[1,36–38] Strict morphologic criteria include formation

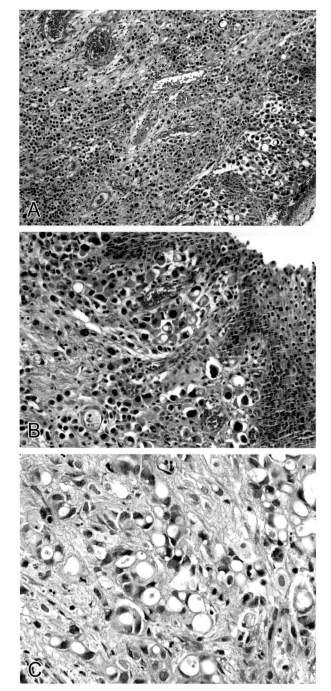

Figure 13-13 Signet ring cell carcinoma (A to C). Tumor has discohesive growth pattern and may have plasmacytoid appearance.

of cords of polygonal cells separated by sinusoids or evidence of bile production and bile canaliculi formation. All reported cases are at least focally positive for α-fetoprotein (AFP) and diffusely positive for α_1-antitrypsin and albumin; carcinoembryonic antigen (CEA) is positive in about one-half of cases, sometimes in a canalicular

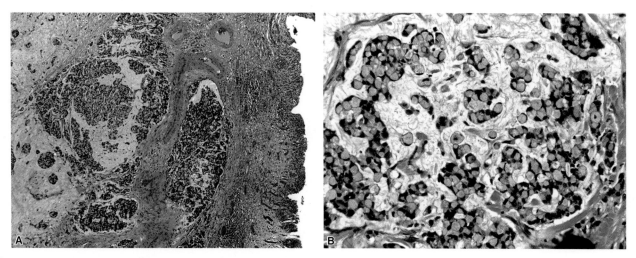

Figure 13-14   Signet ring cell carcinoma with mucin production.

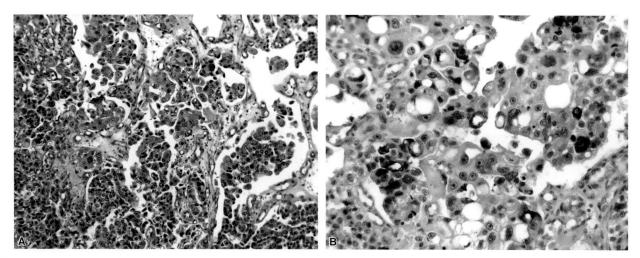

Figure 13-15   Hepatoid adenocarcinoma (A and B). Immunostaining for α-fetoprotein is positive (B).

pattern. Clinically, patients are most often elderly men, with aggressive tumor behavior, including frequent lymph node metastases.[36]

Microscopically, tumor cells are large, polygonal, and poorly differentiated, arranged in solid sheets, nests, and trabeculae, and focally formed glands. The cells may show prominent cytoplasmic clearing, although some have granular eosinophilic cytoplasm. Most tumor cells contain a single large eosinophilic nucleolus. Cancer cells focally display intracytoplasmic PAS-positive, diastase-resistant hyaline globules and bile production.

The immunoprofile of positivity for AFP, low-molecular-weight cytokeratin (CAM5.2), α_1-antitrypsin, albumin, hepatocyte paraffin-1 (HepPar-1), and epithelial membrane antigen (EMA) seem to confirm the apparent hepatic phenotype. A canalicular staining pattern with CEA

and demonstration of the albumin gene mRNA by non-isotopic in situ hybridization affirm genuine hepatocellular differentiation.[36]

The main differential diagnostic considerations include adenocarcinoma with AFP production, germ cell tumor with hepatoid foci, and metastatic hepatocellular carcinoma. Adenocarcinoma with AFP production does not qualify as a hepatoid pattern if it fails to fulfill the strict criteria noted above. Such cases, including an AFP-producing nonhepatoid urachal adenocarcinoma usually stain weakly for AFP, and CEA immunoreactivity is not canalicular but membranous.[39] Hepatoid foci can be seen in yolk sac tumor; however, this has not been described in a bladder tumor. Metastases of hepatocellular carcinoma to the bladder are almost always associated with widespread disseminated cancer, and can usually be excluded by clinical investigation.

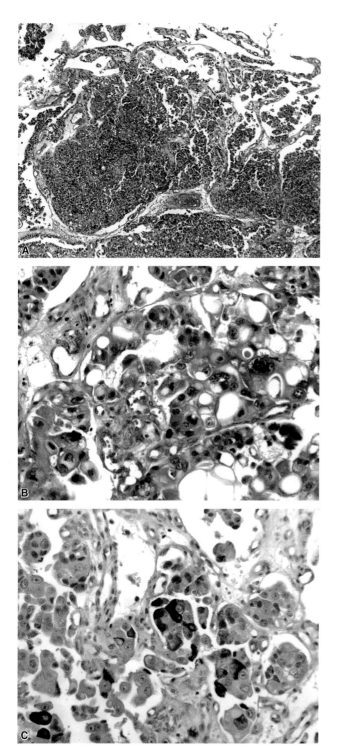

Figure 13-16   Hepatoid adenocarcinoma (A and B) with positive α-fetoprotein staining (C).

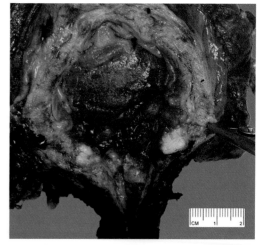

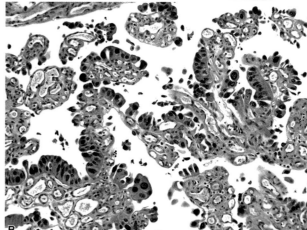

Figure 13-17   Clear cell adenocarcinoma of the bladder. Gross (A) and microscopic appearance (B).

Clear Cell Adenocarcinoma

Clear cell adenocarcinoma is composed of papillary and tubular structures with cytologic features identical to its counterpart in female genital tract.[40-43] It is very rare in the bladder, and only slightly more common in the urethra. Patients are typically females who present with hematuria or dysuria. Occasionally, clear cell adenocarcinoma has been associated with endometriosis or müllerianosis; occurrence in a bladder diverticulum has been reported. Recent molecular genetic data suggest that clear cell adenocarcinoma is probably urothelial in origin.[40]

Macroscopically, clear cell adenocarcinoma is often solid, nodular, or papillary, located in the trigone or posterior wall (Fig. 13-17). Microscopically, it invariably has a tubular component, often with cystic dilatation

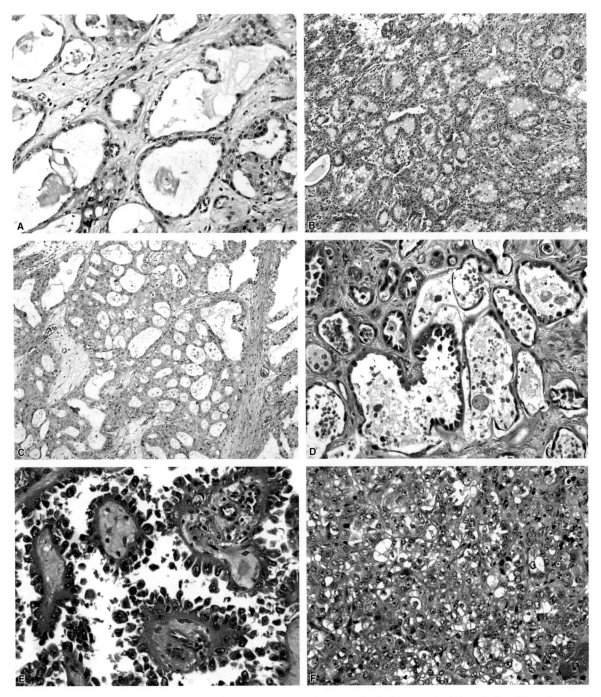

Figure 13-18   Clear cell adenocarcinoma. Various patterns can be seen, including cystic (A), tubular (B), microcystic (C), tubulocystic (D), papillary (E), and solid (F) patterns.

(Figs. 13-17 to 13-22). The lining cells are flat, cuboidal, or columnar; characteristic "hobnail" cells are at least focally present. There is typically significant nuclear pleomorphism with frequent mitotic figures. The cytoplasm is clear due to abundant glycogen and focal cytoplasmic and luminal mucin.

Clear cell adenocarcinoma exhibits a distinctive histologic appearance, with a variety of architectural patterns, forming tubulocystic or papillary structures or growing in diffuse solid sheets. The tubules vary in size and may contain either basophilic or eosinophilic secretions. The papillae are generally small and their fibrovascular cores

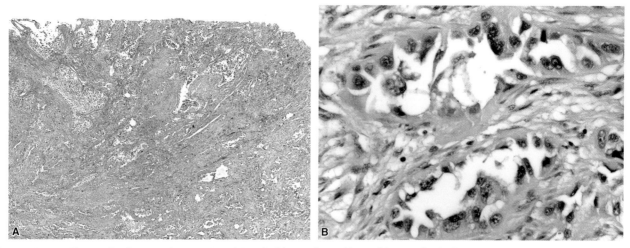

Figure 13-19   Clear cell adenocarcinoma (A and B). Bladder wall is infiltrated by small tubules (A). These tubules are lined by hobnail cells (B).

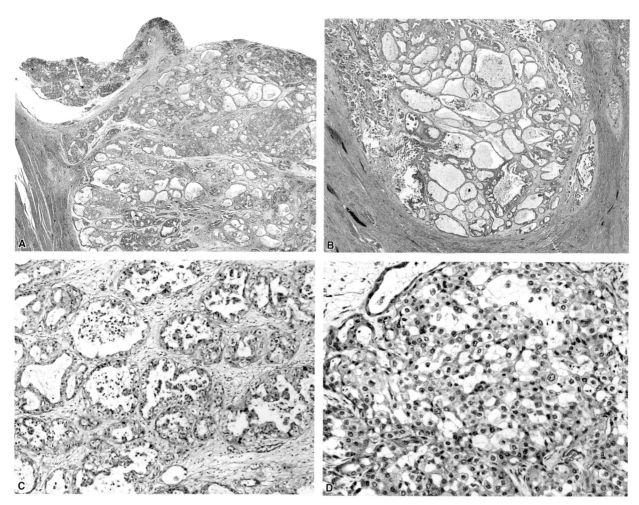

Figure 13-20   Clear cell adenocarcinoma (A to D).

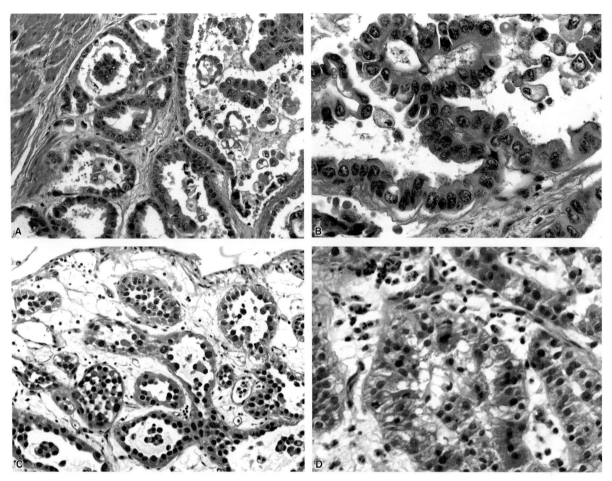

Figure 13-21   Clear cell adenocarcinoma (A to D).

may be extensively hyalinized. The tumor cells range from flat to cuboidal to columnar and they may have either clear or eosinophilic cytoplasm. The cytoplasm often contains glycogen. Hobnail cells are frequently seen. Cytologic atypia is usually moderate to severe, and high mitotic counts are frequently observed. In some cases, clear cell adenocarcinoma is associated with urothelial carcinoma, and rarely with adenocarcinoma, NOS.

The main differential diagnostic consideration for clear cell adenocarcinoma is nephrogenic metaplasia (nephrogenic adenoma) (**Fig. 13-23**; **Table 13-5**). Nephrogenic metaplasia is typically small, consisting of a papillary and tubular proliferation with minimal cytologic atypia, although a variant of nephrogenic metaplasia with cytologic atypia has been reported.[44] A clinical history of trauma or instrumentation may also be helpful in identifying nephrogenic metaplasia. Several immunohistochemical stains have been evaluated for utility in making the distinction between clear cell adenocarcinoma and nephrogenic metaplasia, but only p53 and MIB1 appear useful, with at most focal p53 staining and MIB1 counts of less than 14 per 200 cells in nephrogenic metaplasia and

strong p53 staining and MIB1 counts of greater than 32 per 200 cells in clear cell adenocarcinoma.[45] However, p53 nuclear accumulation (up to 20%), increased MIB1 labeling index (up to 5%), and aneuploid DNA patterns have been observed in atypical nephrogenic metaplasia.[44] All cases of atypical nephrogenic metaplasia display positive immunoreactivity for high molecular weight cytokeratin (34βE12), CK7, and EMA.[44] In contrast to atypical nephrogenic metaplasia, clear cell carcinomas will typically display greater cytologic atypia, a significant mitotic rate, and necrosis.[45] Clear cell adenocarcinoma of the urinary is positive for both CK7 and CK20.[40] Positive α-methylacyl-CoA racemase (AMACR/P504S) immunoreactivity for both clear cell adenocarcinoma and nephrogenic metaplasia has been noted.[40,46] CD10 is focally positive in clear cell adenocarcinoma.[40]

The other differential diagnostic considerations include clear cell variant of urothelial carcinoma, metastatic clear cell renal carcinoma, metastatic clear cell adenocarcinoma of female genital tract, and in males, prostatic adenocarcinoma secondarily involving the bladder (**Fig. 13-24**, **Table 13-6**). Renal cell carcinoma rarely metastasizes to

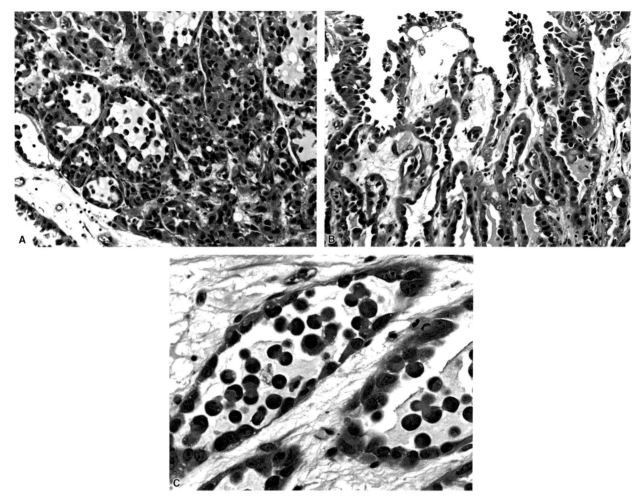

Figure 13-22   Clear cell adenocarcinoma (A to C).

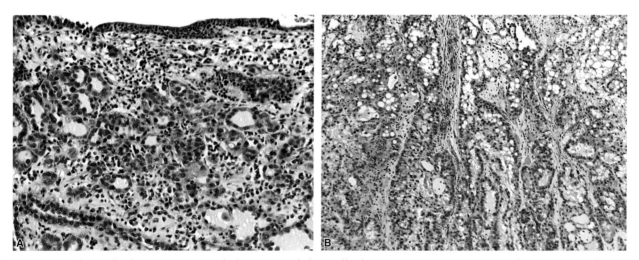

Figure 13-23   Clear cell adenocarcinoma. Tubular pattern of clear cell adenocarcinoma may mimic nephrogenic metaplasia (A). Deeper portion of the same tumor shows typical morphology of clear cell adenocarcinoma (B).

Table 13-5   Differential Diagnosis of Atypical Nephrogenic Metaplasia and Clear Cell Adenocarcinoma[a]

Characteristics	Atypical Nephrogenic Metaplasia	Clear Cell Adenocarcinoma
Gender	Male predominance (male-to-female ratio, 3 : 1)	Female predominance (male-to-female ratio, 1 : 2)
Mean age (years)	62	58
Clinical presentation	Hematuria and voiding symptoms	Hematuria and voiding symptoms
Biological behavior	Benign	Aggressive
Location	No apparent predilection	Predilection for urethra
Size	Small	Large
Microscopic findings		
Necrosis	Absent	Often present (53%)
Mitotic figures	Absent or inconspicuous	Easily identifiable
Stromal edema	Common	Uncommon
Luminal mucin	Common	Common
Clear cell change	May be seen	Common
Hobnail cells	Common	Common
Infiltrative growth	Usually absent	Present
Psammoma bodies	Absent	May be seen
Inflammation	Invariably present	May be present
Cytologic atypia		
Nuclear enlargement	Present	Present
Nuclear hyperchromasia	Present	Present
Prominent nucleoli	Present	Present
Nuclear pleomorphism	Minimal	Present
Immunostaining[b]		
PSA	Negative	Negative
34βE12	Positive	Positive (occasionally negative)
Cytokeratin 7	Positive	Positive
Cytokeratin 20	Negative	Positive
EMA	Positive	Positive
AMACR (P504S)	Often positive	Often positive
MIB labeling index	<5%	Often >15%
p53	Occasional positive	Positive
DNA ploidy	Aneuploid pattern may be seen	Unknown

Source: Modified from Ref. 44, with permission.
[a]Nuclear pleomorphism is more pronounced in clear cell adenocarcinoma.
[b]PSA, prostate-specific antigen; 34βE12, high molecular weight cytokeratin; EMA, epithelial membrane antigen; AMACR, α-methylacyl-CoA racemase.

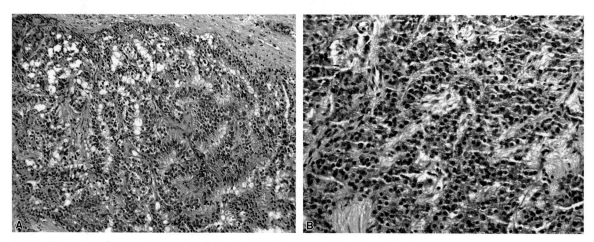

Figure 13-24   Prostatic adenocarcinoma involving the bladder may mimic clear cell adenocarcinoma (A). Immunostaining for PSA is strongly positive (B).

Table 13-6 Differentiating Clinicopathologic Characteristics of Nephrogenic Adenoma (Nephrogenic Metaplasia), Clear Cell Adenocarcinoma, and Prostatic Adenocarcinoma[a]

Nephrogenic adenoma (NA)	Male predilection; minimal cytologic atypia (limited to nuclear enlargement/hyperchromasia and prominent nucleoli in atypical NA); absence of pleomorphism; edematous, inflammatory stroma; infrequent mitotic figures; small to microscopic size; circumscribed growth (may be intermixed with superficial muscle fibers); confinement to lamina propria; absence of necrosis; less frequent abundant clear cytoplasm; minimal, focal p53 staining (up to 20% in atypical NA); Ki67 index <5%; PAX2 positive; negative for PSA
Clear cell adenocarcinoma	Female predilection; significant tumor size; greater cytologic atypia; necrosis; significant mitotic rate; strong p53 staining; Ki67 index >15%; lack of PSA or PSAP staining
Prostatic adenocarcinoma	Male; positivity for PSA and/or PSAP; lacking mixed tubular–papillary components of NA (except in ductal-type prostatic adenocarcinoma); negative for PAX2

[a]Notably, expression of racemase (AMACR/P504S) may be present in all three of these entities.

the bladder and should be excluded; recognition of the typical sinusoidal vascular pattern, lack of tubular differentiation, absence of mucin, and clinical features should resolve this problem. In addition to the immunostaining characteristics noted previously, clear cell adenocarcinoma may show positive staining for CEA and CD15 (LeuM1), but is negative for estrogen and progesterone receptors; these stains may be helpful in the differential. Of note, positivity for AMACR (P504S), a marker commonly used in diagnosis of prostate cancer, may be seen in clear cell adenocarcinoma, representing a potential pitfall. Similarly, nephrogenic metaplasia may also show positivity (**Tables 13-5** and **13-6**).[40,46] Therefore, awareness of these findings is crucial to avoid misinterpretation.

The histogenesis of clear cell adenocarcinoma of the bladder is uncertain. Sung and his colleagues integrated molecular genetic evaluation by fluorescence in situ hybridization (FISH) and X chromosome inactivation with conventional morphological and immunohistochemical analyses in 12 patients with clear cell adenocarcinomas in the urinary tract.[47] Concurrent urothelial carcinoma or urothelial carcinoma in situ were present in six cases (50%) and foci of cystitis glandularis were observed in four cases (33%) (**Fig. 13-25**). Neither intestinal metaplasia nor a müllerian component was identified in any case. Cytoplasmic expression of AMACR was demonstrable in 10 of 12 tumors (83%) (**Fig. 13-26**). Moderate to diffuse immunostaining for CK7 was identified in all 12 tumors (100%), whereas only three of 12 (25%) tumors showed positive immunostaining for CK20. Focal uroplakin III staining was seen in six of 12 tumors (50%). In five cases (42%), focal to moderate CD10 immunoreactivity was observed. Immunostains for OCT4 and CDX-2 were completely negative in all tumors. In UroVysion FISH assays, all tumors displayed chromosomal alterations similar to those commonly found in urothelial carcinoma (**Fig. 13-26**). Identical patterns of nonrandom X chromosome inactivation in concurrent clear cell adenocarcinoma and urothelial

neoplasia were identified in two informative female cases (**Fig. 13-27**). These findings support a urothelial origin for most clear cell adenocarcinomas of the urinary tract, despite their morphologic resemblance to certain müllerian-derived tumors of the female genital tract.[47]

Adenocarcinoma with Mixed Patterns

The mixed pattern refers to adenocarcinoma composed of two or more patterns. The specific patterns should be mentioned in the pathology report.

Urachal Adenocarcinoma

Adenocarcinoma sometimes develops in the setting of urachal remnants, the residual tissue from the embryonic allantoic stalk connecting the umbilicus and bladder (**Fig. 13-28**). Although adenocarcinoma is the characteristic malignancy associated with an urachal remnant, this situation represents only a subset of primary bladder adenocarcinoma, which is already a rare tumor in comparison to urothelial carcinoma.[48–57] Such urachal remnants are reported to occur most frequently in the bladder dome or posterior wall, with adenocarcinoma most frequently developing in the fifth and sixth decades of life, approximately 10 years younger than patients with other primary adenocarcinoma of the bladder.

Urachal adenocarcinoma occurs slightly more often in men, with a ratio of 2:1. Presenting symptoms include hematuria, irritative voiding symptoms, abdominal pain, suprapubic mass, and occasional mucinuria.

Macroscopically, urachal adenocarcinoma is often extensive, infiltrating the bladder wall musculature and extending superiorly toward the abdominal wall in the space of Retzius. The cancer may be gelatinous, depending on the amount of mucin production, and the mucosal surface is often ulcerated. The cancer may be partially or extensively

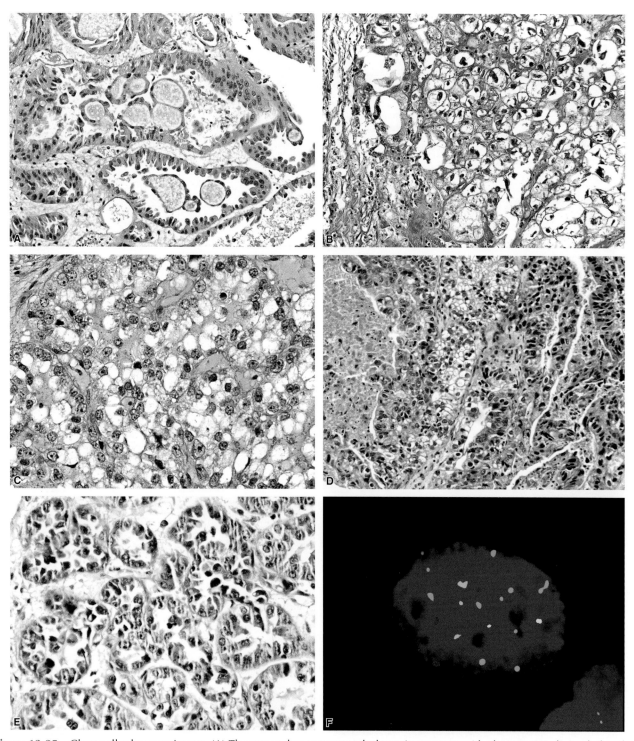

Figure 13-25 Clear cell adenocarcinoma. (A) The tumor demonstrates tubulocystic structure with characteristic lining hobnail cells. (B) Polygonal tumor cells reveals abundant clear cytoplasm. (C) Solid diffuse growth of clear cell adenocarcinoma, exhibiting marked cellular pleomorphism, nucleolar prominence, and mitotical activity. (D) Tumor necrosis is observed within the cystic space. The solid and tubular tumor components shows clear or eosinophilic cytoplasm. (E) Typical tubular formation with inner lining pleomorphic neoplastic cells. (F) A typical tumor cell from clear cell adenocarcinoma of bladder demonstrates chromosomal abnormalities detected by fluorescence in situ hybridization. The cell shows gaining of chromosomes 7 (green) and 17 (aqua), but with normal copy numbers of chromosomes 3 (red) and 9p21 (gold).

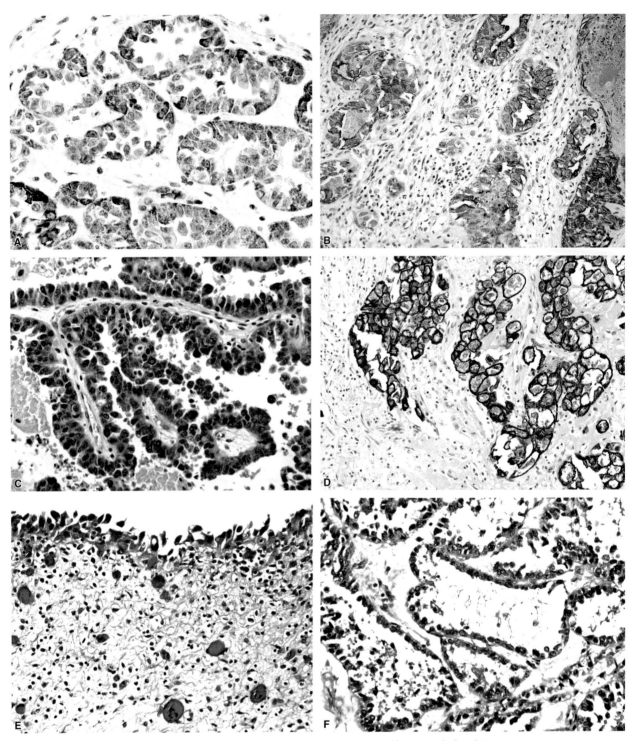

Figure 13-26 Clear cell adenocarcinoma. (A) Tumor cells are positively stained by α-methylacyl-CoA racemase, representing cytoplasmic staining in the tubular components. (B) Diffuse membranous and cytoplasmic expression of CD10. (C) Positive uroplakin III expression in clear cell adenocarcinoma. (D) Cytokeratin 7 is strongly positive. (E and F) A female patient presented with concurrent urothelial carcinoma in situ (E) and clear cell adenocarcinoma (F).

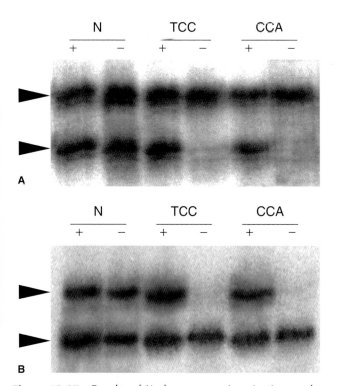

A

B

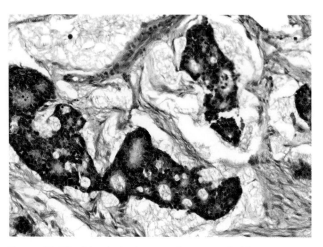

Figure 13-28   Urachal adenocarcinoma, colloid type.

Figure 13-27   Results of X chromosome inactivation analysis in two female patients in whom clear cell adenocarcinoma coexisted with urothelial carcinoma (A) or urothelial carcinoma in situ (B). Concordant patterns of nonrandom inactivation of X chromosome are identified in both components (clear cell adenocarcinoma and urothelial neoplasia) in both patients. Arrows, allelic bands; N, normal control tissue; TCC, urothelial (transitional cell) carcinoma component; CIS, urothelial carcinoma in situ component; CCA, clear cell adenocarcinoma component; —, without Hha1 endonuclease digestion; +, after Hha1 endonuclease digestion. (From Ref. 40; with permission.)

calcified.[56] Grossly, mucin production may be evident, and microscopically, tumors have been classified similarly to bladder adenocarcinoma in general, with signet ring cell, mucinous, NOS types, and so on.[57] Mucinous tumors are most common in this location.

Urachal adenocarcinoma may be associated with cystitis cystica and cystitis glandularis. The cystitis cystica or cystitis glandularis must show no dysplastic changes; when these dysplastic changes of the mucosa or presence of dysplastic intestinal metaplasia are present, this tends to exclude an urachal origin.[19] Urachal adenocarcinoma should also be distinguished from direct extension or metastasis of colorectal carcinoma (see also **Chapters 13, 23, and 27**).

See **Chapter 27** for further discussion.

REFERENCES

1. Williamson SR, Lopez-Beltran A, Montironi R, Cheng L. Glandular lesions of the urinary bladder: clinical significance and differential diagnosis. *Histopathology* 2011;58:811–34.

2. Lopez-Beltran A, Cheng L, Andersson L, Brausi M, de Matteis A, Montironi R, Sesterhenn I, van det Kwast KT, Mazerolles C. Preneoplastic non-papillary lesions and conditions of the urinary bladder: an update based on the Ancona International Consultation. *Virchows Arch* 2002;440:3–11.

3. Cheng L, Lopez-Beltran A, MacLennan GT. Neoplasms of the

Urinary Bladder. Philadelphia: Elsevier/Mosby, 2008.

4. Morton MJ, Zhang S, Lopez-Beltran A, MacLennan GT, Eble JN, Montironi R, Sung MT, Tan PH, Zheng S, Zhou H, Cheng L. Telomere shortening and chromosomal abnormalities in intestinal metaplasia of the urinary bladder. *Clin Cancer Res* 2007;13:6232–6.

4b. Corica FA, Husmann DA, Churchill BM, Young RH, Pacelli A, Lopez-Beltran A, Bostwick DG. Intestinal metaplasia is not a strong risk factor for bladder cancer: study of 53 cases with long-term follow-up. *Urology* 1997;50:427–31.

5. Sung MT, Lopez-Beltran A, Eble JN, MacLennan GT, Tan PH, Montironi R, Jones TD, Ulbright TM, Blair JE, Cheng L. Divergent pathway of intestinal metaplasia and cystitis glandularis of the urinary bladder. *Mod Pathol* 2006;19:1395–1401.

6. Cheng L, Montironi R, Bostwick DG. Villous adenoma of the urinary tract: a report of 23 cases, including 8 with coexistent adenocarcinoma. *Am J Surg Pathol* 1999;23:764–71.

7. Guo CC, Fine SW, Epstein JI. Noninvasive squamous lesions in the urinary bladder: a clinicopathologic analysis of 29 cases. *Am J Surg Pathol* 2006;30:883–91.

8. Lopez-Beltran A, Jimenez RE, Montironi R, Patriarca C, Blanca A, Menendez C, Algaba F, Cheng L. Flat urothelial carcinoma in situ of the bladder with glandular differentiation. *Hum Pathol* 2011;42:1653–9.

9. Miller JS, Epstein JI. Noninvasive urothelial carcinoma of the bladder with glandular differentiation: report of 24 cases. *Am J Surg Pathol* 2009;33:1241–8.

10. Chan TY, Epstein JI. In Situ adenocarcinoma of the bladder. *Am J Surg Pathol* 2001;25:892–9.

11. Cheng L, Lopez-Beltran A, MacLennan GT, Montironi R, Bostwick DG. Neoplasms of the urinary bladder. In: Bostwick DG, Cheng L, eds. Urologic Surgical Pathology, 2nd ed. Philadelphia: Elsevier/Mosby, 2008:259–352.

12. Grignon DJ, Ro JY, Ayala AG, Johnson DE, Ordonez NG. Primary adenocarcinoma of the urinary bladder. A clinicopathologic analysis of 72 cases. *Cancer* 1991;67:2165–72.

13. Lopez-Beltran A, Croghan GA, Croghan I, Matilla A, Gaeta JF. Prognostic factors in bladder cancer. A pathologic, immunohistochemical, and DNA flow-cytometric study. *Am J Clin Pathol* 1994;102:109–14.

14. Bullock PS, Thoni DE, Murphy WM. The significance of colonic mucosa (intestinal metaplasia) involving the urinary tract. *Cancer* 1987;59:2086–90.

15. Lam KY, Ma L, Nicholls J. Adenocarcinoma arising in a diverticulum of the urinary bladder. *Pathology* 1992,24:40 2.

16. Grignon DJ, Ro JY, Ayala AG, Johnson DE. Primary signet-ring cell carcinoma of the urinary bladder. *Am J Clin Pathol* 1991;95:13–20.

17. Bollito ER, Pacchioni D, Lopez-Beltran A, Volante M, Terrone C, Casetta G, Mari M, DePompa R, Cappia S, Papotti M. Immunohistochemical study of neuroendocrine differentiation in primary glandular lesions and tumors of the urinary bladder. *Anal Quant Cytol Histol* 2005;27:218–24.

18. Edge SB, Byrd DR, Compton CC, Fritz AG, Greene FL, Trotti A. American Joint Committee on Cancer Staging Manual, 7th ed. New York: Springer, 2010.

19. Young RH, Bostwick DG. Florid cystitis glandularis of intestinal type with mucin extravasation: a mimic of adenocarcinoma. *Am J Surg Pathol* 1996;20:1462–8.

20. Jacobs LB, Brooks JD, Epstein JI. Differentiation of colonic metaplasia from adenocarcinoma of urinary bladder. *Hum Pathol* 1997;28: 1152–7.

21. Emerson RE, Cheng L. Immunohistochemical markers in the evaluation of tumors of the urinary bladder: a review. *Anal Quant Cytol Histol* 2005;27:301–16.

22. McKenney JK, Amin MB. The role of immunohistochemistry in the diagnosis of urinary bladder neoplasms. *Semin Diagn Pathol* 2005;22:69–87.

23. Werling RW, Yaziji H, Bacchi CE, Gown AM. CDX2, a highly sensitive and specific marker of adenocarcinomas of intestinal origin: and immunohistochemical survey fo 476 primary and metastatic carcinomas. *Am J Surg Pathol* 2003;27:303–10.

24. Kaimaktchiev V, Terracciano L, Tornillo L, Spichtin H, Stoios D, Bundi M, Korcheva V, Mirlacher M, Loda M, Sauter G, Corless CL. The homeobox intestinal differentiation factor CDX2 is selectively expressed in gastrointestinal adenocarcinomas. *Mod Pathol* 2004;17:1392–9.

25. Tamboli P, Mohsin SK, Hailemariam S, Amin MB. Colonic adenocarcinoma metastatic to the urinary tract versus primary tumors of the urinary tract with glandular differentiation: a report of 7 cases and investigation using a limited immunohistochemical panel. *Arch Pathol Lab Med* 2002;126:1057–63.

26. Wang HL, Lu DW, Yerian LM, Alsikafi N, Steinberg G, Hart J, Yang XJ. Immunohistochemical distinction between primary adenocarcinoma of the bladder and secondary colorectal adenocarcinoma. *Am J Surg Pathol* 2001;25:1380–7.

27. Fish DE, Rose DS, Adamson A, Goldin RD, Witherow RO. Neoplastic Paneth cells in a mucinous adenocarcinoma of the bladder. *Br J Urol* 1994;73:105–6.

28. Muthuphei MN. Primary signet-ring cell carcinoma of the bladder. A case report. *S Afr J Surg* 1994;32:107–8.

29. Yorukoglu K, Gencbay A, Cakalagaoglu F, Kirkali Z. Primary signet-ring cell carcinoma of the bladder. *Br J Urol* 1994;73:210–1.

30. Holmang S, Borghede G, Johansson SL. Primary signet ring cell carcinoma of the bladder: a report on 10 cases. *Scand J Urol Nephrol* 1997;31:145–8.

31. Weiss AM, Jeandel R, Lugagne-Delpon PM, Kamalodine T, Barbanel C. [Primary signet ring adenocarcinoma of a diverted neurogenic bladder]. *Ann Pathol* 1995;15:131–3.

32. Torenbeek R, Koot RA, Blomjous CE, De Bruin PC, Newling DW, Meijer CJ. Primary signet-ring cell carcinoma of the urinary bladder. *Histopathology* 1996;28:33–40.

33. Thomas AA, Stephenson AJ, Campbell SC, Jones JS, Hansel DE. Clinicopathologic features and utility of immunohistochemical markers in signet-ring cell adenocarcinoma of the bladder. *Hum Pathol* 2009;40: 108–16.

34. Del Sordo R, Bellezza G, Colella R, Mameli MG, Sidoni A, Cavaliere A. Primary signet-ring cell carcinoma of the urinary bladder: a clinicopathologic and immunohistochemical study of 5 cases. *Appl Immunohistochem Mol Morphol* 2009;17:18–22.

35. Lopez-Beltran A, Amin MB, Oliveira PS, Montironi R, Algaba F, McKenney JK, de Torres I, Mazerolles C, Wang M, Cheng L. Urothelial carcinoma of the bladder, lipid cell variant: clinicopathologic findings and LOH analysis. *Am J Surg Pathol* 2010;34:371–6.

36. Lopez-Beltran A, Luque RJ, Quintero A, Requena MJ, Montironi R. Hepatoid adenocarcinoma of the urinary bladder. *Virchows Arch* 2003;442:381–7.

37. Sinard J, Macleay L Jr, Melamed J. Hepatoid adenocarcinoma in the urinary bladder. Unusual localization of a newly recognized tumor type. *Cancer* 1994;73:1919–25.

38. Yamada K, Fujioka Y, Ebihara Y, Kiriyama I, Suzuki H, Akimoto M. Alpha-fetoprotein producing undifferentiated carcinoma of the bladder. *J Urol* 1994;152:958–60.

39. Lertprasertsuke N, Tsutsumi Y. Neuroendocrine carcinoma of the urinary bladder: case report and review

of the literature. *Jpn J Clin Oncol* 1991;21:203–10.

40. Sung MT, Zhang S, MacLennan GT, Lopez-Beltran A, Montironi R, Wang M, Tan PH, Cheng L. Histogenesis of clear cell adenocarcinoma in the urinary tract: evidence of urothelial origin. *Clin Cancer Res* 2008;14:1947–55.

41. Schultz RE, Bloch MJ, Tomaszewski JE, Brooks JS, Hanno PM. Mesonephric adenocarcinoma of the bladder. *J Urol* 1984;132:263–5.

42. Young RH, Scully R. Clear cell adenocarcinoma of the bladder and urethra: a report of three cases and review of the literature. *Am J Surg Pathol* 1985;9:816–26.

43. Meis JM, Ayala AG, Johnson DE. Adenocarcinoma of the urethra in women. A clinicopathologic study. *Cancer* 1987;60:1038–52.

44. Cheng L, Cheville JC, Sebo TJ, Eble JN, Bostwick DG. Atypical nephrogenic metaplasia of the urinary tract: a precursor lesion? *Cancer* 2000;88:853–61.

45. Gilcrease MZ, Delgado R, Vuitch F, Albores-Saavedra J. Clear cell adenocarcinoma and nephrogenic adenoma of the urethra and urinary bladder: a histopathologic and immunohistochemical comparison. *Hum Pathol* 1998;29.1451–6.

46. Gupta A, Wang IIL, Policarpio-Nicolas ML, Tretiakova MS, Papavero V, Pins MR, Jiang Z, Humphrey PA, Cheng L, Yang XJ. Expression of alpha-methylacyl-coenzyme A racemase in nephrogenic adenoma. *Am J Surg Pathol* 2004;28:1224–9.

47. Sung MT, Zhang S, MacLennan GT, Lopez-Beltran A, Montironi R, Wang M, Tan PH, Cheng L. Histogenesis of clear cell adenocarcinoma in the urinary tract: evidence of urothelial origin. *Clin Cancer Res* 2008;14:1947–55.

48. Loening SA, Jacobo E, Hawtrey CE, Culp DA. Adenocarcinoma of the urachus. *J Urol* 1978;119:68–71.

49. Sheldon CA, Clayman RV, Gonzalez R, Williams RD, Fraley EE. Malignant urachal lesions. *J Urol* 1984;131:1–8.

50. Ghazizadeh M, Yamamoto S, Kurokawa K. Clinical features of urachal carcinoma in Japan: review of 157 patients. *Urol Res* 1983;11:235–8.

51. Mattelaer P, Wolff JM, Jung P, W IJ, Jakse G. Adenocarcinoma of the urachus: 3 case reports and a review of the literature. *Acta Urol Belg* 1997;65:63–7.

52. Gopalan A, Sharp DS, Fine SW, Tickoo SK, Herr HW, Reuter VE, Olgac S. Urachal carcinoma: a clinicopathologic analysis of 24 cases with outcome correlation. *Am J Surg Pathol* 2009;33:659–68.

53. Wright JL, Porter MP, Li CI, Lange PH, Lin DW. Differences in survival among patients with urachal and nonurachal adenocarcinomas of the bladder. *Cancer* 2006;107:721–8.

54. Ashley RA, Inman BA, Sebo TJ, Leibovich BC, Blute ML, Kwon ED, Zincke H. Urachal carcinoma: clinicopathologic features and long-term outcomes of an aggressive malignancy. *Cancer* 2006;107:712–20.

55. Herr HW, Bochner BH, Sharp D, Dalbagni G, Reuter VE. Urachal carcinoma: contemporary surgical outcomes. *J Urol* 2007;178:74–8.

56. Lopez-Beltran A, Nogales F, Donne CH, Sayag JL. Adenocarcinoma of the urachus showing extensive calcification and stromal osseous metaplasia. *Urol Int* 1994;53:110–13.

57. Johnson DE, Hodge GB, Abdul-Karim FW, Ayala AG. Urachal carcinoma. *Urology* 1985;26:218–21.

Chapter 14

Squamous Cell Carcinoma and Other Squamous Lesions

Bladder Pathology, First Edition. Liang Cheng, Antonio Lopez-Beltran, David G. Bostwick.
© 2012 Wiley-Blackwell. Published 2012 by John Wiley & Sons, Inc.

Squamous Cell Carcinoma

Epidemiology, Clinical Features, and Risk Factors

Squamous cell carcinoma of the bladder is uncommon.[1-12] The prevalence of squamous cell carcinoma of the bladder is widely variable around the world, and is highest in areas that are endemic for schistosomiasis, accounting for up to 73% of bladder cancers in those countries. In nonendemic areas such as the United States and Europe, squamous cell carcinoma comprises 1% to 7% of bladder cancers. Patients range in age from 30 years to 90 years (mean, 66 years); it occurs at a younger age when associated with schistosomiasis. Squamous cell carcinoma is more common in men than in women. The male-to-female ratio is approximately 2:1. Risk factors associated with the development of squamous cell carcinoma include tobacco smoking, chronic nonspecific urinary tract infections, and schistosomiasis.[13-18]

Patients typically present with hematuria and lower urinary tract irritative symptoms, and the majority has advanced cancer at the time of diagnosis. Often, there is a long history of bladder irritation caused by infections, calculi, indwelling catheters, intermittent self-catheterization, or urinary retention. Some patients have underlying neurogenic bladder or bladder diverticulum.[19-22] Keratinizing squamous metaplasia may be an important risk factor for the development of squamous cell carcinoma, with cancer occurring from 3 months to 30 years after the diagnosis of metaplasia (mean, 12 years).[23] Squamous metaplasia is present in the adjacent epithelium in 17% to 60% of cases not associated with schistosomiasis.[23] Rarely, squamous cell carcinoma induces hypercalcemia.[24]

Morphologic changes that appear to increase the risk of developing squamous cell carcinoma have been documented. Some of the best characterized changes include the presence of keratinizing squamous metaplasia, squamous dysplasia, and squamous carcinoma in situ of the bladder mucosa,[25] as well as the presence of *Schistosoma* eggs within the bladder wall. Recently, additional mucosal changes that occur either concurrently or preceding the development of invasive squamous cell carcinoma have been reported.[7,26] Verrucous squamous hyperplasia has been documented in several series as a potential precursor lesion in the development of this cancer type. Morphologically, this lesion resembles its counterpart in the oral cavity, including the presence of repetitive upward spiking of the mucosa that resembles "church spires," hyperkeratosis, parakeratosis, and elongation of the rete pegs.[7,26]

Prognostic Features

The most important prognostic indicator for squamous cell carcinoma is pathologic stage. Squamous cell carcinoma of

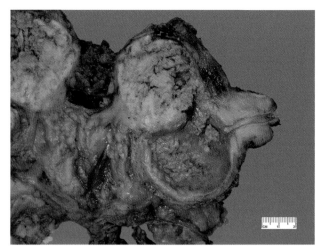

Figure 14-1 Squamous cell carcinoma of the bladder, like urothelial carcinoma, is staged using the American Joint Committee on Cancer tumor, node, metastasis (AJCC TNM) system.

the bladder, like urothelial carcinoma, is staged using the American Joint Committee on Cancer tumor, lymph node, metastasis (AJCC TNM) system.[27] In Eldobky et al.'s study of 154 patients, overall five-year survival was 56%; it was 67% for those patients with organ confined tumor (pT1, pT2) and 19% for nonorgan confined (pT3, pT4) cancers.[28]

The biological behavior of squamous cell carcinoma is somewhat different from that of urothelial carcinoma. In most patients, death results from local recurrence rather than metastatic cancer, and metastases show a striking predilection for bone.[8,29-31] Five-year survival after surgery varies from 35% to 48%. Patients undergoing radical surgery appear to have an improved survival compared to radiation therapy and/or chemotherapy. It is known that squamous cell carcinoma is more resistant than conventional urothelial carcinoma to radiotherapy and chemotherapy.

Macroscopic Pathology

Macroscopically, squamous cell carcinoma is usually bulky, polypoid, solid, and necrotic, often filling the bladder lumen, although it may be flat, irregular, ulcerated, and infiltrating (**Figs. 14-1** and **14-2**). Necrotic material and keratin debris are usually present on the surface. There is an apparent propensity for the lateral wall and trigone.

Microscopic Pathology

Squamous cell carcinoma is defined as a malignant neoplasm that shows a pure squamous cell phenotype.[12] Invasive squamous cell carcinoma of the bladder displays a range of differentiation, from well-differentiated to poorly differentiated, with a histologic spectrum that can vary from

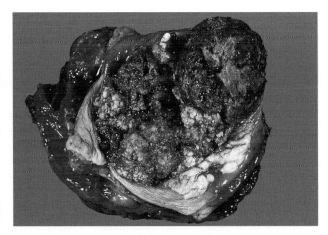

Figure 14-2   Squamous cell carcinoma of the bladder.

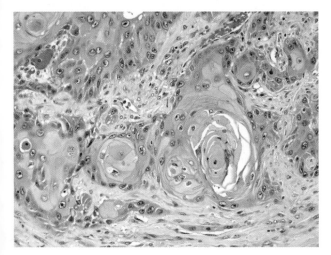

Figure 14-3   Squamous cell carcinoma of the bladder.

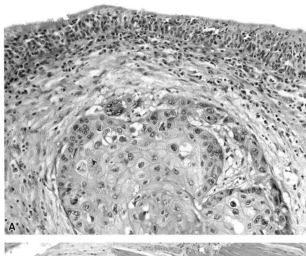

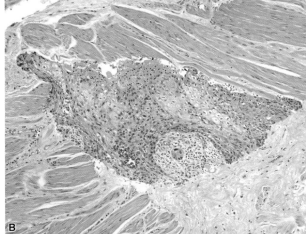

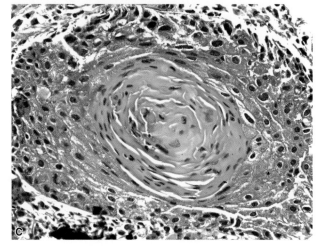

Figure 14-4   Squamous cell carcinoma of the bladder (A to C).

well-defined islands of squamous cells with keratinization, prominent intercellular bridges, and minimal nuclear pleomorphism, to tumors exhibiting marked nuclear pleomorphism and only focal evidence of squamous differentiation.

Histologic grading is similar to that at other sites and is based on the extent of keratinization and degree of nuclear pleomorphism using a three-tiered system (grades 1, 2, and 3) (Figs. 14-3 to 14-6).[8,10,32] Grades 1, 2, and 3 squamous cell carcinoma corresponds to well-differentiated, moderately differentiated, and poorly differentiated tumor, respectively. Well-differentiated squamous cell carcinoma consists of circumscribed islands of squamous cells with extensive keratinization, prominent intercellular bridges, and minimal nuclear pleomorphism. Poorly differentiated cancer displays marked nuclear pleomorphism and focal evidence of squamous differentiation; moderately differentiated squamous cell carcinoma lies in between. Grade correlates with stage and patient outcome. The five-year survival for grades

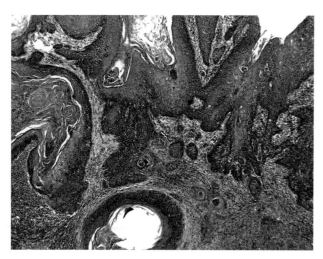

Figure 14-5   Squamous cell carcinoma of the bladder.

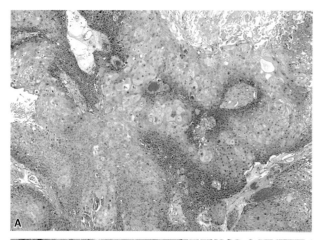

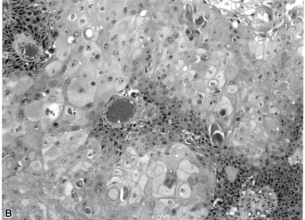

Figure 14-6   Squamous cell carcinoma of the bladder (A and B).

1, 2, and 3 squamous cell carcinoma was 62%, 52%, and 35%, respectively, in one study.[8]

Morphologic variations may be present in a subset of cases and include clear cell change, spindled morphology, large squamous nest formation with central necrosis, and bizarre atypia often associated with giant tumor cells.[7] Common findings associated with the invasive squamous component can include the presence of desmoplastic reaction surrounding the carcinoma, giant cell reaction to keratin, perineural invasion, and angiolymphatic invasion.[7] Verrucous carcinoma and basaloid squamous cell carcinomas are rare and unique variants (see the discussion below). Squamous cell carcinoma may also arise in the setting of diverticulum (Fig. 14-7). Sarcomatoid transformation may also be seen (Fig. 14-8; see Chapter 16 for further discussion).

The major differential diagnostic consideration of squamous cell carcinoma is urothelial carcinoma with extensive squamous differentiation (Fig. 14-9; see Chapter 12 for further discussion). The diagnosis of squamous cell carcinoma of the bladder is reserved for pure tumors. In areas not endemic for schistosomiasis, such tumors should be studied carefully for a urothelial component, including urothelial carcinoma in situ; if found, the tumor is best classified as urothelial carcinoma with squamous differentiation. The presence of keratinizing squamous metaplasia, especially if associated with dysplasia, favors the diagnosis of squamous cell carcinoma. Condyloma acuminatum is also a consideration, but usually is easily distinguished by prominent koilocytotic changes.[33] Squamous papilloma of the bladder is extremely rare.

Secondary invasion of the bladder by squamous cell carcinoma of the cervix or other contiguous primary sites should be excluded. While squamous cell carcinoma is the most typical histology in the cervix, a squamous component is generally associated with urothelial carcinoma in primary bladder tumors. Correlation with clinical and pathologic findings is of paramount importance and thus is critical in any questionable case (see also Chapter 23).[34]

Schistosoma-associated Squamous Cell Carcinoma

Schistosomiasis is known to be associated with squamous cell carcinoma of the bladder (Figs. 14-10 and 14-11). Tumors arising in this setting are typically large, often filling the bladder lumen, and frequently polypoid or solid with visible necrosis and keratin debris; others are ulcerated infiltrating tumors. Histologically, the presence of keratinizing squamous metaplasia in the adjacent flat epithelium is relatively constant and may be associated with dysplasia or carcinoma in situ. The prevalence of associated squamous metaplasia in cases of squamous cell carcinoma of the bladder ranges from 17% to 60% and is widely variable

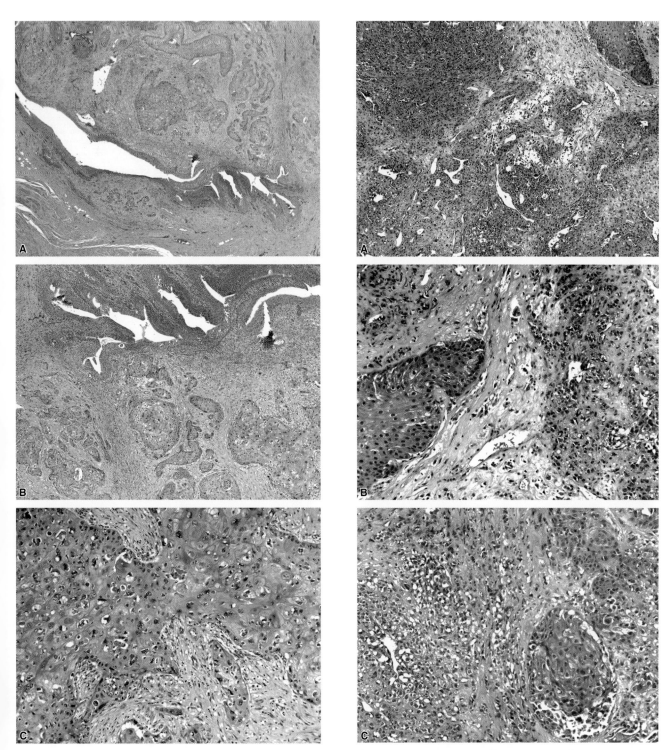

Figure 14-7 Squamous cell carcinoma arising from a diverticulum (A to C).

Figure 14-8 Squamous cell carcinoma with sarcomatoid transformation (A to C; from the same case).

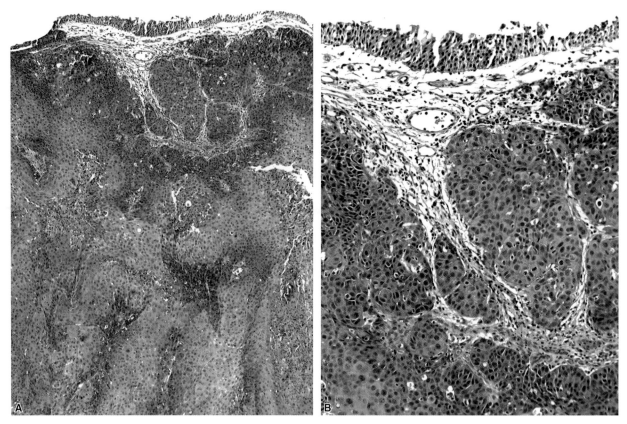

Figure 14-9 Urothelial carcinoma with squamous differentiation (A and B).

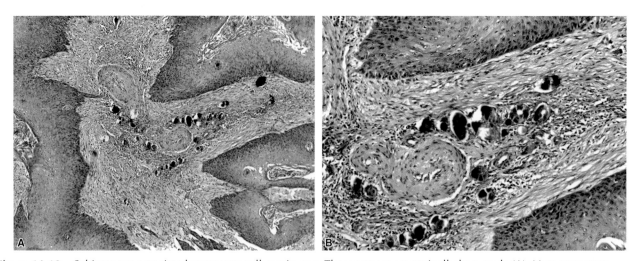

Figure 14-10 *Schistosoma*-associated squamous cell carcinoma. These tumors are typically low grade (A). Note numerous schistosomal eggs (B).

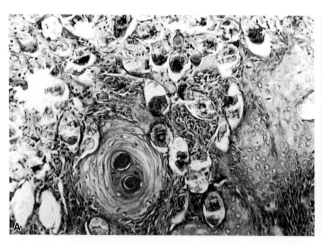
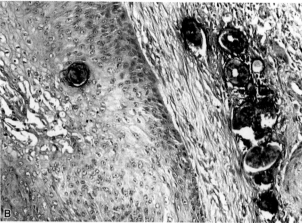

Figure 14-11   *Schistosoma*-associated squamous cell carcinoma (A and B).

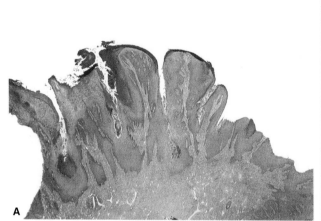
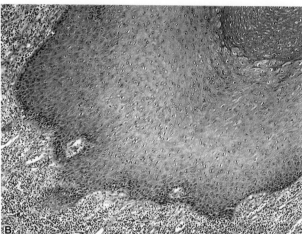

Figure 14-12   Verrucous squamous cell carcinoma. The tumor appears as broad exophytic fronds of squamous mucosa (A). The epithelium is remarkably well differentiated, with evidence of koilocytotic change. There is chronic inflammation at the interface with the stroma (B).

according to geographic location of the patient population. Similar to non–*Schistosoma*-associated squamous cell carcinoma, these tumors range from well-differentiated to poorly differentiated, but most commonly are well differentiated with prominent keratinization and intercellular bridge formation with minimal nuclear pleomorphism. Pathologic stage and lymph node status are significant prognostic and predictive factors, and pathologic grade according to the degree of keratinization and the degree of nuclear pleomorphism is also considered an important prognostic indicator. Radical surgical excision currently is the most widely used treatment option; neoadjuvant radiation has been reported to improve survival in aggressive tumors.

Verrucous Squamous Cell Carcinoma

Verrucous squamous cell carcinoma is a rare low grade, clinically indolent form of squamous cell carcinoma that is usually reported in association with schistosomiasis infection but has also been reported in patients from nonendemic areas.[29,33,35–38] Predisposing factors include recurrent cystitis, bladder diverticula, and especially schistosomiasis.[38] It is morphologically identical to its counterparts at other sites, including the oral cavity. It may appear grossly exophytic, papillary, or as a warty mass.

The tumor is composed of well-differentiated squamous mucosa with complex papillary, exophytic, and endophytic growth (**Figs. 14-12 to 14-15**). It usually has a pushing broad front invasion forming bulbous rete ridges. Cases of squamous carcinoma with verrucous features but which additionally have an infiltrative component have been described; it is recommended by the WHO (2004) not to diagnose such cases as verrucous carcinoma but as regular squamous cell carcinoma.

Sebaceous differentiation has been described in an unusual case, appearing as collections of carcinoembryonic

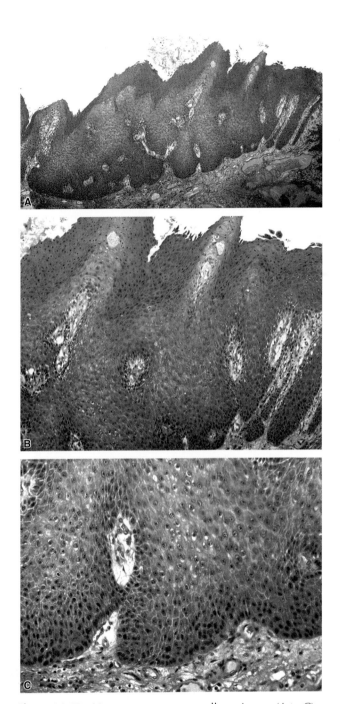

Figure 14-13   Verrucous squamous cell carcinoma (A to C).

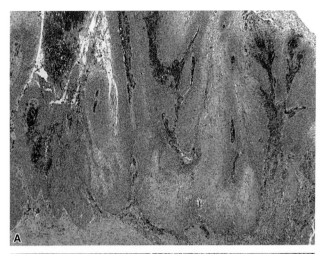

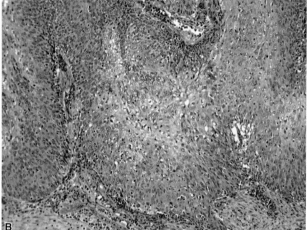

Figure 14-14   Verrucous squamous cell carcinoma.

antigen-immunoreactive clear cells with peculiar glandular spaces at the base.[39]

Verrucous squamous cell carcinoma in the bladder is associated with minimal risk of progression whether or not associated with schistosomiasis. A link to human papillomavirus (HPV) infection has not been established.[33] Local recurrence is frequent, but this cancer does not metastasize early (if ever) to regional lymph nodes. Verrucous

squamous cell carcinoma may undergo transformation to aggressive anaplastic carcinoma after radiation therapy, so this treatment should be avoided.

Condyloma acuminatum is the most common and important differential diagnostic consideration (Table 14-1). Condyloma acuminatum is a squamous epithelial papillary growth that often displays koilocytosis characteristic of HPV infection. Cheng et al.[40] compared three cases of verrucous carcinoma to three cases of condyloma acuminatum and found that condyloma acuminatum contained HPV DNA. All cases of verrucous carcinoma were negative for HPV DNA, indicating that HPV infection does not play a role in the pathogenesis of verrucous carcinoma. Clinical history is helpful because condyloma acuminatum of the bladder is almost always associated with external genitalia lesions.

Basaloid Squamous Cell Carcinoma

Basaloid squamous cell carcinoma has recently been recognized in the urinary bladder, with one case reported.[41]

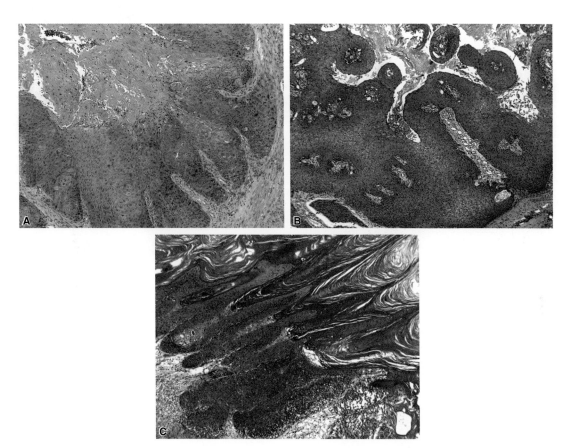

Figure 14-15 Verrucous squamous cell carcinoma (A to C).

Table 14-1 **Differential Diagnosis of Squamous Papilloma, Condyloma Acuminatum, and Verrucous Squamous Cell Carcinoma of the Urinary Bladder[a]**

	Squamous Papilloma	Condyloma Acuminatum	Verrucous Squamous Cell Carcinoma
Age (years)	62 (range, 32–82)	40 (range, 17–76)	66 (range, 43–83)
Gender (male-to-female)	1 : 6	1 : 1.6	1.2 : 1
Clinical history	Nonspecific	External genitalia condyloma or history of immunosuppression	Nonspecific
Clinical presentation	Irritative symptoms	Irritative symptoms	Irritative symptoms
Biological behavior	Rarely recurs	Aggressive	Aggressive
Location	No predilection	No predilection	No predilection
Extent	Small, solitary	Multiple, extensive	Diffuse, extensive
Histologic changes			
Architecture	Papillary	Papillary	Expansive and endophytic
Pushing margin	Absent	Absent	Present
Cytologic atypia	Usually not seen or mild	Usually not seen or mild	May be present
Stromal invasion	Absent	Absent	Present
p53 alteration	−/+	+	+
Human papillomavirus detection	−	+	−
DNA ploidy	Diploid	Aneuploid	Aneuploid

[a]+, usually positive; +/−, variable staining; −, usually negative.

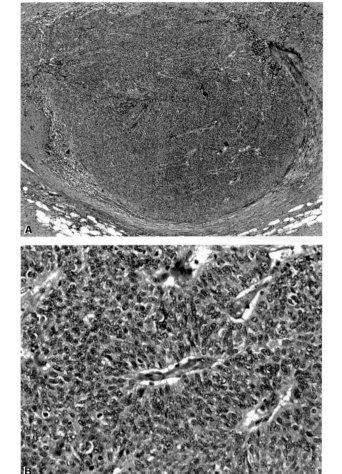

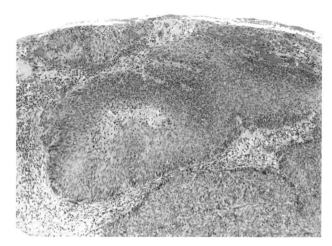

Figure 14-17   Basaloid squamous cell carcinoma.

Figure 14-16   Basaloid squamous cell carcinoma (A and B).

differentiation (basaloid type) until more data are available for this type of tumor.

Other Squamous Lesions

Keratinizing Squamous Metaplasia

Keratinizing squamous metaplasia is considered a putative precursor lesion of squamous cell carcinoma (Fig. 14-18). It may be present in the adjacent epithelium in cases of squamous cell carcinoma of the bladder, and frequently displays the full spectrum of dysplastic lesions and/or carcinoma in situ (Figs. 14-19 to 14-21).[9]

See Chapter 3 for further discussion.

The patient had a long-standing history of recurrent urinary tract infections. Grossly, it was a sessile multilobulated tan-brown mass involving the posterior wall of the bladder. Architecturally, the tumor was characterized by small nests of basaloid cells with minimal cytoplasm arranged with peripheral palisading (Figs. 14-16 and 14-17). Cytologically, the tumor cells had a high nuclear-to-cytoplasmic ratio with dense hyperchromatic nuclei. Central necrosis of the larger nests and pseudoglandular arrangement of the small nests was focally present. The tumor stroma was desmoplastic. Mitotic figures and apoptotic bodies were frequent. The reported case also had microscopic foci of urothelial cell carcinoma with squamous differentiation. Squamous metaplasia was present elsewhere in the bladder in addition to dysplasia and squamous cell carcinoma in situ. The experience with basaloid squamous cell carcinoma in other organs suggests a more aggressive course and a worse prognosis than those of conventional squamous carcinoma.[41] We believe that this tumor should be classified as urothelial carcinoma with squamous cell

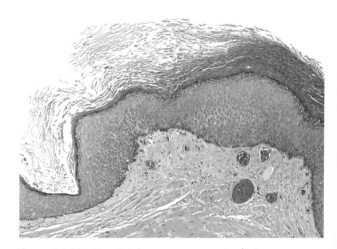

Figure 14-18   Keratinizing squamous metaplasia.

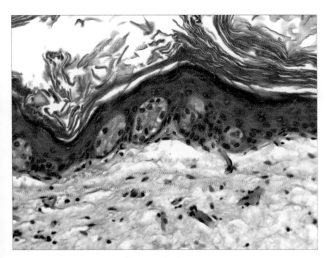

Figure 14-19 Pagetoid spread of carcinoma in situ in keratinizing squamous metaplasia.

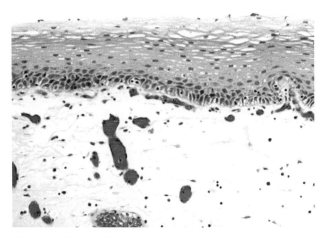

Figure 14-21 Nonkeratinizing squamous metaplasia.

Squamous Cell Carcinoma in Situ

Only a few reports on squamous cell carcinoma in situ of the bladder are available (**Figs. 14-22** to **14-24**).[12,26,42] Histologically, it is identical to squamous cell carcinoma in situ found in other organ sites. It is commonly found in invasive squamous cell carcinoma (**Fig. 14-25**) and is often associated with subsequent or concurrent invasive urothelial carcinoma with squamous differentiation. In a recent report of 11 patients, one patient had no evidence of disease at 8 months; one had residual squamous cell carcinoma in situ at 10 months; one had high grade urothelial carcinoma (not otherwise specified) at rebiopsy after 6 months; three patients were noted to have invasive squamous cell carcinoma at intervals of 2, 3, and 4 months, respectively; and one was found to have invasive urothelial carcinoma with squamous features in the cystectomy specimen at 12 months.[26] A high risk HPV DNA signal was detected in one case. Enhanced expression of epidermal growth factor receptor (EGFR) in these bladder squamous lesions suggests that EGFR may represent a therapeutic target in cases that are difficult to manage surgically.[26]

Squamous Papilloma

Squamous papilloma of the bladder is extremely rare. It occurs in elderly women and follows a benign clinical course with infrequent recurrence. It is diploid, with no or minimal p53 nuclear accumulation, and is HPV negative.[33] Histologically, it is composed of papillary cores with overlying benign squamous epithelium (**Figs. 14-26** and **14-27**). Some demonstrate immunohistochemical expression of EGFR protein.[26] In the bladder or urethra, it has to be differentiated from condyloma acuminatum, an aneuploid benign lesion positive for HPV, increased p53 nuclear accumulation, and prominent koilocytotic

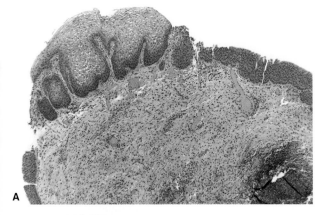

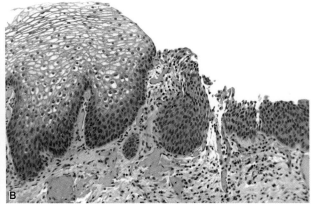

Figure 14-20 Nonkeratinizing squamous metaplasia (A and B). Note the transition between normal urothelium and squamous metaplasia.

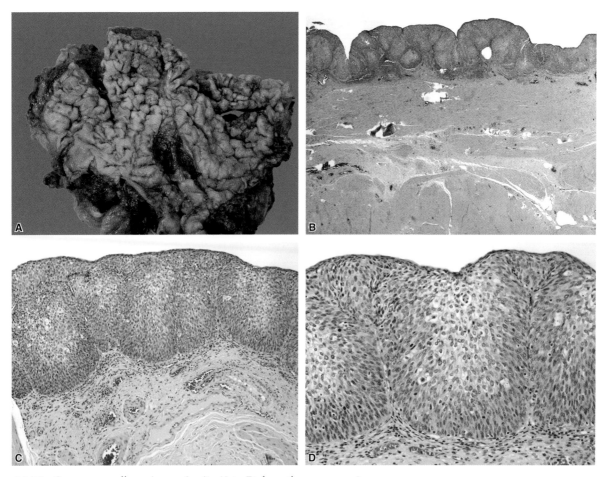

Figure 14-22 Squamous cell carcinoma in situ (A to D; from the same case).

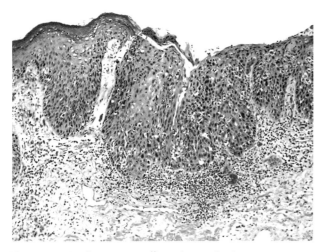

Figure 14-23 Squamous cell carcinoma in situ.

changes. Papillary cystitis, a common reactive lesion in which the urothelium is occasionally replaced by metaplastic squamous epithelium, also enters the differential diagnosis.[33]

See **Chapter 5** for further discussion.

Condyloma Acuminatum

Occasional cases of viral cystitis are associated with HPV infection,[43] but, in our experience, this is extremely uncommon (see also **Chapter 2**).[44]

Condyloma acuminatum of the bladder is associated with HPV infection, is more common in women than in men (2:1 ratio), and affects patients of all ages, although most are younger than 50 years.[33,45] It usually arises in patients with condyloma of the urethra, vulva, vagina, anus, or perineum, but isolated bladder involvement has been reported. Some cases are associated with human immunodeficiency virus (HIV) infection.[46,47] At cystoscopy, condyloma acuminatum typically consists of a solitary lesion, but diffuse involvement has been reported.[48] It usually occurs in the region of the bladder neck and trigone as an exophytic papillary mass, and the major differential diagnostic consideration is papillary urothelial carcinoma (**Fig. 14-28**). Microscopically, it has features similar to those of its counterpart in other organs, including the presence of koilocytotic cells with abundant clear cytoplasm and hyperchromatic wrinkled nuclei with perinuclear halos (**Figs. 14-29** to **14-31**).[49] Condylomata

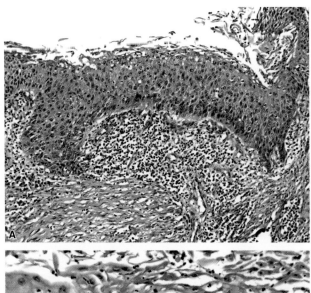

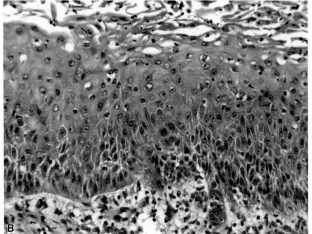

Figure 14-24 Squamous cell carcinoma in situ (A and B).

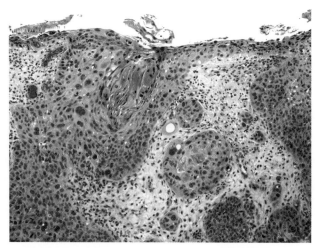

Figure 14-25 Squamous cell carcinoma in situ with microinvasion.

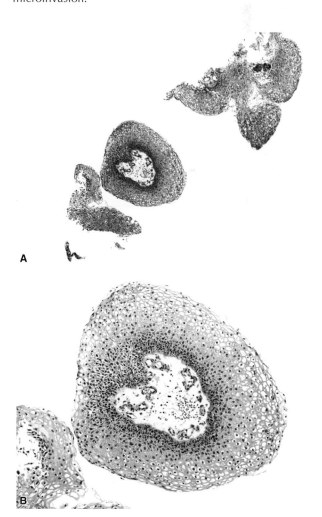

Figure 14-26 Squamous papilloma of the bladder (A and B).

within the bladder, as elsewhere, may undergo malignant transformation,[50] and this may be predicted by the type of HPV involved in its etiology.[44] Urothelial carcinoma may contain foci of koilocytosis, but this is very uncommon. Although condyloma acuminatum is considered by one author to be synonymous with squamous papilloma,[51] we agree with the majority of others and do not consider these to be separate entities, similar to counterpart lesions in many other organs in the body. Cytoplasmic vacuoles may be seen in various urothelial lesions, and caution is warranted in making the diagnosis of condyloma acuminatum of the bladder, which is exceedingly uncommon. The differential diagnosis of condyloma includes squamous metaplasia (**Fig. 14-32**), squamous papilloma, papillary urothelial carcinoma (**Fig. 14-33**), and verrucous squamous cell carcinoma.[33]

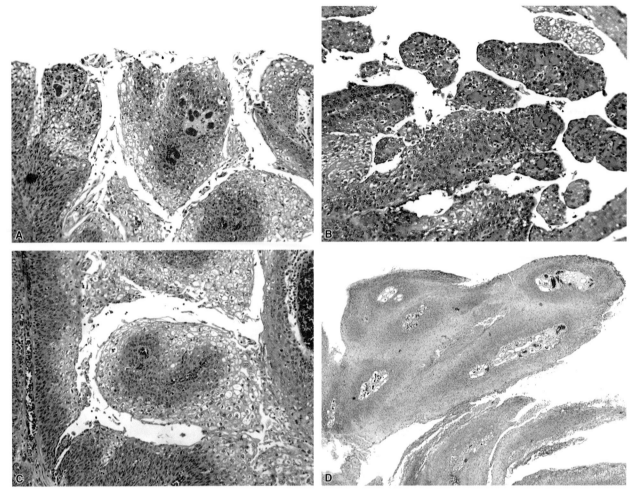

Figure 14-27 Squamous papilloma (A to D).

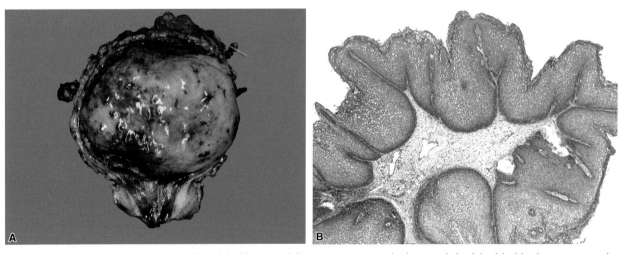

Figure 14-28 Condyloma acuminatum of the bladder. Condyloma is present at the bottom left of the bladder lumen (A). It shows characteristic polypoid configuration (B).

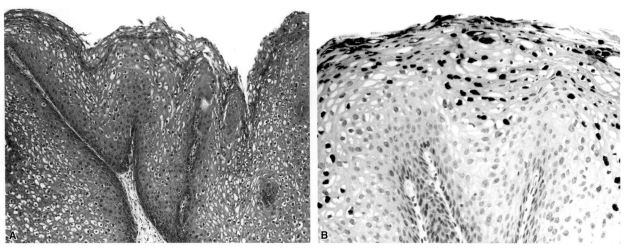

Figure 14-29 Condyloma acuminatum of the bladder. Note the prominent koilocytic atypia (A). Immunostaining for HPV is positive (B).

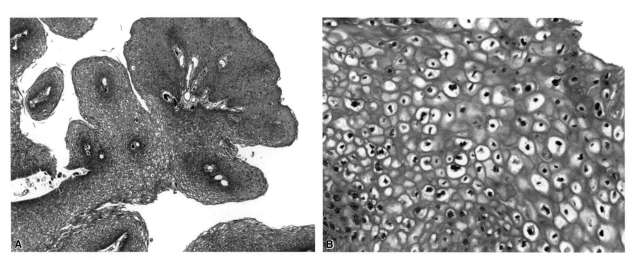

Figure 14-30 Condyloma acuminatum of the bladder (A and B).

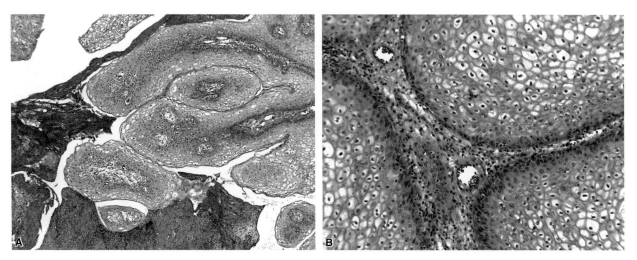

Figure 14-31 Condyloma acuminatum of the bladder (A and B).

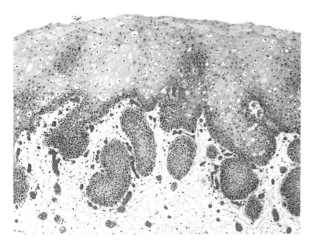

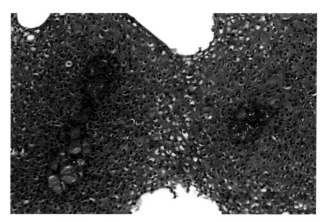

Figure 14-33 Low grade papillary urothelial carcinoma with prominent cytoplasmic vacuoles mimicking koilocytic atypia.

Figure 14-32 Squamous metaplasia with cytoplasmic vacuoles mimicking koilocytic atypia of HPV infection.

REFERENCES

1. Shokeir AA. Squamous cell carcinoma of the bladder: pathology, diagnosis and treatment. *BJU Int* 2004;93:216–20.

2. Ghoneim MA, Abdel-Latif M, el-Mekresh M, Abol-Enein H, Mosbah A, Ashamallah A, el-Baz MA. Radical cystectomy for carcinoma of the bladder: 2,720 consecutive cases 5 years later. *J Urol* 2008;180:121–7.

3. Kassouf W, Spiess PE, Siefker-Radtke A, Swanson D, Grossman HB, Kamat AM, Munsell MF, Guo CC, Czerniak BA, Dinney CP. Outcome and patterns of recurrence of nonbilharzial pure squamous cell carcinoma of the bladder: a contemporary review of The University of Texas M. D. Anderson Cancer Center experience. *Cancer* 2007;110:764–9.

4. Guo CC, Gomez E, Tamboli P, Bondaruk JE, Kamat A, Bassett R, Dinney CP, Czerniak BA. Squamous cell carcinoma of the urinary bladder: a clinicopathologic and immunohistochemical study of 16 cases. *Hum Pathol* 2009;40:1448–52.

5. Rogers CG, Palapattu GS, Shariat SF, Karakiewicz PI, Bastian PJ, Lotan Y, Gupta A, Vazina A, Gilad A, Sagalowsky AI, Lerner SP, Schoenberg MP. Clinical outcomes following radical cystectomy for primary nontransitional cell carcinoma of the bladder compared to transitional cell carcinoma of the bladder. *J Urol* 2006;175:2048–53.

6. Badr KM, Nolen JD, Derose PB, Cohen C. Muscle invasive schistosomal squamous cell carcinoma of the urinary bladder: frequency and prognostic significance of p53, BCL–2, HER2/neu, and proliferation (MIB–1). *Hum Pathol* 2004;35:184–9.

7. Lagwinski N, Thomas A, Stephenson AJ, Campbell S, Hoschar AP, El-Gabry E, Dreicer R, Hansel DE. Squamous cell carcinoma of the bladder: a clinicopathologic analysis of 45 cases. *Am J Surg Pathol* 2007;31:1777–87.

8. Sharfi AR, el Sir S, Beleil O. Squamous cell carcinoma of the urinary bladder. *Br J Urol* 1992;69:369–71.

9. Bessette PL, Abell MR, Herwig KR. A clinicopathologic study of squamous cell carcinoma of the bladder. *J Urol* 1974;112:66–7.

10. Faysal MH. Squamous cell carcinoma of the bladder. *J Urol* 1981;126:598–9.

11. Sarma KP. Squamous cell carcinoma of the bladder. *Int Surg* 1970;53:313–9.

12. Cheng L, Lopez-Beltran A, MacLennan GT, Montironi R, Bostwick DG. Neoplasms of the urinary bladder. In: Bostwick DG, Cheng L, eds. Urologic Surgical Pathology, 2nd ed. Philadelphia: Elsevier/Mosby, 2008:259–352.

13. Brennan P, Bogillot O, Cordier S, Greiser E, Schill W, Vineis P, Lopez-Abente G, Tzonou A, Chang-Claude J, Bolm-Audorff U, Jockel KH, Donato F, Serra C, Wahrendorf J, Hours M, T'Mannetje A, Kogevinas M, Boffetta P. Cigarette smoking and bladder cancer in men: a pooled analysis of 11 case-control studies. *Int J Cancer* 2000;86:289–94.

14. Fortuny J, Kogevinas M, Chang-Claude J, Gonzalez CA, Hours M, Jockel KH, Bolm-Audorff U, Lynge E, t Mannetje A, Porru S, Ranft U, Serra C, Tzonou A, Wahrendorf J, Boffetta P. Tobacco, occupation and non-transitional-cell carcinoma of the bladder: an international case-control study. *Int J Cancer* 1999;80:44–6.

15. Cheever AW. Schistosomiasis and neoplasia. *J Natl Cancer Inst* 1978;61:13–8.

16. IARC. IARC Monographs on the Evaluation of Carcinogenic Risks to Humans. Schistosomes, Liver Flukes, and *Helicobacter Pylori*. Lyon, France: IARC Press, 1994.

17. IARC. IARC Monographs on the Evaluation of Carcinogenic Risks to Humans. Tobacco Smoke and Involuntary Smoking. Lyon, France: IARC Press, 2004.

18. Mostafa MH, Helmi S, Badawi AF, Tricker AR, Spiegelhalder B, Preussmann R. Nitrate, nitrite and volatile N-nitroso compounds in the urine of *Schistosoma haematobium* and *Schistosoma mansoni* infected patients. *Carcinogenesis* 1994;15:619–25.

19. Bickel A, Culkin DJ, Wheeler JS Jr. Bladder cancer in spinal cord injury patients. *J Urol* 1991;146:1240–2.

20. Kaye MC, Levin HS, Montague DK, Pontes JE. Squamous cell carcinoma of the bladder in a patient on intermittent self-catheterization. *Cleve Clin J Med* 1992;59:645–6.

21. Golijanin D, Yossepowitch O, Beck SD, Sogani P, Dalbagni G. Carcinoma in a bladder diverticulum: presentation and treatment outcome. *J Urol* 2003;170:1761–4.

22. Tamas EF, Stephenson AJ, Campbell SC, Montague DK, Trusty DC, Hansel DE. Histopathologic features and clinical outcomes in 71 cases of bladder diverticula. *Arch Pathol Lab Med* 2009;133:791–6.

23. Benson RC Jr, Swanson SK, Farrow GM. Relationship of leukoplakia to urothelial malignancy. *J Urol* 1984;131:507–11.

24. Yoshida T, Suzumiya J, Katakami H, Kimura N, Hisano S, Kikuchi M, Okumura M. Hypercalcemia caused by PTH-rP associated with lung metastasis from urinary bladder carcinoma: an autopsied case. *Intern Med* 1994;33:673–6.

25. Khan MS, Thornhill JA, Gaffney E, Loftus B, Butler MR. Keratinising squamous metaplasia of the bladder: natural history and rationalization of management based on review of 54 years experience. *Eur Urol* 2002;42:469–74.

26. Guo CC, Fine SW, Epstein JI. Noninvasive squamous lesions in the urinary bladder: a clinicopathologic analysis of 29 cases. *Am J Surg Pathol* 2006;30:883–91.

27. Edge S, B, Byrd DR, Compton CC, Fritz AG, Greene FL, Trotti A. American Joint Committee on Cancer Staging Manual, 7th ed. New York: Springer, 2010.

28. Elsobky E, El-Baz M, Gomha M, Abol-Enein H, Shaaban AA. Prognostic value of angiogenesis in schistosoma-associated squamous cell carcinoma of the urinary bladder. *Urology* 2002;60:69–73.

29. Horner SA, Fisher HAG, Barada JH, Eastman AY, Migliozzi J, Ross JS. Verrucous carcinoma of the bladder. *J Urol* 1991;145:1261–3.

30. Utz DC, Schmitz SE, Fugelso PD, Farrow GM. Proceedings: a clinicopathologic evaluation of partial cystectomy for carcinoma of the urinary bladder. *Cancer* 1973;32:1075–7.

31. Richie JP, Waisman J, Skinner DG, Dretler SP. Squamous carcinoma of the bladder: treatment by radical cystectomy. *J Urol* 1976;115:670–2.

32. Newman DM, Brown JR, Jay AC, Pontius EE. Squamous cell carcinoma of the bladder. *J Urol* 1968;100:470–3.

33. Cheng L, Leibovich BC, Cheville JC, Ramnani DM, Sebo TJ, Nehra A, Malek RS, Zincke H, Bostwick DG. Squamous papilloma of the urinary tract is unrelated to condyloma acuminata. *Cancer* 2000;88:1679–86.

34. Morichetti D, Mazzucchelli R, Lopez-Beltran A, Cheng L, Scarpelli M, Kirkali Z, Montorsi F, Montironi R. Secondary neoplasms of the urinary system and male genital organs. *BJU Int* 2009;104:770–6.

35. Oida Y, Yasuda M, Kajiwara H, Onda H, Kawamura N, Osamura RY. Double squamous cell carcinomas, verrucous type and poorly differentiated type, of the urinary bladder unassociated with bilharzial infection. *Pathol Int* 1997;47:651–4.

36. Boxer RJ, Skinner DG. Condylomata acuminata and squamous cell carcinoma. *Urology* 1977;9:72–8.

37. El Sebai I, Sherif M, El Bolkainy MN, Mansour MA, Ghoneim MA. Verrucous squamous carcinoma of bladder. *Urology* 1974;4:407–10.

38. El-Bolkainy MN, Mokhtar NM, Ghoneim MA, Hussein MH. The impact of schistosomiasis on the pathology of bladder carcinoma. *Cancer* 1981;48:2643–8.

39. Michal M, Sulc M, Mukensnabl P. Verrucous carcinoma of the urinary bladder associated with sebaceous differentiation. *J Urol Pathol* 1997;6:153–8.

40. Cheng L, Leibovich B, Cheville J, Ramnani D, Sebo T, Nehra A, Malek R, Zincke H, Bostwick D. Squamous papilloma of the urinary tract is unrelated to condyloma acuminata. *Cancer* 2000;88:1679–86.

41. Vakar-López F, Abrams J. Basaloid squamous cell carcinoma occurring in the urinary bladder. *Arch Pathol Lab Med* 2000;124:455–9.

42. Pierangeli T, Grifoni R, Marchi P, Montironi R, Stefano S. Verrucous carcinoma in situ of the bladder, not associated with urinary schistosomiasis. *Int Urol Nephrol* 1989;21:597–602.

43. Shibutani YF, Schoenberg MP, Carpiniello VL, Malloy TR. Human papillomavirus associated with bladder cancer. *Urology* 1992;40:15–17.

44. Lopez-Beltran A, Munoz E. Transitional cell carcinoma of the bladder: low incidence of human papillomavirus DNA detected by the polymerase chain reaction and in situ hybridization. *Histopathology* 1995;26:565–9.

45. Farrow GM. Significant nonmalignant proliferative and neoplastic lesions of the urinary bladder. *Monogr Pathol* 1992:54–76.

46. Asvesti C, Delmas V, Dauge-Geffroy MC, Grossin M, Boccon-Gibod L, Bocquet L. Multiple condylomata of the urethra and bladder disclosing HIV infection. *Ann Urol* (*Paris*) 1991;25:146–9.

47. Jimenez Lasanta JA, Mariscal A, Tenesa M, Casas D, Gallart A, Olazabal A. Condyloma acuminatum of the bladder in a patient with AIDS: radiological findings. *J Clin Ultrasound* 1997;25:338–40.

48. Bruske T, Loch T, Thiemann O, Wirth B, Janig U. Panurothelial condyloma acuminatum with development of squamous cell carcinoma of the bladder and renal pelvis. *J Urol* 1997;157:620–1.

49. Keating MA, Young RH, Carr CP, Nikrui N, Heney NM. Condyloma acuminatum of the bladder and ureter: Case report and review of the literature. *J Urol* 1985;133:465–7.

50. Libby JM, Frankel JM, Scardino PT. Condyloma acuminatum of the bladder and associated urothelial malignancy. *J Urol* 1985;134:134–6.

51. Murphy WM. Diseases of urinary bladder, urethra, ureters, and renla pelves. In: Murphy WM, ed. Urological Pathology. Philadelphia: W.B. Saunders, 1989:34–146.

Neuroendocrine Tumors

Bladder Pathology, First Edition. Liang Cheng, Antonio Lopez-Beltran, David G. Bostwick.
© 2012 Wiley-Blackwell. Published 2012 by John Wiley & Sons, Inc.

Small Cell Carcinoma

Epidemiology and Clinical Features

Small cell carcinoma of the urinary bladder is a rare but highly aggressive malignancy, accounting for less than 1% of all bladder tumors.[1–21] Demographically, the majority of patients are male, and most patients are in the sixth to seventh decade of life. A recent clinicopathological study of 64 cases by Cheng et al. showed that the mean age at diagnosis is 66 years, ranging from 36 to 85 years, with a male predominance (male-to-female ratio, 3.3 : 1).[1] Many patients have a history of smoking.

Clinical presentations include site-specific and systemic symptoms. Site-specific symptoms are similar to those of urothelial carcinoma. Gross hematuria with or without dysuria is the most common symptom. In Cheng et al.'s study, 88% of patients presented with hematuria.[1] Others had irritative symptoms such as dysuria, nocturia, frequency, urinary obstructive symptoms, or localized abdominal/pelvic pain. Systemic symptoms are nonspecific, including anorexia and weight loss. Occasionally, patients have paraneoplastic syndromes with hypercalcemia, hypophosphatemia, or ectopic secretion of adrenocorticotropic hormone (ACTH).[13–15] One patient was reported to have secretion of ectopic ACTH and Cushing syndrome.[7]

The overall prognosis for small cell carcinoma of the urinary bladder is poor, with a median survival time of one to two years, although a few patients have had long-term survival.[1] In Cheng et al.'s report of 64 cases, the cancer-specific survival rate at five years was 16% (Fig. 15-1),[1] consistent with the 14% rate reported by Choong et al. from the Mayo Clinic.[7] The overall median survival was 1.7 years.[7] Improvement in survival may depend on the identification of new molecular markers for early diagnosis and for the development of novel targeted therapies.[21,22]

Pathologic Findings

Macroscopic Pathology

Small cell carcinoma of the urinary bladder most commonly presents as a large solid polypoid mass, but may also appear sessile and ulcerated (Fig. 15-2). The tumors may infiltrate the bladder wall extensively. The vesical lateral walls and the dome are the most frequent topographies, but rare cases may arise in a diverticulum.

Microscopic Pathology

Small cell carcinoma of the urinary bladder is morphologically similar to its lung counterpart. It typically exhibits both epithelial and neuroendocrine differentiation. However, the diagnosis of small cell carcinoma can be made on the typical morphologic features alone, even if neuroendocrine differentiation cannot be demonstrated.

The tumor consists of sheets or nests of small or intermediate cells with nuclear molding, scant cytoplasm, inconspicuous nucleoli, and evenly dispersed "salt and pepper chromatin" (Figs. 15-3 to 15-10). Mitotic activity is brisk. Punctate or geographical necrosis is common. There may be DNA encrustation of blood vessel walls

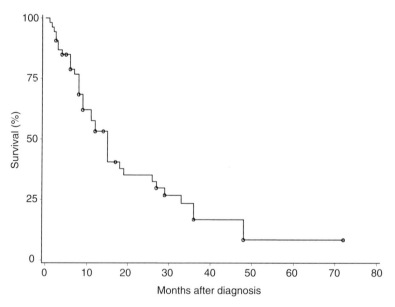

Figure 15-1 Kaplan–Meier survival curves for 64 patients with small cell carcinoma of the urinary bladder. (From Ref. 1; with permission.)

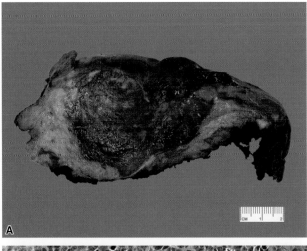

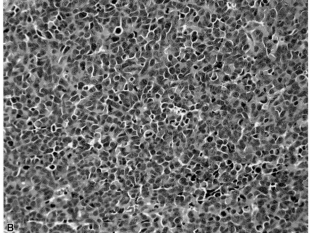

Figure 15-2 Small cell carcinoma of the urinary bladder. Gross (A) and microscopic appearance (B).

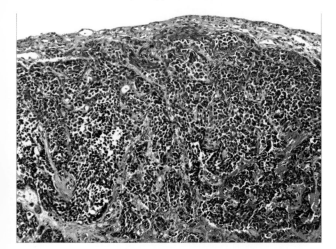

Figure 15-3 Small cell carcinoma of the urinary bladder. Tumors are comprised of sheets, nests, and cords of small cells with scant cytoplasm and hyperchromatic nuclei with nuclear crowding and overlapping. The surface urothelium is denuded. Note the crushing artifact, which is common in neuroendocrine carcinoma.

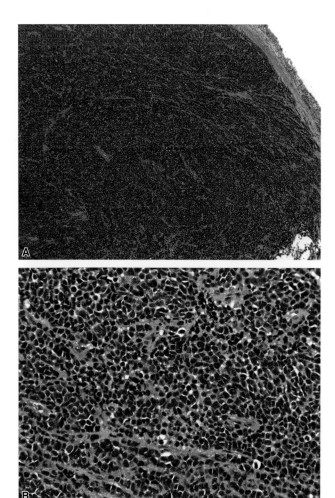

Figure 15-4 Small cell carcinoma of the urinary bladder (A and B). The surface urothelium is intact (A, right upper corner).

(Azzopardi phenomenon). Occasionally, tumor rosettes are present. Vascular invasion is frequent in these tumors. A great majority of tumors infiltrate detrusor muscle extensively. Crush artifact is frequently seen, which can make diagnosis difficult in biopsy specimens.

Coexisting nonsmall cell carcinoma components, including urothelial carcinoma in situ, urothelial carcinoma, adenocarcinoma, squamous cell carcinoma, or sarcomatoid carcinoma, occur in from 12% to 61% of the cases by different studies (**Figs. 15-11** to **15-16**). A study of 64 cases by Cheng et al. showed that 32% were pure small cell carcinoma; 44 cases (68%) consisted of small cell carcinoma admixed with other histological types (urothelial carcinoma in 35 cases, adenocarcinoma in four cases, sarcomatoid urothelial carcinoma in two cases, and both adenocarcinoma and urothelial carcinoma in three cases).[1] In the series of 44 cases, pure small cell carcinoma and mixed small cell carcinoma were present in 27 patients (61%) and 17 patients (39%), respectively.

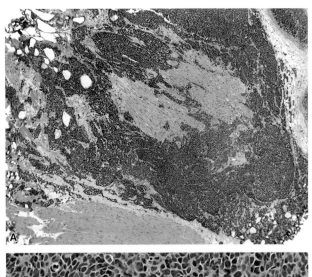

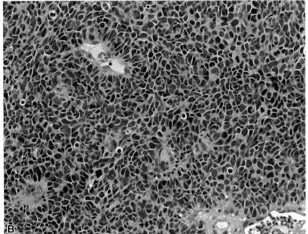

Figure 15-5 Small cell carcinoma of the urinary bladder (A and B). Tumor invades the muscularis propria.

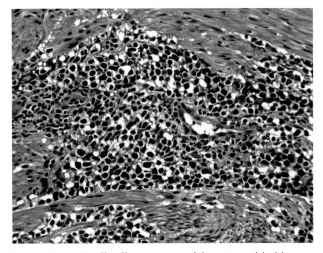

Figure 15-6 Small cell carcinoma of the urinary bladder. Tumor invades the muscularis propria.

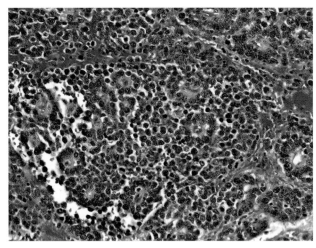

Figure 15-7 Small cell carcinoma with rosette-like formations.

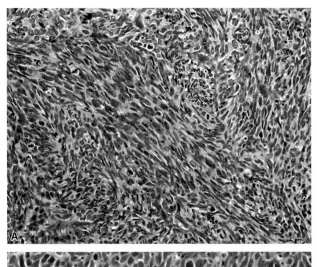

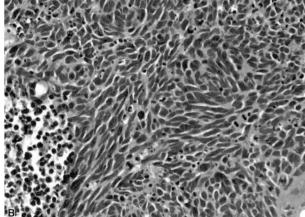

Figure 15-8 Small cell carcinoma with spindle cells (A and B).

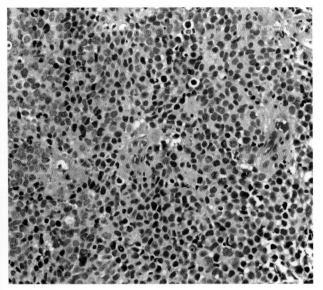

Figure 15-9 Small cell carcinoma with prominent vasculature.

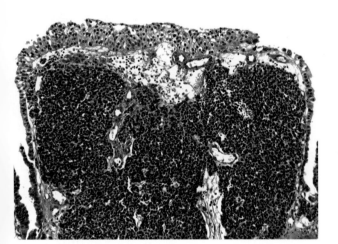

Figure 15-10 Small cell carcinoma of the urinary bladder presenting as a polypoid lesion.

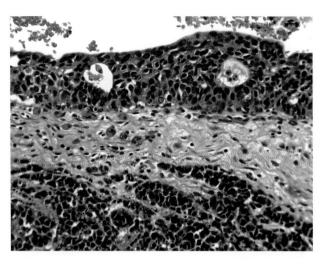

Figure 15-11 Coexisting small cell carcinoma and urothelial carcinoma in situ.

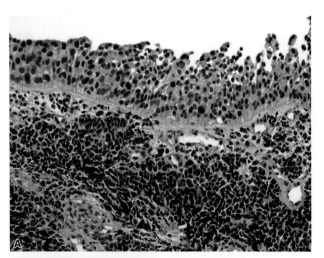

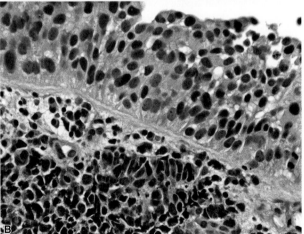

Figure 15-12 Coexisting small cell carcinoma and urothelial carcinoma in situ (A and B).

In another study, only 12% of cases were pure small cell carcinoma, whereas a mixture of small cell carcinoma and urothelial carcinoma was noted in 36 cases (70%), a mixture of small cell carcinoma and adenocarcinoma was present in four cases (8%), and a mixture of small cell carcinoma and squamous cell carcinoma was present in five cases (10%).[5]

Whether the tumor with a predominant component of small cell carcinoma substantially worsens the prognosis as opposed to tumor with a relatively small component has not been ascertained. Current data did not show a survival

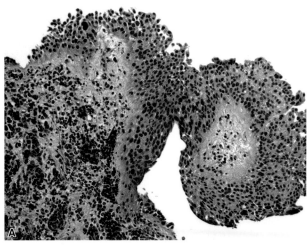

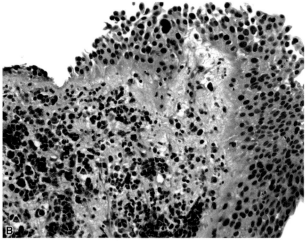

Figure 15-13   Coexisting small cell carcinoma, urothelial carcinoma in situ, and papillary urothelial cacinoma (A and B).

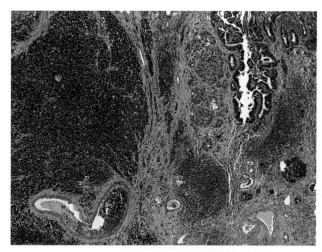

Figure 15-14   Coexisting small cell carcinoma (left), urothelial carcinoma (middle), and adenocarcinoma (right).

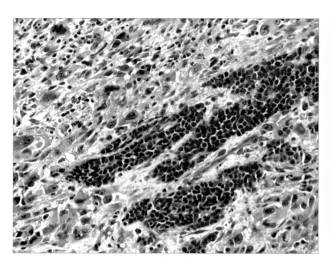

Figure 15-15   Coexisting small cell carcinoma and sarcomatoid carcinoma.

difference between tumors with pure small cell carcinoma and tumors with mixed histology.[1,7]

Ultrastructural Features

Ultrastructurally, tumor cell nuclei are irregular with coarse chromatin. Cytoplasm is scant with sparse organelles including polyribosomes, short segments of rough endoplasmic reticulum, mitochondria, and occasional Golgi complexes. A finding of diagnostic importance is the presence of membrane-limited rounded dense-core granules ranging from 150 nm to 250 nm in diameter, which have been observed in almost all cases examined.[6,19] Tonofilaments and dendrite-like processes are also present in the some of the cases.

Immunohistochemistry

The immunohistochemical profile of small cell carcinoma of the urinary bladder has been investigated extensively (Table 15-1).[5,6,22-29] Markers that have been helpful in confirming neuroendocrine differentiation in small cell carcinoma include neuron-specific enolase (NSE), chromogranin, synaptophysin, Leu 7 (CD57), protein gene product 9.5 (PGP9.5), serotonin, vasoactive intestinal peptide, and others. Neuroendocrine differentiation has been demonstrated in 30% to 100% cases of small cell carcinoma by various markers in different studies. Chromogranin A appears to be a relatively insensitive marker, but very specific, demonstrable immunohistochemically in only a one-third of cases (Fig. 15-17; Table 15-1).

Positive immunostaining for cytokeratin (CK) 7 has been observed in about 60% of cases.[6,17,25,28,30] CK20 and uroplakin III immunostains are negative in small cell carcinoma of the urinary bladder.[25,31-33] Strong and

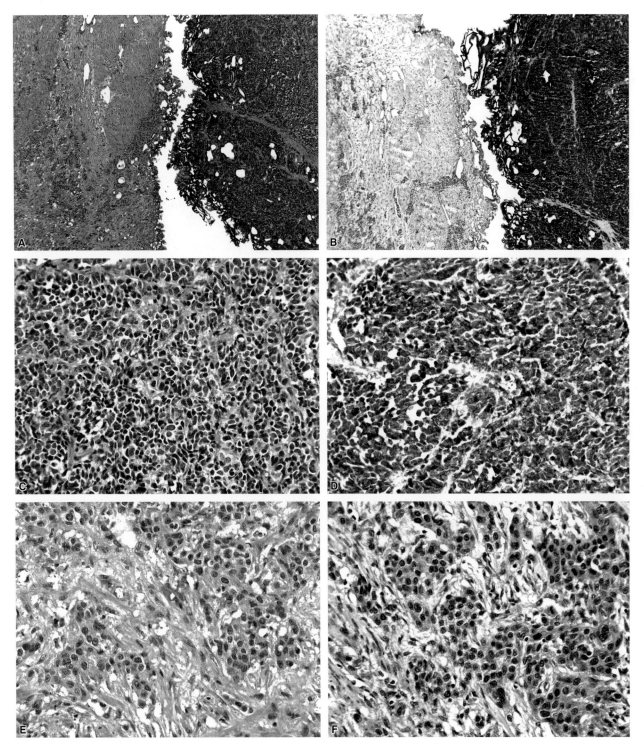

Figure 15-16   Neuroendocrine marker (chromogranin A) staining in small cell carcinoma with coexisting urothelial carcinoma. (A) Left, urothelial carcinoma; right, small cell carcinoma; (B) chromogranin A staining; (C) small cell carcinoma; (D) small cell carcinoma component shows positive cytoplasmic staining for chromogranin A; (E) urothelial carcinoma; and (F) chromogranin A is negative in urothelial carcinoma component. (From Ref. 2; with permission.)

Table 15-1 Immunohistochemistry of Small Cell
Carcinoma of the Urinary Bladder

Markers	% Cases Staining
Neuron-specific enolase	90
Neurofilament	84
Human milk fat globulin	67
Epithelial membrane antigen	63
Cytokeratin AE1/AE3; CAM5.2	61
Carcinoembryonic antigen	50
Synaptophysin	46
LeuM1 (CD15)	43
Chromogranin	41
TTF-1	40
Serotonin	38
Leu 7 (CD57)	35
S100 protein	34
Vasoactive intestinal peptide	17
Vimentin	17
Adrenocorticotropin hormone	9

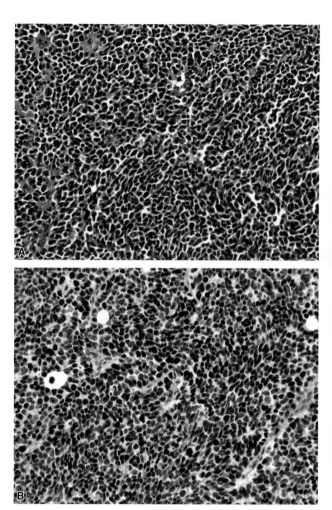

Figure 15-18   Small cell carcinoma of the bladder (A and B) with strong nuclear immunereactivity for TTF-1 (B).

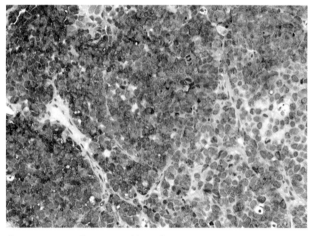

Figure 15-17   Strong positive chromogranin A immunostaining in small cell carcinoma of the bladder.

focally intense cytoplasmic dot-like CAM5.2 reactivity is reported in about two-thirds of cases studied.[5,23] Positive immunostaining for CK 34βE12 has been observed in 40% of cases,[31] and positive epithelial membrane antigen (EMA) immunostaining in about 78% of cases.[6,28] p53 is overexpressed in 52% of cases.[27] Reported frequencies of Ki67 expression have varied from 15 to 80%.[31,32]

CD44v6 may be useful in distinguishing poorly differentiated urothelial carcinoma from small cell carcinoma. CD44, a member of a family of transmembrane glycoproteins, mediates cell–cell and cell–matrix adhesion, the latter by serving as a receptor for hyaluronate binding. CD44v6 splice variant is an isoform conferring metastatic potential and has been correlated with aggressive behavior

in some cancers. CD44v6 immunoreactivity is demonstrable in 60% of cases of urothelial carcinoma, compared with only 7% positivity in small cell carcinoma.[34,35]

Thyroid transcription factor 1 (TTF-1) is considered to be a reliable marker for distinguishing primary adenocarcinomas of the lung from adenocarcinomas of extrapulmonary origin, and for distinguishing pulmonary small cell carcinoma from Merkel cell carcinoma. Jones et al.[25] showed that approximately 40% of cases of small cell carcinoma of the urinary bladder had positive TTF-1 staining (Figs. 15-18 and 15-19). Therefore, TTF-1 immunostaining cannot reliably distinguish between a lung and a urinary bladder primary in cases of metastatic small cell carcinoma of uncertain primary location.

Differential Diagnosis

Small cell carcinoma of the urinary bladder must be distinguished from other primary bladder malignancies, such as

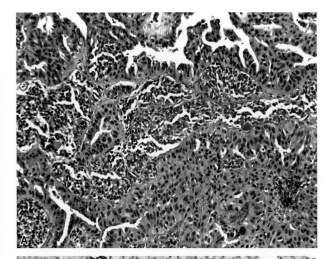

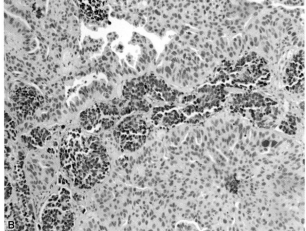

Figure 15-19 Coexisting small cell carcinoma and urothelial carcinoma in situ (A). Small cell carcinoma components are highlighted by TTF-1 nuclear staining (B).

malignant lymphoma, lymphoepithelioma-like carcinoma, plasmacytoid carcinoma, large cell neuroendocrine carcinoma, poorly differentiated urothelial carcinoma, poorly differentiated squamous cell carcinoma, and small cell carcinoma metastatic to the bladder from another site. Ancillary techniques, particularly immunohistochemical staining, can be very helpful in distinguishing these neoplasms (see the discussion above).

Small cell carcinoma can occasionally mimic malignant lymphoma when the tumor cells of small cell carcinoma appear to grow in a discohesive pattern, a finding that may result from artifacts produced by fixation and specimen processing. Lymphoma shows positive immunostaining for leukocyte common antigen, and negative immunostaining for keratin and neuroendocrine markers that typically are positive in small cell carcinoma. Plasmacytoid carcinoma, poorly differentiated urothelial carcinoma, and squamous cell carcinoma do not express neuroendocrine markers

such as synaptophysin or chromogranin as does small cell carcinoma.[36] Large cell neuroendocrine carcinoma is morphologically characterized by large tumor cells with low nuclear-to-cytoplasmic ratios, coarse chromatin, frequent nucleoli, and high mitotic activity with areas of necrosis. Neuroendocrine differentiation can be demonstrated both immunohistochemically and ultrastructurally (see further discussion below).

Small cell carcinoma metastatic to the urinary bladder can be difficult to differentiate from primary bladder tumors without appropriate clinical information. TTF-1 is essentially unhelpful in distinguishing pulmonary from extrapulmonary small cell carcinoma.[25,37] Therefore, appropriate clinical information is essential in establishing a correct diagnosis of metastatic small cell carcinoma involving the urinary bladder. A TTF-1 and p63 immunoprofile may indicate small cell carcinoma originating from the bladder. We have on occasion observed small cell carcinoma of the bladder associated with a more differentiated phenotype resembling atypical carcinoid.

It is notable, however, that almost all the Merkel cell carcinomas are CK20 positive, whereas most small cell carcinomas arising in other sites (including the urinary bladder) are CK20 negative.[38] Therefore, CK20 appears to be useful in distinguishing Merkel cell carcinoma from small cell carcinomas of other origins.

Distinction between small cell carcinoma of the prostate and urinary bladder may be challenging, especially in small biopsy specimens without associated prostatic adenocarcinoma or urothelial carcinoma.[39] Recently, gene fusions between ETS transcription factor genes, particularly *ERG* and *TMPRSS2*, have been identified as a frequent event in prostate cancer. Thus, molecular methods may be helpful in determining the primary site of small cell carcinoma. In a recent study of 30 cases of prostatic small cell carcinoma and 25 cases of bladder small cell carcinoma, Williamson and his colleagues found *TMPRSS2–ERG* gene fusion in 47% (14/30) of prostatic small cell carcinoma (**Figs. 15-20** and **15-21**).[39] Small cell carcinomas of the bladder were negative for *TMPRSS2–ERG* gene fusion. The presence of *TMPRSS2–ERG* gene fusion in small cell carcinoma established prostatic origin.[39]

Histogenesis

Several hypotheses have been proposed to explain the histogenesis of small cell carcinoma of urinary bladder.[1,2] One theory (stem cell theory) is that small cell carcinoma originates from multipotential, undifferentiated stem cells. This is supported by the observation that small cell carcinoma frequently coexists with other histologic types of bladder carcinoma (predominantly urothelial carcinoma, occasionally adenocarcinoma or squamous cell carcinoma).[1,2,6,20,40] At the molecular level, by using laser

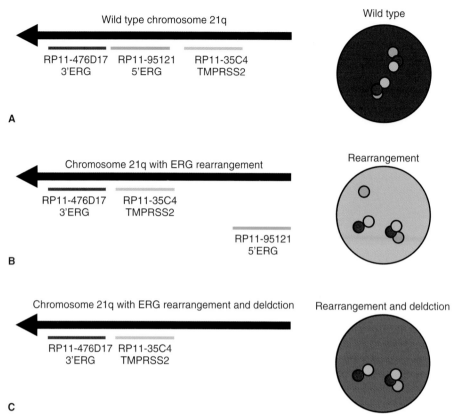

Figure 15-20 Schematic representation of *ERG* rearrangement identification in prostatic small cell carcinoma by tricolor FISH. The red probe hybridizes to the 3′ sequence of *ERG*, the green probe hybridizes to the 5′ sequence of *ERG*, and the aqua probe hybridizes to *TMPRSS2*. (A) Wild type (normal) findings at the 21q22 locus show a triplet of overlapping red and green signals with aqua signals spaced at a variable distance from the red–green pair. (B) Cells with *ERG*–*TMPRSS2* rearrangement exhibit splitting (separation) of the red–green signal pair, accompanied by a fused red–aqua signal for one allele. (C) A subset of cases with rearrangement showed loss of the corresponding green signal for one allele, indicating 5′ *ERG* deletion. (From Ref. 39; with permision.)

capture microdissection and five polymorphic microsatellite markers, Cheng and his colleagues found nearly identical patterns of allelic loss in small cell carcinomas and coexisting urothelial carcinomas, suggesting a common clonal origin (**Figs. 15-22** to **15-24**).[2]

Another theory is that small cell carcinoma originates from neuroendocrine cells in normal or metaplastic urothelium. The occurrence of pure carcinoid tumors of the bladder suggests that neuroendocrine cells of the bladder can become neoplastic.[41] Some authors speculated that Kultschitzky-type neuroendocrine stem cells may exist within the urothelium and may give rise to neuroendocrine tumors, such as small cell carcinoma.[42] Others have suggested that small cell carcinoma of the bladder may be derived from a poorly defined population of submucosal cells of neural crest origin, the same cells from which paragangliomas and neurofibromas arise in the urinary bladder.

Because of frequent findings of glandular metaplasia, adenocarcinoma, and squamous cell carcinoma of the urinary bladder, Cramer et al.[14] suggested that small cell carcinoma in the bladder arises from cells in the urothelium as a result of metaplasia. In addition, a large fraction of patients with small cell carcinoma have concomitant foci of urothelial carcinoma.[1,15,19] Further detailed characterization of genetic changes in biologically and morphologically distinct tumor cell populations, small cell component, and concurrent nonsmall cell carcinoma component (urothelial carcinoma, squamous cell carcinoma, and adenocarcinoma) may provide further insight into the histogenesis.

Molecular Genetics

Only a few studies of the cytogenetic changes and loss of heterozygosity (LOH) in small cell carcinoma of urinary bladder have been reported. The first cytogenetic study by Atkin[43] showed hypertriploidy and hypertetraploidy, associated with extensive chromosomal rearrangements involving chromosomes 1–3, 5–7, 9, 11, and 18. Frequent deletions of 10q, 4q, 5q, and 13q and gains of 8q, 5q, 6p, and 20q have been identified.[44] High level amplifications

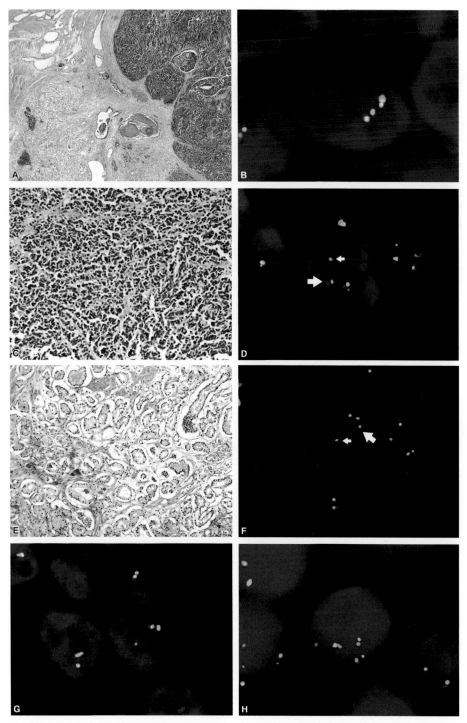

Figure 15-21 Morphology and *ERG* gene rearrangement by FISH in small cell carcinoma and adenocarcinoma of the prostate. (A) Low magnification shows admixed small cell carcinoma and concurrent prostatic acinar adenocarcinoma. (B) The wild type (normal) pattern of *ERG* demonstrates proximate or fused *ERG* 3′ (red) and *ERG* 5′ (green) signals with *TMPRSS2* (aqua) either adjacent to or slightly separated from the red–green signal pair. (C) The small cell carcinoma cells are arranged in cords, nests, or sheets, with the nucleus showing prominent hyperchromasia, nuclear molding, small punctate nucleoli, and brisk mitotic activity. (E) In contrast, the typical prostatic adenocarcinoma component retains the characteristic small, round glands. *ERG* gene rearrangements are detectable by FISH in both small cell (D) and adenocarcinoma components (F). In the typical rearrangement, the green signal (*ERG* 5′, thin arrows) is separated from the red signal with red and aqua signals approximated (*ERG* 3′-*TMPRSS2* fusion, thick arrows, D and F). In other cases, rearrangement is associated with a red–aqua signal doublet, with loss of the corresponding green signal (G). A subset of cases with and without rearrangement demonstrates copy number gain at the 21q22 locus (H). (From Ref. 39; with permission.)

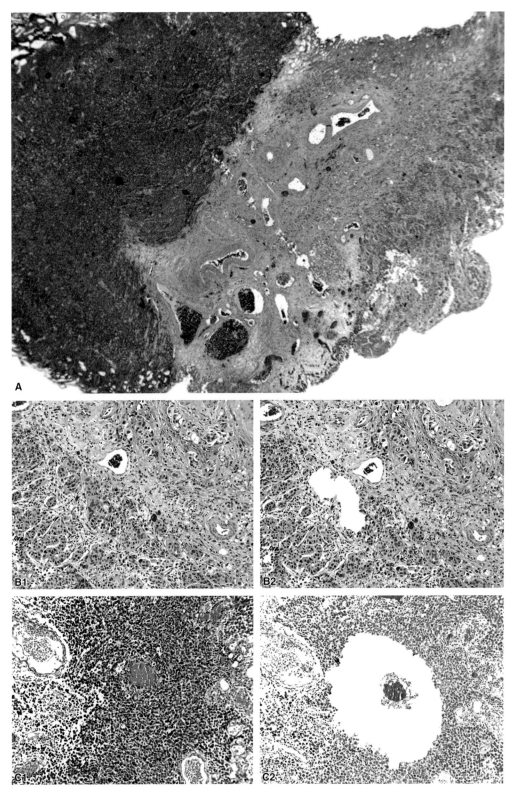

Figure 15-22 Laser microdissection of concomitant small cell and urothelial carcinoma of the urinary bladder. (A) Low-power view of a tumor with coexsting small cell carcinoma and urothelial carcinoma components. (B) Urothelial carcinoma before microdissection (B1) and after microdissection (B2). (C) Urothelial carcinoma before microdissection (C1) and after microdissection (C2). (From Ref. 2; with permission.)

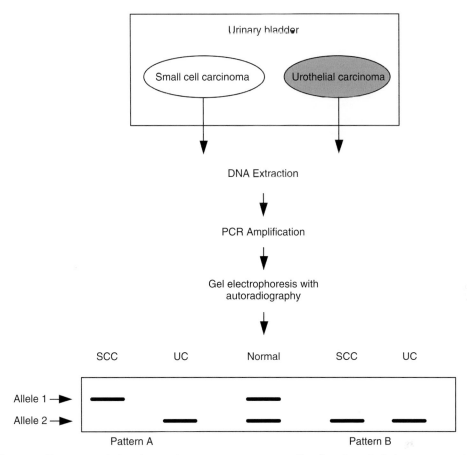

Figure 15-23 Schematic illustration of clonality analysis in concomitant small cell and urothelial carcinoma of bladder. Cells from the distinctly separate small cell and urothelial components were obtained by tissue microdissection, DNA was prepared, and the polymerase chain reaction was used to amplify DNA. DNA sampled from separate small cell and urothelial cells demonstrating identical allelic loss pattern (pattern B) is compatible with a common clonal origin, whereas different patterns of allelic deletions (pattern A) are compatible with independent clonal origins of these two components. SCC, small cell carcinoma; UC, urothelial carcinoma. (From Ref. 2; with permission.)

were found at 1p22–32, 3q26.3, 8q24, and 12q14–21, sites that may harbor oncogenes operative in small cell carcinoma, such as c-myc and MDM2. Monosomy 9, homozygous deletion of p16, and trisomy 7 were found more frequently in small cell carcinoma than in urothelial carcinoma.[45] A study of 20 cases of small cell carcinoma of the urinary bladder by Cheng et al. showed frequent LOH at 3p25–26, 9p21, 9q32–33, and 17p13.[2]

Human papillomavirus (HPV) has been implicated as an etiologic agent for the development of primary small cell carcinoma of the uterine cervix. Wang and Lu demonstrated HPV DNA in all 22 cases of small cell carcinoma of the uterine cervix; however, no HPV DNA was detected in any of the eight cases of urinary bladder small cell carcinomas.[46] This finding suggests that HPV does not play a role in the pathogenesis of small cell carcinoma of urinary bladder.

Prognostic Factors

Small cell carcinoma of the urinary bladder is a highly aggressive neoplasm. A number of investigators have evaluated the usefulness of various immunomarkers in predicting its prognosis. p53, encoded by the TP53 tumor suppressor gene, is a key cell-cycle regulator, involving cell growth and proliferation. Mutations of the TP53 gene have been shown to be the most common genetic alterations in human cancers.[47,48] The abnormal protein coded by mutant TP53 is more stable, has a longer half-life, and subsequently accumulates in the cells. Numerous studies have shown that p53 expression is associated with high grade, high stage, and poor prognosis in malignancies of a variety of organ sites. Several investigators have evaluated p53 expression in small cell carcinoma of the urinary bladder.[23,31,46] TP53 nuclear positivity ranged from 52% to 80% (**Fig. 15-25**).

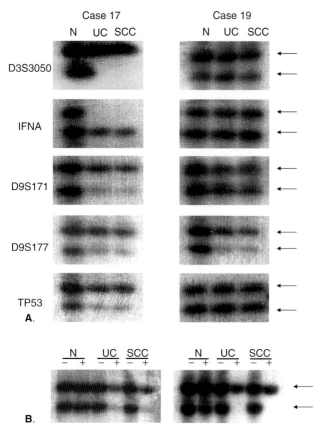

Figure 15-24 Clonality analysis of small cell carcinoma and coexisting urothelial carcinoma. Representative results of loss of heterozygosity (LOH) (A) and X chromosome inactivation analysis (B). DNA was prepared from normal tissue (N), small cell carcinoma (SCC), and urothelial carcinoma (UC) of the combined tumor, amplified by polymerase chain reaction using polymorphic markers D3S3050, IFNA, D9S171, D9S177, and TP53 and separated by gel electrophoresis. Arrows, allelic bands; −, without HhaI digestion; +, with HhaI digestion. (From Ref. 2; with permission.)

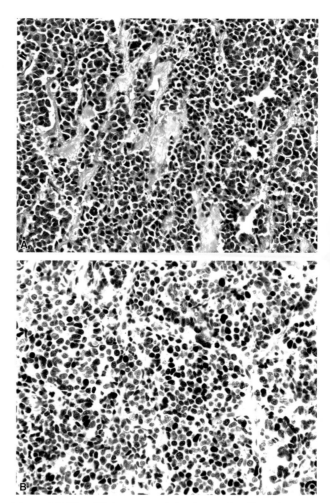

Figure 15-25 p53 immunostaining in small cell carcinoma of the urinary bladder. Small cell carcinoma of the urinary bladder (A) showed nuclear accumulation of p53 protein (B).

However, no correlation between p53 expression and prognosis was demonstrated, possibly due to the overall poor prognosis of this highly aggressive neoplasm.[27]

Ki67 (MIB1) expression has been shown to be an indicator of poor prognosis for numerous malignancies. Reported Ki67 expression frequencies have varied from 15% to 80% in studies of small cell carcinoma of the urinary bladder.[31,32] However, its prognostic significance in the small cell carcinoma of the urinary bladder has not been well defined.

TTF-1 is a nuclear transcriptional factor protein, which is expressed in thyroid and lung epithelium. Although TTF-1 expression has been found to be associated with a better prognosis in nonsmall cell carcinoma of the lung,[49] there is no correlation between TTF-1 expression and prognosis or other clinicopathologic parameters in small cell carcinomas of the urinary bladder or other sites.[25]

Members of the epidermal growth factor receptor (EGFR) superfamily are transmembrane growth factor tyrosine kinases that share similarities in structure and function. They include four distinct receptors (EGFR/erb1, human epidermal growth receptor (HER) 2/erb2, HER3/erb3, and HER4/erb4), which play important roles in tumor cell survival and proliferation. EGFR (HER1, c-erb-B1) is expressed in many human epithelial malignancies, including nonsmall cell carcinoma of the lung.[50] The successful treatment of gastrointestinal stromal tumors and chronic myeloid leukemia utilizing anti-CD117 (Gleevec, STI-571), and the use of monoclonal antibodies against HER1 (Gefitinib) and HER2 (Herceptin, trastuzumab] in the treatment of nonsmall cell carcinoma of the lung and carcinoma of the breast have encouraged investigators to evaluate the potential therapeutic benefit of targeted therapy for other malignancies.[51,52] Several recent studies have focused on the immunohistochemical expression of EGFR in small cell carcinoma of the urinary bladder. Wang et al. analyzed 52 cases of urinary bladder small cell carcinoma and found positive EGFR expression in 14 of 52 (27%) cases.[22] No EGFR gene amplification was observed by fluorescence in situ hybridization (FISH). However, 40 cases had polysomy and the remaining 12 cases displayed disomy (**Fig. 15-26**). These findings raise the possibility that EGFR may be a potential therapeutic target in the treatment of this malignancy.

C-kit (CD117) is a transmembrane tyrosine kinase receptor which is encoded by the protooncogene c-kit. C-kit has been shown to be involved in many physiological and pathological processes, including hematopoiesis and oncogenesis.[53] In a study of small cell carcinoma of the urinary bladder by Pan et al., 14 of 52 cases (27%) showed positive immunostaining for c-kit with more than 10% of tumor cells staining.[26] These data suggest the possibility that c-kit may be a worthwhile therapeutic target in a subset of patients with small cell carcinoma of the urinary bladder.

HER2 is overexpressed in a variety of carcinomas, including those of breast, bladder, ovary, endometrium, and lung. Expression of HER2 is generally associated with a poor prognosis. Typical membranous immunostaining for c-erb-B2 was observed in 50% of cases of small cell carcinoma of the urinary bladder by Soriano et al.,[31] again raising the question of whether therapy against this target molecule might prove beneficial in the management of small cell carcinoma of the urinary bladder.

Staging, Treatment, and Outcome

Data regarding the staging, treatment, and prognosis of small cell carcinoma of the urinary bladder have been derived from more than 200 case reports and patient series of varying sizes. The majority of patients present with metastatic disease at time of diagnosis, including metastases to regional lymph node, bone, liver, and lung.[1,3–5,7,21] Overall prognosis has been shown to be correlated with the stage of disease at the presentation. Other clinicopathologic parameters, such as age, gender, presenting symptoms, and the presence of coexisting nonsmall cell carcinoma component, are not associated significantly with survival.[1]

Cheng et al. studied 64 cases of small cell carcinoma of the urinary bladder and reported that, with only one exception, disease stage was pT2 or higher at the time of initial clinical presentation.[1] Sixty-six percent of patients who underwent lymph node evaluation had lymph node metastases. Thirty-eight patients had cystectomy (37 radical and one partial). Fifty-six percent of the patients received chemotherapy. Cisplatin/etoposide and carboplatin/etoposide combination chemotherapy regimens were those most commonly used in treating the patients in their series. Twenty-five percent of patients received

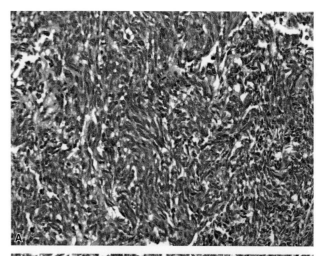

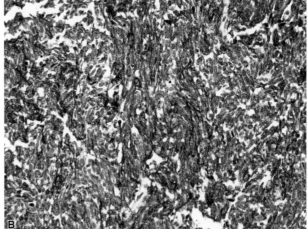

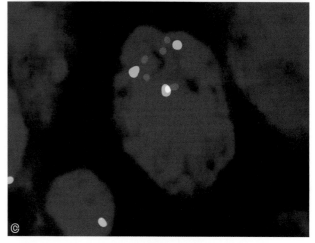

Figure 15-26 Analysis of EGFR expression in small cell carcinoma of the urinary bladder. (A) Small cell carcinoma of the urinary bladder is composed of small round or spindle-shaped cells in compact sheets. (B) Immunohistochemistry showed EGFR expression in a mixed membrane and cytoplasmic distribution. (C) FISH reveals a polysomy pattern. Green, centromere 7 signals; red, EGFR signals.

local radiation therapy. Respectively, one- and five-year cancer-specific survival among patients who underwent cystectomy was 57% and 16%, compared to 55% and 18% among those who were not treated by cystectomy (**Figs. 15-27** and **15-28**). No significant survival difference was found between patients who underwent cystectomy and those not treated by cystectomy ($P = 0.65$). Similarly, chemotherapy and radiation therapy appear to be ineffective in significantly altering the clinical course.[1] In a study of 51 cases by Abrahams et al., [5] 41 cases with clinical and followup data were staged as follows: stage I in two (5%), stage II in 18 (44%), stage III in 10 (24%), and stage IV in 11 (27%) patients. Two stage I patients were treated with transurethral resection. Among 28 patients with surgical resectable disease, nine received preoperative chemotherapy, and 12 proceeded directly to cystectomy. Among 11 patients with metastases at initial presentation, nine received chemotherapy. Despite having metastatic disease at initial presentation, two patients received cystectomy after chemotherapy, with one patient alive and free of disease more than eight years following cystectomy. The overall median survival in their series was 23 months, and the survival rate was 40% at five years. The use of chemotherapy in the preoperative setting may have contributed to the relatively favorable survival of their patients. In a study of 25 cases, Quek et al. demonstrated that patients receiving multimodality therapy had significantly better overall survival than those

treated with cystectomy alone.[54] In meta-analyses by other groups, cystectomy and chemotherapy appeared to confer a more favorable prognosis.[16,55] In the study of 44 cases by Choong et al., 12 (27.3%), 13 (29.6%), and 19 (43.2%) patients had stage II, III, and IV disease, respectively, with five-year survival rates of 63.6%, 15.4%, and 10.5%. Overall median survival was 1.7 years.[7]

Various treatment strategies have been reported in the literature.[1,3,4,21] Current treatment of the disease has been influenced by the experience gained in the management of pulmonary small cell carcinoma. Overall survival is poor and local therapy is usually insufficient for cure. Radical surgery and chemoradiotherapy are currently the favored treatment options.[1,5,7,8] Cytotoxic chemotherapy plays a major therapeutic role in the treatment of limited- and advanced-stage small cell carcinoma of the urinary bladder. Chemotherapy is usually combined with other therapeutic modalities, such as radiation therapy or surgical resection.

Carcinoid Tumor

The full spectrum of neuroendocrine tumors can involve the urinary bladder.[4,56] Carcinoid tumor is morphologically and immunohistochemically similar to its counterpart in the lung or gastrointestinal tract. Less than two dozen cases of carcinoid tumors of the urinary bladder have been

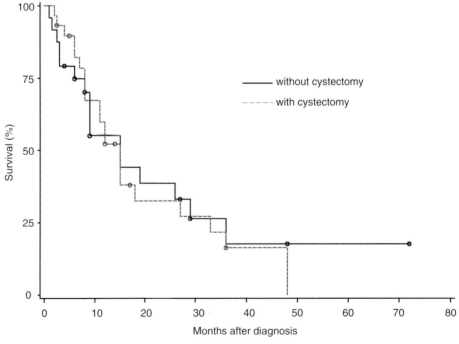

Figure 15-27 Kaplan–Meier survival curves for 64 patients with small cell carcinoma of the urinary bladder stratified according to treatment with cystectomy. Solid black line: treatment without cystectomy; dashed red line: treatment with cystectomy. (From Ref. 1; with permission.)

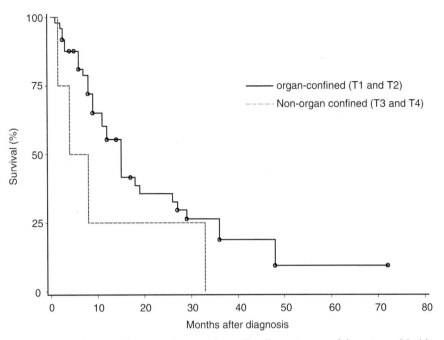

Figure 15-28 Kaplan–Meier survival curves for 64 patients with small cell carcinoma of the urinary bladder stratified according to pathologic tumor classification. Solid black line: organ confined disease (T1 and T2); dashed red line: nonorgan confined disease (T3 and T4). (From Ref. 1; with permission.)

reported.[25,41,57–64] The tumor usually occurs in elderly patients (mean age, 56 years; range, 29 to 75 years), with slight male predominance (male-to-female ratio, 1.8 : 1). Hematuria is the most common clinical presentation, followed by irritative voiding symptoms. Association with carcinoid syndrome has not been reported.

Bladder carcinoid is submucosal with a predilection for the trigone and ranges in size from 3 mm to 3 cm in the largest dimension. The tumor often presents as a polypoid lesion upon cystoscopic examination. Coexistence of carcinoid with other urothelial neoplasms, such as inverted papilloma[61] and adenocarcinoma,[59] has been reported. An association of bladder carcinoid and urothelial carcinoma has not been observed. Pathologists must bear in mind that urothelial high grade neuroendocrine carcinoma may also exhibit focal "carcinoid-like" morphology.

An origin of primary bladder carcinoid from innate or metaplastic mucosal urothelial neuroendocrine cells has been proposed. It is well known that cells with neuroendocrine features may be situated against the basement membrane of normal urothelium in the urethra, as well as in reactive lesions such as von Brunn nests and cystitis cystica/glandularis. Indeed, two cases of primary bladder carcinoid have developed in a background of proliferative cystitis.[41] The prognosis of patients with carcinoid of the bladder is guarded. Approximately 25% of patients will have regional lymph node or distant metastasis, but the majority are cured by excision.

Carcinoid of the bladder is morphologically similar to its counterpart in other organ sites. The tumor cells have abundant amphophilic cytoplasm and are arranged in an insular, acini, trabecular, or pseudoglandular pattern in a vascular stroma. An organoid growth pattern, resembling that seen in paraganglioma, can be seen. Tumor cell nuclei have finely stippled chromatin and inconspicuous nucleoli. Mitotic figures are infrequent. Tumor necrosis is absent.

Differential diagnostic considerations include paraganglioma, nested variant of urothelial carcinoma, and metastatic prostate carcinoma. Immunohistochemistry is helpful. Carcinoid tumors of the bladder typically exhibit strong, diffuse immunohistochemical staining for cytokeratins, NSE, chromogranin, Leu 7 (CD57), and synaptophysin. Rarely, TTF-1 staining can also be seen in carcinoid tumors.

Large Cell Neuroendocrine Carcinoma

The spectrum of neuroendocrine carcinomas of the urinary bladder may include rare examples of large cell neuroendocrine carcinomas, similar to the more common counterpart in the lung (**Figs. 15-29** to **15-31**).[65–68] The age at diagnosis ranges from 32 to 82 years of age. These tumors are either pure or can be associated with other components, such as typical urothelial carcinoma, squamous cell carcinoma, adenocarcinoma, or sarcomatoid

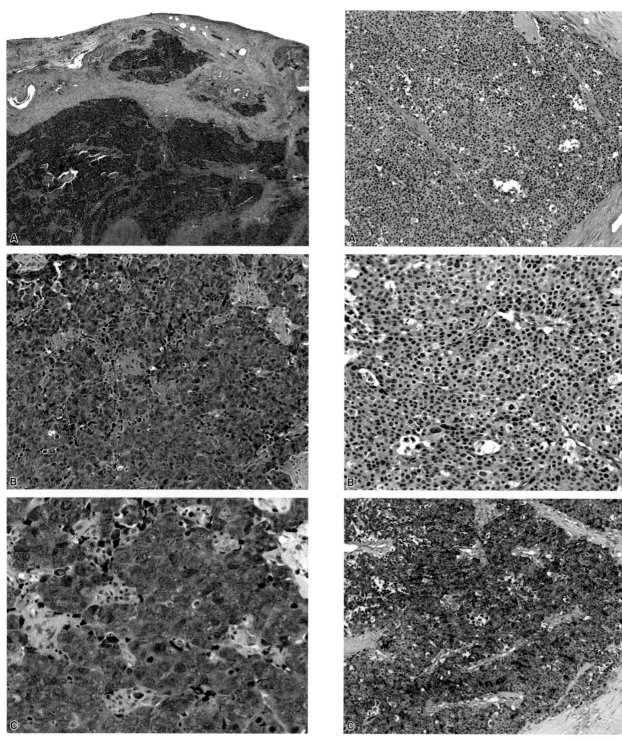

Figure 15-29 Large cell neuroendocrine carcinoma (A to C). Immunostaining for chromogranin A is strongly positive (C).

Figure 15-30 Large cell neuroendocrine carcinoma (A to C). Immunostaining for chromogranin A is strongly positive (C).

carcinoma. Immunohistochemically, the tumor cells frequently show immunoreactivity to chromogranin A, CD56, NSE, and synaptophysin. In addition to neuroendocrine markers, the tumor cells typically show positive immunostaining for cytokeratins CAM5.2 and AE1/AE3

and for EMA, and may show focal positivity for vimentin. In situ hybridization for the detection of Epstein–Barr virus in one reported case was negative. These tumors are aggressive and tend to metastasize systemically despite aggressive adjuvant therapy. Metastasis from a lung

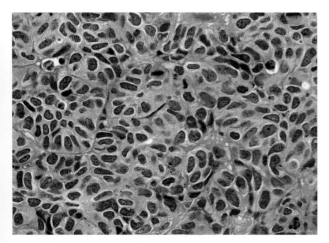

Figure 15-31 Large cell neuroendocrine carcinoma. Note the numerous mitotic figures.

primary should be considered before diagnosing a primary bladder large cell neuroendocrine carcinoma.

Primitive Neuroectodermal Tumors

There are rare case reports of primitive neuroectodermal tumor (PNET) occurring in the urinary bladder. Patients have ranged in age from 15 to 81 years, with a mean age of 43 years.[69] Presenting symptoms have included frequency, dysuria, hematuria, lymphedema of the lower extremities, fatigue, and urge incontinence.[69,70] This tumor is highly malignant, demonstrating rapid growth. It often shows evidence of extension outside the confines of the bladder at the time of diagnosis. Despite this, two patients with this tumor have reportedly been free of disease at 18 months and three years of followup, respectively.[69,70] A patient treated with imatinib following systemic chemotherapy and radical surgery remains alive after fours years of followup.[69]

Histologically, PNET is a highly cellular small round blue cell tumor usually showing numerous mitotic figures (10 to 30 per 10 high power field), rosette-like structures (Homer–Wright rosette), and areas of necrosis. Tumor cells are arranged in lobular sheets surrounded by fibrovascular stroma; tumor cells are monotonously uniform, with scant basophilic cytoplasm (**Figs. 15-32** and **15-33**). Tumor cell nuclei have finely dispersed chromatin; nucleoli are absent or inconspicuous. Some tumor cells demonstrate periodic acid–Schiff (PAS)-positive cytoplasmic granules. A few reticulin fibers may be identified between cells.

PNET is closely related to Ewing sarcoma (EWS), sharing the same chromosomal abnormality: t(11;22) (q12; q24), or a fusion of the *EWS* gene (22q12) with a member of a family of transcription factors, usually *FLI-1* gene (11q24).[69] Lopez-Beltran et al. performed

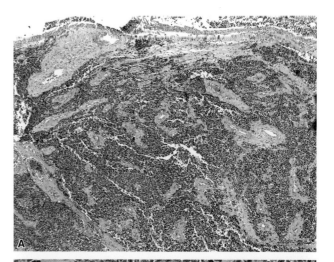

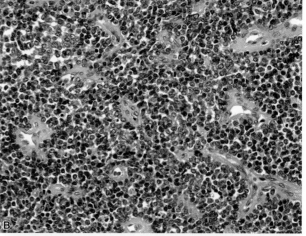

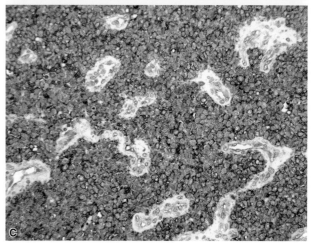

Figure 15-32 Primitive neuroectodermal tumor (PNET) (A to C). The urothelium is focally denuded. Note the presence of rosette-like structures (B). Immunostaining for chromogranin A is strongly positive (C).

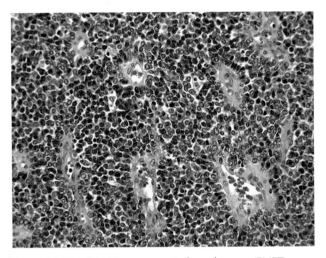

Figure 15-33   Primitive neuroectodermal tumor (PNET).

molecular analysis with reverse transcriptase–polymerase chain reaction (RT-PCR) on a primary PNET of the bladder and demonstrated a type 2 *EWS/FLI-1* fusion transcript, which has been associated with an unfavorable prognosis in such tumors. In contrast, this same tumor, by comparative genomic hybridization (CGH) analysis, showed a genetically balanced tumor without secondary chromosomal changes, a finding that has been associated with a favorable prognosis in these tumors. FISH analysis performed on this tumor showed that most tumor interphase nuclei showed a pattern indicative of rearrangement of one copy of the *EWS* gene.[69] Kruger et al. carried out a similar molecular cytogenetic analysis of PNET primary in the urinary bladder using CGH. Analysis revealed gains of chromosomes 3p, 6, 8q, 12p, 17q, and 21q. No chromosomal losses were identified. The imbalances of 3p and 6 observed have also been reported in single cases of PNET and Ewing sarcoma arising in other locations.[70]

Immunohistochemical staining helps in the identification of PNETs, most of which demonstrate strong immunostaining for CD99, positive immunostaining for vimentin, and membranous immunostaining for CD117 (**Table 15-2**). Focal immunostaining for cytokeratin is seen in up to 57% of cases, as well as focal immunoreactivity for S100 protein.[69] Kruger reported strongly positive immunostaining for NSE.[70] PNET shows no immunoreactivity to

antibodies against α-smooth muscle actin, chromogranin, desmin, EMA, myoglobin, synaptophysin, chromogranin, or leukocyte common antigen.[69,70]

The differential diagnosis includes other small round blue cell tumors such as small cell carcinoma, lymphoma, and rhabdomyosarcoma. Primitive neuroectodermal tumors occasionally stain with chromogranin and synaptophysin, and small cell carcinomas are often cytokeratin positive. In this setting, ultrastructural or genetic studies may be helpful. Lack of staining with lymphoid and muscle markers virtually excludes hematolymphoid malignancy and rhabdomyosarcoma, respectively. Rhabdomyosarcoma typically shows diffuse infiltration of small blue round cells with scant cytoplasm. In the sarcoma botryoides type, the cells are scattered in a loose myxoid stroma with condensation of rhabdomyoblasts beneath the urothelium, creating a cambium layer.

Malignant Peripheral Nerve Sheath Tumor

Malignant peripheral nerve sheath tumor (MPNST) is rare in the urinary bladder. Only a few cases have been documented, predominantly in patients less than 40 years old.[71–73] Some have arisen in the setting of neurofibromatosis type 1, possibly originating in neurofibromas of autonomic nerve plexuses in the bladder wall. It is typically a highly malignant and rapidly growing tumor. Patients present with hematuria, and a suprapubic mass is sometimes noted.[72] The lesion has been seen arising from the trigone, as well as from the lateral and posterior walls of the bladder. It may form multiple large nodules with surface ulceration and areas of necrosis. The tumor may infiltrate the entire thickness of the bladder wall, involving perivesical soft tissues or pelvic peritoneum. Distant metastases may be present at diagnosis. Prognosis is generally poor with local recurrence or distant metastases often evident within 2 months of initial surgical resection.

MPNST is a poorly differentiated tumor that grows in sheets and nodules consisting of interlacing fascicles of malignant spindle cells.[71] The tumor cells are pleomorphic, with variable amounts of eosinophilic cytoplasm.[72] Most have a single nucleus, but multinucleated tumor cells

Table 15-2   Selected Immunohistochemical Profiles of Small Round Blue Cell Tumors of the Urinary Bladder[a]

Small Round Blue Cell Tumors	LCA	CD99	NE Markers	CD117	CK AE1/AE3	SMA/Desmin
PNET	−	+	Variable +	+	Variable +	−
Small cell carcinoma	−	−	+	−	Variable +	−
Lymphoma	+	Variable +	−	−	−	−
Rhabdomyosarcoma	−	−	−	−	−	+

[a]PNET, primitive neuroectodermal tumor; LCA, leukocyte common antigen; NE, neuroendocrine markers (chromogranin A, synaptophysin, and neuron-specific enolase); CK, cytokeratin; SMA, smooth muscle actin.

may be present. Nuclei are round to oval with prominent irregular eosinophilic nucleoli, or elongated and tapered with marked atypia. Mitotic activity may be moderate. An extensive infiltrate of acute and chronic inflammatory cells, including eosinophils, may be present. An epithelioid variant as well as a variant with rhabdomyoblastic differentiation (malignant triton tumor) have been described.[72]

Immunohistochemical stains can help with the identification of this tumor, which typically shows positive immunostaining for S100 protein and vimentin, and focally positive staining for NSE. It usually does not stain for EMA, AE1/AE3, muscle-specific actin, desmin, myoglobin, cytokeratin, chromogranin, or neurofilament.[71,72] In one case, rhabdomyoblastic differentiation with focal immunostaining for myoglobin was identified in a tumor that arose in an infant with neurofibromatosis type 1.[73]

The differential diagnosis of this tumor includes epithelioid sarcoma, undifferentiated carcinoma, melanoma, epithelioid angiosarcoma, rhabdoid tumor, sarcomatoid carcinoma, epithelioid leiomyosarcoma, and rhabdomyosarcoma. Immunoreactivity to HMB45, Melan A, or strong diffuse S100 protein immunoreactivity would favor melanoma. Carcinosarcoma would show evidence of epithelial differentiation with immunoreactivity for cytokeratins and EMA. Unlike epithelioid sarcoma, tumor cells of MPNST are immunoreactive for S100 protein, focally immunoreactive for NSE, and are not immunoreactive for EMA or cytokeratins. Immunohistochemistry can also be used to help rule out endothelial, muscular, and neuroendocrine differentiation as well as anaplastic lymphoma.

Paraganglioma

Primary paraganglioma of the bladder occurs infrequently (Figs. 15-34 to 15-38). The largest series, which included 16 patients followed for a mean of 6.3 years, was reported by Cheng et al.[74] Females are more likely to develop bladder paraganglioma, male-to-female ratio is 1 : 3. The tumor tends to occur in young patients (mean, 45 years) and symptoms are present in over 80% of cases. Presenting symptoms include hematuria, hypertension which may be exacerbated during voiding, and other symptoms of catecholamine excess.[75–95] At cystoscopic examination, small (<3 cm), dome-shaped nodules covered by normal mucosa are found in the trigone, dome, or lateral wall.

In contrast to extraadrenal paragangliomas at other sites, of which approximately 10% exhibits malignant behavior, the frequency of malignancy in bladder paragangliomas is about 20%.[74] No reliable histologic criteria exist to distinguish malignant from benign neoplasms.[80,83,94,96–98]

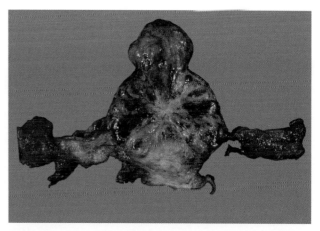

Figure 15-34 Paraganglioma of the bladder, gross appearance. (From Ref. 74; with permission.)

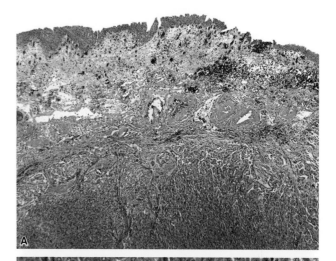

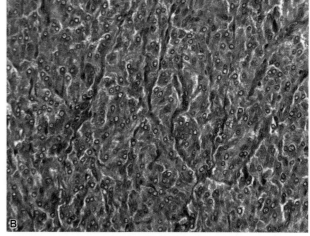

Figure 15-35 Paraganglioma (A and B).

The findings of nuclear pleomorphism, mitotic figures, and necrosis are not a reliable predictor of clinical outcome in patients with paraganglioma of the urinary bladder.[79,83] Malignancy in these tumors can only be confirmed by the

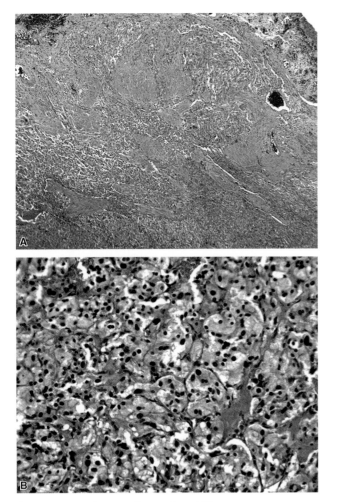

Figure 15-36   Paraganglioma (A and B).

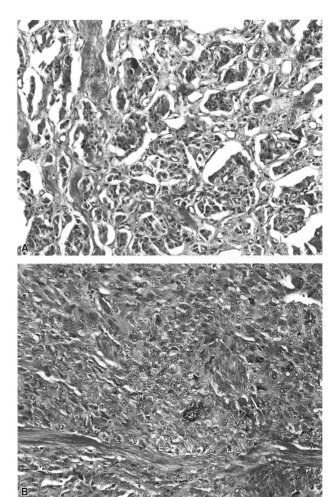

Figure 15-37   Paraganglioma (A and B). Discrete nests of tumor cells are typical (A), although other patterns, including spindle cell pattern (B) may be encountered.

occurrence of regional or distant metastases. No metastases or tumor recurrences have been observed in patients whose tumors were confined within the bladder wall.[74]

Bladder paraganglioma is morphologically similar to its counterparts in other body sites; most are covered by normal urothelium.[74] The tumor consists of round or polygonal epithelioid cells with abundant eosinophilic or granular cytoplasm. Tumor cell nuclei are centrally located and are vesicular with finely granular chromatin. The cells are arranged in discrete nests (Zellballen pattern), with intervening vascular septa. Sustentacular cells may be present. Mitotic figures, necrosis, and vascular invasion are usually absent.[74]

Paraganglioma typically demonstrates immunoreactivity with neuroendocrine markers such as chromogranin, synaptophysin, and NSE (**Fig. 15-39**).[74] The sustentacular cells exhibit immunostaining for S100 protein. Tumor cells are often immunoreactive for vimentin, but usually show no immunoreactivity for CK7, CK20, or pancytokeratin AE1/AE3.[99]

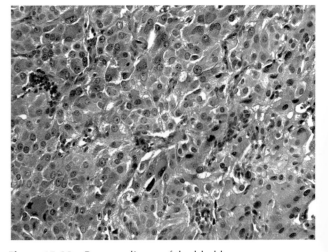

Figure 15-38   Paraganglioma of the bladder.

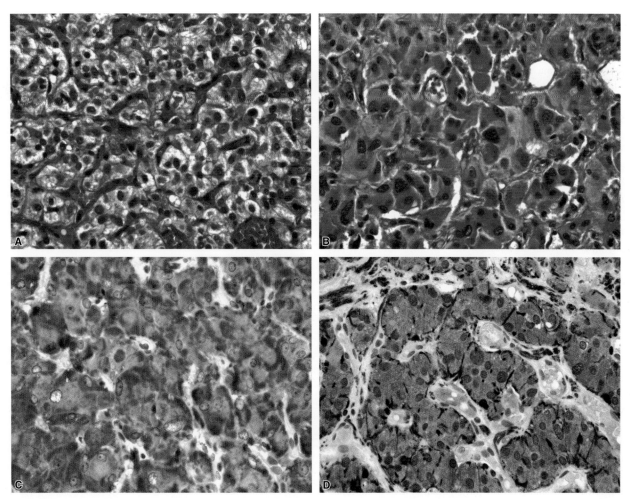

Figure 15-39   Paraganglioma (A-D). Immunostaining for chromogranin A is strongly positive (C). S100 protein staining highlights the sustentacular cells (D).

The differential diagnosis for this tumor includes granular cell tumor, nested variant of urothelial carcinoma, prostatic adenocarcinoma, metastatic large cell neuroendocrine carcinoma, and malignant melanoma.[74,100–104] Granular cell tumor has abundant eosinophilic granular cytoplasm, shows strongly positive immunostaining for S100 protein, and lacks the Zellballen growth pattern, the fine vascular stroma, chromogranin immunoreactivity, and sustentacular cell S100 protein immunostaining.[105–109] The nested variant of urothelial carcinoma also lacks a fine vascular network and is immunohistochemically negative for S100 protein and chromogranin. Metastatic large cell neuroendocrine carcinoma is characterized by necrosis, abundant mitotic activity, and cellular anaplasia. While it is immunoreactive for neuroendocrine markers similar to paraganglioma, it is also immunoreactive for cytokeratin and negative for sustentacular cell S100 protein immunoreactivity. Clinical history is important in differentiating paraganglioma from metastatic carcinoid. Carcinoid tumor is negative for sustentacular cell S100 protein immunoreactivity. Malignant melanoma must be considered in the differential diagnosis since paraganglioma may contain melanin pigment.

The origin of paraganglioma of the bladder is uncertain. It is thought to arise from embryonic rests of chromaffin cells in the sympathetic plexus of the detrusor muscle.[74] It is postulated that small nests of paraganglionic tissue may persist along the aortic axis and in the pelvic regions, and these remnants of paraganglionic tissue may migrate into the urinary bladder wall during fetal development.[110–113] In an autopsy study of 409 patients, Honma identified paraganglia of the urinary bladder in 52% of the cases examined and found that paraganglia were present throughout different layers of the bladder wall, with a predilection for the anterior and posterior walls.[114] The trigone of the bladder was the least common location of paraganglia.[114] In Cheng et al.'s study, the majority of tumors (94%) involved the muscularis propria of the bladder wall, with a predilection for the posterior and lateral walls.[74] A significant number of patients (37%) also had extravesical extension or pelvic involvement. These findings support the hypothesis that paraganglioma of the bladder originates from paraganglionic cells that migrated into the bladder wall.[110] The high prevalence of paraganglionic cells within the muscular wall (63% of all paraganglia of the bladder)[114] is consistent with the frequent occurrence of paraganglioma in this location.

Genomic analyses have identified germline mutations responsible for sporadic as well as familial paraganglioma syndromes.[99,115–121] The susceptibility genes include *SDHB, SDHC*, and *SDHD*. Succinate dehydrogenase (SDH), which consists of four polypeptides [SDHA, SDHB (1p36), SDHC (1q21), and SDHD (11q23)], is the major mitochondrial enzyme linking the aerobic respiratory chain and the Krebs cycle, which oxidizes succinate to fumarate.[99,116] The SDH genes are tumor suppressor genes, the inactivation of which is involved in the hypoxia–angiogenic pathway, activating the transcription factor hypoxia–inducible factor (HIF).[99] Nonsense and missense mutations, insertions, and small and large deletions have been reported in the SDH genes of patients with pheochromocytoma or paraganglioma. These mutations are generally seen in younger patients. *SDHD* mutations have been identified in patients with pheochromocytoma or functional paraganglioma. Patients with these mutations usually have a paternal family history of disease due to maternal imprinting. *SDHB* gene mutations are usually associated with abdominal paragangliomas and are often identified in patients with no family history of the disease. The *SDHB* gene mutation is associated with a high risk of malignancy.[99]

HIF dysregulation is also linked to inactivation of the *VHL* tumor suppressor gene located on chromosome 3p25–26, which is seen in von Hippel–Lindau disease. Pheochromocytomas or paragangliomas may be seen in this disease.[122] Other autosomally dominant diseases associated with pheochromocytomas/paragangliomas include multiple endocrine neoplasia type 2 (due to mutation of the *RET* protooncogene) and neurofibromatosis type 1 (NF1) (due to a mutation in *NF1*, a tumor suppressor gene). Genetic aberrations at other loci (2q and 16p) have also recently been found to be associated with familial pheochromocytoma.[123] Similarly, Lemeta et al. found abnormalities in tumor suppressor genes located at 6q23–24 which may play a role in the tumorigenesis of pheochromocytomas.[124] van Nederveen et al. evaluated 14 benign and 17 malignant pheochromocytoma for phosphatase and tensin homologue (*PTEN*) abnormalities and found LOH in 40% of malignant tumors and 14% of benign tumors, but no mutations of *PTEN*.[125] They concluded that *PTEN* inactivation may play a minor role in the development of malignant pheochromocytomas.

Neurofibroma

Neurofibroma is a rare benign neoplastic tumor of the nerve sheath, composed of Schwann cells, perineurium-like cells, fibroblasts, and intermediate-type cells (**Figs. 15-40 to 15-43**).[126] Although most occur in the setting of NF1, rare cases of isolated sporadic bladder neurofibroma have also been reported.[127] Classically, neurofibromas of the urinary bladder occur in young patients with a slight male predominance.[128] In a recent series of four patients with bladder neurofibroma, the average age at diagnosis was 17 years; male-to-female ratio was 1:1. All patients had NF1. Presenting symptoms included hematuria, irritative voiding symptoms, and symptoms related to pelvic mass effect.[126]

The histologic findings in neurofibroma are the same regardless of site of occurrence. Classically, neurofibroma is a hypocellular proliferation of spindle cells, loosely

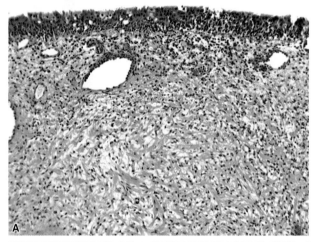

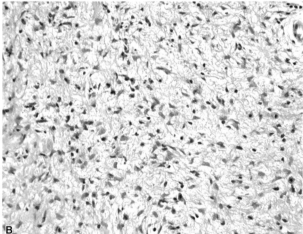

Figure 15-40 Neurofibroma of the bladder (A and B). Note the submucosal involvement (A). The cellularity is increased (B), which should not be mistaken for malignant transformation.

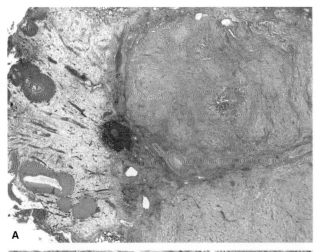

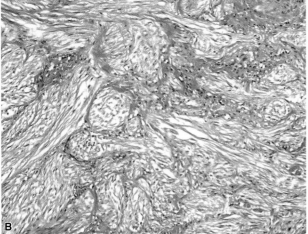

Figure 15-41 Neurofibroma of the bladder (A and B). The tumor displays diffuse and plexiform growth.

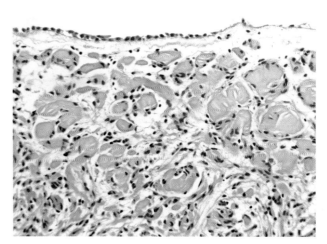

Figure 15-42 Neurofibroma of the bladder. Note the prominent superficial bandlike subepithelial pseudomeissnerian corpuscles; pseudomeissnerian corpuscles are positive for S100 protein (not shown).

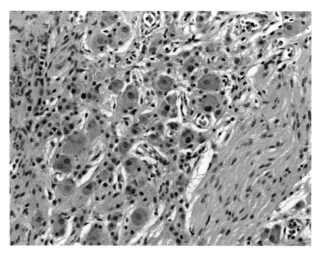

Figure 15-43 Neurofibroma of the bladder with ganglion cell involvement (A and B).

arranged into fascicles with scattered "shredded carrot" bundles of collagen. Individual cells have wavy, bland nuclei. In the series of Cheng et al., three of four were transmural with both diffuse and plexiform growth patterns.[126] Another case had diffuse submucosal involvement with subepithelial pseudomeissnerian corpuscle formation on biopsy examination. Areas of diffuse involvement were hypocellular with small to medium-sized spindle cells having ovoid to elongate nuclei in a collagenized matrix. A few mast cells were present. Immunohistochemical staining was positive in all cases for S100 protein as well as type IV collagen. Three were reactive for neurofilament protein in axons. All were negative for EMA, cytokeratins CAM5.2 and AE1/AE3, and p53 protein.[126] Recently, two neurofibromas have been found not to express ALK-1 protein.[129]

The differential diagnosis of bladder neurofibroma includes other spindle cell tumors, such as leiomyoma, postoperative spindle cell nodule, inflammatory myofibroblastic tumor, low grade leiomyosarcoma, MPNST, and rhabdomyosarcoma. Immunohistochemistry is useful in differentiating these tumors. Atypical neurofibromas may have nuclear atypia; however, they lack mitotic figures, a feature that distinguishes them from MPNST. Cellular neurofibroma differs from MPNST by being composed of smaller cells, and by its lack of mitotic figures, cellular atypia, nuclear pleomorphism, and necrosis. Unfortunately, neurofibromas in adults are occasionally associated with the development of MPNST, sometimes multifocally[71]; therefore, adequate sampling is imperative.[126]

The treatment of choice for bladder neurofibroma is unresolved. Symptomatic patients usually require surgery, sometimes extensive. Continued surveillance for malignant transformation is required. Long-term sequelae include bladder atony, neurogenic bladder, and recurrent urinary tract infection.[126]

Schwannoma

Schwannoma of the urinary bladder is derived from Schwann cells in nerve sheaths. It occurs in both men and women and is often associated with von Recklinghausen disease.[130] The age at presentation ranges from the fourth to sixth decades.[130,131] The presenting symptoms include bladder pressure, suprapubic pain, back pain, urgency, and frequency. No recurrences have been reported during followup periods of one to three years after surgical resection.[130,131]

Grossly, the tumor appears as a circumscribed mass, often arising from the lateral wall, beneath a normal mucosa. It may or may not extend into the perivesical fat. Schwannoma consists of spindle cells with uniform round to oval nuclei arranged in a palisading or organoid pattern. There is no nuclear pleomorphism, and mitotic figures are infrequent.[130,131] Tumor cells show positive immunostaining for S100 protein, NSE, and vimentin. Immunostains for myoglobin, factor VIII, keratins, actin (HHF-35), and desmin are negative.[130,131]

Secondary Neuroendocrine Carcinoma

A key differential diagnostic consideration is direct extension or metastasis from nonurothelial neuroendocrine carcinoma. The difficulty in distinguishing primary from secondary lesions is compounded by immunohistochemical and ultrastructural similarities, including cytoplasmic chromogranin and synaptophysin positivity, "dot-like" cytokeratin positivity. Although initially proposed as a specific marker for pulmonary small cell carcinoma, TTF-1 positivity has subsequently been demonstrated in 25% to 39% of bladder cases, limiting its utility in this differential diagnosis. Given these similarities, high grade pulmonary neuroendocrine carcinoma secondarily involving the bladder must be excluded on clinical and radiological grounds.[3,4] Identification of urothelial carcinoma in situ and coexisting urothelial carcinoma component supports the diagnosis of bladder primary.

Small cell carcinoma originating in the prostate can be difficult to discern pathologically from those originating in the bladder and involving the prostate, and vice versa, especially if a component of conventional urothelial or prostatic carcinoma is absent. Prostatic small cell carcinomas are often negative for prostate-specific antigen and prostate-specific acid phosphatase Recent studies have identified gene fusions between members of the ETS family of genes and transmembrane protease, serine 2 (TMPRSS2) to be a significant event in prostate cancer, in particular fusion of transcriptional regulator ERG (ETS-related gene) and TMPRSS2.[132-134] Williamson and his colleagues evaluated ERG–TMPRSS gene rearrangement in 30 cases of prostatic small cell carcinoma and 25 cases of small cell carcinoma of the urinary bladder by FISH.[39] TMPRSS2–ERG gene fusion was found in 47% of prostatic small cell carcinomas, but not in any of bladder small cell carcinoma examined. Identification of TMPRSS2–ERG gene fusion by FISH is helpful in establishing prostatic origin.

REFERENCES

1. Cheng L, Pan C, Yang XJ, Lopez-Beltran A, MacLennan GT, Lin H, Kuzel TM, Papavero V, Tretiakova M, Nigro K, Koch MO, Eble JN. Small cell carcinoma of the urinary bladder: a clinicopathologic analysis of 64 patients. *Cancer* 2004;101:957–62.

2. Cheng L, Jones TD, McCarthy RP, Eble JN, Wang M, MacLennan GT, Lopez-Beltran A, Yang XJ, Koch MO, Zhang S, Pan CX, Baldridge LA. Molecular genetic evidence for a common clonal origin of urinary bladder small cell carcinoma and coexisting urothelial carcinoma. *Am J Pathol* 2005;166:1533–9.

3. Wang X, MacLennan GT, Lopez-Beltran A, Cheng L. Small cell carcinoma of the urinary bladder—histogenesis, genetics, diagnosis, biomarkers, treatment, and prognosis. *Appl Immunohistochem Mol Morphol* 2007;15:8–18.

4. Mazzucchelli R, Morichetti D, Lopez-Beltran A, Cheng L, Scarpelli M, Kirkali Z, Montironi R. Neuroendocrine tumours of the urinary system and male genital organs: clinical significance. *BJU Int* 2009;103:1464–70.

5. Abrahams NA, Moran C, Reyes AO, Siefker-Radtke A, Ayala AG. Small cell carcinoma of the bladder: a contemporary clinicopathological study of 51 cases. *Histopathology* 2005;46:57–63.

6. Blomjous CE, Vos W, De Voogt HJ, Van der Valk P, Meijer CJ. Small cell carcinoma of the urinary bladder. A clinicopathologic, morphometric, immunohistochemical, and ultrastructural study of 18 cases. *Cancer* 1989;64:1347–57.

7. Choong NW, Quevedo JF, Kaur JS. Small cell carcinoma of the urinary bladder. The Mayo Clinic experience. *Cancer* 2005;103:1172–8.

8. Lohrisch C, Murray N, Pickles T, Sullivan L. Small cell carcinoma of the bladder: long term outcome with integrated chemoradiation. *Cancer* 1999;86:2346–52.

9. Abbas F, Civantos F, Benedetto P, Soloway MS. Small cell carcinoma of the bladder and prostate. *Urology* 1995;46:617–30.

10. Ali SZ, Reuter VE, Zakowski MF. Small cell neuroendocrine carcinoma of the urinary bladder. A clinicopathologic study with emphasis on cytologic features. *Cancer* 1997;79:356–61.

11. Willis D, Canales BK, Cheng L, MacLennan GT. Neural neoplasms of the bladder. *J Urol* 2010;184:1492–3.

12. Yu DS, Chang SY, Wang J, Yang TH, Cheng CL, Lee SS, Ma CM. Small cell carcinoma of the urinary tract. *Br J Urol* 1990;66:590–5.

13. Reyes CV, Soneru I. Small cell carcinoma of the urinary bladder with hypercalcemia. *Cancer* 1985;56:2530–3.

14. Cramer SF, Aikawa M, Cebelin M. Neurosecretory granules in small cell invasive carcinoma of the urinary bladder. *Cancer* 1981;47:724–30.

15. Partanen S, Asikainen U. Oat cell carcinoma of the urinary bladder with ectopic adrenocorticotropic hormone production. *Hum Pathol* 1985;16:313–5.

16. Angulo JC, Lopez JI, Sanchez-Chapado M, Sakr W, Montie JE, Pontes EJ, Redman B, Flaherty L, Grignon DJ. Small cell carcinoma of the urinary bladder: a report of two cases with complete remission and a comprehensive literature review with emphasis on therapeutic decisions. *J Urol Pathol* 1996;5:1–19.

17. Grignon DJ, Ro JY, Ayala AG, Shum DT, Ordonez NG, Logothetis CJ, Johnson DE, Mackay B. Small cell carcinoma of the urinary bladder. A clinicopathologic analysis of 22 cases. *Cancer* 1992;69:527–36.

18. Bastus R, Caballero JM, Gonzalez G, Borrat P, Casalots J, Gomez de Segura G, Marti LI, Ristol J, Cirera L. Small cell carcinoma of the urinary bladder treated with chemotherapy and radiotherapy: results in five cases. *Eur Urol* 1999;35:323–6.

19. Mills SE, Wolfe JT 3rd, Weiss MA, Swanson PE, Wick MR, Fowler JE Jr, Young RH. Small cell undifferentiated carcinoma of the urinary bladder. A light-microscopic, immunocytochemical, and ultrastructural study of 12 cases. *Am J Surg Pathol* 1987;11:606–17.

20. Kim CK, Lin JI, Tseng CH. Small cell carcinoma of urinary bladder. Ultrastructural study. *Urology* 1984;24:384–6.

21. Pan CX, Zhang H, Lara PN, Cheng L. Small-cell carcinoma of the urinary bladder: diagnosis and management. *Expert Rev Anticancer Ther* 2006;6:1707–13.

22. Wang X, Zhang S, MacLennan GT, Eble JN, Lopez-Beltran A, Yang XJ, Pan CX, Zhou H, Montironi R, Cheng L. Epidermal growth factor receptor protein expression and gene amplification in small cell carcinoma of the urinary bladder. *Clin Cancer Res* 2007;13:953–7.

23. Trias I, Algaba F, Condom E, Espanol I, Segui J, Orsola I, Villavicencio H, Garcia Del Muro X. Small cell carcinoma of the urinary bladder. Presentation of 23 cases and review of 134 published cases. *Eur Urol* 2001;39:85–90.

24. Emerson RE, Cheng L. Immunohistochemical markers in the evaluation of tumors of the urinary bladder: a review. *Anal Quant Cytol Histol* 2005;27:301–16.

25. Jones TD, Kernek KM, Yang XJ, Lopez-Beltran A, MacLennan GT, Eble JN, Lin H, Pan CX, Tretiakova M, Baldridge LA, Cheng L. Thyroid transcription factor 1 expression in small cell carcinoma of the urinary bladder: an immunohistochemical profile of 44 cases. *Hum Pathol* 2005;36:718–23.

26. Pan CX, Yang XJ, Lopez-Beltran A, MacLennan GT, Eble JN, Koch MO, Jones TD, Lin H, Nigro K, Papavero V, Tretiakova M, Cheng L. C-kit expression in small cell carcinoma of the urinary bladder: prognostic and therapeutic implications. *Mod Pathol* 2005;18:320–3.

27. Wang X, Jones TD, MacLennan GT, Yang XJ, Lopez-Beltran A, Eble JN, Koch MO, Lin H, Baldridge LA, Tretiakova M, Cheng L. p53 expression in small cell carcinoma of

the urinary bladder: biological and prognostic implications. *Anticancer Res* 2005;25:2001–4.

28. Blomjous CE, Vos W, Schipper NW, De Voogt HJ, Baak JP, Meijer CJ. Morphometric and flow cytometric analysis of small cell undifferentiated carcinoma of the bladder. *J Clin Pathol* 1989;42:1032–9.

29. Hodges KB, Lopez-Beltran A, Emerson RE, Montironi R, Cheng L. Clinical utility of immunohistochemistry in the diagnoses of urinary bladder neoplasia. *Appl Immunohistochem Mol Morphol* 2010;18:401–10.

30. Lopez JI, Angulo JC, Flores N, Toledo JD. Small cell carcinoma of the urinary bladder. A clinicopathological study of six cases. *Br J Urol* 1994;73:43–9.

31. Soriano P, Navarro S, Gil M, Llombart-Bosch A. Small-cell carcinoma of the urinary bladder. A clinico-pathological study of ten cases. *Virchows Arch* 2004;445:292–7.

32. Helpap B. Morphology and therapeutic strategies for neuroendocrine tumors of the genitourinary tract. *Cancer* 2002;95:1415–20.

33. Ordonez NG. Value of thyroid transcription factor-1 immunostaining in distinguishing small cell lung carcinomas from other small cell carcinomas. *Am J Surg Pathol* 2000;24:1217–23.

34. Iczkowski KA, Shanks JH, Allsbrook WC, Lopez-Beltran A, Pantazis CG, Collins TR, Wetherington RW, Bostwick DG. Small cell carcinoma of urinary bladder is differentiated from urothelial carcinoma by chromogranin expression, absence of CD44 variant 6 expression, a unique pattern of cytokeratin expression, and more intense gamma-enolase expression. *Histopathology* 1999;35:150–6.

35. Iczkowski KA, Shanks JH, Bostwick DG. Loss of CD44 variant 6 expression differentiates small cell carcinoma of urinary bladder from urothelial (transitional cell) carcinoma. *Histopathology* 1998;32:322–7.

36. Eble JN, Epstein JI, Sauter G, Sesterhenn IA, eds. WHO

Classification of Tumours: Pathology and Genetics. Tumours of the Urinary and Male Reproductive System. Lyon, France: IARC Press, 2004.

37. Cheuk W, Kwan MY, Suster S, Chan JKC. Immunostaining for thyroid transcription factor 1 and cytokeratin 20 aids in the distinction of small cell carcinoma from Merkel cell carcinoma, but not pulmonary from extrapulmonary small cell carcinomas. *Arch Pathol Lab Med* 2001;125:228–31.

38. Chan JK, Suster S, Wenig BM, Tsang WY, Chan JB, Lau AL. Cytokeratin 20 immunoreactivity distinguishes Merkel cell (primary cutaneous neuroendocrine) carcinomas and salivary gland small cell carcinomas from small cell carcinomas of various sites. *Am J Surg Pathol* 1997;21:226–34.

39. Williamson SR, Zhang S, Yao JL, Huang J, Lopez-Beltran A, Shen S, Osunkoya AO, MacLennan GT, Montironi R, Cheng L. ERG-TMPRSS2 rearrangement is shared by concurrent prostatic adenocarcinoma and prostatic small cell carcinoma and absent in small cell carcinoma of the urinary bladder: evidence supporting monoclonal origin. *Mod Pathol* 2011;24:1120–7.

40. Podesta AH, True LD. Small cell carcinoma of the bladder. Report of five cases with immunohistochemistry and review of the literature with evaluation of prognosis according to stage. *Cancer* 1989;64:710–4.

41. Martignoni G, Eble JN. Carcinoid tumors of the urinary bladder. Immunohistochemical study of 2 cases and review of the literature. *Arch Pathol Lab Med* 2003;127:e22–24.

42. Oesterling JE, Brendler CB, Burgers JK, Marshall FF, Epstein JI. Advanced small cell carcinoma of the bladder. Successful treatment with combined radical cystoprostatectomy and adjuvant methotrexate, vinblastine, doxorubicin, and cisplatin chemotherapy. *Cancer* 1990;65:1928–36.

43. Atkin NB, Baker MC, Wilson GD. Chromosome abnormalities and p53 expression in a small cell carcinoma of the bladder. *Cancer Genet Cytogenet* 1995;79:111–4.

44. Terracciano L, Richter J, Tornillo L, Beffa L, Diener PA, Maurer R, Gasser TC, Moch H, Mihatsch MJ, Sauter G. Chromosomal imbalances in small cell carcinomas of the urinary bladder. *J Pathol* 1999;189:230–5.

45. Leonard C, Huret JL, Gfco, oncologique Gfdc. From cytogenetics to cytogenomics of bladder cancers. *Bull Cancer* 2002;89:166–73.

46. Wang HL, Lu DW. Detection of human papillomavirus DNA and expression of p16, Rb, and p53 proteins in small cell carcinomas of the uterine cervix. *Am J Surg Pathol* 2004;28:901–8.

47. Hollstein M, Sidransky D, Vogelstein B, Harris CC. p53 mutations in human cancers. *Science* 1991;253:49–53.

48. Cheng L, Zhang D. Molecular Genetic Pathology. New York: Humana Press/Springer, 2008.

49. Haque AK, Syed S, Lele SM, Freeman DH, Adegboyega PA. Immunohistochemical study of thyroid transcription factor-1 and HER2/neu in non-small cell lung cancer: strong thyroid transcription factor-1 expression predicts better survival. *Appl Immunohistochem Mol Morphol* 2002;10:103–9.

50. Hirsch FR, Scagliotti GV, Langer CJ, Varella-Garcia M, Franklin WA. Epidermal growth factor family of receptors in preneoplasia and lung cancer: perspectives for targeted therapies. *Lung Cancer* 2003;41 Suppl 1:S29–42.

51. Druker BJ, Talpaz M, Resta DJ, Peng B, Buchdunger E, Ford JM, Lydon NB, Kantarjian H, Capdeville R, Ohno-Jones S, Sawyers CL. Efficacy and safety of a specific inhibitor of the BCR-ABL tyrosine kinase in chronic myeloid leukemia. *N Engl J Med* 2001;344:1031–7.

52. Slamon DJ, Leyland-Jones B, Shak S, Fuchs H, Paton V, Bajamonde A, Fleming T, Eiermann W, Wolter J, Pegram M, Baselga J, Norton L. Use of chemotherapy plus a monoclonal antibody against HER2 for metastatic breast cancer that overexpresses HER2. *N Engl J Med* 2001;344:783–92.

53. Ullrich A, Schlessinger J. Signal transduction by receptors with

tyrosine kinase activity. *Cell* 1990;61:203–12.

54. Quek ML, Nichols PW, Yamzon J, Daneshmand S, Miranda G, Cai J, Groshen S, Stein JP, Skinner DG. Radical cystectomy for primary neuroendocrine tumors of the bladder: the University of Southern California experience. *J Urol* 2005;174:93–6.

55. Mackey JR, Au HJ, Hugh J, Venner P. Genitourinary small cell carcinoma: determination of clinical and therapeutic factors associated with survival. *J Urol* 1998;159:1624–9.

56. Wick MR. Immunohistology of neuroendocrine and neuroectodermal tumors. *Semin Diagn Pathol* 2000;17:194–203.

57. Murali R, Kneale K, Lalak N, Delprado W. Carcinoid tumors of the urinary tract and prostate. *Arch Pathol Lab Med* 2006;130:1693–706.

58. Burgess NA, Lewis DC, Matthews PN. Primary carcinoid of the bladder. *Br J Urol* 1992;69:213–4.

59. Chin NW, Marinescu AM, Fani K. Composite adenocarcinoma and carcinoid tumor of urinary bladder. *Urology* 1992;40:249–52.

60. Colby TV. Carcinoid tumor of the bladder. A case report. *Arch Pathol Lab Med* 1980;104:199–200.

61. Stanfield BL, Grimes MM, Kay S. Primary carcinoid tumor of the bladder arising beneath an inverted papilloma. *Arch Pathol Lab Med* 1994;118:666–7.

62. Sugihara A, Kajio K, Yoshimoto T, Tsujimura T, Iwasaki H, Yamada N, Terada N, Tsuji M, Nojima M, Yabumoto H, Mori Y, Shima H. Primary carcinoid tumor of the urinary bladder. *Int Urol Nephrol* 2002;33:53–7.

63. Walker BF, Someren A, Kennedy JC, Nicholas EM. Primary carcinoid tumor of the urinary bladder. *Arch Pathol Lab Med* 1992;116:1217–20.

64. Yang CH, Krzyzaniak K, Brown WJ, Kurtz SM. Primary carcinoid tumor of urinary bladder. *Urology* 1985;26:594–7.

65. Lee KH, Ryu SB, Lee MC, Park CS, Juhng SW, Choi C. Primary large cell neuroendocrine carcinoma of the urinary bladder. *Pathol Int* 2006;56:688–93.

66. Dundr P, Pesl M, Povysil C, Vitkova I, Dvoracek J, Large cell neuroendocrine carcinoma of the urinary bladder with lymphoepithelioma-like features. *Pathol Res Pract* 2003;199:559–63.

67. Evans AJ, Al-Maghrabi J, Tsihlias J, Lajoie G, Sweet JM, Chapman WB. Primary large cell neuroendocrine carcinoma of the urinary bladder. *Arch Pathol Lab Med* 2002;126:1229–32.

68. Hailemariam S, Gaspert A, Komminoth P, Tamboli P, Amin M. Primary, pure, large-cell neuroendocrine carcinoma of the urinary bladder. *Mod Pathol* 1998;11:1016–20.

69. Lopez-Beltran A, Perez-Seoane C, Montironi R, Hernandez-Iglesias T, Mackintosh C, de Alava E. Primary primitive neuroectodermal tumour of the urinary bladder: a clinico-pathological study emphasising immunohistochemical, ultrastructural and molecular analyses. *J Clin Pathol* 2006;59:775–8.

70. Kruger S, Schmidt H, Kausch I, Bohle A, Holzhausen H, Johannisson R, Feller A. Primitive neuroectodermal tumor (PNET) of the urinary bladder. *Path Res Pract* 2003;199:751–4.

71. Rober PE, Smith JB, Sakr W, Pierce JM Jr. Malignant peripheral nerve sheath tumor (malignant schwannoma) of urinary bladder in von Recklinghausen neurofibromatosis. *Urology* 1991;38:473–6.

72. Eltoum IA, Moore RJ 3rd, Cook W, Crowe DR, Rodgers WH, Siegal GP. Epithelioid variant of malignant peripheral nerve sheath tumor (malignant schwannoma) of the urinary bladder. *Ann Diagn Pathol* 1999;3:304–8.

73. Daimaru Y, Hashimoto H, Enjoji M. Malignant "triton" tumors: a clinicopathologic and immunohistochemical study of nine cases. *Hum Pathol* 1984;15:768–78.

74. Cheng L, Leibovich BC, Cheville JC, Ramnani DM, Sebo TJ, Neumann RM, Nascimento AG, Zincke H, Bostwick DG. Paraganglioma of the urinary bladder: Can biologic potential be predicted? *Cancer* 2000;88:844–52.

75. Yoffa D, Withycombe J. Bladder-pheochromocytoma metastases. *Lancet* 1967;290:422.

76. Pugh R, Gresham G, Mullaney J. Phaeochromocytoma of the urinary bladder. *J Path Bact* 1960;79:89–107.

77. Poirer H, Robinson JO. Pheochromocytoma of the urinary bladder: a male patient. *Br J Urol* 1962;34:88–92.

78. Glucksman MA, Persinger CP. Malignant non-chromaffin paraganglioma of the bladder. *J Urol* 1963;89:822–5.

79. Grignon DJ, Ro JY, Mackay B, Ordonez NG, el-Naggar A, Molina TJ, Shum DT, Ayala AG. Paraganglioma of the urinary bladder: immunohistochemical, ultrastructural, and DNA flow cytometric studies. *Hum Pathol* 1991;22:1162–9.

80. Leestma JE, Price EB Jr. Paraganglioma of the urinary bladder. *Cancer* 1971;28:1063–73.

81. Das S, Lowe P. Malignant pheochromocytoma of the bladder. *J Urol* 1980;123:282–4.

82. Das S, Bulusu NV, Lowe P. Primary vesical pheochromocytoma. *Urology* 1983;21:20–5.

83. Davaris P, Petraki K, Arvanitis D, Papacharalammpous N, Morakis A, Zorzos S. Urinary bladder paraganglioma (U.B.P.). *Pathol Res Pract* 1986;181:101–6.

84. Javaheri P, Raafat J. Malignant phaeochromocytoma of the urinary bladder—report of two cases. *Br J Urol* 1975;47:401–4.

85. Higgins P, Tresidder G. Malignant phaeochromocytoma of the urinary bladder. *Br J Urol* 1980;52:230.

86. Moloney G, Cowdell R, Lewis C. Malignant phaeochromocytoma of the bladder. *Br J Urol* 1966;38:461–70.

87. Shimbo S, Nakano Y. A case of malignant pheochromocytoma producing parathyroid hormone-like substance. *Cal Tissue Res* 1974;15:155.

88. Asbury W, hatcher P, Gould H, Reeves W, Wilson D. Bladder pheochromocytoma with ring calcification. *Abdom Imaging* 1996;21:275–7.

89. Deklerk DP, Catalona WJ, Nime FA, Freeman C. Malignant pheochromocytoma of the bladder: the late development of renal cell carcinoma. *J Urol* 1975;113:864–8.

90. Campbell DR, Mason W, Manchester J. Angiography in pheochromocytomas. *J Can Assoc Radiol* 1974;25:214–23.

91. Lumb B, Gresham G. Phaeochromocytoma of the urinary bladder. *Lancet* 1958;1:81–2.

92. Meyer J, Sane S, Drake R. Malignant paraganglioma (pheochromocytoma) of the urinary bladder: report of a case and review of the literature. *Pediatrics* 1979;63:879–85.

93. Scott W, Eversole S. Pheochromocytoma of the urinary baldder. *J Urol* 1960;83:656–64.

94. Piedrola G, Lopez E, Rueda M, Lopez R, Serrano J, Sancho M. Malignant pheochromocytoma of the bladder: current controversies. *Eur Urol* 1997;31:122–5.

95. Zhou M, Epstein JI, Young RH. Paraganglioma of the urinary bladder: a lesion that may be misdiagnosed as urothelial carcinoma in transurethral resection specimens. *Am J Surg Pathol* 2004;28:94–100.

96. Medeiros L, Wolf B, Balogh K, Federman M. Adrenal pheochromocytoma: a clinicopathologic review of 60 cases. *Hum Pathol* 1985;16:580–9.

97. Albores-Saavedra J, Maldonado ME, Ibarra J, Rodriguez HA. Pheochromocytoma of the urinary bladder. *Cancer* 1969;23:1110–8.

98. Jurascheck F, Egloff H, Buemi A, Laedlein-Greilsammer D. Paraganglioma of urinary bladder. *Urology* 1983;22:659–63.

99. Gimenez-Roqueplo AP. New advances in the genetics of pheochromocytoma and paraganglioma syndromes. *Ann N Y Acad Sci* 2006;1073:112–21.

100. Moyana TN, Kontozoglou T. Urinary bladder paragangliomas. An immunohistochemical study. *Arch Pathol Lab Med* 1988;112:70–2.

101. Drew PA, Furman J, Civantos F, Murphy WM. The nested variant of transitional cell carcinoma: an aggressive neoplasm with innocuous histology. *Mod Pathol* 1996;9:989–94.

102. Murphy WM, Deanna DG. The nested variant of transitional cell carcinoma: a neoplasm resembling proliferation of Brunn's nests. *Mod Pathol* 1992;5:240–3.

103. Talbert ML, Young RH. Carcinomas of the urinary bladder with deceptively benign-appearing foci. A report of three cases. *Am J Surg Pathol* 1989;13:374–81.

104. Moran CA, Albores-Saavedra J, Wenig BM, Mena H. Pigmented extraadrenal paraganlioma: a clinicopathologic and immunohistochemical study of five cases. *Cancer* 1997;79:398–402.

105. Mouradian J, Coleman J, McGovern J, Gray G. Granular cell tumor (myoblastoma) of the bladder. *J Urol* 1974;112:343–5.

106. Mizutani S, Okuda N, Sonoda T. Granular cell myoblastoma of the bladder: report of an additional case. *J Urol* 1973;110:403–5.

107. Seery WH. Granular cell myoblastoma of the bladder: report of a case. *J Urol* 1968;100:735–7.

108. Fletcher MS, Aker M, Hill JT, Pryor JP, Whimster WF. Granular cell myoblastoma of the bladder. *Br J Urol* 1985;57:109–10.

109. Christ M, Ozzello L. Myogenous origin of a granular cell tumor of the urinary bladder. *Am J Clin Pathol* 1971;56:736–49.

110. Zimmerman I, Biron R, MacMahon H. Pheochromocytoma of the urinary bladder. *N Engl J Med* 1953;249:25–6.

111. Dixon J, Gosling J, Canning D, Gearhart J. An immunohistochemical study of human postnatal paraganglia associated with the urinary bladder. *J Anat* 1992;181:431–6.

112. Fletcher T, Bradley W. Neuroanatomy of the bladder-urethra. *J Urol* 1978;119:153–60.

113. Rode J, Bentley A, Parkinson C. Paraganglial cells of urinary bladder and prostate: potential diagnostic problem. *J Clin Pathol* 1990;43:13–16.

114. Honma K. Paraganglia of the urinary bladder. An autopsy study. *Zentralbl Pathol* 1994;139:465–9.

115. Bayley JP, van Minderhout I, Weiss MM, Jansen JC, Oomen PH, Menko FH, Pasini B, Ferrando B, Wong N, Alpert LC, Williams R, Blair E, Devilee P, Taschner PE. Mutation analysis of SDHB and SDHC: novel germline mutations in sporadic head and neck paraganglioma and familial paraganglioma and/or pheochromocytoma. *BMC Med Genet* 2006;7:1.

116. Mannelli M, Simi L, Ercolino T, Gagliano MS, Becherini L, Vinci S, Sestini R, Gensini F, Pinzani P, Mascalchi M, Guerrini L, Pratesi C, Nesi G, Torti F, Cipollini F, Bernini GP, Genuardi M. SDH mutations in patients affected by paraganglioma syndromes: a personal experience. *Ann N Y Acad Sci* 2006;1073:183–9.

117. Braun S, Riemann K, Kupka S, Leistenschneider P, Sotlar K, Schmid H, Blin N. Active succinate dehydrogenase (SDH) and lack of SDHD mutations in sporadic paragangliomas. *Anticancer Res* 2005;25:2809–14.

118. Koch CA, Vortmeyer AO, Zhuang Z, Brouwers FM, Pacak K. New insights into the genetics of familial chromaffin cell tumors. *Ann N Y Acad Sci* 2002;970:11–28.

119. Amar L, Bertherat J, Baudin E, Ajzenberg C, Bressac-de Paillerets B, Chabre O, Chamontin B, Delemer B, Giraud S, Murat A, Niccoli-Sire P, Richard S, Rohmer V, Sadoul JL, Strompf L, Schlumberger M, Bertagna X, Plouin PF, Jeunemaitre X, Gimenez-Roqueplo AP. Genetic testing in pheochromocytoma or functional paraganglioma. *J Clin Oncol* 2005;23:8812–8.

120. Cascon A, Montero-Conde C, Ruiz-Llorente S, Mercadillo F, Leton R, Rodriguez-Antona C, Martinez-Delgado B, Delgado M, Diez A, Rovira A, Diaz JA, Robledo M. Gross SDHB deletions in patients with paraganglioma detected by multiplex PCR: A possible hot spot? *Genes Chromosomes Cancer* 2006;45:213–9.

121. Astuti D, Hart-Holden N, Latif F, Lalloo F, Black GC, Lim C, Moran A, Grossman AB, Hodgson SV, Freemont A, Ramsden R, Eng C, Evans DG, Maher ER. Genetic analysis of mitochondrial complex II subunits SDHD, SDHB and SDHC in paraganglioma and phaeochromocytoma susceptibility. *Clin Endocrinol (Oxf)* 2003;59:728–33.

122. Pollard PJ, El-Bahrawy M, Poulsom R, Elia G, Killick P, Kelly G, Hunt T, Jeffery R, Seedhar P, Barwell J, Latif F, Gleeson MJ, Hodgson SV, Stamp GW, Tomlinson IP, Maher ER. Expression of HIF-1alpha, HIF-2alpha (EPAS1), and their target *genes* in paraganglioma and pheochromocytoma with VHL and SDH mutations. *J Clin Endocrinol Metab* 2006;91:4593–8.

123. Dahia PL. Evolving concepts in pheochromocytoma and paraganglioma. *Curr Opin Oncol* 2006;18:1–8.

124. Lemeta S, Salmenkivi K, Pylkkanen L, Sainio M, Saarikoski ST, Arola J, Heikkila P, Haglund C, Husgafvel-Pursiainen K, Bohling T. Frequent loss of heterozygosity at 6q in pheochromocytoma. *Hum Pathol* 2006;37:749–54.

125. van Nederveen FH, Perren A, Dannenberg H, Petri BJ, Dinjens WN, Komminoth P, de Krijger RR. PTEN gene loss, but not mutation, in benign and malignant phaeochromocytomas. *J Pathol* 2006;209:274–80.

126. Cheng L, Scheithauer BW, Leibovich BC, Ramnani DM, Cheville JC, Bostwick DG. Neurofibroma of the urinary bladder. *Cancer* 1999;86:505–13.

127. Tucker T, Wolkenstein P, Revuz J, Zeller J, Friedman JM. Association between benign and malignant peripheral nerve sheath tumors in NF1. *Neurology* 2005;65:205–11.

128. Eble JN, Sauter G, Epstein JI, Sesterhenn IA, eds. World Health Organization Classification of Tumours: Pathology and Genetics of Tumours of the Urinary System and Male Genital Organs. Lyon, France: IARC Press, 2004.

129. Freeman A, Geddes N, Munson P, Joseph J, Ramani P, Sandison A, Fisher C, Parkinson MC. Anaplastic lymphoma kinase (ALK 1) staining and molecular analysis in inflammatory myofibroblastic tumours of the bladder: a preliminary clinicopathological study of nine cases and review of the literature. *Mod Pathol* 2004;17:765–71.

130. Geol H, Kim DW, Kim TH, Seong YK, Cho WY, Kim SD, Lee KS, Sung GT. Laparoscopic partial cystectomy for schwannoma of urinary bladder: case report. *J Endourol* 2005;19:303–6.

131. Cummings JM, Wehry MA, Parra RO, Levy BK. Schwannoma of the urinary bladder: a case report. *Int J Urol* 1998;5:496–7.

132. Tomlins SA, Rhodes DR, Perner S, Dhanasekaran SM, Mehra R, Sun XW, Varambally S, Cao X, Tchinda J, Kuefer R, Lee C, Montie JE, Shah RB, Pienta KJ, Rubin MA, Chinnaiyan AM. Recurrent fusion of TMPRSS2 and ETS transcription factor *genes* in prostate cancer. *Science* 2005;310: 644–8.

133. Kumar-Sinha C, Tomlins SA, Chinnaiyan AM. Recurrent gene fusions in prostate cancer. *Nat Rev Cancer* 2008;8:497–511.

134. Andreoiu M, Cheng L. Multifocal prostate cancer: biological, prognostic, and therapeutic implications. *Hum Pathol* 2010;41:781–93.

Chapter 16

Sarcomatoid Carcinoma (Carcinosarcoma)

Bladder Pathology, First Edition. Liang Cheng, Antonio Lopez-Beltran, David G. Bostwick.
© 2012 Wiley-Blackwell. Published 2012 by John Wiley & Sons, Inc.

Overview

Uncommonly, bladder carcinomas exhibit the presence of malignant components that morphologically resemble various types of sarcoma. Such tumors have been described under a variety of names, including sarcomatoid carcinoma, carcinosarcoma, malignant mixed mesodermal tumor, and spindle and giant cell carcinoma.[1,2] The current recommendation by the World Health Organization (WHO) is to use the unifying term "sarcomatoid carcinoma" for all biphasic tumors with evidence of both epithelial and mesenchymal differentiation.[3]

Tumors with composite carcinomatous and sarcomatous features have been characterized by a wide range of microscopic appearances.[1,2,4–33] The epithelial component, which may or may not be easily identifiable, may be invasive or in situ carcinoma. The epithelial component is most frequently identified as urothelial carcinoma, small cell carcinoma, squamous cell carcinoma, or adenocarcinoma, whereas the mesenchymal component ranges from an undifferentiated spindle cell malignancy to recognizable heterologous elements such as osteosarcoma, chondrosarcoma, rhabdomyosarcoma, and leiomyosarcoma. The spindle cell component often has marked nuclear pleomorphism and hyperchromasia. Some of these tumors are composed only of sarcomatoid spindle cells and malignant giant cells, and the presence of epithelial differentiation is only appreciated after the performance of immunohistochemical studies. The spindle cell component may appear undifferentiated or may show one or more specific lines of mesenchymal differentiation, such as chondroid or leiomyomatous differentiation. The presence of specific types of apparent differentiation of the spindle cell component does not influence the prognosis. These tumors are usually high grade, biologically aggressive, and associated with a poor prognosis.[1,5]

Although the exact histogenesis of sarcomatoid carcinoma has not been elucidated, two primary theories have been proposed.[1,24,34,35] The monoclonal theory proposes that sarcomatoid carcinoma arises from a single, pluripotential stem cell with divergent differentiation. In contrast, the multiclonal theory suggests that sarcomatoid carcinoma represents a collision tumor composed of the epithelial and mesenchymal derivatives of two different stem cells.[26,27] Recent molecular studies strongly argue for the monoclonal origin of this tumor.[4,8–11] Evidence accumulates that sarcomatoid carcinoma represents the final common pathway of dedifferentiation for all forms of epithelial bladder tumors.[1]

Definition and Terminology

The term "sarcomatoid carcinoma" applies when a malignant neoplasm exhibits morphologic or immunohistochemical evidence of both epithelial and mesenchymal differentiation. These tumors usually have readily identifiable malignant epithelial cells and may contain an admixed component resembling various types of sarcoma. There is considerable confusion and disagreement in the literature regarding nomenclature and histogenesis of these tumors. Various terms have been used for these neoplasms, including carcinosarcoma, sarcomatoid carcinoma, pseudosarcomatous transitional cell carcinoma, malignant mesodermal mixed tumor, spindle cell carcinoma, giant cell carcinoma, and malignant teratoma.[12,27,31] In some reports, both carcinosarcoma and sarcomatoid carcinoma are included under the term "sarcomatoid carcinoma." In others, they are regarded as separate entities. Historically, "sarcomatoid carcinoma" referred to tumors with a mesenchyme-like spindle cell component that retained expression of epithelial markers. The term "carcinosarcoma" was applied to tumors with heterologous elements, or those lacking demonstrable immunohistochemical or ultrastructural evidence of epithelial differentiation in the mesenchymal component. Pathologists have largely discarded the notion of distinguishing between the two tumor types, since both are rapidly growing polypoid neoplasms that present at an advanced stage, confer a similar poor prognosis, and affect patients with similar risk factors. The overlap in clinical and molecular features suggests that these two entities are variations of the same neoplastic transformation process, and both are considered sarcomatoid carcinoma with varying degrees of divergent differentiation.[1]

We prefer to use the term "sarcomatoid carcinoma" for the majority of cases in which there is a spindle cell component with positive cytokeratin and vimentin staining. Some may use the term "carcinosarcoma" for cases with identifiable heterologous elements on hematoxylin and eosin-stained sections or positive staining for markers of specific mesenchymal differentiation. Both diagnostic categories appear to be variations of the same neoplastic transformation process and have the same clinical features and prognosis. The most appropriate term for all of these neoplasms is "sarcomatoid carcinoma."[1] "Sarcomatoid carcinoma" is the umbrella term that most appropriately describes all of these biphasic neoplasms as well as monophasic spindle cell carcinoma.[36–38]

Clinical Presentation

Sarcomatoid carcinoma of the urinary bladder represents approximately 0.3% of all histological types of bladder carcinoma and predominantly affects older adults and elderly, with a predilection for males. The mean age at the diagnosis is 66 years. The male-to-female ratio is 3 : 1.

Sarcomatoid carcinoma of the bladder most commonly causes gross hematuria and, less commonly, is associated with dysuria, pollakiuria, acute urinary retention, lower abdominal pain, or urinary tract infection.[5,13,25,27,31] Cystoscopy reveals broad-based and often polypoid masses with ulcerated and hemorrhagic surfaces. Imaging via computerized tomography and magnetic resonance demonstrates that the broad-based masses usually extend into or beyond the muscularis propria.

The exact etiology is uncertain. A history of radiation therapy or cyclophosphamide therapy, two well-established risk factors for bladder cancer, has been reported in bladder sarcomatoid carcinoma.[1,5,32,38-40] Nonetheless, such cases, apparently induced by radiation or cyclophosphamide exposure, represent only a small fraction of all bladder cancers. Previous treatment with cyclophosphamide and radiation therapy may result in transformation of conventional urothelial carcinoma into sarcomatoid carcinoma.[41] The interval between radiation therapy and cancer development is long, often more than 10 years. Tobacco smoking, another important risk factor for bladder cancer, was noted in five out of eight cases of bladder sarcomatoid carcinoma.[27] Other commonly reported antecedents include previous urothelial carcinoma, recurrent cystitis, diabetes, neurogenic bladder, and bladder diverticulum.[5,29-31]

Pathology

Sarcomatoid carcinoma can present at any site of urothelial epithelium along the urinary tract, including the pelvis, ureters, bladder, and prostatic urethra. Despite this, it is exceedingly rare in those locations outside the bladder.[42,43] It is most frequently found on the lateral walls of the bladder, followed by the dome, trigone, anterior and posterior walls, and even diverticula and prostatic urethra.[13,30,44] The tumors are usually described as polypoid masses, pedunculated or broadly based, projecting into the lumen of the bladder. Occasionally, they may be sessile or intramural. Edema, hemorrhage, and necrosis are often present. Most tumors extend into or beyond the muscularis propria of the bladder. On gross examination, sarcomatoid carcinoma is characteristically "sarcoma-like," with a dull gray, fleshy cut surface, infiltrative margins, and foci of hemorrhage, necrosis, and cysts (Figs. 16-1 and 16-2).

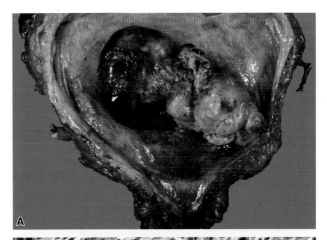
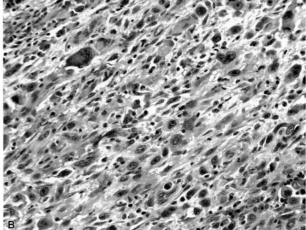

Figure 16-1 Sarcomatoid carcinoma. Gross (A) and microscopic (B) appearance.

Sarcomatoid carcinoma is a biphasic tumor with morphological and immunohistochemical evidence of both epithelial and mesenchymal differentiation (Figs. 16-2 and 16-3). Frequently, sarcomatoid carcinoma of the bladder may have an appearance similar to that of spindle cell tumors, but an epithelial component may be identifiable, or the true nature of the tumor may be revealed by its strong immunoreactivity to epithelial markers such as cytokeratin and/or epithelial membrane antigen (EMA). The carcinomatous and sarcomatous elements may exhibit an abrupt transition resembling a collision tumor, or a gradual transition with an intimate admixture at the interface (Figs. 16-4 to 16-6). The relative proportion of carcinomatous and sarcomatous components is variable, yet the sarcomatous component occupies more than 50% of the tumor area in most cases.[13] Monophasic sarcomatoid carcinoma, referred to as "pure spindle cell carcinoma," represents approximately 20% of cases, and is distinguishable from true sarcoma only by epithelial differentiation on immunohistochemistry or electron microscopy.[5,45]

Sarcomatoid Carcinoma (Carcinosarcoma)

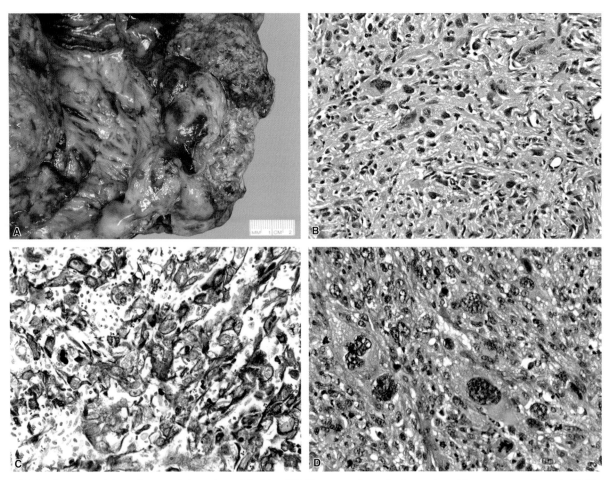

Figure 16-2   Sarcomatoid carcinoma of the urinary bladder. (A) The tumor has a bulky, polypoid appearance (gross). (B) The typical appearance of sarcomatoid carcinoma is that of a malignant spindle cell lesion. (C) Immunostaining of the tumor shown in (B) with antibodies against cytokeratin AE1/AE3 highlights the spindled and pleomorphic cells, supporting a diagnosis of sarcomatoid carcinoma, rather than undifferentiated sarcoma. (D) Anaplastic, pleomorphic giant cells are present. (From Ref. 1; with permission.)

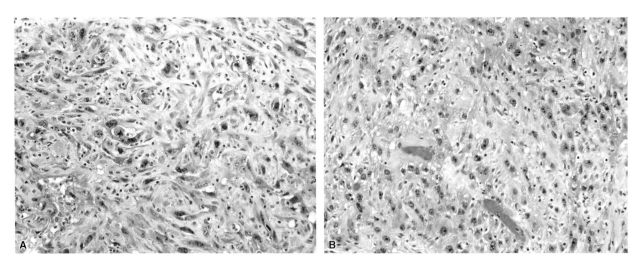

Figure 16-3   Sarcomatoid carcinoma (A and B). The tumor is composed of solid sheets and poorly formed fascicles of predominantly spindled neoplastic cells with marked cellular pleomorphism.

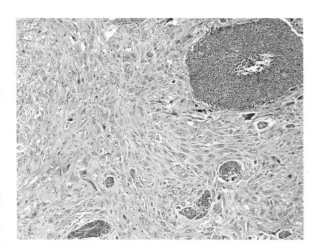

Figure 16-4   Sarcomatoid carcinoma. Note the abrupt transition between sarcomatoid carcinoma and urothelial carcinoma.

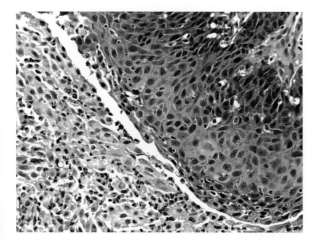

Figure 16-5   Sarcomatoid carcinoma. Note the abrupt transition between sarcomatoid carcinoma and urothelial carcinoma.

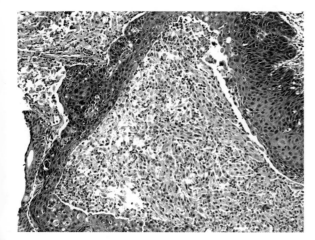

Figure 16-6   Sarcomatoid carcinoma. Note the abrupt transition between sarcomatoid carcinoma and squamous cell carcinoma.

The epithelial and mesenchymal components demonstrate phenotypic variability. In the majority of cases reported, the epithelial component is comprised of moderately to poorly differentiated high grade invasive urothelial carcinoma (**Figs. 16-7** and **16-8**).[5,13] These generally contain brisk (atypical) mitoses and necrosis. While the tumor cells are most frequently spindle shaped, occasionally they tend to be more rounded and epithelioid. Noninvasive papillary urothelial carcinoma and flat carcinoma in situ have been identified in multiple cases, and occasionally, carcinoma in situ is the only epithelial entity (approximately 30% of cases).[27,46] Squamous cell carcinoma, adenocarcinoma, and large and small cell carcinoma are other types of epithelial differentiation frequently described as foci or prominent components of these tumors (**Fig. 16-9**).

It is of primary importance to avoid mistaking sarcomatoid carcinoma for a benign entity, or vice versa, yet this can be rather challenging. Sarcomatoid carcinoma of the urinary bladder is usually biphasic, composed of both epithelial and mesenchymal elements. In cases composed exclusively of spindle cells, the main differential diagnostic consideration is sarcoma, particularly leiomyosarcoma (see the discussion below). A small subset of sarcomatoid carcinomas have prominent myxoid or sclerotic foci with widely dispersed cells, mild atypia, and infrequent mitoses that must not be confused with inflammatory myofibroblastic tumor (**Figs. 16-10** to **16-12**).[25]

Various heterologous components, such as osteosarcoma, chondrosarcoma, rhabdomyosarcoma, leiomyosarcoma, liposarcoma, angiosarcoma, fibrosarcoma, malignant fibrous histiocytoma, or a mixture of sarcoma histologies may be seen (**Figs. 16-13** to **16-17**). The spindle cells may be closely packed or loosely arranged in a diffuse or streaming pattern, and in some cases, the malignant cells may be more rounded or epithelioid in appearance. Some tumors have prominent giant cells (**Fig. 16-18**) or inflammatory cells.[12] Cytologically, the malignant mesenchyme-like cells exhibit pleomorphic and hyperchromatic nuclei, prominent nucleoli, high mitotic activity, and atypical mitotic figures. The presence of the various components should be mentioned in the final pathological report, although the presence or absence and specific types of heterologous components do not have proven clinical impact on prognosis.

Sarcomatoid carcinoma is always a high grade carcinoma (1973 WHO grade 3) and typically presents at a high pathologic stage.[29,30] In a detailed analysis of 26 sarcomatoid carcinomas from the Mayo Clinic, only one (4%) presented with a pT2 tumor and the remaining 96% cases were pT3/4 cancers.[5]

Sarcomatoid Carcinoma (Carcinosarcoma)

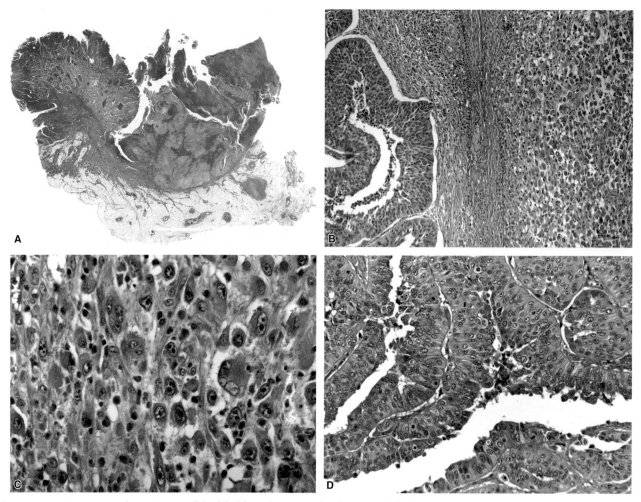

Figure 16-7 Sarcomatoid carcinoma of the bladder. The tumor displays typical biphasic growth pattern. (A) Panoramic view of the tumor. (B) Section from the tumor in (A) shows typical urothelial carcinoma on the left and sarcomatoid carcinoma on the right. (C) Higher power of sarcomatoid carcinoma in tumor shown in (A) and (B). (D) Higher power of high grade urothelial carcinoma in tumor shown in (A) and (B). (From Ref. 1; with permission.)

Ultrastructural Features

On electron microscopy, sarcomatous tissue has features of both mesenchymal and epithelial differentiation. In an undifferentiated spindle cell component, the cells have well-developed endoplasmic reticulum resembling fibroblasts, with a surrounding matrix of collagen fibers and basement membrane material.[12] In tumors with heterologous elements, cells may display varying degrees of specific mesenchymal differentiation, perhaps in inverse proportion to epithelial differentiation. For example, Perret et al. described two cases with elements reminiscent of rhabdomyosarcoma, in which one contained cells with well-developed sarcomeres and the other contained cells with rudimentary sarcomeres with abortive Z bands.[27] More important, all reported cases of sarcomatoid carcinoma, with ultrastructural characterization, have demonstrated

cells with distinct epithelial features, such as desmosomes and tonofilaments, unexpected in true sarcomatous cells, arguing for their epithelial origin.[12,31]

Immunohistochemistry and Differential Diagnosis

It may be rather difficult to distinguish sarcomatoid carcinoma composed exclusively of spindle cells from other spindle-celled neoplasms. Their distinctions from sarcomatoid carcinoma are important, since these entities have differing prognostic as well as therapeutic implications.[46,47] The primary differential diagnostic considerations include leiomyosarcoma, rhabdomyosarcoma, angiosarcoma, malignant fibrous histiocytoma, inflammatory myofibroblastic tumor (IMT), postoperative spindle cell nodule

360

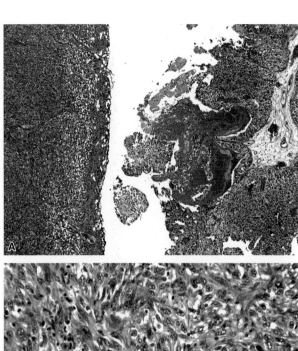

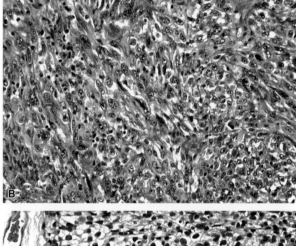

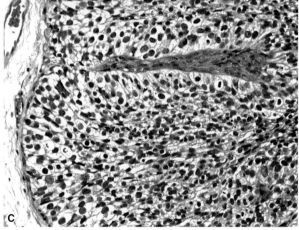

Figure 16-8 Sarcomatoid carcinoma with coexisiting conventional urothelial carcinoma. Tumor displays conventional papillary urothelial on the right and invasive sarcomatoid tumor on the left (A). At higher magnification, the sarcomatoid component is composed of fascicles of pleomorphic spindled neoplastic cells (B), and the carcinomatous component consists of papillary fronds lined by multiple layers of fairly uniform urothelial cells (C). (From Ref. 4; with permission.)

(PSCN), spindle cell malignant melanoma, urothelial carcinoma with pseudosarcomatous stroma, and urothelial carcinoma with osseous or cartilaginous metaplasia (Table 16-1).[31,45–49] Accurate diagnosis is critical given the poor prognosis of sarcomatoid carcinoma in comparison to conventional urothelial carcinoma or benign lesions and often requires utilization of immunohistochemical studies (see also Chapters 19 and 26).

Sarcomatoid carcinoma is characterized by strong staining with cytokeratins (AE1/AE3, CAM5.2) and/or EMA with coexpression of vimentin in the majority of cases (Fig. 16-19). In contrast to smooth muscle neoplasms, actin and desmin are typically negative. However, sarcomatoid carcinomas with heterologous differentiation may rarely be encountered, and in this situation, expression of other mesenchymal markers, such as actin, desmin, and/or S100 protein, may be observed.[31] EMA positivity has been reported in sarcomatoid carcinoma.[3–5] Lopez-Beltran et al. found cytoplasmic immunoreactivity for AE1/AE3, CAM5.2, and vimentin in 41 cases or carcinosarcoma and sarcomatoid carcinoma of the bladder, at least focally.[5] Five tumors with a leiomyosarcomatous component, identified as a specific type of mesenchymal differentiation, were immunoreactive for muscle-specific actin in their series. One tumor, with a rhabdomyosarcoma component, was immunoreactive for desmin and three others, with a chondrosarcoma component, were immunoreactive for S100 protein.[5]

Sarcomatoid carcinoma with prominent myxoid and sclerosing stroma may be mistaken for IMT, postoperative spindle cell nodule, or urothelial carcinoma with pseudosarcomatous stroma.[9,10,14,15] The presence of slit-like vessels and the absence of atypical mitotic figures, necrosis, and significant cytologic atypia favor the diagnosis of benign lesion.

It is noteworthy that IMTs can have considerable morphologic overlap with sarcomatoid carcinoma and leiomyosarcoma, two more ominous lesions, given their tendency toward some more aggressive features on gross and histological examination.[45–47,50] IMTs are benign mesenchymal neoplasms composed of a somewhat monotonous proliferation of myofibroblastic cells in a richly vascularized background with a lymphovascular infiltrate. They may arise either spontaneously or as a result of instrumentation of the bladder. IMTs may contain atypical spindle cells with occasional mitotic figures; however, overt malignant features such as atypical mitoses are absent. Chronic inflammation, usually in the form of a lymphoplasmacytic infiltrate, is typically present. Coffin et al. described three identifiable histologic patterns, including a nodular fasciitis-like pattern with myxoid, vascular, and inflammatory areas; a fibrous histiocytoma-like pattern with compact spindle cells and scattered lymphocytes, plasma cells, and eosinophils; and a scar or desmoid-like

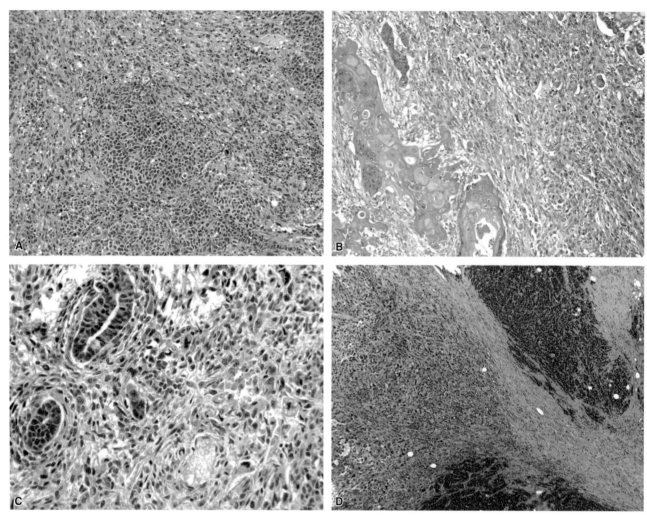

Figure 16-9 Sarcomatoid carcinoma with coexisting urothelial carcinoma (A), squamous cell carcinoma (B), adenocarcinoma (C), and small cell carcinoma (D).

pattern with dense collagen deposition.[51] Immunostaining can be helpful in difficult cases. Most notably, anaplastic lymphoma kinase (ALK) protein, which is associated with the characteristic alteration involving the *ALK* gene by t(2;5), was shown to be overexpressed in 40% to 75% of IMTs but not in sarcomatoid carcinomas.[52–56]

Several large series studies have suggested several markers with certain limitations and caveats.[13,53,57,58] Epithelial markers especially cytokeratins can be strongly positive in both sarcomatoid carcinoma and IMTs.[49] In some cases, cytokeratin AE1/AE3 staining was focal in sarcomatoid carcinoma, requiring the use of a panel of cytokeratin markers to demonstrate epithelial differentiation. Such a panel might include cytokeratin 5/6 (CK5/6), high molecular weight cytokeratin 34βE12, and p63. p63 is positive in approximately 70% of sarcomatoid carcinomas and thus may be helpful in the differential diagnosis (**Fig. 16-20**).[49] CK5/6 and high molecular weight cytokeratin (34βE12) show relative

specificity in sarcomatoid carcinomas, which may be helpful in distinguishing it from IMT and leiomyosarcoma. One should keep in mind that leiomyosarcoma may show focal cytokeratin positivity as well. However, leiomyosarcoma is additionally immunoreactive for SMA and desmin, which are absent in sarcomatoid carcinoma.

PSCN is a benign spindle cell lesion of the bladder, derived from myofibroblast. PSCN is preceded by a traumatic event, such as surgery or instrumentation, and tends to occur in a slightly older age group. The lesions are usually highly vascular with slit-like vessels and prominent infiltrates of lymphocytes and neutrophils. Superficial ulceration is common. These reactive lesions do not show atypical mitoses or severe cytologic atypia, characteristic of the aforementioned malignancies.

It may be rather difficult to distinguish sarcomatoid carcinoma from true sarcoma when it appears as an exclusive

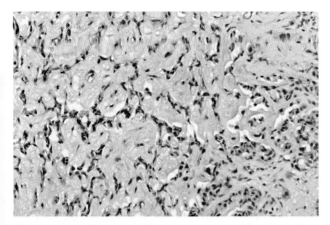

Figure 16-10 Sarcomatoid carcinoma, myxoid variant. The tumor is composed of malignant spindle cells diffusely arrayed in a myxoid stroma.

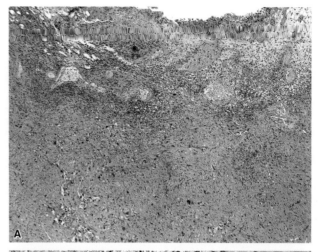

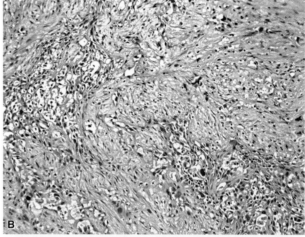

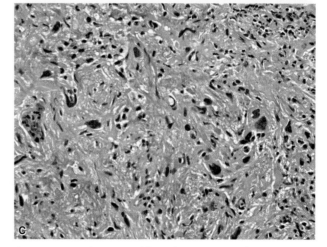

Figure 16-12 Sarcomatoid carcinoma, myxoid variant (A to C).

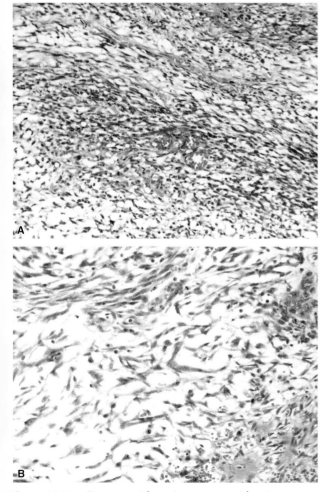

Figure 16-11 Sarcomatoid carcinoma, myxoid variant (A and B).

Sarcomatoid Carcinoma (Carcinosarcoma)

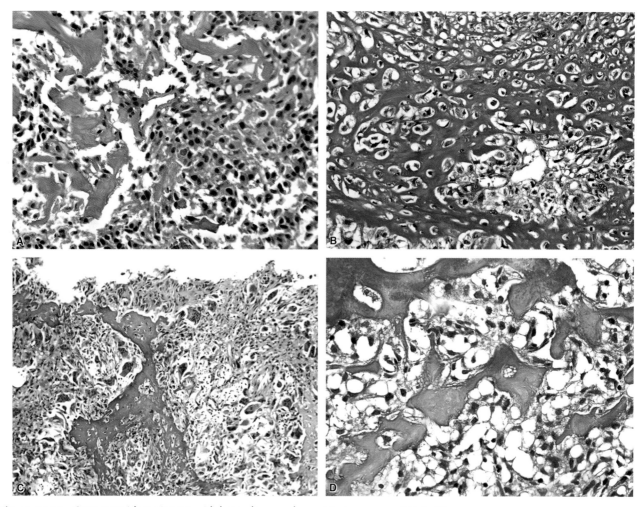

Figure 16-13 Sarcomatoid carcinoma with heterologous element (osteosarcoma) (A to D).

spindle cell malignancy. However, differentiation of sarcomatoid carcinomas from these spindle cell lesions is important, as they have differing prognostic as well as therapeutic implications.[45–47] Apart from clinicopathological characteristics, pure sarcomas usually do not exhibit epithelial markers on immunohistochemistry or desmosomes and tonofilaments on electron microscopy. Vimentin positivity, which is characteristic of sarcomas, is almost uniform in sarcomatoid carcinoma and is not useful in distinguishing the two entities.

The most frequently seen primary sarcoma of bladder is leiomyosarcoma.[59] It, along with sarcomatoid carcinoma, has been associated with cyclophosphamide therapy. These tend to occur 5 to 20 years after exposure to the drug.[60,61] Therefore, patient history of cyclophosphamide exposure does not provide any further distinction between the two tumors. Cytokeratin immunostaining may be helpful in this setting. One should also bear in mind that focal cytokeratin immunoreactivity may be seen in smooth muscle tumors. Leiomyosarcomas are also

immunoreactive for desmin and other muscle differentiation markers, even when they express cytokeratin antigens. Sarcomas lack desmosomes and tonofilaments by electron microscopy.[62]

Primary rhabdomyosarcoma of the bladder is a tumor of childhood and adolescence, which also shows a slight male predominance.[63] A tumor composed of small round or spindled cells, arising in the bladder of a child, will prove to be rhabdomyosarcoma with only very rare exceptions.[64] The most frequent site of involvement is the region of the trigone. Microscopically, rhabdomyosarcoma shows varying degrees of cellularity, with alternating hypercellular areas and loosely packed myxoid areas. There is typically a mixture of unoriented, small, undifferentiated, hyperchromatic round or spindle cells. The cells may show rhabdomyoblastic differentiation with eosinophilic cytoplasm. Immunohistochemically, rhabdomyosarcoma usually shows positivity for desmin, as well as MyoD1 and/or myogenin. In addition, MSA, myoglobin, and myosin immunostains may be positive.

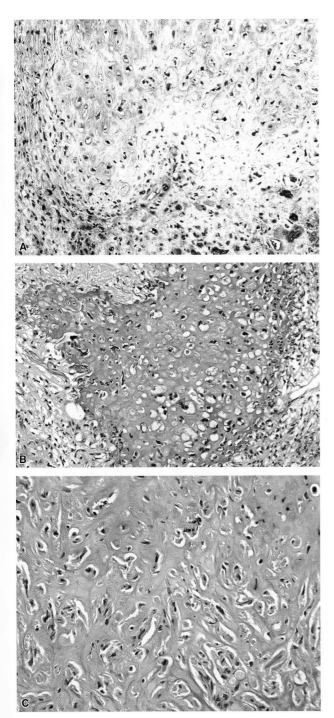

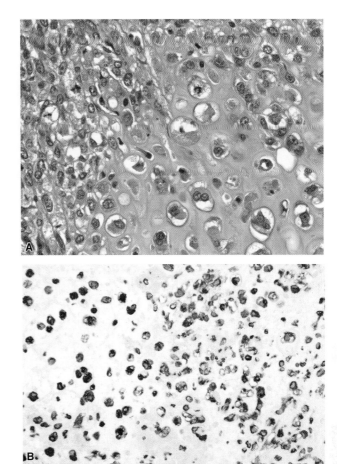

Figure 16-15   Sarcomatoid carcinoma with heterologous element (chondrosarcoma) (A and B). Immunostaining for S100 protein is positive (B).

Figure 16-14   Sarcomatoid carcinoma with heterologous element (chondrosarcoma) (A to C).

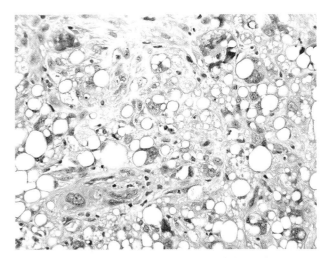

Figure 16-16   Sarcomatoid carcinoma with heterologous element (liposarcoma).

Sarcomatoid Carcinoma (Carcinosarcoma)

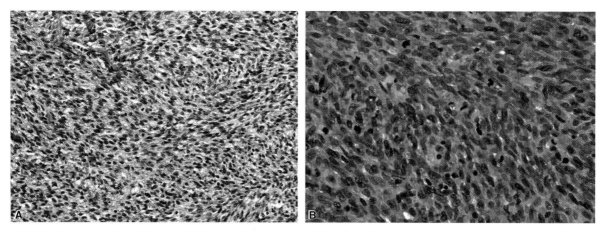

Figure 16-17 Sarcomatoid carcinoma with heterologous element (leiomyosarcoma).

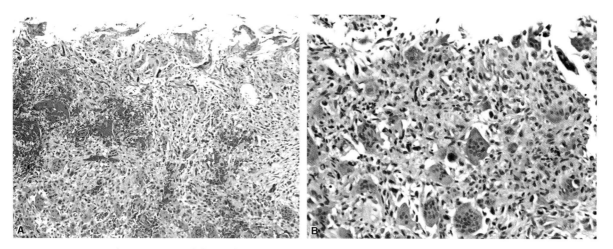

Figure 16-18 Sarcomatoid carcinoma with heterologous element (giant cell tumor) (A and B). Note the numerous giant cells.

Table 16-1 **Key Features to Differentiate Sarcomatoid Carcinoma from Other Spindle Cell Lesions[a]**

	Cytologic Atypia	Mitoses	Tumor Necrosis	Inflammation	Invasion of Muscularis Propria	Coexisting UC/CIS	Immunostaining
Sarcomatoid carcinoma	Present	Present, some atypical	Present	Often present	May be present	Often present	Cytokeratin, EMA
Inflammatory myofibroblastic tumor	Minimal	Few	Surface only	Often prominent	May be present	Absent	ALK-1, actin, vimentin, cytokeratin (patchy)
Leiomyosarcoma	Present	Present, some atypical	Present	Sparse	Present	Absent	Smooth muscle actin, desmin, vimentin
Postoperative spindle cell nodule	Minimal	Variable	Absent	Present	Absent	Absent	Vimentin, cytokeratin, desmin, actin
Rhabdomyosarcoma	Present	Present, some atypical	Varies	Absent	May be present	Absent	Myoglobin, MyoD1, desmin, actin

[a]ALK, anaplastic lymphoma kinase; CIS, urothelial carcinoma in situ; EMA, epithelial membrane antigen; UC, urothelial carcinoma (urothelial carcinoma).

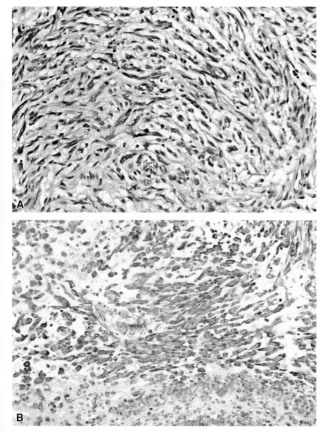

Figure 16-19 Sarcomatoid carcinoma (A and B). The tumor cells display strong cytokeratin AE1/AE3 immunoreactivity (B).

Rhabdomyoblasts may stain for NSE and cytokeratin. The alveolar variant has been reported to stain focally for S100 protein.[65]

Upper Urinary Tract Sarcomatoid Carcinoma

Urothelial carcinomas of the upper urinary tract represent approximately 5% of all urothelial cancers.[66,67] Although the majority of sarcomatoid carcinomas occur in the urinary bladder, upper urinary tract sarcomatoid carcinoma may rarely occur. Fewer than 20 cases have been reported.[12,13,31,43,68–73] The clinical presentation of upper urinary tract sarcomatoid carcinoma is similar to conventional carcinomas in this location, including gross hematuria and signs of ureteral obstruction and hydronephrosis.

Sarcomatoid carcinoma of the upper urinary tract is an aggressive malignancy, with a wide range of differentiations. At the time of diagnosis, sarcomatoid carcinomas in the bladder and in the upper urinary tract are often

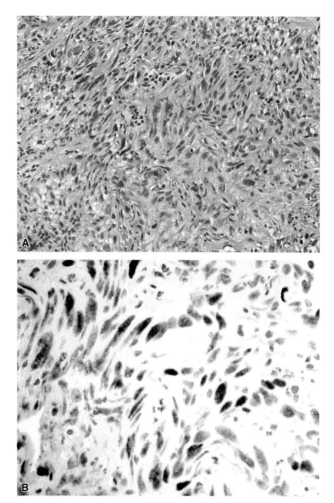

Figure 16-20 Sarcomatoid carcinoma (A and B). The tumor cells show strong p53 positivity (B). (From Ref. 9; with permission.)

at an advanced stage (pT3 or higher). Ureteral sarcomatoid carcinoma seems to arise preferentially in the distal ureter. Only a few cases have been reported in the renal pelvis or proximal ureter.[69,74] Most of the patients are over 60 years of age, and males appeared to be affected more often. In a recent study, Wang et al. analyzed eight patients with upper urinary tract sarcomatoid carcinoma.[43] The mean age at diagnosis was 69 years. Presenting symptoms included gross hematuria, flank mass, urinary obstruction, fever, and/or sepsis. Tumor size ranged from 2 cm to 13 cm. Coexisting urothelial carcinoma was present in all eight cases. Heterologous osteosarcoma was identified in two cases. Pathologic stage was pT4 in five cases and pT3 in three cases. Lymph node metastases were present in five patients at the time of surgery. Most patients died within two years (7/8 patients).[43]

367

Prognosis and Treatment

Sarcomatoid carcinoma of the bladder demonstrates a relatively poor prognosis, and pathologic stage is the only significant prognostic factor.[29,30] Recently, two groups have provided data concerning the clinical implications of sarcomatoid carcinoma by querying the database of the Surveillance, Epidemiology, and End Results (SEER) Program.[29,30] Wang and colleagues[30] reported their findings in 221 cases of sarcomatoid carcinoma of the bladder, and Wright and colleagues[29] compared 135 cases of sarcomatoid carcinoma and 166 cases of carcinosarcoma to 46,515 cases of urothelial carcinomas. The majority of patients presented at an advanced stage in both studies. The mean survival of patients with carcinosarcoma and sarcomatoid carcinoma was 17 months and 10 months, respectively, in one large series from the Mayo Clinic.[5] Pathologic stage appears to be the main predictor of patient survival. Patients with regional and distant spread of disease have a twofold and eightfold increased risk of dying from sarcomatoid carcinoma of the bladder, respectively. A number of other factors, including age, gender, ethnicity, marital status, year of diagnosis, and treatment modality, show no association with disease-specific survival.[30] The median survival for sarcomatoid carcinoma was 14 months overall: 21 months for localized disease, 10 months for regional disease, and 2 months for distant disease. Overall survival rates were 53.9% at one year and 28.4% at five years. Both sarcomatoid carcinoma and carcinosarcoma exhibited worse overall survival rates than high grade urothelial carcinoma (54%, 48%, and 77% at one year, and 37%, 17%, and 47% at five years).[30]

Although some of the authors reported promising data, most of the studies reported a poor outcome, regardless of the type of treatment.[29,30] Patients seldom survive longer than three years.[27,69,73] Aggressive treatment with cystectomy or transurethral resection appears to be the preferred treatment, although radical surgery seems to be the treatment of choice. Adjuvant chemotherapy and radiation therapy have yielded varied results.[13] Although there is no standard treatment for sarcomatoid carcinoma due to the lack of randomized controlled trials, most patients undergo some type of cancer-directed surgery, with or without additional therapies, such as radiotherapy and chemotherapy. The prognosis of patients with sarcomatoid carcinoma of the bladder is poor despite treatment. Reports from the SEER database indicate that surgery varies from transurethral resection for bladder tumor (TURBT) in approximately 40% to 55% of patients to partial, total, or radical cystectomy in 35% to 40% of patients, without significant difference in overall survival between the two approaches.[29,30] Nevertheless, Black and colleagues, after reanalyzing their SEER series and their institutional series at the M.D. Anderson Cancer Center, recommend forgoing TURBT and proceeding directly to cystectomy, since they found no significant difference in overall survival between sarcomatoid carcinoma and urothelial carcinoma when considering only the subset of patients treated with cystectomy.[75] Currently, radical cystectomy is the treatment of choice for both superficial and muscle-invasive disease.[30] Given the high rate of local recurrence and metastasis after radical cystectomy, some authors have advocated for radical cystectomy with lymphadenectomy to be accompanied by various combinations of neoadjuvant or adjuvant chemotherapy and/or radiotherapy.[4]

Multimodality therapy with cystectomy, radiation, and chemotherapy was the common thread amongst the scattered long-term survivors identified in studies by Lopez-Beltran et al. and Ikegami et al.; however, outcomes associated with chemotherapy and radiation therapy are inconsistent in these series and others.[5,13,30] Studies show varying rates of usage of adjuvant radiation and chemotherapy, ranging from approximately 15% to 40% and 5% to 65%, repectively.[5,13,30] Few studies have described specific chemotherapeutic regimens and their associated survival benefit. Case reports indicate that gemcitabine and cisplatin may be a well-tolerated and effective regimen, given its ability to induce complete remission in select patients.[76,77] Neoadjuvant chemotherapy has shown promise in the limited experience with its use. Black et al. reported that five of 11 (45%) patients given neoadjuvant chemotherapy, for clinical T2 or T3 disease, were downstaged to pT0, but this could not be correlated with improved survival, due to insufficient sample size. Multi-institution clinical trials are needed to establish protocols for the treatment of sarcomatoid carcinoma of the urinary bladder.[75] Further characterization of the molecular underpinnings of sarcomatoid carcinoma should foster the development of targeted therapeutics.

Molecular Pathology of Sarcomatoid Carcinoma

Genetic and Molecular Studies

Cytogenetic studies have shown that loss of 9p21 is a known early genetic event in the development of papillary urothelial carcinoma. Increased chromosomal instability and aneuploidy of chromosomes 1, 3, 7, 9, 11, and 17 have been implicated in tumor progression.[10,24,34,35,43,45,78–82] In the study on chromosome alterations by loss of heterozygosity (LOH), including 30 sarcomatoid carcinomas, Sung et al. reported a high incidence of allelic loss from multiple early carcinogenesis-associated loci: 86% at D8S261, 78% at D11S569, 75% at D9S177, and 57% at IFNA.[4]

In a study that included eight sarcomatoid carcinoma patients, Wang et al. investigated the molecular alterations, to include EGFR, HER2, c-kit, and p53 expressions and evaluated the amplification of *EGFR* and *HER2* genes by interphase fluorescence in situ hybridization (FISH).[43] Chromosomes gains of 3, 7, and 17, and loss of 9p21 were analyzed by UroVysion FISH. EGFR immunostaining had moderately to strongly positive results in six of eight cases. Both HER2 and c kit immunostaining had negative results in all cases. p53 immunostaining had positive results in five of eight cases. The EGFR polysomy was demonstrated in seven of eight cases. No amplification of HER2 was present in any case. UroVysion FISH showed abnormalities typical of urothelial carcinoma in all eight cases.[43]

Torenbeek et al. reported that comparative genomic hybridization (CGH) detected a high frequency of chromosome gains and losses from three sarcomatoid carcinomas.[10] The divergent phenotypic components showed a large overlapping of chromosomal aberrations.[10] Volker and colleagues observed the same phenomenon in two cases of upper urinary tract sarcomatoid bladder cancers.[42]

Histogenesis

Sarcomatoid carcinoma is an uncommon malignancy that demonstrates morphological and immunohistochemical evidence of both epithelial and mesenchymal differentiation and occurs in almost every organ capable of developing carcinoma. The exact histogenesis of sarcomatoid carcinoma of the urinary bladder remains a matter of controversy. Two opposing theories, based on clonality, have been proposed to explain the origin of these morphologically diverse biphasic tumors (**Fig. 16-21**). Some investigators believe that it represents a collision tumor of two independent, monoclonal neoplasms occurring simultaneously, whereas others suggest that sarcomatoid carcinoma has a common clonal origin with divergent differentiation into its carcinomatous and sarcomatous elements. The collision theory is based primarily on morphological analysis. Perret et al. noted abrupt transition between the carcinomatous and sarcomatous components without a gradual transition from one morphological entity to another, suggesting a collision of tumor of multiclonal origin.[27] Similar findings have been noted by other investigators.[26]

Recent molecular studies have provided insight into the histogenesis of this tumor. LOH and X chromosome

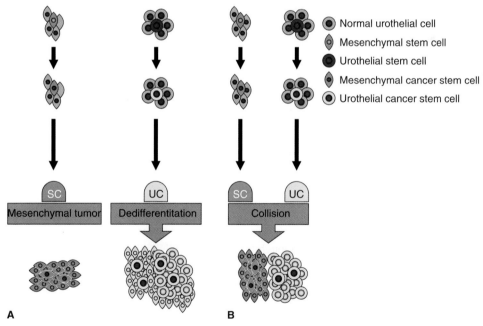

A   B

Figure 16-21   Proposed model for sarcomatoid carcinoma of the urinary bladder. There are two main hypotheses for its histogenesis: divergent differentiation of monoclonal tumor (A), or "collision" of synchronous urothelial and mesenchymal tumors (B). The divergent theory (A) proposes that true sarcoma is derived from mesenchymal stem cells. The carcinomatous and sarcomatous components in sarcomatoid carcinoma are derived from urothelial cancer stem cells with dedifferentiation of a subpopulation of tumor cells into the mesenchymal phenotype. The supporting evidence for this hypothesis is that both the carcinomatous and sarcomatous components retain concordant genetic alterations, and both components express epithelial markers. The collision tumor theory (B) proposes that the carcinomatous and sarcomatous components arise independently from urothelial and mesenchymal stem cells, respectively. These stem cells form carcinoma and sarcoma synchronously and "collide" at the same organ location. SC, sarcoma; UC, urothelial carcinoma. (From Ref. 1; with permission.)

inactivation analysis are two powerful tools for determination of clonality.[79] LOH is based on the analysis of microsatellites (short nucleotide repeats) that are scattered throughout the genome and stably inherited. Because of the variability of these sequences at each locus, individuals usually inherit a different variant from their mother and from their father; two unrelated individuals therefore do not usually contain the same pair of sequences. X chromosome inactivation is the most consistently informative indicator of clonal origin of neoplasms in females. Neoplasms derived from a single progenitor cell are composed of cells in which the same (maternal or paternal) X chromosome is inactivated. Sung et al. analyzed LOH and X chromosome inactivation analysis in 30 sarcomatoid urothelial carcinomas from 10 female patients and 20 male patients.[4] Their results showed a concordant pattern of nonrandom X chromosome inactivation in the informative female patients, supporting the contention that both the carcinomatous and sarcomatous components of this biphasic tumor are of monoclonal origin. High incidences of an identical pattern of allelic loss between the two components were identified at four (D8S261, D9S177, IFNA, and D11S569) of six polymorphic microsatellite markers frequently associated with early urothelial carcinogenesis. In addition, discordant allelic loss of microsatellite markers was found at various loci, suggesting genetic divergence between the two components following initial neoplastic transformation.

Separate analysis of the *TP53* mutation status of 17 sarcomatoid carcinomas using single-strand conformation polymorphisms (SSCP), DNA sequencing, and immunohistochemistry demonstrated identical mutation patterns and nuclear p53 immunohistochemical staining characteristics in a subset of cases.[9] These findings provided further evidence of a common clonal origin for both the phenotypically distinct components of this biphasic tumor. We postulate that sarcomatoid carcinoma is a common final pathway of all forms of epithelial bladder tumors, a hypothesis supported by molecular data and morphologic evidence.

Monoclonal Divergent Differentiation Theory

The monoclonal theory (divergent differentiation) proposes that the carcinomatous and sarcomatous components derive from a single stem cell of urothelial origin with divergent differentiation along separate epithelial and mesenchymal pathways. This theory is supported by morphologic evidence of a gradual transition with intimately intermingled components, as well as immunohistochemical and ultrastructural evidence of sarcomatous cells with epithelial characteristics.[12,26,27] Although Perret et al. noted only two tumors with gradual transition from one cellular type to another and concomitant epithelial and mesenchymal markers on isolated tumor cells,[27] other authors have described small series in which the majority

of cases have composite features consistent with the monoclonal theory.[13,26,31] Because morphological and immunohistochemical evidence for the histogenesis of bladder sarcomatoid carcinoma is inconclusive, a number of investigators have undertaken molecular genetic studies to offer further insight.[4,9–11,27]

Multiclonal Collision Theory

The multiclonal theory (convergence hypothesis) regards sarcomatoid carcinoma as a "collision" tumor, in which two distinct malignancies, carcinoma and sarcoma, arise from two or more different stem cells of separate epithelial and mesenchymal origin.[9,41] The major support for this hypothesis comes from morphological descriptions of sarcomatoid carcinoma with an abrupt transition between the carcinomatous and sarcomatous components. In a study of eight heterologous sarcomatoid carcinomas of the urinary bladder, Perret et al. noted that six of eight cases examined exhibited an abrupt transition and lacked any signs of cross-differentiation in either component, suggestive of true collision tumors.[27] Although the absence of "transition features" is consistent with the multiclonal hypothesis, the authors hypothesized that it might be explained biologically by extreme differentiation along the mesenchymal phenotype with loss of epithelial markers or technically by sampling errors or technical limitations in staining. True collision tumors, resulting from synchronous independent neoplasms, or from metastasis of one tumor into another, are exceedingly rare.

Molecular Genetic Evidence Supportive of Monoclonal Origin

Molecular genetic studies have provided insight into the histogenesis of sarcomatoid carcinoma of the bladder. Carcinogenesis is a multistep process that is a result of an accumulation of genetic alterations, such as activation of oncogenes and/or inactivation of tumor suppressor genes, through mutational events or gains and/or losses of chromosomal segments. Various methods aim to identify shared genetic alterations between phenotypically diverse components of a tumor, especially those known to occur during early carcinogenesis, in order to suggest a common clonal origin.[81,82]

In an effort to further identify concordant genetic alterations between tumor components suggestive of a common clonal origin, our group analyzed the *TP53* mutation status of 17 cases of biphasic sarcomatoid urothelial carcinomas (Fig. 16-22).[9] Mutations in *TP53*, the tumor suppressor gene encoding p53, are common in urothelial carcinomas, especially in high grade or advanced stage cancers. *TP53* exons 5 to 8 harbor most of the point mutations in bladder

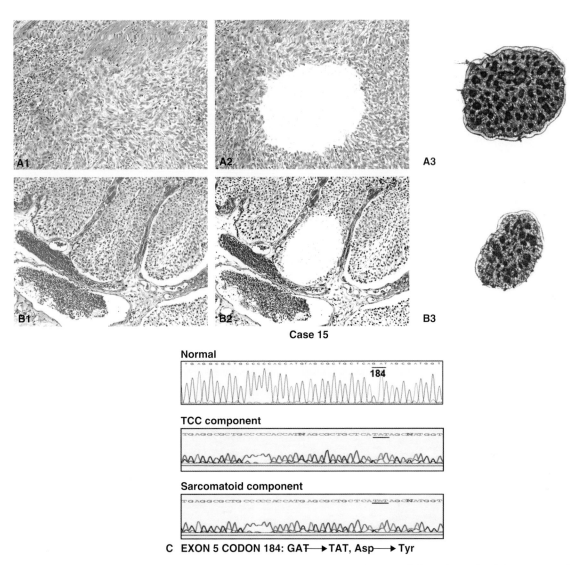

Case 15

Normal

184

TCC component

Sarcomatoid component

C EXON 5 CODON 184: GAT→TAT, Asp→Tyr

Figure 16-22   Laser capture microdissection of sarcomatoid urothelial carcinoma of the urinary bladder (A1 to B3): hematoxylin and eosin–stained sections showing sarcomatoid (A1) and epithelial (B1) components before microdissection; corresponding sarcomatoid component (A2) and epithelial component (B2) after microdissection; and laser-captured sarcomatoid (A3) and epithelial (B3) tumor cells. (C) Case 15: point mutation at exon 5 codon 184: (GAT → TAT, Asp → Tyr) revealing identical mutations in epithelial components (middle panel) and sarcomatoid components (bottom panel); normal tissue did not harbor the mutation in the corresponding codon (top panel). (From Ref. 9; with permission.)

carcinoma. Five out of the 17 tumors contained *TP53* point mutations in exons 5 and 8 on SSCP and DNA sequencing. In all five of these cases, the mutations were identical in the carcinomatous and sarcomatous components. Moreover, these components showed concordant p53 expression patterns in all 17 cases. This study makes a significant contribution to the growing body of literature from molecular genetic pathology in support of the monoclonal theory.[9]

LOH provides another approach for comparing the loss of genetic material between the two components,

but in this case, at specific polymorphic satellite markers relevant to cancer progression rather than along the entire genome. LOH demonstrates the loss of one allele of a heterozygous pair at loci encompassing tumor suppressor genes, and according to the two-hit hypothesis, this loss allows for oncogenesis. Halachmi et al. performed a LOH analysis on six tumors diagnosed as sarcomatoid carcinoma of the urinary bladder.[11] In all six of these tumors, the carcinomatous and sarcomatous components exhibited identical patterns of allelic loss on chromosomes 8p, 8q, 9p, and 9q, corresponding to early events

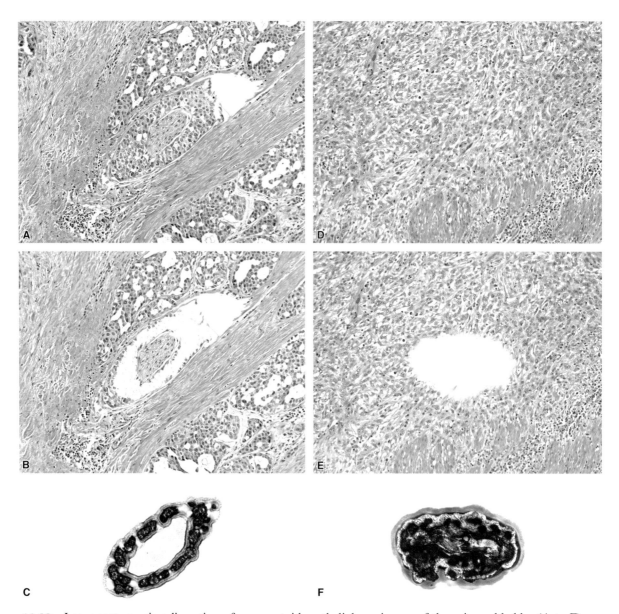

Figure 16-23   Laser capture microdissection of sarcomatoid urothelial carcinoma of the urinary bladder (A to F). Hematoxylin and eosin–stained sections show urothelial carcinoma (UC) component (A) and sarcomatoid component (D) before microdissection. Corresponding UC component (B) and sarcomatoid component (E) after microdissection. Laser-captured UC (C) and sarcomatoid tumor cells (F). (From Ref. 4; with permission.)

in bladder carcinogenesis. Discordant LOHs on other chromosomes were noted more frequently in advanced tumors.[11] Significant homology in LOHs of microsatellite markers, involved in early carcinogenesis, supports the monoclonal origin of sarcomatoid carcinoma.

Because conclusions from these initial molecular genetic studies were limited by the small number of cases, our group recently published two larger studies[4,9] using different molecular approaches to elucidate the clonal origins of sarcomatoid carcinoma of the bladder. In our first study,[4] we investigated the patterns of LOH in

30 cases, as well as X chromosome inactivation in a subset of eight cases from female patients. Using laser capture microdissection, the LOH analysis employed polymorphic microsatellite markers commonly involved in urothelial carcinomas (**Fig. 16-23**).[4] The carcinomatous and sarcomatous components frequently displayed identical patterns of allelic loss at loci in which genetic alterations play critical roles during the early carcinogenesis of urothelial carcinoma: D8S261 (86%), D9S177 (75%), IFNA (57%), and D11S569 (78%) (**Fig. 16-24**). In contrast, the incidence of identical LOH was lower for *TP53* (40%) and D3S3050

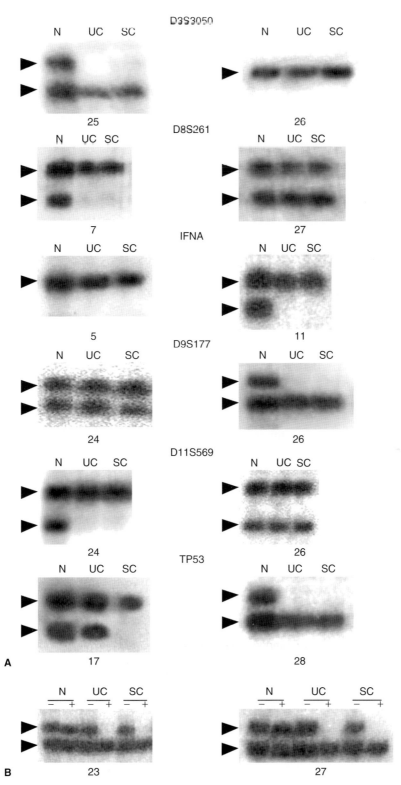

Figure 16-24   Representative results of loss of heterozygosity (A) and X chromosome inactivation analysis (B) in sarcomatoid urothelial carcinoma of the urinary bladder. In (A), DNA was prepared from normal tissue and urothelial carcinoma and sarcomatoid tumor components, amplified by polymerase chain reaction using polymorphic markers D3S3050, D8S261, IFNA, D9S177, D11S569, and TP53 and separated by gel electrophoresis. In (B), nonrandom inactivation of X chromosome was identified. Arrows, allelic bands; N, normal control tissue; UC, urothelial carcinoma component; SC, sarcomatoid component, −, without Hha1 endonuclease digestion; +, after Hha1 endonuclease digestion. (From Ref. 4; with permission.)

(40%), loci encompassing the p53 and von Hippel–Lindau tumor suppressor genes, genes involved in progression to advanced urothelial carcinoma.

Additionally, we analyzed X chromosome inactivation because it is an informative indicator of clonal origin of neoplasms in females, as all the cells of a monoclonal neoplasm will have the same X chromosome inactivated. In our study, tumors were considered to be of the same clonal origin if the same allelic inactivation pattern at the X-linked human androgen receptor (HUMARA) locus was detected in both the carcinomatous and sarcomatous components.[4] The same pattern of nonrandom X chromosome inactivation was indentified in five of eight cases, suggesting that these components came from the same progenitor cell. Although random X chromosome activation in three cases does not provide evidence of monoclonal origin of the two components, it does not completely eliminate this possibility. Previous studies have demonstrated that random X chromosome inactivation may be present in up to 50% of invasive cancers. Of note, there were three cases in which the two components shared the same nonrandom X chromosome inactivation pattern but displayed discordant patterns of LOH in IFNA, D9S177, and TP53, respectively. Although our study does not provide unequivocal evidence that all cases of sarcomatoid carcinoma develop from a single progenitor cell, critical interpretation of the results favors the monoclonal theory with divergent differentiation over the multiclonal theory with collision.[4]

CGH is a powerful tool to compare the gains and losses of all individual chromosomes in distinct tumor cell populations.[83] In a study examining chromosomal aberrations in three cases of sarcomatoid carcinoma of the bladder by CGH, Torenbeek et al. found significant homology in chromosomal aberrations, approximately 20% to 50%, between the carcinomatous and sarcomatous components of each tumor.[10] Another study that used CGH to examine one case of bladder carcinosarcoma revealed losses on the short arm of chromosome 9 and on the long arm of chromosome 11 in both components. Of note, losses on the short arm of chromosome 9, including deletion of tumor suppressor gene TP16, are an early finding in superficial urothelial carcinomas. In both studies, additional aberrations, unique to each component, were detected as well. The CGH studies provide evidence that sarcomatoid carcinoma is derived from a single progenitor cell, probably urothelial in nature, which accumulates genetic alterations and undergoes divergent differentiation during tumor progression.[10]

Epithelial-to-Mesenchymal Transition and Cancer Stem Cells

Sarcomatoid carcinoma of the bladder probably originates as urothelial carcinoma, given similar sites of occurrence

and patient populations, common genetic alterations, and many examples of sarcomatoid carcinoma in recurrences or metastases of conventional carcinoma. Its divergent differentiation exists along a phenotypic spectrum ranging from pure urothelial carcinoma to sarcomatoid carcinoma (malignant spindle cell component) to carcinosarcoma (heterologous component) (**Fig. 16-25**). Current models of carcinogenesis can explain the divergent differentiation and resulting phenotypic heterogeneity. First, sarcomatoid carcinoma may progress through multistep carcinogenesis with the accumulation of genetic alterations, genetic instability, and generation of multiple subclones as supported by the molecular genetic data reviewed.[1,24,34,35,79–82] Second, sarcomatoid carcinoma may represent transdifferentiation from an epithelial to a mesenchymal phenotype, secondary to molecular programs, induced by the stromal microenvironment. An epithelial-to-mesenchymal transition may be responsible for sarcomatoid transformation in urothelial and other carcinomas.[1,24,34,35,79–82,84–87] Ikegami et al. demonstrated decreased expression of E-cadherin and other cell adhesion molecules, a hallmark of epithelial-to-mesenchymal transition, in the sarcomatoid component of sarcomatoid carcinoma of the bladder.[13]

Putative urothelial cancer stem cells have recently been isolated and implicated in the invasiveness and chemoresistance of urothelial carcinoma.[24,84,88] Recently accumulated evidence supports the premise that sarcomatoid carcinoma is derived from a single urothelial progenitor cell with subsequent transformation into a sarcomatoid phenotype.[1,9,24,42,89] It has been shown that both the carcinomatous and sarcomatous components of biphasic urothelial cancers express epithelial markers and retain concordant genetic alterations.[4,9–11] In the current model, true sarcoma is derived from transformed mesenchymal stem cells. However, the sarcomatoid component of sarcomatoid carcinoma (carcinosarcoma) is derived from urothelial stem cells despite sharing morphologic similarity with other mesenchymal tumors. This model is more in alignment with the current epithelial-to-mesenchymal transition theory of tumor progression and metastasis, which has been proposed for similar tumors arising in numerous organ systems (**Figs. 16-26** to **16-30**).[86,87,90] Another hypothesis (collision theory) is that carcinomatous and sarcomatous components arise independently from urothelial and mesenchymal stem cells, respectively. These stem cells synchronously form carcinoma and sarcoma and "collide" at the same organ location. Although plausible, this model is currently falling out of favor. Further studies are necessary to elucidate the role of genetic alterations, epithelial-to-mesenchymal transition, and field cancerization in the conversion of urothelial carcinoma to a sarcomatoid phenotype.

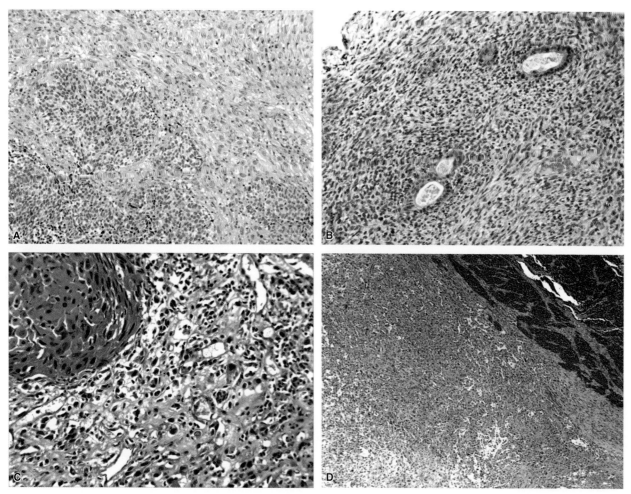

Figure 16-25 Sarcomatoid carcinoma is the final common pathway of dedifferentiation in bladder carcinoma, and may be seen in a background of typical urothelial carcinoma, adenocarcinoma, squamous cell carcinoma, or small cell carcinoma. (A) Urothelial carcinoma intimately intermingled with a spindled sarcomatoid component. (B) Adenocarcinoma intimately intermingled with a spindled sarcomatoid component. (C) Squamous cell carcinoma adjacent to a spindled sarcomatoid component. (D) Small cell carcinoma adjacent to a spindled sarcomatoid component. (From Ref. 1; with permission.)

Summary and Future Perspectives

Sarcomatoid carcinoma of the urinary bladder is an uncommon tumor that must be recognized because of its therapeutic and prognostic implications. Despite the controversy over nomenclature, sarcomatoid carcinoma is the recommended term for any biphasic neoplasm with morphological and immunohistochemical evidence of both epithelial and mesenchymal differentiation. It most commonly affects men in their seventh decade of life and presents at an advanced stage of T3 or higher. It has a relatively poor prognosis, as most patients die within one year. The diagnosis is facilitated by the presence of identifiable urothelial carcinoma or in situ component, but immunohistochemistry may be required in some cases. Accumulated data support the concept of monoclonal origination with divergent

differentiation for most of these biphasic tumors; however, the possibility of a true collision tumor cannot be ruled out completely in a small number of cases.

Sarcomatoid phenotype has been documented in numerous types of human carcinomas, and appears to represent the most aggressive path of tumor progression. The majority of human carcinomas, if they progress long enough without killing the host, might at least theoretically develop sarcomatoid components. Indeed, bladder carcinoma has a tremendous morphologic plasticity. A remarkably wide diversity of histologic patterns may be seen in the same tumor. Interestingly, sarcomatoid carcinoma appears to be uniformly present along those lines of differentiation. Sarcomatoid transformation has been observed in various epithelial tumors of the urinary bladder, including conventional urothelial carcinoma, small cell carcinoma, adenocarcinoma, squamous cell carcinoma, and large cell

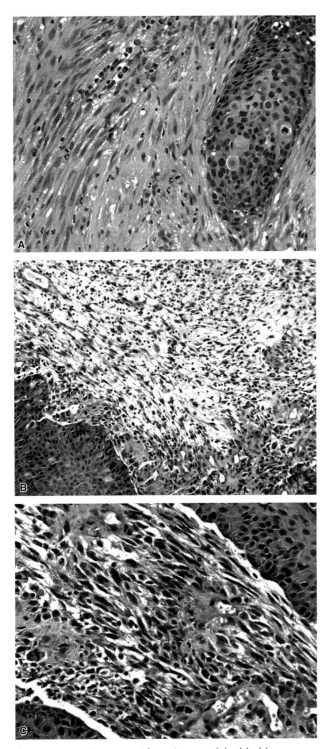

Figure 16-26 Sarcomatoid carcinoma of the bladder as a model for epithelial-to-mesenchymal transition. Note the transition of urothelial carcinoma into mesenchymal (sarcomatoid) component (A to C).

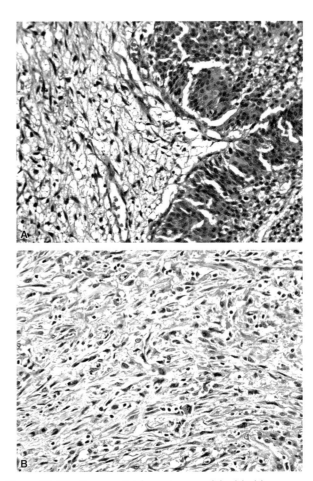

Figure 16-27 Sarcomatoid carcinoma of the bladder as a model for epithelial-to-mesenchymal transition. Note the transition of urothelial carcinoma into myxoid sarcomatoid component (A and B).

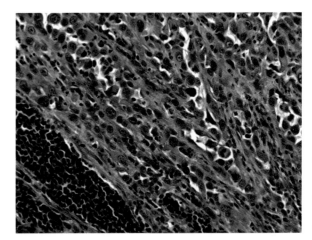

Figure 16-28 Sarcomatoid carcinoma of the bladder as a model for epithelial-to-mesenchymal transition. Note the transition of small cell carcinoma into mesenchymal (sarcomatoid) component.

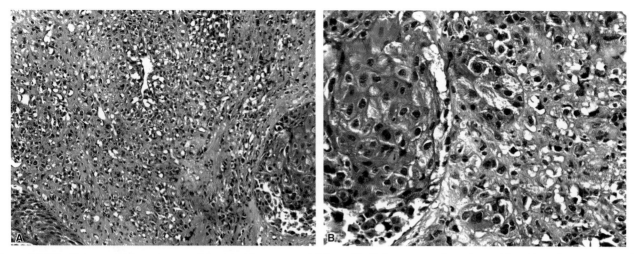

Figure 16-29   Sarcomatoid carcinoma of the bladder as a model for epithelial-to-mesenchymal transition. Note the transition of squamous cell carcinoma into mesenchymal (sarcomatoid) component (A and B).

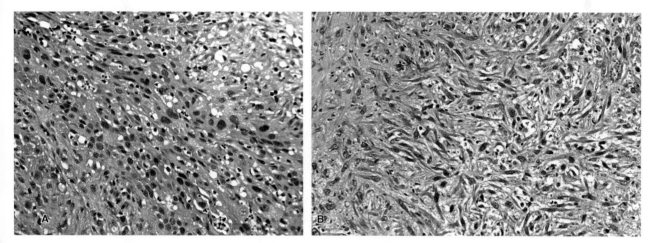

Figure 16-30   Sarcomatoid carcinoma of the bladder as a model for epithelial-to-mesenchymal transition (A and B).

neuroendocrine carcinoma. Sarcomatoid carcinoma appears to represent the final common pathway of human tumor dedifferentiation, including bladder cancer.

Sarcomatoid carcinomas are aggressive variants of urothelial carcinoma, and the full understanding of its histogenesis is lacking. In recent years, molecular genetic methodology has been used increasingly as an effective tool for the analysis of sarcomatoid carcinoma of bladder. These measures will continue to be important diagnostically, and improvements may occur in the near term. Innovative techniques for analyzing sarcomatoid carcinoma of the bladder are currently in development. Some aim to set up the genetic linkage between carcinoma and sarcomatoid components; others continue to focus on clarifying the clonal origin of these tumor components. Searching for protein expression markers remains a significant goal. These methodologies may advance to a level of practicality and cost-effectiveness for routine pathology settings in the next few years. Finally, better understanding of the pathways of tumorigenesis of sarcomatoid carcinoma of the bladder may reveal new agents for its treatment and prevention.

Sarcomatoid Carcinoma (Carcinosarcoma)

REFERENCES

1. Cheng L, Zhang S, Alexander R, MacLennan GT, Hodges KB, Harrison BT, Lopez-Beltran A, Montironi R. Sarcomatoid carcinoma of the urinary bladder: the final common pathway of urothelial carcinoma dedifferentiation. *Am J Surg Pathol* 2011;35:e34–46.

2. Cheng L, Lopez-Beltran A, MacLennan GT, Montironi R, Bostwick DG. Neoplasms of the urinary bladder. In: Bostwick DG, Cheng L, eds. Urologic Surgical Pathology, 2nd ed. Philadelphia: Elsevier/Mosby, 2008;259–352.

3. Eble JN, Sauter G, Epstein JI, Sesterhenn IA, eds. WHO Classification of Tumours: Pathology and Genetics. Tumours of the Urinary and Male Reproductive System. Lyon, France: IARC Press, 2004.

4. Sung MT, Wang M, MacLennan GT, Eble JN, Tan PH, Lopez-Beltran A, Montironi R, Harris JJ, Kuhar M, Cheng L. Histogenesis of sarcomatoid urothelial carcinoma of the urinary bladder: evidence for a common clonal origin with divergent differentiation. *J Pathol* 2007;211:420–30.

5. Lopez-Beltran A, Pacelli A, Rothenberg HJ, Wollan PC, Zincke H, Blute ML, Bostwick DG. Carcinosarcoma and sarcomatoid carcinoma of the bladder: clinicopathological study of 41 cases. *J Urol* 1998;159:1497–1503.

6. Robson SM. Atypical carcinoma of the urinary bladder simulating myosarcoma: report of two cases and review of literature. *J Urol* 1935:638–69.

7. Hirsch EF, Gasser GW. Cancerous mixed tumor of urinary bladder. *Arch Pathol* 1944;37:24–6.

8. Gronau S, Menz CK, Melzner I, Hautmann R, Moller P, Barth TF. Immunohistomorphologic and molecular cytogenetic analysis of a carcinosarcoma of the urinary bladder. *Virchows Arch* 2002;440:436–40.

9. Armstrong AB, Wang M, Eble JN, MacLennan GT, Montironi R, Tan PH, Lopez-Beltran A, Zhang S, Baldridge LA, Spartz H, Cheng L. TP53 mutational analysis supports monoclonal origin of biphasic sarcomatoid urothelial carcinoma (carcinosarcoma) of the urinary bladder. *Mod Pathol* 2009;22:113–8.

10. Torenbeek R, Hermsen MA, Meijer GA, Baak JP, Meijer CJ. Analysis by comparative genomic hybridization of epithelial and spindle cell components in sarcomatoid carcinoma and carcinosarcoma: histogenetic aspects. *J Pathol* 1999;189:338–43.

11. Halachmi S, DeMarzo AM, Chow NH, Halachmi N, Smith AE, Linn JF, Nativ O, Epstein JI, Schoenberg MP, Sidransky D. Genetic alterations in urinary bladder carcinosarcoma: evidence of a common clonal origin. *Eur Urol* 2000;37:350–7.

12. Guarino M, Tricomi P, Giordano F, Cristofori E. Sarcomatoid carcinomas: pathological and histopathogenetic considerations. *Pathology* 1996;28:298–305.

13. Ikegami H, Iwasaki H, Ohjimi Y, Takeuchi T, Ariyoshi A, Kikuchi M. Sarcomatoid carcinoma of the urinary bladder: a clinicopathologic and immunohistochemical analysis of 14 patients. *Hum Pathol* 2000;31:332–40.

14. Terada T. Sarcomatoid carcinoma of the urinary bladder: a case report with immunohistochemical and molecular genetic analysis. *Med Oncol* 2010;27:547–53.

15. Terada T. Urinary bladder carcinoma with triplicate differentiations into giant cell sarcomatoid carcinoma, squamous cell carcinoma, and papillary urothelial transitional cell carcinoma: a case report. *Cases J* 2009;2:9111.

16. Sato K, Ueda Y, Kawamura K, Aihara K, Katsuda S. Plasmacytoid urothelial carcinoma of the urinary bladder: a case report and immunohistochemical study. *Pathol Res Pract* 2009;205:189–94.

17. Paner GP, McKenney JK, Epstein JI, Amin MB. Rhabdomyosarcoma of the urinary bladder in adults: predilection for alveolar morphology with anaplasia and significant morphologic overlap with small cell carcinoma. *Am J Surg Pathol* 2008;32:1022–8.

18. Mekni A, Chelly I, Azzouz H, Ben Ghorbel I, Bellil S, Haouet S, Kchir N, Zitouna M, Bellil K. Extragastrointestinal stromal tumor of the urinary wall bladder: case report and review of the literature. *Pathologica* 2008;100:173–5.

19. Matsuoka Y, Hirokawa M, Chiba K, Hashiba T, Tomoda T, Sugiura S. Biphasic and monophasic sarcomatoid carcinoma of the urinary bladder. *Can J Urol* 2008;15:4106–8.

20. Armah HB, Parwani AV. Sarcomatoid urothelial carcinoma with choriocarcinomatous features: first report of an unusual case. *Urology* 2007;70:812 e11–4.

21. Arenas LF, Fontes DA, Pereira EM, Hering FL. Sarcomatoid carcinoma with osseous differentiation in the bladder. *Int Braz J Urol* 2006;32:563–5.

22. Nimeh T, Kuang W, Levin HS, Klein EA. Sarcomatoid transitional cell carcinoma of bladder managed with transurethral resection alone. *J Urol* 2002;167:641–2.

23. Jemal A, Siegel R, Ward E, Hao Y, Xu J, Thun MJ. Cancer statistics, 2009. *CA Cancer J Clin* 2009;59:225–49.

24. Cheng L, Davidson DD, Maclennan GT, Williamson SR, Zhang S, Koch MO, Montironi R, Lopez-Beltran A. The origins of urothelial carcinoma. *Expert Rev Anticancer Ther* 2010;10:865–80.

25. Jones EC, Young RH. Myxoid and sclerosing sarcomatoid transitional cell carcinoma of the urinary bladder: a clinicopathologic and immunohistochemical study of 25 cases. *Mod Pathol* 1997;10:908–16.

26. Holtz F, Fox JE, Abell MR. Carcinosarcoma of the urinary bladder. *Cancer* 1972;29:294–304.

27. Perret L, Chaubert P, Hessler D, Guillou L. Primary heterologous carcinosarcoma (metaplastic carcinoma) of the urinary bladder: a clinicopathologic, immunohistochemical, and ultrastructural analysis of eight cases and a review of the literature. *Cancer* 1998;82:1535–49.

28. Bloxham CA, Bennett MK, Robinson MC. Bladder carcinosarcomas: three cases with diverse histogenesis. *Histopathology* 1990;16:63–7.

29. Wright JL, Black PC, Brown GA, Porter MP, Kamat AM, Dinney CP, Lin DW. Differences in survival among patients with sarcomatoid carcinoma, carcinosarcoma and urothelial carcinoma of the bladder. *J Urol* 2007;178:2302–7.

30. Wang J, Wang FW, Lagrange CA, Hemstreet GP, Kessinger A. Clinical features of sarcomatoid carcinoma (carcinosarcoma) of the urinary bladder: analysis of 221 cases. *Sarcoma* 2010;2010:4547–92.

31. Torenbeek R, Blomjous CE, de Bruin PC, Newling DW, Meijer CJ. Sarcomatoid carcinoma of the urinary bladder. Clinicopathologic analysis of 18 cases with immunohistochemical and electron microscopic findings. *Am J Surg Pathol* 1994;18:241–9.

32. Lahoti C, Schinella R, Rangwala AF, Lee M, Mizrachi H. Carcinosarcoma of urinary bladder: report of 5 cases with immunohistologic study. *Urology* 1994;43:389–93.

33. Shah SK, Lui PD, Baldwin DD, Ruckle HC. Urothelial carcinoma after external beam radiation therapy for prostate cancer. *J Urol* 2006;175:2063–6.

34. Cheng L, Zhang S, Davidson DD, MacLennan GT, Koch MO, Montironi R, Lopez-Beltran A. Molecular determinants of tumor recurrence in the urinary bladder. *Future Oncol* 2009;5:843–57.

35. Cheng L, Zhang S, Maclennan GT, Williamson SR, Lopez-Beltran A, Montironi R. Bladder cancer: translating molecular genetic insights into clinical practice. *Hum Pathol* 2011;42:455–81.

36. Ro JY, Staerkel GA, Ayala AG. Cytologic and histologic features of superficial bladder cancer. *Urol Clin North Am* 1992;19:435–53.

37. Robey-Cafferty SS, Grignon DJ, Ro JY, Cleary KR, Ayala AG, Ordonez NG, Mackay B. Sarcomatoid carcinoma of the stomach. A report of three cases with immunohistochemical and ultrastructural observations. *Cancer* 1990;65:1601–6.

38. Wick MR, Perrone TL, Burke BA. Sarcomatoid transitional cell carcinomas of the renal pelvis. An ultrastructural and immunohistochemical study. *Arch Pathol Lab Med* 1985;109:55–8.

39. Mukhopadhyay S, Shrimpton AE, Jones LA, Nsouli IS, Abraham NZ Jr. Carcinosarcoma of the urinary bladder following cyclophosphamide therapy: evidence for monoclonal origin and chromosome 9p allelic loss. *Arch Pathol Lab Med* 2004;128:e8–11.

40. Sigel JE, Smith TA, Reith JD, Goldblum JR. Immunohistochemical analysis of anaplastic lymphoma kinase expression in deep soft tissue calcifying fibrous pseudotumor: evidence of a late sclerosing stage of inflammatory myofibroblastic tumor? *Ann Diagn Pathol* 2001;5:10–4.

41. Sigal SH, Tomaszewski JE, Brooks JJ, Wein A, LiVolsi VA. Carcinosarcoma of bladder following long-term cyclophosphamide therapy. *Arch Pathol Lab Med* 1991;115:1049–51.

42. Volker HU, Zettl A, Schon G, Heller V, Heinrich E, Rosenwald A, Handwerker M, Muller-Hermelink HK, Marx A, Strobel P. Molecular genetic findings in two cases of sarcomatoid carcinoma of the ureter: evidence for evolution from a common pluripotent progenitor cell? *Virchows Arch* 2008;452:457–63.

43. Wang X, MacLennan GT, Zhang S, Montironi R, Lopez-Beltran A, Tan PH, Foster S, Baldridge LA, Cheng L. Sarcomatoid carcinoma of the upper urinary tract: clinical outcome and molecular characterization. *Hum Pathol* 2009;40:211–7.

44. Omeroglu A, Paner GP, Wojcik EM, Siziopikou K. A carcinosarcoma/sarcomatoid carcinoma arising in a urinary bladder diverticulum. *Arch Pathol Lab Med* 2002;126:853–5.

45. Cheng L, Zhang S, Alexander R, MacLennan GT, Hodges KB, Harrison BT, Lopez-Beltran A, Montironi R. Sarcomatoid carcinoma of the urinary bladder: the final common pathway of urothelial carcinoma dedifferentiation. *Am J Surg Pathol* 2011;35:e34–46.

46. Lott S, Lopez-Beltran A, Montironi R, MacLennan GT, Cheng L. Soft tissue tumors of the urinary bladder: Part II: Malignant neoplasms. *Hum Pathol* 2007;38:807–23.

47. Lott S, Lopez-Beltran A, Maclennan GT, Montironi R, Cheng L. Soft tissue tumors of the urinary bladder, Part I: myofibroblastic proliferations, benign neoplasms, and tumors of uncertain malignant potential. *Hum Pathol* 2007;38;807–23.

48. Hodges KB, Lopez-Beltran A, Emerson RE, Montironi R, Cheng L. Clinical utility of immunohistochemistry in the diagnoses of urinary bladder neoplasia. *Appl Immunohistochem Mol Morphol* 2010;18:401–10.

49. Westfall DE, Folpe AL, Paner GP, Oliva E, Goldstein L, Alsabeh R, Gown AM, Amin MB. Utility of a comprehensive immunohistochemical panel in the differential diagnosis of spindle cell lesions of the urinary bladder. *Am J Surg Pathol* 2009;33:99–105.

50. Cheng L, Foster SR, MacLennan GT, Lopez-Beltran A, Zhang S, Montironi R. Inflammatory myofibroblastic tumors of the genitourinary tract—single entity or continuum? *J Urol* 2008;180:1235–40.

51. Coffin CM, Watterson J, Priest JR, Dehner LP. Extrapulmonary inflammatory myofibroblastic tumor (inflammatory pseudotumor). A clinicopathologic and immunohistochemical study of 84 cases. *Am J Surg Pathol* 1995;19:859–72.

52. Freeman A, Geddes N, Munson P, Joseph J, Ramani P, Sandison A, Fisher C, Parkinson MC. Anaplastic lymphoma kinase (ALK 1) staining and molecular analysis in inflammatory myofibroblastic tumours of the bladder: a preliminary clinicopathological study of nine cases and review of the literature. *Mod Pathol* 2004;17:765–71.

53. Harik LR, Merino C, Coindre JM, Amin MB, Pedeutour F, Weiss SW. Pseudosarcomatous myofibroblastic proliferations of the bladder: a clinicopathologic study of 42 cases. *Am J Surg Pathol* 2006;30:787–94.

54. Montgomery EA, Shuster DD, Burkart AL, Esteban JM, Sgrignoli A, Elwood L, Vaughn DJ, Griffin CA, Epstein JI. Inflammatory myofibroblastic tumors of the urinary tract: a clinicopathologic study of 46 cases, including a malignant example inflammatory fibrosarcoma and a subset associated with high grade urothelial carcinoma. *Am J Surg Pathol* 2006;30:1502–12.

55. Sukov WR, Cheville JC, Carlson AW, Shearer BM, Piatigorsky EJ, Grogg KL, Sebo TJ, Sinnwell JP, Ketterling RP. Utility of ALK–1 protein expression and ALK rearrangements in distinguishing inflammatory myofibroblastic tumor from malignant spindle cell lesions of the urinary bladder. *Mod Pathol* 2007;20:592–603.

56. Tsuzuki T, Magi-Galluzzi C, Epstein JI. ALK–1 expression in inflammatory myofibroblastic tumor of the urinary bladder. *Am J Surg Pathol* 2004;28:1609–14.

57. Hirsch MS, Dal Cin P, Fletcher CD. ALK expression in pseudosarcomatous myofibroblastic proliferations of the genitourinary tract. *Histopathology* 2006;48:569–78.

58. Lewis JS, Ritter JH, El-Mofty S. Alternative epithelial markers in sarcomatoid carcinomas of the head and neck, lung, and bladder-p63, MOC–31, and TTF–1. *Mod Pathol* 2005;18:1471–81.

59. Martin SA, Sears DL, Sebo TJ, Lohse CM, Cheville JC. Smooth muscle neoplasms of the urinary bladder: a clinicopathologic comparison of leiomyoma and leiomyosarcoma. *Am J Surg Pathol* 2002;26:292–300.

60. Pedersen-Bjergaard J, Jonsson V, Pedersen M, Hou-Jensen K. Leiomyosarcoma of the urinary bladder after cyclophosphamide. *J Clin Oncol* 1995;13:532–3.

61. Tanguay C, Harvey I, Houde M, Srigley JR, Tetu B. Leiomyosarcoma of urinary bladder following cyclophosphamide therapy: report of two cases. *Mod Pathol* 2003;16:512–4.

62. Ogawa K, Kim YC, Nakashima Y, Yamabe H, Takeda T, Hamashima Y. Expression of epithelial markers in sarcomatoid carcinoma: an immunohistochemical study. *Histopathology* 1987;11:511–22.

63. Leuschner I, Harms D, Mattke A, Koscielniak E, Treuner J. Rhabdomyosarcoma of the urinary bladder and vagina: a clinicopathologic study with emphasis on recurrent disease: a report from the Kiel Pediatric Tumor Registry and the German CWS Study. *Am J Surg Pathol* 2001;25:856–64.

64. Arndt C, Rodeberg D, Breitfeld PP, Raney RB, Ullrich F, Donaldson S. Does bladder preservation (as a surgical principle) lead to retaining bladder function in bladder/prostate rhabdomyosarcoma? Results from Intergroup Rhabdomyosarcoma Study IV. *J Urol* 2004;171:2396–403.

65. Kunze E, Theuring F, Kruger G. Primary mesenchymal tumors of the urinary bladder. A histological and immunohistochemical study of 30 cases. *Pathol Res Pract* 1994;190:311–32.

66. Kirkali Z, Chan T, Manoharan M, Algaba F, Busch C, Cheng L, Kiemeney L, Kriegmair M, Montironi R, Murphy WM, Sesterhenn IA, Tachibana M, Weider J. Bladder cancer: epidemiology, staging and grading, and diagnosis. *Urology* 2005;66:4–34.

67. Munoz JJ, Ellison LM. Upper tract urothelial neoplasms: incidence and survival during the last 2 decades. *J Urol* 2000;164:1523–5.

68. Bonsib SM, Cheng L. Renal pelvis and ureter. In: Bostwick DG, Cheng L, eds. Urologic Surgical Pathology, 2nd ed. Philadelphia: Elsevier/Mosby, 2008;173–94.

69. Vermeulen P, Hoekx L, Colpaert C, Wyndaele JJ, Van Marck E. Biphasic sarcomatoid carcinoma (carcinosarcoma) of the renal pelvis with heterologous chondrogenic differentiation. *Virchows Arch* 2000;437:194–7.

70. Volker HU, Scheich M, Holler S, Strobel P, Hagen R, Muller-Hermelink HK, Eck M. Differential diagnosis of laryngeal spindle cell carcinoma and inflammatory myofibroblastic tumor—report of two cases with similar morphology. *Diagn Pathol* 2007;2:1.

71. Byard RW, Bell ME, Alkan MK. Primary carcinosarcoma: a rare cause of unilateral ureteral obstruction. *J Urol* 1987;137:732–3.

72. Perimenis P, Athanasopoulos A, Geraghty J, Speakman M. Carcinosarcoma of the ureter: a rare, pleomorphic, aggressive malignancy. *Int Urol Nephrol* 2003;35:491–3.

73. Johnin K, Kadowaki T, Kushima M, Ushida H, Koizumi S, Okada Y. Primary heterologous carcinosarcoma of the ureter with necrotic malignant polyps. Report of a case and review of the literature. *Urol Int* 2003;70:232–5.

74. Orsatti G, Corgan FJ, Goldberg SA. Carcinosarcoma of urothelial organs: sequential involvement of urinary bladder, ureter, and renal pelvis. *Urology* 1993;41:289–91.

75. Black PC, Brown GA, Dinney CP. The impact of variant histology on the outcome of bladder cancer treated with curative intent. *Urol Oncol* 2009;27:3–7.

76. Damiano R, D'Armiento M, Cantiello F, Amorosi A, Tagliaferri P, Sacco R, Venuta S. Gemcitabine and cisplatin following surgical treatment of urinary bladder carcinosarcoma. *Tumori* 2004;90:458–60.

77. Froehner M, Gaertner HJ, Manseck A, Wirth MP. Durable complete remission of metastatic sarcomatoid carcinoma of the bladder with cisplatin and gemcitabine in an 80-year-old man. *Urology* 2001;58:799.

78. Strefford JC, Lillington DM, Steggall M, Lane TM, Nouri AM, Young BD, Oliver RT. Novel chromosome findings in bladder cancer cell lines detected with multiplex fluorescence in situ hybridization. *Cancer Genet Cytogenet* 2002;135:139–46.

79. Cheng L, Zhang D. Molecular Genetic Pathology. New York: Humana Press/Springer, 2008.

80. Cheng L, Zhang S, Davidson DD. Implications of Cancer Stem Cells for Cancer Therapy. New York: Humana Press/Springer, 2009.

81. Takahashi T, Habuchi T, Kakehi Y, Mitsumori K, Akao T, Terachi T, Yoshida O. Clonal and chronological genetic analysis of multifocal cancers of the bladder and upper urinary tract. *Cancer Res* 1998;58:5835–41.

82. Nowell PC. The clonal evolution of tumor cell populations. *Science* 1976;194:23–8.

83. Kallioniemi A, Kallioniemi OP, Citro G, Sauter G, DeVries S, Kerschmann R, Caroll P, Waldman F. Identification of gains and losses of DNA sequences in primary bladder cancer by comparative genomic hybridization. *Genes Chromosomes Cancer* 1995;12:213–9.

84. McConkey DJ, Lee S, Choi W, Tran M, Majewski T, Siefker-Radtke A, Dinney C, Czerniak B. Molecular

genetics of bladder cancer: emerging mechanisms of tumor initiation and progression. *Urol Oncol* 2010;28:429–40.

85. Polyak K, Weinberg RA. Transitions between epithelial and mesenchymal states: acquisition of malignant and stem cell traits. *Nat Rev Cancer* 2009;9:265–73.

86. Cheng L, Zhang S, Wang M, Davidson DD, Morton MJ, Huang J, Zheng S, Jones TD, Beck SD, Foster RS. Molecular genetic evidence supporting the neoplastic nature of stromal cells in "fibrosis" after chemotherapy for testicular germ cell tumors. *J Pathol* 2007;213:65–71.

87. Paterson RF, Ulbright TM, MacLennan GT, Zhang S, Pan CX, Sweeney CJ, Moore CR, Foster RS, Koch MO, Eble JN, Cheng L. Molecular genetic alterations in the laser-capture-microdissected stroma adjacent to bladder carcinoma. *Cancer* 2003;98:1830–6.

88. Chan KS, Espinosa I, Chao M, Wong D, Ailles L, Diehn M, Gill H, Presti J Jr, Chang HY, van de Rijn M, Shortliffe L, Weissman IL. Identification, molecular characterization, clinical prognosis, and therapeutic targeting of human bladder tumor initiating cells. *Proc Natl Acad Sci U S A* 2009;106:14016–21.

89. Sung MT, Zhang S, MacLennan GT, Lopez-Beltran A, Montironi R, Wang M, Tan PH, Cheng L. Histogenesis of clear cell adenocarcinoma in the urinary tract: Evidence of urothelial origin. *Clin Cancer Res* 2008;14:1947–55.

90. Thiery JP. Epithelial-mesenchymal transitions in tumour progression. *Nat Rev Cancer* 2002;2:442–54.

Chapter 17

Bladder Tumors with Inverted Growth

Bladder Pathology, First Edition. Liang Cheng, Antonio Lopez-Beltran, David G. Bostwick.
© 2012 Wiley-Blackwell. Published 2012 by John Wiley & Sons, Inc.

The potential for misinterpretation of inverted or endophytic urothelial lesions of the bladder is high.[1] The pathologist should be aware of diverse morphologic manifestation of these lesions (**Table 17-1**).

Inverted Papilloma

Clinical Features

Although the term "inverted papilloma" was introduced in 1963 by Potts and Hirst to describe this architecturally distinctive urothelial neoplasm,[2] the Viennese urologist, Paschkis, had previously reported four morphologically identical urothelial tumors in 1927 under the name "adenomatoid polyp."[3] Other terms, such as "urothelial adenoma," "brunnian adenoma," and "inverted urothelial papilloma," were also used in the past. "Inverted papilloma" is the preferred term. Inverted papilloma occurs at all ages, including a few cases in children, and comprises less than 1% of urothelial neoplasms.[4–9] It is more common in men than in women. The male-to-female ratio is 7.3 : 1.[4] The mean age at diagnosis is 60 years (range, 26 to 85 years), with a peak frequency in the sixth decades.[4] A significant number of patients have a history of smoking, suggesting a possible link between tobacco use and inverted papilloma.[4]

Patients usually present with hematuria and irritative symptoms.[4,10–21] The majority of inverted papillomas

Table 17-1 Main Urothelial Lesions and Tumors with Inverted Growth Patterns
Benign lesions Inverted papilloma Florid von Brunn nest proliferations Florid cystitis glandularis Malignant lesions Inverted variant of urothelial carcinoma (urothelial carcinoma with inverted growth) Nested variant of urothelial carcinoma Verrucous squamous cell carcinoma

develop in the region of the trigone and bladder neck (**Fig. 17-1**). Cystoscopically and grossly, inverted papilloma characteristically appears as a sessile or pedunculated lesion with a smooth surface (**Fig. 17-2**). They are usually small (<1 cm in diameter) and single, but large multifocal lesions may occur. The incidence of multiplicity ranges from 1.3% to 4.4%.[4,11]

Using strict diagnostic criteria, inverted papilloma is a benign neoplasm. In the largest series of 75 cases reported by Sung and his colleagues, only one case had recurrence during a mean followup of 68 months.[4] Consequently, transurethral resection of inverted papilloma is adequate treatment, and surveillance protocols as rigorous as those employed in the management of urothelial carcinoma seem unnecessary for this benign entity.

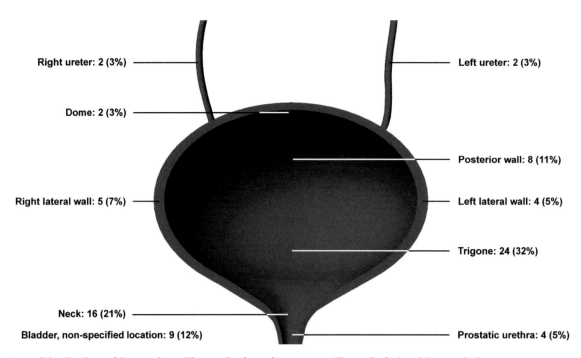

Right ureter: 2 (3%)   Left ureter: 2 (3%)

Dome: 2 (3%)

Posterior wall: 8 (11%)

Right lateral wall: 5 (7%)   Left lateral wall: 4 (5%)

Trigone: 24 (32%)

Neck: 16 (21%)

Bladder, non-specified location: 9 (12%)   Prostatic urethra: 4 (5%)

Figure 17-1 Distribution of inverted papillomas in the urinary tract. (From Ref. 4; with permission.)

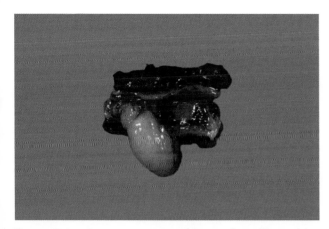

Figure 17-2 Gross appearance of inverted papilloma. Note the polypoid protrusion into the luminal space.

Pathology

Inverted papilloma shows an inverted growth pattern, usually composed of anastomosing islands and trabeculae of histologically and cytologically normal urothelial cells invaginating from the surface urothelium into the subjacent lamina propria but not into the muscularis propria (**Figs. 17-3** to **17-9**; **Table 17-2**). The overlying surface urothelium may be normal, attenuated, or hyperplastic, and, by definition, an exophytic component is either absent or minimal.

Kunze et al. proposed the subdivision of inverted papilloma into two morphologically distinct variants, trabecular and glandular.[10] By their criteria, the trabecular variant is composed of anastomosing cords and trabeculae of urothelial cells invaginating the lamina propria at various angles. These invaginating structures demonstrate mature urothelium centrally, with darker and palisading basal cells peripherally, often surrounded by fibrotic stroma without marked inflammation. The neoplastic cells within the nests and cords of urothelium may have a spindled appearance. Some tumors are punctuated by cystic spaces lined by flattened urothelial cells and containing eosinophilic material, producing an appearance reminiscent of cystitis cystica. The glandular variant is composed of nests of urothelium with either pseudoglandular spaces lined by mature urothelium, or even true glandular elements, containing mucicarminophilic secretions and mucus-secreting cells (**Figs. 17-10** to **17-11**). The glandular variant, as proposed by these investigators, has considerable morphologic overlap with florid cystitis glandularis and is not widely accepted as a diagnostic entity.

Within the spectrum of findings in inverted papilloma, vacuolization and foamy xanthomatous cytoplasmic changes may be seen. These "clear cells" may be concentrated within distinct regions of the tumor, but more frequently are diffusely intermingled with usual inverted papilloma cells. Foci of nonkeratinizing squamous metaplasia and neuroendocrine differentiation may be seen.[20,22] Mitotic figures are either absent or rare. Some cases may demonstrate focal minor cytologic atypia, which is probably degenerative in nature and has no clinical significance.[5] Inverted papillomas with focal papillary features have been described recently, broadening the morphologic spectrum of inverted papillomas.[23] Another uncommon variant, designated "inverted papilloma with atypia," exhibits focal mild cytologic atypia with prominent nucleoli,

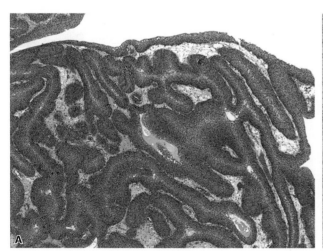
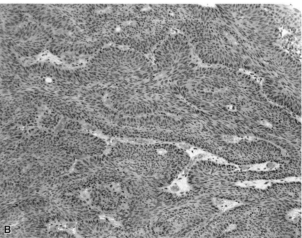

Figure 17-3 Inverted papilloma. (A) The low magnification demonstrates a distinct downward growth pattern of a typical inverted papilloma composed of intact surface lining urothelium and underlying thin anastomosing trabeculae of urothelium in the lamina propria. (B) On a higher magnification, the trabeculae are characterized by central streaming and peripheral palisading without evidence of cytological atypia and mitosis. (From Ref. 4; with permission.)

385

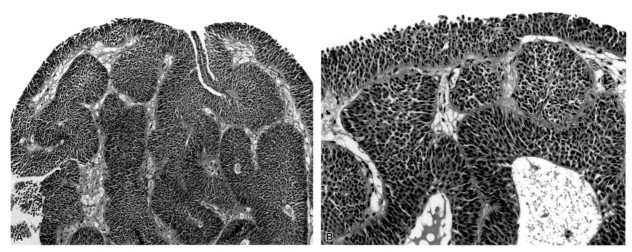

Figure 17-4 Inverted papilloma. (A) This solitary 3.0-cm-diameter mass formed a protruberant nodule in the trigone of a 55-year-old woman. (B) The tumor contains typical anastomosing trabeculae of urothelial cells.

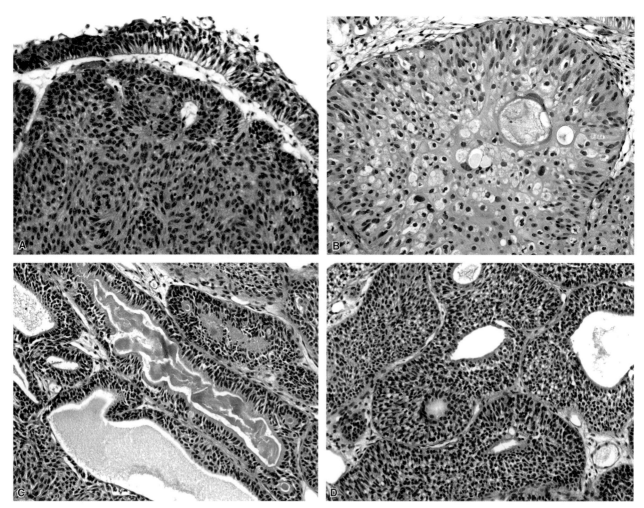

Figure 17-5 Inverted papilloma. The nests may be solid with whorled masses of uniform spindle cells (A), punctuated by small cysts filled with mucin (B), or contain large cysts with variable amounts of proteinacous material (C). Inverted papilloma may also show hyperplastic growth pattern (D).

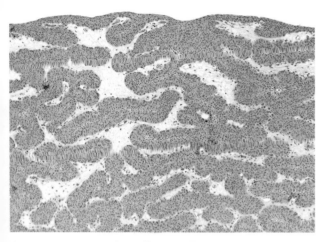

Figure 17-6   Inverted papilloma, trabecular growth.

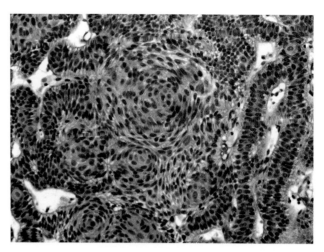

Figure 17-8   Inverted papilloma, spindle cell pattern.

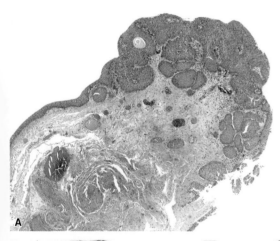

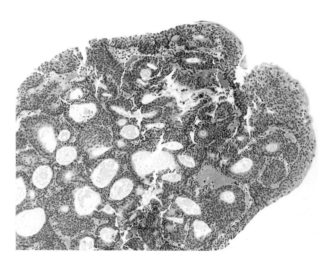

Figure 17-9   Inverted papilloma, microcystic pattern.

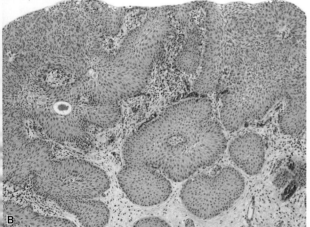

Figure 17-7   Incipient inverted papilloma presents as polypoid lesion (A and B).

Table 17-2   **Key Morphologic Features of Inverted Papilloma**

Relatively smooth surface with absent exophytic
    component
Superficial growth without involvement of muscularis
    propria
Thin trabeculae
Lesional circumscription with smooth base
Lack of stromal desmoplasia
Lack of infiltrative growth
Minimal to no cytologic atypia
Absence of in situ component (urothelial carcinoma in situ
    and/or urothelial dysplasia)

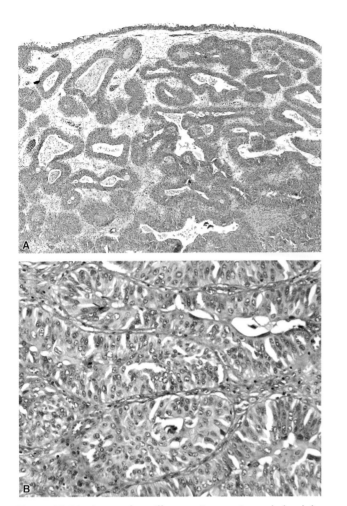

Figure 17-10   Inverted papilloma, microcystic, and glandular pattern (A and B).

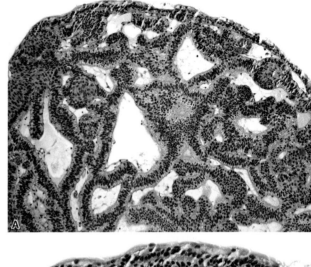

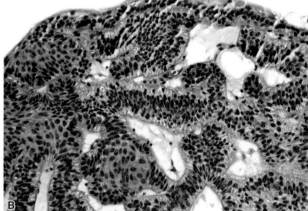

Figure 17-11   Inverted papilloma, glandular pattern (A and B).

atypical squamous features, and degenerate-appearing multinucleated giant cells. These features are not known to have any clinical significance.[10,16] Foci of nonkeratinizing squamous metaplasia are often present, and rare cases may demonstrate neuroendocrine differentiation.[22]

Differential Diagnosis

It is most important to differentiate inverted papilloma from urothelial carcinoma with inverted growth pattern (Table 17-3). Such distinctions may be difficult, especially in limited biopsy specimens or when interpretation is confounded by crush artifact.[5] Inverted papilloma usually exhibits orderly maturation of invaginated trabeculae and cords, composed of spindling and peripherally palisading cells. In contrast, urothelial carcinoma with inverted growth pattern often has thick and irregular tumor columns with transition to more solid nests. Additionally, the presence of an exophytic papillary component and unequivocal tumor invasion in the lamina propria or muscularis propria justifies a diagnosis of inverted urothelial carcinoma. Marked cytological atypia, including nuclear pleomorphism, nucleolar prominence, and abundant mitotic activity, further support a diagnosis of malignancy.

Other differential considerations include florid cystitis glandularis and von Brunn nest proliferations, which are characterized by proliferation of round well-delineated nests of normal-appearing urothelium. Inverted papilloma shows cords with anastomosing growth patterns.

Molecular Pathology

It has been well documented by the finding of nonrandom inactivation of X chromosomes that inverted papilloma is a clonal neoplasm that arises from a single progenitor cell.[24] Sung et al. studied the status of loss of heterozygosity (LOH) in inverted papilloma using microsatellite markers, which are commonly altered in urothelial carcinoma (Figs. 17-12 and 17-13).[24] The incidence of LOH in

Table 17-3   Morphologic, Immunologic, and Molecular Genetic Features of Inverted Papilloma and Urothelial Carcinoma with Inverted Growth[a]

Characteristics	Inverted Papilloma	Urothelial Carcinoma with Inverted Growth
Surface	Smooth, domed shaped, usually intact, cytologically normal	Exophytic papillary lesions usually present
Growth pattern	Endophytic, expansive, sharply delineated, anastomosing cords and thin trabeculae	Endophytic, lesional circumscription variable, thick trabeculae
Cytologic features	Orderly polarized cells, some with spindling and palisading at the periphery; no significant atypia, mitoses rare	Variable, nuclear pleomorphism and atypia present
Immunohistochemistry	Negative CK20 expression	Aberrant CK20 expression
p53 and Ki67	Low or absent p53 expression and Ki67 proliferation index	High p53 expression and Ki67 proliferation index usually present
FGFR3 mutation	Frequent	Variable
UroVysion FISH	Negative	Positive
LOH	Low or absent	High frequency
Clinical behavior	Benign, rare recurrences[b]	Recurrences and progression often depend on grade and stage

[a]CK20, cytokeratin 20; FISH, fluorescence in situ hybridization; LOH, loss of heterozygosity.
[b]Rare recurrences related to incomplete excision.

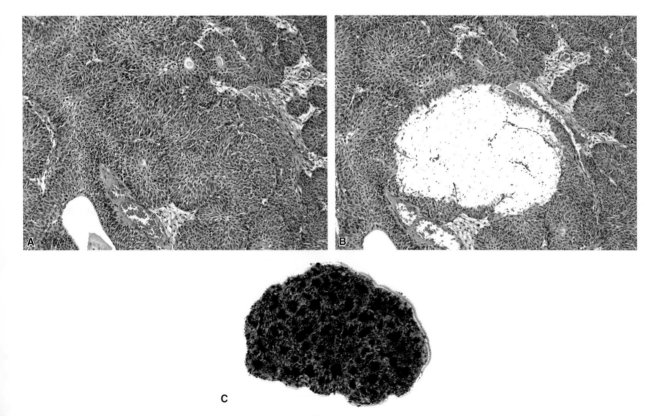

Figure 17-12   Laser capture microdissection of inverted papilloma in urinary bladder. (A) Tumor specimen before microdissection. (B) Tumor specimen after microdissection. (C) Laser-captured tumor cells. (From Ref. 24; with permission.)

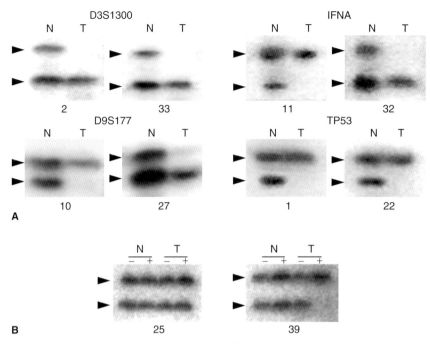

Figure 17-13   Representative results of loss of heterozygosity (A) and X chromosome inactivation analysis (B) in inverted papilloma of the urinary bladder. In (A), DNA was prepared from normal and tumor tissue, amplified by polymerase chain reaction using polymorphic markers D3S1300, IFNA, D9S177, and TP53 and separated by gel electrophoresis. In (B), nonrandom inactivation of X chromosome was identified in case 39. Arrows, allelic bands; N, normal control tissue; T, tumor tissue of inverted papilloma, −, without HhaI endonuclease digestion, +, with HhaI endonuclease digestion. (From Ref. 24; with permission.)

inverted papilloma is low (8% to 10%) and contrasts with the high frequency of LOH (29% to 80%) in urothelial carcinoma and papillary urothelial neoplasm of low malignant potential. The low frequency of allelic loss in inverted papilloma is similar to that of normal urothelium.[25] The markedly reduced frequency of LOH in inverted papilloma as compared to that of urothelial carcinoma suggests that inverted papilloma does not harbor the key genetic abnormalities that predispose to the development of urothelial carcinoma and may indicate that these entities arise through separate and distinct pathogenetic mechanisms.

More recently, Lott et al. analyzed fibroblast growth factor receptor 3 (*FGFR3*) and *TP53* mutation status in 20 cases of inverted papillomas.[26] Point mutations of the *FGFR3* gene were identified in 45% (9 of 20) of inverted papillomas with four cases exhibiting mutations at multiple exons. Seven cases had exon 7 mutations containing R248C, S249T, L259L, P260P, and V266M (**Figs. 17-14** and **17-15**). Two cases had exon 10 and 15 mutations, including A366D, H412H, E627D, D641N, and H643D; five cases had N653H. The most frequent mutation was identified at R248C. None of the inverted papillomas exhibited mutations in *TP53*. These findings support the concept that low grade and low-stage urothelial neoplasms arise in a background of molecular changes that are distinctly different from the molecular changes of high grade and high stage urothelial cancers.

Inverted Variant of Urothelial Carcinoma (Urothelial Carcinoma with Inverted Growth)

Clinical Features and Morphology

This variant has also been referred to as urothelial carcinoma with endophytic (inverted papilloma-like) growth or inverted urothelial carcinoma (**Figs. 17-16** to **17-22**).[5,27–30] In a recent study of 29 patients, the mean age at diagnosis was 65 years (range, 33 to 84 years).[5] The male-to-female ratio was 3 : 1. The pathological stages were Ta (17 patients), T1 (7 patients), and T2 (5 patients).[5] Hematuria and irritative symptoms were typical clinical presentations.

Two histologic patterns may be seen. The endophytic growth pattern in this carcinoma has been described either as interanastomosing cords and columns of urothelium, often with a striking resemblance to inverted papilloma (inverted papilloma-like pattern), or as broad, pushing bulbous invaginations into the lamina propria (broad-front pattern). Unlike inverted papilloma, the trabeculae of inverted urothelial carcinoma are wider and more variable. Most important, the inverted variant of urothelial carcinoma usually exhibits substantial cytologic atypia that is not seen in inverted papilloma. These include nuclear pleomorphism, architectural abnormality, and increased mitotic

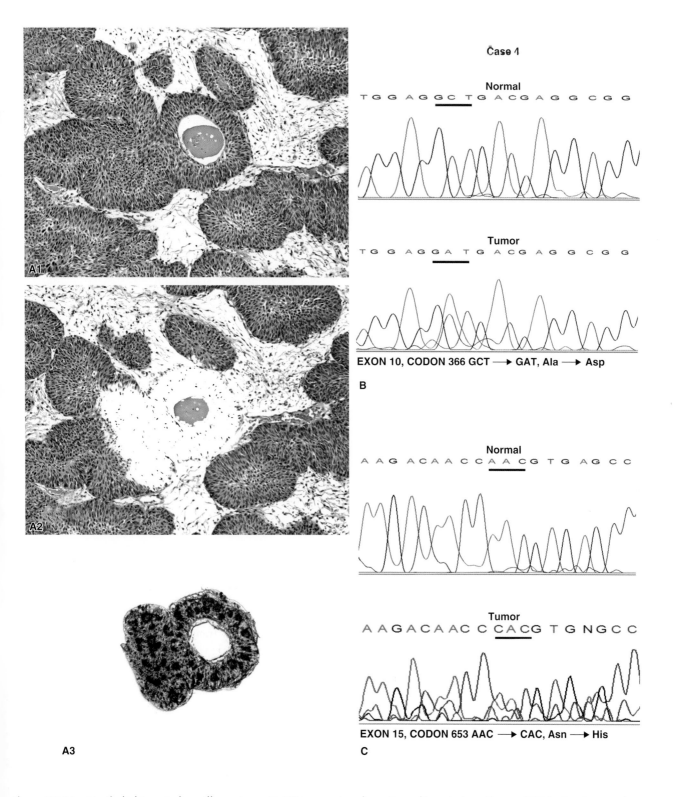

Figure 17-14 Urothelial inverted papilloma (case 4). (A) Laser microdissection of inverted papilloma. (A1) Lesion (inverted papilloma) before microdissection. (A2) Lesion after microdissection. (A3) Laser-captured lesional cells. (B) *FGFR3* gene mutation detected by direct sequencing. Upper panel: normal tissue (control); lower panel: point mutation at exon 10, A366D, GCT → GAT. (C) *FGFR3* gene mutation detected by direct sequencing. Upper panel: normal tissue (control); lower panel: point mutation at exon 15, N653H, AAC → CAC. (From Ref. 26; with permission.)

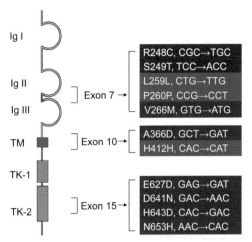

Figure 17-15   Schematic illustration of *FGFR3* mutation positions in the inverted urothelial papillomas. Mutations were presented as the type of mutation and amino acid changes designated to the FGFR3 protein structure. Ig I, Ig II, and Ig III, immunoglobulin-like domains; TM, transmembrane domain; TK1 and TK2, tyrosine kinase domains. Red-coded mutations are activating mutations published previously; blue-coded are missense mutations, which are candidates for activating mutations; green-coded are silent mutations. (From Ref. 26; with permission.)

activity. In most cases, the surface of the neoplasm shows similar abnormalities and is readily recognized as typical urothelial carcinoma. An exophytic papillary or invasive component is often associated with the inverted element. However, in cases of inverted papilloma fragmented during transurethral resection, a pseudoexophytic pattern may result. The identification of urothelial carcinoma in situ or dysplasia in adjacent urothelium supports the diagnosis of inverted urothelial carcinoma.

A diagnosis of invasion requires the unquestionable presence within the lamina propria of irregularly shaped nests or single cells that may have evoked a desmoplastic or inflammatory response (Table 17-4). Desmoplasia and/or a fibrotic stromal response are reliable indicators of invasion. When a stromal response is absent, irregularity of the contours of the invasive nests, architectural complexity, and recognition of single cell invasion is helpful. Paradoxical differentiation can aid in the diagnosis of early invasion. Large papillary tumors with prominent endophytic growth may appear to "invade" the lamina propria with a pushing border. Unless this pattern is accompanied by true destructive stromal invasion, the likelihood of metastasis is minimal, because the basement membrane is not truly breached.

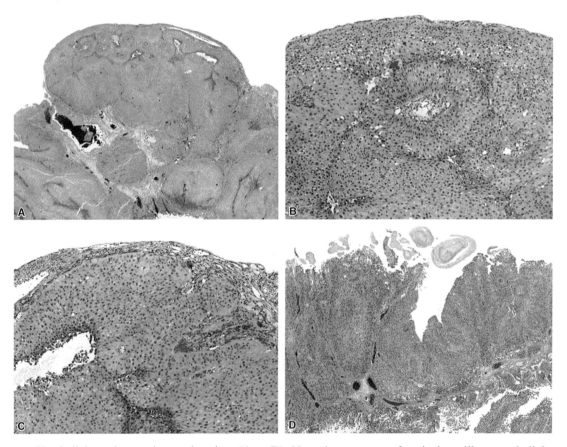

Figure 17-16   Urothelial carcinoma, inverted variant (A to D). Note the presence of typical papillary urothelial carcinoma (D).

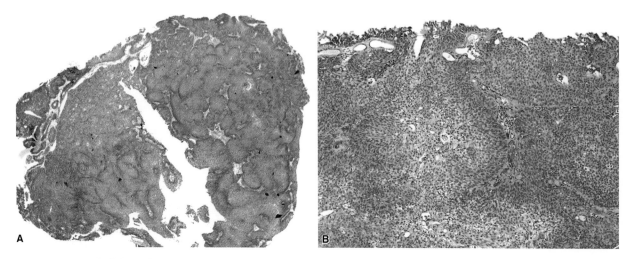

Figure 17-17   Urothelial carcinoma, inverted variant (A and B).

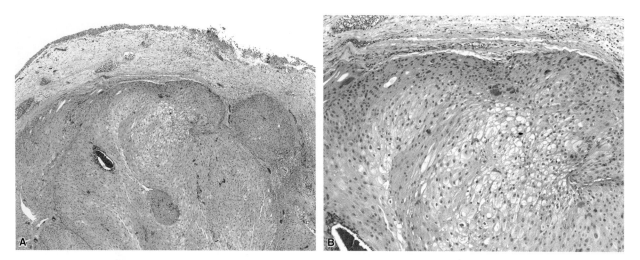

Figure 17-18   Urothelial carcinoma, inverted variant (A and B).

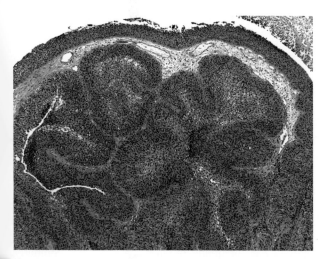

Figure 17-19   Urothelial carcinoma, inverted variant.

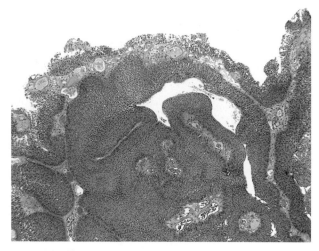

Figure 17-20   Urothelial carcinoma, inverted variant.

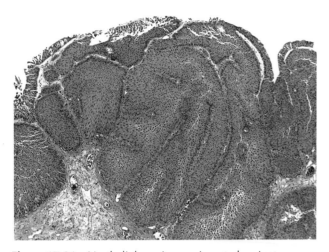

Figure 17-21 Urothelial carcinoma, inverted variant.

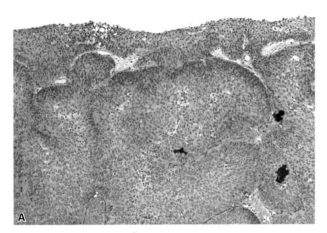

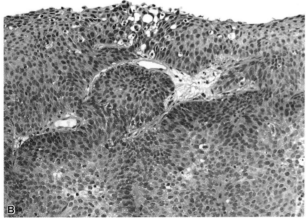

Figure 17-22 Urothelial carcinoma, inverted variant (A and B).

Table 17-4 **Urothelial Carcinoma with Inverted Pattern Criteria for Invasion**

Features	Noninvasive	Invasive
Contours of neoplastic nests/cords	Regular	Irregular
Size and shape of nests	Similar, rounded edges	Variable, irregular, and jagged edges
Inflammatory and desmoplastic stroma	Absent	Present

Grading of these tumors should follow the same criteria for typical urothelial carcinoma (see **Chapter 9** for further discussion). Frequently, components of otherwise typical exophytic or invasive urothelial carcinoma accompany inverted urothelial carcinoma. We require at least 25% of the tumor to have an inverted component to be considered inverted urothelial carcinoma.

Immunohistochemistry and FISH

Inverted urothelial carcinomas are typically positive for cytokeratin 20 (CK20) (**Table 17-5**).[5] The Ki67 labeling index positivity ranged from 2% to 30% of tumor cells (mean, 10%). p53 positivity ranged from 5% to 80% of tumor cells staining (mean, 17%). UroVysion FISH analysis showed alterations in chromosomes 3, 7, 17, and 9p21, commonly seen in conventional urothelial carcinoma of the bladder (gain of chromosomes 3, 7, and 17; and loss of 9p21) (**Fig. 17-23**).[5] LOH at tumor suppressor gene loci is frequent, in contrast to inverted papilloma.[24]

Differential Diagnosis

Urothelial carcinoma with inverted growth pattern may be difficult to distinguish from inverted papilloma.[5] Distinction between these two neoplasms requires strict attention to architectural and cytological features (**Tables 17-3** and **17-5**). Inverted urothelial carcinoma has readily apparent cytologic atypia, increased mitotic figures, and substantial architectural abnormalities consistent with low- or high grade urothelial carcinoma. These features are not seen in inverted papilloma. Urothelial carcinoma in situ, if present in the surface urothelium, provides further support for a diagnosis of inverted urothelial carcinoma. Whereas inverted papillomas usually do not demonstrate immunoreactivity for Ki67, p53, or CK20, urothelial carcinomas with inverted growth pattern frequently express one or more of these biomarkers. Similarly, inverted papillomas do not show the molecular features

Table 17-5   Comparison of Morphologic, Immunohistochemical, and Molecular Features of Inverted-Pattern Urothelial Carcinoma and Inverted Papilloma

	Inverted-Pattern Urothelial Carcinoma	Inverted Papilloma
Cytologic atypia/tumor grade[a]	Grade 1: 9/29 (31%) Grade 2: 14/29 (48%) Grade 3: 6/29 (21%)	0/15 (0%) with significant cytologic atypia
Coexisting exophytic papillary component	22/29 (76%)	0/15 (0%)
Coexisting flat urothelial dysplasia/CIS	0/29 (0%)	0/15 (0%)
Stromal invasion	12/29 (41%)	0/15 (0%)
Peripheral palisading	13/29 (45%)	15/15 (100%)
Mitotic activity	5/29 (17%)	12/15 (80%)
<1/10 hpf	16/29 (55%)	3/15 (20%)
1–5/10 hpf	5/29 (17%)	0/15 (0%)
5–15/10 hpf	3/29 (10%)	0/15 (0%)
>15/10 hpf		
Ki67 immunoreactivity	19/29 (66%)[b]	0/15 (0%)
p53 immunoreactivity	17/29 (59%)[c]	1/15 (7%)
CK20 immunoreactivity	17/29 (59%)	0/15 (0%)
UroVysion FISH positivity	21/29 (72%)	0/15 (0%)

Source: Modified from Ref. 5.
[a]Tumor grades based on 1973 World Health Organization classification. CIS, carcinoma in situ; CK20, cytokeratin 20; FISH, fluorescence in situ hybridization; hpf, high power field.
[b]Ki67 positivity ranged from 2% to 30% of tumor cells (mean, 10%).
[c]p53 positivity ranged from 5% to 80% of tumor cells (mean, 17%).

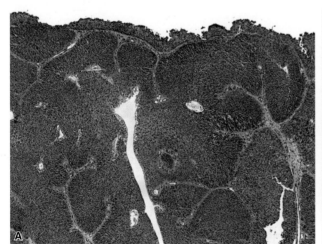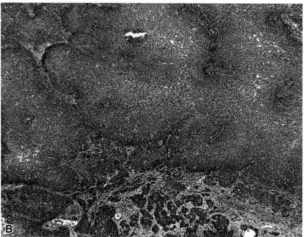

Figure 17-23   (continued on next page) H&E photomicrographs (A, B) and multicolor fluorescence in situ hybridization (FISH) image (C) of urothelial carcinoma with an inverted growth pattern. There are thick columns/cords of neoplastic cells with irregular widths and areas of solid growth. Lamina propria invasion is seen in (B). On FISH, there are gains of chromosomes 3 and 7 (red and green signals, respectively) (C). Inverted pattern of urothelial carcinomas are frequently immunohistochemically positive for Ki67 (D), p53 (E), and cytokeratin 20 (F). By contrast, classic inverted papillomas (G) demonstrate the normal diploid complement of chromosomes 3 (red), 7 (green), 17 (aqua), and 9 (gold) (H). (From Ref. 5; with permission.)

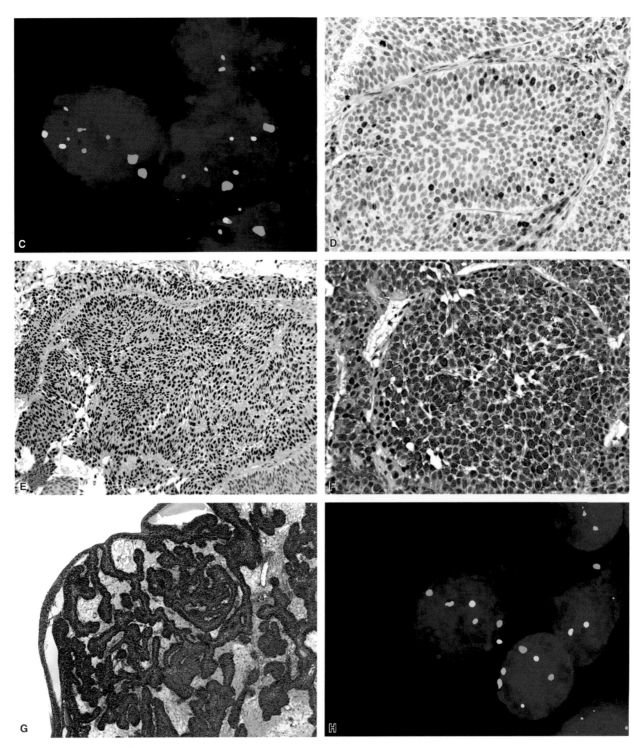

Figure 17-23   (*Continued*)

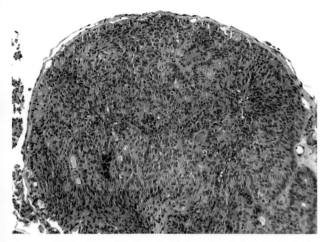

Figure 17-24 Ductal prostatic adenocarcinoma involving the urinary bladder. It may mimic inverted variant of urothelial carcinoma.

of urothelial carcinoma on UroVysion FISH analysis, whereas inverted pattern of urothelial carcinomas often demonstrate genetic alterations that are commonly seen in bladder cancer.[5]

Distinguishing inverted papilloma with atypia from inverted urothelial carcinoma can be challenging. However, inverted papilloma with atypia has only rare mitotic figures and exhibits a very low proliferation rate as estimated by Ki67 immunostaining.

Florid von Brunn nest proliferation should also be considered in the differential diagnosis. Florid von Brunn nest proliferation is characterized by large nests with regular spacing and lobular or linear configurations. Components of cystitis cystica and cystitis glandularis are often present in such proliferations. These benign urothelial proliferations lack cytologic atypia and any appreciable mitotic activities.

Prostatic adenocarcinoma involving the bladder may also have an inverted growth pattern, mimicking inverted urothelial carcinoma (**Fig. 17-24**).

Florid von Brunn Nest Proliferations

See **Chapter 3** for further discussion.

Florid Cystitis Glandularis

See **Chapter 3** for further discussion.

Nested Variant of Urothelial Carcinoma

See **Chapter 12** for further discussion.

Verrucous Squamous Cell Carcinoma

See **Chapter 14** for further discussion.

REFERENCES

1. Cheng L, Bostwick DG. Overdiagnosis of bladder carcinoma. *Anal Quant Cytol Histol* 2008;30:261–4.
2. Potts IF, Hirst E. Inverted Papilloma of the Bladder. *J Urol* 1963;90:175–9.
3. Paschkis R. Über adenoma der harnblase. *Ztschr Urol Chir* 1927;21:315–25.
4. Sung MT, Maclennan GT, Lopez-Beltran A, Montironi R, Cheng L. Natural history of urothelial inverted papilloma. *Cancer* 2006;107:2622–7.
5. Jones TD, Zhang S, Lopez-Beltran A, Eble JN, Sung MT, MacLennan GT, Montironi R, Tan PH, Zheng S, Baldridge LA, Cheng L. Urothelial carcinoma with an inverted growth pattern can be distinguished from inverted papilloma by fluorescence in-situ hybridization, immunohistochemistry, and morphologic analysis. *Am J Surg Pathol* 2007;31:1861–7.
6. Hodges KB, Lopez-Beltran A, MacLennan GT, Montironi R, Cheng L. Urothelial lesions with inverted growth patterns: histogenesis, molecular genetic findings, differential diagnosis and clinical management. *BJU Int* 2011;107:532–7.
7. Montironi R, Lopez-Beltran A, Scarpelli M, Mazzucchelli R, Cheng L. Morphological classification and definition of benign, preneoplastic and non-invasive neoplastic lesions of the urinary bladder. *Histopathology* 2008;53:621–33.
8. Montironi R, Mazzucchelli R, Scarpelli M, Lopez-Beltran A, Cheng L. Morphological diagnosis of urothelial neoplasms. *J Clin Pathol* 2008;61:3–10.
9. Montironi R, Cheng L, Lopez-Beltran A, Scarpelli M, Mazzucchelli R, Mikuz G, Kirkali Z, Montorsi F. Inverted (endophytic) noninvasive lesions and neoplasms of the urothelium: The Cinderella group has yet to be fully exploited. *Eur Urol* 2011;59:225–30.
10. Kunze E, Schauer A, Schmitt M. Histology and histogenesis of two different types of inverted urothelial papillomas. *Cancer* 1983;51:348–58.

11. Cheng CW, Chan LW, Chan CK, Ng CF, Cheung HY, Chan SY, Wong WS, To KF. Is surveillance necessary for inverted papilloma in the urinary bladder and urethra? *ANZ J Surg* 2005;75:213–7.

12. Witjes JA, van Balken MR, van de Kaa CA. The prognostic value of a primary inverted papilloma of the urinary tract. *J Urol* 1997;158:1500–5.

13. Cheville JC, Wu K, Sebo TJ, Cheng L, Riehle D, Lohse CM, Shane V. Inverted urothelial papilloma: Is ploidy, MIB–1 proliferative activity, or p53 protein accumulation predictive of urothelial carcinoma? *Cancer* 2000;88:632–6.

14. Matz LR, Wishart VA, Goodman MA. Inverted urothelial papilloma. *Pathology* 1974;6:37–44.

15. Rozanski TA. Inverted papilloma: an unusual recurrent, multiple and multifocal lesion. *J Urol* 1996;155:1391.

16. Broussard JN, Tan PH, Epstein JI. Atypia in inverted urothelial papillomas: pathology and prognostic significance. *Hum Pathol* 2004;35:1499–1504.

17. Fine SW, Chan TY, Epstein JI. Inverted papillomas of the prostatic urethra. *Am J Surg Pathol* 2006;30:975–9.

18. Fine SW, Epstein JI. Inverted urothelial papillomas with foamy or vacuolated cytoplasm. *Hum Pathol* 2006;37:1577–82.

19. Marquez Moreno AJ, Julve Villalta E, Alonso Dorrego JM, Rubio Garrido FJ, Blanes Berenguel A, Matilla Vicente A. [Multiple bladder inverted papillomas]. *Arch Esp Urol* 2001;54:692–4.

20. Goertchen R, Seidenschnur A, Stosiek P. [Clinical pathology of inverted papillomas of the urinary bladder. A complex morphologic and catamnestic study (2)]. *Pathologe* 1994;15:279–85.

21. Isaac J, Lowichik A, Cartwright P, Rohr R. Inverted papilloma of the urinary bladder in children: case report and review of prognostic significance and biological potential behavior. *J Pediatr Surg* 2000;35:1514–6.

22. Summers DE, Rushin JM, Frazier HA, Cotelingam JD. Inverted papilloma of the urinary bladder with granular eosinophilic cells. An unusual neuroendocrine variant.. *Arch Pathol Lab Med* 1991;115:802–6.

23. Albores-Saavedra J, Chable-Montero F, Hernandez-Rodriguez OX, Montante-Montes de Oca D, Angeles-Angeles A. Inverted urothelial papilloma of the urinary bladder with focal papillary pattern: a previously undescribed feature. *Ann Diagn Pathol* 2009;13:158–61.

24. Sung MT, Eble JN, Wang M, Tan PH, Lopez-Beltran A, Cheng L. Inverted papilloma of the urinary bladder: a molecular genetic appraisal. *Mod Pathol* 2006;19:1289–94.

25. Junker K, Boerner D, Schulze W, Utting M, Schubert J, Werner W. Analysis of genetic alterations in normal bladder urothelium. *Urology* 2003;62:1134–8.

26. Lott S, Wang M, MacLennan GT, Lopez-Beltran A, Montironi R, Sung M-T, Tan P-H, Cheng L. FGFR3 and TP53 mutation analysis in inverted urothelial papilloma: incidence and etiological considerations. *Mod Pathol* 2009;22:627–32.

27. Amin MB, Gomez JA, Young RH. Urothelial transitional cell carcinoma with endophytic growth patterns: a discussion of patterns of invasion and problems associated with assessment of invasion in 18 cases. *Am J Surg Pathol* 1997;21:1057–68.

28. Terai A, Tamaki M, Hayashida H, Tomoyosh T, Takeuchi H, Yoshida O. Bulky transitional cell carcinoma of bladder with inverted proliferation. *Int J Urol* 1996;3:316–9.

29. Sudo T, Irie A, Ishii D, Satoh E, Mitomi H, Baba S. Histopathologic and biologic characteristics of a transitional cell carcinoma with inverted papilloma-like endophytic growth pattern. *Urology* 2003;61:837.

30. Kawachi Y, Ishi K. Inverted transitional cell carcinoma of the ureter. *Int J Urol* 1996;3:313–5.

Chapter 18

Congenital Disorders and Pediatric Neoplasms

Bladder Pathology, First Edition. Liang Cheng, Antonio Lopez-Beltran, David G. Bostwick.
© 2012 Wiley-Blackwell. Published 2012 by John Wiley & Sons, Inc.

Congenital Disorders

Exstrophy

Complete failure of bladder development results in agenesis,[1,2] and incomplete closure of the bladder produces exstrophy.[3] Exstrophy affects about one in 30,000 to 50,000 births.[4] It is usually accompanied by other urinary tract defects, particularly epispadias, similar to agenesis. The common coexistence of exstrophy and epispadias is collectively designated the exstrophy–epispadias complex.[5] Exstrophy may also be associated with cloacal anomalies.

Bladder exstrophy may be incomplete or complete. Both types are recognizable at birth as a mucocutaneous defect in the midline of the infraumbilical region. The macroscopic abnormality results from exposure of the posterior bladder wall without its anterior investiture of mesoderm-derived tissue. Typically, the mucosa is irregular, nodular, and thickened, with a fibrotic wall containing mucin-filled cysts. Urothelial abnormalities result from exposure to the external environment; consequently, surgical repair is recommended early to avoid these changes.[6] Proliferative changes are present in virtually all cases, including cystitis cystica and glandularis, and squamous metaplasia occurs in about 25% (Figs. 18-1 to 18-4).[7-10] Prominent lymphoid hyperplasia in the lamina propria may impart a finely nodular appearance macroscopically. Initially, the lamina propria is edematous and contains a variable amount of acute and chronic inflammation, but eventually, fibrosis develops.

Bladder exstrophy is considered an important risk factor for malignancy and may be associated with adenocarcinoma,[11] squamous cell carcinoma, urothelial carcinoma, and rhabdomyosarcoma.[12] However, a previous

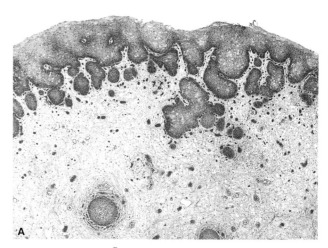
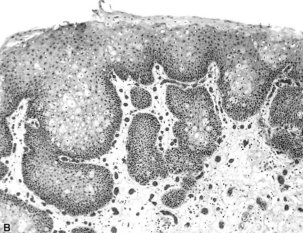

Figure 18-2 Exstrophy of the bladder (A and B). Note the squamous metaplasia.

study challenged bladder exstrophy as a risk factor for developing bladder adenocarcinoma in surgically treated patients.[13]

A less frequent form of exstrophy, cloacal exstrophy or vesicointestinal fissure, consists of an exstrophied portion of intestine from which a distal intestinal segment returns into a blind rectal pouch. A segment of colonic mucosa is exposed on the lower abdominal wall with portions of bladder wall exposed on both sides of the intestinal segment. Males and females are equally prone to cloacal exstrophy, unlike the male predominance with bladder exstrophy (3 : 1 ratio). Cloacal exstrophy is a more severe deformity and usually has coexistent exstrophic bladder with exposed hemibladder along the lateral border of the exstrophic intestine. Urothelial abnormalities in the hemibladder are similar to those in uncomplicated bladder exstrophy.[14,15]

Duplication and Diverticulum

Duplication is rare, characterized by incomplete or complete partitioning of the bladder.[16-20]

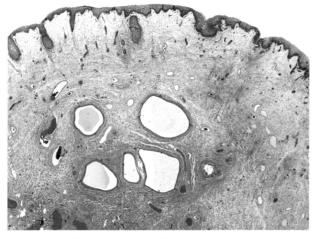

Figure 18-1 Exstrophy of the bladder. Note the squamous metaplasia, stromal edema vascular congestion, and deep dilated glands with periglandular cuffing of myofibroblasts.

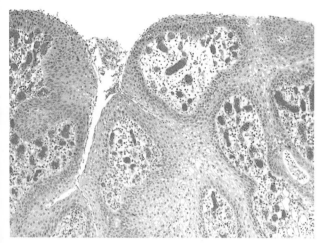

Figure 18-3 Exstrophy of the bladder. Note the squamous metaplasia and vascular congestion.

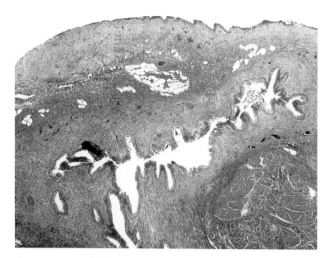

Figure 18-5 Bladder diverticulum.

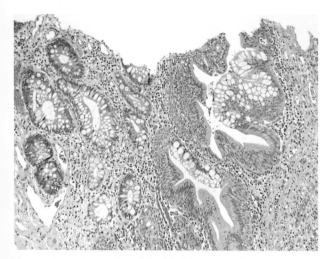

Figure 18-4 Exstrophy of the bladder. Note the intestinal metaplasia, cystitis glandularis, and mucosal erosions.

Bladder diverticulum is classified as "congenital or acquired," including iatrogenic cases.[21] Most congenital diverticula are discovered incidentally without other urologic anomalies (**Fig. 18-5**). Acquired diverticula in children are usually discovered as a complication of bladder neck obstruction, and this may be congenital or associated with neurogenic bladder in patients with meningomyelocele.[22] Acquired diverticula are the most common form in adults and are frequently associated with inflammation, urothelial dysplasia, carcinoma, or sarcoma.[20,23,24] Some cases may be very large and the term "giant diverticulum" may be applied.

Fistula and Cysts

A congenital fistula between the bladder and the anterior abdominal wall may form a superior or inferior vesical fissure and is considered a less severe form of exstrophy than typical exstrophy.[25]

Congenital prepubic sinus is a midline sinus from the skin immediately superior to the pubis that may communicate with the anterior bladder wall. Microscopically, the sinus tract is lined by urothelium and surrounded by a smooth muscle sheath. The sinus is considered a urethral duplication rather than a variant of exstrophy.[26,27]

Trigonal cyst is a developmental anomaly located at or near the trigone that is lined by unremarkable urothelium.

Megacystis

An enlarged bladder may result from any distal anatomic obstruction, often at the bladder neck or urethral valves, or as a manifestation of a syndrome complex such as prune belly syndrome, in that bilateral cryptorchidism is associated with urologic malformations and absence of the abdominal wall musculature. Some authors do not consider it strictly within the category of congenital malformation.[11,28] Megacystis is one component of the syndrome of megacystis–microcolon–intestinal hypoperistalsis.

Congenital Bladder Obstruction (Marion Disease)

Congenital bladder obstruction is an obstructive condition that results in recurrent urinary tract infections in children. Histologically, there is concentric fibromuscular hypertrophy and elastosis of the bladder wall, often with chronic inflammation.

Urachal Anomalies

Anomalies of the urachus in children include mainly patent urachus, persistent urachal remnants, and urachal cysts.

Also, bacterial infections may occur in the presence of a malformation or cyst. Benign neoplasms of the urachus include adenomas and soft tissue tumors. Malignant tumors of the urachus are uncommon, with adenocarcinoma as the most common form. Squamous cell carcinoma and urothelial carcinoma make up only 3% of cancers arising in the urachus, respectively. A number of urachal sarcomas have been reported. The main clinicopathological features of these uncommon lesions are described in **Chapter 27**.

Inflammatory and Related Conditions in Children

Inflammatory and reactive conditions in the bladder of children are encountered most frequently by the pathologist at postmortem examination. Often, these children have an indwelling catheter or have undergone instrumentation. The catheter tip may traumatize the mucosa in the trigone and posterior bladder wall, producing ulceration and secondary epithelial proliferation with atypia and other changes of proliferative cystitis. The catheter may act as a conduit for the introduction of bacteria and other microorganisms. The ileal conduit may be resected and show squamous metaplasia, mucosal ulcer, erosion, and chronic inflammation (**Fig. 18-6**).

Cystitis in a child is histologically identical to that occurring in the adult, and all forms of cystitis have been encountered (see also **Chapter 2**).[29] Inflammation of the bladder is more common in children than would be expected given the small number of bladder biopsies submitted for histologic examination. The indications for bladder biopsy are similar to those in an adult, including unexplained hematuria, voiding difficulties, or a lower abdominal mass.[30] Often, the biopsy reveals nonspecific inflammation and reactive mucosal changes. Nonspecific histologic changes in the bladder in children include edema, focal hemorrhage, vascular ectasia, and variable amounts of acute and chronic inflammation. The inflammation is often less impressive than the other findings. The majority of infections are caused by *Escherichia coli* or other gram-negative organisms.

Hemorrhagic cystitis is an uncommon form of acute cystitis characterized by hemorrhage, fibrin deposition, and necrosis.[31] Occasionally, this may be caused by adenovirus type 11.[32-34] It is often difficult to identify intranuclear inclusions characteristic of the organism because of mucosal sloughing.[35] The lamina propria contains aggregates of lymphocytes surrounded by erythrocytes, reminiscent of follicular cystitis. Hemorrhagic cystitis may also be caused by cytomegalovirus, with typical intranuclear and cytoplasmic inclusions within endothelial cells and macrophages.[32,36] Hemorrhagic cystitis may also

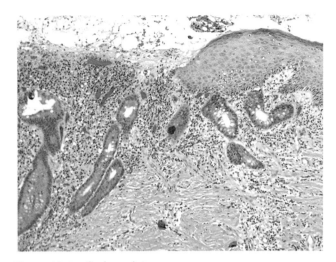

Figure 18-6　Ileal conduit.

result from cyclophosphamide and its metabolites with direct cytotoxic changes within the mucosa.[37] About 8% of children who receive cyclophosphamide weekly for acute lymphocytic leukemia or other diseases develop sterile hematuria. Macroscopically, the bladder wall is thick and boggy, with blood clots in the lumen, and diffusely hemorrhagic, friable, and ulcerated mucosa. Numerous ectatic blood vessels are present in the lamina propria, some with fibrin thrombi or evidence of necrosis. There may be a striking paucity of inflammatory cells, but eosinophils and atypical multinucleated cells may be observed. The urothelium often displays marked cytologic abnormalities that are thought to be regenerative and not neoplastic. A late finding is the presence of interstitial fibrosis within the wall.

Children may also develop eosinophilic or follicular cystitis, usually with no specific causative agent.[38] Eosinophilic cystitis may result from *Toxocara*, but the typical necrotizing eosinophilic granulomas of toxocariasis are absent in the bladder.[39]

Interstitial cystitis (Hunner ulcer) most often occurs in middle-aged women, but has occasionally been observed in children, usually with the same clinical and histologic manifestations.

Granulomatous cystitis in childhood is rare, and patients should be evaluated for the possibility of mycobacterial, fungal, or parasitic infection.[40] In endemic regions, *Schistosoma haematobium* exposure occurs in childhood in a large percentage of the population, resulting in bilharziasis.[41] The ova, frequently calcified, are typically deep in the bladder wall, and superficial biopsy may be negative.

Chronic granulomatous disease in childhood may include chronic cystitis, with characteristic palisading necrotizing granulomas and central collections of neutrophils.[42] Some cases are associated with prominent bullous cystitis.

Crohn disease may occur in children or young adults, involving the bladder by continuous spread of fistulas and inflammatory tracts from the adjacent bowel mucosa. Endoscopy reveals polypoid masses in the dome, and biopsies reveal acute inflammation and edema of the lamina propria with scattered epithelioid histiocytes. Rarely, there may be a terminal ileum stricture.

Malakoplakia is uncommon in children.

Rupture and Calculi in Children

Rupture of the bladder is rare in children. It usually results from blunt trauma with or without pelvic fracture. Although most ruptures occur into the extraperitoneal space in adults, intraperitoneal rupture with disruption of the dome is more common in children. Rarely, rupture presents as neonatal urinary ascites secondary to spontaneous perforation of the bladder. The presence of posterior urethral valves will create increased intravesical pressure in the majority of such infants.

Bladder calculi in children in the United States and Europe are very uncommon.[43,44] Causative factors include foreign body, *Proteus mirabilis* infection, exstrophy, proliferative cystitis, and neurogenic bladder. Most stones are calcium oxalate or a mixture of oxalate and calcium phosphate.

Benign Epithelial and Polypoid Lesions

Children are prone to an uncommon and heterogeneous group of lesions that sometimes form a mass, occasionally with exophytic growth. Proliferative cystitis is one of these lesions, resulting from chronic irritation, exstrophy, or unknown factors. The spectrum of proliferative cystitis includes von Brunn nests, cystitis cystica, and cystitis glandularis.[45,46] These changes may be limited to the trigone; but when large, they may resemble sarcoma botryoides, although they are usually small. Girls with chronic urinary tract infection are most likely to have proliferative cystitis, particularly cystitis cystica, with a frequency ranging from 2.5% to 22% of such patients.

Squamous metaplasia is rare in children, but some of the most dramatic examples reported occurred in children with exstrophy or schistosomiasis.[47] Currently, there is not enough data to identify keratinizing squamous metaplasia of the bladder as a premalignant condition, this term being reserved for those with obvious histological dysplasia. However, at present, all patients should undergo regular followup.[48]

Nephrogenic metaplasia (nephrogenic adenoma) is an uncommon finding in children, usually following manipulation, instrumentation, inflammation, calculi or trauma

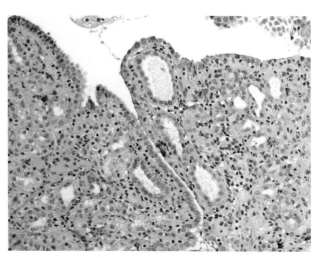

Figure 18-7   Nephrogenic metaplasia (nephrogenic adenoma).

of the bladder,[49-55] or in the background of previous renal transplantation[56] or augmented bladder (**Fig. 18-7**).[57] Patients present with hematuria, urgency, dysuria, and secondary enuresis. Although a male predilection is sometimes cited for adult patients, pediatric nephrogenic adenomas appear to occur more commonly in females, with a male-to-female ratio of $1:5$.[54,58] Microscopically, nephrogenic metaplasia typically displays papillary, exophytic growth. The tubular and papillary components are most often lined by cuboidal to low columnar epithelium, resembling renal tubules, sometimes with a hobnail appearance, or cystic dilation. Typically, the tubules are separated by abundant edematous stroma. In some instances, dilated vessels, calcifications, amyloid-like plaques, or multinucleate giant cells are seen. Reactive changes such as cystitis cystica, cystitis glandularis, or squamous metaplasia are sometimes identifiable in the surrounding tissue. Recurrence of nephrogenic metaplasia is not uncommon in the pediatric population.[54] Transurethral resection is the treatment of choice (see **Chapter 3** for further discussion).

Very few cases of hamartoma of the urinary bladder and prostatic-type polyp have occurred in children.[59,60] One interesting case arose in a 4-year-old girl with Peutz–Jeghers-like lesions in the colon, and two other cases occurred in brothers.[61]

Fibroepithelial polyp is a distinct benign entity commonly involving the bladder neck or prostatic urethra, in contrast to adult patients, in whom involvement of the upper urinary tract is more commonly seen (**Figs. 18-8** and **18-9**).[62] These lesions are completely benign and are believed to be nonneoplastic.[63-76] In one case, the fibroepithelial polyp of the bladder neck arose in an infant with Beckwith–Wiedemann syndrome.[68] Most polyps measure less than 2 cm in diameter and have a smooth surface of normal urothelium and supporting stroma of

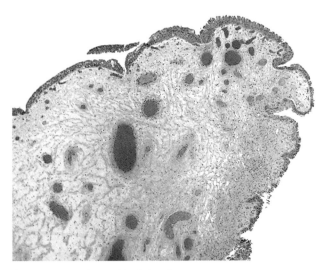

Figure 18-8   Fibroepithelial polyp.

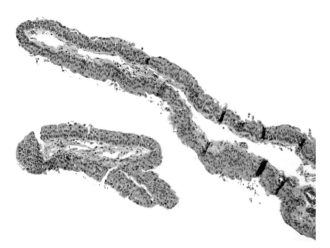

Figure 18-9   Fibroepithelial polyp.

hypocellular fibrous connective tissue; we have seen a case in which the stroma was filled with foamy cell histiocytes. In small biopsies, this lesion may be mistaken for embryonal rhabdomyosarcoma, particularly if the submucosal stromal cells are prominent and condensed in the subepithelial area. However, the stromal cells of fibroepithelial polyp appear benign, although exceptionally they have a pseudosarcomatous appearance. Rarely, adenomatous polyp also occurs in children.[77] (See **Chapter 4** for further discussion.)

Isolated examples of inverted papilloma have also been reported in children.[78–80] (See **Chapter 17** for further discussion.)

Urothelial Papilloma

Urothelial papilloma in pediatric patients is unusual but is reported occasionally.[81–84] Most tumors are solitary and located near the ureteric orifices. The clinical course of these tumors is generally favorable, although some cases in adults are diagnosed with concurrent urothelial carcinoma.[81,82] Papilloma sometimes recurs, although progression is not a feature. In the 2003 study by McKenney and colleagues, one patient presented in childhood (age 8 years), and in all, seven patients were 30 years of age or younger.[82] In another study focusing on urothelial neoplasms in patients under age 21, two patients (8.7%) had tumors that fit the current criteria for urothelial papilloma.[84]

The diagnostic criteria from the 1973[85] and 2004[86] World Health Organization (WHO) classification schemes are restrictive, limiting true urothelial papilloma to a small fraction of epithelial bladder tumors.[81] Microscopically, this lesion is composed of a delicate fibrovascular core covered by architecturally normal urothelium with a normal number of cell layers (approximately two to seven) and no cytologic atypia (**Fig. 18-10**). The larger papillary structures occasionally bud and give rise to smaller fronds or anastomosis of papillae. Mitotic figures are absent to rare and restricted to the basal cell layer. The superficial so-called "umbrella" cells are often prominent and may have vacuolated cytoplasm, eosinophilic syncytial growth, an apocrine-like appearance, or mucinous metaplasia. The stromal component is sometimes edematous with an infiltrate of inflammatory cells; less commonly, it contains dilated lymphatics or foamy histiocytes within the fibrovascular papillae.

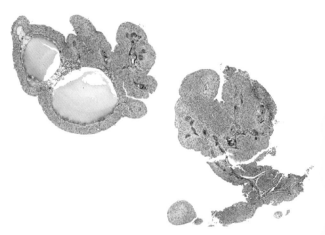

Figure 18-10   Urothelial papilloma.

Urothelial papilloma in pediatric patients has not been found to have any consistent genetic/syndromic associations, although it has been reported in conjunction with *WT1* gene mutation.[83]

Urothelial Carcinoma in Children

Epidemiology and Clinical Features

Urothelial carcinoma is uncommon in children, and the majority of such cases appear between 15 years and 20 years of age.[45,87] Up to 30% of pediatric cases may occur at 10 years of age or younger.[84] Urothelial carcinoma of the upper urinary tract is yet more unusual.[88] Owing to this rarity, several authors have warned that a diagnosis of urothelial tumors in children may be somewhat delayed from the initial onset of symptoms, due to reluctance of many physicians in pursuing an aggressive hematuria workup for these patients.[89-91]

In Javadpour and Mostofi's study, only 40 primary epithelial bladder tumors were identified in the first two decades of life from 10,000 total cases.[92] There was a striking male predilection, with a male-to-female ratio of 9 : 1. Patients in their series ranged from 6 years to 20 years of age, and most presented with gross hematuria.[92] Less frequent presenting symptoms included microscopic hematuria, dysuria, and urinary frequency.

Most arise as solitary papillary lesions in the trigone or lateral wall.[93,94] With rare exceptions, urothelial tumors in childhood are grade 1 or low grade urothelial carcinoma occasionally associated with lymphangiectasia (**Figs. 18-11** and **18-12**).[88,95-99] A recent report showed that urothelial

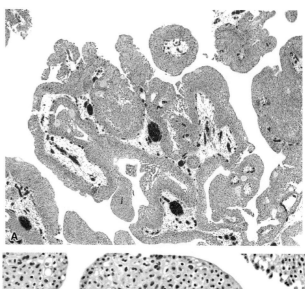

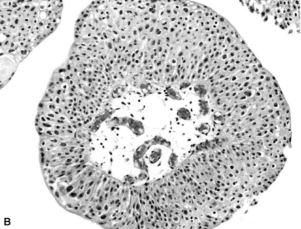

Figure 18-12   Noninvasive papillary urothelial carcinoma, low grade (A and B).

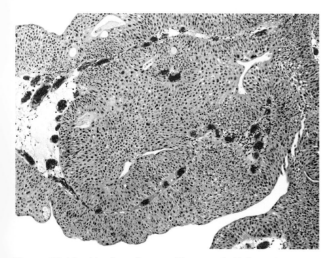

Figure 18-11   Noninvasive papillary urothelial carcinoma, low grade.

neoplasms in individuals younger than 20 years demonstrate very few genetic alterations and have a favorable clinical outcome.[100] Occasionally, urothelial carcinoma may be associated with the epidermal nevus syndrome.

In adult patients, cigarette smoking is highly implicated in the development of urothelial carcinoma,[101] as is exposure to various chemicals in the dye, rubber, textile, and chemical industries,[102] leading some to postulate differing social/occupational circumstances as an explanation for the increased male predilection of urothelial carcinoma. In pediatric patients, this association is somewhat questionable; however, in the Javadpour study, 18 patients of the 40 (primarily those over the age of 14 years) had a documented smoking history of 1.5 packs per day (average). None had known exposure to other carcinogenic agents, although one patient developed squamous cell carcinoma of the bladder related to schistosomiasis.[92] In contrast, in the more modern series by Fine et al., only one patient reported a brief period of cigarette smoking, while one additional patient had secondhand exposure, and none had exposure to carcinogenic agents.[84] Changes in smoking habits over recent decades probably account for these differences, although the possibility that young patients (especially in the late teenage years) are now less likely to report a smoking history is difficult to exclude. In the pediatric population, other etiologic factors may be involved, with or without cigarette smoking, in the development of urothelial tumors, especially so as cumulative pack years for any given patient are likely to be very small compared to those for elderly patients. Additionally, the genetic features of pediatric urothelial carcinoma appear to be distinct, suggesting alternative pathogenetic mechanisms.

The rarity of urothelial tumors in the pediatric population has led to a number of questions regarding their biological behavior. Some authors have found that these tumors are primarily low grade, with infrequent recurrence and more indolent behavior than those of adults[87,92,103]; however, other authors have suggested that pediatric urothelial carcinoma does recur and should be followed carefully.[91,104] It has been posed that in patients with multiple tumors, recurrence may be more likely.[88] As pediatric urothelial tumors include an abundance of low grade lesions, the utility of urinary cytology in establishing the diagnosis has been called into question.[90,103] Recent molecular evidence contrasting abnormalities of urothelial neoplasms in pediatric and adult patients suggests that pediatric tumors indeed are distinct and may develop along different pathways.[105]

Pathology

The majority of cases are low grade noninvasive papillary urothelial carcinoma, morphologically similar to those seen in adult patients. Rarely, some patients may have invasive carcinoma at presentation.[92] Fine and colleagues studied 23 urothelial neoplasms occurring in patients 20 years of age or younger, reclassifying each tumor based on the 2004 WHO and 1998 WHO/International Society of Urological Pathology (ISUP) classification schemes.[84] Tumors included urothelial papilloma (8.7%), papillary urothelial neoplasm of low malignant potential (PUNLMP, 43.5%), noninvasive low grade papillary urothelial carcinoma (34.8%), and noninvasive high grade papillary urothelial carcinoma (13%). Recurrences were identified in three of 21 patients, and all were alive without evidence of disease at 6 months to 13 years (mean, 4.5 years).[84]

The differential diagnostic considerations include nephrogenic adenoma, papillary hyperplasia, papillary polypoid cystitis, fibroepithelial polyp, and, rarely, inverted papilloma.[106]

Immunohistochemistry

A comprehensive immunohistochemistry (IHC) panel of cytokeratin (CK) 20, p53, and Ki67 (MIB1) may have clinical utility in evaluating urothelial carcinoma arising in children and young adults. Wild et al. found that immunohistochemical staining for CK20 demonstrated the normal pattern of expression (only the superficial cell layer) for the majority of the studied pediatric urothelial neoplasms.[105] In particular, all tumors classified as PUNLMP maintained the normal CK20 expression, while two low grade pTa tumors showed abnormal expression. Similarly, IHC for *TP53* was negative in all tumors, with the exception of two noninvasive papillary urothelial carcinoma cases, one low grade (20% staining) and one high grade (5% staining). Ki67 (MIB1) staining reached as high as 10% in the same two cases, with the remainder of tumors showing 1% to 5% staining.[105]

Molecular Features

Urothelial neoplasms in young patients exhibit distinctive molecular and genetic characteristics. In the general adult population, loss of heterozygosity (LOH) of chromosome 9 is reported frequently in noninvasive papillary tumors, while *TP53* gene mutation (located at 17p13.1) is classically described in urothelial carcinoma in situ and high grade invasive cancers.[107–109] Some investigators have found overlap between these abnormalities.[110] More recently, *FGFR3* gene abnormalities have been strongly implicated in the development of papillary tumors.[111]

In contrast to this typical genetic picture for adults, Linn et al. found young patients to have infrequent numerical abnormalities of chromosomes 9 and 17 by interphase cytogenetic analysis, coupled with a surprisingly high nuclear accumulation of p53 protein in low grade, low stage tumors.[112] They acknowledged that use of the centromeric probe method for numerical chromosomal abnormalities may underestimate smaller-scale genetic events while successfully detecting monosomy or aneuploidy.[112] More recently, Wild and colleagues used *FGFR3* and *TP53* mutation screening, comparative genomic hybridization (CGH), UroVysion fluorescence in situ hybridization (FISH) analysis, polymerase chain reaction (PCR) for human papillomavirus, microsatellite instability analysis, and markers for LOH on chromosome arms 9p, 9q, and 17p in a population of patients under age 20 with urothelial neoplasms.[105] Overall, few abnormalities were identified, and there was a notable absence of *FGFR3* gene mutations and 9p deletions, which are characteristically found in adult tumors. In contrast to the Linn study, only one of 14 tumors showed nonsense mutation in the *TP53* gene with accompanying p53 immunoreactivity. Overall, the authors concluded that urothelial neoplasms in patients under age 20 are less frequently associated with the typical genetic alterations of noninvasive urothelial carcinoma in elderly patients, and they represent a biologically distinct and genetically stable subset of bladder tumors.[105]

Soft Tissue Neoplasms

Hemangioma

Most benign tumors in childhood involving the bladder arise in the soft tissue. The most common is hemangioma, which usually arises in the first two decades of life (**Fig. 18-13; Table 18-1**). More than 30% of children with a hemangioma have a similar lesion elsewhere in the body.[113–115] Hemangioma appears as a solitary polypoid lesion in the dome or trigone, but rarely presents as a diffuse multilobular vasoformative proliferation within the wall of the bladder with involvement of the bowel, mesentery, and retroperitoneum. The vascular spaces are variable in appearance, but usually appear as small crowded capillary masses. Cavernous hemangioma consists of large vascular spaces, often with thrombi.[116] Epithelioid hemangioma is rare in childhood, as is diffuse lymphangiomatosis.[117] Hemangioma is benign and may be treated conservatively.[118]

See **Chapter 21** for further discussion.

Neurofibroma

The second most common benign soft tissue tumor of childhood is neurofibroma (**Figs. 18-14 and 18-15**). This

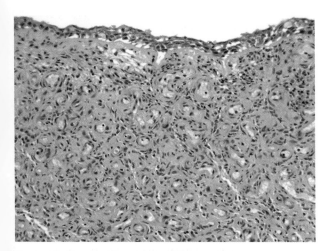

Figure 18-13   Capillary hemangioma.

Table 18-1   **Bladder Tumors in Childhood (in Descending Order of Frequency)**

Rhabdomyosarcoma (>75% of malignant tumors)
Hemangioma
Neurofibroma
Urothelial carcinoma
Leiomyoma
Leukemia/lymphoma (secondary)
Others

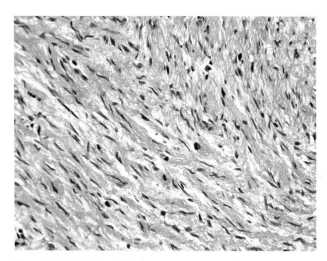

Figure 18-14   Neurofibroma.

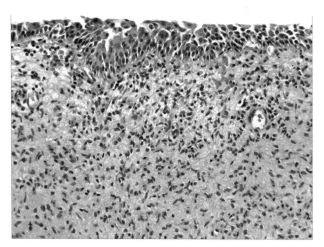

Figure 18-15   Neurofibroma.

is more common in boys than girls and is an expression of von Recklinghausen neurofibromatosis.[118–121] These children often have other sites of genitourinary tract involvement. Cheng et al. reported four patients with bladder neurofibroma, all of whom exhibited features of neurofibromatosis type 1 (NF1). Mean age at diagnosis was 17 years (range, 7 to 28 years), and no patient showed evidence of malignant transformation during a mean followup of 9.6 years.[118] Grossly, the bladder is enlarged and contains multiple glistening nodules in the wall, accompanied by broad polypoid masses protruding into the lumen. Microscopically, the lamina propria shows diffuse replacement by nodules of neurofibroma. Plexiform bundles of neurofibromatous tissue are characteristic and may separate and compress the smooth muscle of the muscularis propria. Another less common histologic pattern of genitourinary neurofibrosis is extensive ganglioneuromatosis similar to that in the intestinal tract.

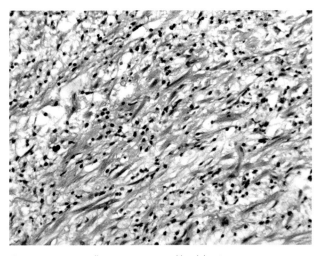

Figure 18-16   Inflammatory myofibroblastic tumor.

See **Chapter 15** for further discussion.

Inflammatory Myofibroblastic Tumor

Inflammatory myofibroblastic tumor (IMT) (inflammatory pseudotumor) of the bladder is another rare lesion that is more common in adults than in children (**Table 18-2**; see also **Chapter 19**).[122–126] When the bladder is involved, the differential diagnostic considerations include postoperative spindle cell nodule, myogenic tumor, sarcoma, and sarcomatoid carcinoma.[127] It often presents as a large intramural or exophytic mass in the bladder. Microscopically, the spindle cell proliferation is variably cellular, with chronic inflammation composed chiefly of lymphocytes and plasma cells with prominent edema and a focally prominent vascular network (**Figs. 18-16** and **18-17**). Some mitotic figures may be identified, but no atypical forms are present.

Ultrastructurally, the spindle cells have the same features as myofibroblasts elsewhere in the body. These cells are immunoreactive for vimentin, cytokeratins, ALK, and muscle-specific actin but do not stain for desmin, myoglobin, or myoD1. We find the inflammatory infiltrate to be diagnostically useful, and embryonal rhabdomyosarcoma is an important diagnostic consideration (see the discussion below), but usually has small neoplastic cells that are uniform, densely hyperchromatic nuclei, and intensely eosinophilic cytoplasm, often with a cambium layer, and lacks the inflammatory infiltrate seen in IMT.

See **Chapter 19** for further discussion.

Rhabdomyosarcoma

Clinical Features

Approximately 75% of malignant tumors of the bladder in children are rhabdomyosarcomas.[45,128–147] The average age at diagnosis is 5 years, and there is a predominance of boys to girls (3 : 2 ratio). Bladder neck obstruction with or without hematuria is the usual presenting symptoms.

Because of the limited anatomic space in the pelvis and the juxtaposition of anatomic structures, it is sometimes difficult to determine whether the sarcoma originated in the prostate and extended superiorly into the bladder neck, or, alternatively, it arose in the retroperitoneum and invaded the bladder, prostate, or vagina.[130] When the tumor presents as multiple polypoid masses in the lumen of the bladder, there is no difficulty in assignment of primary site of origin. A malignant neoplasm composed of small round or spindled cells and arising in the bladder of a child will prove to be rhabdomyosarcoma with only very rare exceptions.[133] Children with NF1 have an increased

Table 18-2   Comparison of Pediatric and Adult Inflammatory Myofibroblastic Tumor (IMT)[a]

	Pediatric	Adult
Location other than genitourinary tract	Gastrointestinal tract	Lung
Multifocality	Absent	Absent
Gender predilection	Male	Male
Location predilection	Dome	Lateral walls
Clinical presentations	Irritative symptoms and hematuria	Irritative symptoms and hematuria
Cytokeratin expression	Possibly less frequent than adults	Frequent
ALK–1 expression by IHC	Variably present	Variably present
ALK–1 expression by FISH	Variably present	Variably present
Recurrence	Infrequent	Infrequent
Metastasis	Rare (possibly ALK-negative cases)	Possibly absent in true IMT
Cancer death	Not clearly documented	Very rare, may occur

[a]Although some authors have proposed that pediatric IMT is a true neoplasm of intermediate malignant potential in contrast to adult pseudosarcomatous proliferations or IMT (some authors prefer the terminology "pseudosarcomatous proliferations"), other authors have integrated both adult and pediatric cases into the same series. The presence of variably frequent ALK–1 abnormalities in both groups suggests that they may represent the same entity.

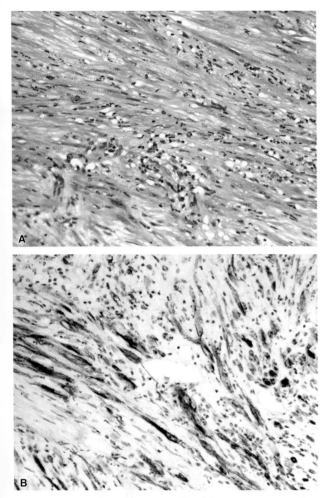

Figure 18-17 Inflammatory myofibroblastic tumor (A and B). ALK staining is positive (B).

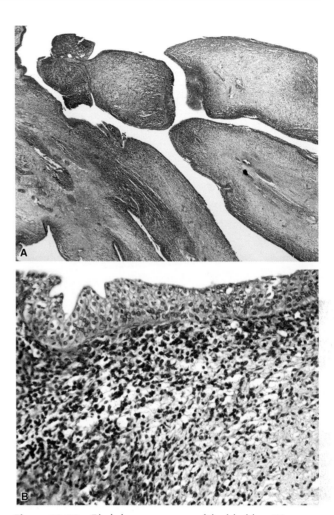

Figure 18-18 Rhabdomyosarcoma of the bladder. (A) Polypoid masses of tumor, characteristic of botryoid growth pattern. (B) Intact urothelium with underlying cambium layer of malignant spindle cells.

prevalence of rhabdomyosarcomas, with a predominance of bladder or prostate primaries.[134]

Macroscopic Pathology

Macroscopically, the characteristic finding is a polypoid mass filling the bladder lumen. The masses may be single or multiple, producing in some instances a sarcoma botryoides (grape-like) appearance. The cut surface is myxoid and gelatinous with variable hemorrhage and necrosis. Most tumors have a covering superficial epithelium. The trigone is the most common location, although rare cases may originate at the bladder dome.[148]

Microscopic Pathology

Both alveolar and embryonal patterns of rhabdomyosarcoma have been described (**Figs. 18-18** to **18-22**). Embryonal rhabdomyosarcoma is the most common type. Embryonal rhabdomyosarcoma shows varying degrees of cellularity, with alternating hypercellular areas and loosely

packed myxoid areas. There is typically a mixture of unoriented, small, undifferentiated, hyperchromatic round or spindle cells. Also present may be rhabdomyoblasts, differentiated cells with eosinophilic cytoplasm. Although rhabdoid or strap cells with cross-striations may be present, this is not necessary for diagnosis. The overall appearance of embryonal rhabdomyosarcoma varies from primitive to well-differentiated, depending on the component of rhabdomyoblasts present. Occasional foci of immature cartilage or bone may be present. Ultrastructural studies may demonstrate rhabdomyoblastic differentiation, but this technique is seldom used.

Botryoid embryonal rhabdomyosarcoma demonstrates a "cambium" layer, or condensed layer of small round blue primitive cells, under the intact epithelium; beneath this cambium layer lies a paucicellular, loose, edematous, or myxoid tumor. Tumor cellularity is often quite variable, as is the degree of bladder wall infiltration. In addition to

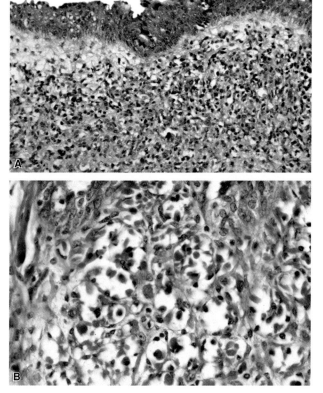

Figure 18-19   Rhabdomyosarcoma of the bladder (A and B). Diagnostic malignant rhabdomyoblasts are present in the cambium layer.

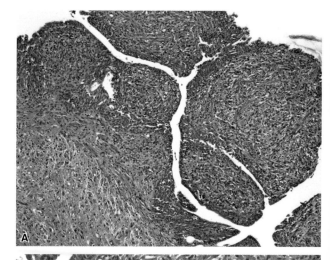

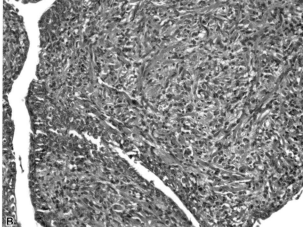

Figure 18-20   Rhabdomyosarcoma with botryoid growth pattern (A and B).

the small round primitive cells that make up the cambium layer, one may observe elongated "strap cells" with cross-striations and hyperchromatic nuclei (**Figs. 18-23** to **18-26**). Typical rhabdomyoblasts, with abundant strongly eosinophilic cytoplasm, may be difficult to identify, especially if a biopsy is taken from a paucicellular area. More poorly differentiated rhabdomyoblasts have been described as medium-sized to large cells with irregularly shaped hyperchromatic nuclei and only a small rim of cytoplasm, often accompanied by readily identified mitotic figures, some of which are atypical.

Alveolar rhabdomyosarcoma, a rare variant, has been reported to occur in the bladder. Its characteristic morphology consists of aggregates of cuboidal or polygonal tumor cells with hyperchromatic nuclei separated by dense, often hyalinized, fibrovascular septa. At the periphery of these aggregates, tumor cells cling to the fibrous tissue; centrally, the tumor cells tend to be very discohesive and appear to be "free-floating," resulting in an overall "alveolar" architecture. Atypical multinucleated giant cells and numerous atypical mitotic figures are often observed. Rhabdomyoblasts and tumor cells with cross-striations are usually absent. The solid type of alveolar rhabdomyosarcoma

grows in confluent sheets, but the cells are similar to those in the classic pattern.

In addition to the embryonal and alveolar subtypes, undifferentiated rhabdomyosarcoma may be difficult to identify definitively without the aid of IHC findings. Such tumors are composed of primitive-appearing small round cells, although preserved expression of muscle markers may assist in discrimination of such lesions from other small blue cell tumors. Unfortunately, the undifferentiated type of rhabdomyosarcoma carries an unfavorable prognosis, like alveolar rhabdomyosarcoma.

Microscopically, the different patterns of rhabdomyosarcoma may merge with each other and appear diffuse. Ultrastructural and immunohistochemical studies are useful as confirmatory tests of the diagnosis but may not be necessary in typical classic cases. Rare cases of rhabdomyosarcoma contain well-differentiated rhabdomyoblasts with deceptively low grade-appearing cytologic features, striking eosinophilic cytoplasm, and well-formed cross-striations. Such tumors may resemble

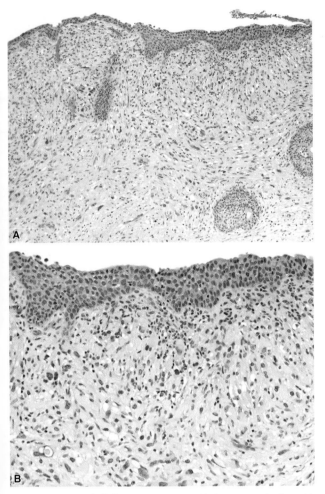

Figure 18-21   Rhabdomyosarcoma with intact urothelium (A and B). Note the malignant spindle cell proliferation underneath the urothelium.

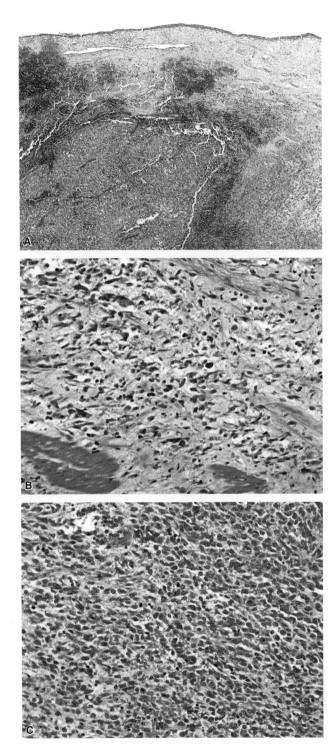

Figure 18-22   Rhabdomyosarcoma (A to C).

rhabdomyoma, but this tumor has not been reported to date in the childhood bladder, and these are considered well-differentiated embryonal rhabdomyosarcomas. Similar findings can be encountered after a full course of chemotherapy (**Figs. 18-27** to **18-29**), with residual sarcoma cells appearing as large rhabdomyoblasts or rhabdomyocytes. In tumor biopsies after treatment, maturing rhabdomyoblasts may be more readily apparent. More poorly differentiated malignant cells in posttreatment biopsies typically exhibit larger hyperchromatic nuclei with an irregular nuclear shape and scant cytoplasm. Mitotic figures may be frequent, including some that are atypical or bizarre.

Immunohistochemistry
Immunohistochemically, rhabdomyosarcoma usually shows positivity for desmin as well as MyoD1 and/or myogenin. In addition, muscle-specific actin, myoglobin, and myosin immunostains may be positive.[132,147,149] Rhabdomyoblasts

may stain for neuron-specific enolase (NSE) and cytokeratin. The alveolar variant has been reported to stain focally for S100 protein.[147]

Differential Diagnosis
Differential diagnostic considerations for rhabdomyosarcoma include leiomyosarcoma, inflammatory

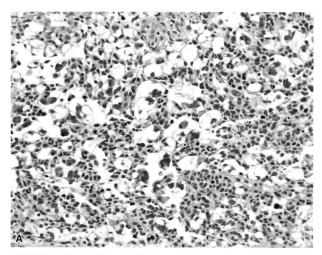

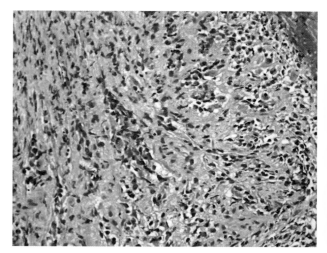

Figure 18-24   Rhabdomyosarcoma. Note the presence of rhabdomyoblasts.

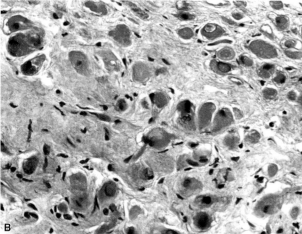

Figure 18-23   Rhabdomyosarcoma (A and B). Note the presence of rhabdomyoblasts.

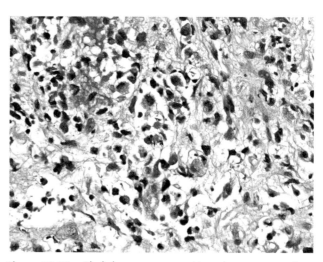

Figure 18-25   Rhabdomyosarcoma. Note the presence of rhabdomyoblasts.

myofibroblastic tumor, postoperative spindle cell nodule, neurofibroma, and sarcomatoid carcinoma (carcinosarcoma).[128] These tumors can often be distinguished on morphologic and clinical grounds. Immunohistochemical stains supporting skeletal muscle differentiation are helpful in establishing a diagnosis of rhabdomyosarcoma.

Leiomyosarcoma can effectively be excluded because it virtually never occurs in the first two decades of life. Further, the histologic findings should be useful in making this separation; in difficult cases, ancillary studies may be of value. Immunohistochemically, the tumor cells of rhabdomyosarcoma show positive staining for markers of muscle differentiation, including desmin, MyoD1 or myogenin, and sometimes muscle-specific actin, myoglobin, and myosin.[140,150] Rhabdomyoblasts may stain for NSE and infrequently for cytokeratin. Inflammatory myofibroblastic tumor often shows prominent inflammatory infiltrates and is positive for ALK and negative for desmin or MyoD1. Postoperative spindle cell nodule occurs weeks to months after instrumentation and is a small nodule with spindle cells arranged in a myxoid vascular stroma, which may infiltrate the muscularis propria of the bladder. Inflammatory cells, usually of chronic type, are present. Postoperative spindle cell nodule may exhibit numerous mitotic figures, but none are atypical, and lesional cells of postoperative spindle cell nodule lack cytologic atypia and ALK-1 immunoreactivity. Sarcomatoid carcinoma typically occurs in adult patients, although rhabdomyosarcoma component can also be seen in these tumors.[127]

Molecular Genetics

Recent molecular genetic studies have helped shed light on the pathogenesis of rhabdomyosarcoma; in fact, FISH can be helpful in establishing the diagnosis in challenging

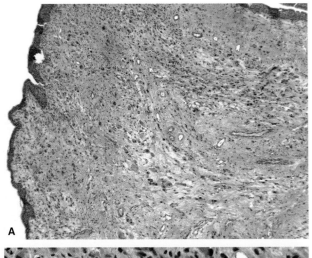

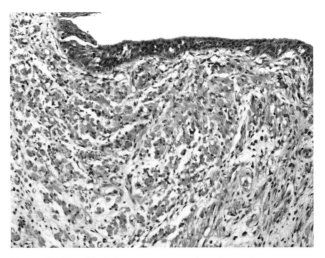

Figure 18-28   Rhabdomyosarcoma after chemotherapy.

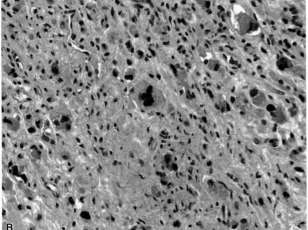

Figure 18-26   Rhabdomyosarcoma (A and B). Note the presence of rhabdomyoblasts.

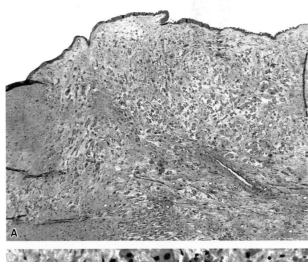

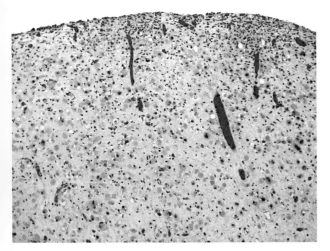

Figure 18-27   Rhabdomyosarcoma after chemotherapy.

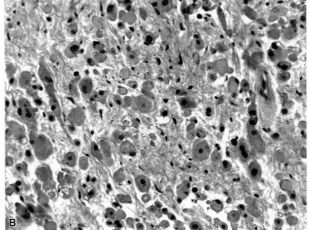

Figure 18-29   Rhabdomyosarcoma after chemotherapy (A and B).

Table 18-3 Molecular Genetics of Pediatric Rhabdomyosarcoma

Alveolar rhabdomyosarcoma
t(2,13)(p35;q14)
70% of all alveolar rhabdomyosarcoma
Fused *PAX3-FKHR* chimeric product
Associated with worse prognosis
t(1,13)(p36:q14)
10% all alveolar rhabdomyosarcoma
Fused *PAX7-FKHR* chimeric product
Associated with better prognosis
Gene amplification of *MDM2, CDK4*
Tetraploidy
TP53 mutation
Embryonal rhabdomyosarcoma
Loss of heterozygosity at 11p15.5
Hyperploidy
TP53 mutation

cases (**Table 18-3**).[140,146,151] Alveolar rhabdomyosarcoma demonstrates distinctive molecular abnormalities, including t(2;13) or t(1;13) translocations, which result in either a *PAX3-FKHR* or *PAX7-FKHR* gene fusion, respectively.[140,146] Identification of *PAX3-FOXO1A* fusion transcripts identifies a high-risk group, while identification of *PAX7-FOXO1A* is associated with a favorable outcome in patients with advanced metastatic alveolar rhabdomyosarcoma.

CGH of embryonal rhabdomyosarcoma showed gains of chromosomes or chromosomal regions 2, 7, 8, 11, 12, 13q21, and 20, and losses of 1p35–36.3m (6m) 9q222, 14q21–32, and 17 most often.[152] Gains of chromosomes 2, 7, 8, 12, and 13 as well as loss of chromosome 14 were also reported in a prior study. Genomic gains in chromosomes 2 and 12 have also been detected in alveolar rhabdomyosarcoma.[153] The *PTCH* gene, a putative tumor suppressor gene, has been mapped to 9q22, a region of genomic loss as detected by CGH or FISH in 33% of the tumors evaluated.[152] This tumor suppressor gene may therefore play a role in embryonal rhabdomyosarcoma. Several genes, which have been mapped to the 12q13–15 region, may be involved in the development or progression of embryonal rhabdomyosarcoma. These genes include the GLI family zinc finger 1 *(GLI1), MDM2, SAS,* and *CHOP*. All of these genes have been shown to be amplified in sarcomas.[152] The chromosomal loss most commonly detected by CGH or FISH in the study by Bridge et al. was loss of 1p35–36.3. This same loss is also frequently detected in neuroblastoma, and it is suggested that neuroblastoma tumor suppressor genes reside here. LOH at the 1p region predicts a poor outcome in neuroblastoma patients. Whether it is predictive of a poor outcome in

rhabdomyosarcoma remains to be determined. 1p36 is also the locus of *PAX7*, which is often fused to *FKHR* in alveolar rhabdomyosarcoma [t(1;13)(p36;q14)].[152] Loss of this gene in embryonal rhabdomyosarcoma indicates that it may play a role in the pathogenesis of this tumor.[152] Oguzkan et al. reported the detection of a large deletion in the *NF1* gene at 17q11.2 in an infant with NF1 and Noonan syndrome who presented with rhabdomyosarcoma of the bladder.[154]

Molecular analysis of posttreatment biopsies for MyoD1 and myogenin by reverse transcription (RT)-PCR to detect minimal residual disease has been reported useful in cases of embryonal rhabdomyosarcoma.[155] Another study evaluating the DNA ploidy and proliferative activity of childhood genitourinary rhabdomyosarcoma found that DNA hyperdiploidy and low cellular proliferative activity are present in a preponderance of childhood rhabdomyosarcoma cases, and these features may predict a favorable outcome.[156]

Recent gene-expressing profiling studies found that as few as five genes can accurately distinguish embryonal rhabdomyosarcoma from alveolar rhabdomyosarcoma with an estimated error rate of less than 5%.[151] The immunostaining data validated the gene expression results. HMGA2 was positive in embryonal rhabdomyosarcoma; negative in alveolar rhabdomyosarcoma. In contrast, TFAP2β was positive in PAX3-FKHR or PAX7-FKHR-positive alveolar rhabdomyosarcoma, and negative in embryonal rhabdomyosarcoma.[151]

Prognosis

Although the prognosis in adults is reportedly poor, advances have been made in the treatment of childhood rhabdomyosarcoma, leading to improved survival with preserved bladder function. Staging is one of the most important prognostic factors (**Table 18-4**). In addition, histologic subtyping has also been shown to correlate with clinical outcome.[157–163] Several histologic classification schemes have been proposed (**Tables 18-5 and 18-6**).[139,164–167] In the International Rhabdomyosarcoma Classification system,[164] histologically recognizable types are assigned to one of three prognostic groups (**Table 18-5**).

In their review of 51 primary bladder rhabdomyosarcoma, Leuschner et al. found that the only feature with a statistically significant influence on survival was growth pattern.[132] The botryoid subtype, which tends not to infiltrate deeply into the detrusor muscle, has a better prognosis overall than either typical embryonal rhabdomyosarcoma or alveolar rhabdomyosarcoma, both of which are often deeply invasive into underlying muscle.[132] Tumors composed of a mixture of alveolar and embryonal subtypes tend to demonstrate biologic behavior typical for that of pure alveolar rhabdomyosarcoma.[128,139,164,168]

Another study evaluating the DNA ploidy and proliferative activity of childhood genitourinary rhabdomyosarcoma

Table 18-4   Tumor, lymph nodes, and metastasis (TNM) Staging of Pediatric Rhabdomyosarcoma[a]

Stage	Sites of Primary Tumor	T Stage	Tumor Size	Regional Lymph Nodes	Distant Metastasis
I	Orbit/eyelid, head and neck (excluding parameningeal), genitourinary (not bladder or prostate)	T1 or T2	Any size	N0, N1, or Nx	M0
II	Bladder/prostate, extremity, cranial parameningeal, other (trunk, retroperitoneal, etc.)	T1 or T2	≤5 cm	N0 or Nx	M0
III	Bladder/prostate, extremity, cranial parameningeal, other (trunk, retroperitoneal, etc.)	T1 or T2	≤5 cm	N1	M0
		T1 or T2	>5 cm	N0, N1, or Nx	M0
		T1 or T2	>5 cm	N0, N1, or Nx	M0
		T1 or T2	>5 cm	N0, N1, or Nx	M0
IV	All	T1 or T2	Any size	N0 or N1	M1

[a]T1, confined to organ of origin; T2, extend beyond organ of origin; M0, absence of metastatic spread; M1, presence of metastatic spread beyond the primary site; N0, absence of nodal spread; N1, presence of nodal spread beyond the primary site; Nx, N status unknown.

Table 18-5   International Classification of Rhabdomyosarcoma

1. Superior prognosis
   A. Botryoid rhabdomyosarcoma
   B. Spindle cell rhabdomyosarcoma
2. Intermediate prognosis
   A. Embryonal rhabdomyosarcoma
3. Poor prognosis
   A. Alveolar rhabdomyosarcoma
   B. Undifferentiated sarcoma
4. Subtypes whose prognosis is not presently evaluable
   A. Rhabdomyosarcoma with rhabdoid features

Source: Ref. 164.

Table 18-6   National Cancer Institute Classification of Rhabdomyosarcoma

Embryonal rhabdomyosarcoma (favorable)
  Conventional
  Pleomorphic
  Leiomyomatous
  With aggressive histologic features
Alveolar rhabdomyosarcoma (unfavorable)
  Conventional
  Solid alveolar
Pleomorphic rhabdomyosarcoma
Rhabdomyosarcoma, "other"

Source: Ref. 165.

found that DNA hyperdiploidy and low cellular proliferative activity are present in a preponderance of childhood rhabdomyosarcoma cases, and these features may predict a favorable outcome.[156]

The Children's Oncology Group (COG) Soft Tissue Sarcoma Study Group, formerly the Intergroup Rhabdomyosarcoma Study (IRS), has observed rhabdomyosarcoma patients, including those with bladder primaries, since 1972.[133,138] By the time of the reporting period for IRS-IV (1991–1997), the rate of retention of a normal-functioning bladder at 6.1 years from the time of diagnosis was approximately 40%, and the survival rate, not including those with disseminated disease when first diagnosed, was 82%.[133] Most patients are treated with conservative surgical resections, chemotherapy, and local

irradiation.[133] Reports of the experiences of European groups treating this malignancy are similar.[132,169] Posttreatment morbidity has been most attributable to radiation therapy.[170] Relapses, when they occur, are usually within five years after treatment, and are generally managed with salvage chemotherapy and sometimes surgery.[132] Posttreatment tumor recurrences often show diminished cellularity, and may also show evidence of maturation or degeneration.[171] There is lack of agreement concerning the significance of the presence of mature-appearing tumor cells in posttreatment biopsies. Leuschner et al. contend that the presence of such cells may portend subsequent tumor recurrence or progression.[132] Heyn et al., however, suggest that the presence of cellular maturation in these treated tumors is an encouraging prognostic sign.[171]

Other Rare Tumors

Squamous cell carcinoma and adenocarcinoma of the bladder are even less common than urothelial carcinoma in children.[172–177]

Primary paraganglioma of the bladder in children is very rare (see also **Chapter 15**).[178–180] Paraganglioma has been identified in the bladder of young patients, ranging from 7 years to 14 years of age. Bladder paraganglioma is often hormonally active, producing episodic hypertension, headache, and diaphoresis, sometimes related to the act of micturition.[180]

Other rare tumors of the bladder include leiomyoma,[181] granular cell tumor, and dermoid cyst.[182] Leiomyoma and leiomyosarcoma both occur in the urinary bladder and are included in the differential diagnosis of mesenchymal-appearing bladder neoplasms. Leiomyoma is rare and seen almost exclusively in adults, for whom it is the most common benign soft tissue bladder neoplasm. Leiomyosarcoma, in contrast, sometimes occurs in young patients and must be distinguished from inflammatory myofibroblastic tumor and rhabdomyosarcoma, using all available ancillary techniques (see also **Chapter 19**).[183]

Germ cell tumors of the bladder in children are exceedingly rare, with reported cases of dermoid cyst[182] and endodermal sinus tumor (yolk sac tumor) (see also **Chapter 22**).[184,185]

Few cases of primary rhabdoid tumor have been described in the bladder, including one with coexistent urothelial carcinoma.[186,187] Rare cases of primitive neuroectodermal tumor arising in the urinary bladder of children and young adults have been reported (see also **Chapter 15**).

The childhood bladder may also be a rare site for involvement by leukemia and lymphoma.[188–191] Very rarely, there may be metastases to the bladder, including Wilms tumor.[192,193]

REFERENCES

1. Palmer JM, Russi MF. Persistent urogenital sinus with absence of the bladder and urethra. *J Urol* 1969;102:590–4.
2. Metoki R, Orikasa S, Ohta S, Kanetoh H. A case of bladder agenesis. *J Urol* 1986;136:662–4.
3. Ives E, Coffey R, Carter CO. A family study of bladder exstrophy. *J Med Genet* 1980;17:139–41.
4. Higgins CC. Exstrophy of the bladder: report of 158 cases. *Am Surg* 1962;28:99–102.
5. Culp DA. The histology of the exstrophied bladder. *J Urol* 1964;91:538–48.
6. Dehner LP. Pediatric Surgical Pathology, 2nd ed., Chapter 10. Baltimore: Williams & Wilkins, 1987.
7. Parker C. Cystitis cystica and glandularis: a study of 40 cases. *Proc R Soc Med* 1970;63:239–42.
8. Beynon J, Zwink R, Chow W, Sturdy DE. The late presentation of adenocarcinoma in bladder exstrophy. *Br J Surg* 1985;72:989.
9. de Riese W, Warmbold H. Adenocarcinoma in extrophy of the bladder. A case report and review of the literature. *Int Urol Nephrol* 1986;18:159–62.
10. Novak TE, Lakshmanan Y, Frimberger D, Epstein JI, Gearhart JP. Polyps in the exstrophic bladder. A cause for concern? *J Urol* 2005;174:1522–6; discussion 1526.
11. Carter TC, Tomskey GC, Ozog LS. Prune-belly syndrome. Review of ten cases. *Urology* 1974;3:279–82.
12. Semerdjian HS, Texter JH Jr, Yawn DH. Rhabdomyosarcoma occurring in repaired exstrophied bladder: a case report. *J Urol* 1972;108:354–6.
13. Corica FA, Husmann DA, Churchill BM, Young RH, Pacelli A, Lopez-Beltran A, Bostwick DG. Intestinal metaplasia is not a strong risk factor for bladder cancer: study of 53 cases with long-term followup. *Urology* 1997;50:427–31.
14. Jeffs RD. Exstrophy and cloacal exstrophy. *Urol Clin North Am* 1978;5:127–40.
15. Diamond DA, Jeffs RD. Cloacal exstrophy: a 22-year experience. *J Urol* 1985;133:779–82.
16. Dunetz GN, Bauer SB. Complete duplication of bladder and urethra. *Urology* 1985;25:179–82.
17. Vaage S, Foerster A, Gerhardt PG, Tveter KJ. A complete pyelo-uretero-vesical duplication. *Scand J Urol Nephrol* 1985;19:309–13.
18. Feins NR, Cranley W. Bladder duplication with one exstrophy and one cloaca. *J Pediatr Surg* 1986;21:570–2.
19. Kapoor R, Saha MM. Complete duplication of the bladder, urethra and external genitalia in a neonate—a case report. *J Urol* 1987;137:1243–4.
20. Cheng EY, Maizels M. Complete duplication of the bladder and urethra in the coronal plane: case report. *J Urol* 1996;155:1414–5.
21. Livne PM, Gonzales ET Jr. Congenital bladder diverticula causing ureteral obstruction. *Urology* 1985;25:273–6.
22. Peterson LJ, Paulson DF, Glenn JF. The histopathology of vesical diverticula. *J Urol* 1973;110:62–4.
23. Rajan N, Makhuli ZN, Humphrey DM, Batra AK. Metastatic umbilical transitional cell carcinoma from a bladder diverticulum. *J Urol* 1996;155:1700.
24. Tamas EF, Stephenson AJ, Campbell SC, Montague DK, Trusty DC, Hansel DE. Histopathologic features and clinical outcomes in 71 cases of bladder diverticula. *Arch Pathol Lab Med* 2009;133:791–6.

25. Chadha R, Agarwal K, Choudhury SR, Debnath PR. The colovesical fistula in congenital pouch colon; a histologic study. *J Pediatr Surg* 2008;43:2048–52.

26. Chatterjee SK, Sarkar SK. Retrovesical cysts in boys. *J Urol* 1973;109:107–10.

27. Herlihy RE, Barnes WF. Neonatal vesical necrosis and perforation secondary to posterior urethral valves. *J Urol* 1985;133:476–7.

28. Inamdar S, Mallouh C, Ganguly R. Vesical gigantism or congenital megacystis. *Urology* 1984;24:601–3.

29. Geist RW, Antolak SJ Jr Interstitial cystitis in children. *J Urol* 1970;104:922–5.

30. Yadin O. Hematuria in children. *Pediatr Ann* 1994;23:474–8, 81–5.

31. Numazaki Y, Shigeta S, Kumasaka T, Miyazawa T, Yamanaka M, Yano N, Takai S, Ishida N. Acute hemorrhagic cystitis in children. Isolation of adenovirus type II. *N Engl J Med* 1968;278:700–4.

32. Chang SC. Urinary cytologic diagnosis of cytomegalic inclusion disease in childhood leukemia. *Acta Cytol* 1970;14:338–43.

33. Goldman RL, Warner NE. Hemorrhagic cystitis and cytomegalic inclusions in the bladder associated with cyclophosphamide therapy. *Cancer* 1970;25:7–11.

34. Mufson MA, Belshe RB, Horrigan TJ, Zollar LM. Cause of acute hemorrhagic cystitis in children. *Am J Dis Child* 1973;126:605–9.

35. Hashida Y, Gaffney PC, Yunis EJ. Acute hemorrhagic cystitis of childhood and papovavirus-like particles. *J Pediatr* 1976;89:85–7.

36. Cos LR, Cockett AT. Genitourinary tuberculosis revisited. *Urology* 1982;20:111–7.

37. Berkson BM, Lome LG, Shapiro I. Severe cystitis induced by cyclophosphamide. Role of surgical management. *JAMA* 1973;225:605–6.

38. Sutphin M, Middleton AW Jr. Eosinophilic cystitis in children: a self-limited process. *J Urol* 1984;132:117–9.

39. Perlmutter AD, Edlow JB, Kevy SV. Toxocara antibodies in eosinophilic cystitis. *J Pediatr* 1968;73:340–4.

40. Ehrlich RM, Lattimer JK. Urogenital tuberculosis in children. *J Urol* 1971;105.461–5.

41. Johnson HW, Elliott GB, Israels S, Balfour J. Granulomatous cystitis of children, bilharzia like, occurring in British Columbia. *Pediatrics* 1967;40:808–15.

42. Cyr WL, Johnson H, Balfour J. Granulomatous cystitis as a manifestation of chronic granulomatous disease of childhood. *J Urol* 1973;110:357–9.

43. Carson CC 3rd, Malek RS. Observations on lower urinary tract calculi in children. *J Urol* 1982;127:977–8.

44. Dalens B, Vanneuville G, Vincent L, Fabre JL. Congenital polyp of the posterior urethra and vesical calculus in a boy. *J Urol* 1982;128:1034–5.

45. Williamson SR, Lopez-Beltran A, Maclennan GT, Montironi R, Cheng L. Unique clinicopathologic and molecular characteristics of urinary bladder tumors in children and young adults. *Urol Oncol* (in press 2012).

46. Aabech HS, Lien EN. Cystitis cystica in childhood: clinical findings and treatment procedures. *Acta Paediatr Scand* 1982;71:247–52.

47. Morgan CL, Grossman H, Trought WS, Oddson TA. Ultrasonic diagnosis of obstructed renal duplication and ureterocele. *South Med J* 1980;73:1016–9.

48. Ahmad I, Barnetson RJ, Krishna NS. Keratinizing squamous metaplasia of the bladder: a review. *Urol Int* 2008;81:247–51.

49. Cheng L, Cheville JC, Sebo TJ, Eble JN, Bostwick DG. Atypical nephrogenic metaplasia of the urinary tract: A precursor lesion? *Cancer* 2000;88:853–61.

50. Oliva E, Clement PB, Young RH. Tubal and tubo-endometrioid metaplasia of the uterine cervix. Unemphasized features that may cause problems in differential diagnosis: a report of 25 cases. *Am J Clin Pathol* 1995;103:618–23.

51. Rahemtullah A, Oliva E. Nephrogenic adenoma: an update on an innocuous but troublesome entity. *Adv Anat Pathol* 2006;13:247–55.

52. Gupta A, Wang HL, Policarpio-Nicolas ML, Tretiakova MS, Papavero V, Pins MR, Jiang Z, Humphrey PA, Cheng L, Yang XJ. Expression of alpha-methylacyl-coenzyme A racemase in nephrogenic adenoma. *Am J Surg Pathol* 2004;28:1224–9.

53. Young RH. Fibroepithelial polyp of the bladder with atypical stromal cells. *Arch Pathol Lab Med* 1986;110:241–2.

54. Heidenreich A, Zirbes TK, Wolter S, Engelmann UH. Nephrogenic adenoma: a rare bladder tumor in children. *Eur Urol* 1999;36:348–53.

55. Schumacher K, Heimbach D, Bruhl P. Nephrogenic adenoma in children. Case report and review of literature. *Eur J Pediatr Surg* 1997;7:115–7.

56. Mazal PR, Schaufler R, Altenhuber-Muller R, Haitel A, Watschinger B, Kratzik C, Krupitza G, Regele H, Meisl FT, Zechner O, Kerjaschki D, Susani M. Derivation of nephrogenic adenomas from renal tubular cells in kidney-transplant recipients. *N Engl J Med* 2002;347:653–9.

57. Goldman HB, Dmochowski RR, Noe HN. Nephrogenic adenoma occurring in an augmented bladder. *J Urol* 1996;155:1410.

58. Vemulakonda VM, Kopp RP, Sorensen MD, Grady RW. Recurrent nephrogenic adenoma in a 10-year-old boy with prune belly syndrome: a case presentation. *Pediatr Surg Int* 2008;24:605–7.

59. Remick DG Jr, Kumar NB. Benign polyps with prostatic-type epithelium of the urethra and the urinary bladder. A suggestion of histogenesis based on histologic and immunohistochemical studies. *Am J Surg Pathol* 1984;8:833–9.

60. Halat S, Eble JN, Grignon DG, Lacy S, Montironi R, MacLennan GT, Lopez-Beltran A, Tan PH, Baldridge LA, Cheng L. Ectopic prostatic tissue: histogenesis and histopathologic characteristics. *Histopathology* 2011;58:750–8.

61. Sommerhaug RG, Mason T. Peutz-Jeghers syndrome and ureteral polyposis. *JAMA* 1970;211:120–2.

62. Williams SV, Sibley KD, Davies AM, Nishiyama H, Hornigold N, Coulter J, Kennedy WJ, Skilleter A, Habuchi T, Knowles MA. Molecular genetic analysis of chromosome 9 candidate tumor-suppressor loci in

bladder cancer cell lines. *Genes Chromosomes Cancer* 2002;34:86–96.

63. Davides KC, King LM. Fibrous polyps of the ureter. *J Urol* 1976;115:651–3.

64. Eilenberg J, Seery W, Cole A. Multiple fibroepithelial polyps in the pediatric age group: case report. *J Urol* 1977;117:793.

65. Van Poppel H, Nuttin B, Oyen R, Stessens R, Van Damme B, Verduyn H. Fibroepithelial polyps of the ureter. Etiology, diagnosis, treatment and pathology. *Eur Urol* 1986;12:174–9.

66. Isaac J, Snow B, Lowichik A. Fibroepithelial polyp of the prostatic urethra in an adolescent. *J Pediatr Surg* 2006;41:e29–31.

67. Tsuzuki T, Epstein JI. Fibroepithelial polyp of the lower urinary tract in adults. *Am J Surg Pathol* 2005;29:460–6.

68. Wolgel CD, Parris AC, Mitty HA, Schapira HE. Fibroepithelial polyp of renal pelvis. *Urology* 1982;19:436–9.

69. Barzilai M, Shinawi M, Ish-Shalom N, Mecz Y, Peled N, Lurie A. A fibroepithelial urethral polyp protruding into the base of the bladder: sonographic diagnosis. *Urol Int* 1996;57:129–31.

70. Al-Ahmadie H, Gomez AM, Trane N, Bove KE. Giant botryoid fibroepithelial polyp of bladder with myofibroblastic stroma and cystitis cystica et glandularis. *Pediatr Dev Pathol* 2003;6:179–81.

71. Zachariou AG, Manoliadis IN, Kalogianni PA, Karagiannis GK, Georgantzis DJ. A rare case of bladder fibroepithelial polyp in childhood. *Arch Ital Urol Androl* 2005;77:118–20.

72. Tayib AM, Al-Maghrabi JA, Mosli HA. Urethral polyp verumontanum. *Saudi Med J* 2004;25:1115–6.

73. Fathi K, Azmy A, Howatson A, Carachi R. Congenital posterior urethral polyps in childhood. A case report. *Eur J Pediatr Surg* 2004;14:215–7.

74. Gleason PE, Kramer SA. Genitourinary polyps in children. *Urology* 1994;44:106–9.

75. Demircan M, Ceran C, Karaman A, Uguralp S, Mizrak B. Urethral polyps in children: a review of the literature and report of two cases. *Int J Urol* 2006;13:841–3.

76. Natsheh A, Prat O, Shenfeld OZ, Reinus C, Chertin B. Fibroepithelial polyp of the bladder neck in children. *Pediatr Surg Int* 2008;24:613–5.

77. Rubin J, Khanna OP, Damjanov I. Adenomatous polyp of the bladder: a rare cause of hematuria in young men. *J Urol* 1981;126:549–50.

78. Lorentzen M, Rohr N. Urinary bladder tumours in children. Case report of inverted papilloma. *Scand J Urol Nephrol* 1979;13:323–7.

79. Isaac J, Lowichik A, Cartwright P, Rohr R. Inverted papilloma of the urinary bladder in children: case report and review of prognostic significance and biological potential behavior. *J Pediatr Surg* 2000;35:1514–6.

80. Tamsen A, Casas V, Patil UB, Elbadawi A. Inverted papilloma of the urinary bladder in a boy. *J Pediatr Surg* 1993;28:1601–2.

81. Cheng L, Cheville JC, Leibovich BC, Weaver AL, Egan KS, Spotts BE, Neumann RM, Bostwick DG. Survival of patients with carcinoma in situ of the urinary bladder. *Cancer* 1999;85:2469–74.

82. McKenney JK, Amin MB, Young RH. Urothelial (transitional cell) papilloma of the urinary bladder: a clinicopathologic study of 26 cases. *Mod Pathol* 2003;16:623–9.

83. Auber F, Lortat-Jacob S, Sarnacki S, Jaubert F, Salomon R, Thibaud E, Jeanpierre C, Nihoul-Fekete C. Surgical management and genotype/phenotype correlations in WT1 gene-related diseases (Drash, Frasier syndromes). *J Pediatr Surg* 2003;38:124–9.

84. Fine SW, Humphrey PA, Dehner LP, Amin MB, Epstein JI. Urothelial neoplasms in patients 20 years or younger: a clinicopathological analysis using the World Health Organization 2004 bladder consensus classification. *J Urol* 2005;174:1976–80.

85. Mostofi FK, Sobin LH, Torloni H. Histological Typing of Urinary Bladder Tumours., Vol. 10 Geneva: World Health Organization, 1973.

86. Eble JN, Sauter G, Epstein JI, Sesterhenn IA, eds. World Health Organization Classification of Tumours: Pathology and Genetics of Tumours of the Urinary System and Male Genital Organs. Lyon, France: IARC Press, 2004.

87. Benson RC Jr, Tomera KM, Kelalis PP. Transitional cell carcinoma of the bladder in children and adolescents. *J Urol* 1983;130:54–5.

88. Yanase M, Tsukamoto T, Kumamoto Y, Takagi Y, Mikuma N, Iwasawa A, Kondo N. Transitional cell carcinoma of the bladder or renal pelvis in children. *Eur Urol* 1991;19:312–4.

89. Yusim I, Lismer L, Greenberg G, Haomud K, Kaneti J. Carcinoma of the bladder in patients under 25 years of age. *Scand J Urol Nephrol* 1996;30:461–3.

90. Madgar I, Goldwasser B, Czerniak A, Many M. Leiomyosarcoma of the ureter. *Eur Urol* 1988;14:487–9.

91. McCarthy JP, Gavrell GJ, LeBlanc GA. Transitional cell carcinoma of bladder in patients under thirty years of age. *Urology* 1979;13:487–9.

92. Javadpour N, Mostofi FK. Primary epithelial tumors of the bladder in the first two decades of life. *J Urol* 1969;101:706–10.

93. Curtis M, Schned A, Hakim S, Cendron M. Papillary transitional cell carcinoma of the bladder with lymphangiectasia in an 8-year-old boy. *J Urol* 1996;156:202.

94. Hoenig DM, McRae S, Chen SC, Diamond DA, Rabinowitz R, Caldamone AA. Transitional cell carcinoma of the bladder in the pediatric patient. *J Urol* 1996;156:203–5.

95. Refsum S Jr, Refsum SB. Bladder papilloma in a child. Case report. *Scand J Urol Nephrol* 1975;9:285–8.

96. Waaler G, Schistad G, Serck-Hanssen A. Papillary urothelial tumor of the bladder in a child. *J Pediatr Surg* 1975;10:841–2.

97. Bruce PT. Bladder papilloma in young patients. *Med J Aust* 1982;1:43–4.

98. Punjani HM. Transitional cell papilloma of the ureter causing hydronephrosis in a child. *Br J Urol* 1983;55:572–3.

99. Williams JL, Cumming WA, Walker RD 3rd, Hackett RL. Transitional cell papilloma of the bladder. *Pediatr Radiol* 1986;16:322–3.

100. Giedl J, Wild PJ, Stoehr R, Junker K, Boehm S, van Oers JM, Zwarthoff EC, Blaszyk H, Fine SW, Humphrey PA, Dehner LP, Amin MB, Epstein JI, Hartmann A. [Urothelial neoplasms in individuals younger than 20 years show very few genetic alterations and have a favourable clinical outcome]. *Verh Dtsch Ges Pathol* 2006;90:253–63.

101. Zeegers MP, Kellen E, Buntinx F, van den Brandt PA. The association between smoking, beverage consumption, diet and bladder cancer: a systematic literature review. *World J Urol* 2004;21:392–401.

102. Johansson SL, Cohen SM. Epidemiology and etiology of bladder cancer. *Semin Surg Oncol* 1997;13:291–8.

103. Androulakakis PA, Davaris P, Karayannis A, Michael V, Aghioutantis C. Urothelial tumors of the bladder. *Child Nephrol Urol* 1992;12:32–4.

104. Paduano L, Chiella E. Primary epithelial tumors of the bladder in children. *J Urol* 1988;139:794–5.

105. Wild PJ, Giedl J, Stoehr R, Junker K, Boehm S, van Oers JM, Zwarthoff EC, Blaszyk H, Fine SW, Humphrey PA, Dehner LP, Amin MB, Epstein JI, Hartmann A. Genomic aberrations are rare in urothelial neoplasms of patients 19 years or younger. *J Pathol* 2007;211:18–25.

106. Francis RR. Inverted papilloma in a 14-year-old male. *Br J Urol* 1979;51:327.

107. Cheng L, Davidson DD, Maclennan GT, Williamson SR, Zhang S, Koch MO, Montironi R, Lopez-Beltran A. The origins of urothelial carcinoma. *Expert Rev Anticancer Ther* 2010;10:865–80.

108. Cheng L, Zhang S, Maclennan GT, Williamson SR, Lopez-Beltran A, Montironi R. Bladder cancer: translating molecular genetic insights into clinical practice. *Hum Pathol* 2011;42:455–81.

109. Cheng L, Montironi R, Davidson DD, Lopez-Beltran A. Staging and reporting of urothelial carcinoma of the urinary bladder. *Mod Pathol* 2009;22 (Suppl 2):S70–95.

110. Hartmann A, Schlake G, Zaak D, Hungerhuber E, Hofstetter A, Hofstaedter F, Knuechel R. Occurrence of chromosome 9 and p53 alterations in multifocal dysplasia and carcinoma in situ of human urinary bladder. *Cancer Res* 2002;62:809–18.

111. Zieger K, Marcussen N, Borre M, Orntoft TF, Dyrskjot L. Consistent genomic alterations in carcinoma in situ of the urinary bladder confirm the presence of two major pathways in bladder cancer development. *Int J Cancer* 2009;125:2095–2103.

112. Linn JF, Sesterhenn I, Mostofi FK, Schoenberg M. The molecular characteristics of bladder cancer in young patients. *J Urol* 1998;159:1493–6.

113. Cheng L, Nascimento AG, Neumann RM, Nehra A, Cheville JC, Ramnani DM, Leibovich BC, Bostwick DG. Hemangioma of the urinary bladder. *Cancer* 1999;86:498–504.

114. Van Dessel J, Michielsen JP. The haemangioma of the bladder. Case report and review of the literature. *Acta Urol Belg* 1978;46:369–77.

115. Nuovo GJ, Nagler HM, Fenoglio JJ Jr. Arteriovenous malformation of the bladder presenting as gross hematuria. *Hum Pathol* 1986;17:94–7.

116. Lee KW, Rodo J, Margarit J, Montaner A, Salarich J. Cavernous haemangioma of the bladder in a child. *Br J Urol* 1995;75:799–801.

117. Caro DJ, Brown JS. Hemangioma of bladder. *Urology* 1976;7:479–81.

118. Cheng L, Scheithauer BW, Leibovich BC, Ramnani DM, Cheville JC, Bostwick DG. Neurofibroma of the urinary bladder. *Cancer* 1999;86:505–13.

119. Clark SS, Marlett MM, Prudencio RF, Dasgupta TK. Neurofibromatosis of the bladder in children: case report and literature review. *J Urol* 1977;118:654–6.

120. Kramer S, Barrett D, Utz D. Neurofibromatosis of the bladder in children. *J Urol* 1981;126:693–4.

121. Willis D, Canales BK, Cheng L, MacLennan GT. Neural neoplasms of the bladder. *J Urol* 2010;184:1492–3.

122. Cheng L, Foster SR, MacLennan GT, Lopez-Beltran A, Zhang S, Montironi R. Inflammatory myofibroblastic tumors of the genitourinary tract–single entity or continuum? *J Urol* 2008;180:1235–40.

123. Varsano I, Savir A, Grunebaum M, Vogel R, Johnston JH. Inflammatory processes mimicking bladder tumors in children. *J Pediatr Surg* 1975;10:909–12.

124. Nochomovitz LE, Orenstein JM. Inflammatory pseudotumor of the urinary bladder—possible relationship to nodular fasciitis. Two case reports, cytologic observations, and ultrastructural observations. *Am J Surg Pathol* 1985;9:366–73.

125. Hojo H, Newton WA Jr, Hamoudi AB, Qualman SJ, Wakasa H, Suzuki S, Jaynes F. Pseudosarcomatous myofibroblastic tumor of the urinary bladder in children: a study of 11 cases with review of the literature. An Intergroup Rhabdomyosarcoma Study. *Am J Surg Pathol* 1995;19:1224–36.

126. Lopez-Beltran A, Lopez-Ruiz J, Vicioso L. Inflammatory pseudotumor of the urinary bladder. A clinicopathological analysis of two cases. *Urol Int* 1995;55:173–6.

127. Cheng L, Zhang S, Alexander R, MacLennan GT, Hodges KB, Harrison BT, Lopez-Beltran A, Montironi R. Sarcomatoid carcinoma of the urinary bladder: the final common pathway of urothelial carcinoma dedifferentiation. *Am J Surg Pathol* 2011;35:e34–46.

128. Lott S, Lopez-Beltran A, Montironi R, MacLennan GT, Cheng L. Soft tissue tumors of the urinary bladder: Part II: Malignant neoplasms. *Hum Pathol* 2007;38:807–23.

129. Fleischmann J, Perinetti EP, Catalona WJ. Embryonal rhabdomyosarcoma of the genitourinary organs. *J Urol* 1981;126:389–92.

130. Geary ES, Gong MC, Shortliffe LM. Biology and treatment of pediatric genitourinary tumors. *Curr Opin Oncol* 1994;6:292–300.

131. Parham DM, Ellison DA. Rhabdomyosarcomas in adults and children: an update. *Arch Pathol Lab Med* 2006;130:1454–65.

132. Leuschner I, Harms D, Mattke A, Koscielniak E, Treuner J. Rhabdomyosarcoma of the urinary bladder and vagina: a clinicopathologic study with emphasis on recurrent disease: a report from the Kiel Pediatric Tumor Registry and the German CWS Study. *Am J Surg Pathol* 2001;25:856–64.

133. Arndt C, Rodeberg D, Breitfeld PP, Raney RB, Ullrich F, Donaldson S. Does bladder preservation (as a surgical principle) lead to retaining bladder function in bladder/prostate rhabdomyosarcoma? Results from Intergroup Rhabdomyosarcoma Study IV. *J Urol* 2004;171:2396–403.

134. Sung L, Anderson JR, Arndt C, Raney RB, Meyer WH, Pappo AS. Neurofibromatosis in children with rhabdomyosarcoma: a report from the Intergroup Rhabdomyosarcoma Study IV. *J Pediatr* 2004;144:666–8.

135. Lauro S, Lalle M, Scucchi L, Vecchione A. Rhabdomyosarcoma of the urinary bladder in an elderly patient. *Anticancer Res* 1995;15:627–9.

136. Aydoganli L, Tarhan F, Atan A, Akalin Z, Yildiz M. Rhabdomyosarcoma of the urinary bladder in an adult. *Int Urol Nephrol* 1993;25:159–61.

137. Hays DM. Bladder/prostate rhabdomyosarcoma: results of the multi-institutional trials of the Intergroup Rhabdomyosarcoma Study. *Semin Surg Oncol* 1993;9:520–3.

138. Hays DM, Raney RB, Wharam MD, Wiener E, Lobe TE, Andrassy RJ, Lawrence W Jr, Johnston J, Webber B, Maurer HM. Children with vesical rhabdomyosarcoma (RMS) treated by partial cystectomy with neoadjuvant or adjuvant chemotherapy, with or without radiotherapy. A report from the Intergroup Rhabdomyosarcoma Study (IRS) Committee. *J Pediatr Hematol Oncol* 1995;17:46–52.

139. Qualman SJ, Coffin CM, Newton WA, Hojo H, Triche TJ, Parham DM, Crist WM. Intergroup Rhabdomyosarcoma Study: update for pathologists. *Pediatr Dev Pathol* 1998;1:550–61.

140. Ferrer FA, Isakoff M, Koyle MA. Bladder/prostate rhabdomyosarcoma: past, present and future. *J Urol* 2006;176:1283–91.

141. Hawkins HK, Camacho-Velasquez JV. Rhabdomyosarcoma in children. Correlation of form and prognosis in one institution's experience. *Am J Surg Pathol* 1987;11:531–42.

142. Hartley AL, Birch JM, Blair V, Kelsey AM, Harris M, Jones PH. Patterns of cancer in the families of children with soft tissue sarcoma. *Cancer* 1993;72:923–30.

143. Heyn R, Haeberlen V, Newton WA, Ragab AH, Raney RB, Tefft M, Wharam M, Ensign LG, Maurer HM. Second malignant neoplasms in children treated for rhabdomyosarcoma. Intergroup Rhabdomyosarcoma Study Committee. *J Clin Oncol* 1993;11:262–70.

144. Raney B Jr, Heyn R, Hays DM, Tefft M, Newton WA Jr, Wharam M, Vassilopoulou-Sellin R, Maurer HM. Sequelae of treatment in 109 patients followed for 5 to 15 years after diagnosis of sarcoma of the bladder and prostate. A report from the Intergroup Rhabdomyosarcoma Study Committee. *Cancer* 1993;71:2387–94.

145. Leuschner I, Newton WA Jr, Schmidt D, Sachs N, Asmar L, Hamoudi A, Harms D, Maurer HM. Spindle cell variants of embryonal rhabdomyosarcoma in the paratesticular region. A report of the Intergroup Rhabdomyosarcoma Study. *Am J Surg Pathol* 1993;17:221–30.

146. Lambert I, Debiec-Rychter M, Dubin M, Sciot R. Solid alveolar rhabdomyosarcoma originating from the urinary bladder in an adult. Diagnostic value of molecular genetics. *Histopathology* 2004;44:508–10.

147. Kunze E, Theuring F, Kruger G. Primary mesenchymal tumors of the urinary bladder. A histological and immunohistochemical study of 30 cases. *Pathol Res Pract* 1994;190:311–32.

148. Royal SA, Hedlund GL, Galliani CA. Rhabdomyosarcoma of the dome of the urinary bladder: a difficult imaging diagnosis. *AJR Am J Roentgenol* 1996;167:524–5.

149. McKenney JK. An approach to the classification of spindle cell proliferations in the urinary bladder. *Adv Anat Pathol* 2005;12:312–23.

150. Morotti RA, Nicol KK, Parham DM, Teot LA, Moore J, Hayes J, Meyer W, Qualman SJ. An immunohistochemical algorithm to facilitate diagnosis and subtyping of rhabdomyosarcoma: the Children's Oncology Group experience. *Am J Surg Pathol* 2006;30:962–8.

151. Davicioni E, Anderson MJ, Finckenstein FG, Lynch JC, Qualman SJ, Shimada H, Schofield DE, Buckley JD, Meyer WH, Sorensen PH, Triche TJ. Molecular classification of rhabdomyosarcoma—genotypic and phenotypic determinants of diagnosis: a report from the Children's Oncology Group. *Am J Pathol* 2009;174:550–64.

152. Bridge JA, Liu J, Weibolt V, Baker KS, Perry D, Kruger R, Qualman S, Barr F, Sorensen P, Triche T, Suijkerbuijk R. Novel genomic imbalances in embryonal rhabdomyosarcoma revealed by comparative genomic hybridization and fluorescence in situ hybridization: an Intergroup Rhabdomyosarcoma Study. *Genes Chromosomes Cancer* 2000;27:337–44.

153. Weber-Hall S, Anderson J, McManus A, Abe S, Nojima T, Pinkerton R, Pritchard-Jones K, Shipley J. Gains, losses, and amplification of genomic material in rhabdomyosarcoma analyzed by comparative genomic hybridization. *Cancer Res* 1996;56:3220–4.

154. Oguzkan S, Terzi YK, Guler E, Derbent M, Agras PI, Saatci U, Ayter S. Two neurofibromatosis type 1 cases associated with rhabdomyosarcoma of bladder, one with a large deletion in the NF1 gene. *Cancer Genet Cytogenet* 2006;164:159–63.

155. Castellino SM, McLean TW. Pediatric genitourinary tumors. *Curr Opin Oncol* 2007;19:248–53.

156. San Miguel-Fraile P, Carrillo-Gijon R, Rodriguez-Peralto JL, Ortiz-Rey JA, Alvarez-Alvarez C, de la Fuente-Buceta A. DNA content and proliferative activity in pediatric genitourinary rhabdomyosarcoma.

Pediatr Pathol Mol Med 2003;22:143–52.

157. Wachtel M, Runge T, Leuschner I, Stegmaier S, Koscielniak E, Treuner J, Odermatt B, Behnke S, Niggli FK, Schafer BW. Subtype and prognostic classification of rhabdomyosarcoma by immunohistochemistry. *J Clin Oncol* 2006;24:816–22.

158. Breneman JC, Lyden E, Pappo AS, Link MP, Anderson JR, Parham DM, Qualman SJ, Wharam MD, Donaldson SS, Maurer HM, Meyer WH, Baker KS, Paidas CN, Crist WM. Prognostic factors and clinical outcomes in children and adolescents with metastatic rhabdomyosarcoma—a report from the Intergroup Rhabdomyosarcoma Study IV. *J Clin Oncol* 2003;21:78–84.

159. Pappo AS, Anderson JR, Crist WM, Wharam MD, Breitfeld PP, Hawkins D, Raney RB, Womer RB, Parham DM, Qualman SJ, Grier HE. Survival after relapse in children and adolescents with rhabdomyosarcoma: a report from the Intergroup Rhabdomyosarcoma Study Group. *J Clin Oncol* 1999;17:3487–93.

160. Crist WM, Anderson JR, Meza JL, Fryer C, Raney RB, Ruymann FB, Breneman J, Qualman SJ, Wiener E, Wharam M, Lobe T, Webber B, Maurer HM, Donaldson SS. Intergroup Rhabdomyosarcoma Study IV: results for patients with nonmetastatic disease. *J Clin Oncol* 2001;19:3091–102.

161. Crist WM, Garnsey L, Beltangady MS, Gehan E, Ruymann F, Webber B, Hays DM, Wharam M, Maurer HM. Prognosis in children with rhabdomyosarcoma: a report of the Intergroup Rhabdomyosarcoma Studies I and II. Intergroup Rhabdomyosarcoma Committee. *J Clin Oncol* 1990;8:443–52.

162. Gaffney EF, Dervan PA, Fletcher CD. Pleomorphic rhabdomyosarcoma in adulthood. Analysis of 11 cases with definition of diagnostic criteria. *Am J Surg Pathol* 1993;17:601–9.

163. Meza JL, Anderson J, Pappo AS, Meyer WH. Analysis of prognostic factors in patients with nonmetastatic rhabdomyosarcoma treated on Intergroup Rhabdomyosarcoma Studies III and IV: the Children's Oncology Group. *J Clin Oncol* 2006;24:3844–51.

164. Newton WA, Gehan EA, Webber BL, Marsden HB, van Unnik AJM, Hamoudi AB, Tsokos MC, Shimada H, Harms D, Schmidt D, Ninfo V, Cavazzana AO, Gonzalez-Crussi F, Parham DM, Reiman HM, Asmar L, Beltangady MS, Sachs NE, Triche TJ, Maurer HM. Classification of rhabdomyosarcomas and related sarcomas. Pathologic aspects and proposal for a new classification—an intergroup rhabdomyosarcoma study. *Cancer* 1995;76:1073–85.

165. Tsokos M, Webber BL, Parham DM, Wesley RA, Miser A, Miser JS, Etcubanas E, Kinsella T, Grayson J, Glatstein E, Pizzo PA, Triche TJ. Rhabdomyosarcoma. A new classification scheme related to prognosis. *Arch Pathol Lab Med* 1992;116:847–55.

166. Qualman SJ, Bowen J, Parham DM, Branton PA, Meyer WH. Protocol for the examination of specimens from patients (children and young adults) with rhabdomyosarcoma. *Arch Pathol Lab Med* 2003;127:1290–7.

167. Coffin CM. The new international rhabdomyosarcoma classification, its progenitors, and consideration beyond morphology. *Adv Anat Pathol* 1997;4:1–16.

168. Parham DM. Pathologic classification of rhabdomyosarcomas and correlations with molecular studies. *Mod Pathol* 2001;14:506–14.

169. Atra A, Ward HC, Aitken K, Boyle M, Dicks-Mireaux C, Duffy PG, Mitchell CD, Plowman PN, Ransley PG, Pritchard J. Conservative surgery in multimodal therapy for pelvic rhabdomyosarcoma in children. *Br J Cancer* 1994;70:1004–8.

170. Fryer CJ. Pelvic rhabdomyosarcoma: paying the price of bladder preservation. *Lancet* 1995;345:141–2.

171. Heyn R, Newton WA, Raney RB, Hamoudi A, Bagwell C, Vietti T, Wharam M, Gehan E, Maurer HM. Preservation of the bladder in patients with rhabdomyosarcoma. *J Clin Oncol* 1997;15:69–75.

172. Castellanos RD, Wakefield PB, Evans AT. Carcinoma of the bladder in children. *J Urol* 1975;113:261–3.

173. Chandy PC, Pai MG, Budihal MR, Kaulgud Sr. Carcinoma of the bladder in young children: report of 2 cases. *J Urol* 1975;113:264–5.

174. Gupta S, Gupta IM. Ectopia vesicae complicated by squamous cell carcinoma. *Br J Urol* 1976;48:244.

175. Raghavaiah NV, Reddy CR. Adenocarcinoma of the bladder in a boy. *J Urol* 1976;116:526–8.

176. Brumskine W, Dragan P, Sanvec L. Transitional cell carcinoma and schistosomiasis in a 5-year-old boy. *Br J Urol* 1977;49:540.

177. Nielsen K, Nielsen KK. Adenocarcinoma in exstrophy of the bladder—the last case in Scandinavia? A case report and review of literature. *J Urol* 1983;130:1180–2.

178. Rhaman SI, Matthews LK, Shaikh H, Townell NH. Primary paraganglioma of the bladder in a 14-year-old boy. *Br J Urol* 1995;75:682–3.

179. Bissada NK, Safwat AS, Seyam RM, Al Sobhi S, Hanash KA, Jackson RJ, Sakati N, Bissada MA. Pheochromocytoma in children and adolescents: a clinical spectrum. *J Pediatr Surg* 2008;43:540–3.

180. Mou JW, Lee KH, Tam YH, Cheung ST, Chan KW, Thakre A. Urinary bladder pheochromocytoma, an extremely rare tumor in children: case report and review of the literature. *Pediatr Surg Int* 2008;24:479–80.

181. Mutchler RW Jr, Gorder JL. Leiomyoma of the bladder in a child. *Br J Radiol* 1972;45:538–40.

182. Bhargava SK, Pal V, Lakhtakia HS, Gupta R, Gogi R. Dermoid cyst of the urinary bladder. *Indian Pediatr* 1977;14:161–2.

183. Lott S, Lopez-Beltran A, Maclennan GT, Montironi R, Cheng L. Soft tissue tumors of the urinary bladder, Part I: myofibroblastic proliferations, benign neoplasms, and tumors of uncertain malignant potential. *Hum Pathol* 2007;38:807–23.

184. Taylor G, Jordan M, Churchill B, Mancer K. Yolk sac tumor of the bladder. *J Urol* 1983;129:591–4.

185. D'Alessio A, Verdelli G, Bernardi M, DePascale S, Chiarenza SF, Giardina C, Cheli M, Rota G, Locatelli G. Endodermal sinus (yolk sac) tumor of the urachus. *Eur J Pediatr Surg* 1994;4:180–1.

186. Harris M, Eyden BP, Joglekar VM. Rhabdoid tumour of the bladder: a histological, ultrastructural and immunohistochemical study. *Histopathology* 1987;11:1083–92.

187. Carter RL, McCarthy KP, al-Sam SZ, Monaghan P, Agrawal M, McElwain TJ. Malignant rhabdoid tumour of the bladder with immunohistochemical and ultrastructural evidence suggesting histiocytic origin. *Histopathology* 1989;14:179–90.

188. Givler RL. Involvement of the bladder in leukemia and lymphoma. *J Urol* 1971;105:667–70.

189. Grooms AM, Morgan SK, Turner WR Jr. Hematuria and leukemic bladder infiltration. *JAMA* 1973;223:193–4.

190. Lewis RH, Mannarino FG, Worsham GF, Martin JE, Javadpour N, O'Connell KJ. Burkitt's lymphoma presenting as urinary outflow obstruction. *J Urol* 1983;130:120–4.

191. Schniederjan SD, Osunkoya AO. Lymphoid neoplasms of the urinary tract and male genital organs: a clinicopathological study of 40 cases. *Mod Pathol* 2009;22:1057–65.

192. Taykurt A. Wilms tumor at lower end of the ureter extending to the bladder: case report. *J Urol* 1972;107:142–3.

193. Candia A, Zegel HG. The occurrence of Wilms tumor in 2 patients with exstrophy of the bladder. *J Urol* 1982;128:589–90.

Chapter 19

Soft Tissue Tumors

Bladder Pathology, First Edition. Liang Cheng, Antonio Lopez-Beltran, David G. Bostwick.
© 2012 Wiley-Blackwell. Published 2012 by John Wiley & Sons, Inc.

Myofibroblastic Proliferations and Neoplasms

Inflammatory Myofibroblastic Tumor

Inflammatory myofibroblastic tumors (IMTs) are rare spindle tumors often mistaken for sarcoma, particularly when they arise in the urinary bladder. Since a bladder sarcoma warrants radical cystectomy, and an IMT of the bladder is generally managed conservatively, distinguishing between the two at this and other sites is of critical importance. IMTs have been described in numerous body sites, and tumors with similar morphology have been assigned many names, including plasma cell pseudotumor, inflammatory pseudotumor, xanthomatous pseudotumor, pseudosarcomatous myofibroblastic proliferation, inflammatory myofibrohistiocytic proliferation, atypical fibromyxoid tumor, and atypical myofibroblastic tumor.[1-3] The relationship between IMTs and the aforementioned tumors has been a matter of debate and controversy. Some investigators have questioned whether IMTs occurring in adult and pediatric patients are the same entity, and whether IMTs are benign, malignant, or part of a spectrum of benign to malignant spindled soft tissue tumors.

Historical Perspective

The earliest reports of lesions possibly representing IMTs and similar entities are those of von Brunn, who in 1939 described two patients, aged 5 and 9 years, respectively, who had lung lesions with constitutional symptoms.[4] von Brunn's diagnosis in one of the cases was "myoma of the lung," with signs of a "lymphocytic infiltrate, small areas of fibrosis and necrosis, and richly vascular stroma," features often seen in IMTs. von Brunn stated that the subacute granulomatous growth clinically seemed to be indicative of a true neoplasm, but that it was difficult to draw a line between neoplasm and granuloma.[4] A similar dilemma regarding the distinction currently exists.

In the genitourinary tract, the first description of such a lesion was by Roth in 1980, who reported "an unusual pseudosarcomatous entity" in the bladder of a 32-year-old woman and concluded that the lesion represented a reactive process.[5] Subsequently, Proppe et al. reported an entity they named "postoperative spindle cell nodule (PSCN)," arising in the lower genital tract of four men and four women 5 weeks to 3 months after instrumentation at the site where the lesion arose.[6] Many of these lesions were mistakenly diagnosed as sarcomas, but in view of the absence of nuclear pleomorphism, hyperchromatism, atypical mitoses, the presence of a plexiform capillary network, and the history of recent surgical procedure, the lesions were regarded as benign and reactive. Use of the term "postoperative

spindle cell nodule" for this clinicopathologic entity persists currently.

The term "inflammatory myofibroblastic tumor" was introduced in 1990 by Pettinato et al. in their report of 20 inflammatory pseudotumors of the lung.[7] Subsequently, Netto et al. suggested the use of this term to describe similar lesions sometimes encountered in the bladders of children, exhibiting an impressive inflammatory infiltrate, proliferation of spindle cell myofibroblasts and fibroblasts, granulation tissue-like vascularity, and absence of significant necrosis, cytologic atypia, and abnormal mitotic figures.[8]

Epidemiology and Clinical Presentation

Following the initial description of their occurrence in the lung, IMTs have been reported in a wide variety of anatomic sites, including the abdomen, retroperitoneum, head and neck region, brain, and extremities.[1] In the genitourinary tract, IMTs have been reported in the kidney, urethra, prostate, ureter, and rete testis, but is most frequently observed in the bladder.[9-15] Although the majority of patients with an IMT of the bladder are teens or young adults, IMTs have also been reported in children and in the elderly. IMTs are much more likely to occur in males, with a 2 to 3 : 1 male predominance.

The most common symptom is painless hematuria. Less often, patients present with dysuria, pelvic pain, or symptoms of urinary tract obstruction or infection, or the lesion may be discernible as a mass lesion during physical or radiologic examination. Other associations with genitourinary IMTs include cigarette smoking, bladder instrumentation, and gynecologic surgery. The occurrence of lesions in other anatomic sites may be accompanied by fever, weight loss, anemia, thrombocytosis, increased erythrocyte sedimentation rate, and increased immune globulins. However, such constitutional symptoms and serologic findings are not common in cases of IMTs of the genitourinary tract.[15]

IMTs are slow growing and rarely exhibit clinically aggressive behavior.[1] There are reports indicating that high-grade invasive urothelial carcinoma arising in patients with an IMT history sometimes exhibits unusually aggressive behavior, resulting in patient death.[12,16] It is unclear whether the occurrence of IMTs in this setting plays any substantial role in the occurrence or behavior of the invasive urothelial carcinoma. Recurrences are reported in 10% to 25% of genitourinary IMT cases; the predilection for recurrence of genitourinary IMTs shows no correlation with anaplastic lymphoma kinase (ALK) expression (see the discussion below).[12] It is unclear whether ALK expression in IMTs arising outside the genitourinary tract influences recurrence rates. Higher recurrence rates were noted in patients with ALK-negative IMTs compared to ALK-positive lesions in one study,[17] whereas other studies suggested that ALK-positive lesions tend to recur more often than ALK-negative lesions.[18] Thus, it is not certain what role ALK plays in prognosis. Moreover, there is no significant difference in gender when it comes to clinical outcomes.

Pathogenesis

The pathogenesis of IMTs is enigmatic, and numerous theories have been proposed. Because IMTs are characterized histologically by an inflammatory infiltrate and because various microbes have been isolated from the lesions, infection has long been suspected to play an important role in their pathogenesis. Microbes such as *Bacteroides corrodens, Klebsiella pneumoniae, Mycobacterium avium-intracellulare, Corynebacterium equi, Campylobacter jejuni, Bacillus sphaericus, Escherichia coli*, and *Coxiella burnetii* have been cultured from IMTs.[19] A study by Arber et al. detected Epstein–Barr virus (EBV) in 40% to 60% of splenic and hepatic inflammatory pseudotumor spindle cells.[20,21] Moreover, there seems to be a connection between tumors expressing EBV and follicular dendritic cells. In three liver cases, follicular dendritic cell tumors developed in a background of inflammatory pseudotumors that expressed the EBV antigen.[20,21]

It has been postulated that cytokines such as IL-1β and IL-6, which are responsible for the constitutional symptoms sometimes associated with IMTs, may reflect other processes, such as viral infection, that are involved in its origin. For example, human herpesvirus-8, which encodes proteins that mimic bcl-2, cyclin D, interferon factors, and IL-6, has been shown to be expressed in pulmonary and ganglion IMTs.[18] Other investigators have postulated an autoimmune origin for IMTs, as suggested by a case report of an IMT of the submandibular gland, in which a patient had polyclonal hypergammaglobulemia, high antinuclear antibody titers, and a positive antithyroid test with no symptoms of systemic autoimmune disease.[22] Autoimmune etiology has also been suggested by reports of IMTs of the spleen associated with thrombocytopenic purpura and IMTs associated with Riedel thyroiditis.[21]

The etiology implicating infection and autoimmune diseases refers primarily to IMTs in other organ sites. Caution is warranted in interpreting the data.

Histopathology

Macroscopic Pathology   An IMT is described grossly as a circumscribed, lobulated, or multinodular firm gray-white or yellow lesion with a whorled or fascicular appearance on sectioning, and sometimes a softer myxoid appearance. Foci of hemorrhage, necrosis, cystic change, and calcification are less commonly seen.[1] Tumor size ranges from 1 cm to 20 cm, with larger lesions seen in the mesentery, intestine, retroperitoneum, and liver. Lesions in the bladder and head and neck region are typically less than 2 cm in greatest dimension. In the bladder they are usually

exophytic and often polypoid, and exhibit no specific site predilection.[11,23–26] They may form large masses that protrude into the bladder lumen and/or invade the muscularis propria of the bladder wall.

Microscopic Pathology   The histologic appearance of the lesion is varied. Characteristically there is a predominance of myofibroblast and fibroblast spindle cells, a variably prominent collagenous or myxoid matrix, and inflammatory cells consisting mainly of plasma cells and lymphocytes with occasional eosinophils (**Figs. 19-1** to **19-10**). IMTs typically exhibit one of three general histologic appearances. The first is the myxoid/vascular pattern, composed of spindle and stellate cells with abundant eosinophilic cytoplasm and vesicular nuclei, which can mimic embryonal rhabdomyosarcoma (RMS). The second is characterized by compact spindle cells arranged in fascicular or storiform patterns, with some ganglion-like cells and varied cellular

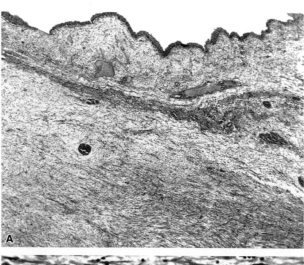

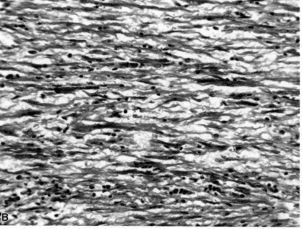

Figure 19-1   Inflammatory myofibroblastic tumor (A and B). The tumor is composed of spindle cells in loose edematous stroma.

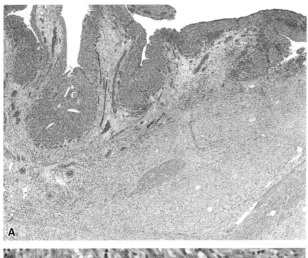

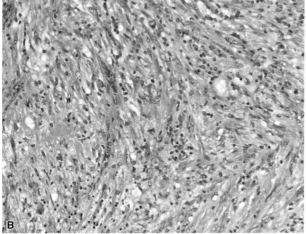

Figure 19-2 Inflammatory myofibroblastic tumor (A and B).

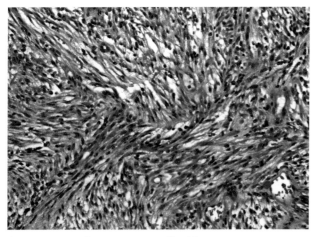

Figure 19-3 Inflammatory myofibroblastic tumor, hypercellular variant.

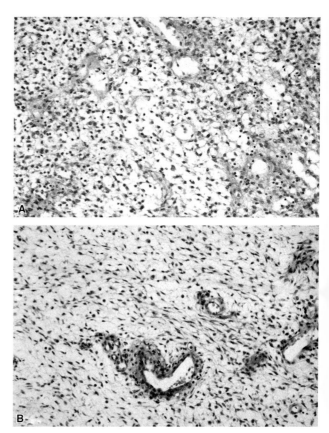

Figure 19-4 Inflammatory myofibroblastic tumor. (A) There is abundant acute and chronic inflammation admixed with the spindle cells, but in some areas (B) the inflammation is sparse or absent.

density (**Figs. 19-11** to **19-13**). The third is a hypocellular fibrous pattern displaying abundant collagen, plasma cells, lymphocytes, and eosinophils. This pattern can be compared to desmoid fibromatosis or scar tissue (**Fig. 19-14**).

Immunohistochemistry

Immunohistochemical findings in cases of IMT overlap those noted in other lesions included in the differential diagnosis, including more than one type of malignancy. IMTs have been reported to stain for vimentin (95% to 100%), desmin (5 to 80%), smooth muscle actin (SMA) (48% to 100%), muscle-specific actin (62%), and keratin (10% to 89%).[1,27–29] IMTs of the bladder are more likely to express keratin than are IMTs at other genitourinary locations, complicating its distinction from sarcomatoid carcinoma, since both lesions characteristically show varying degrees of immunoreactivity for both smooth muscle and epithelial markers.[1,30] IMTs rarely stain for MyoD1 or myogenin, which are skeletal muscle markers expressed by RMS. Approximately one-half of IMTs show positive immunostaining for ALK, thus providing a promising means of differentiating IMTs from other

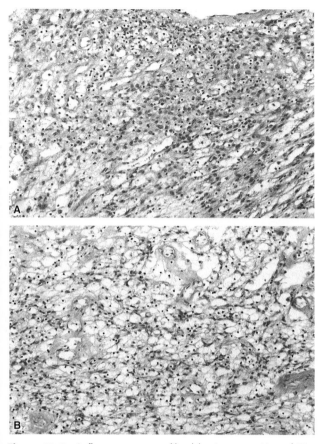

Figure 19-5 Inflammatory myofibroblastic tumor (A and B). Tumor cells are triangular to ovoid, admixed with chronic inflammation (A). Elsewhere, tumor cells have vacuolated cytoplasm (B).

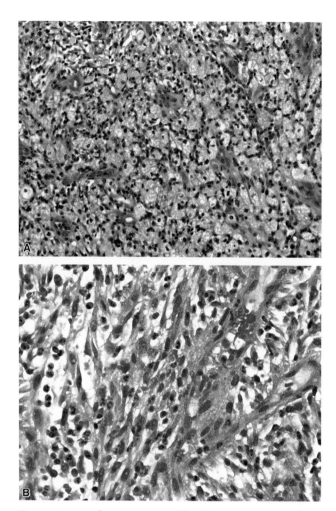

Figure 19-6 Inflammatory myofibroblastic tumor (A and B).

lesions (**Figs. 19-15** and **19-16**). The validity of ALK-1 staining is supported by corresponding fluorescence in situ hybridization (FISH) and cytogenetic studies, with translocation of the *ALK-1* gene on chromosome 2p23 documented in some cases.[1,31] Although the overall histologic and immunohistochemical findings must be taken into account and the sensitivity and specificity of ALK immunostaining for the diagnosis of an IMT has yet to be established, evidence of ALK-1 expression supports the diagnosis of IMTs in individual bladder lesions.[1,2]

Molecular Genetics and ALK
Recent genetic studies of small series of cases have detected karyotypic abnormalities in IMT. About 50% to 60% of IMTs can be shown to have clonal genetic aberrations in the short arm of chromosome 2 in region p21–p23, specifically, a 2p23 rearrangement involving the *ALK* gene, supporting the concept that an IMT is a neoplasm (**Fig. 19-17**).[1] The human *ALK* gene spans a region of about 728 kb on chromosome 2p23 and encodes ALK, a tyrosine kinase

receptor and member of the insulin growth factor receptor superfamily. It is normally expressed in the central nervous system and was first shown to be expressed abnormally in anaplastic large cell lymphoma. *ALK* gene rearrangements lead to fusion with other genes; in IMT, these rearrangements have involved the following genes: *CLTC, RANBP2, TPM3, TPM4, CARS, ATIC,* and *SEC1L1*.[32–34] Rearrangements have been reported in bladder IMTs, the first of which was *ALK-ATIC*.[35] Several translocations have been reported, including t(1;2)(q25;p23), t(2;2)(p23;q13), t(2;11)(p23;p15), t(2;17)(p23;q23), and t(2;19)(p23;p13.1). The translocation t(1;2)(q25;p23) with *TPM3* involvement is most common, and most breakpoints occur in the same intron of *ALK*.

FISH technology can be employed to detect *ALK* break-apart rearrangements. Commercially available dual color probe sets contain *ALK* upstream and downstream probes. The probes hybridize upstream and downstream from the *ALK* breakpoint cluster region and label the two sites with distinctly different fluorescent colors. The

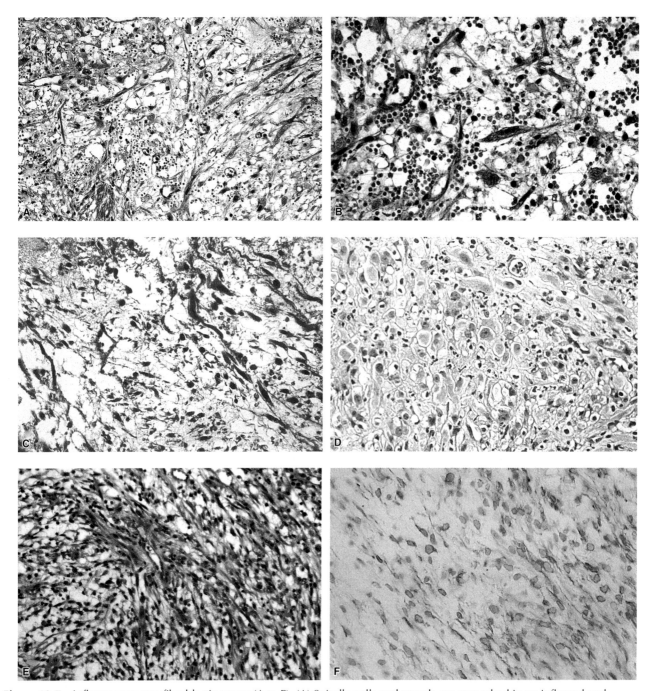

Figure 19-7 Inflammatory myofibroblastic tumor (A to F). (A) Spindle cells and vessels are enmeshed in an inflamed and edematous stroma. (B) At high magnification, atypical myofibroblasts are apparent, together with extravasated red blood cells. (C) Myxoid stroma. (D) In this focus, the myofibroblasts have epithelioid features that may be mistaken for urothelial carcinoma. (E) Note the presence of eosinophils. (F) Intense vimentin immunoreactivity in the spindle cells.

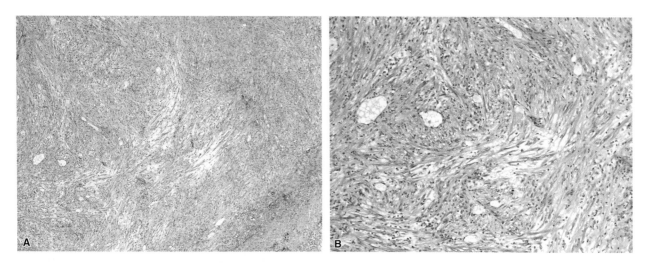

Figure 19-8   Inflammatory myofibroblastic tumor (A and B).

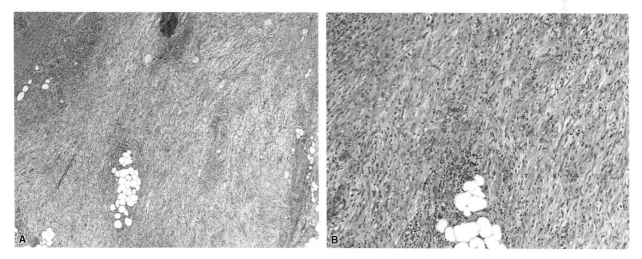

Figure 19-9   Inflammatory myofibroblastic tumor (A and B).

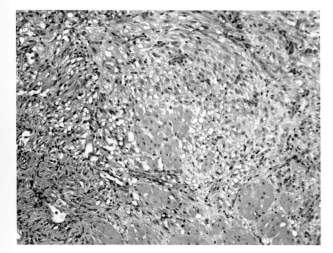

Figure 19-10   Inflammatory myofibroblastic tumor. Tumor invades the muscularis propria.

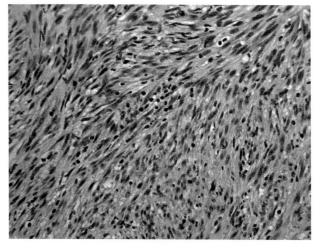

Figure 19-11   Inflammatory myofibroblastic tumor, hypercellular variant.

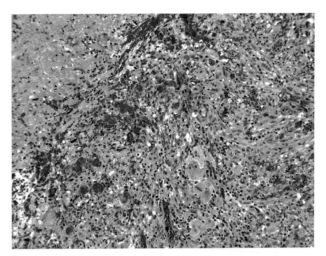

Figure 19-12 Inflammatory myofibroblastic tumor. Note the presence of mitotic figures and ganglion-like cells.

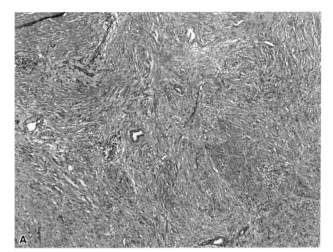

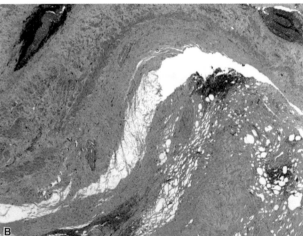

Figure 19-14 Inflammatory myofibroblastic tumor, sclerotic variant (A and B).

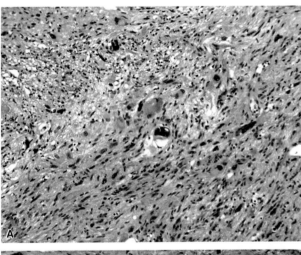

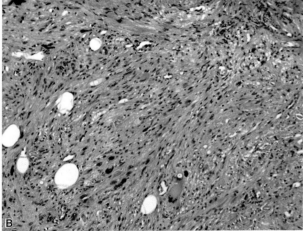

Figure 19-13 Inflammatory myofibroblastic tumor (A and B). Note the presence of cytologic atypia and ganglion-like cells.

chromosome 2p23 *ALK* region in its native state will be seen as two immediately adjacent or fused orange/green signals. If a break-apart occurs at the 2p23 *ALK* breakpoint region, paired orange/green signals split and separate orange and green signals will be seen, while the remaining native *ALK* region will still be visible as an orange/green fusion signal. A number of investigators have used this technology to detect alterations in the *ALK* gene, and it is notable that *ALK* rearrangements are demonstrable in genitourinary IMT lesions occurring both with and without a history of prior instrumentation.

Differential Diagnosis
The differential diagnosis of bladder IMT includes both benign and malignant lesions (**Tables 19-1** and **19-2**). Nodular fasciitis is a benign lesion that can be mimicked by the myxoid/vascular histologic pattern in an IMT. Although rare, leiomyoma is the most common benign soft tissue tumor in the bladder. Leiomyoma has

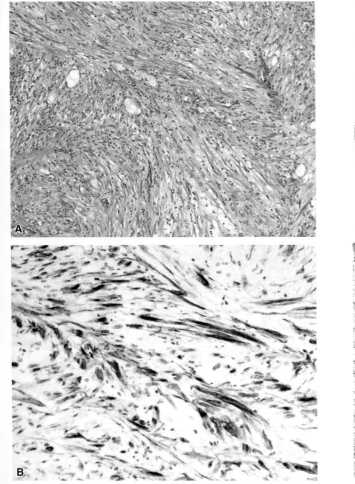

Figure 19-15 Inflammatory myofibroblastic tumor (A and B) displays positive immunostaining for ALK (B).

an immunophenotype similar to that of IMTs, staining positively for vimentin, SMA, and desmin. PSCNs are also benign and have an immunophenotype similar to that of IMTs; however, the clinical scenario includes a history of instrumentation, and PSCNs are typically 1 cm or less in greatest dimension. Some authors consider that PSCNs fall into the continuum spectrum of IMTs.[14]

Malignant lesions in the differential include leiomyosarcoma, sarcomatoid carcinoma, RMS, and urothelial carcinoma with pseudosarcomatous stroma. Leiomyosarcoma is the most common sarcoma in adult bladders. Atypical spindle cells with occasional mitotic figures may be seen in IMTs, but overt malignant feature such as atypical mitoses are absent.

Histologically, leiomyosarcoma and IMTs share certain common findings: both may have components of spindled cells with fibrillar eosinophilic or vacuolated cytoplasm; the background stroma may be extensively myxoid; and

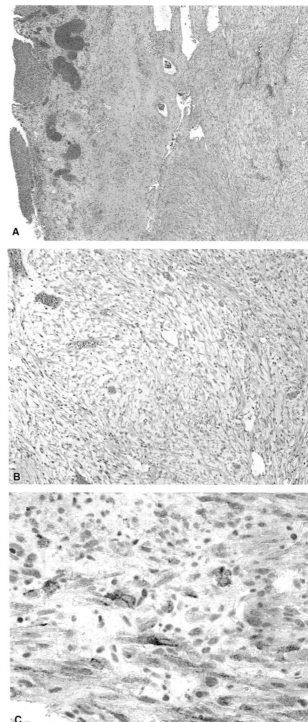

Figure 19-16 Inflammatory myofibroblastic tumor (A to C) displaying positive immunostaining for ALK (C).

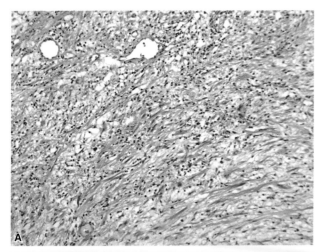

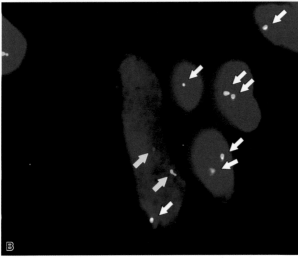

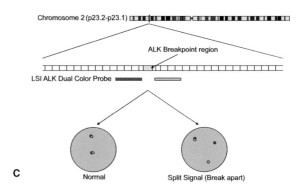

C   Normal   Split Signal (Break apart)

Figure 19-17 (*Continued*)

Figure 19-17 Inflammatory myofibroblastic tumor (IMT) of the urinary bladder. (A) Morphologic appearance of inflammatory myofibroblastic tumor. (B) FISH analysis for the *ALK* gene break-apart rearrangement in IMT of urinary bladder. Typical FISH image of nuclei with the *ALK* gene rearrangement shows the native ALK region as red/green fusion signals (white arrows), whereas the break-apart ALK region is depited as a red and green signal pattern (yellow arrows). The break-apart signal patterns were observed most frequently in the tumor cells with polymorphic morphology. Red signals: ALK upstream; green signals: ALK downstream. C. The human *ALK* gene spanning a region of about 728 kb on chromosome 2p23. LSI ALK dual color probe set contains ALK upstream (Spectrum Orange labeled, red signal) and ALK downstream (Spectrum Green labeled, green signal) probes. The probes hybridize upstream and downstream of the ALK breakpoint cluster region (blue box). The chromosome 2p23 ALK region in its native state will be seen as two immediately adjacent or fused red/green signals (Normal). If a break-apart occurred at the 2p23 ALK breakpoint region, paired red/green signals split and separate red and green signals will be seen (Break-apart), while the remaining native ALK region will still show a red/green fusion signal. (From Ref. 1; with permission.)

both may include aggregates of inflammatory cells, predominantly lymphocytes, and plasma cells. Leiomyosarcoma, however, typically exhibits at least mild to moderate nuclear pleomorphism, necrosis, and atypical mitotic figures.

Both IMTs and urothelial carcinoma with pseudosarcomatous stroma are usually immunoreactive for vimentin and muscle-specific actin, but there may also be aberrant expression of cytokeratins in these lesions. ALK-1 immunostaining and FISH analysis could be valuable in the differential diagnosis, especially in limited small biopsy specimens.

Sarcomatoid carcinoma and low grade sarcoma are important differential diagnostic considerations. The presence of typical fibroblasts, high cellularity and frequent mitoses in IMTs may raise concern for malignancy, but the lack of moderate to severe cytologic atypia, atypical mitotic figures, and extensive necrosis should lead one toward a benign diagnosis.[36,37] Additionally, IMTs often feature a myxoid background, inflammatory infiltrate, and prominent, slit-like vessels that are suggestive of benignity.[37,38] However, there is a subtype of sarcomatoid carcinoma, with myxoid or sclerotic foci, containing widely dispersed, mildly atypical cells that strongly resemble IMTs, further complicating the issue.[39]

IMTs are frequently immunoreactive for pancytokeratin, which is noteworthy when differentiating an IMT from sarcomatoid carcinoma. However, p63 is not expressed in IMTs and, when positive, supports the diagnosis of sarcomatoid carcinoma over IMTs (see also **Chapters 16** and **26**).[30] Westfall et al. investigated the use of a comprehensive immunohistochemical panel—cytokeratin AE1/AE3, high molecular weight cytokeratin 34βE12, cytokeratin 5/6 (CK5/6), SMA, and ALK-1—in the differential diagnosis of 22 sarcomatoid carcinomas, 17 IMTs, and 13 leiomyosarcomas.[40] CK5/6 immunostaining and p63 immunostaining were positive only in the sarcomatoid carcinomas (27% and 70%, respectively), whereas ALK-1 immunostaining was positive only in the IMTs (20%). Another high molecular weight cytokeratin 34βE12, showed results relatively similar to those for CK5/6 and is a good alternative to it. Cytokeratin AE1/AE3 and SMA

Table 19-1 Differential Features of Selected Soft Tissue Tumors of the Urinary Bladder

Tumors	Cytologic Atypia	Mitoses	Atypical Mitoses	Tumor Necrosis	Inflammation	Invasion of Muscle	Other Features
Inflammatory myofibroblastic tumor	Minimal	Few	Absent	Surface only	Often prominent	May be present	Delicate capillaries
Postoperative spindle cell nodule	Minimal	Variable	Absent	Absent	Present	Absent	Delicate capillaries
Leiomyoma	Minimal	Rare	Absent	Absent	Absent	Absent	Well-circumscribed
Neurofibroma	Varies	Absent	Absent	Absent	Sparse	Absent	Strands of collagen
Sarcomatoid carcinoma	Present	Present	Present	Present	Often present	May be present	Concomitant urothelial carcinoma or carcinoma in situ
Leiomyosarcoma	Present	Present	Present	Present	Sparse	Present	Uniform appearance
Angiosarcoma	Present	Present	Present	May be present	Present	May be present	Anastomosing vessels
Malignant fibrous histiocytoma	Present	Present	Present	Present	Present	Present	Multinucleated cells
Rhabdomyosarcoma	Present	Present	Present	Varies	Absent	May be present	Cambium layer in embryonal rhabdomyosarcoma, alveolar appearance

Table 19-2 Immunohistochemistry in Selected Soft Tissue Tumors and Sarcomatoid Carcinoma[a]

	IMT	Leiomyoma	Neurofibroma	PSCN	Sarcomatoid Carcinoma	Leiomyosarcoma	MFH	Rhabdomyosarcoma	Angiosarcoma
ALK-1	pos	—	rare pos	neg	—	—	—	—	—
α_1-Antichymotrypsin	—	—	—	—	—	—	pos	—	—
CD68	—	—	—	—	—	—	pos	—	—
Cytokeratin	pos/neg	—	neg	neg/pos	pos	neg/pos	neg/pos	neg/pos	neg
EMA	pos/neg	—	neg	neg	pos	neg	—	neg	—
h-Caldesmon	—	pos	—	—	—	pos	neg	neg	—
Muscle-specific actin	pos	pos	—	pos	pos/neg	pos	neg/pos	pos	neg
Desmin	pos/neg	pos	—	Pos/neg	neg/pos	pos	neg/pos	pos	neg
MyoD1	—	—	—	—	—	neg	neg	pos	neg
Myogenin	—	—	—	—	—	neg	neg	pos	neg
Myoglobin	neg	—	—	—	—	—	—	pos/neg	neg
Smooth muscle actin	pos	pos	—	Pos/neg	neg/pos	pos	neg/pos	neg/pos	neg
NSE/chromogranin	—	—	pos/neg	—	—	—	—	neg/pos	neg
S100 protein	neg	—	pos	—	—	neg	neg	neg	neg
Vimentin	pos	pos	—	pos	pos/neg	pos	pos	pos	pos
CD31	—	—	—	—	—	—	neg	—	pos
CD34	—	—	—	—	—	Neg/pos	neg	neg	pos
Factor VIII antigen	—	—	—	—	—	—	—	—	pos

[a]IMT, inflammatory myofibroblastic tumor; PSCN, postoperative spindle cell nodule; MFH, malignant fibrous histiocytoma; ALK, anaplastic lymphoma kinase; EMA, epithelial membrane antigen; NSE, neuron-specific enolase. pos/neg, tumors often immunoreactive for antigen; neg/pos, tumors occasionally immunoreactive for antigen; —, no information available or test infrequently used in this setting.

were not as helpful in determining the diagnosis, because both demonstrated significant positivity in all three types of tumors: IMT (70% and 100%, respectively), leiomyosarcoma (58% and 85%, respectively), and sarcomatoid carcinoma (70% and 73%, respectively). SMA positivity in the absence of other markers favors leiomyosarcoma.

RMS, particularly the embryonal subtype, is an important consideration in children, but can be differentiated from IMTs by careful attention to morphologic features and by positive immunohistochemical staining for MyoD1 or myogenin.

Elements of Controversy

There are a number of uncertainties regarding IMTs. For example, how does one define IMTs? Does the definition require a consideration of clinical parameters, such as the age of the patient, or a history of instrumentation? Does the definition hinge upon the immunophenotype of the tumor, or upon the presence or absence of demonstrable gene rearrangements? Is an IMT a single entity or a spectrum of lesions ranging from benign to clearly malignant? Harik et al. have proposed that PSCNs and IMTs are essentially indistinguishable from one another, and should be classified as a single entity with the descriptive name of "pseudosarcomatous myofibroblastic proliferation (PMP).[14]" Review of their 42 cases showed the tumors to be indistinguishable by gross, microscopic, or immunophenotypic criteria. The chief differences between these entities are clinical; a PSCN is preceded by a traumatic event, such as surgery or instrumentation, and tends to occur in a slightly older age group. Other investigators have reported that PSCNs tend to be smaller than PMPs, have a higher mitotic rate, and occasionally have eosinophils present.[41] Furthermore, it has been postulated that IMTs occurring in childhood are distinctly different entities from the lesions occurring in older patients that fall under the designation of PMPs, and that childhood IMTs have a more aggressive course than PMPs.[14] However, there is significant morphologic and genetic overlapping between pediatric and adult IMTs, suggesting that pediatric and adult IMTs may not be fundamentally different from each other.[12,42]

One study sought to compare *ALK* involvement between PMPs and IMTs in the genitourinary tract. Researchers found that 42% of PMPs had cytoplasmic staining for ALK, but no rearrangements were detected by FISH.[41] This contrasts with IMTs, in which more than one-half of cases showed gene alterations. The difficulty with this study was that it was unclear how the investigators subclassified the tumors into two separate groups prior to the performance of the stains and FISH studies. At any rate, the study raises the question of whether the diagnosis of an IMT requires molecular confirmation of *ALK* rearrangement in order to make the diagnosis. The findings also suggest that an IMT

is a neoplastic process, whereas PMPs that lack gene rearrangements may be reactive/reparative in nature.[41]

It has been hypothesized that an IMT in the genitourinary tract is a low grade inflammatory sarcoma.[11] Meis and Enzinger, in 1991, reported lesions in the retroperitoneum, mesentery, mediastinum, and abdominal peritoneum, which they regarded as fibrosarcomas with mature myofibroblasts, fibroblasts, and intense inflammatory infiltrate and distinguished these lesions from morphologically similar IMTs, based on their biologic behavior, noting that the fibrosarcomas were more aggressive than IMTs, with 37% recurring locally, 10% metastasizing, and 18% causing death.[43] Inflammatory fibrosarcoma involving the genitourinary tract is rare. In one case, inflammatory fibrosarcoma developed in the prostate of a patient four years postirradiation for prostate cancer.[12] The fibrosarcoma recurred four months after resection and metastasized to the abdominal cavity, resulting in death nine months later. The lesion was reportedly histologically similar to an IMT except for hyperchromasia of the spindle cell nuclei. Weidner described a case of abdominal inflammatory fibrosarcoma which also involved the bladder.[9] Histologically, the spindle cells had "malignant nuclear features, including irregular coarsely clumped chromatin, large inclusion-like nucleoli, and a more uniform fascicular growth pattern that somewhat resembles leiomyosarcoma and/or malignant fibrous histiocytoma" with rare mitoses. Otherwise, the tumor was considered to be morphologically similar to PSCNs and IMTs. There is also a case where one bladder lesion displayed both IMT and sarcomatoid features, with evidence of *ALK* gene alteration, but behaved clinically like a malignant inflammatory fibrosarcoma.[42] Cases of this sort suggest that IMTs may be part of a continuum, with benign pseudosarcomatous entities at one end and low grade sarcomas at the opposite end.

A number of questions regarding IMTs of the genitourinary tract remain unresolved. It is unclear whether IMTs are separable from PSCNs on morphologic, immunohistochemical, or molecular grounds. Questions concerning the malignant potential of IMTs, and how ALK expression and gene rearrangements can be related to the biologic behavior of such lesions, await further elucidation. Available evidence allows one to hypothesize that IMTs are part of a continuum bordered by benign pseudosarcomatous lesions at one end and low grade sarcomas at the opposite end. Future studies of IMTs will benefit from further use of FISH and other molecular studies in clarifying the significance of abnormalities of the *ALK* gene and possibly other genes as well. Hopefully, such studies will assist in establishing diagnostic and prognostic criteria for these rare, fascinating, and enigmatic lesions.

For practical purposes, an IMT of the genitourinary tract should be considered a neoplasm of uncertain malignant potential, and routine surveillance and close clinical followup are recommended. Aggressive therapy (radical cystectomy, radiation, or chemotherapy) is unwarranted given the indolent and often benign clinical course for the majority of the diseases. In attempting to understanding diagnostic and prognostic implications, future emphasis will be placed on the linkage of genetic abnormalities with clinical course, therapeutic response, and ultimate outcome.

Postoperative Spindle Cell Nodule

Proppe et al. first described PSCNs in a series of eight patients, four women and four men.[6] Following Proppe's report, other cases of PSCNs in the bladder were described.[2,3,6,14,41,42,44–49] It may be seen in both genders months after surgical instrumentation or resection. It is characterized by nodules up to 4 cm in size occurring in the lower genital tract and lower urinary tract.[6] The average size of the lesion in one series was 1.5 cm.[41] Patients ranged in age from 29 years to 79 years, and typically presented with hematuria and/or obstructive voiding symptoms. Some PSCNs were found incidentally by CT scan or at cystoscopy. A tumor may rarely recur, but metastasis has not been reported.

Microscopically, the tumors are uniform, composed of intersecting fascicles of plump spindle cells with delicate vessels, focal hyalinization, and moderate collagen deposition (**Figs. 19-18** and **19-19**). The spindle cells have abundant, tapering, eosinophilic cytoplasm. The nuclei vary only slightly in size, and there is no cytologic atypia. There are numerous mitotic figures, none of which is abnormal. These lesions often have surface mucosal ulceration with acute inflammatory cells in the ulcer bed, as well as scattered chronic inflammatory cells in lamina propria. Moderate edema and small foci of hemorrhage may be identified, but necrosis is absent. Foreign body giant cells and prominent eosinophilia may be seen.[41]

Immunohistochemically, lesional cells of PSCN show positive staining for cytokeratins AE1/AE3, CAM5.2, and vimentin in some nodules; in other nodules, only immunoreactivity for vimentin is present.[46] Iczkowski reported immunohistochemical reactivity for vimentin, desmin, and SMA.[41] Weak reactivity for pancytokeratin and for p53 were also noted in some cases.[41] ALK-1 immunostaining was negative.

The differential diagnoses for PSCNs also includes sarcomatoid carcinoma, myxoid leiomyosarcoma, RMS, and malignant fibrous histiocytoma (MFH) (**Tables 19-1** and **19-2**). Key features of malignant tumors, which are generally absent in myofibroblastic proliferations, include cytologic atypia, atypical mitoses, and tumor necrosis (other than at the surface). PSCNs often show a predominance of chronic over acute inflammation with surface ulceration. In some studies, p53 immunostaining

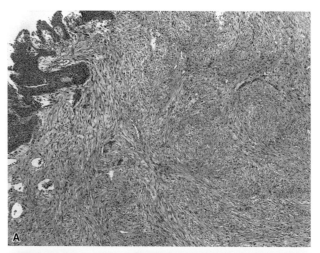

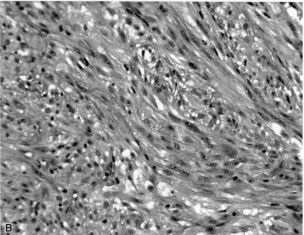

Figure 19-18 Postoperative spindle cell nodule. Elongated spindle cells with eosinophilic cytoplasm are shown (A and B).

was thought to be helpful in distinguishing benign lesions with only rare immunoreactive cells from malignant mesenchymal neoplasms, which showed stronger and more diffuse p53 immunoreactivity.[41,50] Sarcomatoid carcinomas show more pronounced and more diffusely positive immunostaining for cytokeratin, have cytologic atypia, and often have an epithelial component in addition to the mesenchymal proliferation.[30]

Benign Soft Tissue Tumors

Leiomyoma

Although leiomyoma of the bladder is rare, it is the most common benign soft tissue neoplasm of the bladder.[51] Of the 37 cases reported in a recent review, 59% occurred in patients in the third through sixth decades of life, with

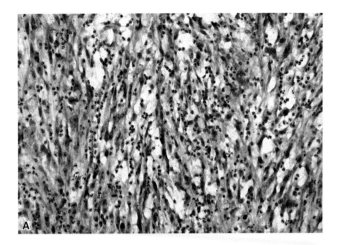

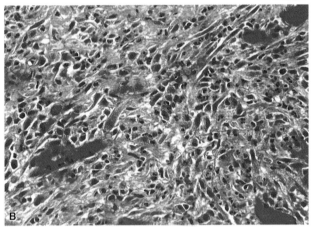

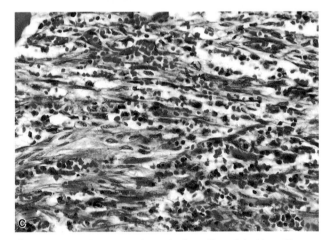

Figure 19-19 Postoperative spindle cell nodule (A to C). Each of these tumors arose in patients within 3 months of transurethral resection of the bladder. The spindle cells with slightly enlarged nuclei are admixed with chronic and acute inflammation.

an average patient age of 44 years. Seventy-six percent of patients were women. Presenting symptoms included obstructive symptoms such as retention and frequency of micturition (49%); irritative symptoms such as burning, dysuria, or urgency (38%), hematuria (11%), and flank pain (13%); and 19% of patients were asymptomatic. Bimanual exam revealed a palpable pelvic mass in 57%. Cystoscopy with biopsy was deemed the most useful diagnostic procedure. Tumors were most often intravesical; a minority were extravesical or predominantly intramural.[52] Excision is usually curative. No recurrences or metastases have been observed.

Grossly, the tumors are typically small, well-circumscribed, white, and fleshy without necrosis (**Fig. 19-20**).[53] Goluboff et al. reported tumor sizes ranging from 1.5 cm to 25 cm, with an average size of 5.8 cm.[52] The 10 bladder leiomyomas in the series of Martin et al. had an average size of 1.6 cm; no site predilection within the bladder was evident in this series.[53]

Microscopically, leiomyomas consist of intersecting fascicles of smooth muscle cells with moderate to abundant eosinophilic cytoplasm (**Figs. 19-21** and **19-22**). They usually display only modest cellularity without evidence of myxoid change. Nuclei are oval to cigar-shaped, centrally located, blunt-ended, and devoid of significant atypical changes such as hyperchromasia, pleomorphism, or individual cell necrosis. Mitotic figures are absent. Kunze described three such tumors with the additional finding of "numerous interspersed medium-sized, thick-walled vessels lined by inconspicuous flat to cuboidal endothelial cells," designating these as angioleiomyomas.[54] Immunohistochemically, most leiomyomas of the bladder exhibit strong diffuse immunoreactivity for SMA, muscle-specific actin, desmin, and vimentin. Martin et al.

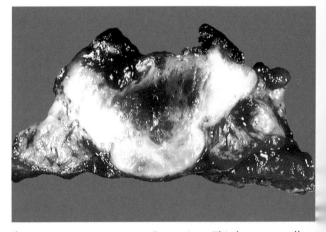

Figure 19-20 Leiomyoma. Gross view. This large centrally hemorrhagic tumor consists entirely of benign smooth muscle cells (B) without cytologic atypia, necrosis, or mitotic figures. The patient is alive and free of recurrence after 11 years.

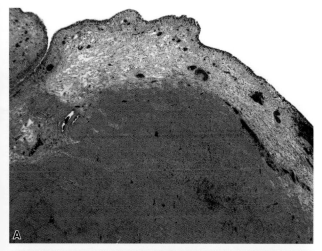

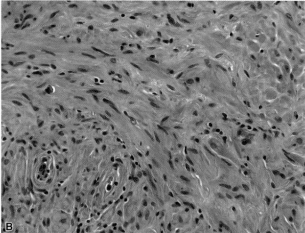

Figure 19-21 Leiomyoma. The tumor is composed of intersecting fascicles of smooth muscle cells with eosinophilic cytoplasm (A). Higher magnification shows cigar-shaped blunt-ended nuclei without atypia (B).

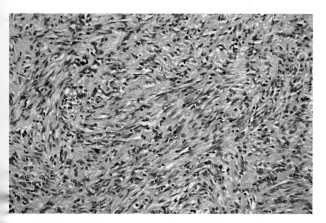

Figure 19-22 Leiomyoma.

reported immunopositivity for CD34 in three of 10 tumors. Leiomyomas are usually negative for cytokeratin and S100 protein.[53]

Hemangioma

Bladder hemangioma is a rare benign lesion (**Figs. 19-23** to **19-27**). The largest series of bladder hemangiomas reported to date, that of Cheng et al., comprised 19 patients with a male-to-female ratio of 3.7 : 1.[55] In this series, the mean age at time of diagnosis was 58 years; previous reports indicated that the lesion occurred in all age groups but was most often diagnosed in patients less than 30 years old.[55] Multiple hemangiomas/lymphangiomas may be associated with syndromes predisposing to their development, including Klippel–Trenaunay–Weber and Sturge–Weber syndromes (**Fig. 19-28**). The most common presenting symptom is gross hematuria; other reported complaints include irritative voiding symptoms and abdominal pain.[55] Effective conservative treatment consists of biopsy with

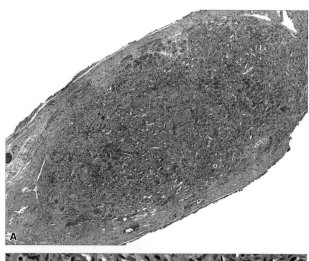

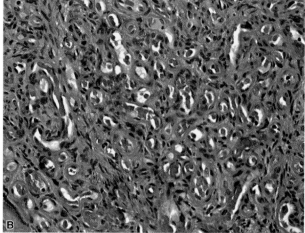

Figure 19-23 Capillary hemangioma (A and B).

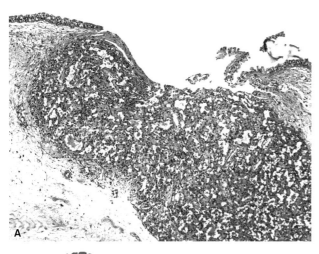

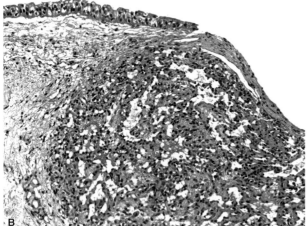

Figure 19-24   Bladder hemangioma (A and B).

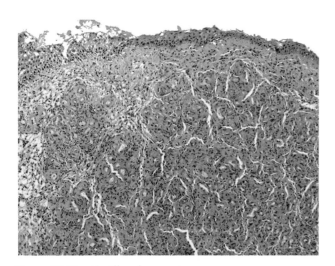

Figure 19-25   Capillary hemangioma.

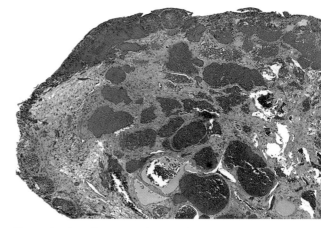

Figure 19-26   Cavernous hemangioma.

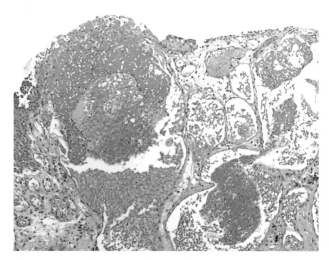

Figure 19-27   Cavernous hemangioma.

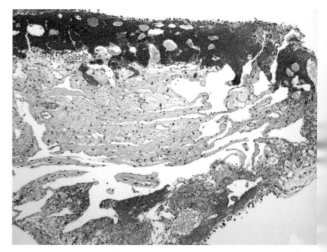

Figure 19-28   Lymphangioma in a patient with
Klippel–Trenaunay–Weber syndrome.

or without fulguration. After such treatment, none of the 19 patients in the series of Cheng et al., with a mean followup of 6.9 years, developed recurrence, nor did any have untoward sequelae.

Cystoscopically, a sessile blue raised mass may be seen, most often on the posterior and lateral walls of the bladder.[55] These lesions are usually small. Cheng et al. reported a median size of 0.7 cm; the majority is reportedly <3 cm.

The most common hemangioma occurring in the bladder is of cavernous type; much less frequent are capillary or arteriovenous types. Histologically, these lesions are identical to hemangiomas found at other sites. Kunze, in a series of 30 primary mesenchymal tumors, identified two hemangiomas, one of which was of capillary type, composed of myriad small blood vessels lined by flat to cuboidal bland-appearing endothelial cells and separated by moderate amounts of fibrous tissue.[54] The other hemangioma in this series was of mixed capillary and cavernous type, composed of innumerable proliferating capillaries admixed with thin-walled, dilated blood-filled vessels lined by flat endothelial cells.[54]

The differential diagnosis for bladder hemangioma includes angiosarcoma and Kaposi sarcoma, both of which exhibit cytologic atypia. Both exuberant granulation tissue and papillary–polypoid cystitis are characterized by prominent inflammation, which is not typically seen in hemangioma.[55] Other entities that warrant consideration in the differential diagnosis include prior biopsy site, chemotherapy effect, or changes secondary to radiation therapy; clearly, clinical history is essential in arriving at a correct diagnosis.[54] It is important to remember that adenovirus-associated hemorrhagic cystitis occurs in children and in immunosuppressed patients; biopsies from such lesions may exhibit viral cytopathic changes and intranuclear inclusions within epithelial cells.

Neurofibroma

Neurofibroma of the urinary bladder is rare. Most of these lesions occur in the setting of neurofibromatosis type 1 rather than as isolated lesions.[56] Classically, neurofibromas of the urinary bladder occur in young patients with a slight male predominance. The average age at diagnosis is 17 years. Presenting symptoms include hematuria, irritative symptoms, and pelvic mass. Neurofibroma is a benign, probably neoplastic tumor of various nerve sheath cells, including Schwann cells, perineurium-like cells, fibroblasts, and intermediate-type cells (**Figs. 19-29 to 19-31**).[57] The histologic findings are the same as in neurofibromas of other organs: tumors are composed of a hypocellular proliferation of spindle cells, loosely arranged into fascicles with scattered "shredded carrot" bundles of collagen. Individual cells have wavy, bland

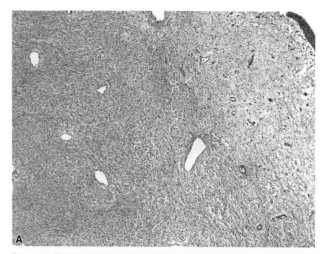
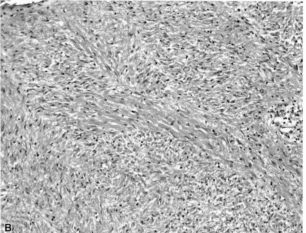

Figure 19-29 Neurofibroma. (A) Submucosal involvement by neurofibroma. (B) Neurofibroma of bladder consisting of a proliferation of spindle cells with scattered bundles of collagen.

nuclei. In a recent series by Cheng et al., three of four bladder neurofibromas were transmural with both diffuse and plexiform growth patterns.[56] Another case had only a diffuse pattern with submucosal involvement and subepithelial pseudomeissnerian corpuscles on biopsy. Areas of diffuse involvement were hypocellular with small to medium-sized spindle cells with ovoid to elongated nuclei in a collagenized matrix. A few mast cells were present. Immunohistochemical staining was reactive in all cases for S100 protein as well as type IV collagen.[56] Three were positive for neurofilament protein in axons. A recent report indicates that bladder neurofibromas do not express ALK-1 protein. The differential diagnosis of bladder neurofibroma includes other spindle cell tumors, such as leiomyoma, PSCN, inflammatory pseudotumor, low grade leiomyosarcoma, other nerve sheet tumors, and rarely, RMS.

See **Chapter 15** for further discussion.

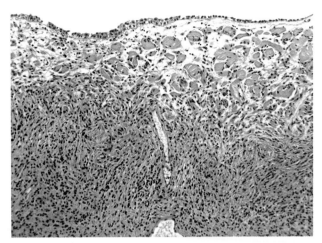

Figure 19-30 Neurofibroma with superficial, band-like subepithelial pseudo-meissnerian corpuscles.

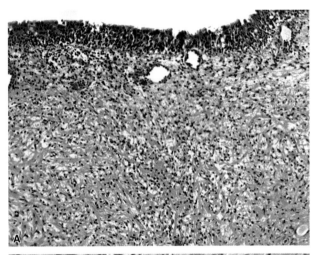

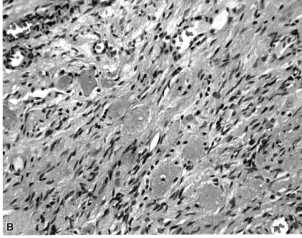

Figure 19-31 Neurofibroma with ganglion cell involvement (A and B).

Schwannoma

See **Chapter 15** for further discussion.

Solitary Fibrous Tumor

Four cases of solitary fibrous tumor of the urinary bladder have been described.[58,59] Three occurred in men and one in a woman, ranging in age from 42 years to 67 years. Two patients experienced genitourinary symptoms including pelvic pressure, while two were found incidentally. Solitary fibrous tumors confined to the bladder have demonstrated no evidence of recurrence after followup ranging from 1 month to 18 months.[58,59] However, Westra et al. reported one genitourinary solitary fibrous tumor, not confined to the bladder, that had atypical features associated with an unfavorable clinical outcome. These features included higher cellularity, cellular pleomorphism, and increased mitotic rate. Followup of this tumor was limited to 9 months.[58]

The tumors ranged in size from 4 cm to 20 cm. Two were described as polypoid with an intact mucosa. Grossly, the tumors were well-circumscribed and yellow-white on the cut surface. Some were solid with a whirling appearance, while one was cystic.[58,59]

Microscopically, the tumors were characterized by a proliferation of cytologically bland spindle cells within a fibrocollagenous background. The cellular arrangement was patternless; some had alternating areas of hypocellularity and hypercellularity. Nuclei were slender with fine chromatin and a pale rim of eosinophilic cytoplasm. Some tumors had nuclear pseudoinclusions. Other areas had plump fusiform and polygonal cells. Prominent vascularity with thin-walled branching vessels and hyalinized thick-walled vessels was identified. One tumor had these benign features focally, while the remainder of the tumor was highly cellular with cellular pleomorphism and 10 mitoses per 10 high power field (hpf).[58] The remaining tumors had fewer than 2 mitoses per 10 hpf and showed little atypia.[58,59]

All tumors displayed diffuse, positive immunohistochemical staining for CD34.[58,59] Two also were immunoreactive for CD99, while one tumor was focally immunoreactive for α-SMA and muscle-specific actin.[59] Immunostains for S100 protein, cytokeratin, and CD31 were negative.[59]

The differential diagnosis for solitary fibrous tumor of the bladder includes other spindle cell lesions, such as PSCN, IMT, malignant peripheral nerve sheath tumor (MPNST), leiomyosarcoma, and MFH. Use of routine light microscopy can usually establish the diagnosis; however, diffuse immunohistochemical staining with CD34 is very useful in distinguishing this tumor from the others mentioned.[58,59]

Paraganglioma

Paraganglioma of the urinary bladder is rare. It is thought to arise from embryonic nests of chromaffin cells in the sympathetic plexus of the detrusor muscle.[60] Although most are indolent, it must be kept in mind that 10% of extraadrenal pheochromocytomas (hormonally active paragangliomas) behave in a malignant fashion.[60] Malignancy in these tumors can only be confirmed by the occurrence of regional or distant metastases. There are no reliable histologic features to distinguish between benign and malignant tumors or to predict biological behavior.

Presenting symptoms of paraganglioma include hematuria, hypertension, and other symptoms of catecholamine excess.[60,61] The tumor is usually intramural and some are multifocal (Fig. 19-32). Tumors are typically located in the lateral and posterior bladder wall.[60] The largest reported series, by Cheng et al., included 16 patients with primary paraganglioma of the bladder, followed for a mean of 6.3 years.[60] The tumor occurred most often in young adult women; the patients ranged in age from 16 years to 74 years, with a mean age of 45 years. The male-to-female ratio was 1 : 3. In 37% of patients, tumors involved perivesical soft tissues or adjacent organs at the time of diagnosis. No metastases or tumor recurrences were observed in patients whose tumors were confined within the mucosa or muscularis propria of the bladder. Of the six patients whose tumors extended beyond the confines of the bladder, one had regional nodal metastasis and another had distant metastases at the time of diagnosis, one developed metastases one year after diagnosis and died of the disease 1.5 years later, and one had a recurrence three years after diagnosis.

Histologically, bladder paraganglioma is similar to its counterparts in other body sites; most are covered by normal urothelium. The tumor consists of round or polygonal epithelioid cells with abundant eosinophilic or granular cytoplasm (Figs. 19-33 and 19-34). The cells are arranged in discrete nests (Zellballen pattern), with intervening vascular septa.[60–62] Sustentacular cells may be present, highlighted by immunostaining for S100 protein.

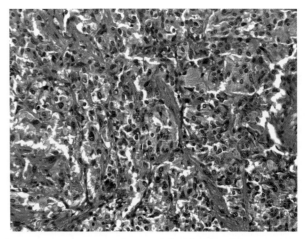

Figure 19-33 Paraganglioma of the bladder. Discrete nests of tumor cells are typical. The tumor is composed of round to polygonal epithelioid cells with central, vesicular nucleus. Cells are arranged in discrete nests (Zellballen pattern) with intervening septa.

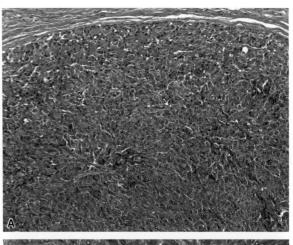
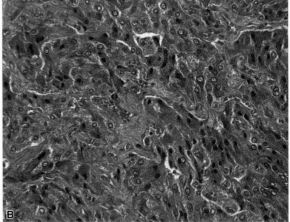

Figure 19-34 Paraganglioma (A and B). Tumor cells have abundant amphophilic cytoplasm. Note the intervening vascular septa.

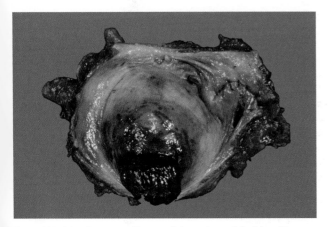

Figure 19-32 Paraganglioma of the urinary bladder. (From Ref. 60; with permission.)

See **Chapter 15** for further discussion.

Granular Cell Tumor

Granular cell tumors, which are of neural origin, are rarely encountered in the urinary bladder. Several cases of benign granular cell tumors, as well as a case of malignant granular cell tumor, appear in the medical literature.[63-69] One case occurred in a patient with neurofibromatosis.[67] Granular cell tumors at all sites occur most often in the fourth to sixth decades, although they may occur at any age. Granular cell tumors of the bladder have been reported to occur in patients ranging from age 23 years to 61 years and measure up to 9 cm in greatest dimension. They may be multifocal.

See **Chapter 22** for further discussion.

Malignant Soft Tissue Tumors

Leiomyosarcoma

Although leiomyosarcoma is the most common malignant mesenchymal tumor of the urinary bladder in adults, it is still relatively very rare, accounting for less than 1% of all bladder malignancies.[53] Patients range in age from 15 years to 75 years, with most patients presenting in the sixth to eighth decades.[54,70] There is a male predominance of over 2 : 1.[71] Some leiomyosarcomas have reportedly developed 5 years to 20 years after the administration of cyclophophamide.[72,73] Acrolein, a degradation product of cyclophosphamide, is thought to be the causative agent in such cases. The most common presenting complaint (in 80%) is gross hematuria; less frequently, patients complain of dysuria or obstructive voiding symptoms, or are noted to have an abdominal mass. Any part of the bladder may be involved by leiomyosarcoma, but the dome, followed by the lateral walls, are the most common tumor sites.[70] A recent review of 18 bladder leiomyosarcomas showed them to be "aggressive neoplasms" with more than 60% of patients developing metastases or dying of recurrent or metastatic tumor.[53] Higher grade tumors had a worse prognosis. Most low grade tumors have a lower risk of recurrence or metastasis.[53,70] When feasible, treatment generally involves surgical excision of the lesion.

Grossly, leiomyosarcomas are often large and polypoid; they are unencapsulated and usually exhibit full-thickness involvement of the bladder wall (**Fig. 19-35**). They are described variously as firm, fleshy, or fibrous masses that may have a mucoid or myxoid consistency, hemorrhagic and/or focally necrotic areas, and often surface ulceration.[10,53]

Suggested criteria for the diagnosis of malignancy in a true smooth muscle neoplasm of the bladder include

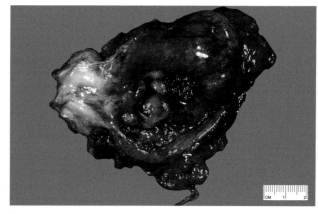

Figure 19-35 Leiomyosarcoma. The bladder lumen is filled and distorted by a large necrotic mass.

the following: significant nuclear pleomorphism with hyperchromasia and irregular nuclear membranes (usually, readily identifiable at low power), coagulative tumor cell necrosis, increased mitotic activity, and infiltration of the muscularis propria (**Figs. 19-36** to **19-39**).[74] It seems reasonable to require the presence of more than just one of these features in a given tumor in order to diagnose leiomyosarcoma. The majority of leiomyosarcomas are moderately or well-differentiated. Several variants, including myxoid (**Fig. 19-40**) and epithelioid histologic subtypes, have been described. Grading is based on the degree of cytologic atypia. The diagnosis of a low grade leiomyosarcoma should be made for a cellular tumor with some mitotic activity (<5 mitotic figures per 10 hpf), mild to moderate cytologic atypia, minimal necrosis, and an infiltrative margin.[10,71] Martin et al. define high grade leiomyosarcoma as having moderate to marked cytologic atypia, with more than 5 mitotic figures per 10 hpf and/or

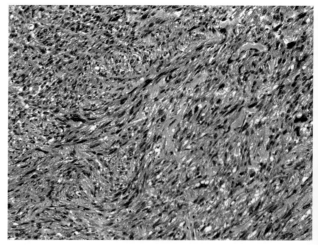

Figure 19-36 Leiomyosarcoma. The tumor is composed of fascicles of malignant spindle cells with significant nuclear pleomorphism and hyperchromasia.

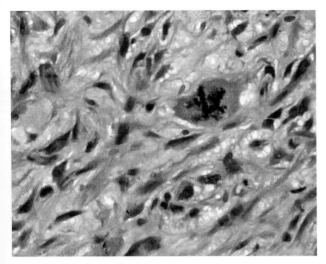

Figure 19-37 Leiomyosarcoma. Note the bizarre atypical mitotic figure.

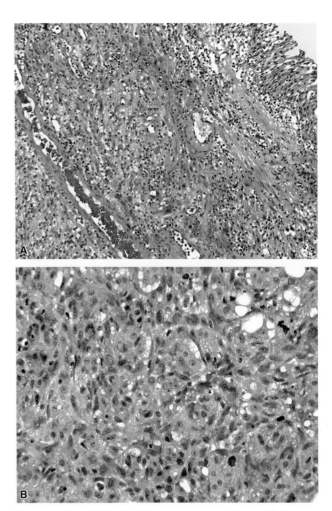

Figure 19-39 Epithelioid leiomyosarcoma (A and B). Tumor with nuclear atypia, atypical mitotic figures, and inflammation.

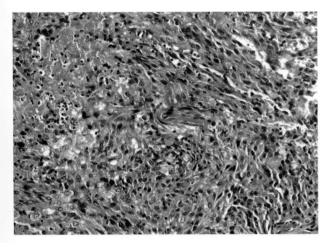

Figure 19-38 Leiomyosarcoma with an area of necrosis.

abundant necrosis.[53] Histologically, well-differentiated tumors have interlacing bundles and fascicles of spindled and elongated cells with eosinophilic cytoplasmic processes, and hyperchromatic nuclei with or without small nucleoli.[53] high grade leiomyosarcomas are typically composed of spindle cells with highly pleomorphic vesicular nuclei, with macronucleoli and often bizarre mitotic figures, sometimes interspersed with multinucleated giant cells.[54] Tumors with prominent myxoid backgrounds may demonstrate slightly atypical spindle cells haphazardly arranged.[70] Surface inflammation in the form of lymphoplasmacytic infiltrates may be present.[70] Myxoid leiomyosarcoma may contain moderate numbers of thin-walled blood vessels. Kunze et al. described two epithelioid leiomyosarcomas as having predominantly rounded tumor cells with clear and often markedly vacuolated cyotoplasm.[54] Other foci had cells with long eosinophilic cytoplasmic processes lying within a myxoid stroma.

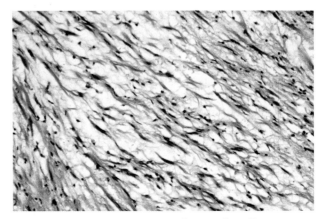

Figure 19-40 Leiomyosarcoma. The spindle cells are arranged in fascicles with a prominent myxoid stroma.

Immunohistochemically, leiomyosarcomas usually stain positively for muscle-specific actin (100%) and vimentin (>90%). Desmin staining may be weak or focal and is reported in 0% to 60% of cases. Leiomyosarcoma infrequently shows scattered positive staining for epithelial markers, including cytokeratins CAM5.2 and AE1/AE3 (10% positivity overall) and epithelial membrane antigen (EMA) (5% positivity overall). ALK-1 immunostains are usually negative.[34,53,70,74,75]

Leiomyosarcoma must be differentiated from several other tumors, including leiomyoma, sarcomatoid carcinoma, RMS, PSCNs, and IMTs (Tables 19-1 and 19-2). The diagnosis of a leiomyoma should be reserved for circumscribed, noninfiltrating lesions demonstrating virtually no mitotic activity and minimal cytologic atypia. Sarcomatoid carcinoma is often accompanied by a history of a high grade urothelial carcinoma or the presence of associated urothelial carcinoma, in situ or invasive.[30] Therefore, extensive tissue sampling is recommended. Immunohistochemical staining in sarcomatoid carcinoma is generally positive for low-molecular-weight cytokeratin and EMA. Sarcomatoid carcinoma usually shows negative immunostaining for myogenous markers such as desmin and muscle-specific actin, although rarely it may be diffusely positive. While leiomyosarcomas may show cytokeratin immunoreactivity, the staining pattern is usually focal or patchy and often weak.[27] RMS may have a myxoid appearance, but this tumor is extremely rare in adults. The presence of cross-striations in tumor cells, a cambium layer, or positive staining for myogenin, all features of RMS, can help differentiate these two tumors. A malignant tumor without an obvious carcinomatous component, strong, diffuse, desmin and actin reactivity, with only focal or absent cytokeratin expression, is probably a leiomyosarcoma. PSCNs, IMTs, and leiomyosarcoma can all exhibit abundant mitotic activity, infiltrative growth patterns, and inflammation; only leiomyosarcoma demonstrates cytologic atypia. PSCNs and IMTs often show positive immunostaining for epithelial markers.[70]

Rhabdomyosarcoma

Approximately 20% of primary RMSs arise in the urinary bladder. RMS is a tumor of childhood and adolescence (see also Chapter 18).[3,76] Indeed, RMS is the most common malignant tumor of the bladder in children, showing a slight male predominance.[54,57,77–93] A handful of reports in the literature have described bladder RMSs in adults.[82,83,93–95] The prognosis of adult RMSs is generally poor; most patients died of diseases within months after the diagnosis.

The classic presenting symptom of RMS is gross hematuria. These tumors may also present with an abdominal mass or obstructive voiding symptoms.[84] The most frequent site of involvement is the region of the trigone, making partial cystectomy difficult. Several histologic variants of RMS are seen in the bladder, with embryonal RMS (including the botryoid subtype), being the most common. Grossly, embryonal RMS, especially the botryoid variant, often appears as a polypoid and lobulated mass protruding into the bladder lumen. A tumor is composed of polypoid masses containing condensed rhabdomyoblasts immediately beneath the epithelium (cambium layer) and an edematous stroma with dispersed malignant spindle cells (Figs. 19-41 to 19-44). Embryonal RMS is the most common histologic type. Well-differentiated rhabdomyoblasts may be difficult to identify; they are elongated spindled cells with hyperchromatic small nuclei with visible cytoplasmic cross-striations. Alveolar RMS appears more often in adults. These tumors exhibit thin fibrovascular septae resembling alveolar airspaces, which are lined by a single layer of cuboida, or hobnail tumor cells with hyperchromatic nuclei. Deceptively, alveolar RMS may grow in confluent sheets; in which case, it may

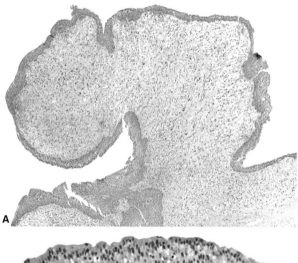

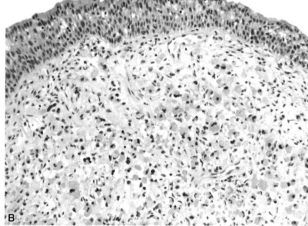

Figure 19-41   Rhabdomyosarcoma with botryoid growth (A and B).

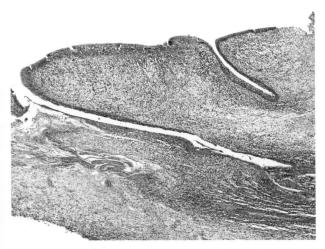

Figure 19-42 Rhabdomyosarcoma with botryoid growth and a cambium layer consisting of condensed rhabdomyoblasts, beneath which is paucicellular tumor.

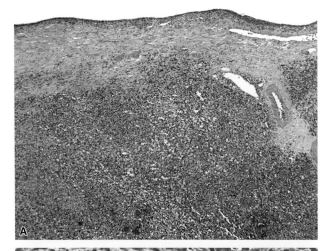

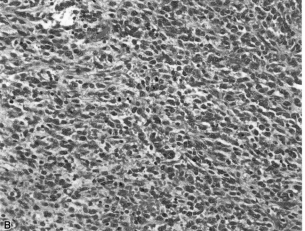

Figure 19-44 Rhabdomyosarcoma with a mixture of small round to spindle cells, strap cells, and rhabdomyoblasts with abundant eosinophilic cytoplasm (A and B).

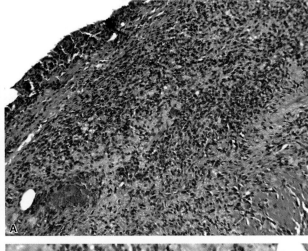

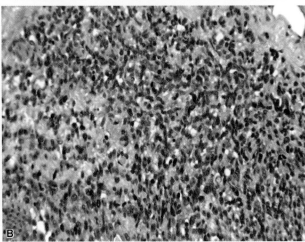

Figure 19-43 Rhabdomyosarcoma with a cambium layer (A and B).

be termed solid alveolar RMS. However, such tumors may be recognized as alveolar RMS, since the cells individually resemble those of the classic pattern.[93] Tumors composed of mixed alveolar and embryonal types sometimes occur, and the biologic behavior of such cases appears to be similar to that of pure alveolar RMS. Tumors exhibiting botryoid growth and only superficial infiltration of the bladder wall behave least aggressively, whereas those with alveolar growth pattern or deeper infiltration carry a poorer prognosis.

In adults, the major diagnostic considerations are sarcomatoid carcinoma with heterologous component (RMS), small cell carcinoma, and primitive neuroectodermal tumor (PNET) (see also **Chapters 15** and **26**).[30] Immunostaining is useful in difficult cases. RMSs are positive for muscle differentiation markers, including desmin, myogenin, MyoD1, as well as muscle-specific actin, myoglobin, and myosin. RMS may also be positive for neuroendocrine markers such as synaptophysin and neuron-specific enolase. Scattered positivity for cytokeratin may also be present.

Angiosarcoma

Angiosarcoma of the bladder, which arises from blood vessel endothelium, is exceedingly rare and carries a very poor prognosis. Fewer than a dozen cases have been reported in the literature.[96-100] Of these, two arose from bladder hemangiomas, two arose in areas of previous radiation therapy, two were preceded by skin lesions, and four occurred de novo without other apparent associations. Angiosarcoma can develop in any part of the bladder. The reported age of occurrence ranges from 38 years to 85 years, with an average of 55 years. There is a male predominance. The development of angiosarcoma has been linked to exposure to certain environmental agents, including vinyl chloride, arsenic, and therapeutic irradiation.[96] All cases have presented with hematuria. Other reported symptoms include flank or groin pain and dysuria. The disease has often extended locally outside the confines of the bladder or has metastasized at the time of presentation. Lung and liver are frequent sites of metastases; lymphatic spread is observed less often. Angiosarcoma originating in the bladder reportedly has a worse prognosis than for similar tumors arising at other sites, with 70% of patients dying within 24 months of diagnosis. Two of the 10 patients reported with bladder angiosarcoma were alive and tumor free at 8 months and 32 months after multimodal therapy.[96,99]

Histologically, angiosarcoma of the bladder is composed of anastomosing vascular channels lined by atypical endothelial cells, often with overlying surface ulceration and inflammation, and typically infiltrating detrusor muscle (**Figs. 19-45** to **19-47**). The poorly differentiated endothelial cells are often pleomorphic with large hyperchromatic nuclei, prominent nucleoli, and frequent mitotic figures. The malignant cells lining the vascular spaces may exhibit a "hobnail" appearance. There is often little or no intervening stroma. Vascular channels range in size from small capillaries to sinusoidal spaces (**Fig. 19-48**). A solid growth pattern consisting of monomorphic cells with vesicular chromatin and moderate amounts of eosinophilic cytoplasm arranged in sheets and nests has been described in some cases, and some tumors have exhibited epithelioid features (**Fig. 19-49**).[96-99]

Immunohistochemically, angiosarcoma stains positively for vimentin, CD31, and CD34, and shows variable immunoreactivity for factor VIII-related antigen. The only epithelioid angiosarcoma of the bladder reported showed negative immunostaining for cytokeratin AE1/AE3, although epithelioid angiosarcoma at other sites may stain positively for cytokeratin.

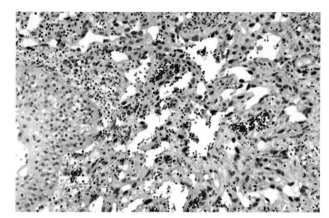

Figure 19-45   Angiosarcoma of the bladder, with typical vascular channels lined by malignant endothelial cells.

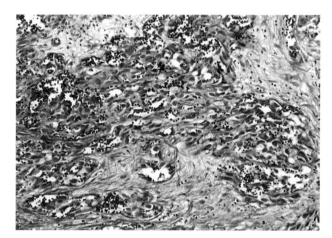

Figure 19-46   Angiosarcoma.

The key differential diagnosis for angiosarcoma of the bladder is hemangioma, which is usually small and lacks cytologic atypia, interanastomosing channels, and solid areas.[55] Kaposi sarcoma may be seen in the urinary bladder, especially in immunocompromised patients. High grade urothelial carcinoma must also be considered in the differential; in such tumors, a focus of obvious in situ or invasive carcinoma may be present, and tumor cells demonstrate positive immunoreactivity for cytokeratin antibodies and lack reactivity for endothelial markers such as CD31 and CD34.

Malignant Fibrous Histiocytoma

Primary MFH of the bladder is rare, although some contend that it is the second most common sarcoma of the adult urinary tract.[54,71,101] It occurs predominantly in men in their fifth to eighth decades of life. In one series of patients with MFH of the urinary bladder, seven of eight tumors occurred

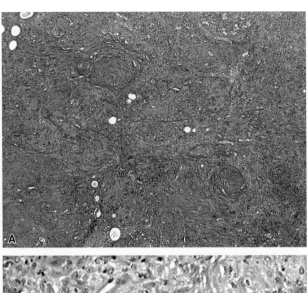

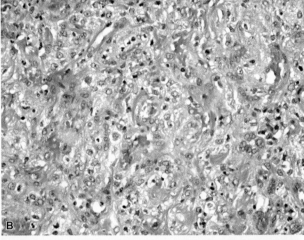

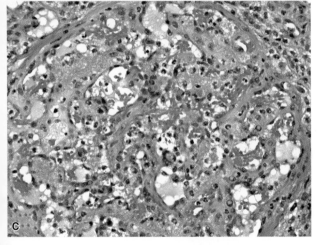

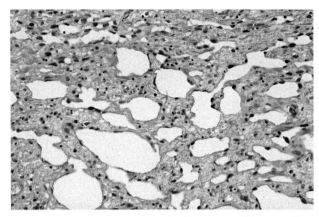

Figure 19-48 Angiosarcoma. The lumens are dilated and the malignant cells may be mistaken for reactive endothelial cells.

Figure 19-47 Angiosarcoma (A to C). Tumor consisting of anastomosing vascular channels lined by atypical endothelial cells. Poorly differentiated endothelial cells have pleomorphic hyperchromatic nuclei with prominent nucleoli and exhibit a "hobnail" appearance.

in men; patients ranged in age from 45 years to 79 years.[54] Patients often present with gross hematuria.

MFH of the urinary bladder is often large at presentation, and most involve the full thickness of the bladder wall (**Figs. 19-50** and **19-51**). The overlying urothelium may be normal or absent, with ulceration. In the series of eight cases of MFH reported by Kunze et al., tumors ranged from 1 cm to 15 cm in greatest dimension. Four morphological variants of MFH are recognized, including myxoid, inflammatory, storiform-fascicular, and pleomorphic (**Figs. 19-52** to **19-54**). Of the eight tumors reported by Kunze et al., three were of the storiform-fascicular type, composed of spindled or polygonal cells with varying degrees of cytologic atypia and variably sized oval to round nuclei displaying coarse chromatin and prominent nucleoli. Mitotic activity was moderate to high. Multinucleated giant cells were often scattered throughout these tumors. Four of eight MFHs in this series were regarded as examples of inflammatory MFH, composed of dense, large polyhedral cells with abundant pale cytoplasm and irregular nuclei. Frequent mitotic figures and isolated multinucleated giant cells were identified. Many inflammatory cells, especially neutrophils, were admixed with the tumor cells, and phagocytic debris was apparent within some tumor cells. The remaining tumor in this series was a pleomorphic MFH, composed of a densely cellular population of pleomorphic, polygonal cells with abundant pale, somewhat vacuolated cytoplasm with very pleomorphic nuclei and, often, bizarre nucleoli. Atypical mitotic figures and multinucleated giant cells were also present.[54] A single case of MFH with focal rhabdoid features arising in the bladder has been reported.[101]

Immunohistochemically, MFH is nonreactive for cytokeratin. It is often reactive for vimentin, α_1-antichymotrypsin, and focally reactive for CD68. Some tumors may be positive for neuron-specific enolase and S100 protein.

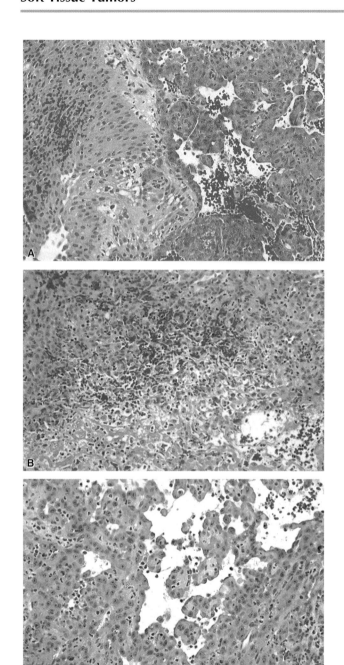

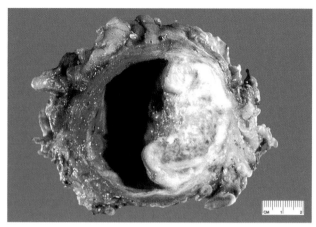

Figure 19-50 Malignant fibrous histiocytoma. This gross image of the bladder reveals a large fleshy mural mass on one side partially filling the lumen.

Figure 19-49 Epithelioid angiosarcoma of the urinary bladder. (A) The sarcoma (right) is present in intimate association with the urothelium (left), and concern was raised for possible sarcomatoid carcinoma. Elsewhere, the angiosarcoma consisted of (B) closely packed vascular structures with extravasated red blood cells, or (C) papillary tufts lined by malignant cells.

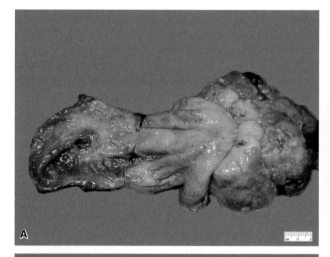

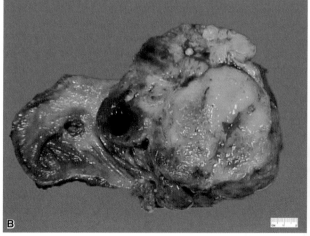

Figure 19-51 Malignant fibrous histiocytoma (A and B).

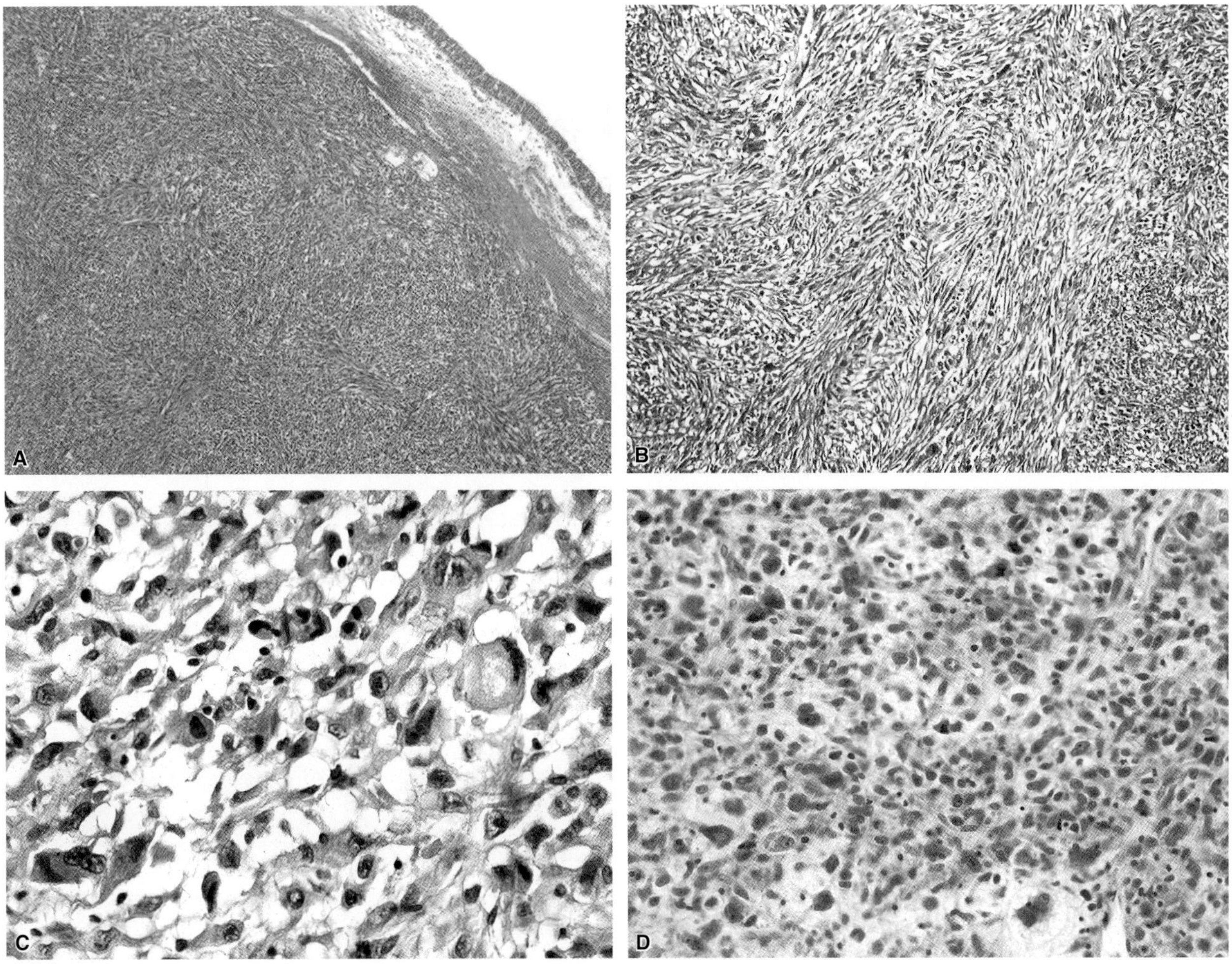

Figure 19-52 Malignant fibrous histiocytoma. The sarcoma is transmural, with an overlying intact urothelium (A). The spindle cells are arranged predominantly in a storiform pattern (B). There is prominent pleomorphism (C). In another case, large multinucleated cells punctuate sheets of smaller tumor cells (D).

Several tumors enter into the differential diagnosis of MFH (**Tables 19-1** and **19-2**). Sarcomatoid carcinoma of the bladder may have a similar appearance, but an epithelial component may be identifiable, or the true nature of the tumor may be revealed by its immunoreactivity to cytokeratin and/or EMA. Differentiating MFHs from IMTs or PSCNs may be difficult. Identifying mixed acute and chronic inflammatory cells and a history of a surgical procedure favors PSCNs. Furthermore, reactive spindle cell proliferations lack cytologic atypia, tumor necrosis, and atypical mitotic figures.

MFHs of the bladder are very aggressive tumors with a high local recurrence rate and frequent metastasis. For example, Egawa et al. reported a case of an 84-year-old woman with inflammatory MFH of the bladder, without evidence of metastases at the time of diagnosis.[101] However, 4 months after surgery and chemotherapy, the patient had a local recurrence. Three months after the

recurrence was treated with radiation, the patient died with widespread metastases.[101] Treatment is usually surgical, combined in some instances with chemotherapy and radiation, but prolonged survival is infrequent. The literature includes one report of a patient with myxoid MFH who survived three years after surgery, chemotherapy, and radiation.[101]

Primitive Neuroectodermal Tumor

PNET of the bladder is an extremely rare, highly aggressive neoplasm belonging to the Ewing family of tumors.[102-104] It is morphologically a small round blue cell tumor that is often associated with extensive necrosis (**Fig. 19-55**). The tumor cells show strong immunoreactivity for CD99 and CD117 (c-kit) and may show focal staining with cytokeratin AE1/AE3 markers and S100 protein. CD99 is not specific for PNETs or Ewing sarcoma, but it is almost

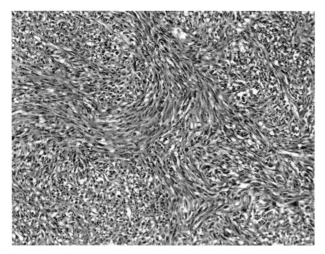

Figure 19-53 Malignant fibrous histiocytoma. Tumor cells are in a storiform/fascicular arrangement and show varying degrees of cytologic atypia with variably sized nuclei and prominent nucleoli.

always present in these tumors. Molecular genetic analysis supports the diagnosis of PNET by showing the *EWS/FLI-1* fusion transcript type 2 by RT-PCR and *EWS* gene rearrangement by FISH.

The differential diagnosis for PNETs includes RMS, lymphoid neoplasms, neuroendocrine carcinoma, and melanoma. Immunohistochemical staining helps in differentiating PNET from the other entities in the differential; negative immunostaining for muscle, lymphoid, melanocytic, and neuroendocrine markers favors PNETs. Metastatic neuroendocrine carcinoma generally expresses epithelial markers more strongly than PNETs.[102,104]

See **Chapter 15** for further discussion.

Malignant Peripheral Nerve Sheath Tumor

Malignant peripheral nerve sheath tumor (MPNST) is rare in the urinary bladder. Only a few cases have been documented.[105–107] The tumor appears to affect patients under 40 years of age, typically with complaints of hematuria; a suprapubic mass is noted in some. Prognosis is poor. Microscopically, MPNST is composed of poorly differentiated tumor cells arranged in sheets or nodules, or of interlacing fascicles of malignant spindle cells.

See **Chapter 15** for further discussion.

Hemangiopericytoma

Rare cases of hemangiopericytoma have been reported in the urinary bladder.[108–113] The tumor typically occurs in adults with an average age of 45 years.[114] It occurs equally in both genders. Intensive exposure to poly(vinyl chloride) was implicated as a causative agent in one case.[108] An

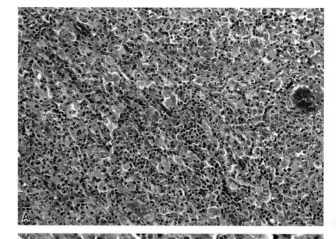

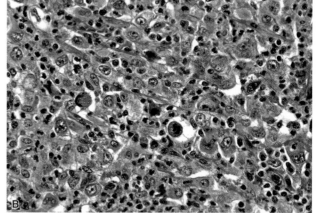

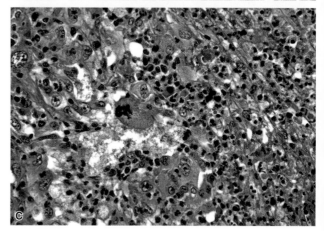

Figure 19-54 Malignant fibrous histiocytoma (A to C). Note the atypical mitotic figures and inflammatory background.

association with hypoglycemia has been reported, possibly mediated by tumor production of insulin-like growth factor.[110,114] Hemangiopericytomas are slowly enlarging painless masses, often presenting late in their course, at which time obstructive symptoms may occur. Groin pain, urinary frequency, dysuria, and acute urinary retention have been reported.[108,109,112,113] Despite its deceptively

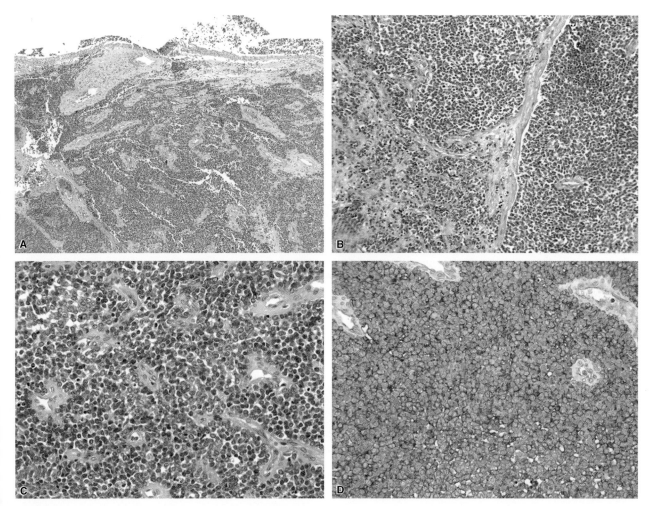

Figure 19-55 Primitive neuroectodermal tumor. (A) The tumor is highly cellular and consists of small, round blue cells in sheets surrounded by fibrovascular stroma. (B) Tumor cells are monomorphic with scant basophilic cytoplasm. (C) Pseudorosette formation is seen. (D) Cells are immunoreactive for CD99.

benign appearance, hemangiopericytoma is associated with a 50% incidence of eventual metastasis.[108]

Grossly, hemangiopericytoma is usually well-circumscribed and covered by a thin, richly vascular pseudocapsule. On cut section, it is gray to red-brown, often with areas of hemorrhage and necrosis.[114]

Microscopically, hemangiopericytoma is composed of an elaborate arrangement of vascular spaces consisting of proliferating blood vessels surrounded by numerous, tightly packed ovoid and spindle-shaped pericytes (Fig. 19-56).[114,115] The vessels vary in caliber and branch into smaller vessels with a "staghorn" configuration.[114] The vessels often are arrayed in a collagenous background. Malignant features include necrosis, increased cellularity, hemorrhage, and increased mitotic activity.[114]

Immunohistochemical reactivity for vimentin is often present in hemangiopericytoma, and some cases show positive immunostaining for CD34. Rarely, focal immunostaining for actin and desmin is observed. CD31 immunostaining

is observed only in the endothelial cells lining the vascular spaces.[114]

The differential diagnosis for hemangiopericytoma in the urinary bladder includes solitary fibrous tumor. Hemangiopericytoma has a prominent pericytic vascular pattern that is only focally evident in solitary fibrous tumor. Solitary fibrous tumor is always immunoreactive for CD34, while hemangiopericytoma displays CD34 immunoreactivity in a smaller percentage of cases and to a lesser degree. Solitary fibrous tumor displays broader zones of hyalinization. MFH may be confused with hemangiopericytoma, but MFH has a more prominent and uniform spindle cell architecture, lacking the elaborate vascular patterns typical of hemangiopericytoma.[114]

The cytogenetic abnormality most commonly associated with hemangiopericytoma is rearrangement of the long arm of chromosome 12, although this abnormality has not, to our knowledge, been reported in tumors originated from the urinary bladder.[114]

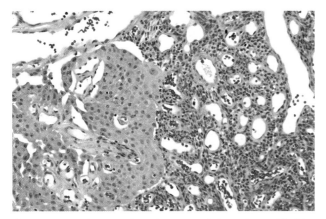

Figure 19-56 Hemangiopericytoma of the urinary bladder. The urothelium (left) stands in contrast with the tumor (right), which consists of a characteristic pattern of anastomosing vessels surrounded by tumor cells with indistinct cellular outlines.

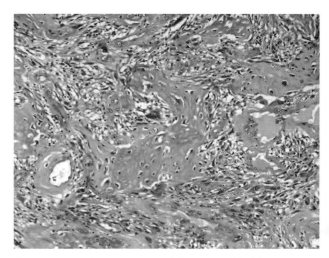

Figure 19-57 Osteosarcoma of the urinary bladder.

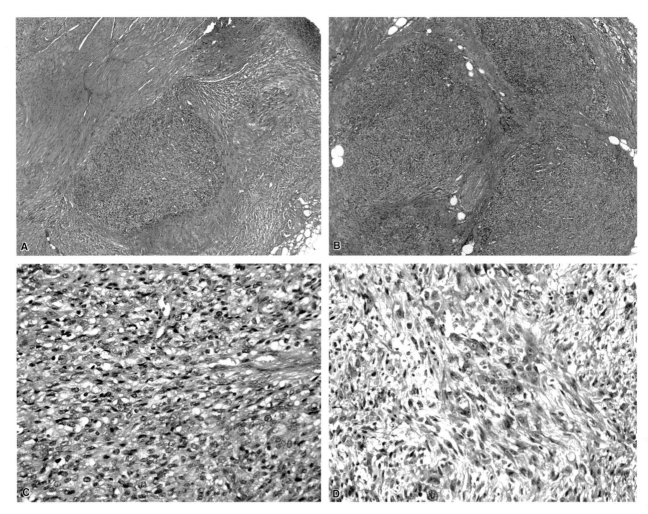

Figure 19-58 Stromal sarcoma of the urinary bladder (A to D).

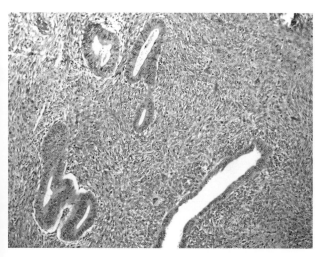

Figure 19-59   Müllerian adenosarcoma of the urinary bladder.

Alveolar Soft Part Sarcoma

Recently, a single case of alveolar soft part sarcoma has been identified in the urinary bladder of a 25-year-old woman.[116] This entity is rare, usually found in the lower extremities of adolescents and young adults, or in the head and neck region of children.[116] The patient presented with dysuria and hematuria. A large intravesical mass was resected. Microscopically, the tumor was composed of sheets and nests of large polygonal to round cells with abundant foamy to clear to finely granular eosinophilic cytoplasm. Nuclei were round with prominent nucleoli, but without pleomorphism or significant mitotic activity. The tumor nests were delineated by fibrovascular trabeculae of varying thickness. Other nests were separated by thin-walled vascular channels. The tumor infiltrated into the muscularis propria and ulcerated the overlying mucosa. The granular cytoplasmic material was found to be periodic acid–Schiff positive with diastase resistance. The tumor did not stain immunohistochemically for desmin, SMA, EMA, cytokeratins, chromogranin, synaptophysin, S100, HMB45, Melan A, CD117, CD34, CD68, CD10, or renal cell carcinoma antibody. However, it showed strong diffuse nuclear immunoreactivity for TFE3. TFE3 is a commercially available antibody directed against the TFE3 protein, which is virtually always seen in alveolar soft part sarcoma. It may also be immunoreactive in Xp11 translocation-associated renal cell carcinoma and benign granular cell tumors. The ASPL-TFE3 fusion protein, detected by the TFE3 antibody, results from a specific translocation, der(17)t(X;17)(p11.2;q25), which is the molecular signature of alveolar soft parts sarcoma.[116] The tumor recurred subsequently as a painful mass protruding from the urethral meatus, and was surgically resected. Grossly, the recurrent tumor was a nonencapsulated well-circumscribed red-tan mass with focal hemorrhage

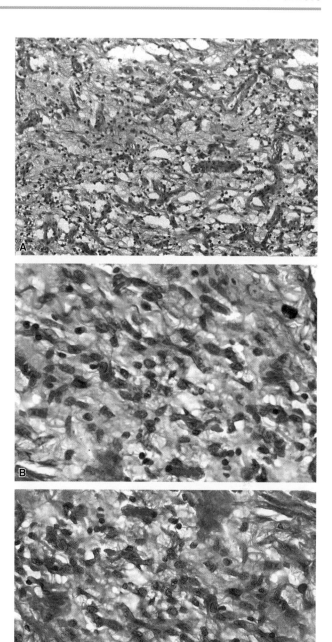

Figure 19-60   Aggressive angiomyxoma arising in the bladder in a patient with Peutz–Jeghers syndrome. (A and B) The tumor consists of spindle cells and stellate cells with thin-walled and thick-walled hyaline vessels in a myxoid stroma. (C) The tumor cells have little or no nuclear atypia and no mitotic activity. (Case courtesy of Dr. Aidan Carney, Rochester, Minnesota.)

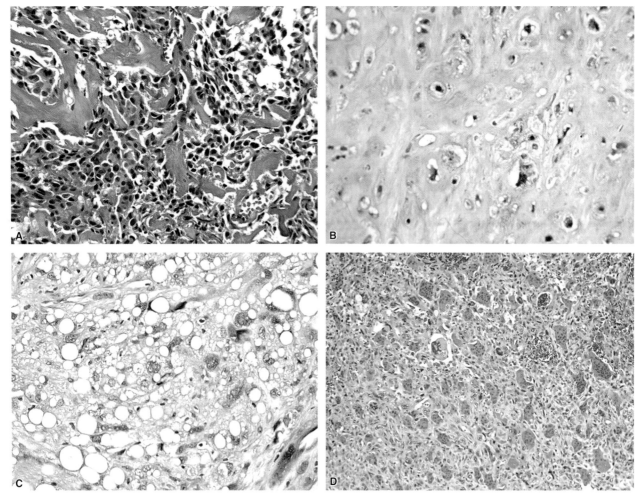

Figure 19-61 Heterologous elements are often seen in sarcomatoid carcinom. (A) The most common is osteosarcoma. (B) The second most common heterologous element in these tumors is chondrosarcoma. (C) Liposarcoma is an infrequent heterologous component of these tumors. (D) Numerous giant cells may be seen in sarcomatoid carcinoma of the bladder. (From Ref. 30; with permission.)

and necrosis. The recurrent tumor was histologically similar to the original tumor except for patchy necrosis as well as areas with cells having central eosinophilic granularity surrounded by a rim of clear cytoplasm.[116] No further recurrence was noted 45 months after the initial presentation.

Included in the differential diagnosis for this tumor are paraganglioma, PEComa, malignant granular cell tumor, and epithelioid leiomyosarcoma. Immunohistochemistry plays a critical role in differentiating these tumors.[29,117] Paragangliomas express neuroendocrine markers, such as chromogranin and synaptophysin. Granular cell tumors are strongly immunoreactive for S100 protein. PEComas express melanocytic markers such as HMB45 and Melan A. PEComa and epithelioid leiomyosarcoma show strong SMA reactivity. The aforementioned immunostains are all absent in alveolar soft parts sarcoma. Desmin expression,

however, may be seen. As stated previously, alveolar soft parts sarcoma expresses TFE3, which, except for granular cell tumor, is absent in the other tumors included in the differential diagnosis.[116]

Other Soft Tissues Neoplasms Arising in the Bladder

Rare examples of other types of sarcoma have been reported to arise in the bladder, including liposarcoma, chondrosarcoma, osteosarcoma, stromal sarcoma, müllerian adenosarcoma, angiomyxoma, and Kaposi sarcoma (**Figs. 19-57** to **19-60**). The diagnosis of primary liposarcoma of the bladder requires that bladder involvement by direct extension from a malignancy in an adjacent site be

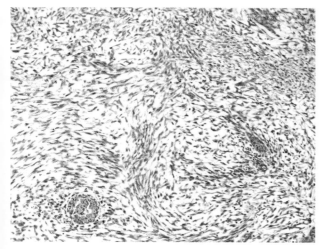

Figure 19-62 Myxoid variant of sarcomatoid carcinoma of the bladder. It should not be mistaken for malignant fibrous histiocytoma. (From Ref. 30; with permission.)

excluded. In the case of primary bladder chondrosarcoma or osteosarcoma, sarcomatoid carcinoma (with heterogonous components) must be excluded (**Figs. 19-61** to **19-62**).[30] Complete sampling is mandatory before the diagnosis can be rendered.

Rare case series of bladder sarcomas in the medical literature describe sarcomas that have not been identifiable as to specific subtype.[118–120] If inadequate tissue or poor preservation of a specimen prevent subtyping, a diagnosis of sarcoma, unclassified, is warranted.[121] In general, these tumors are high grade and are associated with a higher risk of progression and death than that for patients with urothelial carcinoma or squamous cell carcinoma of the bladder.[120] A five-year survival rate of approximately 60% was reported for both sarcoma and leiomyosarcoma of the urinary bladder.[118]

REFERENCES

1. Cheng L, Foster SR, MacLennan GT, Lopez-Beltran A, Zhang S, Montironi R. Inflammatory myofibroblastic tumors of the genitourinary tract—single entity or continuum? *J Urol* 2008;180:1235–40.
2. Lott S, Lopez-Beltran A, Maclennan GT, Montironi R, Cheng L. Soft tissue tumors of the urinary bladder, Part I: myofibroblastic proliferations, benign neoplasms, and tumors of uncertain malignant potential. *Hum Pathol* 2007;38:807–23.
3. Lott S, Lopez-Beltran A, Montironi R, MacLennan GT, Cheng L. Soft tissue tumors of the urinary bladder: Part II: Malignant neoplasms. *Hum Pathol* 2007;38:807–23.
4. Brunn H. Two interesting benign lung tumors of contradictory histopathology. *J Thorac Surg* 1939;9:119–31.
5. Roth JA. Reactive pseudosarcomatous response in urinary bladder. *Urology* 1980;16:635–7.
6. Proppe KH, Scully RE, Rosai J. Postoperative spindle cell nodules of genitourinary tract resembling sarcomas. A report of eight cases. *Am J Surg Pathol* 1984;8:101–8.
7. Pettinato G, Manivel JC, De Rosa N, Dehner LP. Inflammatory myofibroblastic tumor (plasma cell granuloma). Clinicopathologic study of 20 cases with immunohistochemical and ultrastructural observations. *Am J Clin Pathol* 1990;94:538–46.
8. Netto JM, Perez LM, Kelly DR, Joseph DB. Pediatric inflammatory bladder tumors: myofibroblastic and eosinophilic subtypes. *J Urol* 1999;162:1424–9.
9. Weidner N. Inflammatory (myofibroblastic) pseudotumor of the bladder: a review and differential diagnosis. *Adv Anat Pathol* 1995;2:362–75.
10. Young RH. Spindle cell lesions of the urinary bladder. *Histol Histopathol* 1990;5:505–12.
11. Coffin CM, Dehner LP, Meis-Kindblom JM. Inflammatory myofibroblastic tumor, inflammatory fibrosarcoma, and related lesions: an historical review with differential diagnostic considerations. *Semin Diagn Pathol* 1998;15:102–10.
12. Montgomery EA, Shuster DD, Burkart AL, Esteban JM, Sgrignoli A, Elwood L, Vaughn DJ, Griffin CA, Epstein JI. Inflammatory myofibroblastic tumors of the urinary tract: a clinicopathologic study of 46 cases, including a malignant example inflammatory fibrosarcoma and a subset associated with high grade urothelial carcinoma. *Am J Surg Pathol* 2006;30:1502–12.
13. Sirvent N, Hawkins AL, Moeglin D, Coindre JM, Kurzenne JY, Michiels JF, Barcelo G, Turc-Carel C, Griffin CA, Pedeutour F. ALK probe rearrangement in a t(2;11;2)(p23;p15;q31) translocation found in a prenatal myofibroblastic fibrous lesion: Toward a molecular definition of an inflammatory myofibroblastic tumor family? *Genes Chromosomes Cancer* 2001;31:85–90.
14. Harik LR, Merino C, Coindre JM, Amin MB, Pedeutour F, Weiss SW. Pseudosarcomatous myofibroblastic proliferations of the bladder: a clinicopathologic study of 42 cases. *Am J Surg Pathol* 2006;30:787–94.
15. Jones EC, Clement PB, Young RH. Inflammatory pseudotumor of the urinary bladder: a clinicopathological, immunohistochemical, ultrastructural, and flow cytometric study of 13 cases. *Am J Surg Pathol* 1993;17:264–74.
16. Gofrit ON, Pode D, Shapiro A, Zorn KC, Pizov G. Significance of inflammatory pseudotumors in patients with a history of bladder cancer. *Urology* 2007;69:1064–7.

17. Coffin CM, Hornick JL, Fletcher CD. Inflammatory myofibroblastic tumor: comparison of clinicopathologic, histologic, and immunohistochemical features including ALK expression in atypical and aggressive cases. *Am J Surg Pathol* 2007;31:509–20.

18. Gomez-Roman JJ, Ocejo-Vinyals G, Sanchez-Velasco P, Nieto EH, Leyva-Cobian F, Val-Bernal JF. Presence of human herpesvirus–8 DNA sequences and overexpression of human IL–6 and cyclin D1 in inflammatory myofibroblastic tumor (inflammatory pseudotumor). *Lab Invest* 2000;80:1121–6.

19. Horn LC, Reuter S, Biesold M. Inflammatory pseudotumor of the ureter and the urinary bladder. *Pathol Res Pract* 1997;193:607–12.

20. Perez-Ordonez B, Rosai J. Follicular dendritic cell tumor: review of the entity. *Semin Diagn Pathol* 1998;15:144–54.

21. Arber DA, Weiss LM, Chang KL. Detection of Epstein-Barr virus in inflammatory pseudotumor. *Semin Diagn Pathol* 1998;15:155–60.

22. Kojima M, Nakamura S, Itoh H, Suchi T, Masawa N. Inflammatory pseudotumor of the submandibular gland: report of a case presenting with autoimmune disease-like clinical manifestations. *Arch Pathol Lab Med* 2001;125:1095–7.

23. Al-Ahmadie H, Gomez AM, Trane N, Bove KE. Giant botryoid fibroepithelial polyp of bladder with myofibroblastic stroma and cystitis cystica et glandularis. *Pediatr Dev Pathol* 2003;6:179–81.

24. Harper L, Michel JL, Riviere JP, Alsawhi A, De Napoli-Cocci S. Inflammatory pseudotumor of the ureter. *J Pediatr Surg* 2005;40:597–9.

25. Cespedes RD, Lynch SC, Grider DJ. Pseudosarcomatous fibromyxoid tumor of the prostate. A case report with review of the literature. *Urol Int* 1996;57:249–51.

26. Kapusta LR, Weiss MA, Ramsay J, Lopez-Beltran A, Srigley JR. Inflammatory myofibroblastic tumors of the kidney: a clinicopathologic and immunohistochemical study of 12 cases. *Am J Surg Pathol* 2003;27:658–66.

27. Hodges KB, Lopez-Beltran A, Emerson RE, Montironi R, Cheng L. Clinical utility of immunohistochemistry in the diagnoses of urinary bladder neoplasia. *Appl Immunohistochem Mol Morphol* 2010;18:401–10.

28. Coffin CM, Watterson J, Priest JR, Dehner LP. Extrapulmonary inflammatory myofibroblastic tumor (inflammatory pseudotumor). A clinicopathologic and immunohistochemical study of 84 cases. *Am J Surg Pathol* 1995;19:859–72.

29. Emerson RE, Cheng L. Immunohistochemical markers in the evaluation of tumors of the urinary bladder: a review. *Anal Quant Cytol Histol* 2005;27:301–16.

30. Cheng L, Zhang S, Alexander R, MacLennan GT, Hodges KB, Harrison BT, Lopez-Beltran A, Montironi R. Sarcomatoid carcinoma of the urinary bladder: the final common pathway of urothelial carcinoma dedifferentiation. *Am J Surg Pathol* 2011;35:e34–46.

31. Freeman A, Geddes N, Munson P, Joseph J, Ramani P, Sandison A, Fisher C, Parkinson MC. Anaplastic lymphoma kinase (ALK 1) staining and molecular analysis in inflammatory myofibroblastic tumours of the bladder: a preliminary clinicopathological study of nine cases and review of the literature. *Mod Pathol* 2004;17:765–71.

32. Coffin CM, Patel A, Perkins S, Elenitoba-Johnson KS, Perlman E, Griffin CA. ALK1 and p80 expression and chromosomal rearrangements involving 2p23 in inflammatory myofibroblastic tumor. *Mod Pathol* 2001;14:569–76.

33. Patel AS, Murphy KM, Hawkins AL, Cohen JS, Long PP, Perlman EJ, Griffin CA. RANBP2 and CLTC are involved in ALK rearrangements in inflammatory myofibroblastic tumors. *Cancer Genet Cytogenet* 2007;176:107–14.

34. Cessna MH, Zhou H, Sanger WG, Perkins SL, Tripp S, Pickering D, Daines C, Coffin CM. Expression of ALK1 and p80 in inflammatory myofibroblastic tumor and its mesenchymal mimics: a study of 135 cases. *Mod Pathol* 2002;15:931–8.

35. Debiec-Rychter M, Marynen P, Hagemeijer A, Pauwels P. ALK-ATIC fusion in urinary bladder inflammatory myofibroblastic tumor. *Genes Chromosomes Cancer* 2003;38:187–90.

36. Shanks JH, Iczkowski KA. Divergent differentiation in urothelial carcinoma and other bladder cancer subtypes with selected mimics. *Histopathology* 2009;54:885–900.

37. Amin MB. Histological variants of urothelial carcinoma: diagnostic, therapeutic and prognostic implications. *Mod Pathol* 2009;22 (Suppl 2):S96–S118.

38. Lopez-Beltran A, Pacelli A, Rothenberg HJ, Wollan PC, Zincke H, Blute ML, Bostwick DG. Carcinosarcoma and sarcomatoid carcinoma of the bladder: clinicopathological study of 41 cases. *J Urol* 1998;159:1497–503.

39. Jones EC, Young RH. Myxoid and sclerosing sarcomatoid transitional cell carcinoma of the urinary bladder: a clinicopathologic and immunohistochemical study of 25 cases. *Mod Pathol* 1997;10:908–16.

40. Westfall DE, Folpe AL, Paner GP, Oliva E, Goldstein L, Alsabeh R, Gown AM, Amin MB. Utility of a comprehensive immunohistochemical panel in the differential diagnosis of spindle cell lesions of the urinary bladder. *Am J Surg Pathol* 2009;33:99–105.

41. Iczkowski KA, Shanks JH, Gadaleanu V, Cheng L, Jones EC, Neumann R, Nascimento AG, Bostwick DG. Inflammatory pseudotumor and sarcoma of urinary bladder: differential diagnosis and outcome in thirty-eight spindle cell neoplasms. *Mod Pathol* 2001;14:1043–51.

42. Hojo H, Newton WA Jr, Hamoudi AB, Qualman SJ, Wakasa H, Suzuki S, Jaynes F. Pseudosarcomatous myofibroblastic tumor of the urinary bladder in children: a study of 11 cases with review of the literature. An Intergroup Rhabdomyosarcoma Study. *Am J Surg Pathol* 1995;19:1224–36.

43. Meis JM, Enzinger FM. Inflammatory fibrosarcoma of the mesentery and retroperitoneum. A tumor closely simulating inflammatory pseudotumor. *Am J Surg Pathol* 1991;15:1146–56.

44. Angulo JC, Lopez JI, Flores N. Pseudosarcomatous myofibroblastic proliferation of the bladder: report of 2 cases and literature review. *J Urol* 1994;151:1008–12.
45. Hughes DF, Biggart JD, Hayes D. Pseudosarcomatous lesions of the urinary bladder. *Histopathology* 1991;18:67–71.
46. Mottet-Auselo N, Marsollier C, Chapuis H, Costa P, el Sandid M, Louis JF, Marty-Double C, Navratil H. Postoperative pseudosarcomatous nodule: report of one case and review of the literature. *Eur Urol* 1994;25:262–4.
47. Chan JK, Cheuk W, Shimizu M. Anaplastic lymphoma kinase expression in inflammatory pseudotumors. *Am J Surg Pathol* 2001;25:761–8.
48. Jones E, Young R. Nonneoplastic and neoplastic spindle cell proliferations and mixed tumors of the urinary bladder. *J Urol Pathol* 1994;2:105–34.
49. Hirsch MS, Dal Cin P, Fletcher CD. ALK expression in pseudosarcomatous myofibroblastic proliferations of the genitourinary tract. *Histopathology* 2006;48:569–78.
50. Mazzucchelli R, Barbisan F, Tarquini LM, Streccioni M, Galosi AB. Urothelial changes induced by therapeutic procedures for bladder cancer. A review. *Anal Quant Cytol Histol* 2005;27:27–34.
51. Chen M, Lipson SA, Hricak H. MR imaging evaluation of benign mesenchymal tumors of the urinary bladder. *AJR Am J Roentgenol* 1997;168:399–403.
52. Goluboff ET, O'Toole K, Sawczuk IS. Leiomyoma of bladder: report of case and review of literature. *Urology* 1994;43:238–41.
53. Martin SA, Sears DL, Sebo TJ, Lohse CM, Cheville JC. Smooth muscle neoplasms of the urinary bladder: a clinicopathologic comparison of leiomyoma and leiomyosarcoma. *Am J Surg Pathol* 2002;26:292–300.
54. Kunze E, Theuring F, Kruger G. Primary mesenchymal tumors of the urinary bladder. A histological and immunohistochemical study of 30 cases. *Pathol Res Pract* 1994;190:311–32.
55. Cheng L, Nascimento AG, Neumann RM, Nehra A, Cheville JC, Ramnani DM, Leibovich BC, Bostwick DG. Hemangioma of the urinary bladder. *Cancer* 1999;86:498–504.
56. Cheng L, Scheithauer BW, Leibovich BC, Ramnani DM, Cheville JC, Bostwick DG. Neurofibroma of the urinary bladder. *Cancer* 1999;86:505–13.
57. Sung L, Anderson JR, Arndt C, Raney RB, Meyer WH, Pappo AS. Neurofibromatosis in children with rhabdomyosarcoma: a report from the Intergroup Rhabdomyosarcoma Study IV. *J Pediatr* 2004;144:666–8.
58. Westra WH, Grenko RT, Epstein J. Solitary fibrous tumor of the lower urogenital tract: a report of five cases involving the seminal vesicles, urinary bladder, and prostate. *Hum Pathol* 2000;31:63–8.
59. Mentzel T, Bainbridge TC, Katenkamp D. Solitary fibrous tumour: clinicopathological, immunohistochemical, and ultrastructural analysis of 12 cases arising in soft tissues, nasal cavity and nasopharynx, urinary bladder and prostate. *Virchows Arch* 1997;430:445–53.
60. Cheng L, Leibovich BC, Cheville JC, Ramnani DM, Sebo TJ, Neumann RM, Nascimento AG, Zincke H, Bostwick DG. Paraganglioma of the urinary bladder: Can biologic potential be predicted? *Cancer* 2000;88:844–52.
61. Dahm P, Gschwend JE. Malignant non-urothelial neoplasms of the urinary bladder: a review. *Eur Urol* 2003;44:672–81.
62. Zhou M, Epstein JI, Young RH. Paraganglioma of the urinary bladder: a lesion that may be misdiagnosed as urothelial carcinoma in transurethral resection specimens. *Am J Surg Pathol* 2004;28:94–100.
63. Mouradian J, Coleman J, McGovern J, Gray G. Granular cell tumor (myoblastoma) of the bladder. *J Urol* 1974;112:343–5.
64. Fletcher MS, Aker M, Hill JT, Pryor JP, Whimster WF. Granular cell myoblastoma of the bladder. *Br J Urol* 1985;57:109–10.
65. Seery WH. Granular cell myoblastoma of the bladder: report of a case. *J Urol* 1968;100:735–7.
66. Mizutani S, Okuda N, Sonoda T. Granular cell myoblastoma of the bladder: report of an additional case. *J Urol* 1973;110:403–5.
67. Kontani K, Okaneya T, Takezaki T. Recurrent granular cell tumour of the bladder in a patient with von Recklinghausen's disease. *BJU Int* 1999;84:871–2.
68. Yoshida T, Hirai S, Horii Y, Yamauchi T. Granular cell tumor of the urinary bladder. *Int J Urol* 2001;8:29–31.
69. Kondo T, Kajimoto S, Okuda H, Toma H, Tanabe K. A case of granular cell tumor of the bladder successfully managed with extraperitoneal laparoscopic surgery. *Int J Urol* 2006;13:827–8.
70. Mills SE, Bova GS, Wick MR, Young RH. Leiomyosarcoma of the urinary bladder. A clinicopathologic and immunohistochemical study of 15 cases. *Am J Surg Pathol* 1989;13:480–9.
71. Eble JN, Sauter G, Epstein JI, Sesterhenn IA. World Health Organization Classification of Tumours: Pathology and Genetics of Tumours of the Urinary System and Male Genital Organs. Lyon, France: IARC Press, 2004.
72. Pedersen-Bjergaard J, Jonsson V, Pedersen M, Hou-Jensen K. Leiomyosarcoma of the urinary bladder after cyclophosphamide. *J Clin Oncol* 1995;13:532–3.
73. Tanguay C, Harvey I, Houde M, Srigley JR, Tetu B. Leiomyosarcoma of urinary bladder following cyclophosphamide therapy: report of two cases. *Mod Pathol* 2003;16:512–4.
74. McKenney JK. An approach to the classification of spindle cell proliferations in the urinary bladder. *Adv Anat Pathol* 2005;12:312–23.
75. Tsuzuki T, Magi-Galluzzi C, Epstein JI. ALK–1 expression in inflammatory myofibroblastic tumor of the urinary bladder. *Am J Surg Pathol* 2004;28:1609–14.
76. Williamson SR, Lopez-Beltran A, Maclennan GT, Montironi R, Cheng L. Unique clinicopathologic and molecular characteristics of urinary bladder tumors in children and young adults. *Urol Oncol* (in press 2012).

77. Fleischmann J, Perinetti EP, Catalona WJ. Embryonal rhabdomyosarcoma of the genitourinary organs. *J Urol* 1981;126:389–92.

78. Geary ES, Gong MC, Shortliffe LM. Biology and treatment of pediatric genitourinary tumors. *Curr Opin Oncol* 1994;6:292–300.

79. Parham DM, Ellison DA. Rhabdomyosarcomas in adults and children: an update. *Arch Pathol Lab Med* 2006;130:1454–65.

80. Leuschner I, Harms D, Mattke A, Koscielniak E, Treuner J. Rhabdomyosarcoma of the urinary bladder and vagina: a clinicopathologic study with emphasis on recurrent disease: a report from the Kiel Pediatric Tumor Registry and the German CWS Study. *Am J Surg Pathol* 2001;25:856–64.

81. Arndt C, Rodeberg D, Breitfeld PP, Raney RB, Ullrich F, Donaldson S. Does bladder preservation (as a surgical principle) lead to retaining bladder function in bladder/prostate rhabdomyosarcoma? Results from Intergroup Rhabdomyosarcoma Study IV. *J Urol* 2004;171:2396–403.

82. Lauro S, Lalle M, Scucchi L, Vecchione A. Rhabdomyosarcoma of the urinary bladder in an elderly patient. *Anticancer Res* 1995;15:627–9.

83. Aydoganli L, Tarhan F, Atan A, Akalin Z, Yildiz M. Rhabdomyosarcoma of the urinary bladder in an adult. *Int Urol Nephrol* 1993;25:159–61.

84. Hays DM. Bladder/prostate rhabdomyosarcoma: results of the multi-institutional trials of the Intergroup Rhabdomyosarcoma Study. *Semin Surg Oncol* 1993;9:520–3.

85. Hays DM, Raney RB, Wharam MD, Wiener E, Lobe TE, Andrassy RJ, Lawrence W Jr, Johnston J, Webber B, Maurer HM. Children with vesical rhabdomyosarcoma (RMS) treated by partial cystectomy with neoadjuvant or adjuvant chemotherapy, with or without radiotherapy. A report from the Intergroup Rhabdomyosarcoma Study (IRS) Committee. *J Pediatr Hematol Oncol* 1995;17:46–52.

86. Qualman SJ, Coffin CM, Newton WA, Hojo H, Triche TJ, Parham DM, Crist WM. Intergroup Rhabdomyosarcoma Study: update for pathologists. *Pediatr Dev Pathol* 1998;1:550–61.

87. Ferrer FA, Isakoff M, Koyle MA. Bladder/prostate rhabdomyosarcoma: past, present and future. *J Urol* 2006;176:1283–91.

88. Hawkins HK, Camacho-Velasquez JV. Rhabdomyosarcoma in children. Correlation of form and prognosis in one institution's experience. *Am J Surg Pathol* 1987;11:531–42.

89. Hartley AL, Birch JM, Blair V, Kelsey AM, Harris M, Jones PH. Patterns of cancer in the families of children with soft tissue sarcoma. *Cancer* 1993;72:923–30.

90. Heyn R, Haeberlen V, Newton WA, Ragab AH, Raney RB, Tefft M, Wharam M, Ensign LG, Maurer HM. Second malignant neoplasms in children treated for rhabdomyosarcoma. Intergroup Rhabdomyosarcoma Study Committee. *J Clin Oncol* 1993;11:262–70.

91. Raney B Jr, Heyn R, Hays DM, Tefft M, Newton WA Jr, Wharam M, Vassilopoulou-Sellin R, Maurer HM. Sequelae of treatment in 109 patients followed for 5 to 15 years after diagnosis of sarcoma of the bladder and prostate. A report from the Intergroup Rhabdomyosarcoma Study Committee. *Cancer* 1993;71:2387–94.

92. Leuschner I, Newton WA Jr, Schmidt D, Sachs N, Asmar L, Hamoudi A, Harms D, Maurer HM. Spindle cell variants of embryonal rhabdomyosarcoma in the paratesticular region. A report of the Intergroup Rhabdomyosarcoma Study. *Am J Surg Pathol* 1993;17:221–30.

93. Lambert I, Debiec-Rychter M, Dubin M, Sciot R. Solid alveolar rhabdomyosarcoma originating from the urinary bladder in an adult. Diagnostic value of molecular genetics. *Histopathology* 2004;44:508–10.

94. Paner GP, McKenney JK, Epstein JI, Amin MB. Rhabdomyosarcoma of the urinary bladder in adults: predilection for alveolar morphology with anaplasia and significant morphologic overlap with small cell carcinoma. *Am J Surg Pathol* 2008;32:1022–8.

95. Taylor RE, Busuttil A. Case report: adult rhabdomyosarcoma of bladder, complete response to radiation therapy. *J Urol* 1989;142:1321–2.

96. Engel JD, Kuzel TM, Moceanu MC, Oefelein MG, Schaeffer AJ. Angiosarcoma of the bladder: a review. *Urology* 1998;52:778–84.

97. Schindler S, De Frias DV, Yu GH. Primary angiosarcoma of the bladder: cytomorphology and differential diagnosis. *Cytopathology* 1999;10:137–43.

98. Stroup RM, Chang YC. Angiosarcoma of the bladder: a case report. *J Urol* 1987;137:984–5.

99. Ravi R. Primary angiosarcoma of the urinary bladder. *Arch Esp Urol* 1993;46:351–3.

100. Morgan MA, Moutos DM, Pippitt CH Jr, Suda RR, Smith JJ, Thurnau GR. Vaginal and bladder angiosarcoma after therapeutic irradiation. *South Med J* 1989;82:1434–6.

101. Egawa S, Uchida T, Koshiba K, Kagata Y, Iwabuchi K. Malignant fibrous histiocytoma of the bladder with focal rhabdoid tumor differentiation. *J Urol* 1994;151:154–6.

102. Lopez-Beltran A, Perez-Seoane C, Montironi R, Hernandez-Iglesias T, Mackintosh C, de Alava E. Primary primitive neuroectodermal tumour of the urinary bladder: a clinico-pathological study emphasising immunohistochemical, ultrastructural and molecular analyses. *J Clin Pathol* 2006;59:775–8.

103. Ellinger J, Bastian PJ, Hauser S, Biermann K, Muller SC. Primitive neuroectodermal tumor: rare, highly aggressive differential diagnosis in urologic malignancies. *Urology* 2006;68:257–62.

104. Kruger S, Schmidt H, Kausch I, Bohle A, Holzhausen H, Johannisson R, Feller A. Primitive neuroectodermal tumor (PNET) of the urinary bladder. *Path Res Pract* 2003;199:751–4.

105. Eltoum IA, Moore RJ 3rd, Cook W, Crowe DR, Rodgers WH, Siegal GP. Epithelioid variant of malignant peripheral nerve sheath tumor (malignant schwannoma) of the

urinary bladder. *Ann Diagn Pathol* 1999;3:304–8.

106. Daimaru Y, Hashimoto H, Enjoji M. Malignant "triton" tumors: a clinicopathologic and immunohistochemical study of nine cases. *Hum Pathol* 1984;15:768–78.

107. Rober PE, Smith JB, Sakr W, Pierce JM Jr. Malignant peripheral nerve sheath tumor (malignant schwannoma) of urinary bladder in von Recklinghausen neurofibromatosis. *Urology* 1991;38:473–6.

108. Prout MN, Davis HL Jr. Hemangiopericytoma of the bladder after polyvinyl alcohol exposure. *Cancer* 1977;39:1328–30.

109. Bagchi AG, Dasgupta A, Chaudhury PR. Haemangiopericytoma of urinary bladder. *J Indian Med Assoc* 1993;91:211–2.

110. Soran H, Younis N, Joseph F, Hayat Z, Zakhour H, Scott A. A case of haemangiopericytoma-associated hypoglycaemia: beneficial effect of treatment with radiotherapy. *Int J Clin Pract* 2006;60:1319–22.

111. Baglio CM, Crowson CN. Hemangiopericytoma of urachus: report of a case. *J Urol* 1964;91:660–2.

112. Carter RL, McCarthy KP, al-Sam SZ, Monaghan P, Agrawal M, McElwain TJ. Malignant rhabdoid tumour of the bladder with immunohistochemical and ultrastructural evidence suggesting histiocytic origin. *Histopathology* 1989;14:179–90.

113. Kibar Y, Goktas S, Kilic S, Yaman H, Onguru O, Peker AF. Prognostic value of cytology, nuclear matrix protein 22 (NMP22) test, and urinary bladder cancer II (UBC II) test in early recurrent transitional cell carcinoma of the bladder. *Ann Clin Lab Sci* 2006;36:31–8.

114. Enzinger F, Weiss S. Soft Tissue Tumors. St. Louis: Mosby-Year Book, Inc., 1995.

115. Sutton R, Hopper IP, Munson KW. Haemangiopericytoma of the bladder. *Br J Urol* 1989;63:548–9.

116. Amin MB, Patel RM, Oliveira P, Cabrera R, Carneiro V, Preto M, Balzer B, Folpe AL. Alveolar soft-part sarcoma of the urinary bladder with urethral recurrence: a unique case with emphasis on differential diagnoses and diagnostic utility of an immunohistochemical panel including TFE3. *Am J Surg Pathol* 2006;30:1322–5.

117. Davidson DD, Cheng L. Field cancerization in the urothelium of the bladder. *Anal Quant Cytol Histol* 2006;28:337–8.

118. Spiess PE, Kassouf W, Steinberg JR, Tuziak T, Hernandez M, Tibbs RF, Czerniak B, Kamat AM, Dinney CP, Grossman HB. Review of the M.D. Anderson experience in the treatment of bladder sarcoma. *Urol Oncol* 2007;25:38–45.

119. Dotan ZA, Tal R, Golijanin D, Snyder ME, Antonescu C, Brennan MF, Russo P. Adult genitourinary sarcoma: the 25-year Memorial Sloan-Kettering experience. *J Urol* 2006;176:2033–8; discussion 2038–9.

120. Rogers CG, Palapattu GS, Shariat SF, Karakiewicz PI, Bastian PJ, Lotan Y, Gupta A, Vazina A, Gilad A, Sagalowsky AI, Lerner SP, Schoenberg MP. Clinical outcomes following radical cystectomy for primary nontransitional cell carcinoma of the bladder compared to transitional cell carcinoma of the bladder. *J Urol* 2006;175:2048–53.

121. Newton WA, Gehan EA, Webber BL, Marsden HB, van Unnik AJM, Hamoudi AB, Tsokos MG, Shimada H, Harms D, Schmidt D, Ninfo V, Cavazzana AO, Gonzalez-Crussi F, Parham DM, Reiman HM, Asmar L, Beltangady MS, Sachs NE, Triche TJ, Maurer HM. Classification of rhabdomyosarcomas and related sarcomas. Pathologic aspects and proposal for a new classification—an intergroup rhabdomyosarcoma study. *Cancer* 1995;76:1073–85.

Chapter 20

Lymphoid and Hematopoietic Tumors

Bladder Pathology, First Edition. Liang Cheng, Antonio Lopez-Beltran, David G. Bostwick.
© 2012 Wiley-Blackwell. Published 2012 by John Wiley & Sons, Inc.

Malignant Lymphoma

Lymphomas constitute less than 1% of bladder neoplasms.[1-28] More recently, Ploeg et al. reported 75 cases of lymphomas (0.26%) among 28,807 patients with invasive bladder cancer from the Netherlands Cancer Registry from 1995 to 2006.[29] Patients with malignant lymphoma of can be divided into three distinct groups: those with primary lymphoma localized in the bladder, lymphoma presenting in the bladder as the first sign of disseminated disease (nonlocalized lymphoma), and recurrent bladder involvement by lymphoma in patients with a history of malignant lymphoma (secondary lymphoma).[2] Primary lymphoma is defined by the following criteria: presenting symptoms attributable to bladder involvement; involvement of the bladder without involvement of adjacent tissue; and absence of involvement of liver, spleen, lymph nodes, peripheral blood, and bone marrow within 6 months of the diagnosis of bladder involvement.[2]

Primary malignant lymphoma in the bladder is very rare, accounting for only 0.14% of extranodal lymphomas (Figs. 20-1 to 20-3).[1-3] In an analysis of 1467 extranodal

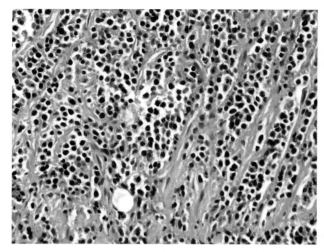

Figure 20-2 Small lymphocytic lymphoma involving the wall of the bladder.

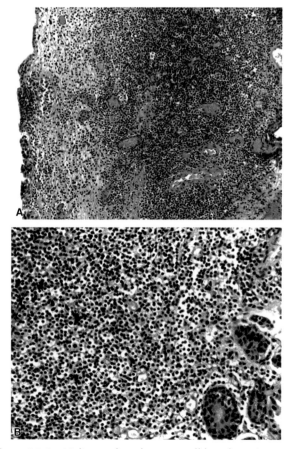

Figure 20-1 Malignant lymphoma, small lymphocytic type (A and B).

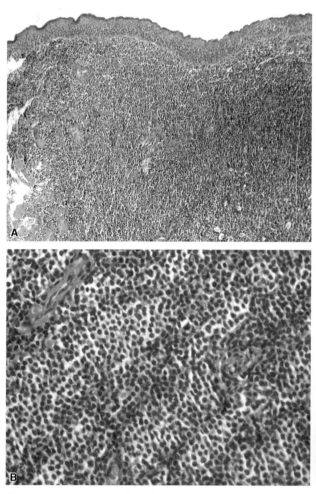

Figure 20-3 Malignant lymphoma, small lymphocytic type (A and B).

lymphomas, only two cases were primary in the bladder.[3] However, secondary involvement of lymphoma is not uncommon. The urinary bladder is secondary in 13% to 17% of cases of systemic lymphoma at autopsy, and most patients have no bladder symptoms.[30,31] Only 1% of these are clinically apparent.[3,4]

Primary lymphoma is far more common in females than in males, with a male-to-female ratio of approximately 1 : 4.[2,24,25] However, a recent report by Schniederjan and Osunkoya found a male predominance in primary bladder lymphomas.[11] The median age at the diagnosis was 58 years (range, 12 to 85 years).[2] Signs and symptoms include gross hematuria, dysuria, irritative symptoms, and incontinence. Rare cases may be associated with Epstein–Barr virus.[10]

Cystoscopically, lymphoma appears as single or multiple masses that are sessile or polypoid. Primary lymphoma has a predilection for the dome and trigone. Posterior and lateral wall may also be involved. The tissue specimen for examination is usually a biopsy or transurethral resection. The mucosa overlying the mass is usually intact, and this is a useful diagnostic clue. Occasionally, there may be diffuse thickening of the bladder wall. Ulceration is uncommon in primary lymphoma, but frequent in secondary lesions. Frank hemorrhagic changes of the mucosa have been observed.

Most examples of bladder lymphoma have been reported as single cases, and histologic classification has varied greatly, with only a small number having modern immunohistochemical workup to phenotype the lymphoma. Immunohistochemically, almost all bladder lymphomas are of B cell origin and display monoclonality.[12] The most frequent type of primary lymphoma is extranodal marginal zone lymphoma of mucosa-associated lymphoid tissue (MALT) type (MALT lymphoma) (**Figs. 20-4** to **20-7**).[2,25] Diffuse large B cell lymphoma is the most common type in a recent series.[11]

Other types of primary bladder lymphoma, such as Burkitt lymphoma, T cell lymphoma, Hodgkin lymphoma,

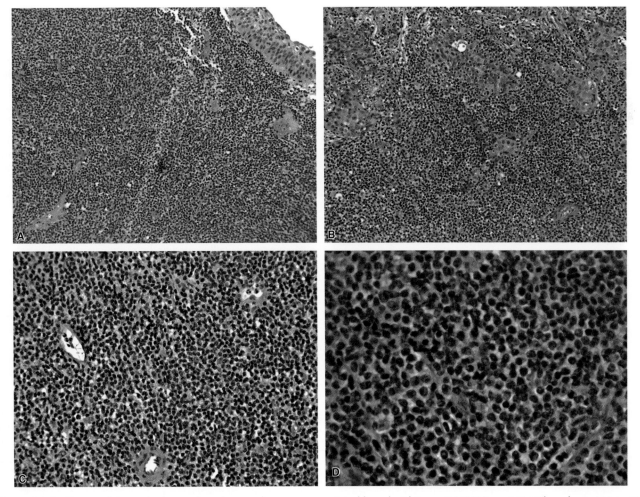

Figure 20-4 Extranodal marginal zone lymphoma of mucosa-associated lymphoid tissue (MALT) type (MALT lymphoma) (A to D).

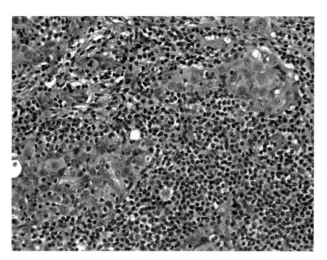

Figure 20-5 MALT lymphoma of the bladder. Note the lymphoepithelial lesions.

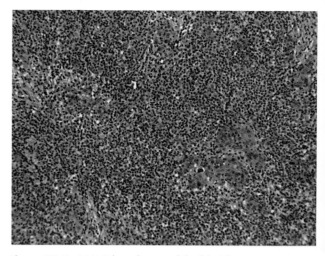

Figure 20-7 MALT lymphoma of the bladder.

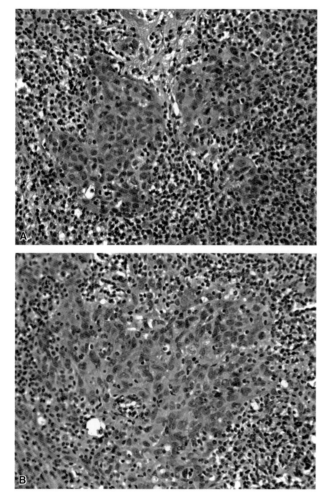

Figure 20-6 MALT lymphoma of the bladder (A and B).

and plasmacytoma are extremely rare.[13] Involvement of bladder by lymphomatoid granulomatosis and Burkitt lymphoma have been reported and typically cause bladder outflow obstruction and gross hematuria.[15,16,32] Among secondary bladder lymphomas, diffuse large B cell lymphoma is the single most frequent histological subtype, followed by follicular, small cell low grade MALT, mantle cell, Burkitt and Hodgkin lymphoma.

The etiology of bladder lymphoma remains unclear. Schistosomiasis is associated with a T cell lymphoma of the bladder. Rare cases of lymphoma arise synchronously in association with adenocarcinoma and urothelial carcinoma. Papillary urothelial tumors may present simultaneously with bladder lymphoma, either primary or secondary. Primary marginal zone B cell MALT lymphoma of the bladder has an excellent prognosis after therapy.[2] Histologically, the tumor consists of a diffuse infiltrate of lymphoid cells surrounding and permeating normal structures. Architectural effacement of the bladder wall by centrocyte-like cells accompanied by plasma cells and nonneoplastic germinal centers is typically present in MALT lymphoma involving the bladder. Lymphoepithelial lesions may be seen in areas of cystitis cystica and cystitis glandularis, and they should not be confused with lymphoepithelioma-like carcinoma or lymphoid-rich variant urothelial carcinoma. Since the bladder is an embryonic derivative of the cloaca, bladder lymphomas might arise from inherent lymphoid tissue that is related to Peyer patches in the gut. Alternatively, MALT lymphomas of the urinary bladder could also arise in MALT acquired as the result of an inflammatory process such as chronic cystitis related to a bacterial infection. Further investigation is warranted to clarify the pathogenesis of primary bladder lymphoma.

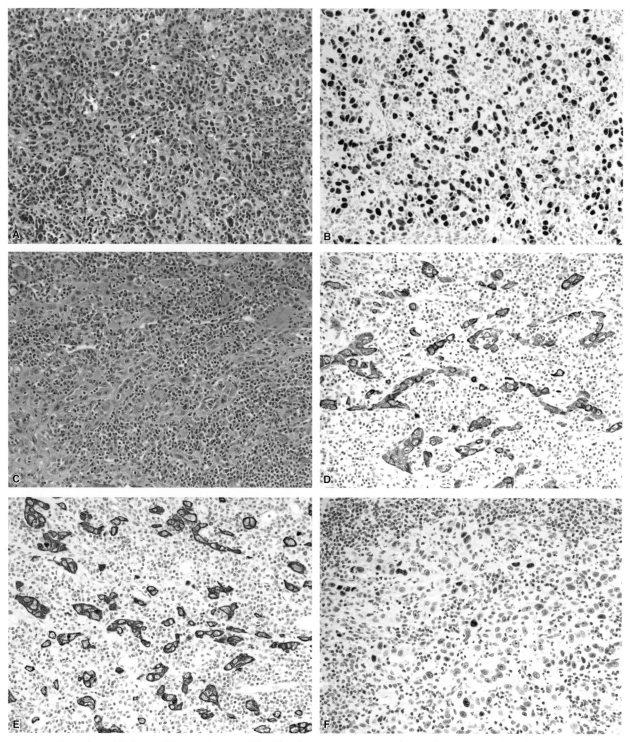

Figure 20-8   Lymphoepithelioma-like carcinoma of the bladder (A to F). Syncytial growth may mimic lymphoepithelial lesions of MALT lymphoma (A and C). Immunostaining for p53 (B and F), cytokeratin 7 (D), high molecular weight cytokeratin 34βE12 (E) is positive in lymphoepithelioma-like carcinoma.

Lymphoid and Hematopoietic Tumors

Overall survival for bladder lymphoma is estimated to be 68% to 73% at one year and 27% to 64% at five years.[2,11,17,24,26,28] Patients with nonlocalized bladder involvement without a prior history of lymphoma who presented with symptoms attributable only to the bladder had a mean cancer-specific survival of four years. For primary bladder lymphoma, the type of treatments include surgery, radiation, and chemotherapy.[2,18,28] Due to the rarity of the disease, no standard treatment is available.[28] In Kempton et al.'s report, none of patients with primary lymphoma of the bladder died of disease or had tumor recurrence after resection and radiation therapy.[2]

The major differential diagnostic considerations are lymphoepithelioma-like carcinoma (Fig. 20-8), plasmacytoid and lymphoid-rich variant of urothelial carcinoma, small cell carcinoma, follicular or florid chronic cystitis, and other inflammatory processes.[33-37] It is particularly problematic in limited biopsy samples. Attention to histologic features, together with clinical history and appropriate immunohistochemical studies, should help distinguish lymphoma from its mimickers. Lymphoepithelioma-like carcinoma is an important variant of bladder cancer that has diagnostic, prognostic, and therapeutic significance. It often shows nests, sheets, and cords of undifferentiated malignant cells, arranged in syncytia with ill-defined cytoplasmic borders, resembling nasopharyngeal lymphoepithelioma. Nuclear features include large vesicular nuclei with prominent nucleoli and frequent mitotic figures. The accompanying lymphoid component includes mature lymphocytes, plasma cells, histiocytes, neutrophils, and eosinophils. These tumors can be readily distinguished from lymphoma by identification of coexisting urothelial carcinoma and urothelial carcinoma in situ. The epithelial cells of lymphoepithelioma-like carcinoma are positive for cytokeratin 7, p53, p63, and high molecular weight cytokeratin 34βE12 and show molecular abnormalities detected by UroVysion FISH.[34]

Leukemia

Granulocytic sarcoma (chloroma, myeloid sarcoma) rarely involves the urinary bladder (Fig. 20-9).[14,30,38-40] Other types of hematopoietic tumors may also secondarily involve the urinary bladder. At autopsy, fewer than 18% of patients who died of chronic lymphocytic leukemia and chronic myelogenous leukemia have bladder involvement.[30] The frequency is somewhat higher in patients with acute leukemia. Grossly, there are mucosal nodules or foci of hemorrhagic thickening. Histologically, these tumors are similar to those from other organ sites. Relevant clinical data and high index of suspicion are critical to avoid misdiagnosis.

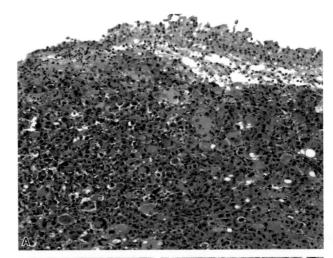
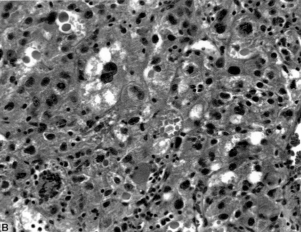

Figure 20-9   Granulocytic sarcoma involving the bladder (A and B).

Multiple Myeloma/Plasmacytoma

The bladder is rarely involved with multiple myeloma or solitary plasmacytoma (Figs. 20-10 and 20-11).[23,41-45] There is no apparent gender predilection, and adult patients of all ages may be affected (range, 28 to 89 years). Most patients present with hematuria, and urine cytology may reveal malignant plasma cells.[43] The tumor forms solid polypoid or pedunculated masses composed of sheets of plasma cells with varying degrees of atypia. The mucosa is typically intact.

In the urinary bladder, the main differential diagnostic considerations include benign conditions such as chronic cystitis with prominent plasma cell infiltrate, as well as other malignant tumors, such as signet ring cell adenocarcinoma and metastatic carcinoma from other primary sites, specifically breast and stomach (Table 20-1).[35,36] Myofibroblastic proliferations enter the differential diagnosis since they may have a prominent plasma cell infiltrate.

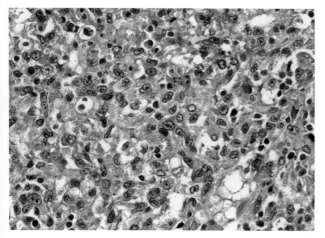

Figure 20-10 Anaplastic plasmacytoma involving the bladder.

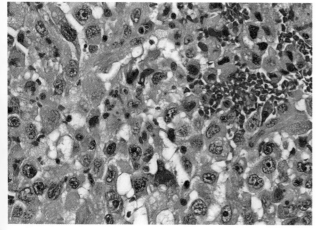

Figure 20-11 Anaplastic plasmacytoma involving the bladder.

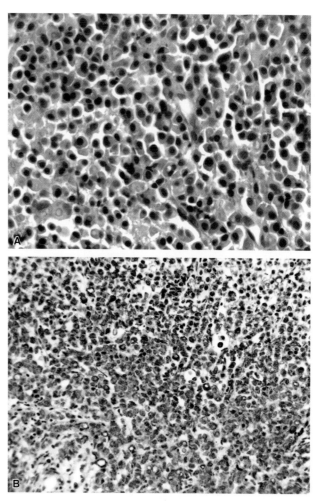

Figure 20-12 Plasmacytoid variant of urothelial carcinoma (A and B). Immunostaining for cytokeratin is strongly positive (B).

Table 20-1   Main Differential Features of Bladder Tumors with Plasmacytoid Cells[a]

	Cytologic Features			Immunohistochemical Features									
	Nuclear Shape	Nucleolus	Cytoplasm	Pan-CK	Vim	CK7	CK20	S100	LCA	HMB45	Syn/Chr	CD138	Desmin
Lymphoma/plasmacytoma	Round	±	Eosino/ampho	±	+	−	−	−	+	−	−	+	−
Plasmacytoid carcinoma	Round	±	Eosino/ampho	+	−	+	+	−	−	−	−	±	−
Rhabdoid carcinoma	Round	+	Eosino	±	+	±	±	−	−	−	−	−	−
Signet ring cell carcinoma	Indented	±	Ampho/clear	+	−	+	+	−	−	−	−	−	−
Neuroendocrine carcinoma/small cell carcinoma	Round	+	Scant/eosino	±	+	±	−	+	−	−	+	−	−
Paraganglioma	Round	+	Ampho/clear	±	+	±	+[b]	+	−	−	+	−	−
Melanoma	Round	+	Eosino	±	+	−	−	+	−	+	−	−	−
Rhabdomyosarcoma	Round/fusiform	±	Scant/eosino	±	+	−	−	−	−	−	±	−	+

[a]Ampho, amphophilic; eosino, eosinophilic; CK, cytokeratin; Vim, vimentin; LCA, leukocyte common antigen; Syn/Chr, synaptophysin/chromogranin A.
[b]Sustentacular cells staining for S100 protein.

Plasmacytoid urothelial carcinoma, a rare variant of urothelial carcinoma with histologic appearance similar to that of plasma cells, may pose a significant differential diagnostic problem, particularly if it is the predominant or exclusive pattern in a limited biopsy sample (**Fig. 20-12**). The finding of some plasmacytoid urothelial carcinomas of the bladder immunoreactive for CD138, a marker of plasma cells, represents an important challenge in daily practice.[35,36]

Immunohistochemically, plasmacytoid variant is also positive for cytokeratin 7, cytokeratin 20, and AE1/AE3. Primary signet ring cell adenocarcinoma enters into the differential diagnosis due to the occasional presence of intracytoplasmic vacuoles and the noncohesive nature of the tumor cells. Urothelial carcinoma with rhabdoid phenotype should also be considered in the differential diagnosis. It is distinguished from plasmacytoma by the presence of prominent nucleoli and positive immunostaining for vimentin in rhabdoid cells.

Primary plasmacytoma of the bladder is rare, but in patients with a prior history of multiple myeloma, where there is no identifiable surface urothelial component, it is necessary to maintain a level of suspicion to avoid misdiagnosis of a plasmacytoma as urothelial carcinoma with plasmacytoid features. There have been cases of extramedullary plasmacytoma involving the bladder in patients with no demonstrable systemic involvement by multiple myeloma; however, reports such as these are still rare and the majority of patients present with systemic disease. In a clinical scenario where this is a diagnostic concern, ancillary immunohistochemical testing for cytokeratin, vimentin, CD138, and kappa and lambda light chains may further confirm the diagnosis.

REFERENCES

1. Simpson RH, Bridger JE, Anthony PP, James KA, Jury I. Malignant lymphoma of the lower urinary tract. A clinicopathological study with review of the literature. *Br J Urol* 1990;65:254–60.
2. Kempton CL, Kurtin PJ, Inwards DJ, Wollan P, Bostwick DG. Malignant lymphoma of the bladder: evidence from 36 cases that low grade lymphoma of the MALT-type is the most common primary bladder lymphoma. *Am J Surg Pathol* 1997;21:1324–33.
3. Freeman C, Berg JW, Cutler SJ. Occurrence and prognosis of extranodal lymphomas. *Cancer* 1972;29:252–60.
4. Clarke NW, Maxwell AJ. Primary lymphoma of the urinary bladder. *Br J Radiol* 1991;64:761–2.
5. Grooms AM, Morgan SK, Turner WR Jr. Hematuria and leukemic bladder infiltration. *JAMA* 1973;223:193–4.
6. Siegelbaum MH, Edmonds P, Seidmon EJ. Use of immunohistochemistry for identification of primary lymphoma of the bladder. *J Urol* 1986;136:1074–6.
7. Kuhara H, Tamura Z, Suchi T, Hattori R, Kinukawa T. Primary malignant lymphoma of the urinary bladder. A case report. *Acta Pathol Jpn* 1990;40:764–9.
8. Pawade J, Banerjee SS, Harris M, Isaacson P, Wright D. Lymphomas of mucosa-associated lymphoid tissue arising in the urinary bladder. *Histopathology* 1993;23:147–51.
9. Ohsawa M, Aozasa K, Horiuchi K, Kanamaru A. Malignant lymphoma of bladder. Report of three cases and review of the literature. *Cancer* 1993;72:1969–74.
10. Sundaram S, Zhang K. Epstein-Barr virus positive B-cell lymphoproliferative disorder/polymorphous B-cell lymphoma of the urinary bladder: A case report with review of literature. *Indian J Urol* 2009;25:129–31.
11. Schniederjan SD, Osunkoya AO. Lymphoid neoplasms of the urinary tract and male genital organs: a clinicopathological study of 40 cases. *Mod Pathol* 2009;22:1057–65.
12. Abraham NZ Jr, Maher TJ, Hutchison RE. Extra-nodal monocytoid B-cell lymphoma of the urinary bladder. *Mod Pathol* 1993;6:145–9.
13. Bocian JJ, Flam MS, Mendoza CA. Hodgkin's disease involving the urinary bladder diagnosed by urinary cytology: a case report. *Cancer* 1982;50:2482–5.
14. Forrest JB, Saypol DC, Mills SE, Gillenwater JY. Immunoblastic sarcoma of the bladder. *J Urol* 1983;130:350–1.
15. Feinberg SM, Leslie KO, Colby TV. Bladder outlet obstruction by so-called lymphomatoid granulomatosis (angiocentric lymphoma). *J Urol* 1987;137:989–90.
16. Lewis RH, Mannarino FG, Worsham GF, Martin JE, Javadpour N, O'Connell KJ. Burkitt's lymphoma presenting as urinary outflow obstruction. *J Urol* 1983;130:120–4.
17. Guthman DA, Malek RS, Chapman WR, Farrow GM. Primary malignant lymphoma of the bladder. *J Urol* 1990;144:1367–9.
18. Hernández Alcaraz D, Gómez Pascual JA, Soler Martínez J, Vozmediano Chicharro R, Morales Jiménez P, Vivas Vargas E, Baena González V. [Bilateral obstructive uropathy as clinical presentation of primary bladder lymphoma]. *Arch Esp Urol* 2009;62:230–2.
19. Weaver MG, Abdul-Karim FW. The prevalence and character of the muscularis mucosae of the human urinary bladder. *Histopathology* 1990;17:563–6.
20. Kurtman C, Andrieu MN, Baltaci S, Gogus C, Akfirat C. Conformal radiotherapy in primary non-Hodgkin's lymphoma of the male urethra. *Int Urol Nephrol* 2001;33:537–9.
21. Mearini E, Zucchi A, Costantini E, Fornetti P, Tiacci E, Mearini L. Primary Burkitt's lymphoma of bladder in patient with AIDS. *J Urol* 2002;167:1397–8.

22. Krober SM, Aepinus C, Ruck P, Muller-Hermelink HK, Horny HP, Kaiserling E. Extranodal marginal zone B cell lymphoma of MALT type involving the mucosa of both the urinary bladder and stomach. *J Clin Pathol* 2002;55:554–7.

23. Lemos N, Melo CR, Soares IC, Lemos RR, Lemos FR. Plasmacytoma of the urethra treated by excisional biopsy. *Scand J Urol Nephrol* 2000;34:75–6.

24. Al-Maghrabi J, Kamel-Reid S, Jewett M, Gospodarowicz M, Wells W, Banerjee D. Primary low grade B-cell lymphoma of mucosa-associated lymphoid tissue type arising in the urinary bladder: report of 4 cases with molecular genetic analysis. *Arch Pathol Lab Med* 2001;125:332–6.

25. Bates AW, Norton AJ, Baithun SI. Malignant lymphoma of the urinary bladder: a clinicopathological study of 11 cases. *J Clin Pathol* 2000;53:458–61.

26. Hughes M, Morrison A, Jackson R. Primary bladder lymphoma: management and outcome of 12 patients with a review of the literature. *Leuk Lymphoma* 2005;46:873–7.

27. Mourad WA, Khalil S, Radwi A, Peracha A, Ezzat A. Primary T-cell lymphoma of the urinary bladder. *Am J Surg Pathol* 1998;22:373–7.

28. Horasanli K, Kadihasanoglu M, Aksakal OT, Ozagari A, Miroglu C. A case of primary lymphoma of the bladder managed with multimodal therapy. *Nat Clin Pract Urol* 2008;5:167–70.

29. Ploeg M, Aben KK, Hulsbergen-van de Kaa CA, Schoenberg MP, Witjes JA, Kiemeney LA. Clinical epidemiology of nonurothelial bladder cancer: analysis of the Netherlands Cancer Registry. *J Urol* 2010;183:915–20.

30. Givler RL. Involvement of the bladder in leukemia and lymphoma. *J Urol* 1971;105:667–70.

31. Sufrin G, Keogh B, Moore RH, Murphy GP. Secondary involvement of the bladder in malignant lymphoma. *J Urol* 1977;118:251–3.

32. Fujiwara H, Odawara J, Hayama B, Takanashi Y, Iwama K, Yamakura M, Takeuchi M, Matsue K. Gross hematopyuria presenting as a first symptom due to the bladder infiltration of extranodal Burkitt's lymphoma. *J Clin Oncol* 2010;28:e252–3.

33. Zukerberg LR, Harris NL, Young RH. Carcinomas of the urinary bladder simulating malignant lymphoma. A report of five cases. *Am J Surg Pathol* 1991;15:569–76.

34. Williamson SR, Zhang S, Lopez-Beltran A, Shah RB, Montironi R, Tan PH, Wang M, Baldridge LA, MacLennan GT, Cheng L. Lymphoepithelioma-like carcinoma of the urinary bladder: clinicopathologic, immunohistochemical, and molecular features. *Am J Surg Pathol* 2011;35:474–83.

35. Lopez-Beltran A, Cheng L. Histologic variants of urothelial carcinoma: differential diagnosis and clinical implications. *Hum Pathol* 2006;37:1371–88.

36. Lopez-Beltran A, Requena MJ, Montironi R, Blanca A, Cheng L. Plasmacytoid urothelial carcinoma of the bladder. *Hum Pathol* 2009;40:1023–8.

37. Wronski S, Marszalek A. Diagnostic pitfalls of rare urinary bladder tumors: differential diagnosis of lymphoma-like carcinoma of the bladder—a clinicopathologic study and literature review. *J Clin Oncol* 2011;29:e196–9.

38. Al-Quran SZ, Olivares A, Lin P, Stephens TW, Medeiros LJ, Abruzzo LV. Myeloid sarcoma of the urinary bladder and epididymis as a primary manifestation of acute myeloid leukemia with inv(16). *Arch Pathol Lab Med* 2006;130:862–6.

39. Hasegeli UA, Altundag K, Saglam A, Tekuzman G. Granulocytic sarcoma of the urinary bladder. *Am J Hematol* 2004;75:262–3.

40. Aki H, Baslar Z, Uygun N, Ozguroglu M, Tuzuner N. Primary granulocytic sarcoma of the urinary bladder: case report and review of the literature. *Urology* 2002;60:345.

41. Gesme D Jr, Boatman D, Weinman G, Tewfik H. Extramedullary plasmacytoma of skin, bowel and bladder. *Iowa Med* 1994;84:354–5.

42. Ho DS, Patterson AL, Orozco RE, Murphy WM. Extramedullary plasmacytoma of the bladder: case report and review of the literature. *J Urol* 1993;150:473–4.

43. Neal MH, Swearingen ML, Gawronski L, Cotelingam JD. Myeloma cells in the urine. *Arch Pathol Lab Med* 1985;109:870–2.

44. Thornhill JA, Dervan P, Otridge BW, Fitzpatrick JM, Smith JS. Symptomatic plasmacytoma (myeloma) involving the bladder. *Br J Urol* 1990;65:542–3.

45. Yang C, Motteram R, Sandeman TF. Extramedullary plasmacytoma of the bladder: a case report and review of literature. *Cancer* 1982;50:146–9.

Chapter 21

Urothelial Carcinoma Following Augmentation Cystoplasty

Bladder Pathology, First Edition. Liang Cheng, Antonio Lopez-Beltran, David G. Bostwick.
© 2012 Wiley-Blackwell. Published 2012 by John Wiley & Sons, Inc.

Overview

Mikulicz first proposed using the small intestine to augment the urinary bladder in the late nineteenth century.[1] Since then, augmentation cystoplasty incorporating gastrointestinal segments to reconstruct the urinary bladder has been widely used in the management of a variety of urological disorders. This technique has demonstrated utility in prevention of renal disease that otherwise would result from high pressure urine storage, as well as restoration of storage function and quality of life.[2–5] However, a few inherent complications of this surgical procedure have been recognized during the last several decades, including bladder perforation, infection, urolithiasis, and malignancy.[2,5] In a study by Soergel and collaborators, malignancy was diagnosed in three of 483 bladder augmentation patients.[4] The development of malignancies from the native bladder or incorporated segments has raised a serious concern in urological practice, with isolated cases of developing urothelial carcinoma having been described in patients receiving this surgical intervention (Table 21-1).[2,5–18]

The exact pathological characteristics and underlying molecular genetic alterations of neoplasms following augmentation cystoplasty have remained unknown until recently. A relatively large series has been reported, evaluating the morphological features, immunohistochemical characteristics, chromosomal abnormalities by UroVysion fluorescence in situ hybridization (FISH) tests, and gene mutations of fibroblast growth factor receptor 3 (FGFR3) and the TP53 gene in urothelial carcinomas after augmentation cystoplasty.[5]

A detailed analysis of the cases reported suggested that neoplasms occurring in patients receiving bladder augmentation had unusual clinical presentations and an ominous prognosis. In addition, these tumors demonstrated distinct pathological characteristics and genetic alterations not commonly present in conventional urothelial carcinomas and appeared to represent a rare variant of urothelial carcinoma.[5]

Clinical Features

The formation of an epithelial malignancy after augmentation cystoplasty represents a small but present risk associated with this procedure. Augmentation cystoplasty-associated urothelial carcinomas occur in a population of relative young age (mean, 37 years at diagnosis; range, 29 to 44 years) at a long-term latency (mean, 19 years; range, 17 to 21 years) after receiving bladder augmentation for managing their nonneoplastic urinary disorders.[5] No other significant risk factors responsible for urothelial

carcinogenesis, such as tobacco smoking and occupational exposure or particular drug usage, were identified in these patients. Differences in clinicopathologic and molecular characteristics of urothelial carcinoma in adult, pediatric, and augmentation cystoplasty patients are highlighted in Table 21-2.

In Sung et al.'s report, the patient population consisted of two men and two women; three were born with myelomeningocele and the fourth suffered from an obstructive urinary disorder.[5] Two patients underwent ileocecal augmentation and the two others received cecal augmentations for managing urinary disorders. The initial symptoms/signs of the subsequent malignancy included hematuria (three cases), urinary tract infection (one case), and bladder neck contracture (one case). Three neoplasms were located in the native urinary bladder and the remaining tumor arose from the junction between the native bladder and the ileal segment. One patient underwent cystectomy alone for treatment; one patient was managed with cystectomy and adjuvant chemotherapy and radiotherapy, and the remaining two by transurethral resection with subsequent chemotherapy.

All tumors behaved in an extremely aggressive manner, rarely seen in conventional vesical urothelial carcinoma, and all patients developed metastasis shortly after initial diagnosis.[5] All patients died of cancer within months of initial diagnosis (mean, 5 months; range, 1.5 to 8 months), despite the intense treatment comprising cystectomy combined with adjuvant chemotherapy and radiotherapy (Table 21-1).

Optimal clinical followup and management of such patients remains to be fully elucidated. Soergel and colleagues have suggested careful endoscopic surveillance of such patients beginning 10 years after surgery.[4] Hamid et al. have suggested, however, that surveillance cystoscopy is not necessary for at least the first 15 years, as it has not been shown to detect cancer during this timeframe. These authors do note, however, that hematuria or other worrisome symptoms should prompt an immediate evaluation including cystoscopy and imaging.[19] The utility of urinary cytology and molecular assays (such as UroVysion FISH test) in surveillance is not completely clear.

Histopathology

Histologically, these neoplasms are typically invasive high grade urothelial carcinomas accompanied by brisk mitotic activities, capabilities of lymphovascular invasion, and the existence of tumor necrosis (Figs. 21-1 to 21-3), which correlated with their extremely aggressive biological behavior evident by widespread metastasis and ominous prognosis.[5]

Table 21-1   Literature Review of Urothelial Carcinoma (Transitional Cell Carcinoma) Following Augmentation Cystoplasty[a]

Reference	Publication Year	Gender	Age	Type of Augmentation	Latency	Pathological Diagnosis (Stage)	Metastasis	Tumor Site	Treatment	Outcome (Length of Followup)
Smith and Hardy[9]	1971	F	43	Ileocystoplasty	17	PD UC SD (NR)	NR	NA	Wide excision	NR (NR)
Stone et al.[10]	1987	F	54	Ileocystoplasty	5	UC SD CIS (NR)	Neg	NA	Cystectomy	NED (NR)
Golomb et al.[11]	1989	M	69	Sigmoidocystoplasty	24	G3 UC (pT4N0)	Neg	A	Partial cystectomy	NED (3Y)
Gregoire et al.[12]	1993	M	72	Cecocytoplasty	7	UC GD CIS (pT1N0)	Neg	NA	Cystectomy	AWD (2Y)
Shokeir[13]	1995	F	42	Colocystoplasty	19	G2 UC (NR)	Neg	A	Cystectomy	Alive (3Y)
Barrington et al.[14]	1997	F	46	Ileocystoplasty	5	CIS (pTis)	Neg	A	Cystectomy	NED (NR)
Lane and Shah[15]	2000	M	72	Ileocystoplasty	2	G3 UC (pT1)	Neg	Bladder	Cystectomy	NED (3Y)
Ali-El-Dein et al.[16]	2002	F	43	Ileocystoplasty	24	G2 UC (pT3aNo)	Neg	A	Cystectomy	NR (9Y)
Qiu et al.[17]	2003	F	73	Gastrocytoplasty	14	UC SD CIS (NR)	NR	NA	Cystectomy	NR
Castellan et al.[18]	2007	M	20	Gastrocytoplasty	14	PD UC (pT4N2)	Pos	Whole reservoir	Cystectomy CT	DOD (1M)
Sung et al.[15]		F	29	Ileocystoplasty	21	HG G3 UC SD (pT3Nx)	Pos	Left bladder wall	Cystectomy	DOD (8M)
		M	44	Cecocystoplasty	21	HG G3 UC GD (pT2Nx)	Pos	Bladder	Cystectomy CT RT	DOD (8M)
		F	37	Ileocystoplasty	13	HG G3 UC GD (pT3N1)	Pos	A	TUR CT	DOD (3M)
		M	39	Cecocystoplasty	28	HG G3 UC GD CIS (pT1Nx)	Pos	Bladder	TUR CT	DOD (1M)

[a]A, anastomosis; CIS, carcinoma in situ; CT, chemotherapy; DOD, died of disease; FISH, fluorescence in situ hybridization; HG, high grade; G, grade; GD, glandular differentiation; M, month; NA, near anastomosis; Neg, negative; NR, not reported; PD, poorly differentiated; Pos, positive; UC, urothelial (transitional cell); TUR, transurethral resection; SD, squamous differentiation; Y, year.

Table 21-2 Clinicopathologic and Molecular Characteristics of Urothelial Carcinoma in Adult, Pediatric, and Augmentation Cystoplasty Patients

	Adult	Pediatric	Augmentation Cystoplasty
Incidence	Common	Rare	Rare
Association with cigarette smoking	Strong	Conflicting data, probably absent	Absent
Association with occupational exposure	Strong	Absent	Absent
Gender predilection	Male	Male	Males and females affected equally
Tumor grade	Variable	Primarily low grade	High grade
Tumor stage	Variable (typically, low stage)	Noninvasive (pTa)	Advanced stage
Multifocality	Common	Uncommon	Unifocal
Location predilection	Trigone	Trigone	Adjacent to enterovesical anastomosis
Clinical presentations	Irritative symptoms and hematuria	Irritative symptoms and hematuria	Hematuria/metastatic disease
Association with dysplasia/carcinoma in situ	Associated with invasive carcinoma	Uncommon	May be present
Upper urinary tract involvement	Frequent	Very rare	Very rare
Biological behavior			Aggressive
Recurrence	Frequent	Infrequent	Frequent
Progression	Infrequent	Very infrequent	Frequent
Metastasis	Infrequent	Very infrequent	Frequent
Molecular features	FGFR3 and TP53 mutations, and chromosome 9 and 17 abnormalities are common	Molecular abnormalities frequently absent	Amplifications of 2q, 5q, 10p, 21p, 21q and deletions of 5p and 16p
UroVysion testing	Useful	May be useful	Useful

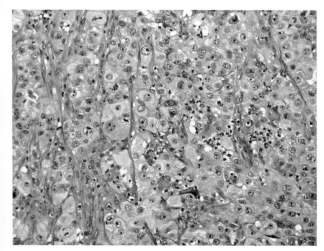

Figure 21-1 High grade urothelial carcinoma following augmentation cystoplasty. Note the atypical mitotic figures and nuclear pleomorphism.

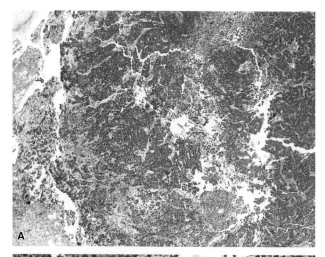

Figure 21-2 High grade urothelial carcinoma following augmentation cystoplasty (A and B). Note the tumor necrosis.

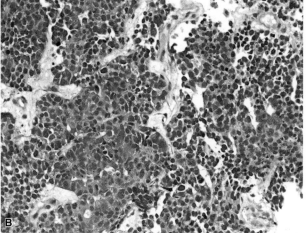

Figure 21-3 High grade urothelial carcinoma following augmentation cystoplasty. Note the tumor necrosis.

Based on the World Health Organization (WHO) classification system, all tumors were categorized as grade 3 (1973) or high grade (2004) tumors (Table 21-1). All were invasive neoplasms; two invaded into the perivesical soft tissue microscopically (pT3a), one to muscularis propria (pT2), and the remaining one to the lamina propria (pT1) of the transurethral resection specimen.

A wide spectrum of histopathologic changes can be seen in association with urothelial carcinoma following augmentation cystoplasty (Figs. 21-4 to 21-6). In addition to the presence of papillary tumor fronds seen in conventional papillary urothelial carcinoma (Fig. 21-7), these tumors comprised diverse architectures, including nests, cords, tubules, and solid tumor sheets; and exhibited unusual frequent glandular differentiation and occasional squamous differentiation (Figs. 21-8 to 21-13; Table 21-3). The exceptional tendency of glandular evolution highlighted the distinct morphological presentation of these neoplasms.[5] Two tumors harbored exophytic papillary components. Invasive cords and nests were identified in three and two cases, respectively. One neoplasm had a tubular formation and one consisted of diffuse solid tumor sheets. In situ urothelial carcinoma of the lining urothelium was present in two cases.

Cytologically, all neoplasms had vesicular tumor nuclei with clumping chromatin, and additional hyperchromatic tumor nuclei were found focally in two cases. Nuclear pleomorphism was evident in all tumors. Nucleolar prominence was present in two neoplasms. There were components of tumor cells with eosinophilic or basophilic cytoplasm in all four cases, but an area of tumor cells harboring clear cytoplasm appeared in one neoplasm. Glandular differentiation was observed in three tumors; squamous differentiation was present in one case. Tumor necrosis was found in all four cases. Angiolymphatic invasion

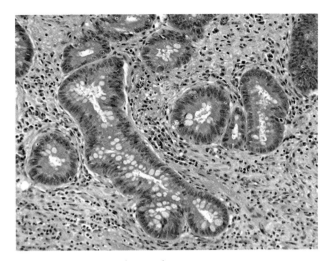

Figure 21-4 Intestinal metaplasia.

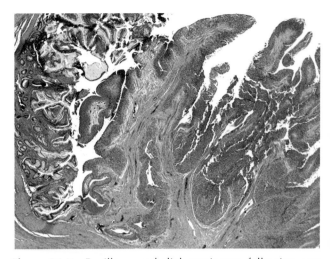

Figure 21-7 Papillary urothelial carcinoma following augmentation cystoplasty.

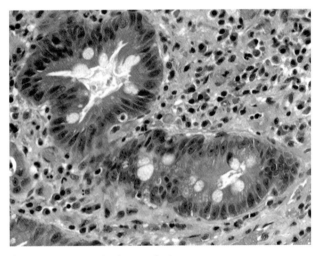

Figure 21-5 Intestinal metaplasia.

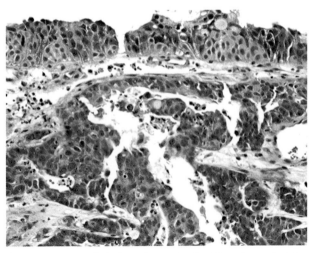

Figure 21-6 Urothelial carcinoma in situ. Note the underlying poorly differentiated urothelial carcinoma.

and perineural invasion were present in three and one patients, respectively. All tumors were mitotically active, with a mean mitotic count of 12 (range, 4 to 17) per 10 high power fields within the most mitotically active regions.

Immunohistochemistry

Cytokeratin (CK) 7 is an intermediate filament that is found in the majority of urothelial neoplasias of the urinary bladder and serves as a sensitive marker for diagnosing urothelial carcinomas. In comparison, the incidence of positive expression of CK20 is relatively lower in urothelial neoplasia.[20,21] In urothelial carcinomas after bladder augmentation, three tumors demonstrated strong CK7 expression, but only one tumor exhibited CK20 staining in Sung et al.'s study (**Fig. 21-14; Table 21-4**).[5] This trend of expression of the cytokeratins is somewhat similar to the one in conventional urothelial carcinoma, although the lower CK20 expression might reflect that its particular evolution deviated from the ordinary urothelial carcinoma. Moderate cytoplasmic and membranous staining for uroplakin III was identified in 10% of tumor cells in one case.[5]

In urothelial carcinomas following augmentation cystoplasty, 50% of tumors revealed CDX2 expression, which is similar to the incidence in primary vesical adenocarcinoma (47%). Moderate to strong staining for CDX2 was observed in tumor nuclei with variable staining percentages at the areas of glandular or solid tumor components (**Fig. 21-15**). These observations suggest that intestinal differentiation, evident by both morphologically glandular involution and immunohistochemical CDX2 expression, may play an important role in the pathogenesis of urothelial carcinoma

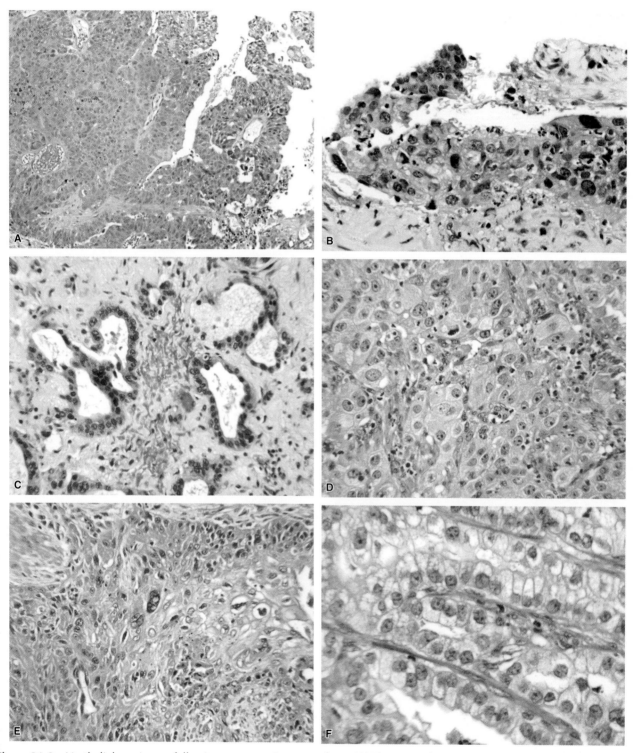

Figure 21-8 Urothelial carcinoma following augmentation cystoplasty. (A) The tumor demonstrates conventional papillary structures comprising central fibrovascular cores and lining neoplastic cells bearing pleomorphic nuclei and eosinophilic cytoplasm. (B) Flat in situ carcinoma revealing cellular pleomorphism in the lining urothelium. (C) Tumor cells forming small tubules scattered in the lamina propria of the bladder. (D) Solid diffuse tumor sheets exhibiting vesicular nuclei, prominent nucleoli, basophilic cytoplasm, and brisk mitotic figures. (E) Squamous differentiation evident by the presence of an intercellular bridge and keratinous cytoplasm in tumor cells. (F) Glandular tumor structure with distinct clear cytoplasm in urothelial carcinoma. (From Ref 5; with permission.)

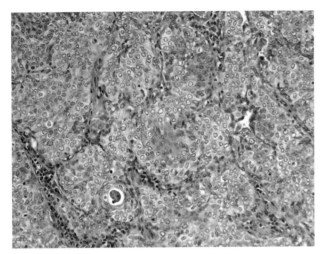

Figure 21-9 High grade urothelial carcinoma following augmentation cystoplasty. Note the solid growth pattern.

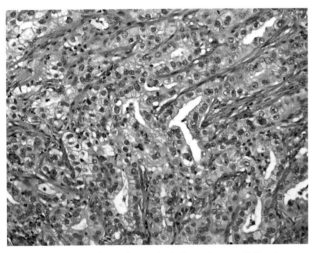

Figure 21-10 High grade urothelial carcinoma following augmentation cystoplasty. Note the glandular differentiation.

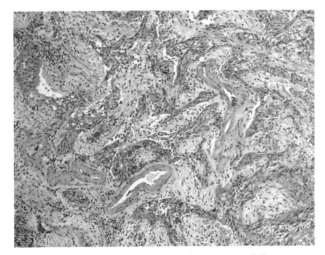

Figure 21-11 High grade urothelial carcinoma following augmentation cystoplasty. Note the infiltrative cords of tumor cells in desmoplastic stroma.

Table 21-3 Clinicopathological Characteristics of Four Urothelial Carcinomas Following Augmentation Cystoplasty

Characteristics	Number
Gender	
Male	2
Female	2
Age	Mean: 37 years (range, 29–44)
Type of augmentation cystoplasty	
Ileocystoplasty	2
Cecocystoplasty	2
Disease for cystoplasty	
Myelomeningocele	3
Obstructive disorder	1
Symptoms	
Hematuria	3
Urinary tract infection	1
Bladder neck contracture	1
Latency period	Mean, 19 years (range, 17–21)
Surgery procedure	
Cystectomy	2
Transurethral resection	2
Adjuvant therapy	
Chemotherapy	2
Combined chemo- and radiotherapy	1
Followup	Mean, 5 months (range, 1.5–8)
Distant metastasis	
Present	4
Absent	0
Died of cancer	4
Tumor location	
Native bladder	3
Anastomosis site	1
Histologic grade	
2004 WHO high grade	4
1973 WHO grade 3	4
Pathologic stage	
pT1	1
pT2	1
pT3a	2
Tumor architecture	
Papilla	2
Nest	3
Cord	2
Tubule	1
Solid	1
Tumor cytology	
Vesicular nuclei	4
Hyperchromatic nuclei	2
Prominent nucleoli	2
Eosinophilic cytoplasm	4
Clear cytoplasm	1

Table 21-3 (*Continued*)

Characteristics	Number
Urothelial carcinoma in situ	
Present	2
Absent	2
Tumor necrosis	
Present	4
Absent	0
Mixed differentiation	
Glandular differentiation	3
Squamous differentiation	1
Tumor invasion	
Angiolymphatic invasion	3
Perineural invasion	1
Mitosis	Mean, 12 (range, 4–17)/10 hpf

hpf, high power field;
Source: Modified from Ref. 5.

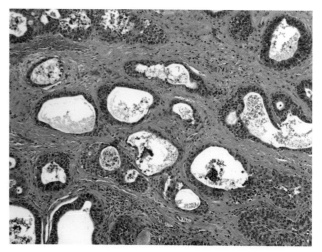

Figure 21-13 High grade urothelial carcinoma following augmentation cystoplasty, microcystic pattern.

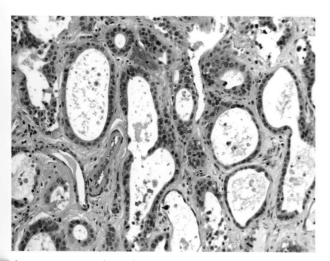

Figure 21-12 High grade urothelial carcinoma following augmentation cystoplasty. Note the tubular and cystic structures lined by malignant urothelial cells.

in patients incorporated with intestinal segments in native bladders.

Abnormal β-catenin expression (decreasing membranous staining) was identified in all these neoplasms, suggesting that the dysfunction of the cadherin–catenin complex with consequent disruption of intercellular interaction might contribute to the development or progression of this distinct neoplasm. In addition, the abnormal β-catenin immunohistochemistry in these patients is in accordance with former reports describing the correlation between decreasing β-catenin expression and both advanced stage and poor outcome in the subset of urothelial carcinoma.

Molecular Genetics

The *FGFR3* gene mapping on chromosome 4p16 is a member of a family of tyrosine kinase receptors and plays a significant role in cell signaling pathways for cell proliferation, development, and differentiation.[22] Ligand binding activates intracellular tyrosines, and mutations

Table 21-4 Immunostaining Results in Four Urothelial Carcinomas Following Augmentation Cystoplasty

Percentage of Positive Cells (%)	Markers[a]				
	CDX2	Uroplakin III	β-Catenin	CK7	CK20
0	2	3	0	1	3
1–25	1	1	0	1	1
26–50	0	0	3	0	0
51–100	1	0	1	2	0

[a]CK7, cytokeratin 7; CK20, cytokeratin 20.

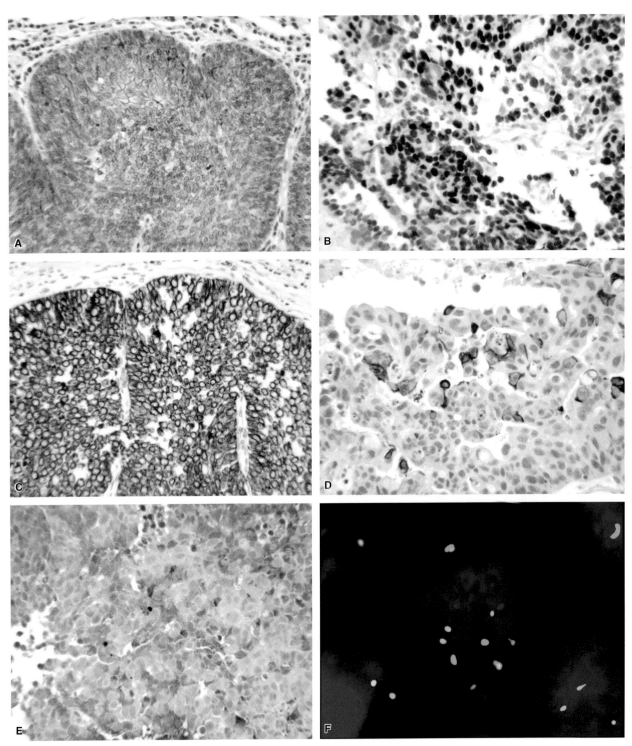

Figure 21-14 High grade urothelial carcinoma following augmentation cystoplasty. (A) Tumor cells are positively stained by β-catenin, representing moderate membranous staining in tumor nests. (B) Strong CDX2 expression in tumor nuclei. (C) Diffuse membranous and cytoplasmic staining of cytokeratin 7. (D) Strong cytokeratin 20 expression in a few isolated tumor cells. (E) Focal membranous and cytoplasmic staining of uroplakin III in urothelial carcinoma. (F) UroVysion fluorescence in situ hybridization (FISH) analysis of tumor developed following augmentation cystoplasty. Chromosomal alteration was detected by interphase FISH by using the UroVysion probe set containing CEP3 (red), CEP 7 (green), CAP17 (aqua), and 9p21 (gold). The representative tumor cell exhibited gains of chromosome 3 (three signals), 7 (four signals), 17 (five signals), and loss of a 9p21 (one signal). (From Ref. 5; with permission.)

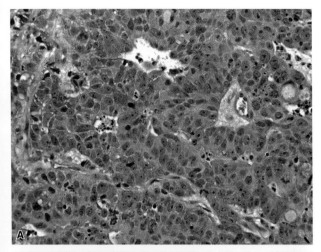

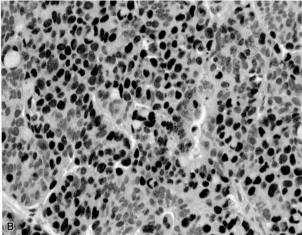

Figure 21-15 High grade urothelial carcinoma following augmentation cystoplasty. Note the glandular differentiation. The tumor cells show strong nuclear immunoreactivity for CDX2.

in the *FGFR3* gene lead to constitutive activation of the receptor.[23] Urothelial carcinomas harboring *FGFR3* mutations tend to be of both lower histologic grade and pathologic stage, and consequently are associated with a more favorable clinical outcome.[24–28] In contrast,

mutations of the *TP53* gene, located on chromosome 17q23 and encoding proteins as a key gatekeeper in cell cycle regulation, were identified frequently in either invasive urothelial carcinoma or high grade superficial urothelial carcinoma and regarded as a hallmark of aggressiveness of urothelial neoplasia.[29] Recent studies focusing on the roles of *FGFR3* and *TP53* in pathogenesis of urothelial carcinoma have observed that most urothelial carcinomas possessed either one mutation or the other.[30,31] Interestingly, they occurred almost always mutually exclusively, and concurrency developed exceptionally in only a minority of tumors, which suggested that *FGFR3* and *TP53* characterize two distinct pathogenetic pathways in the evolution of the majority of urothelial carcinomas.[30,31]

In mutational analysis of urothelial carcinoma following bladder augmentation, all but one case was free of gene mutations of *FGFR3* or *TP53*, and the remaining one simultaneously harbored mutations at both loci.[5] *FGFR3* mutation at exon 15 codon 646 was identified in one tumor (25%) with a concurrent *TP53* mutation at exon 7 codon 237 (**Fig. 21-16**). The remaining three tumors were negative for *FGFR3* or *TP53* gene mutations. These unusual genetic alterations, different from the classic presentations observed in the majority of conventional urothelial carcinoma, indicate that the roles of both gene mutations may not be significant in this subset of urothelial neoplasia, and they may evolve through different carcinogenetic pathways, leading to their aggressive biological behaviors and distinct histopathological characteristics.

In UroVysion FISH assay, all four tumors displayed characteristic chromosomal aberrations (**Table 21-5**).[5] Gains of chromosome 3 were observed in all four tumors, and gains of chromosomes 7 and 17 in tumor cells were identified in two and three cases, respectively. In addition, loss of chromosome 9p21 was observed in one tumor. These findings suggest that the UroVysion FISH assay serves as a potential utility to monitor patients in this unique clinical setting.

Ivil et al. performed FISH studies on touch preparations obtained from tissue taken from near the enterovesical anastomosis of ileocystoplasty patients.[32] They found

Table 21-5 Chromosomal Alterations Detected by Fluorescence In Situ Hybridization UroVysion Assay in Four Urothelial Carcinomas Following Augmentation Cystoplasty[a]

Case	Chromosome Gain			Chromosome Loss
	Chromosome 3	Chromosome 7	Chromosome 17	Chromosome 9p21
1	+	−	+	−
2	+	−	−	−
3	+	+	+	+
4	+	+	+	−

Source: Modified from Ref. 5.
[a]+, positive; −, negative.

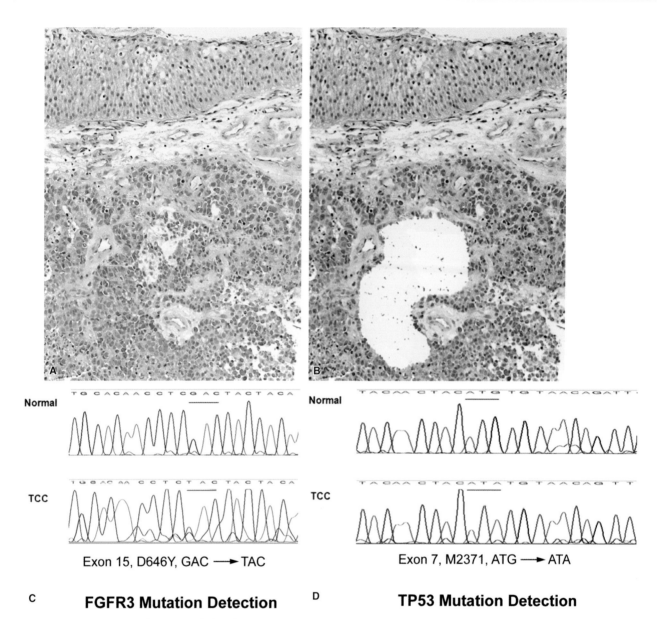

Exon 15, D646Y, GAC ⟶ TAC

Exon 7, M2371, ATG ⟶ ATA

C   FGFR3 Mutation Detection   D   TP53 Mutation Detection

Figure 21-16   Gene mutation analysis for fibroblast growth factor receptor 3 (*FGFR3*) and *TP53* in urothelial carcinoma following augmentation cystoplasty. (A and B) Laser capture microdissection of urothelial carcinoma cells. (A) Hematoxylin and eosin-stained sections showed urothelial carcinoma before microdissection. (B) Corresponding tumor component after microdissection. (C) Mutation analysis of *FGFR3* in urothelial carcinoma (transitional cell carcinoma, TCC). The chromatogram reveals a point mutation at exon 15, D646Y, GAC → TAC. The top chromatogram is sequenced from normal tissue; the bottom chromatogram sequenced from urothelial carcinoma. (D) Mutation analysis of *TP53* in urothelial carcinoma. The chromatogram revealed a point mutation at exon 7, M237I, ATG → ATA. The top chromatogram is sequenced from normal tissue; the bottom chromatogram is sequenced from urothelial carcinoma. (From Ref. 5; with permission.)

significant aneusomy despite the absence of histologic dysplastic changes. The most common finding was alteration of copy numbers of chromosome 18 (monosomy or trisomy), followed by monosomy of chromosome 9 and monosomy/trisomy of chromosome 8. These findings support the notion that genetic instability is present in even

morphologically normal tissue of some augmentation cystoplasty patients, particularly adjacent to the enterovesical anastomosis.

More recently, Appanna and colleagues investigated the genetic abnormalities in augmentation cystoplasty mucosa by comparative genomic hybridization (CGH), to identify those patients at increased risk for tumor formation.[3] In patients without evidence of malignancy, increased amplifications of 2p, 3q, 8q, 9p, 17p, 18pq, and 20pq were noted in bladder biopsies from areas near the enterovesical anastomosis, as compared to those obtained more distant from it, suggesting that urothelium adjacent to the bowel anastomosis is genetically unstable. CGH analysis of tumor DNA from augmentation cystoplasty tumors revealed amplifications at 2q, 5q, 10p, and 21pq, and deletions of 5p and 16p.[3]

REFERENCES

1. Mikulicz J. Zur Operation der angeborenen Blasenspalte. *Centralbl Chir* 1899;26:641−3.
2. Williamson SR, Lopez-Beltran A, Maclennan GT, Montironi R, Cheng L. Unique clinicopathologic and molecular characteristics of urinary bladder tumors in children and young adults. *Urol Oncol* (in press, 2012).
3. Appanna TC, Doak SH, Jenkins SA, Kynaston HG, Stephenson TP, Parry JM. Comparative genomic hybridization (CGH) of augmentation cystoplasties. *Int J Urol* 2007;14:539−44.
4. Soergel TM, Cain MP, Misseri R, Gardner TA, Koch MO, Rink RC. Transitional cell carcinoma of the bladder following augmentation cystoplasty for the neuropathic bladder. *J Urol* 2004;172:1649−52.
5. Sung MT, Zhang S, Lopez-Beltran A, Montironi R, Wang M, Davidson DD, Koch MO, Cain MP, Rink RC, Cheng L. Urothelial carcinoma following augmentation cystoplasty: an aggressive variant with distinct clinicopathological characteristics and molecular genetic alterations. *Histopathology* 2009;55:161−73.
6. Austen M, Kalble T. Secondary malignancies in different forms of urinary diversion using isolated gut. *J Urol* 2004;172:831−8.
7. Metcalfe PD, Cain MP, Kaefer M, Gilley DA, Meldrum KK, Misseri R, King SJ, Casale AJ, Rink RC. What is the need for additional bladder surgery after bladder augmentation in childhood? *J Urol* 2006;176:1801−5.
8. Filmer RB, Spencer JR. Malignancies in bladder augmentations and intestinal conduits. *J Urol* 1990;143:671−8.
9. Smith P, Hardy GJ. Carcinoma occurring as a late complication of ileocystoplasty. *Br J Urol* 1971;43:576−9.
10. Stone AR, Davies N, Stephenson TP. Carcinoma associated with augmentation cystoplasty. *Br J Urol* 1987;60:236−8.
11. Golomb J, Klutke CG, Lewin KJ, Goodwin WE, deKernion JB, Raz S. Bladder neoplasms associated with augmentation cystoplasty: report of 2 cases and literature review. *J Urol* 1989;142:377−80.
12. Gregoire M, Kantoff P, DeWolf WC. Synchronous adenocarcinoma and transitional cell carcinoma of the bladder associated with augmentation: case report and review of the literature. *J Urol* 1993;149:115−8.
13. Shokeir AA. Bladder cancer following ileal ureter. Case report. *Scand J Urol Nephrol* 1995;29:113−5.
14. Barrington JW, Fulford S, Griffiths D, Stephenson TP. Tumors in bladder remnant after augmentation enterocystoplasty. *J Urol* 1997;157:482−5; discussion 485−6.
15. Lane T, Shah J. Carcinoma following augmentation ileocystoplasty. *Urol Int* 2000;64:31−2.
16. Ali-El-Dein B, El-Tabey N, Abdel-Latif M, Abdel-Rahim M, El-Bahnasawy MS. Late uro-ileal cancer after incorporation of ileum into the urinary tract. *J Urol* 2002;167:84−8.
17. Qiu H, Kordunskaya S, Yantiss RK. Transitional cell carcinoma arising in the gastric remnant following gastrocystoplasty: a case report and review of the literature. *Int J Surg Pathol* 2003;11:143−7.
18. Castellan M, Gosalbez R, Perez-Brayfield M, Healey P, McDonald R, Labbie A, Lendvay T. Tumor in bladder reservoir after gastrocystoplasty. *J Urol* 2007;178:1771−4; discussion 1774.
19. Hamid R, Greenwell TJ, Nethercliffe JM, Freeman A, Venn SN, Woodhouse CR. Routine surveillance cystoscopy for patients with augmentation and substitution cystoplasty for benign urological conditions: Is it necessary? *BJU Int* 2009;104:392−5.
20. Hodges KB, Lopez-Beltran A, Emerson RE, Montironi R, Cheng L. Clinical utility of immunohistochemistry in the diagnoses of urinary bladder neoplasia. *Appl Immunohistochem Mol Morphol* 2010;18:401−10.
21. Jiang J, Ulbright TM, Younger C, Sanchez K, Bostwick DG, Koch MO, Eble JN, Cheng L. Cytokeratin 7 and cytokeratin 20 in primary urinary bladder carcinoma and matched lymph node metastasis. *Arch Pathol Lab Med* 2001;125:921−3.
22. Chellaiah AT, McEwen DG, Werner S, Xu J, Ornitz DM. Fibroblast growth factor receptor (FGFR) 3. Alternative splicing in immunoglobulin-like domain III creates a receptor highly specific for acidic FGF/FGF− *J Biol Chem* 1994;269:11620−7.
23. Passos-Bueno MR, Wilcox WR, Jabs EW, Sertie AL, Alonso LG, Kitoh H. Clinical spectrum of fibroblast growth factor receptor mutations. *Hum Mutat* 1999;14:115−25.
24. Cheng L, Zhang S, Maclennan GT, Williamson SR, Lopez-Beltran A, Montironi R. Bladder cancer: translating molecular genetic insights into clinical practice. *Hum Pathol* 2011;42:455−81.
25. Cheng L, Davidson DD, Maclennan GT, Williamson SR, Zhang S, Koch MO, Montironi R, Lopez-Beltran A. The origins of urothelial carcinoma. *Expert Rev Anticancer Ther* 2010;10:865−80.

26. van Rhijn BW, Vis AN, van der Kwast TH, Kirkels WJ, Radvanyi F, Ooms EC, Chopin DK, Boeve ER, Jobsis AC, Zwarthoff EC. Molecular grading of urothelial cell carcinoma with fibroblast growth factor receptor 3 and MIB−1 is superior to pathologic grade for the prediction of clinical outcome. *J Clin Oncol* 2003;21:1912–21.

27. van Rhijn BW, Montironi R, Zwarthoff EC, Jobsis AC, van der Kwast TH. Frequent FGFR3 mutations in urothelial papilloma. *J Pathol* 2002;198:245–51.

28. Kimura T, Suzuki H, Ohashi T, Asano K, Kiyota H, Eto Y. The incidence of thanatophoric dysplasia mutations in FGFR3 gene is higher in low grade or superficial bladder carcinomas. *Cancer* 2001;92:2555–61.

29. Fujimoto K, Yamada Y, Okajima E, Kakizoe T, Sasaki H, Sugimura T, Terada M. Frequent association of p53 gene mutation in invasive bladder cancer. *Cancer Res* 1992;52:1393–8.

30. Bakkar AA, Wallerand H, Radvanyi F, Lahaye JB, Pissard S, Lecerf L, Kouyoumdjian JC, Abbou CC, Pairon JC, Jaurand MC, Thiery JP, Chopin DK, de Medina SG. FGFR3 and TP53 gene mutations define two distinct pathways in urothelial cell carcinoma of the bladder. *Cancer Res* 2003;63:8108–12.

31. van Rhijn BW, van der Kwast TH, Vis AN, Kirkels WJ, Boeve ER, Jobsis AC, Zwarthoff EC. FGFR3 and P53 characterize alternative genetic pathways in the pathogenesis of urothelial cell carcinoma. *Cancer Res* 2004;64:1911–4.

32. Ivil KD, Doak SH, Jenkins SA, Parry EM, Kynaston HG, Parry JM, Stephenson TP. Fluorescence in-situ hybridisation on biopsies from clam ileocystoplasties and on a clam cancer. *Br J Cancer* 2006;94:891–5.

Chapter 22

Other Rare Tumors

Bladder Pathology, First Edition. Liang Cheng, Antonio Lopez-Beltran, David G. Bostwick.
© 2012 Wiley-Blackwell. Published 2012 by John Wiley & Sons, Inc.

Malignant Melanoma

Primary malignant melanoma is rare in the bladder.[1–12] It occurs with equal frequency in men and women, and the age ranges from 44 years to 81 years. Gross hematuria is the most frequent presenting symptom, but some patients with bladder melanoma have presented with symptomatic metastases. Two-thirds of the patients have died of metastatic melanoma within three years of diagnosis. Followup of those alive at the time of other reports has been less than two years.[8,13]

Macroscopically, melanoma is dark brown to black, polypoid or fungating, and solid or infiltrating (**Fig. 22-1**). Some cases have a flat or "macular" appearance. It may arise anywhere in the bladder, and histologically resembles melanoma at other sites, with a variable amount of pigment. Occasionally, melanocytes may be present in the adjacent urothelium. Two cases of spindle cell melanoma of the bladder have been reported.[1]

The generally accepted criteria for determining that melanoma is primary in the bladder are lack of a cutaneous lesion history, failure to find a regressed melanoma of the skin with a Woods lamp examination, failure to find a different visceral primary, and a pattern of spread consistent with bladder primary. Almost all of the tumors appeared darkly pigmented at cystoscopy and on gross pathologic examination. Their sizes range from less than 1 cm to 8 cm. Histologically, the tumors show classic features of malignant melanoma: pleomorphic nuclei, spindle and polygonal cytoplasmic contours, and intracytoplasmic melanin pigment (**Figs. 22-2** to **22-4**). Pigment production is variable and may be absent. One example of clear cell melanoma has been reported. A few tumors were associated with melanosis of the vesical epithelium.[14] One malignant melanoma arose in a bladder diverticulum.

The major differential diagnostic concern is metastatic melanoma to the bladder (**Table 22-1**).[3] Metastatic melanoma in the bladder is much more common than melanoma primary in the bladder. One unique case of melanoma metastasized to a urothelial carcinoma.[7] Immunohistochemical procedures have shown positive reactions with antibodies to S100 protein and with HMB45 or Melan A.[8]

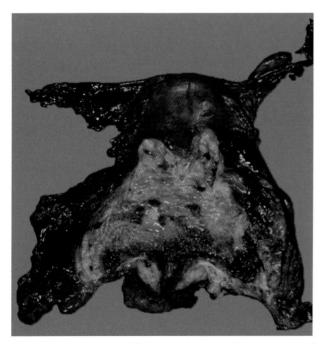

Figure 22-1 Primary malignant melanoma of the urethra and bladder neck. Grossly, part of the tumor displays jet-black pigment.

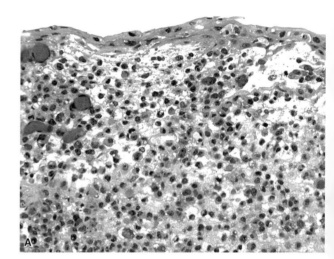

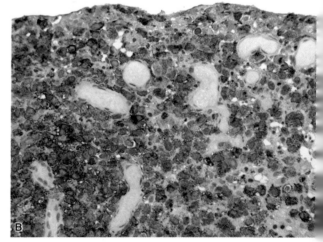

Figure 22-2 Malignant melanoma. The tumor has a discohesive growth pattern (A). It mimics plasmacytoid variant urothelial carcinoma. Immunostaining for HMB45 is strongly positive (B).

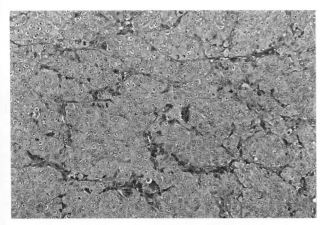

Figure 22-3   Malignant melanoma. Typical features of melanoma, with a mixture of pigmented and nonpigmented cells. The tumor displayed intense cytoplasmic immunoreactivity for S100 protein and HMB45 (not shown).

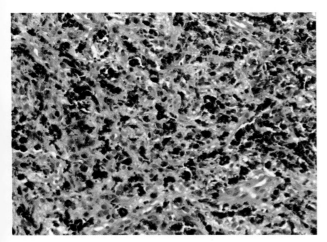

Figure 22-4   Malignant melanoma with prominent melanin depositions.

Table 22-1   Diagnostic Criteria for Separation of Primary and Metastatic Malignant Melanoma of the Urinary Bladder

- No prior history of melanoma of skin or other site.
- Careful examination of the entire skin surface, including use of a Woods light to exclude a depigmented area that may represent regressed melanoma.
- Clinical studies to exclude an ophthalmic or other visceral primary site.
- The pattern of metastases or recurrence should be consistent with a primary bladder tumor rather than metastatic melanoma.
- No widespread metastasis 16 months after the primary tumor diagnosis.
- Atypical melanocytes should be present in the mucosia adjacent to the tumor nodule.

Germ Cell Tumors

A number of germ cell neoplasms may arise rarely in the bladder, including teratoma, seminoma, choriocarcinoma, and yolk sac tumor.[15 23]

Yolk Sac Tumor

Although exceedingly rare, yolk sac tumor has been reported to occur in the bladder and in the setting of urachal remnants.[15–17] Taylor et al. reported a 1-year-old male Caucasian who presented with hematuria and was found to have a large bladder mass.[15] Grossly, the tumor was polypoid, hemorrhagic, gelatinous, and necrotic. Microscopically, it contained solid and cystic areas with cuboidal and columnar cells displaying eosinophilic to clear cytoplasm. Schiller–Duval bodies and hyaline globules were present. The patient underwent partial cystectomy, pelvic lymph node dissection, and chemotherapy, and at 4 months showed no evidence of recurrence.[15]

Another case, in a 2-year-old, arose in apparent urachal remnants and was entirely removed; the boy was tumor-free after three years.[16] In a report by Huang et al., urachal yolk sac tumor may microscopically demonstrate a reticular, microcystic/macrocystic architectural pattern with myxoid stroma, focal solid growth, and glandular areas (**Figs. 22-5** and **22-6**).[17] Similar to testicular tumors, Schiller–Duval bodies may be appreciated. Differentiation from primary urachal adenocarcinoma may sometimes be challenging, especially as positivity for α-fetoprotein has been identified in urachal adenocarcinoma. A key distinguishing feature is the typical patient age, which is young (<2 years) for yolk sac tumor and older than 50 years for urachal adenocarcinoma.

Choriocarcinoma

Pure choriocarcinoma of the bladder in the absence of recognizable papillary or solid urothelial carcinoma is rare, and is associated with an aggressive clinical course. Diagnostic features include syncytiotrophoblastic giant cells and cytotrophoblast cells that display human chorionic gonadotropin (hCG) immunoreactivity (**Fig. 22-7**). Choriocarcinoma should not be confused with urothelial carcinoma with syncytiotrophoblastic giant cells (**Fig. 22-8**; see also **Chapter 12**).[24–29] One reported case had isochromosome 12 by fluorescence in situ hybridization.[20] Patients usually have symptoms typical of other bladder cancers, including hematuria, dysuria, and frequency. Some male patients may have gynecomastia. Increased serum levels of hCG may be present.[19–21,30,31]

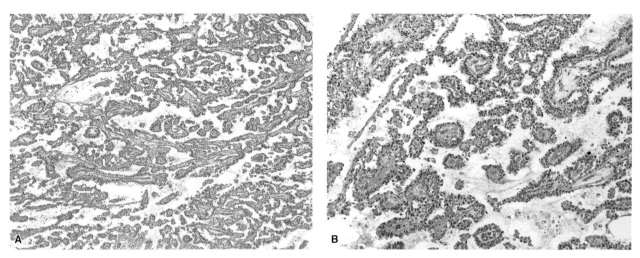

Figure 22-5   Yolk sac tumor of the bladder (A and B). (Photo courtesy of Dr. Sung.)

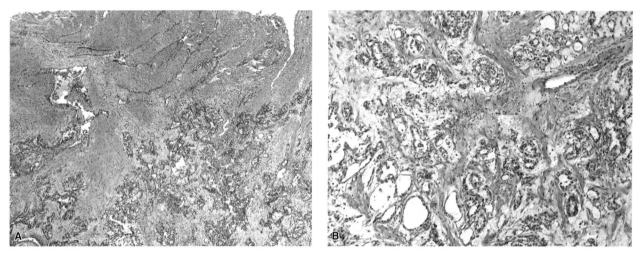

Figure 22-6   Yolk sac tumor of the bladder (A and B). Tumor invades the muscularis propria. (Photo courtesy of Dr. Sung.)

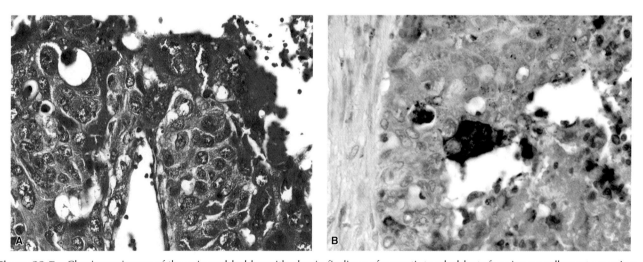

Figure 22-7   Choriocarcinoma of the urinary bladder with classic findings of syncytiotrophoblasts forming an adherent covering over the cytotrophoblasts (A) Immunoreactivity for hCG is limited to the syncytiotrophoblasts (B).

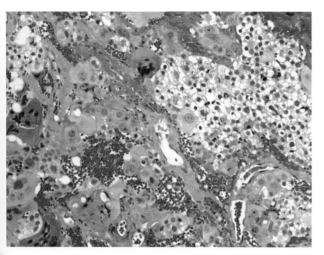

Figure 22-8   Urothelial carcinoma with syncytiotrophoblast differentiation. It should not be confused with choriocarcinoma of the bladder, which is exceedingly rare.

Other Germ Cell Tumors

Rare cases of teratoma arising in the bladder have been described in both adults and children,[32] including one arising in an 8-year-old that was cured by complete excision.[22] A unique case of seminoma involving the bladder has also been reported.[23]

Dermoid Cyst

Rarely, dermoid cysts arise in the bladder of women between 30 and 49 years old, all presenting with non-specific symptoms.[32-34] Typical pathologic features of dermoid cyst are present, including hair, teeth, and calcifications. The possibility of direct extension from ovarian teratoma should be considered.

Rhabdoid Tumor

A small number of cases of primary rhabdoid tumor of the bladder have been reported.[35-37] The first case arose in a 46-year-old woman and contained a mixture of urothelial carcinoma, high grade sarcoma, and rhabdoid tumor, apparently representing a case of sarcomatoid carcinoma.[36] The other cases developed in two girls aged 6 and 14 years old, with typical histologic, immunohistochemical, and ultrastructural features of rhabdoid tumor.[35,37] Key diagnostic features include characteristic rhabdoid morphology, constant expression of vimentin, and variable coexpression of cytokeratin. Patients are young, and ultrastructural features include whorled cytoplasmic intermediate filaments adjacent to the nucleus.

Perivascular Epithelioid Cell Tumor

Perivascular epithelioid cell tumors (PEComas) are low grade mesenchymal tumors composed of histologically and immunohistochemically distinctive perivascular cells.[38-42] The PEComa family consists of entities such as angiomyolipoma, clear cell ("sugar") tumor of the lung, and lymphangioleiomyoma. PEComas have alternatively been termed "clear cell myomelanocytic tumors."[43] These tumors characteristically exhibit an epithelioid morphology arranged radially around blood vessels and a more spindled morphology distant from the blood vessels, and coexpress muscle and melanocytic immunohistochemical markers (**Figs. 22-9 to 22-11**). Few well-documented examples of this tumor arising primarily in the bladder have been reported.[38,43-46] Patients with the PEComas of the bladder often present with dysuria and hematuria. The mean age at diagnosis is approximately 36 years.

The largest series of PEComas, reported by Sukov and colleagues, consisted of three cases.[46] One of the cases showed principally a spindle cell pattern. The second case was principally an epithelioid pattern, and the third case demonstrated a mixed pattern. In another report,[44] the tumor was described as being composed of epithelioid and occasionally spindled cells, containing abundant cytoplasm that varied from clear to granular and eosinophilic. Nuclei were round and generally uniform; inconspicuous nucleoli and nuclear inclusions were observed. Mitotic figures were rare to absent, and necrosis was not seen.[44] Another tumor exhibited perivascularly arranged cells with granular eosinophilic cytoplasm, round to oval vesicular nuclei, and prominent nucleoli. Focal cytologic atypia and a few mitotic figures were identified (**Fig. 22-12**).[45] Both of these tumors demonstrated intracytoplasmic glycogen in some tumor cells by prostate-specific antigen (PAS) staining with and without diastase digestion.[44,45] The other tumor, which was designated as a clear cell myomelanocytic tumor, had clear to eosinophilic epithelioid and spindle cells arranged in fascicles or packets with delicate vascular stoma among the nests.[43] Interestingly, a normal counterpart to the perivascular epithelioid cell has not been identified in the urinary bladder.

PEComas demonstrate divergent immunoreactivity.[38,41,46,47] Tumor cells may show immunoreactivity to antibodies against melanocytic markers such as HMB45, Melan A, tyrosinase, and microphthalmia transcription factor, as well as weakly positive immunostaining for myoid markers, including smooth muscle actin, smooth muscle myosin heavy chain, desmin, calponin, and CD117. The vasculature is highlighted by reticulin and CD31. The tumor cells typically show no immunostaining for S100 protein, cytokeratin AE1/AE3, myoglobin, synaptophysin, or chromogranin. Immunoreactivity for vimentin is usually

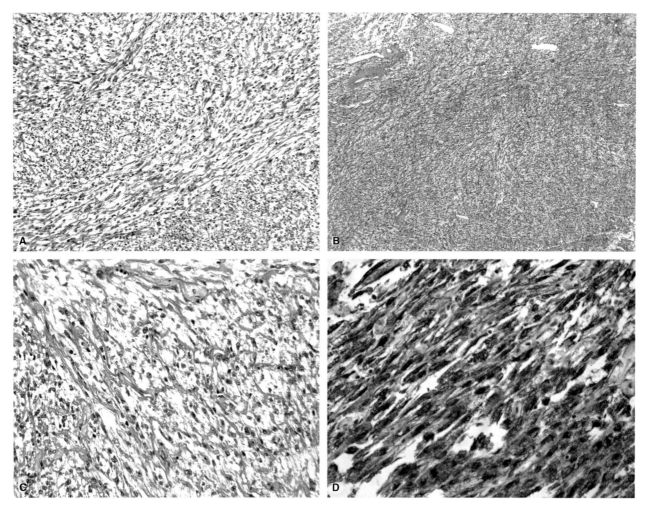

Figure 22-9   Perivascular epithelioid cell tumor of the bladder (A to D). PEComa of the urinary bladder consists of a proliferation of epithelioid cells that display HMB45 immunoreactivity (D). The tumor has a fascicular arrangement of cells. (Photo courtesy of Dr. Pan.)

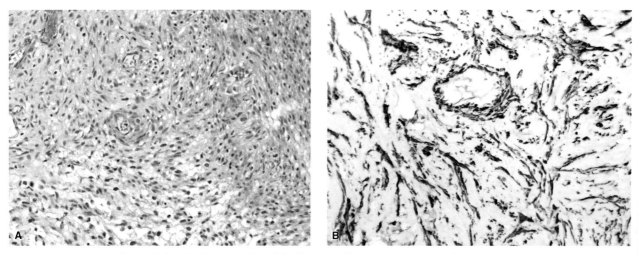

Figure 22-10   Perivascular epithelioid cell tumor of the bladder (A and B). Immunostaining for smooth muscle actin is positive (B). (Photo courtesy of Dr. Pan.)

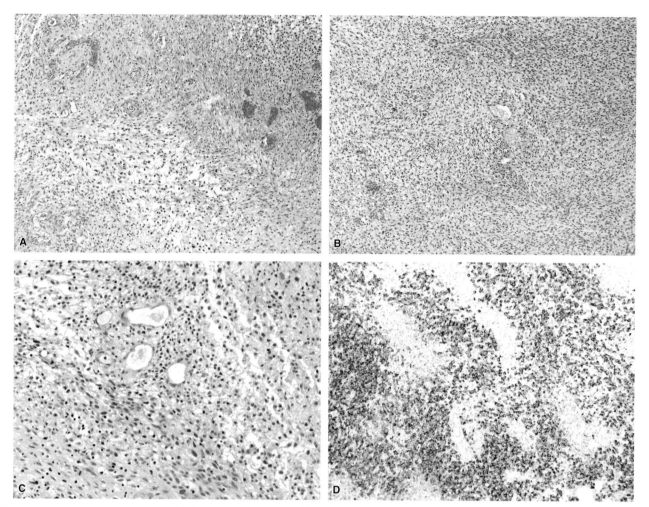

Figure 22-11 Perivascular epithelioid cell tumor of the bladder (A to D). Note prominent vasculature. PEComa of the urinary bladder is positive for HMB45 (D).

inconspicuous. Interestingly, PEComas are thought to be capable of modulating their immunophenotype according to morphology. For example, a PEComa with prominent spindle cell morphology expresses smooth muscle actin more strongly than HMB45. In contrast, a purely epithelioid PEComa displays HMB45 immunoreactivity and only focal actin positivity. PEComas with spindle cell morphology may display immunoreactivity for progesterone receptors, suggesting a role for this hormone in morphologic and immunophenotypic modulation.

A recent study by Pan et al. involved comparative genomic hybridization studies of nine perivascular epithelioid cell tumors, including one from the urinary bladder.[48,49] All exhibited gross chromosomal aberrations. Frequent imbalances included losses on chromosome 19 (eight cases), 16p (six cases), 17p (six cases), 1p (five cases), and 18p (four cases). Gains were seen on chromosome X (six cases), 12q (six cases), 3q (five cases), 5q (four cases), and 2q (four cases). The single bladder tumor exhibited chromosomal gains at 3p12, 10p15, 12p11.2–p12, and 12q21 and chromosomal loss at 19q13.1. Chromosomal gain on 12q13–q21 has been identified in different types of sarcomas. Although not identified in the bladder PEComa, deletions in chromosome 16p, where the *TSC2* gene is located, were frequently identified in such tumors at other sites. These recurrent chromosomal aberrations provide evidence that the PEComa is a distinctive tumor entity at any anatomic location.

Although primary epithelial tumors are by far the most common urinary bladder neoplasms in adults, a wide spectrum of soft tissue lesions can occur in the bladder,[3,4] sometimes creating the false impression of an aggressive urothelial malignancy due to extravesical growth. In particular, perivascular epithelioid cell tumor, or PEComa, is a rare soft tissue lesion that may generate a broad differential diagnosis at the histopathologic level, due to its biphasic light microscopic and immunohistochemical

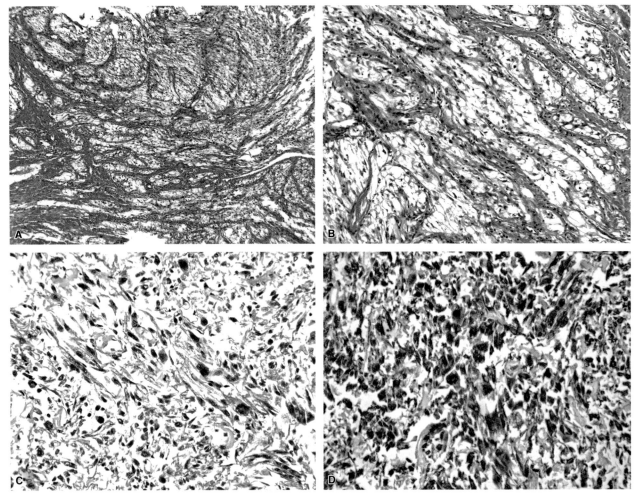

Figure 22-12 Perivascular epithelioid cell tumor of the bladder (A to D). Note the cytologic atypia. Tumor cells are positive for HMB45 (D).

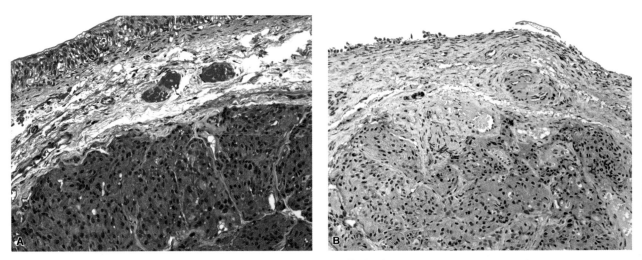

Figure 22-13 Granular cell tumor of the bladder (A and B). Tumor cells display strong immunoreactivity for S100 protein (B).

features.[38,41,46,50–53] Tumors included in the differential diagnoses of PEComa include leiomyoma, leiomyosarcoma, paraganglioma, melanoma, clear cell sarcoma of soft parts, epithelioid sarcoma, postoperative spindle cell nodule, inflammatory myofibroblastic tumor, sarcomatoid carcinoma, and metastatic carcinoma. Smooth muscle tumor cells are typically more eosinophilic and are not arranged in packets; similarly, they do not typically express melanocytic markers. Primary malignant melanoma is rare in the bladder. It typically develops from the urothelium, is often focally melanotic, and does not demonstrate immunoreactivity for actin. The mixture of spindled and epithelioid morphology in PEComa may also raise consideration of metastatic malignant melanoma, especially in combination with the expression of melanocytic markers. However, in contrast to melanoma, expression of S100 protein is seen in only a subset of PEComas.[1] Although very rare, extragastrointestinal stromal tumor (EGIST) may also show mixed epithelioid and spindled features. Clear cell melanoma is similar to clear cell sarcoma of soft parts. It shares some overlapping histologic features with PEComa, but the thin vascular stroma among tumor nests seen in PEComa is not seen in clear cell sarcoma of soft parts, which, instead, has nests separated by collagenous, avascular stroma. Whereas clear cell sarcoma of soft parts is immunoreactive for HMB45 and S100, it is negative for actin. Postoperative spindle cell nodule and inflammatory myofibroblastic tumor, as well as sarcomatoid carcinoma, can be excluded by reference to their characteristic histologic and immunohistochemical features.[38,50,53]

All reported cases of bladder PEComas have demonstrated indolent biologic behavior, but such tumors occurring at other sites have, in rare instances, behaved in a malignant fashion.[44] We have also seen a case of PEComa that behaved in malignant fashion. One patient was lost to followup, and neither of the other patients had evidence of recurrence at four and six years.[43,44] Recently, criteria for prediction of malignant behavior in PEComa in general (of all organ sites) have been proposed, including two or more of the following: size greater than 5 cm, infiltrative growth, high cellularity, high nuclear grade, necrosis, vascular invasion, and mitotic rate greater than or equal to 1 per 50 high power fields. Tumors with only nuclear pleomorphism ("symplastic" features), or size greater than 5 cm, are classified as having uncertain malignant potential.[38,41,46,51]

Granular Cell Tumor

Several cases of benign granular cell tumors, as well as a case of malignant granular cell tumor have been reported.[54–61] One case occurred in a patient with neurofibromatosis.[58] The patients range in age from 23 years to 61 years. The most common presenting symptom was painless hematuria, sometimes accompanied by a palpable mass.[54–57] One tumor presented with pain with micturition, while another was discovered incidentally.[59,60]

Granular cell tumors of the urinary bladder are usually cured by local excision, particularly if removal includes a rim of normal bladder tissue.[55–57] One patient received postoperative radiation therapy.[57] Recurrence at 10 months and 17 months status postexcision was reported in one patient, but subsequent followup at 2.5 years revealed the patient to be free of disease.[54] Yoshida reported recurrence at 6 months with no subsequent recurrence at three years following reexcision.[59] Most cases have had no recurrence at followup of 1 to 18 years.[54,56–58,60]

Macroscopically, the tumors are variously described as an encapsulated yellow-white smooth mass, an "unusual appearing ulcer," or an irregular mass with a nodular surface and focal hemorrhagic degeneration. They may be multifocal, with tumor size up to 9 cm in greatest dimension.

Microscopically, the tumor is composed of large polyhedral, spindle, or round cells arranged in columns and pseudoalveolar formations, separated by slender fibrous connective tissue septa (**Fig. 22-13**). The tumor may compress focally and stretch the overlying urothelium.[54] The overlying mucosa may ulcerate or remain intact. Tumor cell cytoplasm is abundant and contains numerous pink-stained granules of varying sizes. The nuclei are centrally located, small, and uniform, although focal atypia is reported to occur in granular cell tumors at other sites. Mitotic figures are inconspicuous.

Granular cell tumors stain positively for S100 protein and CD68, a panmacrophage antigen. Positive immunostaining for neuron-specific enolase and keratin sulfate has been reported.[58–60] Histochemically, the cytoplasmic granules in these tumors are periodic acid–Schiff positive, diastase resistant.

Malignant granular cell tumor is exceedingly rare in the urinary bladder. Ravich et al. reported one case of granular cell "myoblastoma" in a 31-year-old male, which was felt to arise from the urinary bladder.[61] The tumor was large at 12 cm × 11 cm × 9 cm, but grossly and microscopically appeared to be a granular cell tumor. A nodular pattern of small nuclei and finely acidophilic cytoplasmic granules was present without cross-striations or mitoses. Slender connective tissue strands separated the cords. However, the tumor recurred after excision and metastasized widely, causing death 17 months later. Interestingly, most of the metastatic tumor at autopsy resembled the primary, but the recurrent tumor and the pulmonary metastases had different-appearing cells with larger, more hyperchromatic nuclei and decreased cytoplasm. No mitoses were identified, but some "chondriosome" formation was seen.[61] The diagnosis of malignant granular cell tumor should follow the same criteria as those used in other organ sites.[51] These tumors have three or more of the following: necrosis, spindling, vesicular nuclei with prominent nucleoli, mitotic rate of more than 2 mitoses per 10 high power fields, high nuclear-to-cytoplasmic ratio, and pleomorphism. Tumors with fewer than three of these features are "atypical granular cell tumors," having an excellent prognosis and no risk of metastases.

REFERENCES

1. De Torres I, Fortuno MA, Raventos A, Tarragona J, Banus JM, Vidal MT. Primary malignant melanoma of the bladder: immunohistochemical study of a new case and review of the literature. *J Urol* 1995;154:525–7.

2. Ironside JW, Timperley WR, Madden JW, Royds JA, Taylor CB. Primary melanoma of the urinary bladder presenting with intracerebral metastases. *Br J Urol* 1985;57:593–4.

3. Ainsworth AM, Clark WH, Mastrangelo M, Conger KB. Primary malignant melanoma of the urinary bladder. *Cancer* 1976;37:1928–36.

4. Khalbuss WE, Hossain M, Elhosseiny A. Primary malignant melanoma of the urinary bladder diagnosed by urine cytology: a case report. *Acta Cytol* 2001;45:631–5.

5. Pacella M, Gallo F, Gastaldi C, Ambruosi C, Carmignani G. Primary malignant melanoma of the bladder. *Int J Urol* 2006;13:635–7.

6. Tainio HM, Kylmala TM, Haapasalo HK. Primary malignant melanoma of the urinary bladder associated with widespread metastases. *Scand J Urol Nephrol* 1999;33:406–7.

7. Arapantoni-Dadioti P, Panayiotides J, Kalkandi P, Christodoulou C, Delides GS. Metastasis of malignant melanoma to a transitional cell carcinoma of the urinary bladder. *Eur J Surg Oncol* 1995;21:92–3.

8. Akbas A, Akman T, Erdem MR, Antar B, Kilicarslan I, Onol SY. Female urethral malignant melanoma with vesical invasion: a case report. *Kaohsiung J Med Sci* 2010;26:96–8.

9. Siroy AE, Maclennan GT. Primary melanoma of the bladder. *J Urol* 2011;185:1096–7.

10. Van Ahlen H, Nicolas V, Lenz W, Boldt I, Bockisch A, Vahlensieck W. Primary melanoma of urinary bladder. *Urology* 1992;40:550–4.

11. Tajima Y, Aizawa M. Unusual renal pelvic tumor containing transitional cell carcinoma, adenocarcinoma and sarcomatoid elements (so-called sarcomatoid carcinoma of the renal pelvis). A case report and review of the literature. *Acta Pathol Jpn* 1988;38:805–14.

12. Katz EE, Suzue K, Wille MA, Krausz T, Rapp DE, Sokoloff MH. Primary malignant melanoma of the urethra. *Urology* 2005;65:389.

13. Morichetti D, Mazzucchelli R, Lopez-Beltran A, Cheng L, Scarpelli M, Kirkali Z, Montorsi F, Montironi R. Secondary neoplasms of the urinary system and male genital organs. *BJU Int* 2009;104:770–6.

14. Sanborn SL, MacLennan G, Cooney MM, Zhou M, Ponsky LE. High grade transitional cell carcinoma and melanosis of urinary bladder: case report and review of the literature. *Urology* 2009;73:928 e13–5.

15. Taylor G, Jordan M, Churchill B, Mancer K. Yolk sac tumor of the bladder. *J Urol* 1983;129:591–4.

16. D'Alessio A, Verdelli G, Bernardi M, DePascale S, Chiarenza SF, Giardina C, Cheli M, Rota G, Locatelli G. Endodermal sinus (yolk sac) tumor of the urachus. *Eur J Pediatr Surg* 1994;4:180–1.

17. Huang HY, Ko SF, Chuang JH, Jeng YM, Sung MT, Chen WJ. Primary yolk sac tumor of the urachus. *Arch Pathol Lab Med* 2002;126:1106–9.

18. Melicow M. Tumors of the urinary bladder: A clinico-pathological analysis of over 2500 specimens and biopsies. *J Urol* 1955;74:498–521.

19. Yokoyama S, Hayashida Y, Nagahama J, Nakayama I, Kashima K, Ogata J. Primary and metaplastic choriocarcinoma of the bladder. A report of two cases. *Acta Cytol* 1992;36:176–82.

20. Hanna NH, Ulbright TM, Einhorn LH. Primary choriocarcinoma of the bladder with the detection of isochromosome 12p. *J Urol* 2002;167:1781.

21. Cho JH, Yu E, Kim KH, Lee I. Primary choriocarcinoma of the urinary bladder—a case report. *J Korean Med Sci* 1992;7:369–72.

22. Misra S, Agarwal PK, Tandon RK, Wakhlu AK, Misra NC. Bladder teratoma: a case report and review of literature. *Indian J Cancer* 1997;34:20–1.

23. Khandekar JD, Holland JM, Rochester D, Christ ML. Extragonadal seminoma involving urinary bladder and arising in the prostate. *Cancer* 1993;71:3972–4.

24. Shah VM, Newman J, Crocker J, Chapple CR, Collard MJ, O'Brien JM, Considine J. Ectopic beta-human chorionic gonadotropin production by bladder urothelial neoplasia. *Arch Pathol Lab Med* 1986;110:107–11.

25. Seidal T, Breborowicz J, Malmstrom P. Immunoreactivity to human chorionic gonadotropin in urothelial carcinoma: correlation with tumor grade, stage, and progression. *J Urol Pathol* 1993;1:397–410.

26. Martin JE, Jenkins BJ, Zuk RJ, Oliver RT, Baithun SI. Human chorionic gonadotrophin expression and histological findings as predictors of response to radiotherapy in carcinoma of the bladder. *Virchows Arch A Pathol Anat Histopathol* 1989;414:273–7.

27. Grammatico D, Grignon DJ, Eberwein P, Shepherd RR, Hearn SA, Walton JC. Transitional cell carcinoma of the renal pelvis with choriocarcinomatous differentiation. Immunohistochemical and immunoelectron microscopic assessment of human chorionic gonadotropin production by transitional cell carcinoma of the urinary bladder. *Cancer* 1993;71:1835–41.

28. Campo E, Algaba F, Palacin A, Germa R, Sole-Balcells FJ, Cardesa A. Placental proteins in high grade urothelial neoplasms. An immunohistochemical study of human chorionic gonadotropin, human placental lactogen, and pregnancy-specific beta-1-glycoprotein. *Cancer* 1989;63:2497–504.

29. Yamase HT, Wurzel RS, Nieh PT, Gondos B. Immunohistochemical demonstration of human chorionic gonadotropin in tumors of the urinary bladder. *Ann Clin Lab Sci* 1985;15:414–7.

30. Obe JA, Rosen N, Koss LG. Primary choriocarcinoma of the urinary bladder. Report of a case with probable epithelial origin. *Cancer* 1983;52:1405–9.

31. Fowler AL, Hall E, Rees G. Choriocarcinoma arising in transitional cell carcinoma of the bladder. *Br J Urol* 1992;70:333–4.

32. Sabnis RB, Bradoo AM, Desai RM, Bhatt RM, Randive NU. Primary benign vesical teratoma. A case report. *Arch Esp Urol* 1993;46:444–5.

33. Cauffield EW. Dermoid cysts of the bladder. *J Urol* 1956;75:801–4.

34. Valizadeh A, Arend P, Diallo B, Kotowitz A, Pontus T. [Dermoid cyst of the bladder. Case report]. *Acta Urol Belg* 1991;59:79–83.

35. Harris M, Eyden BP, Joglekar VM. Rhabdoid tumour of the bladder: a histological, ultrastructural and immunohistochemical study. *Histopathology* 1987;11:1083–92.

36. Egawa S, Uchida T, Koshiba K, Kagata Y, Iwabuchi K. Malignant fibrous histiocytoma of the bladder with focal rhabdoid tumor differentiation. *J Urol* 1994;151:154–6.

37. McBride JA, Ro JY, Hicks J, Ordóñez NG, Raney RB, Ayala AG. Malignant rhabdoid tumor of the bladder in an adolescent. Case report and discussion of extrarenal rhabdoid tumor. *J Urol Pathol* 1994;2:255–63.

38. Williamson SR, Cheng L. Perivascular epithelioid cell tumor of the urinary bladder. *J Urol* 2011;185:1473–4.

39. Martignoni G, Pea M, Reghellin D, Zamboni G, Bonetti F. PEComas: the past, the present and the future. *Virchows Arch* 2008;452:119–32.

40. Hornick JL, Fletcher CD. PEComa: What do we know so far? *Histopathology* 2006;48:75–82.

41. Folpe AL, Kwiatkowski DJ. Perivascular epithelioid cell neoplasms: pathology and pathogenesis. *Hum Pathol* 2010;41:1–15.

42. Martignoni G, Pea M, Reghellin D, Zamboni G, Bonetti F. Perivascular epithelioid cell tumor (PEComa) in the genitourinary tract. *Adv Anat Pathol* 2007;14:36–41.

43. Pan C-C, Yu I-T, Yang A-H, Chiang H. Clear cell myomelanocytic tumor of the urinary bladder. *Am J Surg Pathol* 2003;27:689–92.

44. Parfitt JR, Bella AJ, Wehrli BM, Izawa JI. Primary PEComa of the bladder treated with primary excision and adjuvant interferon-alpha immunotherapy: a case report. *BMC Urol* 2006;6:20.

45. Kalyanasundaram K, Parameswaran A, Mani R. Perivascular epithelioid tumor of urinary bladder and vagina. *Ann Diagn Pathol* 2005;9:275–8.

46. Sukov WR, Cheville JC, Amin MB, Gupta R, Folpe AL. Perivascular epithelioid cell tumor (PEComa) of the urinary bladder: report of 3 cases and review of the literature. *Am J Surg Pathol* 2009;33:304–8.

47. Hodges KB, Lopez-Beltran A, Emerson RE, Montironi R, Cheng L. Clinical utility of immunohistochemistry in the diagnoses of urinary bladder neoplasia. *Appl Immunohistochem Mol Morphol* 2010;18:401–10.

48. Pan CC, Chung MY, Ng KF, Liu CY, Wang JS, Chai CY, Huang SH, Chen PC, Ho DM. Constant allelic alteration on chromosome 16p (TSC2 gene) in perivascular epithelioid cell tumour (PEComa): genetic evidence for the relationship of PEComa with angiomyolipoma. *J Pathol* 2008;214:387–93.

49. Pan CC, Jong YJ, Chai CY, Huang SH, Chen YJ. Comparative genomic hybridization study of perivascular epithelioid cell tumor: molecular genetic evidence of perivascular epithelioid cell tumor as a distinctive neoplasm. *Hum Pathol* 2006;37:606–12.

50. Cheng L, Foster SR, MacLennan GT, Lopez-Beltran A, Zhang S, Montironi R. Inflammatory myofibroblastic tumors of the genitourinary tract—single entity or continuum? *J Urol* 2008;180:1235–40.

51. Lott S, Lopez-Beltran A, Maclennan GT, Montironi R, Cheng L. Soft tissue tumors of the urinary bladder, Part I: Myofibroblastic proliferations, benign neoplasms, and tumors of uncertain malignant potential. *Hum Pathol* 2007;38:807–23.

52. Lott S, Lopez-Beltran A, Montironi R, MacLennan GT, Cheng L. Soft tissue tumors of the urinary bladder: Part II: Malignant neoplasms. *Hum Pathol* 2007;38:807–23.

53. Cheng L, Zhang S, Alexander R, MacLennan GT, Hodges KB, Harrison BT, Lopez-Beltran A, Montironi R. Sarcomatoid carcinoma of the urinary bladder: the final common pathway of urothelial carcinoma dedifferentiation. *Am J Surg Pathol* 2011;35:e34–46.

54. Mouradian J, Coleman J, McGovern J, Gray G. Granular cell tumor (myoblastoma) of the bladder. *J Urol* 1974;112:343–5.

55. Fletcher MS, Aker M, Hill JT, Pryor JP, Whimster WF. Granular cell myoblastoma of the bladder. *Br J Urol* 1985;57:109–10.

56. Seery WH. Granular cell myoblastoma of the bladder: report of a case. *J Urol* 1968;100:735–7.

57. Mizutani S, Okuda N, Sonoda T. Granular cell myoblastoma of the bladder: report of an additional case. *J Urol* 1973;110:403–5.

58. Kontani K, Okaneya T, Takezaki T. Recurrent granular cell tumour of the bladder in a patient with von Recklinghausen's disease. *BJU Int* 1999;84:871–2.

59. Yoshida T, Hirai S, Horii Y, Yamauchi T. Granular cell tumor of the urinary bladder. *Int J Urol* 2001;8:29–31.

60. Kondo T, Kajimoto S, Okuda H, Toma H, Tanabe K. A case of granular cell tumor of the bladder successfully managed with extraperitoneal laparoscopic surgery. *Int J Urol* 2006;13:827–8.

61. Ravich A, Stout AP, Ravich RA. Malignant granular cell myoblastoma invovling the urinary bladder. *Ann Surg* 1945;121:361–72.

Chapter 23

Secondary Tumors

Overview

The urinary bladder is involved secondarily by a wide spectrum of malignancies.[1–5] Secondary tumors represent up to 14% of bladder neoplasms. In a retrospective study of 282 tumors, secondary bladder neoplasms represented 2.3% of all malignant bladder tumors in surgical specimens at one institution.[1]

The majority represent direct invasion from cancer arising in adjacent organs. The most common primary sites and their relative frequencies include colon (21%), prostate (19%), rectum (12%), and cervix (11%).[1] Most tumors from these sites involved the bladder by direct extension.

Metastases to the bladder from distant organs are less common than contiguous spread. Overall, distant metastases account for up to 3.5% of secondary tumors. The most common distant sites of origin of tumors metastatic to the bladder and their relative frequencies are stomach (4.3%), skin (melanoma) (3.9%), lung (2.8%), and breast (2.5%).[1] Infrequently, renal cell carcinoma may also metastasize to the bladder.[3]

Secondary tumor deposits are almost always solitary (96.7%), and 54% of these are located in the bladder neck or trigone.[1] Over one-half of secondary tumors are adenocarcinomas. Metastases should be suspected in any bladder tumor with unusual histology and in cases of pure adenocarcinoma or squamous cell carcinoma. Occasional cases of pelvic lipomatosis can simulate a neoplasm extending to the bladder.[6]

In terms of differential diagnosis, few secondary tumors have distinctive histological features, making it difficult to make the appropriate diagnosis. Hence, knowledge of the history and clinical setting is particularly important in these cases. Practicing pathologists should be aware of the incidence and histological appearances of secondary neoplasms of the urinary bladder, with emphasis on the points of distinction from primary tumors and their histological variants.[1,7] Immunohistochemistry is useful for distinguishing primary tumors of the urinary bladder from metastases or direct extension from other sites.[8,9]

Secondary Adenocarcinoma

Secondary involvement of the urinary bladder by a glandular malignancy from an adjacent organ is more common than primary bladder adenocarcinoma. Metastasis or direct extension of tumors originating in the colon, prostate, and female genital tract are probable culprits for bladder involvement.[10] In some circumstances, these tumors can be indistinguishable from primary bladder adenocarcinoma by light microscopic examination, placing utmost importance on a number of additional findings, including clinical information and immunohistochemical studies.[11]

Colorectal Adenocarcinoma Extension to the Bladder

Histologically, 54% of secondary tumors are adenocarcinomas. Colorectal adenocarcinoma is the most frequent secondary malignancy to involve the urinary bladder (**Figs. 23-1** to **23-3**). Accurate diagnosis is essential because of potentially differing prognosis and therapeutic approaches. Clinical history and comparison of morphology are of paramount importance.[4,12] Spread from colonic or rectal primary could represent a diagnostic challenge in bladder transurethral resection and biopsy samples. Differentiating a secondary adenocarcinoma from primary adenocarcinoma of bladder may not be possible on a morphologic

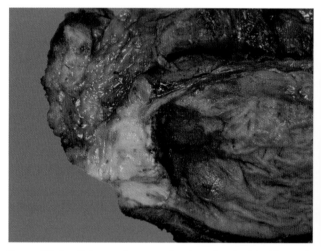

Figure 23-1 Colorectal cancer that invades the bladder and prostate.

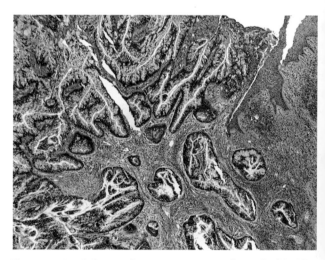

Figure 23-2 Colonic adenocarcinoma involving the bladder.

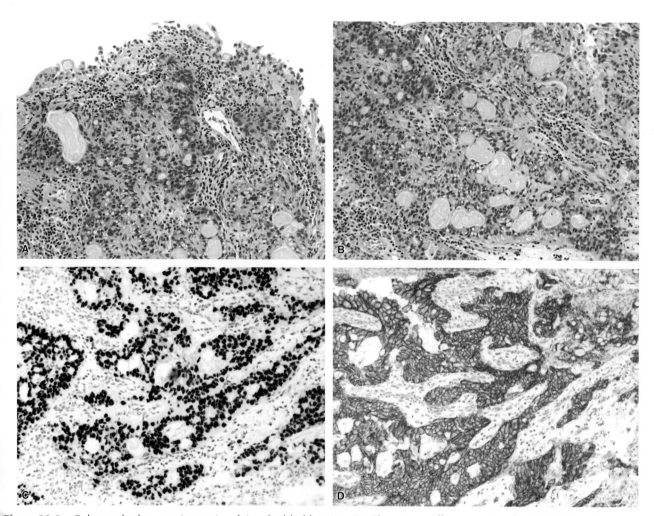

Figure 23-3   Colorectal adenocarcinoma involving the bladder (A to D). The tumor cells are positive for CDX2 (C) and β-catenin (D).

basis. At a number of levels, including light microscopy, histochemistry,[13] immunohistochemistry,[10,11,14] and electron microscopy,[10] the tumors from both primary sites may have similar characteristics. The presence of a background of urothelial intestinal metaplasia with associated glandular dysplasia favors a primary origin. However, one should be aware of the possibility of colonization of the bladder urothelial mucosa by a secondary well-differentiated colonic adenocarcinoma mimicking intestinal metaplasia and glandular dysplasia background.[8,9,11,15–17] Colorectal carcinoma involving the bladder may demonstrate villous projections indistinguishable from those seen in villous adenoma of either the bladder or colon. Similarly, within these villous projections, intraepithelial changes of adenocarcinoma in situ may be present, such as cribriform architecture or significant cytologic atypia. So-called "dirty necrosis," the characteristic luminal debris associated with colon cancer, may be seen. The invasive component may sometimes undermine the overlying urothelium.

Nonetheless, morphologic features may not always be reliable in proving colonic origin.

Primary adenocarcinoma of the urinary tract shares a similar immunohistochemical profile with primary and metastatic colonic adenocarcinoma. Therefore, the utility of an immunohistochemical panel in differentiating between primary and metastatic tumors is somewhat limited (**Fig. 23-3**; **Table 23-1**; see also **Chapters 13 and 26**). Wang and colleagues studied this challenging diagnostic dilemma, evaluating cases of bladder adenocarcinoma that included enteric type (well to moderately differentiated), signet ring cell type, and clear cell type.[10] Nuclear staining for β-catenin was evident in 13 of 16 (81%) colorectal adenocarcinoma cases, while cytoplasmic, membranous, or absent staining was seen in primary bladder adenocarcinoma. Thrombomodulin and cytokeratin (CK) 7 were negative in colorectal tumors, while primary bladder tumors exhibited variable staining (59% and 65%, respectively), suggesting that they may be of some utility

Table 23-1 Primary Adenocarcinoma of the Bladder versus Colorectal Adenocarcinoma[a]

	CK7	CK20	CDX2	Villin	β-Catenin	Uroplakin III
Bladder adenocarcinoma	Pos	Pos	Pos	Pos	Pos (cytoplasmic)	Pos
Colorectal adenocarcinoma	Neg	Pos	Pos	Pos	Pos (nuclear)	Neg

[a]Pos, positive; Neg, negative, CK7, cytokeratin 7, CK20, cytokeratin 20.

in resolving the differential diagnosis. CK20 staining was present in 94% of colorectal tumors and 53% of bladder tumors, leaving it with somewhat limited usefulness by itself.[10] In contrast, other authors have found occasional CK7 staining in colorectal tumors.[14] Although villin has shown some utility in the differentiation of enteric-type bladder adenocarcinoma from urothelial carcinoma with glandular differentiation, it does not appear useful in differentiation between enteric-type bladder cancer and involvement by colorectal malignancy.[11] Some authors have found combined absence of villin and CDX2 staining to suggest a bladder primary,[18] although a significant number of bladder primary tumors are CDX2 positive,[19] as is intestinal metaplasia of the bladder.[8,9,20]

In some cases, despite extensive workup, it may still not be possible to ascertain if the tumor is primary adenocarcinoma of the bladder or an extension from colorectal adenocarcinoma. It is important that the pathologists make a recommendation to the urologists to rule out spread from a colorectal primary. Radical cystectomy is usually not indicated in cases of secondary involvement of bladder by colorectal adenocarcinoma.

Prostate Adenocarcinoma Extension to the Bladder

The second most common source of secondary tumor involvement of the bladder is prostatic adenocarcinoma (Figs. 23-4 to 23-7). Distinction of prostatic versus urothelial origin has important prognostic and therapeutic implications since androgen deprivation therapy is commonly employed for advanced stage prostate cancer. Bladder carcinoma is more responsive than prostate cancer to chemotherapy.

Most cases of secondary involvement by prostatic adenocarcinoma are readily recognized by the distinctive histology of the tumor and an immunohistochemistry approach will assure proper classification (Tables 23-2 and 23-3).[8,17] However, superimposed morphologic changes, such as squamous differentiation due to prior hormonal or radiation treatment effect, could pose a difficulty in distinguishing prostatic carcinoma recurrence from primary urothelial carcinoma in small bladder biopsy specimens. Furthermore, this may become problematic when the tumor is poorly differentiated or when a neoplasm of urothelial origin demonstrates a prominent tubular component or more extensive glandular differentiation. Poorly differentiated prostate cancers may have enlarged nuclei and prominent nucleoli, yet there is little variability in nuclear shape or size from one nucleus to another. High grade urothelial carcinoma often displays marked nuclear pleomorphism with occasional nuclear anaplasia. Urothelial carcinoma tends to grow in nests, even when poorly differentiated, but usually lacks the cribriforming and cord-like architecture of prostate cancer. In addition, inflammatory background favors the diagnosis of urothelial carcinoma.

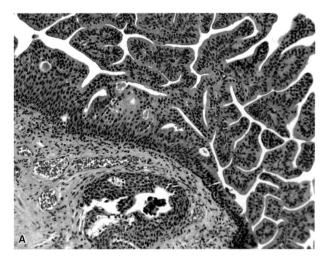
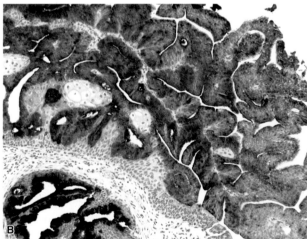

Figure 23-4 Ductal-type prostatic adenocarcinoma involving the bladder (A and B). Immunostaining for prostate-specific antigen is strongly positive (B).

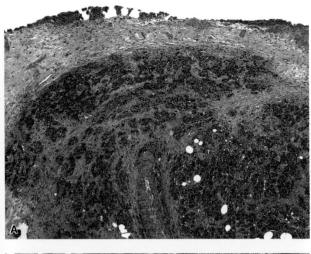

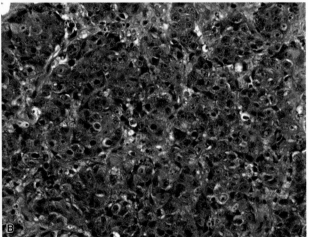

Figure 23-5 Prostatic adenocarcinoma involving the bladder (A and B). The tumor cells are relatively uniform and have abundant eosinophilic cytoplasm and prominent nucleoli.

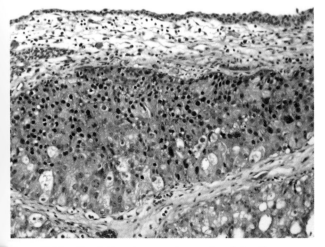

Figure 23-6 Prostatic adenocarcinoma involving the bladder.

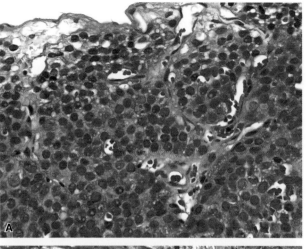

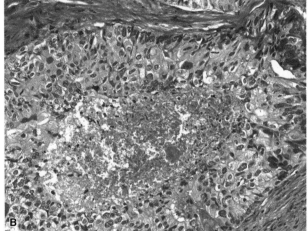

Figure 23-7 Prostatic adenocarcinoma involving the bladder (A and B). Note the central comedonecrosis (B).

A panel consisting of prostate-specific antigen (PSA), prostate-specific acid phosphatase (PSAP) and α-methylacyl-CoA racemase (AMACR; P504S), which are commonly positive in adenocarcinoma of the prostate, is useful in difficult cases (**Fig. 23-8**; **Table 23-2**). If these studies are inconclusive, high molecular weight cytokeratin (34βE12), p63, uroplakin III, and thrombomodulin may also be used. Together, these immunostains will generally resolve the vast majority of cases. In the setting of poorly differentiated tumors, Genega et al. examined the immuno-histochemical profiles of prostatic adenocarcinoma and urothelial carcinoma, finding positivity for PSA, PSAP, or Leu 7 to support the former and positivity with 34βE12, CK7, or p53 to support the latter.[21] Although PSA and PSAP are uniformly negative in urothelial carcinoma, their positivity varies with the degree of tumor differentiation in prostatic adenocarcinoma.[22] Mhawech and colleagues found positivity for one or more of the two markers to have a sensitivity of 95% and specificity of 100% for prostatic origin.[22] Uroplakin III, a membrane glycoprotein

Table 23-2   **Prostatic Adenocarcinoma Versus Urothelial Carcinoma**[a]

	PSA/PSAP/P501S	HWMCK	p63	AMACR	CK7	CK20	Uroplakin III
Urothelial carcinoma	Neg	Pos	Pos	Pos/Neg	Pos	Pos	Pos
Prostatic adenocarcinoma	Pos	Neg	Neg	Pos	Pos	Neg	Neg

[a]PSA/PSAP/P501S, prostate-specific antigen/prostate-specific acid phosphatase/prostein; HWMCK, high molecular weight cytokeratin 34βE12; AMACR, α-methylacyl-CoA racemase (P504S); CK7, cytokeratin 7; CK20, cytokeratin 20.

Table 23-3   **Selected Immunochemical Biomarkers for Establishing Tumor Origin**

Urothelial carcinoma: uroplakin III, thrombomodulin, CK7, CK20, GATA3, p63, and high molecular weight cytokeratin (34βE12), S100P (placental S100)

Colorectal adenocarcinoma: CDX2 (nuclear staining), β-catenin (nuclear staining), and CK20

Prostatic adenocarcinoma: prostate-specific antigen (PSA), prostate-specific acid phosphatase (PSAP), prostate-specific membrane antigen (PSMA), prostein (P501S), PIN4 cocktail [high molecular weight cytokeratin (34βE12), p63, and α-methylacyl-CoA racemase (AMACR; P504S)]

Squamous cell carcinoma of female genital tract: CK7, high molecular weight cytokeratins (34βE12), p63, Mac387, and human papillomavirus (HPV)

Lung adenocarcinoma: thyroid transcription factor 1 (TTF-1), Napsin A

Breast carcinoma: estrogen and progesterone receptors, gross cystic disease fluid protein-15 (GCDFP-15)

Renal cell carcinoma: CD10, PAX2, and PAX8, RCC marker (RCC Ma), carbonic anhydrase-IX (CA9), α-methylacyl-CoA racemase (AMACR; P504S) (for papillary renal cell carcinoma)

Melanoma: HMB45, Melan A/MART-1, tyrosinase, S100 protein

Thyroid carcinoma: thyroglobulin, thyroid transcription factor 1 (TTF-1), galectin-3, and HBME1 (papillary thyroid carcinoma)

Hepatocellular carcinoma: glypican 3, CD10, polyclonal carcinoembryonic antigen (CEA)

Germ cell tumors: OCT4 (seminoma and embryonal carcinoma), c-kit (seminoma), CD30 (embryonal carcinoma), glypican 3 (yolk sac tumor), human chorionic gonadotrophin (hCG) (choriocarcinoma)

[a]CK7, cytokeratin 7; CK20, cytokeratin 20; RCC, renal cell carcinoma

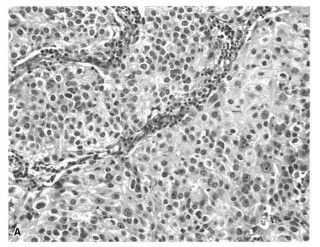 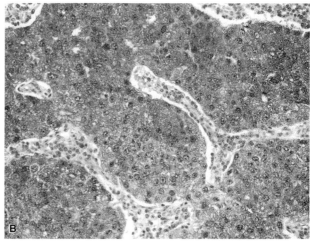

Figure 23-8   Prostatic adenocarcinoma involving the bladder (A and B). High grade prostatic adenocarcinoma (Gleason score 5+5) mimicking urothelial carcinoma with contiguous spread to the bladder (A). A prostatic origin was confirmed by diffuse immunoreactivity for prostate-specific antigen (B).

expressed in normal urothelium, demonstrates an apical staining pattern in urothelial carcinoma. In the same study, this marker was found to have 60% sensitivity and 100% specificity for urothelial origin. Similarly, thrombomodulin demonstrated a moderate sensitivity and excellent specificity. Combined, however, the two markers may reasonably be used together to support urothelial origin with a sensitivity of 80% and specificity of 100%. CK7 and CK20 alone may be insufficient for complete distinction of prostatic from urothelial carcinoma; however, negativity for both may be used as supportive evidence of prostatic origin and positivity for both may be supportive evidence of urothelial origin.[22]

Carcinomas of the Female Genital Tract Extension to the Bladder

Squamous Cell Carcinoma Extension to the Bladder

Direct spread of cervical cancer is one of the most common nonprimary squamous cell carcinomas of the bladder. Only rarely is it difficult to differentiate primary bladder cancer from secondary involvement by cervical cancer, since these tumors can easily be distinguished morphologically and clinically.

In bladder cancer, squamous differentiation is associated with typical urothelial carcinoma. The diagnosis of primary squamous cell carcinoma of the urinary bladder is restricted to pure tumors. Obtaining a proper clinical history and the use of immunohistochemistry will help reach a proper diagnosis in difficult cases. Finding cervical carcinoma in situ in cervical primaries is of diagnostic value. Uroplakin III and thrombomodulin expression is present in urothelial carcinoma. CK7 is positive in both urothelial and cervical carcinomas. CK20 and 34βE12 are usually negative in cervical carcinoma and positive in urothelial bladder carcinoma (Table 23-3). Recently, Lopez-Beltran et al. investigated the utility of Mac387 on 145 urothelial tumors with squamous differentiation.[23] The authors found that Mac387 may be a reliable marker for squamous differentiation in primary urothelial tumors and therefore may be potentially useful in distinguishing primary squamous cell carcinoma from direct spread from the cervix. Human papillomavirus (HPV) positivity supports the diagnosis of cervical squamous cell carcinoma.

Bladder involvement by squamous cell carcinoma of the vagina poses the same clinicopathological issues.

Bladder Involvement by Malignancy of the Female Genital Tract

Aside from squamous cell carcinoma, other malignancies originating from the female genital tract may sometimes involve the urinary bladder by either direct extension or metastasis.[4,14] Positivity for vimentin may be helpful in demonstrating endometrial origin, as it correctly classified 100% of cases of bladder adenocarcinoma and 81% of cases of endometrial adenocarcinoma in one study.[14] Metastasis from ovarian cancer should be considered in elderly women. Awareness of clinical history in most cases is the most integral diagnostic tool available to the pathologist.[24]

Secondary Lobular Carcinoma of the Breast

The possibility of a breast carcinoma metastasis should be raised when the bladder neoplasm displays discohesive or a single cell growth pattern without overlying urothelial abnormalities (dysplasia or carcinoma in situ) (Fig. 23-9). In such cases, the differential presents with an epithelial infiltration in the form of cords or individual cells involving the lamina propria, and should also include rare variants of urothelial carcinoma: namely, plasmacytoid/signet ring variant and urothelial carcinoma with lobular carcinoma-like features (a form of plasmacytoid bladder carcinoma).[25] Similar to breast lobular carcinoma, this rare urothelial carcinoma variant shows areas where the tumor is composed of uniform cells with a discohesive single cell diffusely invasive growth pattern. In areas the tumor cells are arranged in linear single cell patterns and, in separate areas, in solid sheets of discohesive cells. In all the cases, some tumor cells show prominent intracytoplasmic vacuoles. In addition to this pattern, some cases show typical urothelial carcinoma or carcinoma in situ. The majority of the tumors express CK20 but not estrogen and progesterone receptors. It is important to recognize this rare variant to avoid misdiagnosis of metastatic lobular carcinoma of the breast, especially in small biopsies.

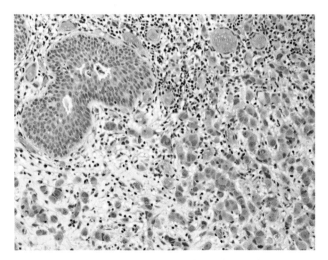

Figure 23-9 Breast carcinoma involving the bladder.

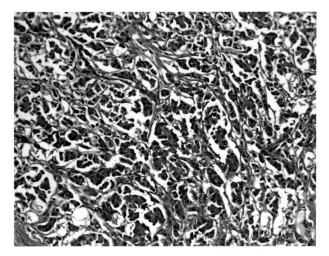

Figure 23-10 Micropapillary carcinoma.

Obtaining a proper clinical history and the use of immunohistochemistry, such as antibodies to estrogen and progesterone receptors, uroplakin III, and thrombomodulin, will help reach a proper diagnosis (**Table 23-3**).[4,26]

Invasive Micropapillary Carcinoma: Primary versus Secondary

Invasive micropapillary carcinoma is generally an aggressive morphologic variant that has been described in the bladder, lung, breast, salivary gland, gastrointestinal tract, and ovary (**Fig. 23-10**).[7,27,28] Given the morphologic similarities between invasive micropapillary carcinomas arising from different organ systems and the high propensity of this histologic subtype for lymphatic metastasis, it may be necessary to use immunohistochemical markers to determine the primary site of an invasive micropapillary carcinoma.

Few studies have compared the immunohistochemical profiles of invasive micropapillary carcinoma originating from different sites. Lotan et al.[28] recently tested a panel of 11 immunohistochemical markers for their ability to distinguish urothelial, lung, breast, and ovarian invasive micropapillary carcinoma using a tissue microarray constructed of primary tumor tissue from 47 patients with invasive micropapillary carcinoma (16 breast, 13 bladder, 12 ovarian, and 6 lung). For each tumor, correct classification as invasive micropapillary carcinoma was verified by reverse-polarity MUC1 expression (see also **Chapter 12**). It was found that immunostaining for uroplakin, CK20, thyroid transcription factor 1 (TTF-1), estrogen receptor, Wilms tumor gene 1 (WT1) and/or paired box homeotic 8 (PAX8), and mammaglobin was the best panel for determining the most likely primary site of invasive micropapillary carcinoma. The best markers to identify urothelial invasive micropapillary carcinoma were uroplakin III and CK20, whereas p63, high molecular weight cytokeratin, and thrombomodulin were less sensitive and specific. Invasive micropapillary carcinoma of the lung was uniformly TTF-1 positive. Breast-invasive micropapillary carcinoma was estrogen receptor positive, mammaglobin positive, and WT1/PAX8 negative; whereas, ovarian-invasive micropapillary carcinoma was estrogen receptor positive, mammaglobin negative, and WT1/PAX8 positive.[28]

In the metastatic setting, or when invasive micropapillary carcinoma occurs without an associated in situ or conventional carcinoma component, staining for uroplakin III, CK20, TTF-1, estrogen receptor, WT1/PAX8, and mammaglobin is the best panel for accurately classifying the likely primary site of invasive micropapillary carcinoma.[28]

Metastasis from Other Organs

Other malignancies to involve the urinary bladder include those of the skin (melanoma), stomach, and lung,[4] all of which may display morphologic characteristics seen in primary bladder carcinomas. Signet ring cell carcinoma may be the most challenging, as such tumors exhibit a similar immunophenotype regardless of bladder or gastrointestinal origin. Knowledge of clinical information is critical for the diagnosis. Immunohistochemical studies and other ancillary tests are an integral part of the diagnostic workup (see **Chapter 26** for further discussion).

REFERENCES

1. Bates AW, Baithun SI. The significance of secondary neoplasms of the urinary and male genital tract. *Virchows Arch* 2002;440:640–7.

2. Okaneya T, Inoue Y, Ogawa A. Solitary urethral recurrence of sigmoid colon carcinoma. *Urol Int* 1991;47:105–7.

3. Goldstein AG. Metastatic carcinoma to the bladder. *J Urol* 1967;98:209–15.

4. Morichetti D, Mazzucchelli R, Lopez-Beltran A, Cheng L, Scarpelli M, Kirkali Z, Montorsi F, Montironi R. Secondary neoplasms of the urinary system and male genital organs. *BJU Int* 2009;104:770–6.

5. Velcheti V, Govindan R. Metastatic cancer involving bladder: a review. *Can J Urol* 2007;14:3443–8.

6. Fogg LB, Smyth JW. Pelvic lipomatosis: a condition simulating pelvic neoplasm. *Radiology* 1968;90:558–64.

7. Lopez-Beltran A, Cheng L. Histologic variants of urothelial carcinoma: differential diagnosis and clinical implications. *Hum Pathol* 2006;37:1371–88.

8. Hodges KB, Lopez-Beltran A, Emerson RE, Montironi R, Cheng L. Clinical utility of immunohistochemistry in the diagnoses of urinary bladder neoplasia. *Appl Immunohistochem Mol Morphol* 2010;18:401–10.

9. Emerson RE, Cheng L. Immunohistochemical markers in the evaluation of tumors of the urinary bladder: a review. *Anal Quant Cytol Histol* 2005;27:301–16.

10. Wang HL, Lu DW, Yerian LM, Alsikafi N, Steinberg G, Hart J, Yang XJ. Immunohistochemical distinction between primary adenocarcinoma of the bladder and secondary colorectal adenocarcinoma. *Am J Surg Pathol* 2001;25:1380–7.

11. Tamboli P, Mohsin SK, Hailemariam S, Amin MB. Colonic adenocarcinoma metastatic to the urinary tract versus primary tumors of the urinary tract with glandular differentiation: a report of 7 cases and investigation using a limited immunohistochemical panel. *Arch Pathol Lab Med* 2002;126:1057–63.

12. Williamson SR, Lopez-Beltran A, Montironi R, Cheng L. Glandular lesions of the urinary bladder: clinical significance and differential diagnosis. *Histopathology* 2011;58:811–34.

13. Nakanishi K, Tominaga S, Kawai T, Torikata C, Aurues T, Ikeda T. Mucin histochemistry in primary adenocarcinoma of the urinary bladder (of urachal or vesicular origin) and metastatic adenocarcinoma originating in the colorectum. *Pathol Int* 2000;50:297–303.

14. Torenbeek R, Lagendijk JH, van Diest PJ, Bril H, van de Mollengraft FJM, Meijer CJ. Value of a panel of antibodies to identify the primary origin of adenocarcinomas presenting as bladder carcinoma. *Histopathology* 1998;32:20–7.

15. Raspollini MR, Nesi G, Baroni G, Girardi LR, Taddei GL. Immunohistochemistry in the differential diagnosis between primary and secondary intestinal adenocarcinoma of the urinary bladder. *Appl Immunohistochem Mol Morphol* 2005;13:358–62.

16. Silver SA, Epstein JI. Adenocarcinoma of the colon simulating primary urinary bladder neoplasia. A report of nine cases. *Am J Surg Pathol* 1993;17:171–8.

17. Chuang AY, Demarzo AM, Veltri RW, Sharma RB, Bieberich CJ, Epstein JI. Immunohistochemical differentiation of high grade prostate carcinoma from urothelial carcinoma. *Am J Surg Pathol* 2007;31:1246–55.

18. Suh N, Yang XJ, Tretiakova MS, Humphrey PA, Wang HL. Value of CDX2, villin, and alpha-methylacyl coenzyme A racemase immunostains in the distinction between primary adenocarcinoma of the bladder and secondary colorectal adenocarcinoma. *Mod Pathol* 2005;18:1217–22.

19. Werling RW, Yaziji H, Bacchi CE, Gown AM. CDX2, a highly sensitive and specific marker of adenocarcinomas of intestinal origin: and immunohistochemical survey of 476 primary and metastatic carcinomas. *Am J Surg Pathol* 2003;27:303–10.

20. Sung MT, Lopez-Beltran A, Eble JN, MacLennan GT, Tan PH, Montironi R, Jones TD, Ulbright TM, Blair JE, Cheng L. Divergent pathway of intestinal metaplasia and cystitis glandularis of the urinary bladder. *Mod Pathol* 2006;19:1395–401.

21. Genega EM, Hutchinson B, Reuter VE, Gaudin PB. Immunophenotype of high grade prostatic adenocarcinoma and urothelial carcinoma. *Mod Pathol* 2000;13:1186–91.

22. Mhawech P, Uchida T, Pelte MF. Immunohistochemical profile of high grade urothelial bladder carcinoma and prostate adenocarcinoma. *Hum Pathol* 2002;33:1136–40.

23. Lopez-Beltran A, Requena MJ, Alvarez-Kindelan J, Quintero A, Blanca A, Montironi R. Squamous differentiation in primary urothelial carcinoma of the urinary tract as seen by MAC387 immunohistochemistry. *J Clin Pathol* 2007;60:332–5.

24. Mazzucchelli R, Morichetti D, Lopez-Beltran A, Cheng L, Scarpelli M, Kirkali Z, Montironi R. Neuroendocrine tumours of the urinary system and male genital organs: clinical significance. *BJU Int* 2009;103:1464–70.

25. Baldwin L, Lee AH, Al-Talib RK, Theaker JM. Transitional cell carcinoma of the bladder mimicking lobular carcinoma of the breast: a discohesive variant of urothelial carcinoma. *Histopathology* 2005;46:50–6.

26. Zagha RM, Hamawy KJ. Solitary breast cancer metastasis to the bladder: an unusual occurrence. *Urol Oncol* 2007;25:236–9.

27. Lopez-Beltran A, Montironi R, Blanca A, Cheng L. Invasive micropapillary urothelial carcinoma of the bladder. *Hum Pathol* 2010;41:1159–64.

28. Lotan TL, Ye H, Melamed J, Wu XR, Shih Ie M, Epstein JI. Immunohistochemical panel to identify the primary site of invasive micropapillary carcinoma. *Am J Surg Pathol* 2009;33:1037–41.

Chapter 24

Treatment Effects

Bladder Pathology, First Edition. Liang Cheng, Antonio Lopez-Beltran, David G. Bostwick.
© 2012 Wiley-Blackwell. Published 2012 by John Wiley & Sons, Inc.

Overview

The bladder and, in particular, the urothelium react to different therapies applied to the bladder itself (intravesically) or as a result of secondary affectation in systemic therapies. Bacillus Calmette–Guérin (BCG) granulomatous cystitis and postsurgical necrobiotic granulomas of the bladder, the most common therapy-associated change, are covered in **Chapter 2**. Antineoplastic agents used in the bladder or systemically, such as thiotepa (triethylenethiophosphoramide), mitomycin C, cyclophosphamide, BCG, and radiation therapy, produce urothelial changes that can mimic cancer histologically. Pathologists must be aware of the diagnostic pitfalls and exercise caution when evaluating urothelial atypia following treatment.[1–4] The damaged mucosa may become ulcerated, with adjacent atypical regenerating urothelium showing pseudocarcinomatous epithelial hyperplasia (peudoepitheliomatous hyperplasia). In most cases, knowledge of the prior treatment is crucial to a correct diagnosis of the epithelial and stromal changes present. If the distinction between treatment-induced atypia and dysplasia/carcinoma in situ is uncertain, a conservative approach with repeat cystoscopy and biopsy is indicated, preferably after the inflammation has subsided.

A handful of traditional and newer therapeutic procedures, such as chemotherapy, immunotherapy, radiotherapy, photodynamic and laser treatment, and gene therapy, are used to treat bladder cancer. These treatment modalities, used either intravesically or systemically, produce pronounced morphological changes that can be mistaken for carcinoma. The pathologist must be able to separate toxic and drug-related alterations from neoplastic processes. The clinical history is invaluable in this assessment.

Chemotherapy-related Changes

Systemic Cyclophosphamide (Cytoxan)

This alkylating agent is used in the treatment of nonurothelial malignancies and diseases such as systemic lupus erythematosus, rheumatoid arthritis, nephrotic syndrome, and lymphoproliferative disorders.[2,5,6] The active metabolites acrolein and phosphoramide mustard are concentrated in the urine, where they can be in contact with the urothelium for prolonged periods. The drug is toxic to the urinary bladder mucosa and increases the risk of urinary bladder cancer.

Cyclophosphamide therapy may induce stromal fibrosis, vascular changes (intimal thickening, mural fibrin deposition, and ectasia), urothelial atypia, and hemorrhagic cystitis (**Figs. 24-1 to 24-6; Table 24-1**).[7,8] Cyclophosphamide induces epithelial necrosis, followed by rapid

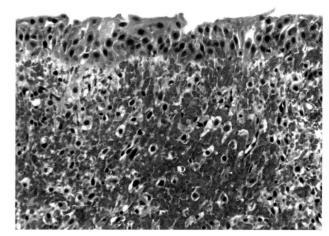

Figure 24-1 Hemorrhagic cystitis after cyclophosphamide (cytoxan) therapy. Note the cytologic atypia of urothelial cells.

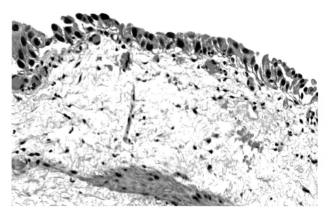

Figure 24-2 Reactive urothelial atypia after cyclophosphamide therapy. It should not be mistaken for urothelial carcinoma in situ. Pertinent clinical history is important in the diagnosis.

atypical regeneration of the urothelium. These atypical features can be misdiagnosed as urothelial dysplasia or carcinoma in situ. Pseudocarcinomatous epithelial hyperplasia may also be seen (**Fig. 24-7**) and should not be mistaken for invasive carcinoma. Clinical information is critical for accurate diagnosis.

The metabolic effects of cyclophosphamide, including arrest of cell and nuclear division, produce binucleated and multinucleated cells, often with large bizarre nuclei resembling the changes of radiation injury.[9,10] This radiomimetic effect creates cellular changes that can be mistaken for malignancy. There is marked but variable cellular and nuclear enlargement. Nuclei are often eccentric, slightly irregular in outline, and usually markedly

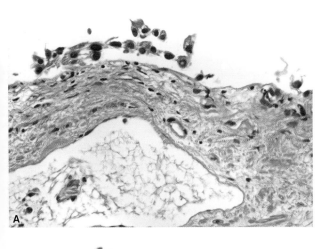

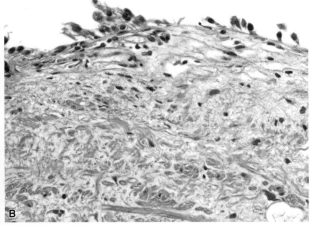

Figure 24-3   Reactive urothelial atypia after cyclophosphamide therapy (A and B), mimicking clinging-type urothelial carcinoma in situ.

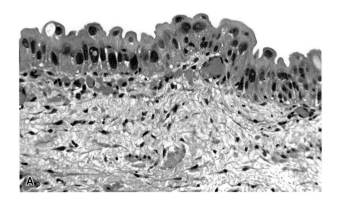

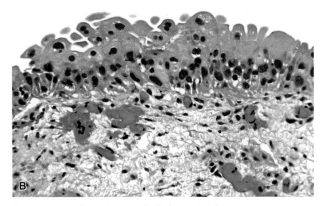

Figure 24-4   Reactive urothelial atypia after cyclophosphamide therapy (A and B).

hyperchromatic.[11] Chromatin may be coarse, but is usually evenly distributed. Nuclear pyknosis is a common late effect that results in loss of chromatin texture. Nucleoli are single or double, and occasionally large and distorted with irregular and sharp edges.

In patients with muscle-invasive bladder cancer, systemic chemotherapy, in which cyclophosphamide may be given in combination with other agents, has been added to locoregional treatment in an attempt to downstage the primary tumor and reduce micrometastases and, in some instances, as a radiosensitizer. The morphological changes are basically characterized by tumor cell necrosis.[12] A similar effect can be seen following perioperative chemotherapy.

Hemorrhagic cystitis can be caused by systemic cyclophosphamide treatment and appears to be dose independent (**Figs. 24-8** and **24-9**; see also **Chapter 3**).[7,11,13-16] The histological changes include vascular ectasia with severe

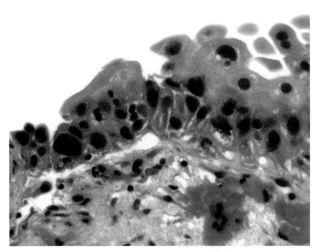

Figure 24-5   Reactive urothelial atypia after cyclophosphamide therapy.

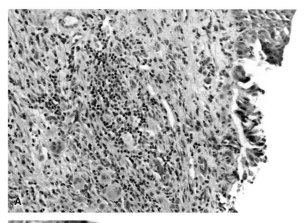

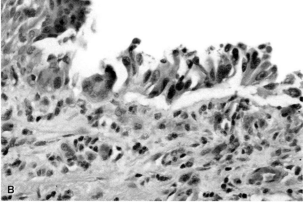

Figure 24-6 Reactive urothelial atypia after cyclophosphamide therapy (A and B). The urothelium is distorted and hyperchromatic and is separating from the underlying inflamed submucosa following cyclophosphamide therapy. Note the prominent eosinophil infiltrates in the lamina propria.

Table 24-1 **Pathological Alterations Associated with Systemic Cyclophosphamide Treatment**

- Large binucleated and multinucleated urothelial cells
- Degenerative changes to large bizarre nuclei resembling changes of radiation injury
- Vascular changes, including intimal thickening, mural fibrin deposition, and telangiectasia
- Hemorrhagic cystitis
- Reactivation of polyomavirus infection
- Encrusted cystitis (rare)
- Bladder cancer following cyclophosphamide treatment (rare)

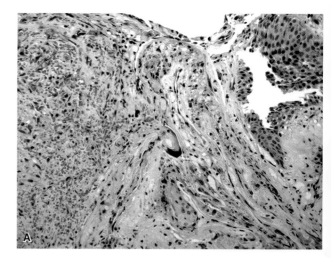

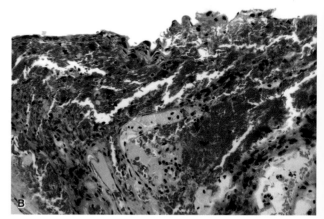

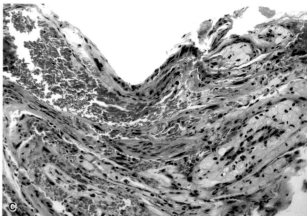

Figure 24-7 Hemorrhagic cystitis after cyclophosphamide therapy in a 15-year-old boy with acute myeloid leukemia (A to C).

edema and hemorrhage of the lamina propria, usually associated with necrosis of the epithelial lining and mucosal ulceration. Fibrosis of the lamina propria and the muscularis propria is present in 25% of cases examined at necropsy. Bladder wall calcification has been seen in occasional cases.[17,18]

Systemic cyclophosphamide treatment may also induce reactivation of polyomavirus (BK virus) infection (Fig. 24-10). Early in the reactivation process, cells shedding from the bladder may mimic dysplasia or urothelial carcinoma. DNA aneuploidy or a hyperdiploid

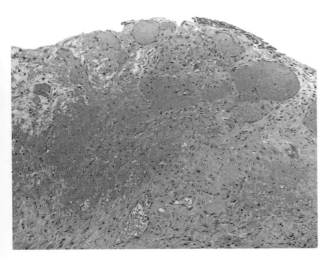

Figure 24-8 Hemorrhagic cystitis after cyclophosphamide therapy.

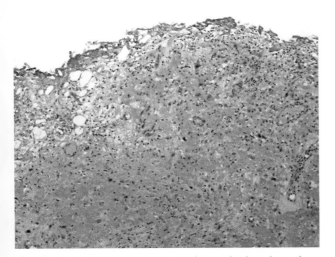

Figure 24-9 Hemorrhagic cystitis after cyclophosphamide therapy.

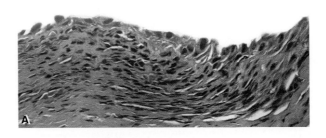

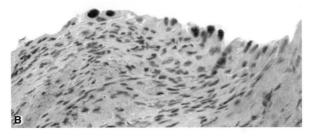

Figure 24-10 Polyomavirus (BK virus) infection after cyclophosphamide therapy (A). Immunostaining for polyomavirus is positive (B).

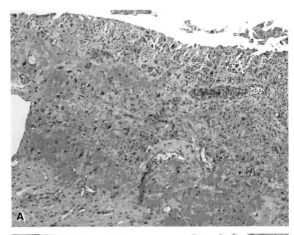

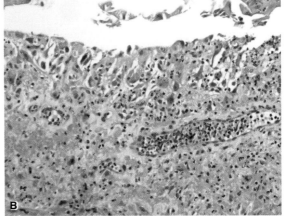

Figure 24-11 Cytomegalovirus (CMV) infection after cyclophosphamide therapy (A and B). Immunostaining for CMV is positive (not shown).

DNA content may be encountered as a false-positive indicator of urothelial carcinoma in patients with reactivated polyomavirus associated with urothelial atypia and no evidence of urothelial carcinoma. Cytomegalovirus (CMV) infection may also be seen after cyclophosphamide treatment (**Figs. 24-11** and **24-12**).

The evidence that cyclophosphamide increases the risk of bladder cancer is based primarily on case reports, but there is some evidence that the risk increases with the cumulative total dose of cyclophosphamide.[19,20] Bladder cancer occurs most commonly in patients receiving cyclophosphamide for immunosuppression after organ transplantation or treatment of lymphoproliferative or myeloproliferative disorder, particularly multiple myeloma and Hodgkin disease. The risk of bladder cancer associated with cyclophosphamide is apparently increased in patients

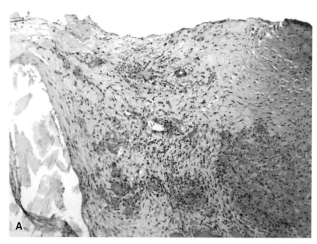

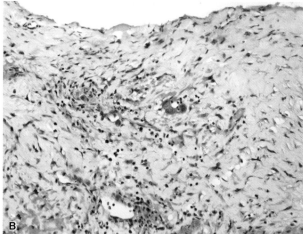

Figure 24-12   Cytomegalovirus (CMV) infection after cyclophosphamide therapy (A and B).

with a history of cystitis. In this setting, urothelial carcinoma is the most common cancer, although squamous cell carcinoma, adenocarcinoma, undifferentiated carcinoma, fibrosarcoma, leiomyosarcoma, and sarcomatoid carcinoma have also been reported.[21-24] This occurs in a minority of patients following prolonged administration. The average interval from primary tumor to bladder cancer is variable, although usually lengthy, and may be as long as 11 years.

Intravesical Therapy

Mitomycin C

Mitomycin C, an antitumor antibiotic, is an intravesical chemotherapeutic agent that reduces the likelihood of tumor recurrences in patients with bladder cancer.[25,26] It induces interstrand and intrastrand cross-links in many types of DNA, depending on the base composition of the DNA. It has been shown to degrade DNA and inhibit DNA synthesis, thus making it effective during the late G1 and S phases of the cell cycle.

Mitomycin C increases exfoliation and denudation, multi-inucleation, cytoplasmic vacuolation, and the appearance of bizarre, nonmalignant nuclei in the superficial layer of the urothelium (**Figs. 24-13** to **24-16**; **Table 24-2**). Exfoliation of preserved cells is followed within 48 hours by the appearance of degenerated cells. Toxic effects do not become more severe with continued exposure, and tend to subside after removal of the drug. Urothelial denudation makes recurrences difficult to detect cystoscopically and to document histologically; urine cytology is important for followup.[27] **Table 24-3** lists features that are helpful in distinguishing intravesical therapy-induced changes from low grade urothelial carcinoma.

A marked necroinflammatory process follows administration of topical mitomycin C. Isolated single and clustered macrophages are seen. The histiocytic response may extend deep into the bladder wall, suggesting an

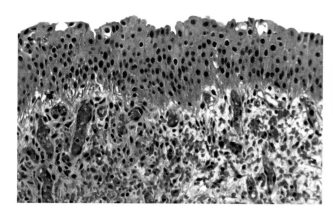

Figure 24-13   Reactive urothelial atypia after mitomycin therapy. Note the mitotic figure and stromal hemorrhage.

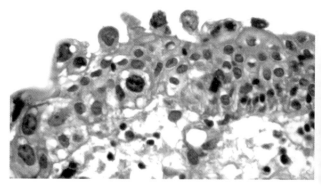

Figure 24-14   Reactive urothelial atypia after mitomycin therapy.

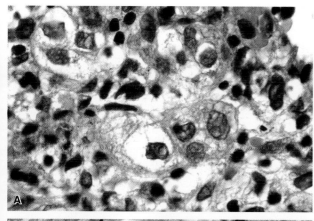

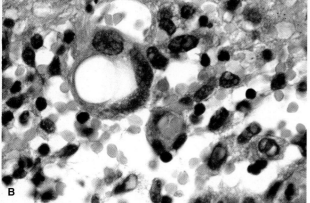

Figure 24-15 Mitomycin C–induced changes, including stromal atypia, acute and chronic inflammation (A and B).

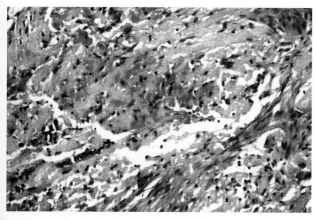

Figure 24-16 Mitomycin C–induced changes. Note necrosis of the muscularis propria (detrusor muscle).

inflammatory neoplasm (such as inflammatory myofibroblastic tumor). Mitomycin C may also initiate nonallergic eosinophilic cystitis.[27,28] These agents are not metabolic inhibitors of DNA replication, and thus typically do not produce full-thickness urothelial atypia such as that seen after cyclophosphamide.

Table 24-2 Pathological Alterations Associated with Intravesical Chemotherapy (Mitomycin C and Thiotepa)

- Denudation of the surface urothelium
- Atypical changes in the superficial umbrella cells
- Large cells with nuclear enlargement, multinucleation, and eosinophilic cytoplasm
- Eosinophilic cystitis (rare)
- Hemorrhagic cystitis (rare)
- Encrusted cystitis (rare)

A form of truncated papillae can be seen in some cases of low grade bladder cancer treated with intravesical chemotherapy.

Thiotepa

Triethylene thiophosphoramide (thiotepa), a polyfunctional alkylating agent, is the oldest of the intravesical chemotherapeutic agents still in active use today. Its mechanism of action involves the formation of covalent bonds between DNA, RNA, nucleic acids, and proteins. The result is the inhibition of nucleic acid synthesis. In addition to this effect, thiotepa reduces cell adherence, with a direct cytotoxic effect.

Thiotepa produces histologic and cytologic changes similar to those of mitomycin C. Like mitomycin C, thiotepa is not a metabolic inhibitor of DNA and thus does not produce the atypical cells seen after cyclophosphamide therapy. It appears to affect only normal and nonneoplastic urothelium. Superficial cells are large and often fused, with vacuolated cytoplasm and enlarged hyperchromatic nuclei, indicative of degeneration and regeneration. Typically, the cells have slightly or moderately enlarged nuclei, but there is no significant increase in chromatin density. When mild to moderate hyperchromasia occurs, it usually appears with smudged chromatin that lacks a sharply detailed pattern. Nuclei are round or ovoid, with smooth, thin, chromatic rims, or wrinkled rims because of degeneration. Large multinucleated superficial cells frequently contain multiple small nucleoli and display cytoplasmic vacuolization with frayed borders.[29] These changes occur almost exclusively in superficial cells, recognized by their abundant cytoplasm and convex outer borders.

It should be kept in mind that the cytologic changes produced by thiotepa are not specific for topical chemotherapy and can be produced by chronic inflammation, catheterization, and instillation of saline. Morphologic features of malignancy, whether low or high grade, are not altered by these forms of therapy.

Thiotepa and mitomycin C suppress tumor growth and progression, but they do not eradicate cancer. Apparently, they act as surface abrasives to destroy the tips of papillary fronds, resulting in stubby papillae lined by neoplastic cells. Urothelial denudation makes recurrences difficult

Table 24-3   Intravesical Therapy-associated Atypia and Low Grade Urothelial Carcinoma

Feature	Therapy-associated Atypia (Mitomycin C, Thiotepa)	Low Grade Carcinoma
Cellularity	Early: high Late: low	Usually high
Cell size	Enlarged	Normal to minimal enlargement
Nuclear-to-cytoplasmic ratio	Normal	Increased
Staining	Hyperchromatic	Hyperchromatic
Nuclear borders	Irregular	Irregular
Chromatin	Fine, regular	Fine, regular
Nucleoli	Variable	Variable
Architecture	Loose, discohesive	Papillary and loose clusters
Ploidy	Diploid	Usually diploid

to detect cystoscopically and to document histologically. Despite denudation of the urothelium, urothelial dysplasia and carcinoma in situ may still be found in von Brunn nests.

Other Chemotherapeutic Agents

Doxorubicin hydrochloride (Adriamycin), epirubicin, ethoglucid (epodyl), cisplatin, and mitoxantrone are known to cause alterations in the bladder mucosa.[30–32] The frequency varies from agent to agent. For instance, there is a 21% and 25% incidence of epirubicin- and doxorubicin-induced cystitis, respectively. A frequency of cystitis ranging from 3% to 56% has been seen with ethoglucid. Doxorubicin hydrochloride causes chemical cystitis. Danazol (a synthetic anabolic steroid) and ortho-toluidine (a skin-absorbed chemical) may produce severe vesical hemorrhage.[30] Analgesic abuse with phenacetin, a drug with a chemical structure similar to that of aniline dyes, is associated with an increased risk of urothelial carcinoma of the renal pelvis and bladder.[31] Busulfan-induced hemorrhagic cystitis rarely occurs, but can be clinically significant.[32]

A rare form of cystitis in patients receiving ketamine has recently been described.[33] The authors described seven cases and concluded that ketamine can lead to reactive urothelial changes that can mimic carcinoma in situ, but the long-term cancer risk remains unknown.[33]

Immunotherapy

Bacillus Calmette–Guérin Therapy   Ideally, intravesical treatment should eradicate residual disease and prevent tumor recurrence, thus ultimately averting the serious consequences of muscle invasion and metastasis. The immunotherapeutic agent BCG offers high rates of early and durable complete response. However, although several studies have demonstrated a decrease in cancer progression by intravesical BCG therapy, conclusive evidence of a survival advantage is still lacking.[25,34,35] Complications are more frequent than with topical drugs, and rarely include systemic infections with tubercle bacilli (TB).[36]

BCG is a pleiotropic immune stimulator oriented toward cellular immunity. In particular, BCG has been shown to activate macrophages, natural killer cells, B cells, and various T cells (CD4+, CD8+, and $\gamma\delta$T cells) in vitro and in vivo. The analysis of cytokine production from human urine during BCG treatment has shown that BCG can stimulate the expression of interleukins (IL-1, IL-2, IL-4, IL-6, IL-8, IL-10, and IL-12), tumor necrosis factor α, granulocyte–macrophage colony-stimulating factor, the antiangiogenic chemokine IP-10, and interferon gamma (IFN-γ). Of these, IFN-γ appears to be a crucial mediator of the antimycobacterial infection response. Although the exact mechanism of BCG action in bladder cancer remains incompletely understood, BCG antitumor efficacy appears to depend on a cell-mediated T helper cell immune response.

The histopathologic hallmark of BCG treatment is noncaseating granulomas (**Fig. 24-17**; see **Chapter 2** for further discussion). Other changes may also be observed (**Table 24-4**).

Immunotherapeutic Agents other than BCG   Several immunotherapeutic agents other than BCG have been investigated for the prophylaxis of superficial bladder cancer, including recombinant interferon-alpha (IFN-α).[25,34,37–39]

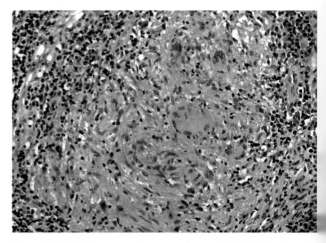

Figure 24-17   Noncaseating granuloma after BCG treatment.

Table 24-4   Pathological Alterations Associated with Intravesical Immunotherapy (BCG, Interferon α)

Denudation and ulceration of urothelium
Noncaseating granulomas
Reactive epithelial atypia
Degenerated urothelial cells
Inflammatory background with histiocytes and rare multinucleated giant cells
Stromal edema (especially after interferon α treatment)
Perivascular inflammation with lymphocytes, eosinophils, plasma cells, and dendritic cells (interferon α)
Persistence of carcinoma in situ in von Brunn nests, and denuding cystitis

IFNs are known to have antiviral and direct antiproliferative activity and to inhibit angiogenesis, regulate differentiation, activate immune effector cells, induce cytokine production, and enhance tumor-associated antigen expression. The precise role of recombinant IFN-α in the treatment of superficial bladder cancer is still under investigation.

Bladder cancer cells express large numbers of the IFN-α receptors, and greater receptor densities are found in high grade lesions. The indirect antitumor effects of IFNs are probably mediated via the stimulation of a cellular immune response. Intravesical recombinant IFN-α increases the cytotoxic activity of T cells and natural killer cells by increasing the infiltration of these cells into the bladder wall, and this improved immune cell activity persists for 3 to 6 months. This increases the susceptibility of urothelial carcinoma cells to attack from cytotoxic T cells and directly inhibits the proliferation of tumor cells.

The pathological changes associated with IFN-based treatment are not specific and are characterized by edema of the lamina propria and perivascular collections of inflammatory cells: mainly lymphocytes, neutrophils, and eosinophils.

Intravesical vaccinia virus is also considered as a promising immunotherapeutic agent for bladder cancer.[40] The limited number of cases tested has shown a significant mucosal and submucosal inflammatory infiltration, characterized by lymphocytes, eosinophils, plasma cells, and dendritic cells. The tumor cells show some nuclear features that suggest a viral effect.

Radiation-induced Changes

Radiation therapy produces a variety of bladder lesions associated with diverse symptoms and pathologic findings.[2–4,21,41–47] The clinical course is divided into three reaction patterns according to the time of onset of symptoms: acute, less than 6 months; subacute, 6 months to 2 years; and chronic, 2 to 5 years. Bladder lesions are caused by mucosal, stromal, and vascular damage, and include acute and chronic radiation cystitis with mucosal ulceration and bladder contracture as a late complication. Chronic radiation cystitis occurs in patients who received radiation therapy for cervical (**Fig. 24-18**) or prostate cancer (**Fig. 24-19**).

Acute changes include denudation of urothelium, stroma edema, hemorrhage, and surface ulceration with fibrin deposition (**Figs. 24-20** to **24-26**; **Table 24-5**). Depending on the duration and severity of vesical injury, the urine sediment contains cellular debris and degenerated or necrotic urothelial cells, variable hemorrhage, and other inflammatory cells, including histiocytes. Urothelial cells are enlarged and may show striking gigantism with or

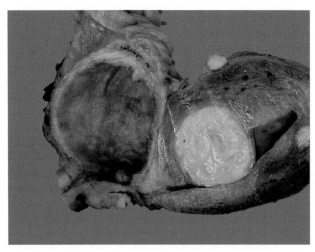

Figure 24-18   Radiation cystitis from a 55-year-old women who received radiation therapy for cervical cancer.

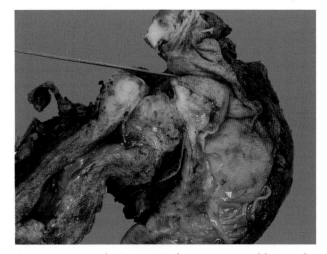

Figure 24-19   Radiation cystitis from a 77-year-old man who received radiation therapy for prostate cancer. The patient also developed rectourethral fistula.

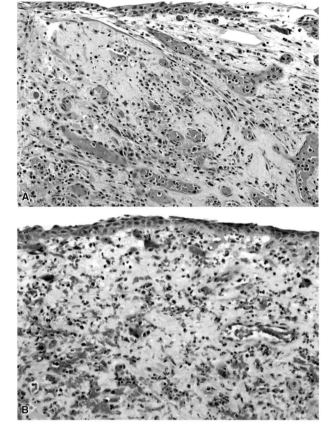

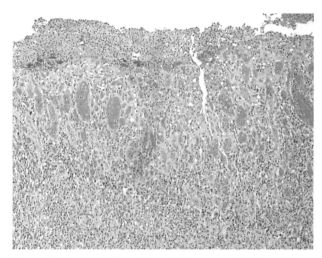

Figure 24-20   Radiation-induced changes, including mucosal atrophy, inflammation of the lamina propria, and marked vascular congestion (A and B).

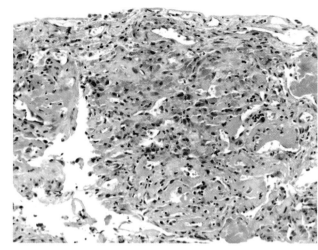

Figure 24-22   Radiation-induced changes. Note the urothelial denudation and atypical stroma cells.

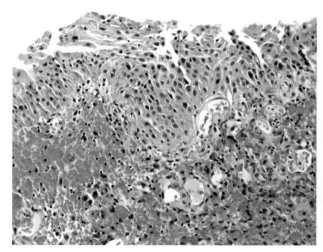

Figure 24-23   Radiation-induced changes. Note the urothelial atypia and submucosal hemorrhage.

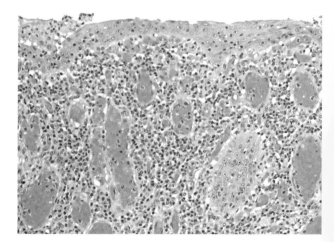

Figure 24-21   Radiation-induced changes. Note the surface ulcer and granulation tissue, and acute and chronic inflammation.

Figure 24-24   Reactive urothelial atypia after radiation therapy.

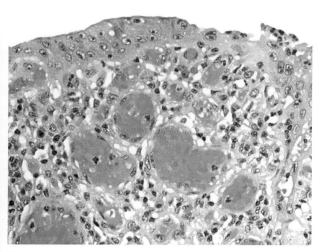

Figure 24-25 Reactive urothelial atypia after radiation therapy.

without binucleation or multinucleation. Nuclear enlargement is also present, but the nuclear-to-cytoplasmic ratio is low. Enlarged nuclei may contain macronucleoli, but degenerative changes, including vacuolization, chromatin clearing, karyorrhexis, and loss of chromatin texture, are usually present. Nuclear irregularities and hyperchromasia reflect varying degrees of pyknosis. Cytoplasmic vacuolization and polychromasia are characteristic findings, and frayed borders indicate cellular degeneration. Cytologic changes may persist in the urine sediment for years. Pseudocarcinomatous epithelial hyperplasia, a lesion uncommonly seen after radiation and/or chemotherapy, should be distinguished from tumor recurrence (**Figs. 24-27** and **24-28**).

Vascular changes include endothelial swelling and necrosis, vessel wall thickening and hyalinization, telangiectasia, and thrombosis of blood vessels (**Figs. 24-29** and **24-30**). Stromal edema is common, and may occasionally be accompanied by bizarre stromal cells, similar to those seen in giant cell cystitis (**Figs. 24-31** and **24-32**; see also

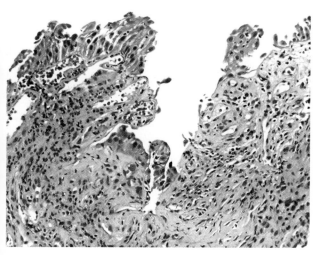

Figure 24-26 Reactive urothelial atypia after radiation therapy. Note the focal mucosal erosion and reactive urothelial cells with abundant eosinophilic cytoplasm.

Table 24-5   Radiation-Induced Changes

Surface ulceration and denudation
Urothelial cell enlargement, mutinucleation, and
    cytoplasmic vacuolization
Nodules of squamoid epithelium (reactive) and
    pseudoepitheliomatous hyperplasia
Stromal edema, acute and chronic inflammation
Mural thickening, hyalinization, and calcification of blood
    vessels
Bladder wall fibrosis (late stage)

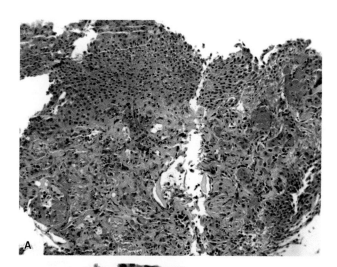

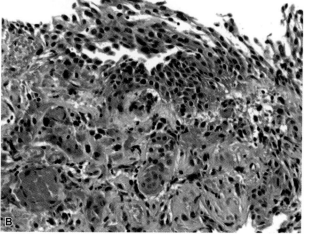

Figure 24-27 Pseudocarcinomatous epithelial hyperplasia after radiation therapy (A and B).

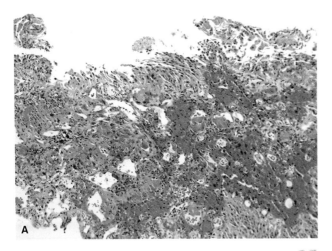

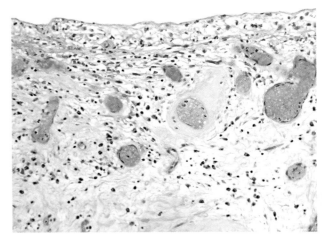

Figure 24-30   Radiation-induced changes. Note the hyalinized vessels.

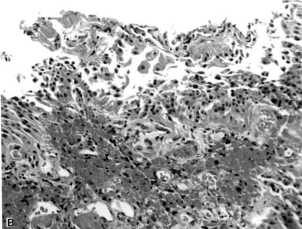

Figure 24-28   Pseudocarcinomatous epithelial hyperplasia after radiation therapy (A and B).

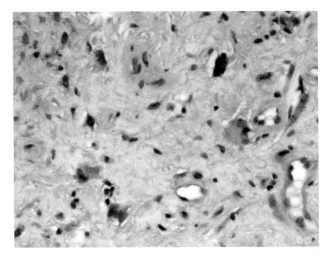

Figure 24-31   Radiation-induced changes. Note the atypical stromal cells.

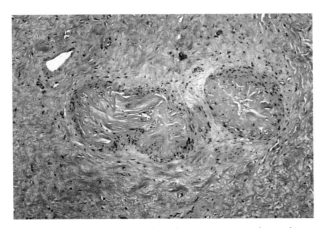

Figure 24-29   Radiation-induced prominent accelerated arteriolosclerotic changes.

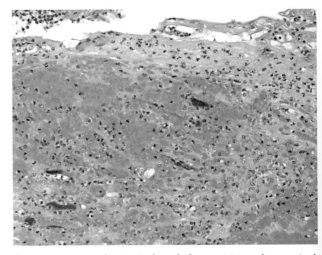

Figure 24-32   Radiation-induced changes. Note the atypical stromal cells in a hemorrhagic background.

Chapter 2). Ulceration, mucosal denudation, acute and chronic inflammation, hemorrhage, fibrin and hemosiderin depositions, and stromal fibrosis and calcifications are often seen after radiation therapy (**Figs. 24-33** to **24-36**).

Late complications of radiation injury include ulcers, marked contraction of the bladder due to fibrosis, and ureteral stricture.[46] An important long-term effect of radiotherapy is the development of de novo radiation-induced bladder cancer, which usually is urothelial carcinoma but occasionally is squamous cell carcinoma. Rare examples of sarcomatoid carcinoma (or carcinosarcoma) and sarcoma of the urinary bladder have been reported (**Fig. 24-37**).[2–4,21,41,42]

See **Chapter 2** for further discussion.

Chemical Cystitis

Ether cystitis is very uncommon, and occurs when ether is introduced into the bladder to dissolve a catheter balloon that resists mechanical deflation. Formalin, instilled vesically to control bleeding, and turpentine ingestion, excreted by the kidney, creates ether-type injury, including hemorrhagic urothelial necrosis, edema, and leukocytic infiltration. Bonney blue is frequently instilled in the bladder during gynecologic surgery, but failure to dilute the concentrate to 0.5% solution incites a severe chemical cystitis.

Gene Therapy

The discovery that many cancers develop in concert with the loss of function of tumor suppressor genes suggests that the combined regimen of gene replacement and chemotherapy may be therapeutically useful.[34,39,48–54]

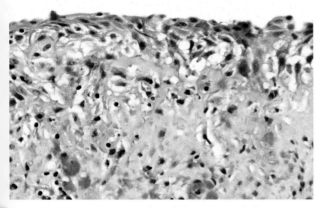

Figure 24-33 Radiation-induced changes, including cytologic abnormalities, chronic inflammation, and submucosal fibrosis.

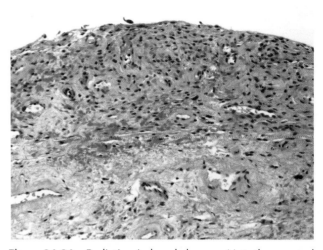

Figure 24-34 Radiation-induced changes. Note the mucosal denudation and submucosal hemorrhage.

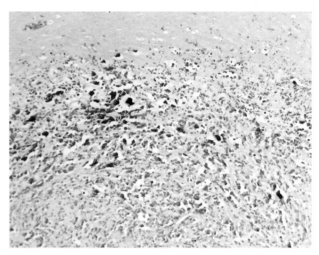

Figure 24-35 Radiation-induced changes. Note the stromal calcifications.

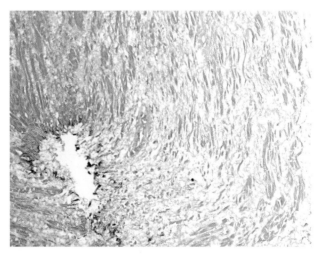

Figure 24-36 Radiation-induced changes. Note the necrosis and calcifications.

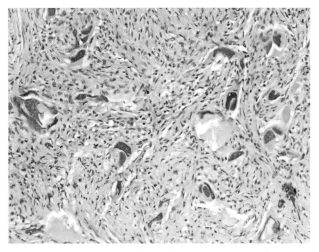

Figure 24-37 Sarcomatoid (urothelial) carcinoma after radiation therapy. Cytokeratin immunostaining is strongly positive (not shown).

Studies of bladder cancer have yielded several candidate genes for therapeutic replacement. Among these are the cell cycle-related genes *RB, TP53, p21/WAF1,* and *p16.*

Tumor suppressor gene therapy is well suited for intravesical administration. Gene-correcting and tumor vaccination studies have been shown to be effective in animals, in particular by increasing the sensitivity of bladder cancer cells to chemotherapeutic agents. These findings suggest that the combined regimen of gene replacement and chemotherapy may become an efficient and powerful tool for the treatment of bladder cancer.

Very few morphological studies of cytopathological effects of gene therapy have been published. Various degrees of necrosis, more commonly seen in high grade lesions, are present in cancer foci (Table 24-6). Nuclear changes include the loss of chromatin detail and nucleoli in the earlier stages. In the late stages, the nuclei shrink, become pyknotic, and acquire a spindled morphology, in contrast to the normal round/ovoid shape. The resulting nucleus, found in dead cells, is dark, dense, pyknotic, and comma shaped, with no nuclear detail. Hyperchromatic bizarre nuclei are occasionally seen.

Table 24-6   Pathological Changes Associated with Gene Therapy

Various degrees of necrosis in cancer foci with loss of chromatin detail and nucleoli in the earlier phases following treatment
In the late phases, the nuclei shrink, become pyknotic, and acquire a spindled morphology
Normal urothelial mucosa is rarely affected by necrosis
Intense chronic inflammatory infiltrate composed predominantly of B cells in the lamina propria

The normal urothelial mucosa is rarely affected by necrosis, but contains an intense chronic inflammatory infiltrate composed predominantly of B cells. Some lymphocytic infiltration is present at the tumor–normal bladder interface or inside the tumor itself. Macrophages are abundant within tumor foci, mostly in areas of necrosis. Injection sites with hemorrhagic foci and a foreign body type of giant cell reaction may be observed.

Photodynamic and Laser Therapy

Photodynamic and laser treatment for bladder cancer produces acute mucosal inflammation, with sloughing and edema (Table 24-7).[55–67] Other findings include coagulative necrosis that may contain dystrophic calcification and spindle cell artifact of cells at the periphery of necrotic tissues.[60,66,67]

Photodynamic Therapy

Photodynamic treatment using hematoporphyrin derivatives is a form of novel diagnosis and treatment for bladder cancer.[55–60,62] It is based on the systemic or local administration of photosensitizers. These substances accumulate in tumor tissue but not, or to some extent only, in normal tissue. When the photosensitizer is activated by light, it produces tumor necrosis, preserving normal structures. The response is noted 1 or 2 days after the treatment is applied.

It can achieve a high initial complete response rate, especially against urothelial carcinoma in situ, but generalized cutaneous photosensitivity remains limiting. Moreover, severe local irritative symptoms persisting for months are not uncommon, in addition to occasional bladder contractures.

The photosensitizer also accumulates in the stroma and in the vessel wall, suggesting tumor ischemia as a possible mechanism of action. In fact, early morphological changes show intravascular coagulation and adjacent tumor cell necrosis.

Histologically, it is characterized by coagulation necrosis, sometimes with hemorrhagic necrosis clearly demarcated from the nonneoplastic tissue Adjacent nonneoplastic tissues may show morphological changes ranging

Table 24-7   Pathological Alterations Associated with Photodynamic and Laser Treatment

Coagulation necrosis, sometimes with hemorrhagic necrosis, clearly demarcated from nonneoplastic tissue
Spindle cell artifact of urothelial cells
Intravascular coagulation
Stromal edema
Fibrosis and dystrophic calcification

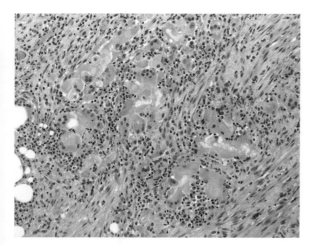

Figure 24-38 Granuloma after transurethral resection. Note the prominent eosinophils.

from moderate to severe edema, but necrosis is rare. Other findings include spindle cell artifact of urothelial cells and dystrophic calcification.

Laser Therapy

Laser treatment has been used to ablate bladder tumors.[55,64,68-74] Lasers are usually reserved for patients with recurrent low grade tumors, because tissue is not usually available for histological evaluation. It is believed that the lack of biopsy tissue in such circumstances does not compromise patient care because these lesions are usually low grade Ta lesions. The neodymium:YAG laser has been most commonly used. Flexible fibers can usually be inserted through standard cystoscopes or through cystoscopic equipment modified for use with laser fibers.

One advantage of the laser is that it allows for transmural coagulative necrosis without perforation and extravasation. The boundary between the necrotic tissue and the surrounding tissue is sharp. The endothelial cells in the tissue adjacent to cancer may looks atypical. The pathologists should avoid considering these cells as residual cancer.

Treatment-related Granulomatous Cystitis

Postsurgical Necrobiotic Granuloma

See **Chapter 2** for further discussion (**Fig. 24-38**).

Suture Granuloma

See **Chapter 2** for further discussion.

BCG-induced Granulomatous Cystitis

See discussion above and **Chapter 2** for further discussion.

Surgery-related Pathologic Lesions

Postoperative Spindle Cell Nodule

See **Chapter 19** for further discussion.

Malignancy Associated with Bladder Augmentations and Intestinal Conduits

See **Chapter 21** for further discussion.

REFERENCES

1. Lopez-Beltran A, Luque RJ, Mazzucchelli R, Scarpelli M, Montironi R. Changes produced in the urothelium by traditional and newer therapeutic procedures for bladder cancer. *J Clin Pathol* 2002;55:641–7.
2. Lopez-Beltran A. Bladder treatment. Immunotherapy and chemotherapy. *Urol Clin North Am* 1999;26:535–54.
3. Lopez-Beltran A, Cheng L, Andersson L, Brausi M, de Matteis A, Montironi R, Sesterhenn I, van det Kwast KT, Mazerolles C. Preneoplastic non-papillary lesions and conditions of the urinary bladder: an update based on the Ancona International

Consultation. *Virchows Arch* 2002;440:3–11.
4. Lopez-Beltran A. Urothelial changes induced by therapeutic procedures for bladder cancer. *Anal Quant Cytol Histol* 2006;28:339.
5. Plotz PH, Klippel JH, Decker JL, Grauman D, Wolff B, Brown BC, Rutt G. Bladder complications in patients receiving cyclophosphamide for systemic lupus erythematosus or rheumatoid arthritis. *Ann Intern Med* 1979;91:221–3.
6. Lawrence HJ, Simone J, Aur RJ. Cyclophosphamide-induced

hemorrhagic cystitis in children with leukemia. *Cancer* 1975;36:1572–6.
7. Berkson BM, Lome LG, Shapiro I. Severe cystitis induced by cyclophosphamide. Role of surgical management. *JAMA* 1973;225:605–6.
8. Johnson WW, Meadows DC. Urinary-bladder fibrosis and telangiectasia associated with long-term cyclophosphamide therapy. *N Engl J Med* 1971;284:290–4.
9. Forni AM, Koss LG, Geller W. Cytological study of the effect of cyclophosphamide on the epithelium of the urinary bladder in man. *Cancer* 1964;17:1348–55.

10. Helin I, Okmian L. Haemorrhagic cystitis complicating cyclophosphamide treatment in children. *Acta Paediatr Scand* 1973;62:497–500.
11. Goldman RL, Warner NE. Hemorrhagic cystitis and cytomegalic inclusions in the bladder associated with cyclophosphamide therapy. *Cancer* 1970;25:7–11.
12. Moulder SL, Roth BJ. Systemic chemotherapy for urothelial transitional cell carcinoma: an overview of toxicity. *Semin Urol Oncol* 2001;19:194–201.
13. Cox PJ, Abel G. Cyclophosphamide cystitis. Studies aimed at its minimization. *Biochem Pharmacol* 1979;28:3499–502.
14. deVries CR, Freiha FS. Hemorrhagic cystitis: a review. *J Urol* 1990;143:1–9.
15. Marshall FF, Klinefelter HF. Late hemorrhagic cystitis following low-dose cyclophosphamide therapy. *Urology* 1979;14:573–5.
16. Stillwell TJ, Benson RC Jr. Cyclophosphamide-induced hemorrhagic cystitis. A review of 100 patients. *Cancer* 1988;61:451–7.
17. Pollack HM, Banner MP, Martinez LO, Hodson CJ. Diagnostic considerations in urinary bladder wall calcification. *AJR Am J Roentgenol* 1981;136:791–7.
18. Francis RS, Shackelford GD. Cyclophosphamide cystitis with bladder wall calcification. *J Can Assoc Radiol* 1974;25:324–6.
19. Wall RL, Clausen KP. Carcinoma of the urinary bladder in patients receiving cyclophosphamide. *N Engl J Med* 1975;293:271–3.
20. Rowland RG, Eble JN. Bladder leiomyosarcoma and pelvic fibroblastic tumor following cyclophosphamide therapy. *J Urol* 1983;130:344–6.
21. Kanno J, Sakamoto A, Washizuka M, Kawai T, Kasuga T. Malignant mixed mesodermal tumor of bladder occurring after radiotherapy for cervical cancer: report of a case. *J Urol* 1985;133:854–6.
22. Siddiqui A, Melamed MR, Abbi R, Ahmed T. Mucinous (colloid) carcinoma of urinary bladder following long-term cyclophosphamide therapy for Waldenstrom's macroglobulinemia. *Am J Surg Pathol* 1996;20:500–4.

23. Talar-Williams C, Hijazi YM, Walther MM, Linehan WM, Hallahan CW, Lubensky I, Kerr GS, Hoffman GS, Fauci AS, Sneller MC. Cyclophosphamide-induced cystitis and bladder cancer in patients with Wegener granulomatosis. *Ann Intern Med* 1996;124:477–84.
24. Fernandes ET, Manivel JC, Reddy PK, Ercole CJ. Cyclophosphamide associated bladder cancer—a highly aggressive disease: analysis of 12 cases. *J Urol* 1996;156:1931–3.
25. Barlow LJ, Seager CM, Benson MC, McKiernan JM. Novel intravesical therapies for non-muscle-invasive bladder cancer refractory to BCG. *Urol Oncol* 2010;28:108–11.
26. Murphy WM, Soloway MS, Lin CJ. Morphologic effects of thio-TEPA on mammalian urothelium. Changes in abnormal cells. *Acta Cytol* 1978;22:550–4.
27. Choe JM, Kirkemo AK, Sirls LT. Intravesical thiotepa-induced eosinophilic cystitis. *Urology* 1995;46:729–31.
28. Ulker V, Apaydin E, Gursan A, Ozyurt C, Kandiloglu G. Eosinophilic cystitis induced by mitomycin-C. *Int Urol Nephrol* 1996;28:755–9.
29. Murphy WM, Soloway MS, Finebaum PJ. Pathological changes associated with topical chemotherapy for superficial bladder cancer. *J Urol* 1981;126:461–4.
30. Scharf J, Nahir M, Eidelman S, Jacobs R, Levin D. Carcinoma of the bladder with azathioprine therapy. *JAMA* 1977;237:152.
31. Piper JM, Tonascia J, Matanoski GM. Heavy phenacetin use and bladder cancer in women aged 20 to 49 years. *N Engl J Med* 1985;313:292–5.
32. Pode D, Perlberg S, Steiner D. Busulfan-induced hemorrhagic cystitis. *J Urol* 1983;130:347–8.
33. Oxley JD, Cottrell AM, Adams S, Gillatt D. Ketamine cystitis as a mimic of carcinoma in situ. *Histopathology* 2009;55:705–8.
34. Chiong E, Esuvaranathan K. New therapies for non-muscle-invasive bladder cancer. *World J Urol* 2010;28:71–8.
35. Cheng L, Davidson DD, Maclennan GT, Williamson SR, Zhang S, Koch MO, Montironi R, Lopez-Beltran A. The origins of urothelial carcinoma.

Expert Rev Anticancer Ther 2010;10:865–80.
36. Betz SA, See WA, Cohen MB. Granulomatous inflammation in bladder wash specimens after intravesical bacillus Calmette-Guérin therapy for transitional cell carcinoma of the bladder. *Am J Clin Pathol* 1993;99:244–8.
37. Belldegrun AS, Franklin JR, O'Donnell MA, Gomella LG, Klein E, Neri R, Nseyo UO, Ratliff TL, Williams RD. Superficial bladder cancer: the role of interferon-alpha. *J Urol* 1998;159:1793–801.
38. Shintani Y, Sawada Y, Inagaki T, Kohjimoto Y, Uekado Y, Shinka T. Intravesical instillation therapy with bacillus Calmette-Guérin for superficial bladder cancer: study of the mechanism of bacillus Calmette-Guérin immunotherapy. *Int J Urol* 2007;14:140–6.
39. Adam L, Black PC, Kassouf W, Eve B, McConkey D, Munsell MF, Benedict WF, Dinney CP. Adenoviral mediated interferon-alpha 2b gene therapy suppresses the pro-angiogenic effect of vascular endothelial growth factor in superficial bladder cancer. *J Urol* 2007;177:1900–6.
40. Gomella LG, Mastrangelo MJ, McCue PA, Maguire HJ, Mulholland SG, Lattime EC. Phase I study of intravesical vaccinia virus as a vector for gene therapy of bladder cancer. *J Urol* 2001;166:1291–5.
41. Lopez-Beltran A, Pacelli A, Rothenberg HJ, Wollan PC, Zincke H, Blute ML, Bostwick DG. Carcinosarcoma and sarcomatoid carcinoma of the bladder: clinicopathological study of 41 cases. *J Urol* 1998;159:1497–503.
42. Pazzaglia S, Chen XR, Aamodt CB, Wu SQ, Kao C, Gilchrist KW, Oyasu R, Reznikoff CA, Ritter MA. In Vitro radiation-induced neoplastic progression of low grade uroepithelial tumors. *Radiat Res* 1994;138:86–92.
43. Antonakopoulos GN, Hicks RM, Berry RJ. The subcellular basis of damage to the human urinary bladder induced by irradiation. *J Pathol* 1984;143:103–16.
44. Marks LB, Carroll PR, Dugan TC, Anscher MS. The response of the urinary bladder, urethra, and ureter to radiation and chemotherapy. *Int J*

Radiat Oncol Biol Phys 1995;31:1257–80.

45. Hietala SO, Winblad B, Hassler O. Vascular and morphological changes in the urinary bladder wall after irradiation. *Int Urol Nephrol* 1975;7:119–29.

46. Fajardo LF, Berthrong M. Radiation injury in surgical pathology. Part I. *Am J Surg Pathol* 1978;2:159–99.

47. Chan TY, Epstein JI. Radiation or chemotherapy cystitis with "pseudocarcinomatous" features. *Am J Surg Pathol* 2004;28:909–13.

48. Dumey N, Mongiat-Artus P, Devauchelle P, Lesourd A, Cotard JP, Le Duc A, Marty M, Cussenot O, Cohen-Haguenauer O. In Vivo retroviral mediated gene transfer into bladder urothelium results in preferential transduction of tumoral cells. *Eur Urol* 2005;47:257–63.

49. Irie A, Matsumoto K, Anderegg B, Kuruma H, Kashani-Sabet M, Scanlon KJ, Uchida T, Baba S. Growth inhibition efficacy of an adenovirus expressing dual therapeutic *genes*, wild-type p53, and anti-erbB2 ribozyme, against human bladder cancer cells. *Cancer Gene Ther* 2006;13:298–305.

50. Kikuchi E, Menendez S, Ozu C, Ohori M, Cordon-Cardo C, Logg CR, Kasahara N, Bochner BH. Highly efficient gene delivery for bladder cancers by intravesically administered replication-competent retroviral vectors. *Clin Cancer Res* 2007;13:4511–8.

51. Lojo Rial C, Wilby D, Sooriakumaran P. Role and rationale of gene therapy and other novel therapies in the management of NMIBC. *Expert Rev Anticancer Ther* 2009;9:1777–82.

52. Malmstrom PU, Loskog AS, Lindqvist CA, Mangsbo SM, Fransson M, Wanders A, Gardmark T, Totterman TH. AdCD40L immunogene therapy for bladder carcinoma—the first phase I/IIa trial. *Clin Cancer Res* 2010;16:3279–87.

53. Miyake H, Hara I, Hara S, Arakawa S, Kamidono S. Synergistic chemosensitization and inhibition of tumor growth and metastasis by adenovirus-mediated p53 gene transfer in human bladder cancer model. *Urology* 2000;56:332–6.

54. Miyake H, Yamanaka K, Muramaki M, Hara I, Gleave ME. Therapeutic

efficacy of adenoviral-mediated p53 gene transfer is synergistically enhanced by combined use of antisense oligodeoxynucleotide targeting clusterin gene in a human bladder cancer model. *Neoplasia* 2005;7:171–9.

55. Svatek RS, Kamat AM, Dinney CP. Novel therapeutics for patients with non-muscle-invasive bladder cancer. *Expert Rev Anticancer Ther* 2009;9:807–13.

56. Laihia JK, Pylkkanen L, Laato M, Bostrom PJ, Leino L. Protodynamic therapy for bladder cancer: in vitro results of a novel treatment concept. *BJU Int* 2009;104:1233–8.

57. Juarranz A, Jaen P, Sanz-Rodriguez F, Cuevas J, Gonzalez S. Photodynamic therapy of cancer. Basic principles and applications. *Clin Transl Oncol* 2008;10:148–54.

58. Muller M, Reich E, Steiner U, Heicappell R, Miller K. Photodynamic effects of sulfonated aluminum chlorophthalocyanine in human urinary bladder carcinoma cells in vitro. *Eur Urol* 1997;32:339–43.

59. Kelly JF, Snell ME. Hematoporphyrin derivative: a possible aid in the diagnosis and therapy of carcinoma of the bladder. *J Urol* 1976;115:150–1.

60. Fanning CV, Staerkel GA, Sneige N, Thomsen S, Myhre MJ, Von Eschenbach AC. Spindling artifact of urothelial cells in post-laser treatment urinary cytology. *Diagn Cytopathol* 1993;9:279–81.

61. Smith JA Jr. Laser treatment of bladder cancer. *Semin Urol* 1985;3:2–9.

62. Prout GR Jr, Lin CW, Benson R Jr, Nseyo UO, Daly JJ, Griffin PP, Kinsey J, Tian ME, Lao YH, Mian YZ, et al. Photodynamic therapy with hematoporphyrin derivative in the treatment of superficial transitional-cell carcinoma of the bladder. *N Engl J Med* 1987;317:1251–5.

63. Shanberg AM, Baghdassarian R, Tansey LA. Use of Nd:YAG laser in treatment of bladder cancer. *Urology* 1987;29:26–30.

64. Vicente J, Salvador J, Laguna P, Algaba F. Histological evaluation of superficial bladder tumors treated by Nd-YAG laser and transurethral resection. *Eur Urol* 1991;20:192–6.

65. Keane TE, Petros JA, Velimirovich B, Yue KT, Graham SD Jr.

Methoxypsoralen phototherapy of transitional cell carcinoma. *Urology* 1994;44:842–6.

66. Pisharodi LR, Bhan R. Spindling artefact of urothelial cells. *Diagn Cytopathol* 1995;12:195.

67. Wong AK, Lupu AN, Shanberg AM. Laser ablation of renal pelvic transitional cell carcinoma in a solitary kidney: a 9-year followup. *Urology* 1996;48:298–300.

68. Bader MJ, Sroka R, Gratzke C, Seitz M, Weidlich P, Staehler M, Becker A, Stief CG, Reich O. Laser therapy for upper urinary tract transitional cell carcinoma: indications and management. *Eur Urol* 2009;56:65–71.

69. Gao X, Ren S, Xu C, Sun Y. Thulium laser resection via a flexible cystoscope for recurrent non-muscle-invasive bladder cancer: initial clinical experience. *BJU Int* 2008;102:1115–8.

70. Ruszat R, Seitz M, Wyler SF, Abe C, Rieken M, Reich O, Gasser TC, Bachmann A. GreenLight laser vaporization of the prostate: single-center experience and long-term results after 500 procedures. *Eur Urol* 2008;54:893–901.

71. Smith JA Jr. Laser surgery for transitional-cell carcinoma. Technique, advantages, and limitations. *Urol Clin North Am* 1992;19:473–83.

72. Soler-Martinez J, Vozmediano-Chicharro R, Morales-Jimenez P, Hernandez-Alcaraz D, Vivas-Vargas E, Santos Garcia-Vaquero I, Baena-Gonzalez V. Holmium laser treatment for low grade, low stage, noninvasive bladder cancer with local anesthesia and early instillation of mitomycin C. *J Urol* 2007;178:2337–9.

73. Yang Y, Wei ZT, Zhang X, Hong BF, Guo G. Transurethral partial cystectomy with continuous wave laser for bladder carcinoma. *J Urol* 2009;182:66–9.

74. Zhu Y, Jiang X, Zhang J, Chen W, Shi B, Xu Z. Safety and efficacy of holmium laser resection for primary nonmuscle-invasive bladder cancer versus transurethral electroresection: single-center experience. *Urology* 2008;72:608–12.

Chapter 25

Handling and Reporting of Bladder Specimens

Bladder Pathology, First Edition. Liang Cheng, Antonio Lopez-Beltran, David G. Bostwick.
© 2012 Wiley-Blackwell. Published 2012 by John Wiley & Sons, Inc.

Specimen Handling

Efforts have been made recently to standardize the handling and reporting of bladder specimens.[1-23] The most common bladder specimens are endoscopic biopsies and transurethral resections (TURs) of the bladder. Other specimens include cystectomy (partial or total), cystoprostatectomy, pelvic exenteration (en bloc resection), and diverticulum resections. Surgical excision of an urachal carcinoma usually includes the bladder dome, urachus, and umbilicus.

Biopsy and Transurethral Resection Specimens

Small noninvasive papillary neoplasms are often excised using biopsy with cold-cup forceps, diathermy forceps, or a small diathermy loop (Fig. 25-1). Excellent biopsy results are obtained in the urinary bladder using computerized tomography–guided transmural needle biopsy with a 1.2-mm cutting needle.[24] Thermal artifact may render the specimen uninterpretable (Fig. 25-2). In such cases, repeat biopsy should be obtained. To avoid tissue distortion, these specimens should be carefully transferred to fixative immediately upon resection. Tissue may be fixed in formalin or formol-saline, but picric acid-based fixatives may provide better tissue preservation of bladder biopsies.[25] Deeper levels should be obtained when clinically suspicious lesions are sampled (Fig. 25-3).

Larger neoplasms are often sampled by TUR with a diathermy loop that produces strips of tissue approximately 6 mm in width and of variable length. Additional resection of the tumor base may be obtained to assess the depth of invasion and the presence or absence of muscularis propria invasion (see Chapters 10 and 11 for further discussion).

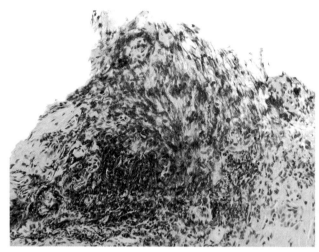

Figure 25-2 Cold-cup biopsy of the bladder markedly distorted by thermal artifact. This finding is uninterpretable, and additional biopsy is recommended.

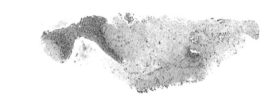

A

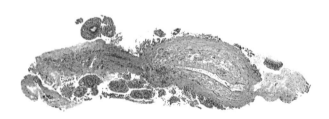

B

Figure 25-3 Deeper levels are helpful in small bladder biopsies. (A) The original slide did not show any significant pathology. (B) Deeper levels (from the same block) revealed a low grade papillary urothelial carcinoma.

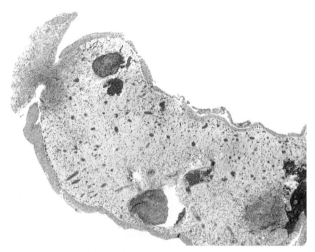

Figure 25-1 Cold-cup biopsy specimen with excellent histology.

Any erythematous or velvety area of urothelium is sampled to exclude carcinoma in situ. Random biopsies are also taken from cystoscopically normal urothelium distant from the tumor site to determine the extent of involvement. It has been suggested that random biopsy samples be obtained from predetermined sites in four quadrants of the urinary bladder.[26-31] Some urologists also submit biopsy specimens of the urethra to assess the extent of disease, particularly in patients with grade 2 or 3 (high grade) papillary urothelial carcinoma or carcinoma in situ (Table 25-1).[28,32,33]

Bladder TUR and bladder biopsy specimens are to provide diagnostic and prognostic information for urologists to plan surveillance and treatment, and to predict tumor response to therapy. Tissues from biopsy specimens should be entirely embedded for histologic examination. Biopsy specimens obtained through the cystoscope often vary in size. At least two levels of sectioning should be obtained on each small biopsy. Proper orientation of bladder tumor biopsy specimens is difficult, even with a dissecting microscope. It may be necessary to reembed and reorient the tissue to facilitate assessment of the depth of invasion.

TUR specimens should be weighed in aggregate. The number of tissue chips with involvement and gross tumor size should be recorded. Overfilling of specimen cassettes should be avoided. Papillary tumors may be grossly recognizable in these specimens and should be documented and submitted for histologic examination. We recommend complete submission of the specimen for histopathologic examination, but some laboratories prefer to submit only representative samples. In partially sampled specimens, an effort should be made to select fragments that contain muscle; also, the proportion of the specimen processed for examination should be stated if only partially sampled. When there is no evaluable muscularis propria in the sample, all of the tissue should be processed (or, minimally, 10 blocks should be submitted).

If the tumor is noninvasive, submitting any residual specimen may be necessary to firmly rule out stromal invasion. If there is invasion into the lamina propria in the initial sampling, additional sampling is recommended to rule out muscularis propria invasion. We recommend that the urologist submit superficial and deep tumor base specimens in separate containers to facilitate the detection of muscularis propria invasion. Recently, it has been recommended that any pT1 tumor be restaged by doing an additional re-TUR 3 months following the initial TUR.[34,35] The same criteria as those described above apply to this material.[1]

Routine reporting of presence or absence of muscularis propria in the specimen when there is no cancer present may be useful for surgical quality control, but is not included uniformly by all pathologists; we consider this a useful

Table 25-1 Reporting of Bladder Biopsy/Transurethral Resection Specimens

Gross findings
  Cold-cup biopsy
    Estimated number of tissue fragments, aggregate dimensions
    Presence or absence of papillary growth
    All tissue fragments should be submitted
  Transurethral resection of the bladder
    Estimated number of tissue fragments, aggregate dimensions
    Total weight of resected tissue fragments
    Proportion of tissue embedded, if not completely embedded[a]

Microscopic findings
  General assessment
    Epithelial surface (intact, ulcerated, denuded)
    Presence or absence of muscularis propria (detrusor muscle)
    Comment on cautery artifact if it compromises evaluation
  Tumor assessment
    Anatomic location (if available)
    Histologic diagnosis
      Specify invasive or noninvasive urothelial carcinoma
    Histologic grade (we recommend using both the 1973 and 2004 WHO grading systems)
    Overall architecture (e.g., papillary, flat, ulcerated, solid, or nodular)
    Pattern of invasion (nodular, trabecular, or infiltrative)
    Presence or absence of lymphovascular invasion
    Extent of invasion (specify if stromal invasion is present or not and the level of invasion)
    Invasion into lamina propria
      Extent and/or depth of invasion should be provided
      Reporting of muscularis mucosae invasion is optional since muscularis mucosae is not uniformly present in the biopsy specimens
    Invasion into muscularis propria (detrusor muscle)
    T2 substaging (pT2a vs. T2b) cannot be performed on biopsy specimens
    Statements of tumor stage should be provided (e.g., at least T1, or T2)
      Comment that accurate staging may require complete resection of the tumor
      T2 substaging (pT2a vs. T2b) cannot be performed on biopsy specimens
      Fat invasion in biopsy is not necessarily indicative of extravesical invasion (pT3) since fat can be present throughout the bladder wall
    Findings in the adjacent mucosa
      Presence or absence of dysplasia, carcinoma in situ
      Other findings: intestinal metaplasia, cystitis glandularis, keratinizing squamous metaplasia

[a]We recommend that a minimum of 10 cassettes be submitted for initial evaluation. If lamina propria invasion is identified, the entire specimen may be submitted to rule out muscularis propria invasion and to further assess the extent of invasion.

statement to include in the report. The level of muscularis propria invasion (outer vs. inner one-half of muscularis propria wall invasion) is impossible to assess in TUR specimens, and the only reasonable statement may be "at least stage pT2." The presence of adipose tissue in biopsy specimens is not a clear indication of extravesical sampling because fat may be present within the lamina propria or the muscle layers.[36,37]

Cystectomy, Cystoprostatectomy, and Pelvic Exenteration (en Bloc Resection) Specimens

The way these specimens are processed may be summarized in three steps: (1) orientation of the specimen and identification of relevant anatomic structures (e.g., ureters); (2) fixation of the specimen; and (3) dissection of the specimen (Fig. 25-4; Table 25-2). Peritoneum covering the surface of the bladder is a reliable anatomic landmark. In both male and female patients, the peritoneum descends farther along the posterior wall of the bladder than it does along the anterior wall. Other pelvic organs, if present, may also be used to orient the specimen. In the male, the bladder adjoins the rectum and seminal vesicle posteriorly, the prostate

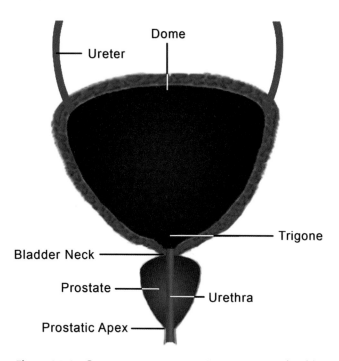

Figure 25-4 Cystoprostatectomy specimen. Sections should be taken from tumor, bladder neck, trigone, anterior wall, posterior wall, lateral walls, dome, ureteral orifices (including intramural portion), margins (ureteral, urethral, and perivesical soft tissue), and any abnormal-appearing bladder mucosa. The prostate should be sampled using the standard protocol for radical prostatectomy specimens. (From Ref 1; with permission.)

Table 25-2 Reporting of Cystectomy Specimens

Gross findings
  Fresh or fixed specimen
  Nature of the specimen: partial cystectomy, radical cystectomy, cystoprostatectomy, pelvic exenteration
  Three-dimensional measurements of recognizable anatomic structures, and of tumors or other recognizable lesions
  Site of involvement
  Growth pattern (papillary, flat, ulcerated, solid/nodular, infiltrative, indeterminate)
  Gross assessment of invasion (into lamina propria or muscularis propria)
  Gross extravesical fat extension
  Gross invasion into adjacent organs, such as prostate, ureter, urethra, uterus, vagina, or pelvic and abdominal wall
  Gross assessment of margin status
Lymph nodes
  Location and the number of lymph nodes sampled
    Report if the lymph nodes are bisected or completely embedded
    Report if the lymph nodes are grossly involved by cancer

Microscopic findings
  Anatomic location of the tumor
  Histologic diagnosis
  Tumor size and multifocality
  Histologic grade (we recommend using both the 1973 and 2004 WHO grading systems)
  Pattern of invasion (nodular, trabecular, or infiltrative)
  Extent of invasion (pathologic staging)
    No invasion (pTa or pTis)
    Invasion into the lamina propria (pT1)
    Invasion into inner or outer half of muscularis propria (pT2)
    Invasion into perivesical soft tissue (pT3)
    Tumor arising in a diverticulum (specify whether detrusor muscle is present)
  Surgical margins
    Ureteral margin
    Urethral margins
    Perivesical soft tissue margin
    Pelvic soft tissue margin (for pelvic exenteration specimens)
  Presence or absence of lymphovascular invasion
  Other intraepithelial abnormalities
    Presence or absence of dysplasia and carcinoma in situ in adjacent mucosa, including pagetoid spread of carcinoma in situ
    Location and multifocality
    Other findings, such as intestinal metaplasia, squamous metaplasia, therapeutic treatment effects

(continued)

Table 25-2 (*Continued*)

Extent of tumor invasion into adjacent organs
  Prostate
    Involvement of the prostatic urethra with or
      without stromal invasion
    Involvement of prostatic ducts/acini without
      stromal invasion
    Prostatic stromal invasion
    Direct extension into the prostate from
      carcinoma through the bladder neck
    Direct extravesical extension into the prostatic
      parenchyma
    Seminal vesicle invasion through intraprostatic
      epithelium or by direct perivesical extension
  Ureter and urethra
    Report any dysplastic/neoplastic change of the
      mucosa, including pagetoid spread of
      carcinoma in situ
    Report invasion into adjacent lamina propria or
      muscularis propria
  Seminal vesicles
    Report spread of carcinoma in these organs
      either through epithelium or by direct
      extension of an infiltrative carcinoma
  Vagina/uterus
    Report direct extension or metastases to either
      organ
  Rectum, pelvic and abdominal wall
    Report direct extension or metastases
  Lymph node status
    Report the number of lymph nodes sampled
    Report the presence or absence of metastases
    If metastases are present, state the following in
      the report:
      Number of positive nodes
      Diameter of the largest metastasis
      Presence or absence of extranodal extension
Final pathologic staging (using the 2010 TNM staging)
Results of ancillary studies (if performed)
Correlation with frozen section diagnosis (if
  performed)

inferiorly, and the pubis and peritoneum anteriorly. In the female, the vagina is located posteriorly, and the uterus is located superiorly. Once the specimen is oriented, both ureters and, when present, the vasa deferentia should be identified. Location and dissection of the ureters is easier after fixation. The outer dimensions of the urinary bladder, as well as the length and diameter of ureters, should be recorded. The external surface of the bladder should be inked.

Adequate fixation of the specimens is a prerequisite for adequate histologic evaluation. We recommend that large bladder specimens be fixed in formalin overnight. Some prefer to expand the bladder with formalin. Injection of formalin into the urinary bladder cavity is accomplished either through the urethra via a Foley catheter or through the bladder dome using a large-gauge needle after the urethra has been clamped. We prefer to open the bladder before formalin fixation. It should be opened anteriorly from the urethra to the bladder dome, and the bladder mucosa everted for close examination. Any subtle alteration of the mucosa, such as granularity, ulceration, hemorrhage, or erythema, should be carefully documented. If a grossly visible tumor is identified, the size, location, configuration (flat, papillary, solid/nodular, sessile, exophytic, endophytic, or ulcerated), color, and consistency of the tumor should be documented.

After the specimen is well fixed, the dissection is resumed by shaving the margins from each ureter and from the urethra. When the specimen includes the prostate, the distal urethral margin is the distal end of the prostate at the apex. The ureters are opened at their trigone orifices and examined for strictures, dilatations, ulcerations, diverticula, or exophytic lesions. If a tumor is identified in the bladder, a full-thickness cut should be made through the tumor and bladder wall. The tumor should be sampled generously for accurate staging, grading, and histologic typing. For a large tumor, at least one section should be taken for each centimeter of tumor diameter. Sections are taken in such a way as to demonstrate the relationship of tumor to adjacent urothelium, its maximal level of penetration, and external soft tissue margin. For large exophytic tumors, several sections are taken from the tumor base to adequately assess the extent of invasion. Normal-appearing mucosa is also sampled to detect occult multifocal carcinomas due to the field effect of bladder carcinogenesis. The entire bladder is transversely step-sectioned at 5-mm intervals from the bladder neck to the dome. Perivesical fat is carefully searched for lymph nodes. The presence or absence of gross fat invasion should be documented.

The minimum number of sections to be taken are as follows: tumor (more than three, depending on tumor size); bladder neck (one), trigone (two), anterior wall (two), posterior wall (two), lateral walls (two), dome (two), ureteral orifices (including intramural portion), margins (ureteral, urethral, and perivesical soft tissue), any abnormal-appearing bladder mucosa, and any perivesical lymph nodes.[38] At least one block per centimeter of tumor diameter, up to 10 cassette blocks, should be submitted at the initial sampling.

Preoperative treatments or repeat TUR may render residual tumors grossly invisible. As TUR techniques have improved, there is increasing incidence of pT0 carcinoma at cystectomy (see also **Chapter 11**). For such cases, the bladder should be sampled extensively, with particular attention to abnormal-appearing mucosa and to sites of previously documented tumor resection.

For a cystoprostatectomy specimen, the bladder is opened anteriorly by an incision from the prostatic urethra to the dome. The urethral mucosa is examined carefully for evidence of tumor extension into the prostatic urethra. The prostate should be examined by the established protocol for pathological evaluation and reporting of radical prostatectomy specimens. The prostate is transversely sectioned from apex to base at 5-mm intervals, with the plane of the sections perpendicular to the posterior surface of the gland. If a tumor is grossly visible, it is important to document whether the tumor arises centrally from the prostatic urethra or more peripherally in the common location for prostate cancer (peripheral zone). It is important to take sections from the bladder neck since this is an important route for urothelial carcinoma to invade prostatic stroma.[39] Recent whole-mount analysis of large numbers of cystoprostatectomy specimens emphasizes the importance of thorough prostate sampling.[40]

For pelvic exenteration specimens, the rectum, uterus, and vagina should be evaluated according to the standardized protocols for these organs. Pelvic soft tissue margins should be documented. Since the uterus and rectum are located posterior to the bladder, an anterior opening of the bladder is preferred to facilitate the documentation of urothelial tumors and to evaluate the tumor's relationship to these other organs for staging. Sections should be taken to confirm the presence of each pelvic organ and to demonstrate the relationship between the tumor and each of these structures. These sections also document the resection margins for each organ and examine each organ for primary disease.

Partial Cystectomy and Urachal Resection Specimens

Partial cystectomy specimens (including resections of diverticula) should be fixed and dissected according to the guidelines for radical cystectomy (see the previous discussion). The edges of the specimen are inked because these represent the surgical margins of the bladder wall. A variation of the partial cystectomy is performed for resections of urachal tract neoplasms. These specimens consist of the dome of the bladder in continuity with the urachal tract, including the umbilicus. After inking the soft tissue margin, the urachal tract should be sectioned serially at right angles to the long axis from the bladder to the umbilicus. Submit for histology a number of these urachal tract cross sections as well as the standard bladder sections. Appropriate samples of the soft tissue margin surrounding the urachus and of the skin margin around the umbilicus should be submitted for histology.

Lymph Node Dissection

The regional lymph nodes of the bladder are the pelvic lymph nodes below the bifurcation of the common iliac arteries. These include the hypogastric, obturator, iliac (internal, external, not otherwise specified), perivesical, pelvic (not otherwise specified), sacral (lateral, sacral promontory), and presacral lymph nodes. The common iliac nodes are considered sites of distant metastasis and are coded as M1.[41] Current nodal classification is based on the number and size of positive nodes.

Recent studies have emphasized the importance of lymph node density,[42] and we recommend that the number of lymph nodes sampled be clearly stated in the report. Unlike colon cancer, the minimum number of lymph nodes that should be sampled has not been established. We recommend at least eight lymph nodes be sampled. In difficult cases, a clearing solution may be used to aid in the detection of lymph nodes. These may, on occasion, be detected in the perivesical fat, so a thorough search should be made of this area in addition to other pelvic node-bearing structures. Lymph node revealing solution (LNRS) is helpful in recovering the hidden lymph nodes from fatty tissue (Figs. 25-5 and 25-6).

Pathology Reporting

Overview

The pathology report should include clinically relevant historical information as well as clinically useful gross and microscopic information.[1,2,4-9,11,14,16] Bladder cancer reports must include the specimen type, anatomic location of the tumor, tumor size, tumor configuration, histologic type, histologic grade, TNM (tumor, lymph nodes, and metastases) staging, tumor growth pattern, surgical margin status, treatment effect, lymphovascular invasion, and any other intraepithelial lesions (Tables 25-1 and 25-2). These parameters are listed in Tables 25-1 and 25-2, which illustrate synoptic formats for biopsy and cystectomy cancer specimen reports. The 2010 TNM staging system should be used in pathology reporting of bladder cancer regardless of tumor type (see Chapter 11 for further discussion).[41]

The biopsy report should record which tissues are present. Separately submitted biopsies, including random biopsies, should receive separate diagnoses. In patients with urothelial malignancy, a report of "denuded biopsy" is significantly different from one stating that "no tumor is seen."[10] Similarly, invasion of the lamina propria may have different implications depending on the presence or absence of muscularis propria. Care must be taken to distinguish the thin and often incomplete muscularis mucosae within the lamina propria from the muscularis propria (Figs. 25-7 to 25-10; see also Chapter 10). The designation of mere muscle invasion in the report is inadequate. The type of muscle being invaded, whether muscularis

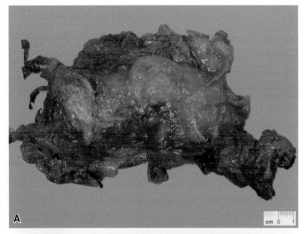

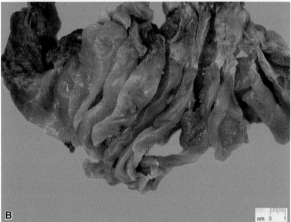

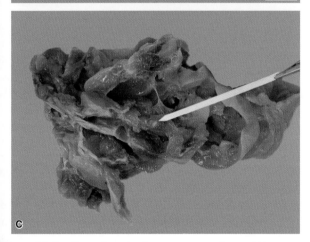

Figure 25-5 Gross lymphadenectomy specimen. (A) Demonstrated here is the appearance of a separated node packet removed during a radical cystectomy. This picture was taken after formalin fixation. Note the fatty nature of the specimen and the lack of any easily identifiable lymph nodes. (B) This picture demonstrates the effects of lymph node revealing solution (Carnoy solution, in this case) on the tissue after 12-hour fixation. Notice the lightening of the fatty tissue. (C) After thorough sectioning, a node is located (arrow) and identified by its brighter white color compared to that of adjacent fatty soft tissue.

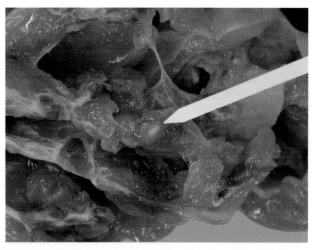

Figure 25-6 Lymph node revealing solution is helpful in recovering the hidden lymph nodes from fatty tissue. The arrow points to a revealed lymph node.

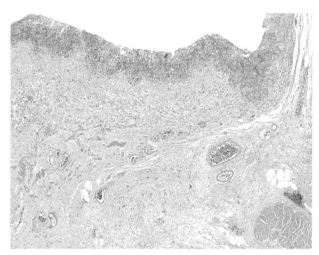

Figure 25-7 Lamina propria of the bladder wall. Note the presence of muscularis mucosae (left middle field), contrasting with thick bundled muscularis propria (detrusor muscle) in the right lower corner.

mucosae (T1 carcinoma) or detrusor muscle invasion (T2 carcinoma), should be clearly stated. Although staging based on the level of muscularis mucosae invasion is not recommended,[43] an indication of the extent of invasion is of clinical interest and should be reported. The use of an ocular micrometer to measure depth of invasion may be considered.[44–46] Patients with invasion of less than 1.5 mm have a better prognosis than other T1 bladder cancer patients.[46]

The presence or absence of muscularis propria (detrusor muscle), regardless of whether there is invasion, should also be reported as an indication of the resection adequacy.

531

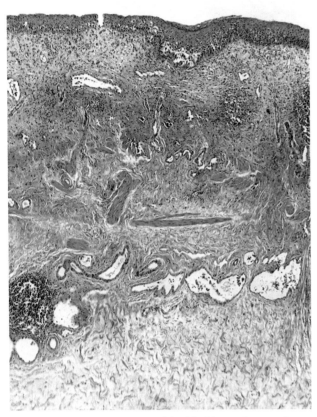

Figure 25-8 Lamina propria of the bladder wall. Note the presence of muscularis mucosae (middle field).

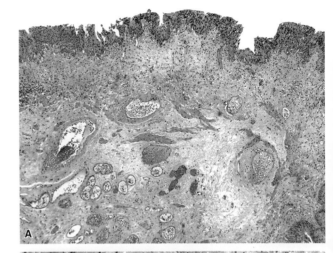

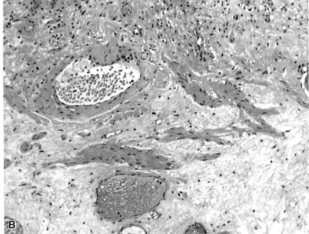

Figure 25-9 Muscularis mucosae (A and B).

Substaging of T2 bladder cancer (T2a vs. T2b) is not feasible in bladder biopsy or TUR specimens, since the entire thickness of the detrusor muscle is not present. The term "superficial muscle invasion" in the pathology report leads to confusion. Therefore, it should be avoided. For biopsy and TUR of invasive bladder carcinoma, some urologists prefer a statement of pathologic stage (T1 or T2) in the report. In such an instance, we recommend that tumor stage be indicated as "at least" pT1 or pT2.

Adipose tissue is present in the lamina propria and muscularis propria of the bladder wall (Fig. 25-11). Therefore, the presence of fat invasion in the biopsy or TUR specimen does not necessarily indicate higher stage (pT3) cancer. Currently, there is no reliable method to predict extravesical extension with a TUR specimen.[47] However, a tumor with a 4-mm or greater depth of invasion in the TUR specimen is most likely to have extravesical extension.[48]

For biopsy and TUR specimens, it is particularly important to mention the presence or absence of lymphovascular invasion and to comment on certain histologic variants, such as micropapillary and nested variants of urothelial carcinoma.[1,2,49] Aggressive therapies may be considered for those patients with lymphovascular invasion, micropapillary variant, or nested variant of urothelial carcinoma.

Recommendations for the reporting of specimens from urinary bladder have been published (Tables 25-3 and 25-4). Laboratories accredited by the College of American Pathologists (CAP) are required to use CAP cancer reporting guidelines.

Tumor Size

The pathology report should include the largest tumor dimension and information about multifocality. In an analysis of 249 patients with stage Ta and T1 cancer, Heney et al. found that tumor size was a significant predictor of cancer progression.[50] Thirty-five percent of patients with tumor size ≥ 5 cm developed muscularis propria invasion or metastasis. On the other hand, only 9% of patients with tumor size below 5 cm developed cancer progression.[50] One study found that tumor size was an independent predictor of distant metastasis-free survival

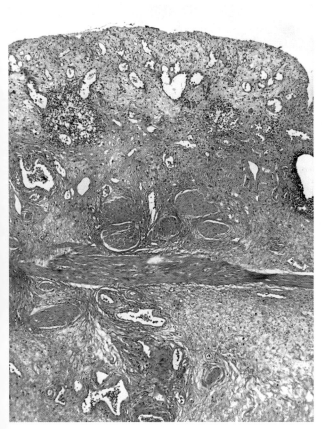

Figure 25-10 Hypertrophic muscularis mucosae. It may be difficult to distinguish from muscularis propria (detrusor muscle) in poorly oriented or fragmented biopsy specimens.

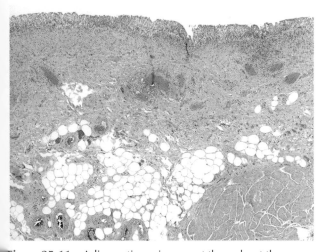

Figure 25-11 Adipose tissue is present throughout the bladder wall. The presence of fat invasion in biopsy or TUR specimens does not indicate extravesical extension (pT3 bladder cancer).

Table 25-3 Protocol for the Examination of Biopsy and Transurethral Resection Specimens from Patients with Carcinoma of the Urinary Bladder (CAP Checklist, 2011)

Procedure
_____ Biopsy
_____ TURBT
_____ Other (specify)
_____ Not specified

Histologic type
_____ Urothelial (transitional cell) carcinoma
_____ Urothelial (transitional cell) carcinoma with squamous differentiation
_____ Urothelial (transitional cell) carcinoma with glandular differentiation
_____ Urothelial (transitional cell) carcinoma with variant histology (specify)
_____ Squamous cell carcinoma, typical
_____ Squamous cell carcinoma, variant histology (specify)
_____ Adenocarcinoma, typical
_____ Adenocarcinoma, variant histology (specify)
_____ Small cell carcinoma
_____ Undifferentiated carcinoma (specify)
_____ Mixed cell type (specify)
_____ Other (specify)
_____ Carcinoma, type cannot be determined

Associated epithelial lesions (select all that apply)
_____ None identified
_____ Urothelial (transitional cell) papilloma [World Health Organization (WHO) 2004/ International Society of Urologic Pathology (ISUP)]
_____ Urothelial (transitional cell) papilloma, inverted type
_____ Papillary urothelial (transitional cell) neoplasm, low malignant potential (WHO 2004/ISUP)
_____ Cannot be determined

Histologic grade
_____ Not applicable
_____ Cannot be determined

Urothelial carcinoma (WHO 2004/ISUP)
_____ Low grade
_____ High grade
_____ Other (specify)

Adenocarcinoma and squamous cell carcinoma
_____ GX: Cannot be assessed
_____ G1: Well differentiated
_____ G2: Moderately differentiated
_____ G3: Poorly differentiated
_____ Other (specify)

(*continued*)

Table 25-3 (*Continued*)

Tumor configuration (select all that apply)
____ Papillary
____ Solid/nodule
____ Flat
____ Ulcerated
____ Indeterminate
____ Other (specify)

Adequacy of material for determining muscularis propria invasion
____ Muscularis propria (detrusor muscle) not identified
____ Muscularis propria (detrusor muscle) present
____ Presence of muscularis propria indeterminate

Lymphovascular invasion
____ Not identified
____ Present
____ Indeterminate

Microscopic extent of tumor (select all that apply)
____ Cannot be assessed
____ Noninvasive papillary carcinoma
____ Flat carcinoma in situ
____ Tumor invades subepithelial connective tissue (lamina propria)
____ Tumor invades muscularis propria (detrusor muscle)
____ Urothelial carcinoma in situ involving prostatic urethra in prostatic chips sampled by TURBT
____ Urothelial carcinoma in situ involving prostatic ducts and acini in prostatic chips sampled by TURBT
____ Urothelial carcinoma invasive into prostatic stroma in prostatic chips sampled by TURBT

Additional pathologic findings (select all that apply)
____ Urothelial dysplasia (low grade intraurothelial neoplasia)
____ Inflammation/regenerative changes
____ Therapy-related changes
____ Cautery artifact
____ Cystitis cystica/glandularis
____ Keratinizing squamous metaplasia
____ Intestinal metaplasia
____ Other (specify)

Table 25-4 **Protocol for the Examination of Cystectomy (Partial, Total, or Radical; Anterior Exenteration) Specimens from Patients with Carcinoma of the Urinary Bladder (CAP Checklist, 2011)**

Specimen
____ Bladder
____ Other (specify)
____ Not specified

Procedure
____ Partial cystectomy
____ Total cystectomy
____ Radical cystectomy
____ Radical cystoprostatectomy
____ Anterior exenteration
____ Other (specify)
____ Not specified

Tumor site (select all that apply)
____ Trigone
____ Right lateral wall
____ Left lateral wall
____ Anterior wall
____ Posterior wall
____ Dome
____ Other (specify)
____ Not specified

Tumor size
Greatest dimension: ____ cm
Additional dimensions: ____ × ____ cm
____ Cannot be determined (see comment)

Histologic type
____ Urothelial (transitional cell) carcinoma
____ Urothelial (transitional cell) carcinoma with squamous differentiation
____ Urothelial (transitional cell) carcinoma with glandular differentiation
____ Urothelial (transitional cell) carcinoma with variant histology (specify)
____ Squamous cell carcinoma, typical
____ Squamous cell carcinoma, variant histology (specify)
____ Adenocarcinoma, typical
____ Adenocarcinoma, variant histology (specify)
____ Small cell carcinoma
____ Undifferentiated carcinoma (specify)
____ Mixed cell type (specify)
____ Other (specify)
____ Carcinoma, type cannot be determined

(*continued*)

but not of overall survival.[51] In a recent cystectomy series, tumor size was an independent predictor of distant metastasis-free survival, cancer-specific survival, and overall survival.[52,53] The use of a 3-cm largest tumor diameter cutoff appeared to stratify patients into distinct prognostic groups (**Fig. 25-12**).[52,53]

Table 25-4   (*Continued*)

Associated epithelial lesions (select all that apply)
____ None identified
____ Urothelial (transitional cell) papilloma [World Health Organization (WHO) 2004/ International Society of Urologic Pathology (ISUP)]
____ Urothelial (transitional cell) papilloma, inverted type
____ Papillary urothelial (transitional cell) neoplasm, low malignant potential (WHO 2004/ISUP)
____ Cannot be determined

Histologic grade
____ Not applicable
____ Cannot be determined

Urothelial carcinoma (WHO 2004/ISUP)
____ Low grade
____ High grade
____ Other (specify)

Adenocarcinoma and squamous cell carcinoma
____ GX: Cannot be assessed
____ G1: Well differentiated
____ G2: Moderately differentiated
____ G3: Poorly differentiated
____ Other (specify)

Tumor configuration (select all that apply)
____ Papillary
____ Solid/nodule
____ Flat
____ Ulcerated
____ Indeterminate
____ Other (specify)

Microscopic tumor extension (select all that apply)
____ None identified
____ Perivesical fat
____ Rectum
____ Prostatic stroma
____ Seminal vesicle (specify laterality)
____ Vagina
____ Uterus and adnexae
____ Pelvic sidewall (specify laterality)
____ Ureter (specify laterality)
____ Other (specify)

Margins (select all that apply)
____ Cannot be assessed
____ Margins uninvolved by invasive carcinoma
    Distance of invasive carcinoma from closest margin: ____ mm
    Specify margin
____ Margin(s) involved by invasive carcinoma
    Specify margin(s)
____ Margin(s) uninvolved by carcinoma in situ
____ Margin(s) involved by carcinoma in situ
    Specify margin(s)

Table 25-4   (*Continued*)

Lymphovascular invasion
____ Not identified
____ Present
____ Indeterminate

Pathologic staging (pTNM)
TNM descriptors (required only if applicable) (select all that apply)
____ m (multiple primary tumors)
____ r (recurrent)
____ y (posttreatment)

Primary tumor (pT)
____ pTX: Primary tumor cannot be assessed
____ pT0: No evidence of primary tumor
____ pTa: Noninvasive papillary carcinoma
____ pTis: Carcinoma in situ: "flat tumor"
____ pT1: Tumor invades subepithelial connective tissue (lamina propria)
pT2: Tumor invades muscularis propria (detrusor muscle)
____ pT2a: Tumor invades superficial muscularis propria (inner half)
____ pT2b: Tumor invades deep muscularis propria (outer half)
pT3: Tumor invades perivesical tissue
____ pT3a: Microscopically
____ pT3b: Macroscopically (extravesicular mass)
pT4: Tumor invades any of the following: prostatic stroma, seminal vesicles, uterus, vagina, pelvic wall, abdominal wall
____ pT4a: Tumor invades prostatic stroma or uterus or vagina
____ pT4b: Tumor invades pelvic wall or abdominal wall

Regional lymph nodes (pN)
____ pNX: Lymph nodes cannot be assessed
____ pN0: No lymph node metastasis
____ pN1: Single regional lymph node metastasis in the true pelvis (hypogastric, obturator, external iliac or presacral lymph node)
____ pN2: Multiple regional lymph node metastasis in the true pelvis (hypogastric, obturator, external iliac or presacral lymph node metastasis)
____ pN3: Lymph node metastasis to the common iliac lymph nodes
____ No nodes submitted or found
Number of lymph nodes examined
Specify: ____
____ Number cannot be determined (explain)
Number of lymph nodes involved (*any size*)
Specify: ____
____ Number cannot be determined (explain)

(*continued*)

Table 25-4   (*Continued*)

Distant metastasis (pM)
____ Not applicable
____ pM1: Distant metastasis
Specify site(s), if known

Additional pathologic findings (select all that apply)
____ Adenocarcinoma of prostate (use protocol for
carcinoma of prostate)
____ Urothelial (transitional cell) carcinoma involving
urethra, prostatic ducts, and acini with or without
stromal invasion (use protocol for carcinoma of
urethra)
____ Urothelial dysplasia (low grade intraurothelial
neoplasia)
____ Inflammation/regenerative changes
____ Therapy-related changes
____ Cystitis cystica glandularis
____ Keratinizing squamous metaplasia
____ Intestinal metaplasia
____ Other (specify)

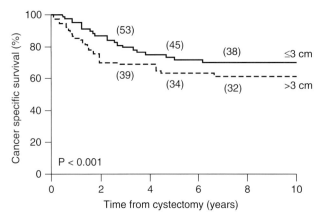

Figure 25-12 Cancer-specific survival for 218 patients treated by radical cystectomy according to tumor size ($P < 0.001$). Tumor sizes were analyzed as continuous variables, and the median (3 cm) was used for the purpose of presenting. Numbers in parentheses represent numbers of patients under observation at three, five, and seven years. (From Ref. 53; with permission.)

Gross Tumor Configuration

The CAP Cancer Protocols and Checklist has included the following tumor configuration that should be reported: papillary, solid/nodule, flat, ulcerated, indeterminate, other (specify). The clinical utility and prognostic value of these parameters have not been clearly demonstrated.

Tumor Multifocality

Development of multifocal tumors in the same patient, either synchronous or metachronous, is a common characteristic of urothelial malignancy.[54–57] Premalignant changes, such as dysplasia or carcinoma in situ, often are found in urothelial mucosa aside from an invasive bladder cancer.[58,59] Studies of urothelial genetic alterations and of atypia mapping in cystectomy specimens confirm the importance of field cancerization in the development of multifocal urothelial tumors, especially in early-stage cancer. There is evidence that multifocal urothelial carcinoma arises through independent concurrent genetic events at multiple locations in the lower urinary tract.[60,61] Other studies, however, have suggested a monoclonal origin for multifocal urothelial carcinoma.[62,63] In cases with multifocal cancer, the location and size of each tumor should be documented in the gross description. Some studies have suggested that tumor multifocality is associated with poor outcome for patients with urothelial carcinoma.[50,56,57,64] Cohorts in these studies were limited to early-stage (Ta and T1) bladder cancer. In a recent study of cystectomy specimens that included more advanced stage cancers, tumor multifocality did not have prognostic significance.[53]

Histologic Type

Histologic types and variants should be clearly indicated in the report (see **Chapters 6** and **12** to **23** for appropriate classifications).

Histologic Grading

The greatest utility of histologic grading is for noninvasive urothelial carcinoma. Either the 1973[65] or the 2004[66] World Health Organization (WHO) grading system may be used for this purpose. We recommend using both the 1973 and the 2004 WHO grading systems in the reporting.[1,2,67] We have proposed a four-tiered grading system that may have the advantages of both the 1973 and the 2004 grading systems (see **Chapter 9** for further discussion) (**Fig. 25-13**). Histologic grading for invasive bladder carcinoma is of limited utility since the majority of these tumors are high grade or grade 3 urothelial carcinoma (see **Chapter 9** for further discussion).[47,68]

Tumor Growth Pattern

Different growth patterns are commonly seen in bladder cancer. Jimenez et al. proposed a classification of invasive bladder tumors based on pattern of growth. They noted three common patterns: nodular, trabecular, and infiltrative.[69] In the infiltrative pattern, there are

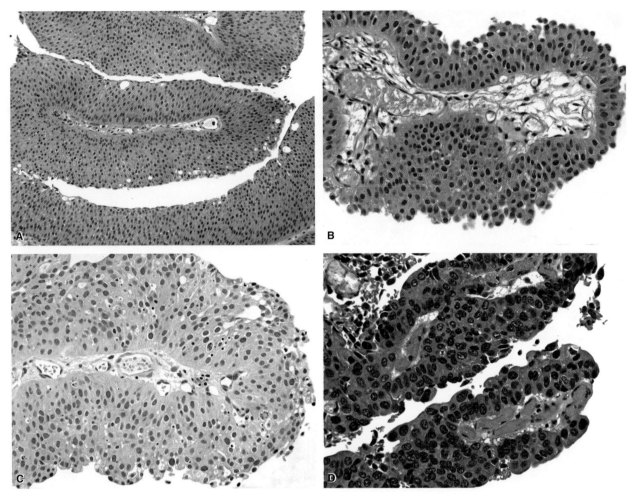

Figure 25-13   Histologic grading according to the new proposal (see Chapter 9 for further discussion). (A) Grade 1 urothelial carcinoma (low grade); (B) grade 2 urothelial carcinoma (low grade); (C) grade 3 urothelial carcinoma (high grade); (D) grade 4 urothelial carcinoma (high grade).

narrow cords or single cells permeating the stroma. These tumor cells are either highly pleomorphic or small and undifferentiated. Desmoplasia and necrosis are common with this pattern. Tumors with an infiltrative growth pattern are associated with a worse prognosis (median survival of 29 months) than that of tumors displaying a noninfiltrative (nodular or trabecular) growth pattern (median survival of 85 months).[69] The significance of assessing tumor growth pattern has been highlighted in a recent study.[70] The five-year metastasis-free survival rates for urothelial carcinomas with nodular, trabecular, and infiltrative invasion pattern were 94%, 74%, and 12%, respectively.[70]

Lymphovascular Invasion

The incidence of lymphovascular invasion is variable and has been reported to be as high as 42% (**Figs. 25-14**

to **25-16**).[71] The presence of lymphovascular invasion in both bladder TUR and cystectomy specimens predicts poor outcome, and this finding should be included in the pathology report.[71–80] The five-year cancer-specific survival was 87% and 65%, respectively, for those without and with lymphovascular invasion.[78] In another study of 283 radical cystectomy specimens, vascular invasion, pathologic stage, and lymph node metastasis were independent predictors of cancer-specific survival.[77] In the most recent study of radical cystectomy specimens with stratification for lymphovascular invasion, this parameter was the most significant predictor of cancer-specific survival ($P = 0.009$), surpassing even the pT stage ($P = 0.03$).[79]

Identification of lymphovascular invasion is often difficult due to artifactual clefting around nests of invasive carcinoma.[13,81] Retraction artifact is prominent and almost uniformly present in the micropapillary variant of urothelial carcinoma.[49] In suspicious cases, endothelial-lined vessels

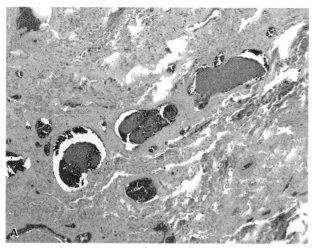

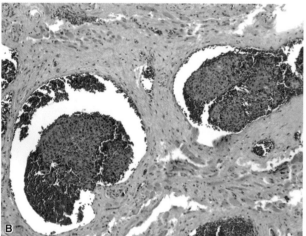

Figure 25-14   Lymphovascular invasion (A and B).

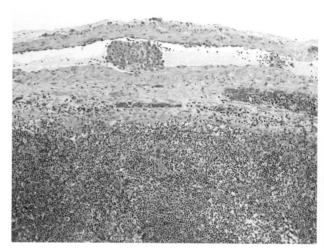

Figure 25-16   Lymphovascular invasion in the sinusoidal vessel of a lymph node.

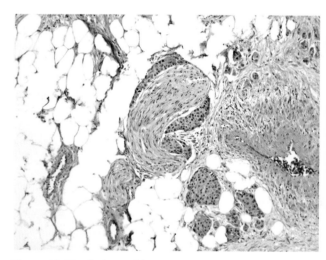

Figure 25-17   Perineural invasion.

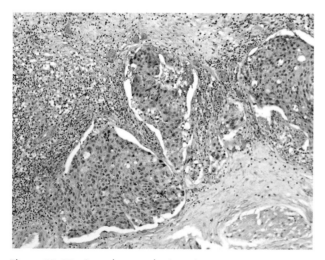

Figure 25-15   Lymphovascular invasion.

can be highlighted by immunohistochemical staining for CD31 or CD34. The presence of vascular or lymphatic invasion, and whether immunohistochemical stains assisted in identifying this finding, should be included in the report. Immunohistochemical studies directed against endothelial cells have found that fewer than 40% of cases with purported vascular invasion on routine hematoxylin and eosin examination are definitively confirmed.[9]

Perineural Invasion

The incidence of perineural invasion is high in advanced stage bladder carcinoma (**Figs. 25-17** to **25-19**). Leissner et al. found perineural invasion in 47% of 283 radical cystectomy specimens.[77] Perineural invasion is often present at fronts of fatty infiltration by urothelial carcinoma. The

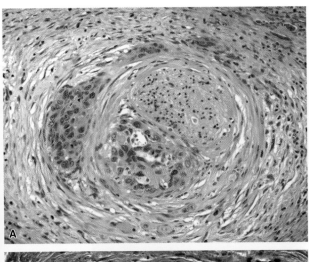

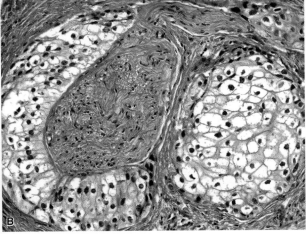

Figure 25-18 Perineural invasion (A and B).

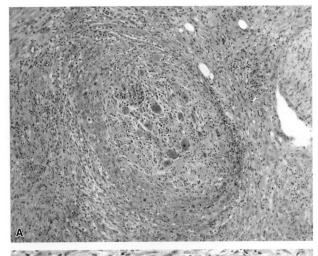

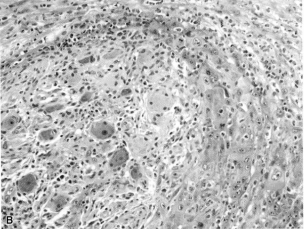

Figure 25-19 Perineural invasion (A and B).

prognostic significance of perineural invasion is uncertain. In multivariate analyses, perineural invasion was not an independent predictor of patient outcome.[77,82]

Surgical Margins

A positive soft tissue surgical margin is a significantly adverse prognostic factor.[39,53,73] Tumor present at the resection margin is assumed to indicate residual tumor in the patient (**Figs. 25-20** to **25-22**). A positive margin should be classified as macroscopic or microscopic according to the findings at gross examination and at the microscopic study of inked margins. The incidence of positive soft tissue margins is 4% in modern series, and a positive soft tissue margin is associated with poor cancer survival.[39,53] Five-year cancer-specific survival rates of 32% and 72% were found for those with and without positive surgical margins, respectively (**Fig. 25-23**).[53] None of the patients with positive margins survived after 10 years.[53]

The resection margins should be specified individually in the pathology report, especially when positive. The following margins should be reported separately: ureteral (right and left), urethral, perivesical soft tissue, and pelvic soft tissue margins (for pelvic exenteration specimens). In cases of urachal adenocarcinoma in which partial cystectomy with excision of the urachal tract and umbilicus is performed, the margins of the urachal tract (i.e., the soft tissue surrounding the urachus and the skin around the umbilical margin) should be specified.

Consistent and standardized pathologic evaluation is essential for comparison of treatment results between clinical trials and for translational research endeavors.

Tissue Artifacts

Pathologists should alert surgeons when important tissue artifacts are encountered, including mechanical distortion that occurs when tissues are transferred from biopsy forceps

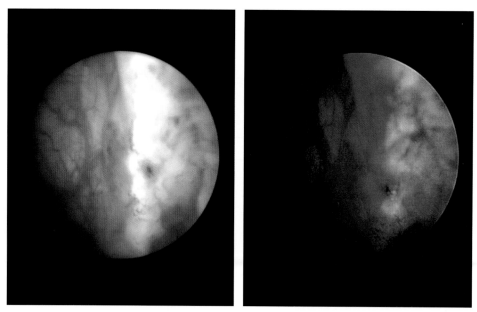

Figure 25-20 Positive margins visualized by standard white light cystoscopy (left) and fluorescence cystoscopy (right). Hexaminolevulinate causes photoactive porphyrins to accumulate preferentially in rapidly proliferating tumor cells. These porphyrins emit red fluorescence when exposed to blue light. (Photo courtesy of Dr. Montironi.)

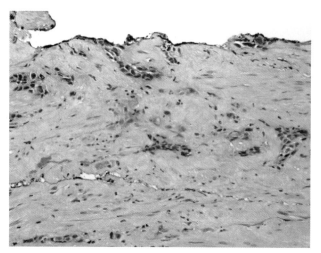

Figure 25-21 Positive surgical margins. Tumor cells are at the inked margin.

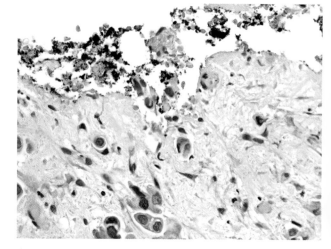

Figure 25-22 Positive surgical margins.

to fixative with the aid of a gauze swab, and thermal distortion that occurs when tissue is overheated by the diathermy loop (**Figs. 25-24** to **25-26**; see also **Chapter 10**). The epithelium of carcinoma in situ is particularly delicate and prone to partial or complete (denuding cystitis) detachment from the lamina propria. Occasionally, carcinoma in situ is identified in von Brunn nests, even when the overlying urothelium is denuded.[83]

Treatment Effect

The pathologists should be aware of a variety of histologic changes associated with different therapeutic regimens (see **Chapter 24** for further discussion). Pathology reports should comment on the presence or absence of treatment effect.

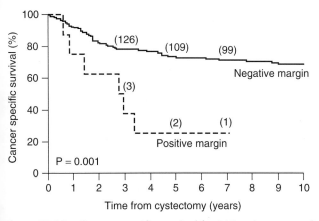

Figure 25-23 Cancer-specific survival for 218 patients treated by radical cystectomy is shown according to surgical margin status ($P = 0.001$). Numbers in parentheses represent numbers of patients under observation at three, five, and seven years. (From Ref. 53; with permission.)

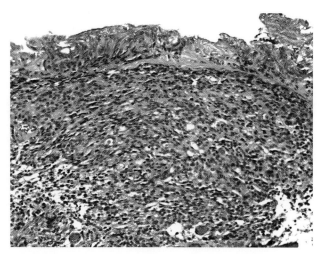

Figure 25-25 Crushing artifact. Despite crushing artifact, immunostaining for prostate-specific antigen confirms the diagnosis of prostatic adenocarcinoma.

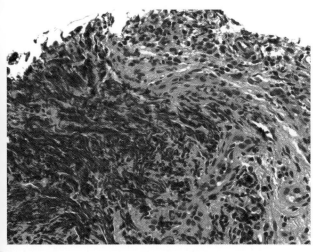

Figure 25-24 Crushing artifact. This biopsy specimen is uninterpretable.

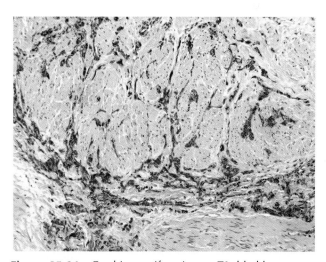

Figure 25-26 Crushing artifact in a pT2 bladder cancer. Tumor infiltrates the muscularis propria

REFERENCES

1. Cheng L, Montironi R, Davidson DD, Lopez-Beltran A. Staging and reporting of urothelial carcinoma of the urinary bladder. *Mod Pathol* 2009;22(Suppl 2):S70–95.
2. Cheng L, Lopez-Beltran A, MacLennan GT, Montironi R, Bostwick DG. Neoplasms of the urinary bladder. In: Bostwick DG, Cheng L, eds. Urologic Surgical Pathology, 2nd ed. Philadelphia: Elsevier/Mosby, 2008;259–352.
3. Lopez-Beltran A, Algaba F, Berney DM, Boccon-Gibod L, Camparo P, Griffiths D, Mikuz G, Montironi R, Varma M, Egevad L. Handling and reporting of transurethral resection specimens of the bladder in Europe: a Web-based survey by the European Network of Uropathology (ENUP). *Histopathology* 2011;58:579–85.
4. Lopez-Beltran A, Bassi P, Pavone-Macaluso M, Montironi R. Handling and pathology reporting of specimens with carcinoma of the urinary bladder, ureter, and renal pelvis. *Eur Urol* 2004;45:257–66.
5. Amin MB, Srigley JR, Grignon DJ, Reuter VE, Humphrey PA, Cohen MB, Hammond ME. Updated protocol for the examination of specimens from patients with carcinoma of the urinary bladder, ureter, and renal pelvis. *Arch Pathol Lab Med* 2003;127:1263–79.
6. Recommendations for the reporting of urinary bladder specimens containing bladder neoplasms. Association of Directors of Anatomic and Surgical Pathology. *Hum Pathol* 1996;27:751–3.

7. Herr HW, Faulkner JR, Grossman HB, Crawford ED. Pathologic evaluation of radical cystectomy specimens: a cooperative group report. *Cancer* 2004;100:2470–5.
8. Murphy WM, Crissman JD, Johansson SL, Ayala AG. Recommendations for the reporting of urinary bladder specimens that contain bladder neoplasms. *Mod Pathol* 1996;9:796–8.
9. Bostwick DG, Ramnani D, Cheng L. Diagnosis and grading of bladder cancer and associated lesions. *Urol Clin North Am* 1999;26:493–507.
10. Parkinson MC, Fisher C. Gross examination of bladder specimens. *J Clin Pathol* 1991;44:890–5.
11. Lopez-Beltran A, Bollito E, Luque RJ, Montironi R. A practical approach to bladder sampling and diagnostic reporting of pathological findings. *Pathologica* 2001;93:688–92.
12. Lapham RL, Grignon D, Ro JY. Pathologic prognostic parameters in bladder urothelial biopsy, transurethral resection, and cystectomy specimens. *Semin Diagn Pathol* 1997;14:109–22.
13. Lopez-Beltran A, Cheng L. Stage pT1 bladder carcinoma: diagnostic criteria, pitfalls and prognostic significance. *Pathology* 2003;35:484–91.
14. Hammond EH, Henson DE. Practice protocol for the examination of specimens removed from patients with carcinoma of the urinary bladder, ureter, renal pelvis, and urethra. *Arch Pathol Lab Med* 1996;120:1103–10.
15. Murphy WM, Grignon DG, Perlman EJ, eds. Tumors of the kidney, bladder, and related urinary structures. Washington D.C.: American Registry of Pathology, 2004.
16. Murphy WM. ASCP survey on anatomic pathology examination of the urinary bladder. *Am J Clin Pathol* 1994;102:715–23.
17. Montironi R, Mazzucchelli R, Scarpelli M, Lopez-Beltran A, Cheng L. Morphological diagnosis of urothelial neoplasms. *J Clin Pathol* 2008;61:3–10.
18. Montironi R, Lopez-Beltran A, Scarpelli M, Mazzucchelli R, Cheng L. Morphological classification and definition of benign, preneoplastic and non-invasive neoplastic lesions of the urinary bladder. *Histopathology* 2008;53:621–33.
19. Chandra A, Griffiths D, McWilliam LJ. Best practice: gross examination and sampling of surgical specimens from the urinary bladder. *J Clin Pathol* 2010;63:475–9.
20. Manyak MJ, Nochomovitz LE. Cystourethroscopy, biopsy, and tissue preparation. In: Nochomovitz LE, ed. Bladder Biopsy Interpretation. New York: Raven Press, 1992.
21. Murphy WM, Beckwith JB, Farrow GM. Tumors of the kidney, bladder, and related urinary structures. In: Rosai J, ed. Atlas of Tumor Pathology, 3rd ed., Fascicle 11. Washington, DC: Armed Forces Institute of Pathology, 1994:202–48.
22. Recommendations for the reporting of urinary bladder specimens containing bladder neoplasms. Association of Directors of Anatomic and Surgical Pathology. *Am J Clin Pathol* 1996;106:568–70.
23. Lesourd A, Billerey C. [Protocol for the pathologic examination of cystectomy and cystoprostatectomy specimens. Proposal for a standardized form]. *Ann Pathol* 2000;20:85–90.
24. Malmstrom PU, Lonnemark M, Busch C, Magnusson A. Staging of bladder carcinoma by computer tomography-guided transmural core biopsy. *Scand J Urol Nephrol* 1993;27:193–8.
25. Murphy WM, Ramsey J, Soloway MS. A better nuclear fixative for diagnostic bladder and prostate biopsies. *J Urol Pathol* 1993;1:79–87.
26. Kirkali Z, Chan T, Manoharan M, Algaba F, Busch C, Cheng L, Kiemeney L, Kriegmair M, Montironi R, Murphy WM, Sesterhenn IA, Tachibana M, Weider J. Bladder cancer: epidemiology, staging and grading, and diagnosis. *Urology* 2005;66:4–34.
27. Parsons KF, Scott AG, Traer S. Endoscopic biopsy in the diagnosis of peripheral denervation of the bladder. *Br J Urol* 1980;52:455–9.
28. Sakamoto N, Tsuneyoshi M, Naito S, Kumazawa J. An adequate sampling of the prostate to identify prostatic involvement by urothelial carcinoma in bladder cancer patients. *J Urol* 1993;149:318–21.
29. Soloway MS, Murphy W, Rao MK, Cox C. Serial multiple-site biopsies in patients with bladder cancer. *J Urol* 1978;120:57–9.
30. Vicente Rodriguez J, Laguna Pes P, Salvador Bayarri J, Algaba F, Santaularia Segura JM, Villavicencio Mavrich H. [Endoscopic biopsy in the staging of infiltrating tumor of the bladder]. *Arch Esp Urol* 1994;47:24–30.
31. Wallace DM, Hindmarsh JR, Webb JN, Busuttil A, Hargreave TB, Newsam JE, Chisholm GD. The role of multiple mucosal biopsies in the management of patients with bladder cancer. *Br J Urol* 1979;51:535–40.
32. Coloby PJ, Kakizoe T, Tobisu K, Sakamoto M. Urethral involvement in female bladder cancer patients: mapping of 47 consecutive cysto-urethrectomy specimens. *J Urol* 1994;152:1438–42.
33. Kunze E, Weidhase A, Schulz H. Incidence and morphology of concurrent primary carcinomas of the urinary bladder and prostate in transurethral resection specimens. *Zentralbl Pathol* 1994;140:113–22.
34. van Rhijn BW, Burger M, Lotan Y, Solsona E, Stief CG, Sylvester RJ, Witjes JA, Zlotta AR. Recurrence and progression of disease in non-muscle-invasive bladder cancer: from epidemiology to treatment strategy. *Eur Urol* 2009;56:430–42.
35. Montie JE, Abrahams NA, Bahnson RR, Eisenberger MA, El-Galley R, Herr HW, Hudes GR, Kuzel TM, Lange PH, Patterson A, Pollack A, Richie JP, Sexton WJ, Shipley WU, Small EJ, Trump DL, Walther PJ, Wilson TG. Bladder cancer. Clinical guidelines in oncology. *J Natl Compr Canc Netw* 2006;4:984–1014.
36. Philip AT, Amin MB, Tamboli P, Lee TJ, Hill CE, Ro JY. Intravesical adipose tissue: a quantitative study of its presence and location with implications for therapy and prognosis. *Am J Surg Pathol* 2000;24:1286–90.
37. Bochner BH, Nichols PW, Skinner DG. Overstaging of transitional cell carcinoma: clinical significance of lamina propria fat within the urinary bladder. *Urology* 1995;45:528–31.
38. Rosai J. Appendix E Guidelines for handling of most common and important surgical specimens. Rosai and Ackerman's Surgical Pathology, 9th ed. Philadelphia: Mosby/Elsevier, 2004;2911–77.

39. Dotan ZA, Kavanagh K, Yossepowitch O, Kaag M, Olgac S, Donat M, Herr HW. Positive surgical margins in soft tissue following radical cystectomy for bladder cancer and cancer specific survival. *J Urol* 2007;178:2308–12.

40. Montironi R, Cheng L, Mazzucchelli R, Scarpelli M, Kirkali Z, Montorsi F, Lopez-Beltran A. Critical evaluation of the prostate from cystoprostatectomies for bladder cancer: insights from a complete sampling with the whole mount technique. *Eur Urol* 2009;55:1305–9.

41. Edge S, B, Byrd DR, Compton CC, Fritz AG, Greene FL, Trotti A. American Joint Committee on Cancer Staging Manual, 7th ed. New York: Springer, 2010.

42. Kassouf W, Agarwal PK, Herr HW, Munsell MF, Spiess PE, Brown GA, Pisters L, Grossman HB, Dinney CP, Kamat AM. Lymph node density is superior to TNM nodal status in predicting disease-specific survival after radical cystectomy for bladder cancer: analysis of pooled data from MDACC and MSKCC. *J Clin Oncol* 2008;26:121–6.

43. Epstein JI, Amin MB, Reuter VR, Mostofi FK. The World Health Organization/International Society of Urological Pathology consensus classification of urothelial (transitional cell) neoplasms of the urinary bladder. Bladder Consensus Conference Committee. *Am J Surg Pathol* 1998;22:1435–48.

44. Cheng L, Weaver AL, Neumann RM, Scherer BG, Bostwick DG. Substaging of T1 bladder carcinoma based on the depth of invasion as measured by micrometer. A new proposal. *Cancer* 1999;86:1035–43.

45. Cheng L, Bostwick DG. Progression of T1 bladder tumors: better staging or better biology. *Cancer* 1999;86:910–2.

46. Cheng L, Neumann RM, Weaver AL, Spotts BE, Bostwick DG. Predicting cancer progression in patients with stage T1 bladder carcinoma. *J Clin Oncol* 1999;17:3182–7.

47. Cheng L, Neumann RM, Weaver AL, Cheville JC, Leibovich BC, Ramnani DM, Scherer BG, Nehra A, Zincke H, Bostwick DG. Grading and staging of bladder carcinoma in transurethral resection specimens. Correlation with 105 matched cystectomy specimens. *Am J Clin Pathol* 2000;113:275–9.

48. Cheng L, Weaver AL, Bostwick DG. Predicting extravesical extension of bladder carcinoma: a novel method based on micrometer measurement of the depth of invasion in transurethral resection specimens. *Urology* 2000;55:668–72.

49. Lopez-Beltran A, Cheng L. Histologic variants of urothelial carcinoma: differential diagnosis and clinical implications. *Hum Pathol* 2006;37:1371–88.

50. Heney NM, Ahmed S, Flanagan MJ, Frable W, Corder MP, Hafermann MD, Hawkins IR. Superficial bladder cancer: progressioin and recurrence. *J Urol* 1983;130:1083–6.

51. Fung CF, Shipley WU, Young RH, Griffin PP, Convery KM, Kaufman DS, Althausen AF, Heney NM, Prout GR. Prognostic factors in invasive bladder carcinoma in a prospective trial of preoperative adjuvant chemotherapy and radiotherapy. *J Clin Oncol* 1991;9:1533–42.

52. Cheng L, Neumann RM, Scherer BG, Weaver AL, Nehra A, Zincke H, Bostwick DG. Tumor size predicts the survival of patients with pathologic stage T2 bladder carcinoma: a critical evaluation of the depth of muscle invasion. *Cancer* 1999;85:2638–47.

53. Cheng L, Weaver AL, Leibovich BC, Ramnani DM, Neumann RM, Scherer BG, Nehra A, Zincke H, Bostwick DG. Predicting the survival of bladder carcinoma patients treated with radical cystectomy. *Cancer* 2000;88:2326–32.

54. Koss LG, Tiamson EM, Robbins MA. Mapping cancerous and precancerous bladder changes. A study of the urothelium in ten surgically removed bladders. *JAMA* 1974;227:281–6.

55. Weinstein RS. Origin and dissemination of human urinary bladder carcinoma. *Semin Oncol* 1979;6:149–56.

56. Lutzeyer W, Rubben H, Dahm H. Prognostic parameters in superficial bladder cancer: an analysis of 315 cases. *J Urol* 1982;127:250–2.

57. Kiemeney LA, Witjes JA, Heijbroek RP, Verbeek AL, Debruyne FM. Predictability of recurrent and progressive disease in individual patients with primary superficial bladder cancer. *J Urol* 1993;150:60–4.

58. Koss LG. Mapping of the urinary bladder: its impact on the concepts of bladder cancer. *Hum Pathol* 1979;10:533–48.

59. Koss LG, Nakanishi I, Freed SZ. Nonpapillary carcinoma in situ and atypical hyperplasia in cancerous bladders: further studies of surgically removed bladders by mapping. *Urology* 1977;9:442–55.

60. Jones TD, Wang M, Eble JN, MacLennan GT, Lopez-Beltran A, Zhang S, Cocco A, Cheng L. Molecular evidence supporting field effect in urothelial carcinogenesis. *Clin Cancer Res* 2005;11:6512–19.

61. Hartmann A, Rosner U, Schlake G, Dietmaier W, Zaak D, Hofstaedter F, Knuechel R. Clonality and genetic divergence in multifocal low grade superficial urothelial carcinoma as determined by chromosome 9 and p53 deletion analysis. *Lab Invest* 2000;80:709–18.

62. Sidransky EA, Frost P, von Eschenbach A, Oyasu R, Preisinger AC, Vogelstein B. Clonal origin of bladder cancer. *N Engl J Med* 1992;326:737–40.

63. Simon R, Eltze E, Schafer KL, Burger H, Semjonow A, Hertle L, Dockhorn-Dworniczak B, Terpe HJ, Bocker W. Cytogenetic analysis of multifocal bladder cancer supports a monoclonal origin and intraepithelial spread of tumor cells. *Cancer Res* 2001;61:355–62.

64. Parmar MK, Freedman LS, Hargreave TB, Tolley DA. Prognostic factors for recurrence and followup policies in the treatment of superficial bladder cancer: report from the British Medical Research Council Subgroup on Superficial Bladder Cancer (Urological Cancer Working Party). *J Urol* 1989;142:284–8.

65. Mostofi FK, Sobin LH, Torloni H. Histological Typing of Urinary Bladder Tumours, Vol. 10. Geneva: World Health Organization, 1973.

66. Eble JN, Sauter G, Epstein JI, Sesterhenn IA, eds. World Health Organization Classification of Tumours: Pathology and Genetics of Tumours of the Urinary System and Male Genital Organs. Lyon, France: IARC Press, 2004.

67. Montironi R, Lopez-Beltran A, Scarpelli M, Mazzucchelli R, Cheng L. 2004 World Health Organization classification of the noninvasive urothelial neoplasms: Inherent problems and clinical reflections. *Eur Urol* 2009;Suppl 8:453–7.

68. Cheng L, Maclennan GT, Lopez-Beltran A. Histologic grading of urothelial carcinoma: A reappraisal. *Hum Pathol* 2012 (in press).

69. Jimenez RE, Gheiler E, Oskanian P, Tiguert R, Sakr W, Wood DP Jr, Pontes JE, Grignon DJ. Grading the invasive component of urothelial carcinoma of the bladder and its relationship with progression-free survival. *Am J Surg Pathol* 2000;24:980–7.

70. Langner C, Hutterer G, Chromecki T, Rehak P, Zigeuner R. Patterns of invasion and histological growth as prognostic indicators in urothelial carcinoma of the upper urinary tract. *Virchows Arch* 2006;448:604–11.

71. Saito K, Kawakami S, Fujii Y, Sakura M, Masuda H, Kihara K. Lymphovascular invasion is independently associated with poor prognosis in patients with localized upper urinary tract urothelial carcinoma treated surgically. *J Urol* 2007;178:2291–6.

72. Andius P, Johansson SL, Holmang S. Prognostic factors in stage T1 bladder cancer: tumor pattern (solid or papillary) and vascular invasion more important than depth of invasion. *Urology* 2007;70:758–62.

73. Tilki D, Svatek RS, Karakiewicz PI, Novara G, Seitz M, Sonpavde G, Gupta A, Kassouf W, Fradet Y, Ficarra V, Skinner E, Lotan Y, Sagalowsky AI, Stief CG, Reich O, Shariat SF. pT3 Substaging is a prognostic indicator for lymph node negative urothelial carcinoma of the bladder. *J Urol* 2010;184:470–4.

74. Cho KS, Seo HK, Joung JY, Park WS, Ro JY, Han KS, Chung J, Lee KH. Lymphovascular invasion in transurethral resection specimens as predictor of progression and metastasis in patients with newly diagnosed T1 bladder urothelial cancer. *J Urol* 2009;182:2625–30.

75. Larsen MP, Steinberg GD, Brendler CB, Epstein JI. Use of Ulex Europaeus Agglutinin I (UEAI) to distinguish vascular and "pseudovascular" invasion in transitional cell carcinoma of bladder with lamina propria invasion. *Mod Pathol* 1990;3:83–8.

76. Raghavan D, Shipley WU, Garnick MB, Russell PJ, Richie JP. Biology and management of bladder cancer. *N Engl J Med* 1990;322:1129–38.

77. Leissner J, Koeppen C, Wolf HK. Prognostic significance of vascular and perineural invasion in urothelial bladder cancer treated with radical cystectomy. *J Urol* 2003;169:955–60.

78. Lotan Y, Gupta A, Shariat SF, Palapattu GS, Vazina A, Karakiewicz PI, Bastian PJ, Rogers CG, Amiel G, Perotte P, Schoenberg MP, Lerner SP, Sagalowsky AI. Lymphovascular invasion is independently associated with overall survival, cause-specific survival, and local and distant recurrence in patients with negative lymph nodes at radical cystectomy. *J Clin Oncol* 2005;23:6533–9.

79. Quek ML, Stein JP, Nichols PW, Cai J, Miranda G, Groshen S, Daneshmand S, Skinner EC, Skinner DG. Prognostic significance of lymphovascular invasion of bladder cancer treated with radical cystectomy. *J Urol* 2005;174:103–6.

80. Türkölmez K, Tokgöz H, Resorlu B, Köse K, Bedük Y. Muscle-invasive bladder cancer: predictive factors and prognostic difference between primary and progressive tumors. *Urology* 2007;70:477–81.

81. Lopez JI, Angulo JC. The prognostic significance of vascular invasion in stage T1 bladder cancer. *Histopathology* 1995;27:27–33.

82. Hong SK, Kwak C, Jeon HG, Lee E, Lee SE. Do vascular, lymphatic, and perineural invasion have prognostic implications for bladder cancer after radical cystectomy? *Urology* 2005;65:697–702.

83. Murphy WM, Beckwith JB, Farrow GM. Tumors of the kidney, urinary bladder, and related structures. In: Atlas of Tumor Pathology, 3rd ed., Fascicle 11. Washington DC: Armed Forces Institute of Pathology, 1994:193–288.

Chapter 26

Diagnostic Immunohistochemistry

Bladder Pathology, First Edition. Liang Cheng, Antonio Lopez-Beltran, David G. Bostwick.
© 2012 Wiley-Blackwell. Published 2012 by John Wiley & Sons, Inc.

Urothelial carcinomas represent a diverse group of challenging diagnostic entities. Most urothelial neoplasms are diagnosed based on morphology alone; however, ancillary immunohistochemistry (IHC) may be needed in some cases. The utility of IHC continues to improve when biomarkers are used in a panel approach.

Markers Useful for the Determination of Urothelial Origin

The diagnosis of urothelial carcinoma is usually straightforward based on morphology alone. However, some poorly differentiated urothelial carcinomas can mimic nonurothelial carcinomas. Therefore, sensitive and specific markers of urothelial origin are needed, especially in the setting of metastatic tumors. A panel of immunomarkers should be used to establish urothelial origin (**Fig. 26-1**; **Table 26-1**). In the authors' experience, cytokeratin 20 (CK20), high molecular weight cytokeratin (HMWCK) 34βE12, and p63 are the most useful markers in establishing urothelial origin.

The apical surface of superficial umbrella cells of urothelium is covered by rigid-appearing urothelial plaques, also known as asymmetric unit membranes. These plaques are composed of uroplakins, a group of integral transmembranous proteins synthesized by mammalian urothelia as their major differentiated products.[1–4] Four uroplakins have been identified, including uroplakin Ia, uroplakin Ib, uroplakin II, and uroplakin III. Uroplakin III has been validated as a highly specific immunohistochemical marker for urothelial tumor, although with moderate sensitivity.[1,5,6] Kaufmann et al. reported that 57% of urothelial carcinomas were positively stained by uroplakin III, but all of the other 318 nonurothelial carcinomas were consistently negative.[5] In a microarray study, Parker and his colleagues observed a similar result, in which all 498 nonurothelial tumors and normal tissue were negative for uroplakin III, but 64 of 112 (57%) urothelial tumors displayed uroplakin expression.[6] It has been noted that the sensitivity of uroplakin III expression decreases during the progression from noninvasive to invasive urothelial carcinoma.[7–9]

Thrombomodulin is another sensitive and specific urothelial marker with a sensitivity of 69% and a specificity of 96% for urothelial lesions.[6] Another study found thrombomodulin expression in 91% of primary urothelial carcinomas.[10]

Cytokeratin 7 (CK7) is present in a wide variety of simple epithelia, including the lung, cervix, breast, bile ducts, collecting ducts of the kidney, urothelium, and mesothelium. However, it is largely absent in gastrointestinal epithelium, hepatocytes, proximal and distal tubules of the kidney, and squamous cell epithelia. Conversely, CK20

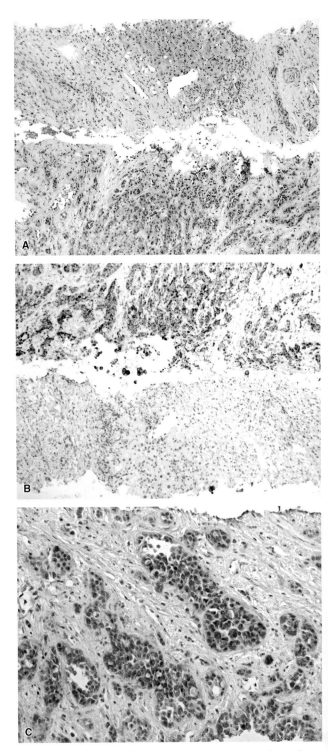

Figure 26-1 Metastatic urothelial carcinoma involving the liver (A). Positive immunostaining for cytokeratin 20 (B) and uroplakin III (C) confirms the bladder primary.

Table 26-1 Markers Useful in Establishing Urothelial Origins

CK7 and CK20
High molecular weight cytokeratin 34βE12
p63
Uroplakin III
Thrombomodulin
Placental S100 (S100P)
GATA-binding protein 3 (GATA3)

Table 26-2 Establishing Tumor Origins Using CK7 and CK20 Markers[a]

	CK7	CK20
Predominantly CK7+/CK20+		
Urothelial carcinoma	+	+/−
Ovarian mucinous tumors	+	+
Endocervical adenocarcinoma	+	+/−
Small intestinal adenocarcinoma	+/−	+/−
Cholangiocarcinoma	+/−	+/−
Pancreatic adenocarcinoma	+/−	+/−
Gastric adenocarcinoma	−/+	+/−
Predominantly CK7−/CK20+		
Colorectal adenocarcinoma[b]	−/+	+
Appendiceal adenocarcinoma	−	+
Appendiceal goblet cell carcinoid	−	+
Merkel cell carcinoma	−	+
Predominantly CK7−/CK20−		
Prostatic adenocarcinoma	−/+	−
Clear cell renal cell carcinoma	−	−
Adrenal cortical carcinoma	−	−
Germ cell tumor	−	−
Esophageal squamous cell carcinoma	−/+	−
Head and neck squamous cell carcinoma	−/+	−
Hepatocellular carcinoma	−	−
Gastrointestinal and lung carcinoid	−	−
high grade neuroendocrine carcinoma	−	−
Small cell carcinoma	−/+	−
Lung squamous cell carcinoma	−/+	−
Lung carcinoid	−/+	−
Lung high grade neuroendocrine carcinoma	−	−
Thymoma	−	−
Predominantly CK7+/CK20−		
Primary seminal vesicle adenocarcinoma	+	−
Ovarian nonmucinous carcinoma	+	−
Uterine adenocarcinoma	+	−
Cervical squamous cell carcinoma	+	−
Breast carcinoma	+	−
Breast colloid adenocarcinoma	+	−
Esophageal adenocarcinoma	+	−
Lung adenocarcinoma	+	−
Mesothelioma	+/−	−
Thyroid papillary and follicular carcinoma	+	−
Salivary gland neoplasms	+	−
Papillary renal cell carcinoma	+	−

[a]+, positive; −, negative.
[b]CK7 positivity more common in rectal carcinoma.

is present in human intestinal epithelium, gastric foveolar cells, urothelial umbrella cells, and Merkel cells of the epidermis. This relatively limited tissue distribution of CK20 is useful in the differential diagnosis of carcinoma of unknown primary, especially in combination with CK7 (**Table 26-2**). Urothelial carcinomas characteristically coexpress CK7 and CK20 in 40% to 80% of cases (**Table 26-2**).[6,11] Conversely, hepatocellular carcinoma, prostatic adenocarcinoma, renal cell carcinoma, squamous cell carcinoma, and neuroendocrine carcinoma are usually negative for both CK7 and CK20. The immunophenotype CK7−/CK20+ is highly specific for colorectal adenocarcinomas, whereas CK7+/CK20− is found in the vast majority of carcinomas arising from other sites, including ovary, endometrium, breast, lung, and malignant mesothelioma (**Table 26-2**).[12]

HMWCKs are typically expressed in a wide variety of epithelia, including the urinary bladder and prostate gland (**Fig. 26-2**). Monoclonal antibody clone 34βE12 is specific for HMWCK 1, 5, 10, and 14 in Moll's catalog, corresponding to molecular weight 68, 58, 56.5, and 50 kDa, respectively.[13] It has been reported that HMWCK antibody clone 34βE12 is a very sensitive marker for high grade invasive urothelial carcinoma, particularly when used with microwave heat retrieval.[14] Parker et al.[6] demonstrated HMWCK in 80% of urothelial neoplasms, which is consistent with previous studies.[6,11,15,16] The 34βE12 staining should be interpreted with caution in carcinomas with squamous differentiation. While diffuse HMWCK immunoreactivity in typical high grade carcinoma would indicate urothelial carcinoma rather than prostate cancer, HMWCK positivity restricted to areas of squamous differentiation would not exclude prostate cancer.[17]

p63 is a relatively new biomarker used for identifying urothelium. The *p63* gene, located on chromosome 3q27–28, is a member of the *TP53* gene family. p63 is expressed predominantly in basal and squamous cell carcinoma and urothelial carcinoma, but not in adenocarcinoma. When used as part of a panel of immunohistochemical stains, p63 increases the sensitivity and specificity for identifying neoplasms of urothelial origin.

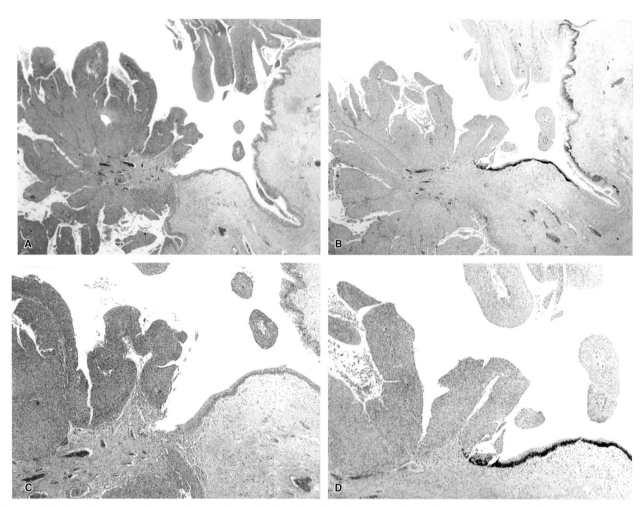

Figure 26-2 Papillary urothelial carcinoma of the bladder (A to D). High molecular weight cytokeratin 34βE12 stainings is typically restricted to basal and intermediate cell layers of normal urothelium (B and D).

Placental S100 (S100P) and GATA-binding protein 3 (GATA3) are markers recently identified for urothelial carcinoma. Higgins et al. analyzed expression patterns in prostate and bladder cancer tissue using complementary DNA microarrays and IHC.[18] They found that S100P stained 78% ($n = 300$) of urothelial carcinomas and only 2% ($n = 256$) of prostatic adenocarcinomas. GATA3 stained 67% ($n = 308$) of urothelial carcinomas, but none of the prostate carcinomas. When S100P and p63 were combined, 95% of urothelial carcinomas were labeled by one or both markers. Taken together, their study indicates that both S100P and GATA3 may be novel biomarkers useful in identifying tumors of urothelial origin.

Because of the limitation of a single marker, a panel of markers has been used to confirm urothelial origin. A panel consisting of antibodies to uroplakin III, thrombomodulin, HMWCK (1, 5, 10, and 14), and CK20 was investigated in 112 urothelial tumors.[6] The overall positive staining results were as follows: uroplakin III, 64 of 112 (57%); thrombomodulin, 77 of 112 (69%); HMWCK, 88 of 110 (80%); and CK20, 53 of 110 (48%). The authors suggest that the coexpression of thrombomodulin, HMWCK, and CK20 strongly suggests urothelial origin. The coexpression of two of three nonuroplakin III markers (thrombomodulin, HMWCK, CK20) suggests urothelial origin but requires clinicopathologic correlation.[6]

Distinguishing Muscularis Propria from Muscularis Mucosae

Distinguishing muscularis propria from muscularis mucosae, particularly in transurethral resections can be a potential problem in staging bladder cancer.[19] Council and Hameed investigated the role of several immunohistochemical markers in distinguishing smooth muscle cells of the muscularis propria from the muscularis mucosae, including vimentin and smoothelin.[20] Smoothelin is a novel smooth muscle-specific contractile protein expressed only by fully

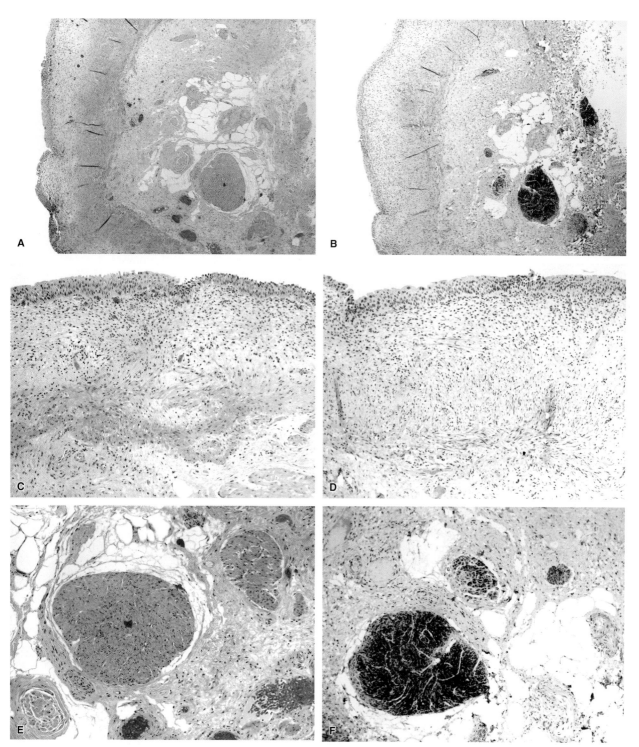

Figure 26-3   Utility of smoothelin in distinguishing muscularis mucosae from muscularis propria (A to F). Smoothelin staining is negative or weak in muscularis mucosae (D). Muscularis propria (detrusor muscle) is strongly positive for smoothelin (B and F).

differentiated smooth muscle cells, and not by proliferative or noncontractile smooth muscle cells or myofibroblasts (**Fig. 26-3**). The authors found that differential expression of smoothelin and vimentin could distinguish between the two muscle layers. The sensitivity and specificity of strong smoothelin expression was 100% for muscularis propria, whereas sensitivity and specificity for vimentin expression was 93% and 82%, respectively. Muscularis propria displayed moderate smoothelin expression in one (9%) of 11 cases studied. Paner et al. made similar findings in their study of 10 transurethral resection specimens, suggesting that the relatively distinct immunohistochemical staining pattern of smoothelin between muscularis propria and muscularis mucosa makes it a robust marker to be used in staging bladder urothelial carcinoma.[21]

Distinguishing Dysplasia and Carcinoma in Situ from Reactive Atypia

The expression of CK20 is restricted to superficial "umbrella" cells and occasional intermediate cells in the benign and reactive urothelium, even in the presence of severe inflammation.[4,22] However, there is usually loss of this cellular restriction, at least focally, in dysplasia and carcinoma in situ (CIS), with positive expression in all layers of the urothelium in 31 of 36 cases.[23] Thus, abnormal expression of CK20 is a useful adjunct to morphology in the diagnosis of dysplasia and may be of greatest utility in the distinction from reactive states in which diagnostic difficulties are greatest (**Fig. 26-4**). Abnormal expression of CK20 also predicted recurrence in patients with urothelial dysplasia, although this finding has not been confirmed independently.[24] Aberrant CK20 and HWMCK 34βE12 expression may also be predictive of bladder cancer recurrences.[25]

Previous reports have described the utility of CK20, p53, Ki67, and CD44 in distinguishing normal urothelium from dysplasia and CIS (**Figs. 26-5** to **26-7**; **Table 26-3**).[4,26–28] CK20 is limited to the superficial umbrella cells in normal urothelium, whereas CD44 staining is limited to the basal and parabasal urothelial cells, and p53 nuclear staining is absent to focal. In urothelium with reactive atypia, CD44 shows increased reactivity in all layers of the urothelium. CK20 and p53 staining patterns are identical to normal conditions in reactive atypia. In cases of CIS, CK20 shows diffuse, strong cytoplasmic reactivity, and p53 is observed throughout the urothelium. Ki67 is absent or only focally positive in normal urothelium, but its expression is increased in urothelial dysplasia and CIS. Recently, Yin et al. investigated a panel including CK20 and Ki67 immunostains to distinguish CIS from flat nonneoplastic urothelium.[29] The authors found that

CIS showed CK20 staining of deep urothelial cells in 88% of CIS cases compared to restricted staining of the surface cells of nonneoplastic urothelium. Additionally, CIS had a significantly increased Ki67 index compared to nonneoplastic urothelium. These findings suggest that aberrant expression of either CK20 or Ki67 should raise the suspicion for dysplasia or CIS. *p16*^{ink4} is a tumor suppressor gene that plays an important role in the cell cycle. Recently, Yin et al. showed increased expression of p16 in CIS compared to normal and reactive atypia, suggesting that p16 immunoreactivity may be a reliable marker of urothelial CIS.[30]

Expression of RNA-binding protein IMP3 (KOC) also appears to be useful in the diagnosis of urothelial CIS as well as high grade papillary tumors and invasive urothelial carcinoma.[31] Li et al. showed that IMP3 is generally not expressed in benign and/or low grade urothelial tumors, whereas it is frequently overexpressed in high grade urothelial lesions, including CIS.[31] Including p53 immunostaining with IMP3 appears to further improve the diagnostic accuracy.

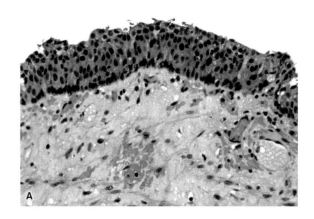

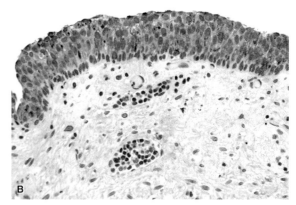

Figure 26-4   Urothelial dysplasia (A and B). Cytokeratin 20 (CK20) is usually confined in the superficial cells of normal urothelium. Aberrant CK20 expression is useful in the diagnosis of urothelial dysplasia (B).

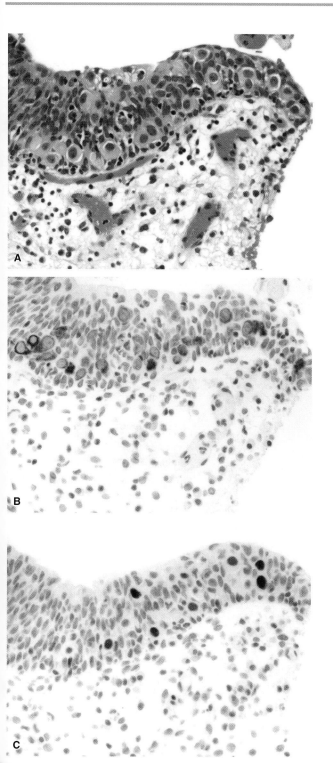

Figure 26-5 Urothelial carcinoma in situ (CIS), pagetoid spread (A). Immunostainings for cytokeratin 20 (B) and p53 (C) highlight malignant CIS cells.

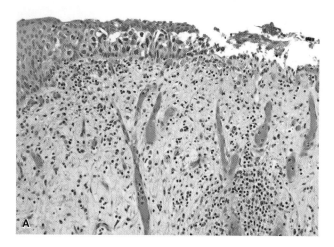

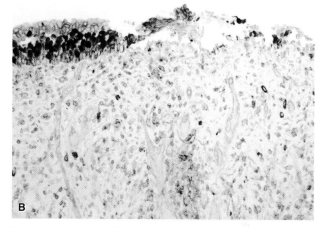

Figure 26-6 Urothelial dysplasia (A and B). URO-3 triple stain (B): (CD44, p53, and CK20) (A and B). CD44 (blue) cytoplasmic, p53 (brown) nuclear, and CK20 (red) cytoplasmic staining.

Distinguishing Urothelial Carcinoma from Prostatic Adenocarcinoma

Prostatic adenocarcinoma may represent a differential diagnostic problem when extending into the bladder and may sometimes be morphologically indistinguishable from poorly differentiated urothelial carcinoma (**Fig. 26-8**). Furthermore, urothelial carcinoma with glandular differentiation or clear cell features may rarely resemble prostate adenocarcinoma. Immunohistochemical analysis may be warranted in these situations (**Table 26-4**).[4,27] Kunju et al. evaluated prostate-specific antigen (PSA), prostate-specific acid phosphatase (PSAP), HMWCK (34βE12), CK7, CK20, and p63 as a possible panel to reliably distinguish poorly differentiated prostate carcinoma from urothelial carcinoma.[32] They found that 95% of documented prostate carcinomas and 97% of urothelial carcinomas expressed a

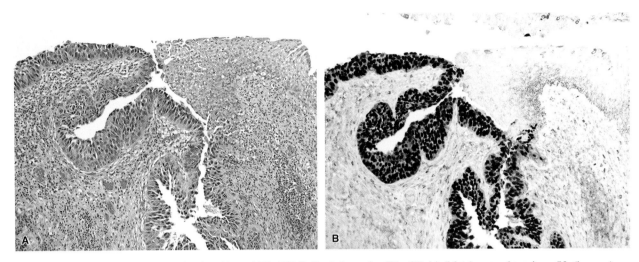

Figure 26-7   Urothelial carcinoma in situ (A and B). URO-3 triple stain (B): CD44 (blue) cytoplasmic, p53 (brown) nuclear, and CK20 (red) cytoplasmic staining.

Table 26-3   Immunohistochemical Features of Selected Flat Urothelial Lesions

	Normal	Reactive Atypia	Dysplasia	Carcinoma in Situ
CK20	Limited to umbrella cells	Limited to umbrella cells	Increased reactivity in deeper layers	May be full thickness
CD44	Limited to basal cells	Increased reactivity in all cell layers	Absent	Absent
p53	Absent	Absent	Positive	Positive

diagnostic immunohistochemical profile: prostate cancer was PSA+/HMWCK− and/or p63−negative, whereas urothelial carcinoma was PSA−HMWCK+ and/or p63+. It should be emphasized that PSA and PSAP expression may become decreased or absent with increasing Gleason score. Inclusion of thrombomodulin and uroplakin III may be helpful in some instances. Both uroplakin III and thrombomodulin expression support urothelial origin, whereas prostate adenocarcinoma is negative for these biomarkers. Although CK7+/CK20+ or CK7+/CK20− supports urothelial carcinoma and CK7−/CK20− supports prostate origin, results frequently overlap. Thus, a cytokeratin immunoprofile may not be helpful in distinguishing urothelial carcinoma from prostate carcinoma. Newer markers, such as prostein (P501S), prostate-specific membrane antigen (PSMA), proPSA (pPSA), and NKX3 may be of added utility.[33] We currently use a panel consisting of PSA, PSAP, and α-methylacyl-CoA racemase (AMACR; P504S), which are commonly positive in adenocarcinoma of the prostate. If these studies are inconclusive, we followup with uroplakin III, thrombomodulin, and p63. Together, these immunostains will generally resolve the vast majority of cases (Table 26-4).

Differentiating Primary Squamous Cell Carcinoma of the Bladder from Secondary Tumors

Carcinomas with squamous differentiation pose a great challenge. The diagnosis of primary squamous cell carcinoma of the urinary bladder is restricted to pure tumors lacking a urothelial component.[34] The majority of primary squamous cell carcinomas of the bladder and secondary squamous cell carcinomas of cervical origin are positive for both HMWCK and p63, limiting their diagnostic utility in this situation. Recently Lopez-Beltran et al. investigated the utility of Mac387 on 145 urothelial tumors with squamous differentiation.[35] Mac387 detects the myelomonocytic L1 antigen, which is a member of the calgranulin family shared by epithelial cells and keratinocytes. The authors found that Mac387 may be a reliable marker for squamous differentiation in primary urothelial tumors, and helpful in distinguishing squamous cell carcinoma of the cervix secondarily involving the bladder. Human papillomavirus (HPV) in situ hybridization and/or IHC may also be

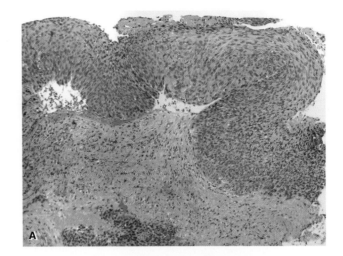

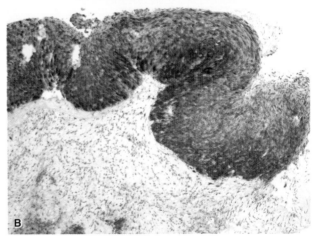

Figure 26-9 Squamous cell carcinoma in situ of the cervix extending into the bladder (A and B). p16, a surrogate marker for HPV infection, is strongly positive (B).

helpful (**Fig. 26-9**). Primary squamous cell carcinoma of the urinary bladder is typically negative for HPV.

Glandular Tumors

Differential diagnosis of glandular lesions of the bladder is quite broad, and distinguishing primary bladder adenocarcinoma from secondary involvement could be challenging (see also **Chapter 13**).[36] The immunohistochemical profile

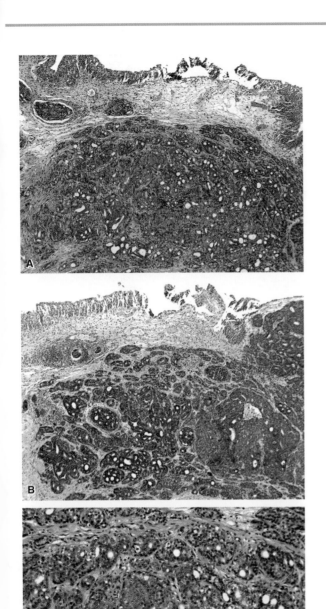

Figure 26-8 Ductal-type prostatic adenocarcinoma involving the urinary bladder (A to C). Immunostaining for prostate-specific antigen is strongly positive (B).

Table 26-4   Immunohistochemical Panel to Distinguish Prostate from Urothelial Carcinoma[a]

	PSA	PSAP	34βE12	p63	Uroplakin III	Thrombomodulin
Prostate carcinoma	+	+	−	−	−	−
Urothelial carcinoma	−	−	+	+	+	+

[a]PSA, prostate-specific antigen; PSAP, prostate-specific acid phosphatase.
[b]+, positive; −, negative.

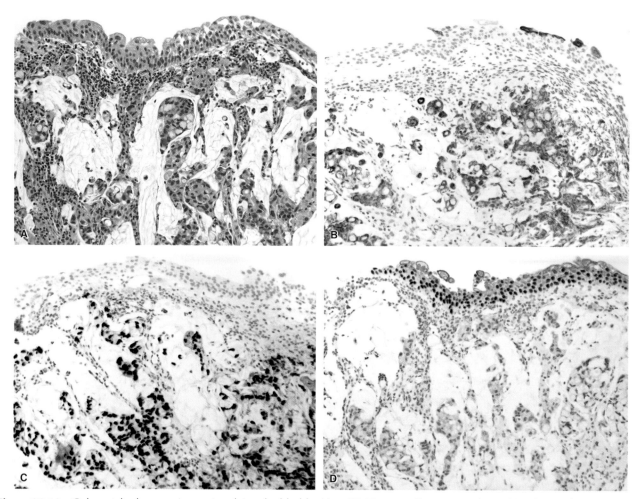

Figure 26-10 Colorectal adenocarcinoma involving the bladder (A to D). Tumor cells are strongly positive for cytokeratin 20 (B), CDX2 (C), and negative for p63 (D). p63 stains the basal and intermediate cells in normal urothelium.

of primary adenocarcinoma of the bladder is variable, with a significant degree of overlap with traditional markers CK7, CK20, villin, β-catenin, and CDX2 (**Fig. 26-10**). In general, the immunophenotype resembles that of colonic adenocarcinoma.[4,36]

β-catenin is a cadherin-binding protein that plays a critical role in both signal transduction and intercellular adhesion.[37] The dysfunction of β-catenin has recently been recognized as related to the development of urothelial malignancy.[38–40] Hanlin et al. investigated the immunohistochemical distinction between primary adenocarcinoma of the bladder and secondary colorectal adenocarcinoma.[41] Immunohistochemical studies utilizing β-catenin demonstrated positive nuclear staining in 81% of the colorectal adenocarcinomas secondarily involving the bladder, but none in the primary adenocarcinomas of the bladder. Thrombomodulin was positive in 59% of primary adenocarcinomas of the bladder. Villin is positive in the enteric type of adenocarcinoma of the bladder.[42]

Taken together, these findings suggest that a panel of immunostains including CK7, CK20, thrombomodulin, and β-catenin is of diagnostic value in distinguishing primary adenocarcinoma of the bladder from secondary colorectal adenocarcinoma.

The *CDX2* gene is a homeobox gene involved in regulating the differentiation and maintenance of intestinal epithelium.[43] Several studies have demonstrated significant expression of CDX2 in adenocarcinomas and intestinal metaplasia at various sites.[44,45] In the urinary tract, immunoreactivity to CDX2 has been reported in up to 83% of cases of intestinal metaplasia[46] and in 47% of primary adenocarcinomas.[47]

Primary signet ring cell carcinoma of the bladder is an extremely rare, high grade neoplasm with a poor prognosis.[48,49] Thomas et al. evaluated the utility of immunohistochemical markers, including CK7, CK20, villin-1, CDX2, and β-catenin, in nine tumors with signet ring cell morphology.[48] They found that the absence of

CDX2 and villin appeared to be the most robust markers in the determination of primary bladder origin. E-cadherin expression was identified in a subset of tumors with signet ring cell features, which could be misinterpreted as indicating metastatic lobular carcinoma from the breast. The authors pointed out that the small number of cases studied limited their ability to perform adequate statistical analysis. Del Sordo et al. used an immunohistochemical panel to discriminate five cases of primary urinary bladder signet ring cell carcinoma from secondary origin.[49] They found that three of their cases showed diffuse staining for CK20, but that two cases had a CK7+/CK20− pattern. They pointed out that stomach, lung, and breast have a similar profile and that this pattern did not support a primary bladder neoplasm. Future studies that examine the role of IHC in primary signet ring cell carcinoma of the bladder are needed.

Morphologically, clear cell adenocarcinoma of the urinary bladder resembles its counterpart in the female genital tract.[50] Although the immunohistochemical findings vary, most tumors are positive for pancytokeratin AE1/AE3, CK7, CK20, and CA-125, suggesting müllerian origin. CA-125 expression, however, may be seen in typical urothelial carcinoma and carcinoma from a variety of other sites. Thus, CA-125 positivity does not prove müllerian origin. The primary differential diagnostic consideration is nephrogenic adenoma (nephrogenic metaplasia). Nephrogenic adenomas are positive for EMA and low-molecular-weight cytokeratin CAM5.2 and negative for CEA. In contrast, clear cell adenocarcinoma is positive for CAM5.2, EMA, and CEA. Positive AMACR (P504S) has been reported in both nephrogenic adenoma and clear cell adenocarcinoma (Fig. 26-11).[50,51] Thus, AMACR may not be helpful in making a distinction. Herawi et al. compared cases of clear cell adenocarcinoma to nephrogenic adenoma and found that Ki67 nuclear expression averaged 50% in clear cell adenocarcinoma and only 2% in nephrogenic adenoma.[52] Similarly, p53 nuclear expression was higher (20%) in clear cell adenocarcinoma than in nephrogenic adenoma (4%). Gilcrease et al. evaluated the immunohistochemical features of four cases of clear cell adenocarcinoma and 13 cases of nephrogenic adenoma.[53] They found that MIB1 positivity in greater than 30 per 200 cells, and strong staining for p53 supports the diagnosis of clear cell adenocarcinoma over nephrogenic adenoma. In difficult cases, the diagnosis of nephrogenic adenoma can be supported by its unique positivity for PAX2 and PAX8.[54,55]

Secondary tumors may involve the urinary bladder either by direct extension from other organs or via angiolymphatic spread from distant lesions (see also **Chapter 23**).[56] Bates and Baithun examined 282 cases of tumors secondarily involving the bladder by direct extension and found

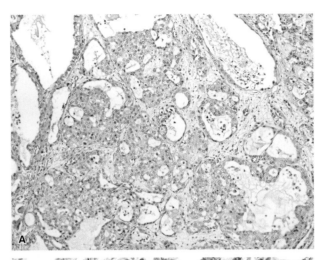
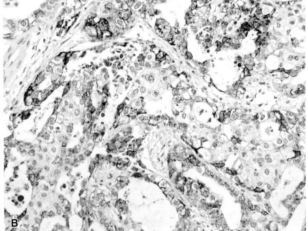

Figure 26-11   Clear cell adenocarcinoma (A and B) with positive immunostaining for α-methylacyl-CoA racemase (P504S) (B).

that prostate, colorectum, and cervix are the most common sites of tumors.[57] Common primary sites for tumors metastatic to the bladder are stomach, lung, and breast. Colorectal adenocarcinoma accounts for approximately one-third of secondary neoplasms of the bladder. Distinction between secondary colorectal adenocarcinoma and primary adenocarcinoma of the bladder can be difficult based on morphology alone. Immunohistochemical studies are often critical in making the distinction. Unfortunately, traditional markers such as CK7, CK20, villin, and CDX2 have a significant degree of overlap between primary adenocarcinoma of the bladder and secondary tumors. For example, CDX2 is positive in 33% to 100% of primary enteric-type adenocarcinoma of the bladder.[58] Wang et al. analyzed the immunostaining pattern of 17 primary adenocarcinomas of the bladder and 16 secondary colorectal carcinomas for CK7, CK20, and thrombomodulin to determine whether this panel could distinguish between the two tumors.[41] They found that CK7 and thrombomodulin were expressed variably in primary adenocarcinomas of the bladder and were negative in all secondary colorectal adenocarcinomas. In contrast, CK20 was frequently expressed in secondary colorectal adenocarcinomas (94%) but was less frequently expressed in primary adenocarcinomas of the bladder (53%). They concluded that using a panel of immunohistochemical staining for CK7, CK20, and thrombomodulin could reliably distinguish primary bladder adenocarcinoma from secondary adenocarcinoma of colorectal origin.

Neuroendocrine Tumors

The full spectrum of neuroendocrine tumors can involve the urinary bladder (see also Chapter 15).[59–61] Histologically, small cell carcinoma of the bladder is similar to its counterparts in the lung or gastrointestinal tract,[60,62] and shares a common clonal origin with urothelial carcinoma.[63] CIS, conventional urothelial carcinoma, adenocarcinoma, or sarcomatoid carcinoma may coexist with small cell carcinoma of the bladder in 12% to 61% of cases.[59,62] Molecular genetic studies suggest common clonal origin of small cell carcinoma and coexisting urothelial carcinoma.[63] The immunohistochemical profile of small cell carcinoma of the bladder has been studied extensively (Table 26-5).[4,27,59,64,65] Iczkowski et al. evaluated 46 small cell carcinomas of the bladder for the expression of chromogranin A, CD44 variant 6 (CD44v6), cytokeratin CAM5.2, γ-enolase, and synaptophysin (Fig. 26-12).[66] Small cell and urothelial carcinoma were mixed in 21 (46%) cases. The two immunohistochemical markers with the best ability to discriminate between small cell carcinoma and poorly differentiated urothelial carcinoma with small cell features were chromogranin A and CD44v6. Chromogranin A had 97% specificity for small cell carcinoma, staining 65% of cases: only one case (5%) of urothelial carcinoma was weakly positive. CD44v6 was 80% specific for urothelial carcinoma, with immunoreactivity in 60% of cases, compared with 7% of small cell carcinoma cases. Thyroid transcription factor 1

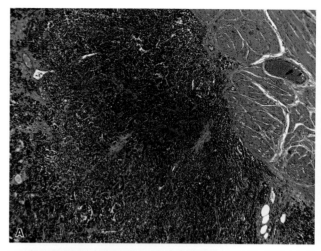

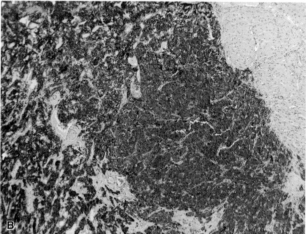

Figure 26-12   Small cell carcinoma of the bladder (A and B) with positive immunostaining for synaptophysin (B). Note the muscularis propria invasion.

(TTF-1) is considered a reliable marker for distinguishing adenocarcinoma of the lung from extrapulmonary sites and small cell carcinoma of the lung from Merkel cell carcinoma. However, Jones et al. found that approximately 40% of small cell carcinomas of the urinary bladder may show TTF-1 positivity (Fig. 26-13).[65] Therefore, TTF-1 immunostaining cannot distinguish primary small

Table 26-5   **Immunohistochemical Features in the Differential Diagnosis of Small Round Blue Cell Tumors of the Urinary Bladder[a]**

	LCA	CD99	MD	NE	CD117	TTF-1	CK AE1/AE3
PNET	−	+	−	Variable +	+	−	Variable +
SCC	−	−	−	+	−/+	+/−	Variable +
Lymphoma	+	Variable +	−	−	−	−	−
Rhabdomyosarcoma	−	−	+	−/+	−	−	−

[a]PNET, primitive neuroectodermal tumor; SCC, small cell carcinoma; LCA, leukocyte common antigen; MD, muscle differentiation markers; NE, neuroendocrine markers; TTF-1, thyroid transcription factor 1; CK, cytokeratin; +, positive; −, negative.

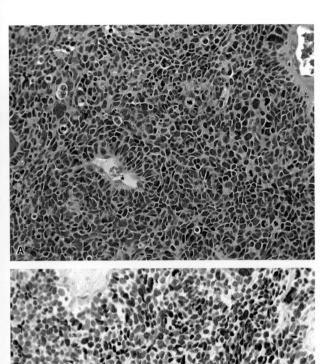

Figure 26-13 Small cell carcinoma of the bladder (A and B) with positive immunostaining for TTF-1 (B). TTF-1 staining can be seen in small cell carcinoma of various organs, and is not specific for lung primary.

cell carcinoma of the urinary bladder from metastatic small cell carcinoma from other sites. TTF-1 positivity is also seen in cervical small cell carcinoma and ovarian adenocarcinomas.[59]

Carcinoid tumor is morphologically and immunohistochemically similar to its counterpart in the lung or gastrointestinal tract.[67,68] These tumors exhibit strong, diffuse immunohistochemical staining for cytokeratins, neuron-specific enolase (NSE), chromogranin, CD57, and synaptophysin.[67] Rarely, TTF-1 staining can be seen in carcinoid tumors, but the significance is uncertain.[65,68]

Large cell neuroendocrine carcinoma is also morphologically identical to its counterpart in the lung.[69,70] These tumors may be pure or coexist with other components, such as typical urothelial carcinoma, squamous cell carcinoma, adenocarcinoma, or sarcomatoid carcinoma.[62] Large cell neuroendocrine carcinomas typically show immunoreactivity for cytokeratins CAM5.2, AE1/AE3, and EMA as

well as the neuroendocrine markers chromogranin A, CD56, NSE, and synaptophysin.[69] Given their rarity, metastasis from a lung primary should be strongly considered before making the diagnosis of primary large cell neuroendocrine carcinoma of the urinary bladder.

Primitive neuroectodermal tumor of the bladder (PNET) is an extremely rare, highly aggressive neoplasm belonging to the Ewing family of tumors.[71,72] Morphologically, it is a small round blue cell tumor that is often associated with extensive necrosis. The tumor cells show strong immunoreactivity for CD99 and CD117 (c-kit), and may show focal staining with cytokeratin AE1/AE3 markers and S100 protein.[71] CD99 is not specific for PNET or Ewing sarcoma, but it is almost always present in these tumors. The differential diagnosis includes other small round blue cell tumors, such as small cell carcinoma, lymphoma, and rhabdomyosarcoma (Table 26-5). PNETs occasionally stain with chromogranin and synaptophysin, and small cell carcinomas are often cytokeratin positive. In this setting, ultrastructural or genetic studies may be helpful. Lack of staining with lymphoid and muscle markers virtually excludes hematolymphoid and rhabdomyosarcoma, respectively.[73]

Spindle Cell Tumors

Spindle cell lesions may pose a difficult diagnostic challenge when encountered in clinical practice because the differential diagnoses are broad and there is considerable morphologic and immunologic overlap (see also **Chapters 16, 19, and 22**).[74-77] Sarcomatoid carcinoma is typically a biphasic tumor exhibiting morphologic and/or immunologic evidence of epithelial and mesenchymal differentiation.[74,78,79] Sarcomatoid carcinoma frequently contains a conventional urothelial carcinoma component that is pancytokeratin and uroplakin III positive (**Table 26-6**). Rare cases may be associated with small cell carcinoma, as confirmed by chromogranin and/or synaptophysin positivity. The mesenchymal component is usually an undifferentiated high grade spindle cell neoplasm, which is vimentin positive. Osteosarcoma is the most common heterologous element, followed by chondrosarcoma, rhabdomyosarcoma, leiomyosarcoma, liposarcoma, or angiosarcoma. The spindle cell components react with vimentin and/or specific markers corresponding to the type of mesenchymal differentiation. Some cases of sarcomatoid carcinoma may be composed almost exclusively of spindle cells, raising the differential diagnosis of leiomyosarcoma. However, in view of the rarity of primary bladder sarcoma, any malignant spindle cell tumor in the urinary bladder in an adult is considered sarcomatoid carcinoma until proven otherwise (**Fig. 26-14**).[4] Apart from clinicopathological

Table 26-6   **Immunohistochemistry of Selected Spindle Cell Lesions of the Bladder[a]**

	CK	p63	SMA/MSA/desmin	EMA	Vimentin	ALK-1	p53
Postoperative spindle cell nodule	−/+	−	+/−	−	+	−	−/+
Inflammatory myofibroblastic tumor	−/+	−	+/−	−	+	+	−
Malakoplakia and caruncle	−	−	−	−	+	−	−
Sarcomatoid carcinoma	+	+	+/−	+	+	−	+/−
Leiomyosarcoma	−	−	+	−	+	−	+/−
Rhabdomyosarcoma	−	−	+	−	+	−	−/+

[a]CK, cytokeratin; SMA, smooth muscle actin; MSA, muscle-specific actin; EMA, epithelial membrane antigen; ALK-1, anaplastic lymphoma kinase 1.

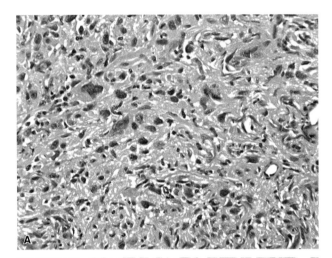
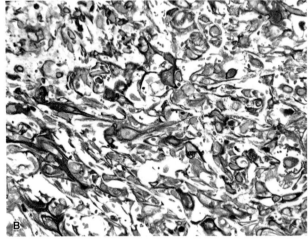

Figure 26-14   Sarcomatoid carcinoma of the bladder (A and B) with positive immunostaining for cytokeratin AE1/AE3 (B).

characteristics, pure sarcomas usually do not exhibit epithelial markers on IHC, or desmosomes and tonofilaments on electron microscopy. Vimentin positivity, which is characteristic of sarcomas, is almost uniform in sarcomatoid carcinoma and is not useful for distinguishing the two entities.[80]

Westfall et al. studied the utility of a comprehensive immunohistochemical panel consisting of AE1/AE3, HMWCK 34βE12, CK5/6, p63, SMA, and anaplastic lymphoma kinase (ALK-1) in the differential diagnosis of 45 (10 inflammatory myofibroblastic tumor, 22 sarcomatoid urothelial carcinomas, and 13 leiomyosarcomas) spindle cell lesions of the urinary bladder.[81] CK5/6 immunostaining showed relative specificity with positivity in 27% of sarcomatoid carcinomas; no immunoreactivity was found in either the inflammatory myofibroblastic tumors (IMTs) or leiomyosarcomas. Although the sensitivity with CK5/6 is relatively low, it is helpful in distinguishing sarcomatoid carcinoma from IMTs and leiomyosarcoma. A previous study by Kaufmann et al. showed a similar rate of CK5/6 staining in sarcomatoid carcinoma.[82] HMWCK 34βE12 showed similar results and therefore appears to be a good alternative for CK5/6.[81] Substantial smooth muscle actin (SMA) immunostaining was demonstrated in IMTs (100%), sarcomatoid carcinoma (73%), and leiomyosarcoma (85%), suggesting that this marker is not particularly helpful in the differential diagnosis. The authors also observed positivity with pancytokeratin marker AE1/AE3 in IMTs and sarcomatoid carcinomas (78% and 70%, respectively). Only 20% ALK-1 expression was demonstrated in IMTs, which is generally lower than previous studies that report ranges between 8% and 89% ALK-1 positivity in IMTs (Fig. 26-15).[75,83–85] ALK-1 reactivity was not observed in either the sarcomatoid carcinomas or leiomyosarcomas. p63 was positive in 70% of sarcomatoid carcinomas, whereas all IMTs were negative for p63. When positive, p63 immunostaining supports the diagnosis of sarcomatoid carcinoma over IMT. Taken together, diffuse immunoreactivity with p63 may be discriminatory between sarcomatoid carcinoma and IMTs or leiomyosarcoma. A combination of pancytokeratin, SMA, and ALK-1 positivity favors IMT; expression of HMWCK 34βE12 and CK5/6 with p63 favors sarcomatoid carcinoma. SMA positivity with overall absence of other markers favors leiomyosarcoma (Table 26-6).

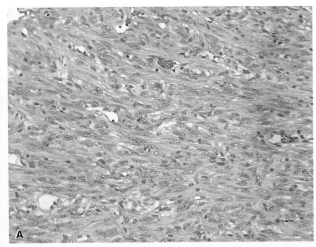
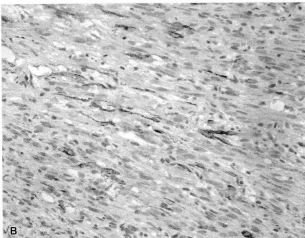

Figure 26-15 Inflammatory myofibroblastic tumor of the bladder (A and B) with positive immunostaining for ALK-1 (B).

Postoperative spindle cell nodule (PSCN) may be seen months after surgical instrumentation. Immunohistochemically, PSCNs show positive staining for AE1/AE3, CAM5.2, and vimentin in some cases, similar to the findings in IMTs (**Table 26-6**). However, some cases show immunoreactivity only for vimentin.[86] The differential diagnoses of PSCN include sarcomatoid carcinoma, myxoid leiomyosarcoma, rhabdomyosarcoma, and malignant fibrous histiocytoma. p53 immunostaining may be helpful in distinguishing these lesions, being noted only rarely in PSCN but stronger and more diffuse in malignant mesenchymal neoplasms.[66]

Leiomyosarcoma is a primary differential consideration, particularly in perivascular epithelioid cell tumors (PEComas) with significant spindle cell morphology. Immunohistochemically, both tumors are likely to be positive for SMA. Leiomyosarcomas in the gynecologic tract may show aberrant immunoreactivity to HMB45; however, leiomyosarcomas do not express other markers

of melanocytic differentiation. In contrast, PEComas express myogenic and melanocytic markers, including HMB45 (**Fig. 26-16**), Melan A/Mart1, microphthalmia transcription factor (Mitf), SMA, and rarely, desmin (see also **Chapter 22**). Other spindle cell neoplasms, such as sarcomatoid carcinoma or IMT of the urinary bladder, can usually be distinguished based on morphology and immunohistochemical profile.

Metastatic Urothelial Carcinoma

When urothelial carcinoma presents at other sites, recognition of urothelial origin may be difficult, particularly since squamous and glandular differentiation are common in high grade urothelial carcinoma. Uroplakin III is a highly specific marker for urothelial origin,[1,5,6,87] but its sensitivity is limited in our experience. Differential cytokeratin expression may be of value in the confirmation of metastatic urothelial carcinoma.[11,88–90] Expression of the combination of thrombomodulin, HMWCK 34βE12, and CK20 is strongly suggestive of urothelial origin in the setting of metastatic carcinoma of unknown primary, while the expression of two of these three is still suggestive, albeit more weakly (**Table 26-1**).[6]

Ovarian Brenner tumors, which histologically resemble urothelial neoplasms, may stain with uroplakin III and, therefore, may be included as a possible alternative primary site for uroplakin III+ metastatic carcinomas in female patients.[5,87] Some immunophenotypic differences between Brenner tumors and urothelial carcinomas of the bladder do exist. Urothelial carcinomas are frequently positive for thrombomodulin and CK20, while Brenner tumors typically do not stain with these antibodies.[91] Ovarian transitional cell carcinomas rarely (6%) express uroplakin III and typically have a uroplakin III−/CK20−/WT1+ phenotype in contrast to the uroplakin III+ phenotype observed in 82% of Brenner tumors.[87] In fact, the differences in staining with uroplakin III and other markers suggest that Brenner tumors are the only true urothelial neoplasms of the ovary, with ovarian transitional cell carcinomas representing a pattern of poorly differentiated adenocarcinoma.[92]

Other Applications

Bladder cancer has diverse morphologic manifestations and histologic variants (**Figs. 26-17** to **26-19**); see also **Chapters 12** to **24**). IHC is essential in modern the practice of urologic surgical pathology.[93,94]

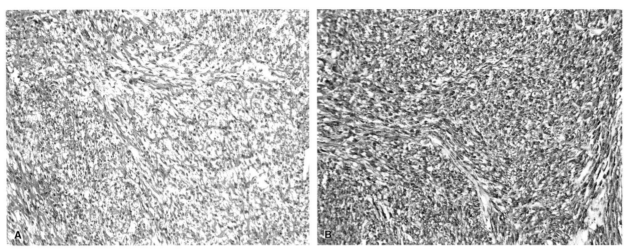

Figure 26-16   Perivascular epithelioid cell tumors (PEComas) of the bladder (A and B) with positive immunostaining for HMB45 (B).

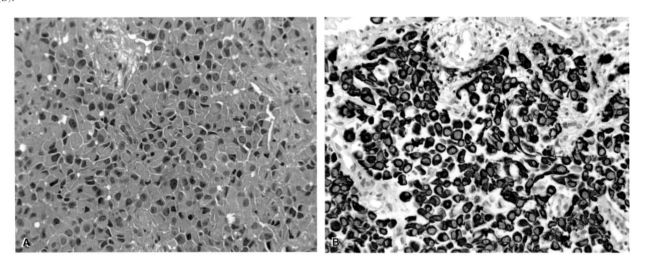

Figure 26-17   Plasmacytoid variant of urothelial carcinoma (A and B) with positive immunostaining for cytokeratin 7 (B).

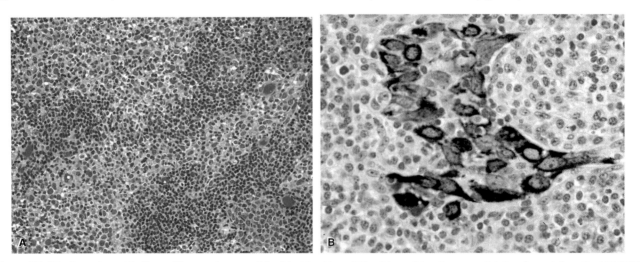

Figure 26-18   Lymphoepithelioma-like carcinoma of the bladder (A and B) with positive immunostaining for cytokeratin AE1/AE3 (B). Discrete or irregular islands of malignant urothelial cells punctuate sheets of lymphocytes, mimicking MALT lymphoma. The epithelial component displays intense immunoreactivity for broad-spectrum cytokeratin AE1/AE3.

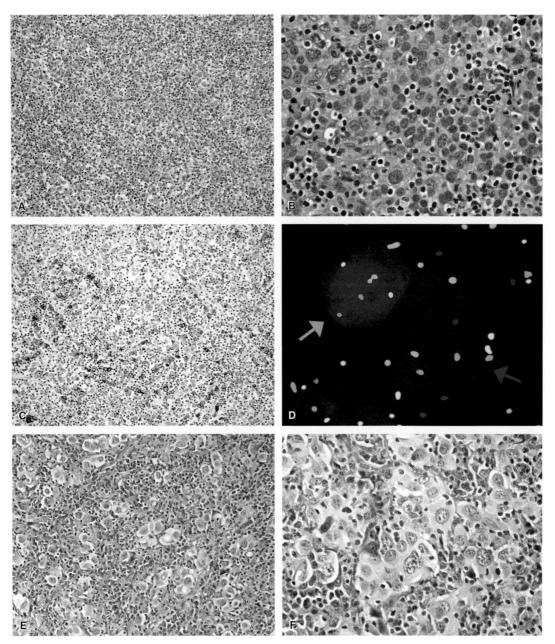

Figure 26-19 (*Continued on next page*) Lymphoepithelioma-like carcinoma (LELC) of the bladder (A to F). (A) A case of urinary tract LELC, showing diffusely scattered single tumor cells and small clusters, admixed with a brisk mixed inflammatory cell component. (B) High magnification, showing syncytially arranged tumor cells intimately admixed with lymphocytes and eosinophils. (C) Immunohistochemistry (IHC) for high molecular weight cytokeratin 34βE12, highlighting the epithelial component. (D) UroVysion fluorescence in situ hybridization (FISH) analysis of LELC. Chromosomal alterations detected using interphase FISH. UroVysion probe set contains CEP3 (red), CEP7 (green), CEP17 (aqua), and 9p21 (gold). The representative LELC tumor cell (red arrow) exhibits gains of chromosome 3 (three signals), 7 (three signals), 17 (four signals), and 9p21 (three signals). In contrast, the lymphocyte (green arrow) shows normal copy numbers of each chromosome (two signals with each probe). (E and F) Another case, showing somewhat larger aggregates of epithelial cells with vesicular nuclei and prominent nucleloli. (G) IHC for CK7, highlighting the epithelial component. (H) IHC for p53, showing intense nuclear staining in the majority of the tumor cells. (From Ref. 93; with permission.)

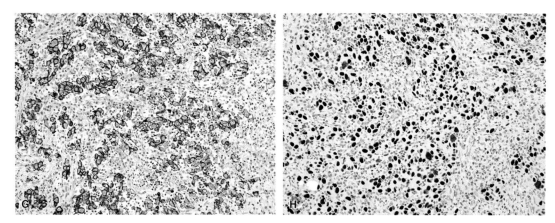

Figure 26-19   (*Continued*)

REFERENCES

1. Moll R, Wu XR, Lin JH, Sun TT. Uroplakins, specific membrane proteins of urothelial umbrella cells, as histological markers of metastatic transitional cell carcinomas. *Am J Pathol* 1995;147:1383–97.
2. Yuasa T, Yoshiki T, Isono T, Tanaka T, Okada Y. Molecular cloning and expression of uroplakins in transitional cell carcinoma. *Adv Exp Med Biol* 2003;539:33–46.
3. Olsburgh J, Harnden P, Weeks R, Smith B, Joyce A, Hall G, Poulsom R, Selby P, Southgate J. Uroplakin gene expression in normal human tissues and locally advanced bladder cancer. *J Pathol* 2003;199:41–9.
4. Hodges KB, Lopez-Beltran A, Emerson RE, Montironi R, Cheng L. Clinical utility of immunohistochemistry in the diagnoses of urinary bladder neoplasia. *Appl Immunohistochem Mol Morphol* 2010;18:401–10.
5. Kaufmann O, Volmerig J, Dietel M. Uroplakin III is a highly specific and moderately sensitive immunohistochemical marker for primary and metastatic urothelial carcinomas. *Am J Clin Pathol* 2000;113:683–7.
6. Parker DC, Folpe AL, Bell J, Oliva E, Young RH, Cohen C, Amin MB. Potential utility of uroplakin III, thrombomodulin, high molecular weight cytokeratin, and cytokeratin 20 in noninvasive, invasive, and metastatic urothelial (transitional cell) carcinomas. *Am J Surg Pathol* 2003;27:1–10.
7. Kageyama S, Yoshiki T, Isono T, Tanaka T, Kim CJ, Yuasa T, Okada Y. High expression of human uroplakin Ia in urinary bladder transitional cell carcinoma. *Jpn J Cancer Res* 2002;93:523–31.
8. Mhawech P, Iselin C, Pelte MF. Value of immunohistochemistry in staging T1 urothelial bladder carcinoma. *Eur Urol* 2002;42:459–63.
9. Xu X, Sun TT, Gupta PK, Zhang P, Nasuti JF. Uroplakin as a marker for typing metastatic transitional cell carcinoma on fine-needle aspiration specimens. *Cancer* 2001;93:216–21.
10. Ordonez NG. Thrombomodulin expression in transitional cell carcinoma. *Am J Clin Pathol* 1998;110:385–90.
11. Jiang J, Ulbright TM, Younger C, Sanchez K, Bostwick DG, Koch MO, Eble JN, Cheng L. Cytokeratin 7 and cytokeratin 20 in primary urinary bladder carcinoma and matched lymph node metastasis. *Arch Pathol Lab Med* 2001;125:921–3.
12. Folpe AL, Gown AM, Lamps LW, Garcia R, Dail DH, Zarbo RJ, Schmidt RA. Thyroid transcription factor–1: immunohistochemical evaluation in pulmonary neuroendocrine tumors. *Mod Pathol* 1999;12:5–8.
13. Moll R, Franke WW, Schiller DL, Geiger B, Krepler R. The catalog of human cytokeratins: patterns of expression in normal epithelia, tumors and cultured cells. *Cell* 1982;31:11–24.
14. Varma M, Morgan M, Amin MB, Wozniak S, Jasani B. High molecular weight cytokeratin antibody (clone 34betaE12): a sensitive marker for differentiation of high grade invasive urothelial carcinoma from prostate cancer. *Histopathology* 2003;42:167–72.
15. Genega EM, Hutchinson B, Reuter VE, Gaudin PB. Immunophenotype of high grade prostatic adenocarcinoma and urothelial carcinoma. *Mod Pathol* 2000;13:1186–91.
16. Oliai BR, Kahane H, Epstein JI. A clinicopathologic analysis of urothelial carcinomas diagnosed on prostate needle biopsy. *Am J Surg Pathol* 2001;25:794–801.
17. Varma M, Morgan M, Amin MB, Wozniak S, Jasani B. High-molecular-weight cytokeratin antibody (clone 34betaE12) as a urothelial marker: a note of caution. *Histopathology* 2004;44:189–90.
18. Higgins JP, Kaygusuz G, Wang L, Montgomery K, Mason V, Zhu SX, Marinelli RJ, Presti JC Jr, van de Rijn M, Brooks JD. Placental S100 (S100P) and GATA3: markers for transitional epithelium and urothelial carcinoma discovered by complementary DNA microarray. *Am J Surg Pathol* 2007;31:673–80.

19. Cheng L, Montironi R, Davidson DD, Lopez-Beltran A. Staging and reporting of urothelial carcinoma of the urinary bladder. *Mod Pathol* 2009;22 (Suppl 2):S70–95.

20. Council L, Hameed O. Differential expression of immunohistochemical markers in bladder smooth muscle and myofibroblasts, and the potential utility of desmin, smoothelin, and vimentin in staging of bladder carcinoma. *Mod Pathol* 2009;22:639–50.

21. Paner GP, Shen SS, Lapetino S, Venkataraman G, Barkan GA, Quek ML, Ro JY, Amin MB. Diagnostic utility of antibody to smoothelin in the distinction of muscularis propria from muscularis mucosae of the urinary bladder: a potential ancillary tool in the pathologic staging of invasive urothelial carcinoma. *Am J Surg Pathol* 2009;33:91–8.

22. Hodges KB, Lopez-Beltran A, Davidson DD, Montironi R, Cheng L. Urothelial dysplasia and other flat lesions of the urinary bladder: clinicopathologic and molecular features. *Hum Pathol* 2010;41:155–62.

23. Harnden P, Eardley I, Joyce AD, Southgate J. Cytokeratin 20 as an objective marker of urothelial dysplasia. *Br J Urol* 1996;78:870–5.

24. Harnden P, Mahmood N, Southgate J. Expression of cytokeratin 20 redefines urothelial papillomas of the bladder. *Lancet* 1999;353:974–7.

25. Ramos D, Navarro S, Villamon R, Gil-Salom M, Llombart-Bosch A. Cytokeratin expression patterns in low grade papillary urothelial neoplasms of the urinary bladder. *Cancer* 2003;97:1876–83.

26. Kunju LP, Lee CT, Montie J, Shah RB. Utility of cytokeratin 20 and Ki–67 as markers of urothelial dysplasia. *Pathol Int* 2005;55:248–54.

27. Emerson RE, Cheng L. Immunohistochemical markers in the evaluation of tumors of the urinary bladder: a review. *Anal Quant Cytol Histol* 2005;27:301–16.

28. Requena MJ, Alvarez-Kindelan J, Blanca A. Immunohistochemical markers in the evaluation of tumors of the urinary bladder: a review. *Anal Quant Cytol Histol* 2007;29:380–2.

29. Yin H, He Q, Li T, Leong AS. Cytokeratin 20 and Ki–67 to

30. distinguish carcinoma in situ from flat non-neoplastic urothelium. *Appl Immunohistochem Mol Morphol* 2006;14:260–5.

30. Yin M, Bastacky S, Parwani AV, McHale T, Dhir R. p16ink4 immunoreactivity is a reliable marker for urothelial carcinoma in situ. *Hum Pathol* 2008;39:527–35.

31. Li L, Xu H, Spaulding BO, Cheng L, Simon R, Yao JL, di Sant'Agnese PA, Bourne PA, Huang J. Expression of RNA-binding protein IMP3 (KOC) in benign urothelium and urothelial tumors. *Hum Pathol* 2008;39:1205–11.

32. Kunju LP, Mehra R, Snyder M, Shah RB. Prostate-specific antigen, high-molecular-weight cytokeratin (clone 34betaE12), and/or p63: an optimal immunohistochemical panel to distinguish poorly differentiated prostate adenocarcinoma from urothelial carcinoma. *Am J Clin Pathol* 2006;125:675–81.

33. Chuang AY, Demarzo AM, Veltri RW, Sharma RB, Bieberich CJ, Epstein JI. Immunohistochemical differentiation of high grade prostate carcinoma from urothelial carcinoma. *Am J Surg Pathol* 2007;31:1246–55.

34. Cheng L, Lopez-Beltran A, MacLennan GT, Montironi R, Bostwick DG. Neoplasms of the urinary bladder. In: Bostwick DG, Cheng L, eds. Urologic Surgical Pathology, 2nd ed. Philadelphia: Elsevier/Mosby, 2008:259–352.

35. Lopez-Beltran A, Requena MJ, Alvarez-Kindelan J, Quintero A, Blanca A, Montironi R. Squamous differentiation in primary urothelial carcinoma of the urinary tract as seen by MAC387 immunohistochemistry. *J Clin Pathol* 2007;60:332–5.

36. Williamson SR, Lopez-Beltran A, Montironi R, Cheng L. Glandular lesions of the urinary bladder: clinical significance and differential diagnosis. *Histopathology* 2011;58:811–34.

37. Behrens J, Vakaet L, Friis R, Winterhager E, Van Roy F, Mareel MM, Birchmeier W. Loss of epithelial differentiation and gain of invasiveness correlates with tyrosine phosphorylation of the E-cadherin/beta-catenin complex in cells transformed with a

temperature-sensitive v-SRC gene. *J Cell Biol* 1993;120:757–66.

38. Bilim V, Kawasaki T, Katagiri A, Wakatsuki S, Takahashi K, Tomita Y. Altered expression of beta-catenin in renal cell cancer and transitional cell cancer with the absence of beta-catenin gene mutations. *Clin Cancer Res* 2000;6:460–6.

39. Shimazui T, Schalken JA, Giroldi LA, Jansen CF, Akaza H, Koiso K, Debruyne FM, Bringuier PP. Prognostic value of cadherin-associated molecules (alpha-, beta-, and gamma-catenins and p120cas) in bladder tumors. *Cancer Res* 1996;56:4154–8.

40. Syrigos KN, Harrington K, Waxman J, Krausz T, Pignatelli M. Altered gamma-catenin expression correlates with poor survival in patients with bladder cancer. *J Urol* 1998;160:1889–93.

41. Wang HL, Lu DW, Yerian LM, Alsikafi N, Steinberg G, Hart J, Yang XJ. Immunohistochemical distinction between primary adenocarcinoma of the bladder and secondary colorectal adenocarcinoma. *Am J Surg Pathol* 2001;25:1380–7.

42. Tamboli P, Mohsin SK, Hailemariam S, Amin MB. Colonic adenocarcinoma metastatic to the urinary tract versus primary tumors of the urinary tract with glandular differentiation: a report of 7 cases and investigation using a limited immunohistochemical panel. *Arch Pathol Lab Med* 2002;126:1057–63.

43. Silberg DG, Sullivan J, Kang E, Swain GP, Moffett J, Sund NJ, Sackett SD, Kaestner KH. Cdx2 ectopic expression induces gastric intestinal metaplasia in transgenic mice. *Gastroenterology* 2002;122:689–96.

44. Ko S, Chu KM, Luk JM, Wong BW, Yuen ST, Leung SY, Wong J. CDX2 co-localizes with liver-intestine cadherin in intestinal metaplasia and adenocarcinoma of the stomach. *J Pathol* 2005;205:615–22.

45. Osawa H, Kita H, Satoh K, Ohnishi H, Kaneko Y, Mutoh H, Tamada K, Ido K, Sugano K. Aberrant expression of CDX2 in the metaplastic epithelium and inflammatory mucosa of the gallbladder. *Am J Surg Pathol* 2004;28:1253–4.

46. Sung MT, Lopez-Beltran A, Eble JN, MacLennan GT, Tan PH, Montironi R, Jones TD, Ulbright TM, Blair JE, Cheng L. Divergent pathway of intestinal metaplasia and cystitis glandularis of the urinary bladder. *Mod Pathol* 2006;19:1395–401.

47. Suh N, Yang XJ, Tretiakova MS, Humphrey PA, Wang HL. Value of CDX2, villin, and alpha-methylacyl coenzyme A racemase immunostains in the distinction between primary adenocarcinoma of the bladder and secondary colorectal adenocarcinoma. *Mod Pathol* 2005;18:1217–22.

48. Thomas AA, Stephenson AJ, Campbell SC, Jones JS, Hansel DE. Clinicopathologic features and utility of immunohistochemical markers in signet-ring cell adenocarcinoma of the bladder. *Hum Pathol* 2009;40:108–16.

49. Del Sordo R, Bellezza G, Colella R, Mameli MG, Sidoni A, Cavaliere A. Primary signet-ring cell carcinoma of the urinary bladder: a clinicopathologic and immunohistochemical study of 5 cases. *Appl Immunohistochem Mol Morphol* 2009;17:18–22.

50. Sung MT, Zhang S, MacLennan GT, Lopez-Beltran A, Montironi R, Wang M, Tan PH, Cheng L. Histogenesis of clear cell adenocarcinoma in the urinary tract: evidence of urothelial origin. *Clin Cancer Res* 2008;14:1947–55.

51. Gupta A, Wang HL, Policarpio-Nicolas ML, Tretiakova MS, Papavero V, Pins MR, Jiang Z, Humphrey PA, Cheng L, Yang XJ. Expression of alpha-methylacyl-coenzyme A racemase in nephrogenic adenoma. *Am J Surg Pathol* 2004;28:1224–9.

52. Herawi M, Drew PA, Pan CC, Epstein JI. Clear cell adenocarcinoma of the bladder and urethra: cases diffusely mimicking nephrogenic adenoma. *Hum Pathol* 2010.

53. Gilcrease MZ, Delgado R, Vuitch F, Albores-Saavedra J. Clear cell adenocarcinoma and nephrogenic adenoma of the urethra and urinary bladder: a histopathologic and immunohistochemical comparison. *Hum Pathol* 1998;29:1451–6.

54. Tong GX, Melamed J, Mansukhani M, Memeo L, Hernandez O, Deng FM, Chiriboga L, Waisman J. PAX2: a reliable marker for nephrogenic

adenoma. *Mod Pathol* 2006;19:356–63.

55. Tong GX, Weeden EM, Hamele-Bena D, Huan Y, Unger P, Memeo L, O'Toole K. Expression of PAX8 in nephrogenic adenoma and clear cell adenocarcinoma of the lower urinary tract: evidence of related histogenesis? *Am J Surg Pathol* 2008;32:1380–7.

56. Morichetti D, Mazzucchelli R, Lopez-Beltran A, Cheng L, Scarpelli M, Kirkali Z, Montorsi F, Montironi R. Secondary neoplasms of the urinary system and male genital organs. *BJU Int* 2009;104:770–6.

57. Bates AW, Baithun SI. Secondary neoplasms of the bladder are histological mimics of nontransitional cell primary tumours: clinicopathological and histological features of 282 cases. *Histopathology* 2000;36:32–40.

58. Werling RW, Yaziji H, Bacchi CE, Gown AM. CDX2, a highly sensitive and specific marker of adenocarcinomas of intestinal origin: and immunohistochemical survey fo 476 primary and metastatic carcinomas. *Am J Surg Pathol* 2003;27:303–10.

59. Wang X, MacLennan GT, Lopez-Beltran A, Cheng L. Small cell carcinoma of the urinary bladder—histogenesis, genetics, diagnosis, biomarkers, treatment, and prognosis. *Appl Immunohistochem Mol Morphol* 2007;15:8–18.

60. Pant-Purohit M, Lopez-Beltran A, Montironi R, MacLennan GT, Cheng L. Small cell carcinoma of the urinary bladder. *Histol Histopathol* 2010;25:217–21.

61. Wick MR. Immunohistology of neuroendocrine and neuroectodermal tumors. *Semin Diagn Pathol* 2000;17:194–203.

62. Cheng L, Pan CX, Yang XJ, Lopez-Beltran A, MacLennan GT, Lin H, Kuzel TM, Papavero V, Tretiakova M, Nigro K, Koch MO, Eble JN. Small cell carcinoma of the urinary bladder: a clinicopathologic analysis of 64 patients. *Cancer* 2004;101:957–62.

63. Cheng L, Jones TD, McCarthy RP, Eble JN, Wang M, MacLennan GT, Lopez-Beltran A, Yang XJ, Koch MO, Zhang S, Pan CX, Baldridge LA. Molecular genetic evidence for a

common clonal origin of urinary bladder small cell carcinoma and coexisting urothelial carcinoma. *Am J Pathol* 2005;166:1533–9.

64. Abrahams NA, Moran C, Reyes AO, Siefker-Radtke A, Ayala AG. Small cell carcinoma of the bladder: a contemporary clinicopathological study of 51 cases. *Histopathology* 2005;46:57–63.

65. Jones TD, Kernek KM, Yang XJ, Lopez-Beltran A, MacLennan GT, Eble JN, Lin H, Pan CX, Tretiakova M, Baldridge LA, Cheng L. Thyroid transcription factor 1 expression in small cell carcinoma of the urinary bladder: an immunohistochemical profile of 44 cases. *Hum Pathol* 2005;36:718–23.

66. Iczkowski KA, Shanks JH, Allsbrook WC, Lopez-Beltran A, Pantazis CG, Collins TR, Wetherington RW, Bostwick DG. Small cell carcinoma of urinary bladder is differentiated from urothelial carcinoma by chromogranin expression, absence of CD44 variant 6 expression, a unique pattern of cytokeratin expression, and more intense gamma-enolase expression. *Histopathology* 1999;35:150–6.

67. Murali R, Kneale K, Lalak N, Delprado W. Carcinoid tumors of the urinary tract and prostate. *Arch Pathol Lab Med* 2006;130:1693–706.

68. Martignoni G, Eble JN. Carcinoid tumors of the urinary bladder. Immunohistochemical study of 2 cases and review of the literature. *Arch Pathol Lab Med* 2003;127:e22–24.

69. Lee KH, Ryu SB, Lee MC, Park CS, Juhng SW, Choi C. Primary large cell neuroendocrine carcinoma of the urinary bladder. *Pathol Int* 2006;56:688–93.

70. Evans AJ, Humphrey PA, Belani J, van der Kwast TH, Srigley JR. Large cell neuroendocrine carcinoma of prostate: a clinicopathologic summary of 7 cases of a rare manifestation of advanced prostate cancer. *Am J Surg Pathol* 2006;30:684–93.

71. Lopez-Beltran A, Perez-Seoane C, Montironi R, Hernandez-Iglesias T, Mackintosh C, de Alava E. Primary primitive neuroectodermal tumour of the urinary bladder: a clinico-pathological study emphasising immunohistochemical, ultrastructural and molecular analyses. *J Clin Pathol* 2006;59:775–8.

72. Ellinger J, Bastian PJ, Hauser S, Biermann K, Muller SC. Primitive neuroectodermal tumor: rare, highly aggressive differential diagnosis in urologic malignancies. *Urology* 2006;68:257–62.

73. Cheng L, Pan C, Yang XJ, Lopez-Beltran A, MacLennan GT, Lin H, Kuzel TM, Papavero V, Tretiakova M, Nigro K, Koch MO, Eble JN. Small cell carcinoma of the urinary bladder: a clinicopathologic analysis of 64 patients. *Cancer* 2004;101:957–62.

74. Cheng L, Zhang S, Alexander R, MacLennan GT, Hodges KB, Harrison BT, Lopez-Beltran A, Montironi R. Sarcomatoid carcinoma of the urinary bladder: the final common pathway of urothelial carcinoma dedifferentiation. *Am J Surg Pathol* 2011;35:e34–46.

75. Cheng L, Foster SR, MacLennan GT, Lopez-Beltran A, Zhang S, Montironi R. Inflammatory myofibroblastic tumors of the genitourinary tract—single entity or continuum? *J Urol* 2008;180:1235–40.

76. Lott S, Lopez-Beltran A, Maclennan GT, Montironi R, Cheng L. Soft tissue tumors of the urinary bladder, Part I: Myofibroblastic proliferations, benign neoplasms, and tumors of uncertain malignant potential. *Hum Pathol* 2007;38:807–23.

77. Lott S, Lopez-Beltran A, Montironi R, MacLennan GT, Cheng L. Soft tissue tumors of the urinary bladder: Part II: Malignant neoplasms. *Hum Pathol* 2007;38:807–23.

78. Sung MT, Wang M, MacLennan GT, Eble JN, Tan PH, Lopez-Beltran A, Montironi R, Harris JJ, Kuhar M, Cheng L. Histogenesis of sarcomatoid urothelial carcinoma of the urinary bladder: evidence for a common clonal origin with divergent differentiation. *J Pathol* 2007;211:420–30.

79. Lopez-Beltran A, Pacelli A, Rothenberg HJ, Wollan PC, Zincke H, Blute ML, Bostwick DG. Carcinosarcoma and sarcomatoid carcinoma of the bladder: clinicopathological study of 41 cases. *J Urol* 1998;159:1497–503.

80. Guarino M, Tricomi P, Giordano F, Cristofori E. Sarcomatoid carcinomas: pathological and histopathogenetic considerations. *Pathology* 1996;28:298–305.

81. Westfall DE, Folpe AL, Paner GP, Oliva E, Goldstein L, Alsabeh R, Gown AM, Amin MB. Utility of a comprehensive immunohistochemical panel in the differential diagnosis of spindle cell lesions of the urinary bladder. *Am J Surg Pathol* 2009;33:99–105.

82. Kaufmann O, Fietze E, Mengs J, Dietel M. Value of p63 and cytokeratin 5/6 as immunohistochemical markers for the differential diagnosis of poorly differentiated and undifferentiated carcinomas. *Am J Clin Pathol* 2001;116:823–30.

83. McKenney JK, Amin MB. The role of immunohistochemistry in the diagnosis of urinary bladder neoplasms. *Semin Diagn Pathol* 2005;22:69–87.

84. Harik LR, Merino C, Coindre JM, Amin MB, Pedeutour F, Weiss SW. Pseudosarcomatous myofibroblastic proliferations of the bladder: a clinicopathologic study of 42 cases. *Am J Surg Pathol* 2006;30:787–94.

85. Freeman A, Geddes N, Munson P, Joseph J, Ramani P, Sandison A, Fisher C, Parkinson MC. Anaplastic lymphoma kinase (ALK 1) staining and molecular analysis in inflammatory myofibroblastic tumours of the bladder: a preliminary clinicopathological study of nine cases and review of the literature. *Mod Pathol* 2004;17:765–71.

86. Montgomery EA, Shuster DD, Burkart AL, Esteban JM, Sgrignoli A, Elwood L, Vaughn DJ, Griffin CA, Epstein JI. Inflammatory myofibroblastic tumors of the urinary tract: a clinicopathologic study of 46 cases, including a malignant example inflammatory fibrosarcoma and a subset associated with high grade urothelial carcinoma. *Am J Surg Pathol* 2006;30:1502–12.

87. Logani S, Oliva E, Amin MB, Folpe AL, Cohen C, Young RH. Immunoprofile of ovarian tumors with putative transitional cell (urothelial) differentiation using novel urothelial markers: histogenetic and diagnostic implications. *Am J Surg Pathol* 2003;27:1434–41.

88. Chu P, Wu E, Weiss LM. Cytokeratin 7 and cytokeratin 20 expression in epithelial neoplasms: a survey of 435 cases. *Mod Pathol* 2000;13:962–72.

89. Wang NP, Zee S, Zarbo RJ, Bacchi CE, Gown AM. Coordinate expression of cytokeratins 7 and 20 defines unique subsets of carcinomas. *Appl Immunohistochem* 1995;3:99–107.

90. Moll R, Lowe A, Laufer J, Franke WW. Cytokeratin 20 in human carcinomas: a new histodiagnostic marker detected by monoclonal antibodies. *Am J Pathol* 1992;140:427–47.

91. Ordonez NG. Transitional cell carcinomas of the ovary and bladder are immunophenotypically different. *Histopathology* 2000;36:433–8.

92. Riedel I, Czernobilsky B, Lifschitz-Mercer B, Roth LM, Wu XR, Sun TT, Moll R. Brenner tumors but not transitional cell carcinomas of the ovary show urothelial differentiation: immunohistochemical staining of urothelial markers, including cytokeratins and uroplakins. *Virchows Arch* 2001;438:181–91.

93. Williamson SR, Zhang S, Lopez-Beltran A, Shah RB, Montironi R, Tan PH, Wang M, Baldridge LA, MacLennan GT, Cheng L. Lymphoepithelioma-like carcinoma of the urinary bladder: clinicopathologic, immunohistochemical, and molecular Features. *Am J Surg Pathol* 2011;35:474–83.

94. Bostwick DG, Cheng L, eds. Urologic Surgical Pathology, 2nd ed. Philadelphia: Elsevier/Mosby, 2008.

Chapter 27

Pathology of the Urachus

Bladder Pathology, First Edition. Liang Cheng, Antonio Lopez-Beltran, David G. Bostwick.
© 2012 Wiley-Blackwell. Published 2012 by John Wiley & Sons, Inc.

Overview

Embryologically, the urachus is a canal connecting the apex of the bladder to the umbilicus, which serves to remove waste from the fetal urinary bladder.[1-3] It may be either distinct from or interconnected with the umbilical arteries, and typically becomes obsolete over time. A variety of lesions may be seen in the urachus.[4-13] Anomalies of the urachus mainly include patent urachus, persistent urachal remnants, and urachal cysts. These are reported to occur in the dome (54%), posterior wall (44%), and anterior wall midline (2%) of the bladder.[8,14] Also, bacterial infections may occur in the presence of a malformation or cyst of the urachal remnants. Benign neoplasms of the urachus include adenomas and soft tissue tumors. Malignant tumors of the urachus

are uncommon with adenocarcinoma as the most common form. Squamous cell carcinoma and urothelial carcinoma may also occur. A number of urachal sarcomas have been described. The main clinicopathologic features of these uncommon lesions are described below.

Congenital Anomalies

Patent Urachus

Patent urachus usually presents at birth, and may be complete or incomplete (**Fig. 27-1**). In its complete form, patent urachus results in urine flow from the umbilical stump or umbilicus due to patency of the lumen from the bladder to the umbilicus at birth.[15] It occurs at any age and is twice as

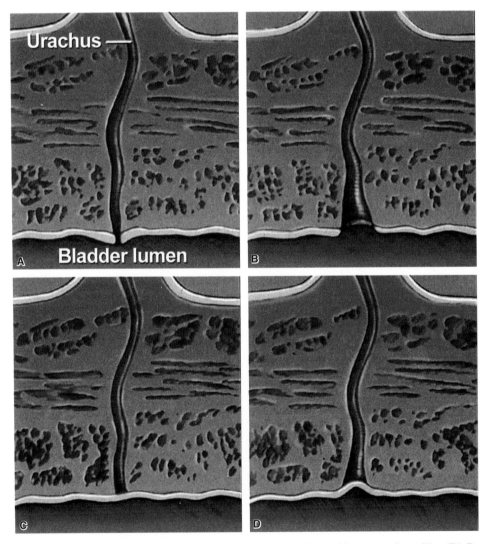

Figure 27-1 Urachal openings into the bladder (A to D). (A) Patent urachus with mucosal papilla. (B) Patent urachus with wide opening. (C) Imperforate urachus with mucosal covering. (D) Imperforate urachus with mucosal depression.

likely in males than in females. The umbilicus is often swollen and inflamed. Most patients have no other developmental anomaly, but some may have congenital deficiency of the abdominal musculature as part of prune belly syndrome.

There are multiple incomplete forms of patent urachus in which the lumen is closed at least focally, resulting in umbilicourachal sinus, vesicourachal sinus, or bladder diverticulum. In the blind variant, the urachus is closed at both ends but remains patent in the middle segment. Rarely, calculi form in the resulting cavities or urachal malformations. In patients with vesicourachal sinus, the stone is chemically similar to usual vesical calculi. The surgical pathologist rarely encounters biopsy or tissue specimens of patent urachus.

Urachal Remnant

Urachal remnant is the residual tissue from the embryonic allantoic stalk connecting the umbilicus and bladder (Figs. 27-2 and 27-3).[1-3] Urachal remnant may typically present during late childhood or adulthood and may persist in up to 33% of adults.[2,4,5,8-11,13,16] Urachal remnants are typically asymptomatic, although symptomatic cases may be seen in young children. The most common problems with urachal remnants are infection and cyst formation. Patients present with abdominal pain and symptoms of urinary tract infection; the latter symptoms are particularly common when there is communication of the urachal remnant with the bladder or umbilicus. Severe cases may present with rupture of an infected urachal cyst in the peritoneal cavity with resulting peritonitis.[12] The most common organism cultured in urachal cyst fluid is *Staphylococcus aureus*. A recent study suggests that urachal remnant is a risk factor for urachal cancer, and urachal lesions in pediactric patients should be excised to prevent problems in adulthood.[13]

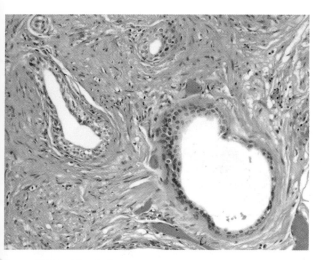

Figure 27-2   Urachal remnant.

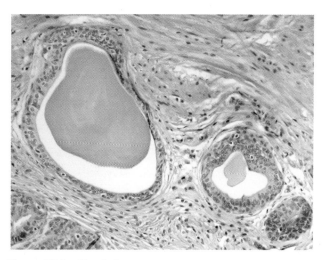

Figure 27-3   Urachal remnant.

On the mucosal surface of the bladder, the urachal remnant may have a flush luminal opening or a small papilla; however, in most cases an opening is absent. Histologically, the urachal remnant is most commonly lined by urothelial cells, although columnar mucus-secreting cells may sometimes be seen. Polypoid hamartoma of the urachal remnant was reported in a 45-year-old woman.[17]

Indication for surgical excision of asymptomatic cases is somewhat unclear. Copp et al. investigated this issue, hypothesizing that, in particular, those remnants without an epithelial lining are unlikely to develop carcinoma and may not warrant surgical treatment.[5] In the study, urachal remnants lined by urothelium were most common (38%), followed by those without an intact lining, termed "fibrostromal" (31%). Other types of urachal tract lining included gastrointestinal, squamous, metaplastic, and mixed (urothelial and gastrointestinal, or urothelial with squamous metaplasia).[5] Carcinoma is the most common type of malignancy arising from the urachal remnant. The authors hypothesized that incidentally identified urachal remnants would be less likely to demonstrate a true epithelial lining, and thus less likely to require excision. However, they found no association between incidental presentation and absence of epithelial lining, leaving the decision to excise these lesions somewhat unclear.[5]

In the differential diagnosis of glandular bladder lesions, urachal remnants may be occasionally histologically identified in bladder carcinoma resection specimens. Thus, knowledge of the anatomic location and histologic appearance of these specimens may be helpful in avoiding the false impression of glandular differentiation of bladder neoplasms or confusion with endocervicosis, which typically causes a symptomatic mass lesion. More frequently, however, the epithelial lining of urachal remnants is urothelial, or less frequently squamous. Carcinoma of the urachus is discussed below with malignant lesions.

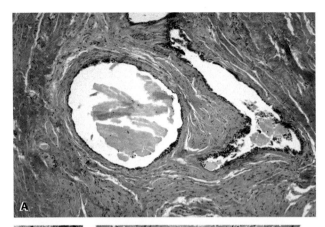

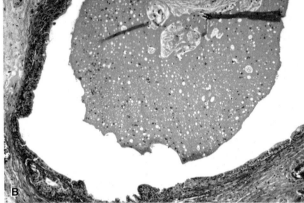

Figure 27-4   Urachal cyst (A and B). (A) This intramural segment of urachus with mild cystic dilatation was an incidental finding at autopsy. (B) A symptomatic urachal cyst with marked dilatation.

Urachal Cysts

Urachal cyst may occur at any level of the urachus and may be small and incidental or large and compressive (**Figs. 27-4** to **27-8**). The cyst may be intramural and unilocular or multilocular. Smaller cysts are commonly lined by urothelium or cuboidal cells, but columnar epithelium may also be seen.[12] Larger cysts usually are lined by flattened atrophic epithelium. When infected, the cyst lining may be lost, and the wall replaced by granulation tissue and scar. Large urachal diverticula such as those in prune belly syndrome may require resection due to urethral obstruction. The urachus and its remnants may also be involved with tuberculosis, echinococcus, and actinomycosis.

Infectious Conditions

Bacterial infections of the urachus usually occur in the presence of a malformation or cyst. Purulent bacteria infections related to umbilicourachal sinus, vesicourachal sinus,

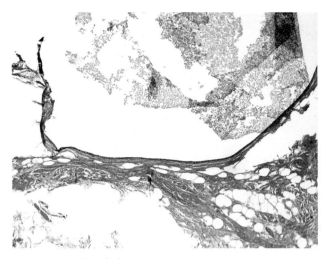

Figure 27-5   Urachal cyst.

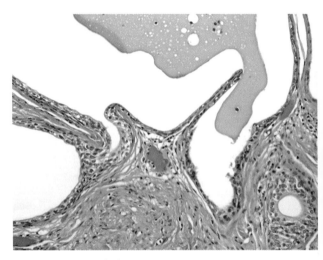

Figure 27-6   Urachal cyst.

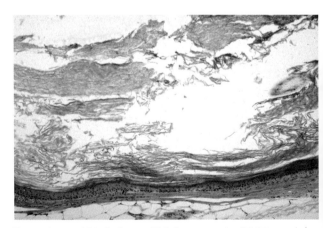

Figure 27-7   Urachal cyst. This large cyst in the dome of the bladder was lined by keratinizing squamous epithelium. Clinically, it was thought to be urachal in origin.

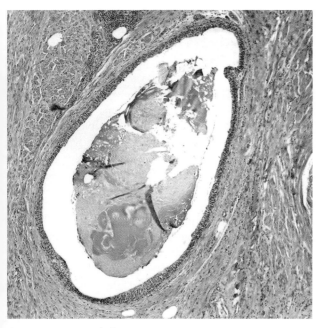

Figure 27-8 Urachal cyst.

blind urachus, or urachal cyst have been reported. These infections often develop into abscesses and may drain spontaneously through the umbilicus or into the bladder. Rupture through the peritoneum is a serious complication. In some cases, it may be difficult to determine the exact nature of the associated urachal anomaly. More rarely, tuberculous, actinomycotic, echinococcal, and tineal infections have been reported to involve the urachus.[18,19] Xanthogranulomatous inflammation has been reported.

Benign Neoplasms of the Urachus

Adenoma and Villous Adenoma

Benign epithelial neoplasms of the urachus are rare; most of them are adenomas.[5,13,20-33] These lesions are found most often in the lower third of the urachus. The average reported size ranges from less than 1 cm to 8 cm. Mucinuria is a common finding in these patients.

Macroscopically, these neoplasms present as mucin-filled cavitary or cystic lesions and may be multilocular. Microscopically, the epithelium consists of tall columnar cells and goblet cells, often with a striking resemblance to colonic glandular epithelium. Accordingly, these tumors are often referred to as villous, tubulovillous, or tubular adenoma. The epithelium may be papillary or flat, sometimes admixed with urothelium.

Villous adenoma of the urachus is an uncommon benign glandular epithelial neoplasm with exophytic growth that may be seen associated with urachal adenocarcinoma and

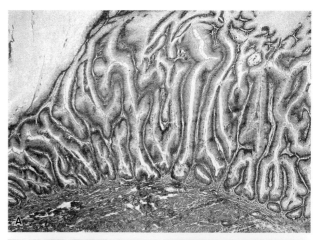

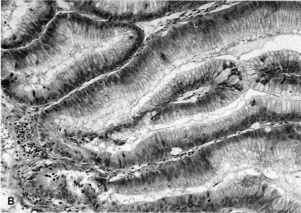

Figure 27-9 Villous adenoma of the urachus (A and B). (A) The bladder dome is partially replaced by this villiform growth, which on high magnification (B) displays typical features of villous adenoma with low grade dysplasia. Resection revealed extension into the urachal canal.

may be seen elsewhere in the bladder.[23] Histologically it is identical to villous adenoma of the colon, showing columnar mucinous cells and goblet cells lining delicate fibrovascular stalks with nuclear stratification, crowding, and hyperchromasia (Figs. 27-9 to 27-11). Villous adenomas are positive for cytokeratin (CK)20 (100% of cases), CK7 (56%), carcinoembryonic antigen (89%), epithelial membrane antigen (22%), and acid mucin with Alcian blue periodic acid–Schiff (78%).[23]

The differential diagnosis includes urachal remnant, urachal cyst, adenocarcinoma, and papillary urothelial carcinoma with villous-like morphology. Villous adenoma is a benign glandular neoplasm of the urinary bladder that histologically mimics its enteric counterpart. Invasion may be difficult to evaluate in superficial specimens, and repeat biopsy or transurethral resection may be of value. In some cases, cuboidal epithelium and urothelium have also been found, and distinction between a multilocular urachal cyst and adenoma may be difficult when the lesion

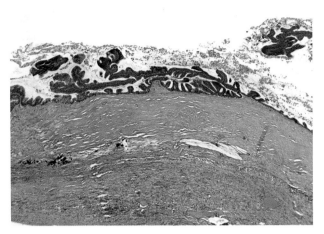

Figure 27-10   Villous adenoma of the urachus.

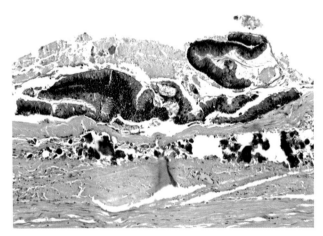

Figure 27-11   Villous adenoma of the urachus.

is not complex and the epithelium is simple and without evidence of proliferative activity.

Benign Soft Tissue Tumors

These tumors occur rarely in the urachus and most frequently represent fibromas, leiomyomas, or fibromyomas, with a patient age range of 45 years to 80 years and with higher frequency in women. Some cases reported as fibroadenomas of the urachus have also been described[34]; so has a single case of mature teratoma.[35]

Malignant Neoplasms

Malignancy of the urachus is rare and carries a poor prognosis.[16,36-40] The incidence of urachal carcinoma

varies from 0.07% to 0.7% of bladder carcinomas in North America and Europe, but as high as 1.2% in Japan.[41] One case was reported out of the 5 million people in the Swedish Cancer Registry, and two cases of urachal carcinoma were reported in a survey of 17,688 patients hospitalized in Massachusetts.[42,43]

Since the great majority of urachal malignancies involve the urinary bladder, the most difficult problems of classification for the practicing pathologist are those involved in distinguishing neoplasms of the urachus from neoplasms of the urinary bladder proper. It is particularly problematic when the dome is involved. Wheeler and Hill proposed criteria for separating adenocarcinoma of the urinary bladder and urachus[44]; these criteria were later modified by Mostofi and his colleagues (Table 27-1).[45]

Although these criteria are helpful in many cases, advanced cancers cannot always be reliably distinguishable as vesical or urachal in origin. Unless the evidence of urachal origin is strong, they are generally assumed to be of bladder nonurachal origin. Similar criteria are applied for sarcoma arising in the dome of the bladder.[46]

The staging of urachal carcinoma is similar regardless of histologic subtype (Table 27-2).[47]

Table 27-1   Diagnostic Criteria for Urachal Origin of Adenocarcinoma

Cancer located in the dome or anterior wall of the bladder
Absence of cystitis cystica or cystitis glandularis in the region of the dome
Predominant involvement of the muscularis propria by cancer rather than the lamina propria (submucosa); the vesical mucosal surface may be intact or ulcerated
Urachal remnant connected with cancer
Presence of a suprapubic mass
Cancer infiltrating through the bladder wall, with contiguous spread through the space of Retzius in the anterior abdominal wall
Sharp demarcation between the cancer and the overlying urothelium of the bladder dome
Is demonstrated not to be secondary carcinoma

Table 27-2   Staging of Urachal Tumors

Stage I	Carcinoma confined to the urachal mucosa
Stage II	Invasion confined to the urachus
Stage III	Local extension
IIIA	Extension into the urinary bladder
IIIB	Extension into the abdominal wall
IIIC	Extension into the peritoneum
IIID	Extension into other viscera
Stage IV	Metastasis
IVA	Metastasis to regional lymph nodes
IVB	Metastasis to distant sites

Urachal Adenocarcinoma

Urachal adenocarcinoma is far less common than non-urachal adenocarcinoma of the bladder, but it is the most common cancer of the urachus, accounting for 85% to 90% of cases.[16,37–41,47–51] More than 70% arise in patients between 20 years and 84 years, with a male-to-female ratio of 2:1. Urachal adenocarcinoma has a poorer survival rate than adenocarcinoma of the bladder. Most cases of urachal adenocarcinoma occur in the fifth and sixth decades of life, which is about 10 years younger than patients with adenocarcinoma arising in the bladder proper.

Hematuria is the most common symptom (71%), followed by pain (42%), irritative symptoms (40%), and umbilical discharge (2%). The patient may present with a suprapubic mass. Mucinuria occurs in about 25% of the cases reported. At cystoscopy, the tumor protrudes from the dome or anterior surface of the bladder as a polypoid or papillary mass, sometimes creating a gelatinous or bloody discharge from the urachal orifice. Transurethral biopsy is often helpful in establishing the diagnosis.

Radiographically, adenocarcinoma creates a filling defect in the dome of the bladder. Early in the disease process, the tumor size may be small; although, in some cases, urachal carcinoma may form a substantial mass, invading the retropubic space of Retzius or extending to the anterior abdominal wall. Notably, calcification identified by radiographic imaging studies may be an initial clinical presentation, as mucinous areas often develop calcification over time.[40] Stippled calcifications are strongly suggestive of neoplasm of urachal origin.[40]

Urachal adenocarcinoma usually involves the muscular wall of the bladder dome, and it may or may not destroy the overlying mucosa (**Figs. 27-12** and **27-13**). The mass may be discrete, but it may follow the route of the urachal remnants, forming a relatively large mass that invades the Retzius space and reaches the anterior abdominal wall.

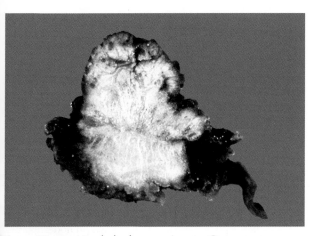

Figure 27-12   Urachal adenocarcinoma. Gross appearance of the exophytic mass.

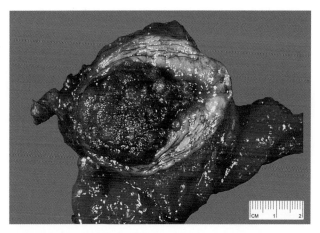

Figure 27-13   Urachal adenocarcinoma, gross appearance.

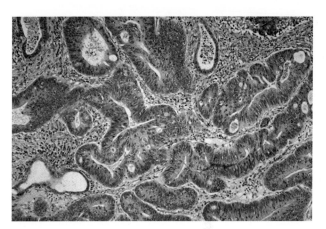

Figure 27-14   Urachal adenocarcinoma.

Mucinous lesions tend to calcify, and these calcifications may be detected on plain x-ray films of the abdomen. The mucosa of the urinary bladder is not destroyed in early stages of the disease, but it eventually becomes ulcerated as the tumor reaches the bladder cavity. The cut surface of this tumor exhibits a glistening light tan appearance, reflecting its mucinous contents. Although urachal adenocarcinoma has been staged as a bladder carcinoma using the tumor, lymph nodes, and metastases (TNM) staging system, a specific staging system for this neoplasm was proposed by Sheldon et al.[47] (**Table 27-2**), a system that seems to correlate well with prognosis in urachal adenocarcinoma.[37]

Microscopically, urachal adenocarcinoma has a varied appearance (**Figs. 27-14** to **27-18**). Urachal adenocarcinomas are subdivided into mucinous, enteric, not otherwise specified, signet ring cell, and mixed types; these subtypes are similar to variants of adenocarcinoma of the urinary bladder proper (see also **Chapter 13**). Most are mucinous.[52] Nonmucinous types often resemble conventional adenocarcinoma of the colon, but other

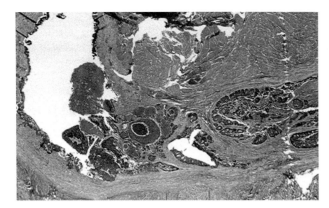

Figure 27-15   Urachal adenocarcinoma.

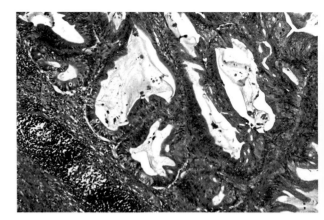

Figure 27-17   Urachal adenocarcinoma.

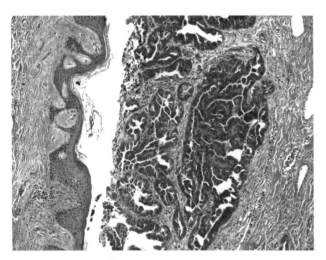

Figure 27-16   Urachal adenocarcinoma.

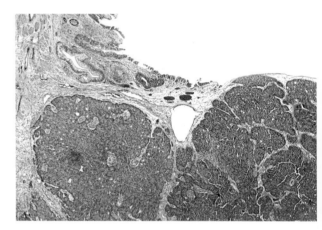

Figure 27-18   Urachal adenocarcinoma.

types include colloid mucinous carcinoma (**Figs. 27-19** to **27-21**), signet ring cell carcinoma, and high grade poorly differentiated adenocarcinoma. Osseous metaplasia of the stroma may be present.[40,53] In one study with 24 cases of urachal carcinoma, 12 (50%) tumors were mucinous, seven (29%) were enteric, four (17%) were mixed, and one (4%) was a signet ring cell carcinoma.[54] Mucinous carcinomas are characterized by pools or lakes of extracellular mucin with single cells or nests of columnar or signet ring cells floating in them; rarely, it may be the cause of a pseudomyxoma peritonei.[55] The enteric type closely resembles a colonic type of adenocarcinoma and may be difficult to differentiate from it.[56]

Pure signet ring cell carcinoma rarely occurs in the urachus; most commonly, signet ring cell differentiation is present within a mucinous carcinoma. Signet ring cell adenocarcinoma of the urachus is considered by many authors as a separate histopathologic subtype of adeno-carcinoma because of its distinctive invasiveness.[57–60] Most cases are mixed with typical adenocarcinoma, and the signet ring cells may be present within glands or in

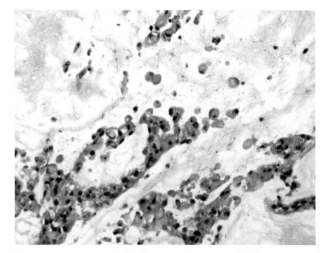

Figure 27-19   Urachal adenocarcinoma, colloid (mucinous) type.

mucus lakes of typical colloid carcinoma. The diffusely infiltrative pattern resembles linitis plastica.[50] Pure signet ring cell pattern accounts for less than 10% of cases of urachal adenocarcinoma. Inclusion criteria for signet

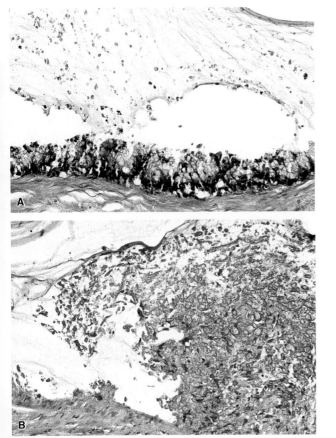

Figure 27-20 Urachal adenocarcinoma, colloid (mucinous) type (A and B). There is marked cystic dilation with luminal mucin (A). The lining of the cyst is lost.

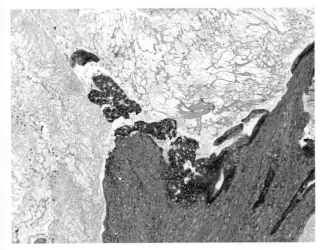

Figure 27-21 Urachal adenocarcinoma, colloid (mucinous) type.

ring cell carcinoma of the urachus are similar to those for the bladder, including at least a focal component of diffuse linitis plastica-like growth and absence of urothelial carcinoma.[59] The male-to-female ratio (3 : 1) is similar to

that of typical urachal adenocarcinoma, and mean patient age varies from 48 years to 54 years.[54,59] Local recurrence is frequent and usually precedes metastases. Sites of recurrence include the pelvis and urinary bladder, surgical wound, and abdominal wall. The most common sites for metastases in descending order are lymph nodes, lung, peritoneum, omentum, mesentery, liver, bone, and small intestine.

The normal urachus also contains argyrophilic cells.[61] Urachal adenocarcinoma is presumably derived from urachal remnant and may display neuroendocrine differentiation. These cells express neuroendocrine markers such as chromogranin A and synaptophysin. The significance of these neuroendocrine cells in urachal adenocarcinoma remains uncertain. Two cases of urachal adenocarcinoma admixed with large cell neuroendocrine carcinoma have been described.[62] One additional case of adenocarcinoma admixed with small cell neuroendocrine carcinoma of the urachus has been reported. In addition, two cases of adenocarcinoma with focal components of lymphoepithelioma-like carcinoma have also been reported.[63] One case consisted of a composite of colonic-type adenocarcinoma and large cell neuroendocrine carcinoma.[64] Immunohistochemical studies reveal expression of chromogranin, serotonin, somatostatin, neuron-specific enolase, and carcinoembryonic antigen in cases with neuroendocrine differentiation.[50,65]

At immunohistochemistry, the cells of urachal adenocarcinoma stain for carcinoembryonic antigen and CD15. A recent report found these tumors positive for CK20, and variable positivity for CK7 and high molecular weight cytokeratin 34βE12. The majority showed a cytoplasmic membranous staining pattern for β-catenin, although in one case, focal nuclear immunoreactivity was identified.[37] Urachal adenocarcinoma and bladder adenocarcinoma display immunoreactivity for a colonic epithelial protein recognized by monoclonal antibody 7E12H12, unlike urothelial carcinoma.[66] Paner and his colleagues found the expression levels of p63, CK7, CK20, CDX2, nuclear β-catenin, claudin-18, and Reg IV were 3%, 50%, 100%, 85%, 6%, 53%, and 85%, respectively.[67] Nuclear β-catenin staining, typically seen in colonic adenocarcinoma, is rarely seen in urachal adenocarcinoma.

Bladder adenocarcinoma may be difficult to rule out because it has the same histologic and immunohistochemical features as urachal adenocarcinoma. However, distinction between bladder adenocarcinoma and urachal adenocarcinoma is critical since treatment may differ. The original diagnostic criteria for urachal adenocarcinoma included a site in the bladder dome, the absence of cystitis cystica/glandularis, the invasion of muscle with intact or ulcerated overlying epithelium, the presence of urachal remnant, a suprapubic mass, a sharp demarcation between the tumor and surface epithelium, and growth in the bladder wall extending into the space of Retzius.[44] However, as urachal remnants may occur outside the bladder dome and tumor may develop to such an extent that benign urachal remnants are no longer identifiable, Johnson and colleagues in 1985 proposed that less restrictive criteria might reasonably be used, limited to three: (1) tumor in the bladder dome, (2) sharp demarcation between the tumor and surface epithelium, and (3) exclusion of secondary involvement of the bladder by tumor of another organ.[50] Cases with adjacent or distant cystitis cystica and cystitis glandularis may then be included by these criteria, given that a transition from dysplasia to malignancy is absent.[50] When dysplastic changes of the mucosa or dysplastic intestinal metaplasia are present, this tends to exclude an urachal origin.[68] Immunohistochemistry may be helpful in the differential diagnosis. Nonurachal bladder adenocarcinoma shows positive expression of carcinoembryonic antigen in 29% to 67% of cases and LeuM1 (CD15) in 73% of cases. Urachal adenocarcinoma, in contrast, stains consistently with both markers.[69-72]

An interesting and suggestive feature of urachal carcinoma is its involvement of the muscular wall of the bladder dome, sometimes without disruption of the overlying mucosa. This finding, however, may be mimicked by both primary and secondary adenocarcinoma, depending on the plane of histologic sectioning and therefore is not entirely specific. Preservation of an intact urothelium overlying the tumor is most often present in early stages of the disease, with the mucosa becoming ulcerated as the tumor impinges on the bladder lumen.

Differential diagnostic considerations also include metastases or contiguous spread from colorectal adenocarcinoma; this is usually easily distinguished clinically (see also **Chapters 13** and **23**).[44,51,73] Unlike colonic adenocarcinoma, urachal and urinary bladder cancers do not produce sulfated acid mucopolysaccharides.[74] Unusual metastases from urachal adenocarcinoma include involvement of the orbit and the ovary.[75,76] Malignant lymphoma may also rarely simulate signet ring cell carcinoma of the urachus.[77]

Management of urachal adenocarcinoma may include consideration of partial cystectomy, with resection of the umbilicus, including the entire urachal remnant.[16,37-39,50] Recurrences are common, especially in partial cystectomy-treated cases. The five-year survival rate has been reported to range from 25% to 61%, and signet ring cell adenocarcinoma seems to be the most aggressive form; in fact, some authors include in this group adenocarcinoma with a minor component of signet ring cells as well as those composed purely of signet ring cells. Diffusely infiltrative patterns resembling linitis plastica have been observed.

Urothelial Carcinoma

Urothelial carcinoma of the urachus comprises less than 5% of reported cases of urachal cancer.[16,37-40] These have occurred most frequently in men over the age of 40, with typical symptoms of hematuria and pain. Microscopically, they resemble urothelial carcinomas occurring elsewhere in the bladder. Urachal carcinoma may also contain mixed differentiation, including one case with adenocarcinoma, squamous cell carcinoma, and urothelial carcinoma.[73] A metachronous urothelial carcinoma of the bladder and urachus has been reported.[78]

Partial or radical cystectomy, including the resection of the umbilicus, is the treatment of choice.

Squamous Cell Carcinoma

Squamous cell carcinoma accounts for about 4% of cancers arising in the urachus.[79-84] The mean patient age is 50 years (range, 27 to 77 years). They are more frequent in men than in women and seem to be aggressive neoplasms. The cancer may be supravesical or intramural, and is typically squamous cell carcinoma, similar to that in the urinary bladder.

Partial cystectomy may be performed but may carry an increased risk of recurrence.

Sarcoma Arising in the Urachus

Sarcomas of the urachus make up less 10% of urachal cancers and occur in a much younger population than carcinomas (mean, 22 years of age).[47,85,86] Sarcomas occur nearly equally in males and females. Common symptoms include pain, umbilical discharge, or irritative bladder symptoms, but hematuria has not been reported. Most reported cases are fibrosarcoma, rhabdomyosarcoma, leiomyosarcoma, hemangiopericytoma, spindle cell sarcoma, or sarcoma not otherwise specified.

Other Malignant Tumors Arising in the Urachus

Extragonadal germ cell tumors, primarily of the urachus, are an extremely rare finding.[87-89] A primary yolk sac tumor of the urachus in an adult has recently been described in a 44-year-old woman, who presented with six months of pelvic pain associated with a sensation of progressive mass growth.[89] At the time of tumor resection, the tumor was attached by a pedicle to the dome of the bladder, with no injury to the adjacent organs. Microscopic examination revealed a neoplasm with epithelioid cells, pseudocysts, a myxomatous background, and Schiller–Duval body formations. Immunohistochemistry stains showed positivity to AE1/AE3, α-fetoprotein, and α_1-antitrypsin.

Differentiation from primary urachal adenocarcinoma may sometimes be challenging, especially as positivity for α-fetoprotein has been identified in urachal adenocarcinoma. A key distinguishing feature is the typical patient age, which is young (<2 years) for yolk sac tumor and older than 50 years for urachal adenocarcinoma.[89]

REFERENCES

1. Begg RC. The urachus: its anatomy, histology and development. *J Anat* 1930;64:170–83.
2. Marshall FF. Embryology of the lower genitourinary tract. *Urol Clin North Am* 1978;5:3–15.
3. Bauer SB, Retik AB. Urachal anomalies and related umbilical disorders. *Urol Clin North Am* 1978;5:195–211.
4. Eble JN. Abnormalities of the urachus. In: Young RH, ed. Pathology of the Urinary Bladder. New York: Churchill Livingstone, 1989.
5. Copp HL, Wong IY, Krishnan C, Malhotra S, Kennedy WA. Clinical presentation and urachal remnant pathology: implications for treatment. *J Urol* 2009;182:1921–4.
6. Young RH. Non-neoplastic disorders of the urinary bladder. In: Bostwick DG, Cheng L, eds. Urologic Surgical Pathology, 2nd ed. Philadelphia: Elsevier/Mosby, 2008;215–58.
7. Williamson SR, Lopez-Beltran A, Montironi R, Cheng L. Glandular lesions of the urinary bladder:clinical significance and differential diagnosis. *Histopathology* 2011;58:811–34.
8. Schubert GE, Pavkovic MB, Bethke-Bedurftig BA. Tubular urachal remnants in adult bladders. *J Urol* 1982;127:40–2.
9. Sterling JA, Goldsmith R. Lesions of urachus which appear in the adult. *Ann Surg* 1953;137:120–8.
10. Berman SM, Tolia BM, Laor E, Reid RE, Schweizerhof SP, Freed SZ. Urachal remnants in adults. *Urology* 1988;31:17–21.
11. Newman BM, Karp MP, Jewett TC, Cooney DR. Advances in the management of infected urachal cysts. *J Pediatr Surg* 1986;21:1051–4.
12. Nair KP. Mucous metaplasia and rupture of urachal cyst as a rare cause of acute abdomen. *Br J Urol* 1987;59:281–2.
13. Ashley RA, Inman BA, Routh JC, Rohlinger AL, Husmann DA, Kramer SA. Urachal anomalies: a longitudinal study of urachal remnants in children and adults. *J Urol* 2007;178:1615–8.
14. Gearhart JP, Jeffs RD. Urachal abnormalities. In: Walsh PC, Retik AB, Stamey TA, Vaughan ED, eds. Campbell's Urology, 6th ed. Philadelphia: W.B. Saunders, 1992; 1815–21.
15. Nix JT, Menville JG, Albert M, Wendt DL. Congenital patent urachus. *J Urol* 1958;79:264–73.
16. Ashley RA, Inman BA, Sebo TJ, Leibovich BC, Blute ML, Kwon ED, Zincke H. Urachal carcinoma: clinicopathologic features and long-term outcomes of an aggressive malignancy. *Cancer* 2006;107:712–20.
17. Park C, Kim H, Lee YB, Song JM, Ro JY. Hamartoma of the urachal remnant. *Arch Pathol Lab Med* 1989;113:1393–5.
18. Sakamoto S, Ogata J, Sakazaki Y, Ikegami K. Fungus ball formation of *Aspergillus* in the bladder: an unusual case report. *Eur Urol* 1978;4:388–9.
19. King DT, Lam M. Actinomycosis of the urinary bladder: association with an intrauterine contraceptive device. *J Am Med Assoc* 1978;240:1512–3.
20. Eble JN, Young RH. Benign and low grade papillary lesions of the urinary bladder: a review of the papilloma-papillary carcinoma controversy and a report of five typical papillomas. *Semin Diagn Pathol* 1989;6:351–71.
21. Eble JN, Hull MT, Rowland RG, Hostetter M. Villous adenoma of the urachus with mucusuria: a light and electron microscopic study. *J Urol* 1986;135:1240–4.
22. Hamm FC. Benign cytadenoma of the bladder probably of urachal origen. *J Urol* 1940;44:227–30.
23. Cheng L, Montironi R, Bostwick DG. Villous adenoma of the urinary tract: a report of 23 cases, including 8 with coexistent adenocarcinoma. *Am J Surg Pathol* 1999;23:764–71.
24. Miller DC, Gang DL, Gavris V, Alroy J, Ucci AA, Parkhurst EC. Villous adenoma of the urinary bladder: a morphologic or biologic entity? *Am J Clin Pathol* 1983;79:728–31.
25. Trotter SE, Philp B, Luck R, Ali M, Fisher C. Villous adenoma of the bladder. *Histopathology* 1994;24:491–3.
26. Seibel JL, Prasad S, Weiss RE, Bancila E, Epstein JI. Villous adenoma of the urinary tract: a lesion frequently associated with malignancy. *Hum Pathol* 2002;33:236–41.
27. Adegboyega PA, Adesokan A. Tubulovillous adenoma of the urinary bladder. *Mod Pathol* 1999;12:735–8.
28. Val-Bernal JF, Mayorga M, Garijo MF. Villous adenoma of the urinary tract: a lesion frequently associated with malignancy. *Hum Pathol* 2002;33:1150.
29. Tamboli P, Ro JY. Villous adenoma of urinary tract: a common tumor in an uncommon location. *Adv Anat Pathol* 2000;7:79–84.
30. Rubin J, Khanna OP, Damjanov I. Adenomatous polyp of the bladder: a rare cause of hematuria in young men. *J Urol* 1981;126:549–50.

31. Husain AS, Papas P, Khatib G. Villous adenoma of the urinary bladder presenting as gross hematuria. *Pathol.* 1996;4:299–306.
32. Billis A, Lima AC, Queiroz LS, Cia EM, Oliveira ER, Pinto W Jr. Adenoma of bladder in siblings with renal dysplasia. *Urology* 1980;16:299–302.
33. West DC, Orihuela E, Pow-sang M, Adekosan A, Cowan DF. Villous adenoma-like lesions associated with invasive transitional cell carcinoma of the bladder. *Urol Pathol* 1995;3:263–8.
34. Loening S, Richardson JR Jr. Fibroadenoma of the urachus. *J Urol* 1974;112:759–61.
35. Defabiani N, Iselin CE, Khan HG, Pache JC, Rohner S. Benign teratoma of the urachus. *Br J Urol* 1998;81:760–1.
36. Lane V. Prognosis in carcinoma of the urachus. *Eur Urol* 1976;2:282–3.
37. Gopalan A, Sharp DS, Fine SW, Tickoo SK, Herr HW, Reuter VE, Olgac S. Urachal carcinoma: a clinicopathologic analysis of 24 cases with outcome correlation. *Am J Surg Pathol* 2009;33:659–68.
38. Wright JL, Porter MP, Li CI, Lange PH, Lin DW. Differences in survival among patients with urachal and nonurachal adenocarcinomas of the bladder. *Cancer* 2006;107:721–8.
39. Herr HW, Bochner BH, Sharp D, Dalbagni G, Reuter VE. Urachal carcinoma: contemporary surgical outcomes. *J Urol* 2007;178:74–8; discussion 78.
40. Lopez-Beltran A, Nogales F, Donne CH, Sayag JL. Adenocarcinoma of the urachus showing extensive calcification and stromal osseous metaplasia. *Urol Int* 1994;53:110–3.
41. Ghazizadeh M, Yamamoto S, Kurokawa K. Clinical features of urachal carcinoma in Japan: review of 157 patients. *Urol Res* 1983;11:235–8.
42. von Garrelts B, Moberg A, Ohman U. Carcinoma of the urachus. Review of the literature and report of two cases. *Scand J Urol Nephrol* 1971;5:91–5.
43. Cornil C, Reynolds CT, Kickham CJ. Carcinoma of the urachus. *J Urol* 1967;98:93–5.
44. Wheeler JD, Hill WT. Adenocarcinoma involving the urinary bladder. *Cancer* 1954;7:119–35.
45. Mostofi FK, Thomson RV, Dean AL Jr. Mucous adenocarcinoma of the urinary bladder. *Cancer* 1955;8:741–58.
46. Hayman J. Carcinoma of the urachus. *Pathology* 1984;16:167–71.
47. Sheldon CA, Clayman RV, Gonzalez R, Williams RD, Fraley EE. Malignant urachal lesions. *J Urol* 1984;131:1–8.
48. Loening SA, Jacobo E, Hawtrey CE, Culp DA. Adenocarcinoma of the urachus. *J Urol* 1978;119:68–71.
49. Mattelaer P, Wolff JM, Jung P, WIJ, Jakse G. Adenocarcinoma of the urachus: 3 case reports and a review of the literature. *Acta Urol Belg* 1997;65:63–7.
50. Johnson DE, Hodge GB, Abdul-Karim FW, Ayala AG. Urachal carcinoma. *Urology* 1985;26:218–21.
51. Whitehead ED, Tessler AN. Carcinoma of the urachus. *Br J Urol* 1971;43:468–76.
52. Burnett AL, Epstein JI, Marshall FF. Adenocarcinoma of urinary bladder: classification and management. *Urology* 1991;37:315–21.
53. Okamoto K, Fukuyama T, Okamoto E, Yoshida O, Hiai H. Adenocarcinoma of the urachus associated with stromal osseous metaplasia. *Urol Int* 1993;51:240–2.
54. Grignon DJ, Ro JY, Ayala AG, Johnson DE, Ordonez NG. Primary adenocarcinoma of the urinary bladder. A clinicopathologic analysis of 72 cases. *Cancer* 1991;67:2165–72.
55. Jacobs LB, Brooks JD, Epstein JI. Differentiation of colonic metaplasia from adenocarcinoma of urinary bladder. *Hum Pathol* 1997;28:1152–7.
56. Fish DE, Rose DS, Adamson A, Goldin RD, Witherow RO. Neoplastic Paneth cells in a mucinous adenocarcinoma of the bladder. *Br J Urol* 1994;73:105–6.
57. Alonso-Gorrea M, Mompo-Sanchis JA, Jorda-Cuevas M, Froufe A, Jimenez-Cruz JF. Signet ring cell adenocarcinoma of the urachus. *Eur Urol* 1985;11:282–4.
58. Jakse G, Schneider HM, Jacobi GH. Urachal signet-ring cell carcinoma, a rare variant of vesical adenocarcinoma: incidence and pathological criteria. *J Urol* 1978;120:764–6.
59. Grignon DJ, Ro JY, Ayala AG, Johnson DE. Primary signet-ring cell carcinoma of the urinary bladder. *Am J Clin Pathol* 1991;95:13–20.
60. Loggie BW, Fleming RA, Hosseinian AA. Peritoneal carcinomatosis with urachal signet-cell adenocarcinoma. *Urology* 1997;50:446–8.
61. Satake T, Takeda A, Matsuyama M. Argyrophil cells in the urachal epithelium and urachal adenocarcinoma. *Acta Pathol Jpn* 1984;34:1193–9.
62. Abenoza P, Manivel C, Sibley RK. Adenocarcinoma with neuroendocrine differentiation of the urinary bladder. Clinicopathologic, immunohistochemical, and ultrastructural study. *Arch Pathol Lab Med* 1986;110:1062–6.
63. Williamson SR, Zhang S, Lopez-Beltran A, Shah RB, Montironi R, Tan PH, Wang M, Baldridge LA, MacLennan GT, Cheng L. Lymphoepithelioma-like carcinoma of the urinary bladder: clinicopathologic, immunohistochemical, and molecular Features. *Am J Surg Pathol* 2011;35:474–83.
64. Abenoza P, Manivel C, Fraley EE. Primary adenocarcinoma of urinary bladder. Clinicopathologic study of 16 cases. *Urology* 1987;29:9–14.
65. Melamed MR, Farrow GM, Haggitt RC. Urologic neoplasma. In: Proceedings of the 50th Annual Antomic Pathology Slide Seminar of the American Society of Clinical Pathologists. Chicago: ASCP Press, 1987.
66. Pantuck AJ, Bancila E, Das KM, Amenta PS, Cummings KB, Marks M, Weiss RE. Adenocarcinoma of the urachus and bladder expresses a unique colonic epithelial epitope: an immunohistochemical study. *J Urol* 1997;158:1722–7.
67. Paner GP, McKenney JK, Barkan GA, Yao JL, Frankel WL, Sebo TJ, Shen SS, Jimenez RE. Immunohistochemical analysis in a morphologic spectrum of urachal epithelial neoplasms: diagnostic implications and pitfalls. *Am J Surg Pathol* 2011;35:787–98.
68. Young RH, Bostwick DG. Florid cystitis glandularis of intestinal type with mucin extravasation: a mimic of adenocarcinoma. *Am J Surg Pathol* 1996;20:1462–8.

69. Hodges KB, Lopez-Beltran A, Emerson RE, Montironi R, Cheng L. Clinical utility of immunohistochemistry in the diagnoses of urinary bladder neoplasia. *Appl Immunohistochem Mol Morphol* 2010;18:401–10.

70. Grignon D, Ro J, Ayala A, Johnson D, Ordonez N. Primary adenocarcinoma of the urinary bladder: a clinicopathologic analysis of 72 cases. *Cancer* 1990;67:2165–72.

71. Emerson RE, Cheng L. Immunohistochemical markers in the evaluation of tumors of the urinary bladder: a review. *Anal Quant Cytol Histol* 2005;27:301–16.

72. Torenbeek R, Lagendijk JH, van Diest PJ, Bril H, van de Mollengraft FJM, Meijer CJ. Value of a panel of antibodies to identify the primary origin of adenocarcinomas presenting as bladder carcinoma. *Histopathology* 1998;32:20–7.

73. Kitami K, Masuda N, Chiba K, Kumagai H. [Carcinoma of the urachus with variable pathological findings: report of a case and review of literature]. *Hinyokika Kiyo* 1987;33:1459–64.

74. Tiltman AJ, Maytom PA. Adenocarcinoma of the urinary bladder. Histochemical distinction between urachal and metastatic carcinomas. *S Afr Med J* 1977;51:74–5.

75. Giordano GG. Orbital metastasis from a urachal tumor. *Arch Ophthalmol* 1995;113:413–5.

76. Young RH. Urachal adenocarcinoma metastatic to the ovary simulating primary mucinous cystadenocarcinoma of the ovary: report of a case. *Virchows Arch* 1995;426:529–32.

77. Siegel RJ, Napoli VM. Malignant lymphoma of the urinary bladder. A case with signet-ring cells simulating urachal adenocarcinoma. *Arch Pathol Lab Med* 1991;115:635–7.

78. Satake I, Nakagomi K, Tari K, Kishi K. Metachronous transitional cell carcinoma of the urachus and bladder. *Br J Urol* 1995;75:244.

79. Chow YC, Lin WC, Tzen CY, Chow YK, Lo KY. Squamous cell carcinoma of the urachus. *J Urol* 2000;163:903–4.

80. Shaaban AA, Orkubi SA, Said MT, Yousef B, Abomelha MS. Squamous cell carcinoma of the urinary bladder. *Ann Saudi Med* 1997;17:115–9.

81. Lin RY, Rappoport AE, Deppisch LM, Natividad NS, Katz W. Squamous cell carcinoma of the urachus. *J Urol* 1977;118:1066–7.

82. Jimi A, Munaoka H, Sato S, Iwata Y. Squamous cell carcinoma of the urachus. A case report and review of literature. *Acta Pathol Jpn* 1986;36:945–52.

83. Utz DC, Schmitz SE, Fugelso PD, Farrow GM. Proceedings: A clinicopathologic evaluation of partial cystectomy for carcinoma of the urinary bladder. *Cancer* 1973;32:1075–7.

84. Richie JP, Waisman J, Skinner DG, Dretler SP. Squamous carcinoma of the bladder: treatment by radical cystectomy. *J Urol* 1976;115:670–2.

85. Powley PH. Sarcoma of the urachus. *Br J Surg* 1961;48:649–50.

86. Butler DB, Rosenberg HS. Sarcoma of the urachus. *Arch Surg* 1959;79:724–8.

87. D'Alessio A, Verdelli G, Bernardi M, DePascale S, Chiarenza SF, Giardina C, Cheli M, Rota G, Locatelli G. Endodermal sinus (yolk sac) tumor of the urachus. *Eur J Pediatr Surg* 1994;4:180–1.

88. Romero-Rojas A, Messa-Botero OA, Melo-Uribe MA, Diaz-Perez JA, Chinchilla-Olaya SI. Primary yolk sac tumor of the urachus. *Int J Surg Pathol* 2011;19:658–61.

89. Huang HY, Ko SF, Chuang JH, Jeng YM, Sung MT, Chen WJ. Primary yolk sac tumor of the urachus. *Arch Pathol Lab Med* 2002;126:1106–9.

Bladder Pathology, First Edition. Liang Cheng, Antonio Lopez-Beltran, David G. Bostwick.
© 2012 Wiley-Blackwell. Published 2012 by John Wiley & Sons, Inc.

Pathology of Renal Pelvis, Ureter, and Urethra

The clinical, macroscopic, and microscopic features, as well as the differential diagnosis of the most common lesions and tumors seen in a routine surgical pathology practice of the renal pelvis, ureter, and the urethra, are reviewed in this chapter. Most of these lesions are similar to those of the bladder. The current classification of tumors and the appropriated tumor, node, and metastases (TNM) staging system according to the 2010 revision are also included.[1] Applicable ancillary testing modalities, including immunohistochemistry and other molecular findings, are discussed.

Congenital Anomalies

Renal Pelvis and Ureter

A number of congenital anomalies occur in the renal pelvis and/or the ureter.[2] Duplication, ectopia, ureteral agenesis, ureterocele, and obstructive lesions are the most common ureteral malformations (**Fig. 28-1**). More than one abnormality may be present, resulting in a complex anomaly.

The double ureter (ureteral duplication) is the most common anomaly, seen in approximately 0.8% of autopsies. It is frequently associated with a double renal pelvis. Ureteral duplication is most likely to be partial and unilateral.

Ureteral ectopia with or without duplication is a common cause of vesicoureteral reflux. The ectopic insertion may be located in the rectum, vagina, urethra, or abnormally situated in the bladder. Ureteral agenesis virtually always accompanies renal agenesis.

Megaureter (primary or secondary to reflux) can also be seen and it is characterized by the near-absence of the longitudinal muscle fibers, preponderance of circular muscle, or fibrosis of muscle and adventitia (**Figs. 28-2** to **28-3**). In cases of renal dysplasia, the ureter is usually dysplastic.

Ureterocele (congenital dilatation of intramural portion of the ureter) is a marked dilatation of the intravesical

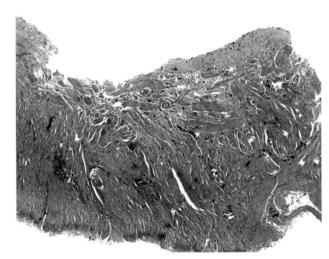

Figure 28-2 Megaureter.

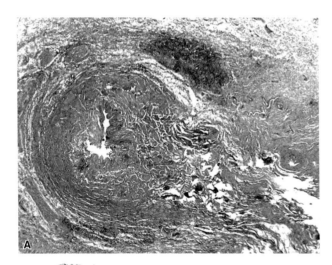

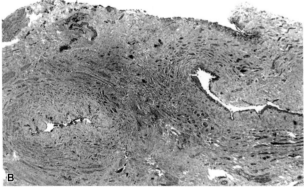

Figure 28-1 Duplex ureter (A and B).

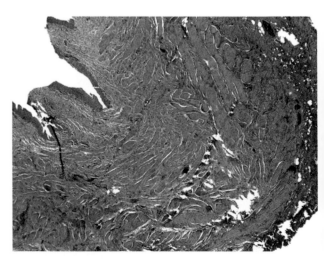

Figure 28-3 Megaureter.

portion of the distal ureter at its orifice. Ureterocele may be seen in some cases, resulting in obstruction or reflux.

Ureteral obstruction may involve any portion of the urinary tract, but it is most frequent at the ureteropelvic junction. Childhood ureteropelvic junction obstruction is the most important cause of intrinsic urinary blockage. Ureteral diverticulum and inflammation can also cause obstruction (**Figs. 28-4** and **28-5**).

Urethra

A number of congenital anomalies have been reported to occur in the urethra. The most common include duplication, congenital urethral polyps (usually in the prostatic urethra), and urethral valves, which frequently result in obstructive symptoms. Duplication of the urethra may occur with complex rectal and urogenital malformations. Obstructive lesions of the lower urinary tract include posterior urethral valves, urethral stenosis, or atresia.

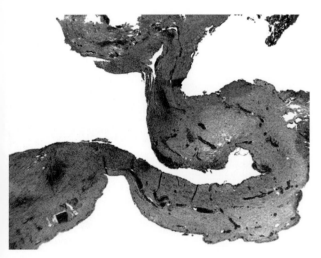

Figure 28-4   Ureteral diverticulum.

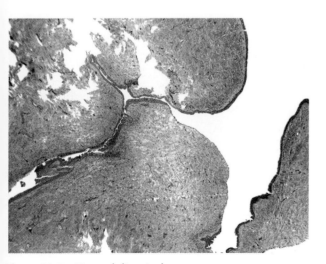

Figure 28-5   Ureteral diverticulum.

Pyelitis, Ureteritis, and Urethritis

Inflammatory lesions of the renal pelvis and ureter are generally an extension of pyelonephritis or reflux nephropathy. Descriptive and often nonspecific terms refer to a variety of benign acute or chronic inflammatory lesions anywhere in the urinary tract, but they are more common in the bladder (**Figs. 28-6** to **28-10**; see **Chapter 2** for further discussion). Peyronie disease is seen in penile urethral resection specimens, which are characterized by collagen disorganization and perivascular lymphocytic infiltration (**Figs. 28-11** and **28-12**).[3]

Benign Lesions and Mimics of Cancer

Most benign lesions and mimics of cancer are more common in the bladder (**Table 28-1**; see also **Chapters 3, 4**, and **5** for further discussion). However, some entities deserve mention since they are more common in the upper urinary tract.

Idiopathic Retroperitoneal Fibrosis

Retroperitoneal fibrosis is an uncommon disease characterized by encasement of retroperitoneal structures, such as the ureters and abdominal aorta, by fibrosis and chronic inflammation (**Figs. 28-13** and **28-14**).[4,5] Clinically, there is a medial deviation of the ureter on radiological examination. The ureter is encased in firm fibrotic tissue. There are varying amounts of fibrosis with collagen deposition. In areas, the lesion shows a chronic inflammatory infiltrate with lymphocytes and plasma cells with occasional formation of lymphoid nodules. Stromal edema is also seen and, in selected cases, imparts a myxoid appearance to the lesion, raising a concern of myxoid liposarcoma.

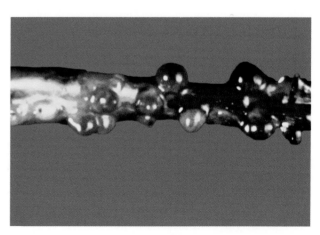

Figure 28-6   Ureteritis cystica (gross appearance).

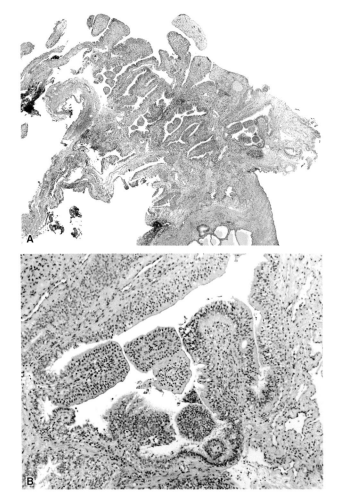

Figure 28-7 Papillary urethritis (A and B).

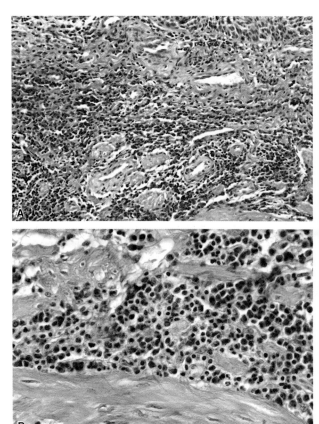

Figure 28-8 Idiopathic eosinophilic ureteritis (A and B). (A) The mucosa is intact, but there is dense inflammation in the submucosa with an abundance of eosinophils. (B) The muscular wall is involved.

Recently, idiopathic retroperitoneal fibrosis has been linked to an IgG4-driven autoimmune process.[4,6–12] IgG4-related sclerosing disease is a recently recognized entity that encompasses many organ systems, including autoimmune pancreatitis.[13–15] These patients may have multiple organ involvement. Approximately 50% of idiopathic retroperitoneal fibrosis cases are IgG4 positive and should be included within the IgG4-related spectrum of sclerosing diseases.[6]

Fibroepithelial Polyp

Fibroepithelial polyp is an uncommon benign lesion of the ureter that usually occurs in young adult men and presents with hematuria and intermittent flank pain or with obstructive symptoms. The polyp arises most commonly in the region of verumontanum or posterior urethra. It also occurs in the proximal ureter, more frequently in the left side and rarely in other locations. Microscopically, there is a polypoid projection of edematous vascular stroma with

Figure 28-9 Peyronie disease. Note the disorganization of the collagen.

overlying atrophic or hyperplastic urothelium (**Fig. 28-15**). Light chronic inflammatory infiltrate is usually present in the stroma. Rare cases may have a prominent histiocytic component.

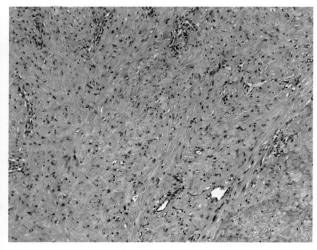

Figure 28-10   Peyronie disease.

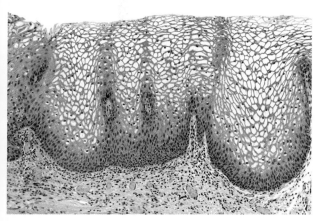

Figure 28-11   Squamous metaplasia of the urethra.

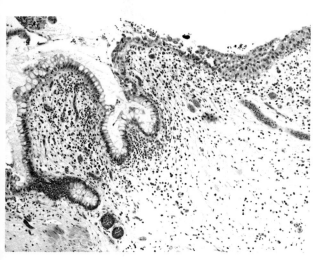

Figure 28-12   Intestinal metaplasia of the urethra.

Table 28-1   Histological Classification of Tumors of Renal Pelvis and Ureter

Epithelial tumors
  Benign
    Urothelial papilloma
    Inverted papilloma
    Squamous cell papilloma
    Villous adenoma
  Malignant
    Urothelial carcinoma
      Micropapillary
      Nested
      Microcystic
      Inverted
      Clear cell
      With squamous differentiation
      With glandular differentiation
      Lymphoepithelioma-like
      Sarcomatoid
      Giant cell
    Squamous cell carcinoma
    Adenocarcinoma
    Small cell carcinoma
    Undifferentiated carcinoma
Nonepithelial tumors
  Benign
    Fibroepithelial polyp
    Leiomyoma
    Fibrous histiocytoma
    Neurofibroma
    Hemangioma
    Lipoma
    Hibernoma
  Malignant
    Leiomyosarcoma
    Rhabdomyosarcoma
    Fibrosarcoma
    Angiosarcoma
    Osteosarcoma
    Malignant peripheral nerve sheath tumor
Miscellaneous
  Pheochromocytoma
  Carcinoid
  Wilms tumor
  Choriocarcinoma
  Malignant melanoma
  Lymphoma
  Plasmacytoma

Endometriosis

Clinically, endometriosis occurs more frequently in the bladder, but the lesion may also occur in the upper urinary tract, with the ureter being the most common location (see also **Chapter 4**).[16] It typically occurs in women of reproductive age, and up to 50% have a history of

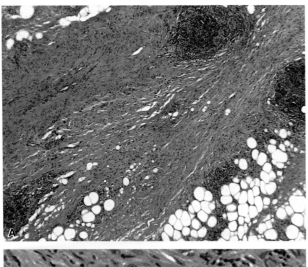

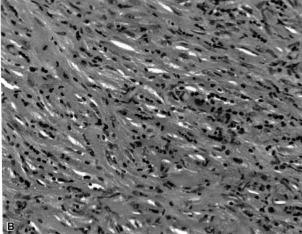

Figure 28-13 Idiopathic retroperitoneal fibrosis (A and B).

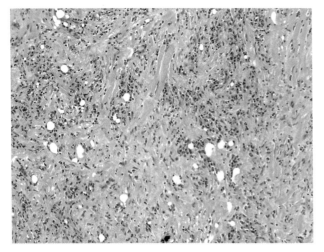

Figure 28-14 Idiopathic retroperitoneal fibrosis.

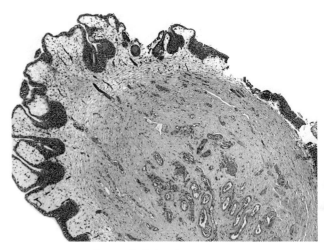

Figure 28-15 Fibroepithelial polyp.

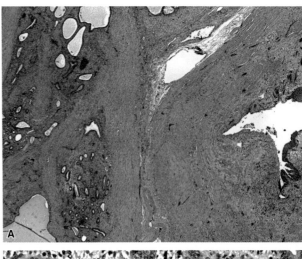

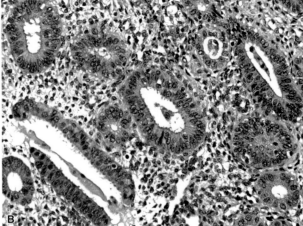

Figure 28-16 Ureteral endometriosis (A and B).

pelvic surgery. Clinical manifestations include frequency, dysuria, and hematuria; in 75% of cases, these symptoms have catamenial exacerbations. Microscopically, the lesion is composed of endometriotic glands and stroma with

hemosiderin deposition (requires two of these three elements to make the diagnosis) (Figs. 28-16 and 28-17). The endometrial glands are typically lined by cuboidal cells with eosinophilic cytoplasm and pseudostratified nuclei

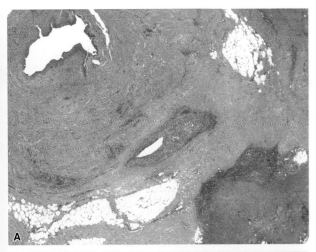

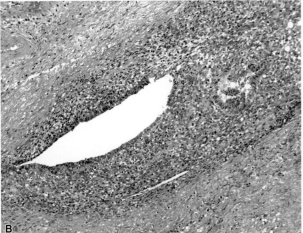

Figure 28-17   Ureteral endometriosis (A and B).

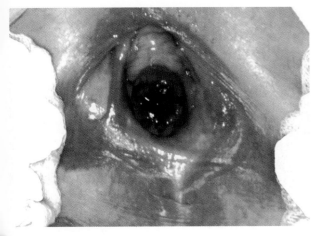

Figure 28-18   Urethral caruncle.

that may show mitotic activity, depending on the phase of the cycle. The stroma may contain foamy histiocytes with some chronic inflammatory cells. The stroma may be focally absent around some of the glands; in

postmenopausal women who are not on estrogen replacement, the diagnosis of endometriosis may be made in the absence of endomctrial stroma.[16] In such instances, the glands still retain their endometriotic appearance. In some cases, the endometrial stroma may be replaced by elastotic stroma similar to that seen in radial scars of the breast.

Urethral Inflammatory Polyp

Urethral inflammatory polyp is usually composed of inflamed and vascular stroma lined by normal or hyperplastic urothelium, with an extensive inflammatory cell component extending to the urothelium.

Urethral Caruncle

Urethral caruncle usually occurs in postmenopausal women at a mean age of 68 years.[17] It typically presents as a red painful mass at the external ureteral meatus (**Fig. 28-18**). The etiology remains uncertain. It may be asymptomatic or present with hematuria, dysuria, and pain. They usually present as a nodular or pedunculated erythematous lesion in the posterior or lateral distal urethral wall. At histology, there is an exuberant proliferation of fibroblasts and endothelial cells in an inflammatory background; it is similar to granulation tissue (**Figs. 28-19** to **28-21**). Urethral caruncle lacks significant cytologic atypia, and mitotic figures are inconspicuous. Atypical stromal cells may occasionally be present, raising the possibility of malignancy in rare cases. At immunohistochemistry, caruncle is cytokeratin negative. The urothelium may show hyperplasia, metaplasia, or be denuded. Carcinosarcoma or myofibroblastic proliferations enter the differential diagnosis occasionally (**Fig. 28-22**). Recently, the disease has been linked to an autoimmune process.[17] A substantial number of cases (30%) showed positive IgG4 staining (**Fig. 28-23**).[17]

Urethral Diverticula

Urethral diverticula usually affect women and are often asymptomatic. Most are lined by urothelium, but squamous and glandular metaplasia can be seen. Nephrogenic adenoma (nephrogenic metaplasia) or carcinoma may develop in urethral diverticula.

Ectopic Prostatic Tissue

Ectopic prostatic tissue occurs in adolescents or young adults and presents with hematuria or irritative symptoms (see also **Chapter 4**).[18] In some cases, atypical cells may be shed in the urine. Most commonly, these lesions are located in the posterior portion of prostatic urethra; it is composed of benign prostatic glands with overlying intact urothelium (**Figs. 28-24** to **28-26**). Secretory cells are prostate-specific antigen (PSA)

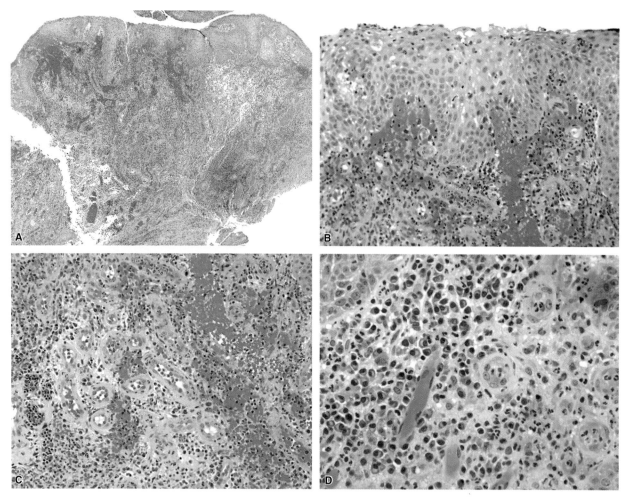

Figure 28-19   Urethral caruncle (A to D).

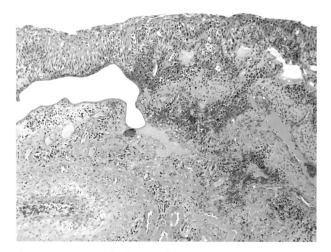

Figure 28-20   Urethral caruncle.

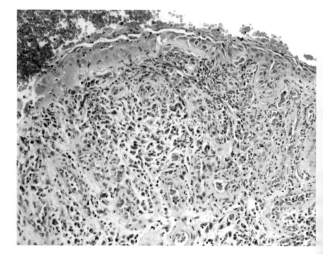

Figure 28-21   Urethral caruncle. Note the reactive stromal atypia.

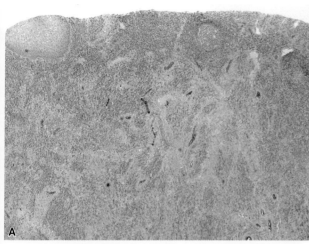

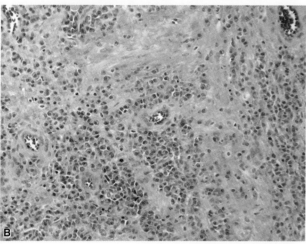

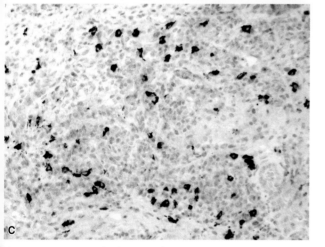

Figure 28-22 Urethral caruncle (A to C). IgG4 staining is positive (C), linking the disease to the autoimmune process.

positive; high molecular weight cytokeratin positively stains the basal cell layer. Also, in the prostatic urethra verumontanum gland, hyperplasia is important since it can be confused with prostatic adenocarcinoma on a biopsy, as it shows an increased number of crowded and small prostatic

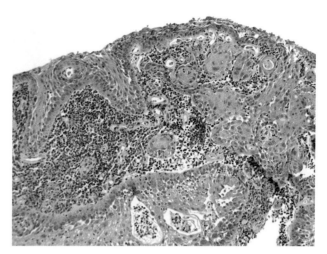

Figure 28-23 Urethral caruncle. Note the pseudocarcinomatous epithelial hyperplasia.

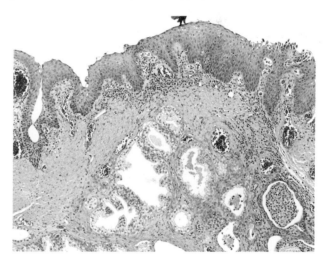

Figure 28-24 Ectopic prostate.

acini. However, the epithelial cells frequently have cuboidal eosinophilic or, even more frequently, pale cytoplasm with small nuclei and small to absent nucleoli. In verumontarium gland hyperplasia, the basal cell layer is preserved. Corpora amylacea with concentric laminations and occasional fragmentation are commonly seen.

Subepithelial Hematoma of the Renal Pelvis

Subepithelial hematoma of the renal pelvis can clinically mimic cancer.[19] Microscopically, it is characterized by subepithelial hemorrhage and urothelial denudation and erosion (**Figs. 28-27** and **28-28**).

Neoplasms of the Renal Pelvis and Ureter

Tumors arising in the renal pelvis and the ureter are morphologically similar to those in the bladder (**Table 28-1**).

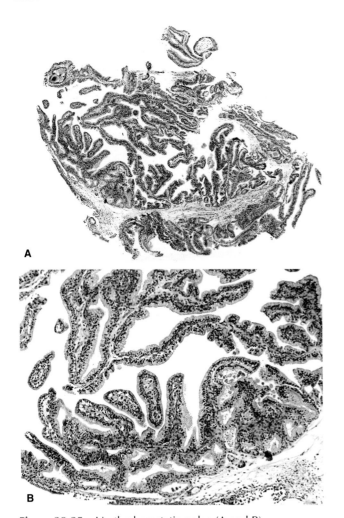

A

B

Figure 28-25   Urethral prostatic polyp (A and B).

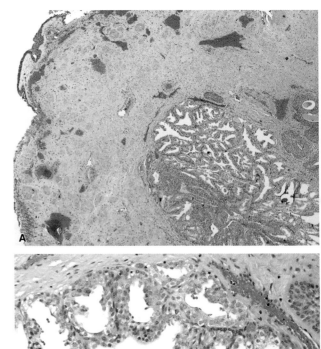

A

B

Figure 28-26   Ectopic prostatic tissue in female urethra. (A) Low power view of a focus of ectopic prostatic tissue in the female urethra in a subepithelial location. (B) High power view showing the complex architecture of the glands, which is reminiscent of the central zone. Note the slight nuclear enlargement with occasional nucleoli. We consider these as reactive changes and should not be interpreted as high grade prostatic intraepithelial neoplasia.

The incidence of these tumors ranges from 0.7 to 1.1 per 100,000 and there is a male-to-female ratio of 1.7:1, with an increasing incidence in females.[20–24] Tumors of the ureter and renal pelvis account for 8% of all urinary tract neoplasms and are more common in older patients (mean, 70 years).[25] More than 90% are urothelial carcinomas. Hematuria and flank pain are the chief presenting symptoms.[20,26–34]

Benign Urothelial Neoplasms

Most benign epithelial tumors are urothelial papilloma, inverted papilloma, villous adenoma, or squamous papilloma.[35–39] These lesions are usually incidental findings and show histology similar to that of bladder cases. Synchronous inverted papilloma of the urinary bladder and the renal pelvis may occur.[38] Rarely, nephrogenic adenoma may occur in the renal pelvis and the ureter. Benign epithelial tumors are rare in the upper urinary tract (see Chapter 5 for further discussion).

Flat Urothelial Lesions with Atypia

There are similar categories to those seen in the bladder (see Chapters 6 and 7 for further discussion).

Urothelial Carcinoma

Clinical Features

Carcinomas arising in the renal pelvis and calyces are twice as common as those of the ureter (Figs. 28-29 and 28-30).[2] Multifocality is frequent. Bilateral synchronous or metachronous ureteral and renal pelvic carcinomas may occur. Etiologic and predisposing factors additional to those for bladder malignancy include phenacetin abuse, kidney

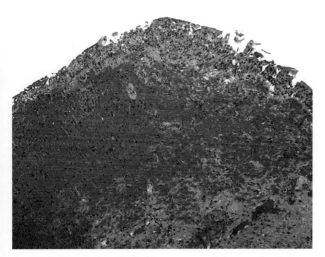

Figure 28-27 Subepithelial hematoma of the renal pelvis that clinically mimics cancer.

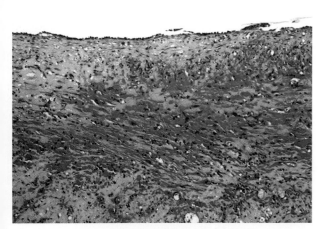

Figure 28-28 Subepithelial hematoma of the renal pelvis.

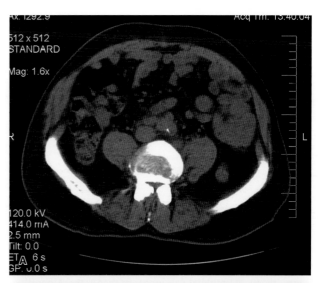

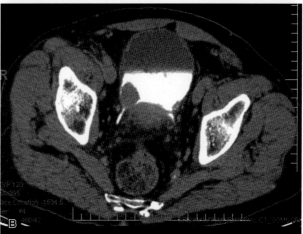

Figure 28-29 Urothelial carcinoma of the ureter. CT scan shows retroperitoneal adenopathy (A). The same patient also has ureteral carcinoma overlying the ureteral orifice (B). (Photo courtesy of Dr. Koch.)

papillary necrosis, Balkan nephropathy, thorium containing radiologic contrast material, urinary tract infections, or nephrolithiasis.[30–32,34,40,41] Some tumors of the ureter are associated with hereditary nonpolyposis colon cancer syndrome (Lynch syndrome).[41,42] Hydronephrosis and stones may be present in renal pelvic tumors, while hydroureter and/or stricture may accompany ureteral neoplasms.[43] Prior histories of bladder and upper tract tumor multifocality are the most important risk factors for bladder tumor recurrence following treatment of upper urinary tract urothelial carcinoma.[44]

Urothelial carcinoma behaves identically in the upper and lower urinary tract after controlling for pathologic stage and histologic grade.[45]

Macroscopic Pathology
Grossly, tumors may be papillary, polypoid, nodular, ulcerative, or infiltrative (**Figs. 28-31** and **28-32**). Some tumors distend the entire pelvis, while others ulcerate and infiltrate,

causing thickening of the wall.[26,28,31,46] A high grade tumor may appear as an ill-defined mass that involves the renal parenchyma, mimicking a primary renal cell carcinoma.

Microscopic Pathology
The renal pelvic malignancies mirror bladder urothelial neoplasia and therefore occur with similar histology, including papillary noninvasive or invasive tumors, carcinoma in situ (CIS), and solid invasive carcinoma (**Figs. 28-33** to **28-38**).[20,27,28,30,31,47,48] The entire morphologic spectrum of urothelial carcinoma and its variants may be seen in the upper tract. Tumor types include those showing squamous and glandular differentiation, inverted growth, different morphologic variants (nested, microcystic, micropapillary, clear cell, plasmacytoid), and poorly differentiated or undifferentiated carcinoma (lymphoepithelioma-like, sarcomatoid, and pleomorphic

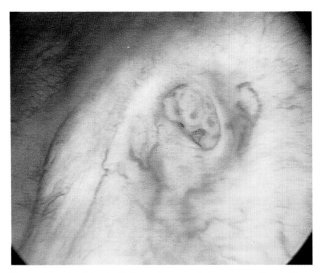

Figure 28-30 Urothelial carcinoma of the ureter. A papillary ureteral tumor can be seen emanating from the left ureteral orifice. (Photo courtesy of Dr. Koch.)

giant cell) (**Figs. 28-39** and **28-40**).[28,40,48–64] Sarcomatoid carcinoma is rare in the pelvis and ureter, has a poor prognosis, and may show either homologous or heterologous stromal elements (**Fig. 28-41**).[55,57,65] Rare cases of choriocarcinoma reported in this location are currently viewed as high grade urothelial carcinoma with trophoblastic

differentiation.[66,67] There is a separate TNM staging system for tumors of the renal pelvis and ureter according to the American Joint Committee on Cancer (AJCC) TNM (tumor, lymph nodes, and metastases) staging system, 2010 revision (**Table 28-2**).[1]

The most important prognostic factor is tumor stage.[1,28] In evaluating these specimens, it is important to avoid overstaging as pT3 tumors that invade the muscularis (pT2) but with extension into renal tubules in a pagetoid or intramucosal pattern.[68] Survival for patients with pTa/pTis lesions is essentially 100% but declines up to 75% in patients with pT2. Survival for patients with pT3 and pT4 tumors, tumors with nodal involvement, and patients with residual tumor after surgery is poor.[34] Other prognostic factors include patient age and type of treatment.[28,46] The characteristics of invading neoplastic nests (infiltrative vs. nodular or trabecular), vascular invasion, and tumor necrosis could be of prognostic significance.[28,46,69,70] Recently, it has been noticed that extensive coagulative tumor necrosis (>10% of the tumor area under microscopic examination) is an independent predictor of poor survival in patients with tumors of the renal pelvis and ureter.[70] It has been suggested that Ki67 overexpression might also be of prognostic value and that ErbB2 expression could be a predictor of disease progression and disease-related survival in upper urothelial carcinoma.[71,72]

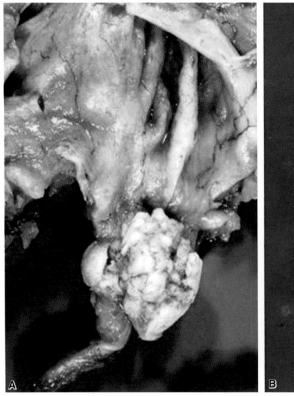
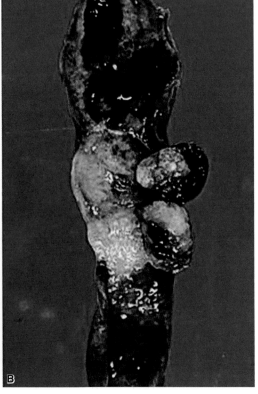

Figure 28-31 Papillary urothelial carcinoma of the the ureteropelvic junction (A) and of the ureter (B).

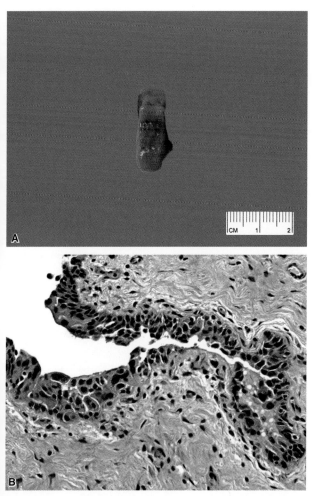

Figure 28-32   Urothelial carcinoma in situ of the ureter (A and B).

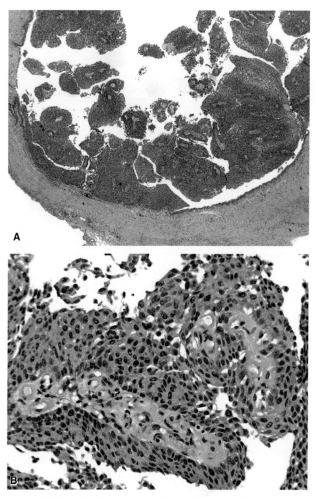

Figure 28-34   Papillary urothelial carcinoma of the ureter (A and B).

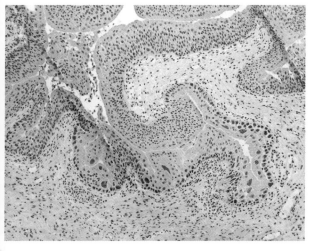

Figure 28-33   Urothelial carcinoma in situ of the ureter.

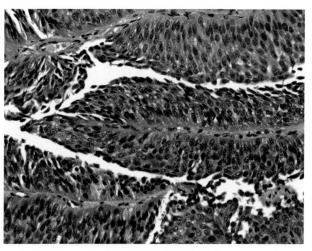

Figure 28-35   Papillary urothelial carcinoma of the ureter.

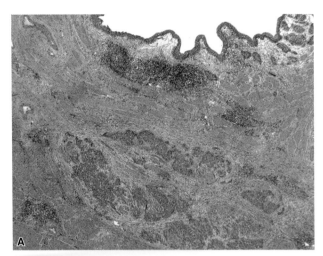

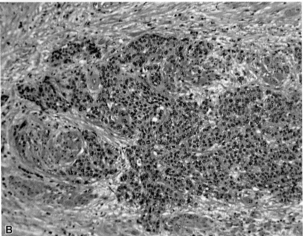

Figure 28-36 Invasive urothelial carcinoma of the ureter (A and B). Tumor invades the muscularis propria.

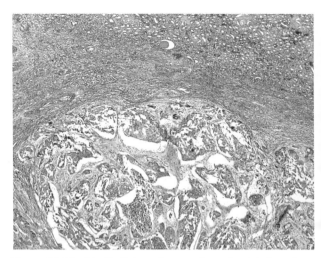

Figure 28-38 Urothelial carcinoma of renal pelvis invading the renal parenchyma.

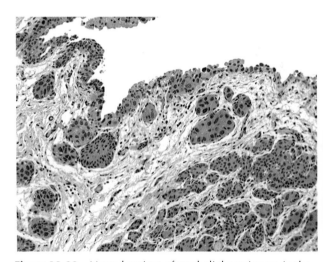

Figure 28-39 Nested variant of urothelial carcinoma in the ureter.

Lymphovascular invasion is also a poor prognostic factor in upper urinary tract urothelial carcinoma and is an independent predictor of shortened recurrence-free survival.

Grading Urothelial Carcinoma

Urothelial tumors should be graded following the proposal for the bladder urothelial tumors made by the World Health Organization (WHO) in 1973 or, until validated, both the 1973 WHO grade and the 2004 WHO grade can be stated in the final pathology report (see **Chapter 9** for further discussion).[28,30,36,68] The existence of papillary urothelial neoplasia of low malignant potential (PUNLMP) in the upper urinary tract has recently been challenged.[28,30,36,68]

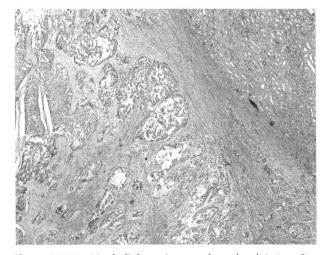

Figure 28-37 Urothelial carcinoma of renal pelvis invading the renal parenchyma.

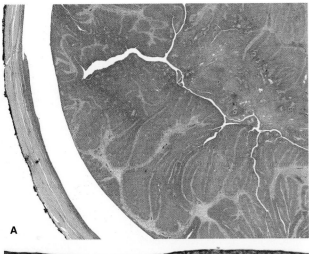

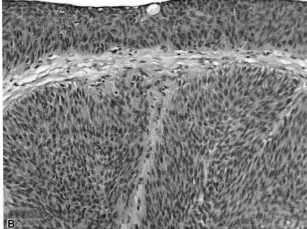

Figure 28-40 Inverted variant of urothelial carcinoma in the ureter (A and B).

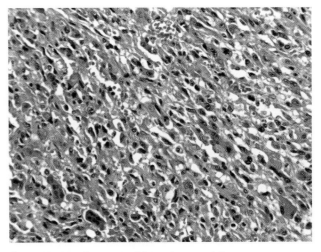

Figure 28-41 Sarcomatoid carcinoma of the ureter.

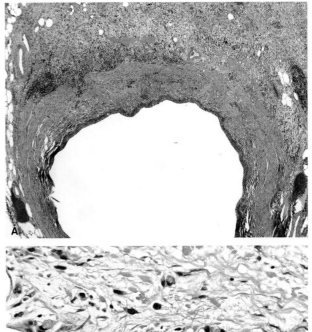

Figure 28-42 Signet ring cell adenocarcinoma of the ureter (A and B).

Immunohistochemistry and Molecular Pathology

Some urothelial carcinomas in this location display α-fetoprotein or cyclooxygenase-2 expression by immunohistochemistry.[63,73] Synchronous renal cell carcinoma and urothelial cell carcinoma may coexist. p63 and high molecular weight cytokeratin (34βE12) are relevant in the differential diagnosis of urothelial carcinoma with poorly differentiated renal cell carcinoma. Urothelial carcinomas of the renal pelvis, ureter, and urinary bladder show molecular similarities to bladder carcinoma, but microsatellite instability (MSI) is more common in upper urinary tract cancers.[74–78] Deletions on chromosome 9p and 9q occur in 50% to 75% of all patients, and frequent deletions at 17p in addition to *TP53* mutations are seen in advanced invasive tumors of the upper urinary tract. Twenty percent to 30% of all upper urinary tract cancers demonstrate MSI and loss of the mismatch repair proteins MSH2, MLH1, or MSH6.[74] Mutations in the sequences

Table 28-2   **TNM Classification of Tumors of the Renal Pelvis and Ureter (2010 Revision)**

T: Primary tumor		
	TX	Primary tumor cannot be assessed
	T0	No evidence of primary tumor
	Ta	Papillary noninvasive carcinoma
	Tis	Carcinoma in situ
	T1	Tumor invades subepithelial connective tissue
	T2	Tumor invades the muscularis propria
	T3	(*For renal pelvis only*) Tumor invades beyond muscularis into peripelvic fat or renal parenchyma
		(*For ureter only*) Tumor invades beyond muscularis into periureteric fat
	T4	Tumor invades adjacent organs or through the kidney into perinephric fat
N: Regional lymph nodes		
	NX	Regional lymph nodes cannot be assessed
	N0	No regional lymph node metastasis
	N1	Metastasis in a single lymph node 2 cm or less in greatest dimension
	N2	Metastasis in a single lymph node more than 2 cm but not more than 5 cm in greatest dimension, or multiple lymph nodes, none more than 5 cm in greatest dimension
	N3	Metastasis in a lymph node more than 5 cm in greatest dimension
M: Distant metastasis		
	M0	No distant metastasis
	M1	Distant metastasis

of TGFβ-RII, *Bax, MSH3,* and *MSH6* genes are found in 20% to 33% of cases with MSI, indicating a molecular pathway of carcinogenesis that is similar to some mismatch repair-deficient colorectal cancers. Tumors with MSI have different clinical and histological features, including low tumor stage and grade, papillary growth, and a higher prevalence in female patients; some of these tumors exhibit an inverted growth pattern.[74–78]

Adenocarcinoma

Pure adenocarcinoma of the renal pelvis and ureter is rare, showing morphologic types similar to those in the bladder (enteric, mucinous, or signet ring cell) (**Fig. 28-42**).[55,60,79] Glandular (intestinal) metaplasia, nephrolithiasis, and repeated infections are predisposing factors. Most adenocarcinomas are high grade and are widely invasive at presentation. In the ureter, florid cystitis glandularis may occur, raising concern in the differential diagnosis with well-differentiated adenocarcinoma. Pathologic characteristics of adenocarcinoma are similar to those of the bladder (see **Chapter 13** for further discussion).[80,81]

Squamous Cell Carcinoma

Squamous cell carcinoma is very rare but may occur in the renal pelvis, where it follows urothelial carcinoma in frequency.[54,61,82] Squamous differentiation in an otherwise urothelial carcinoma is seen in about 40% cases in the renal pelvis.[39,47] Pure squamous cell carcinomas are usually high grade and high stage tumors and frequently invade the kidney; they usually occur in the background of nephrolithiasis, chronic inflammation, or being associated with squamous metaplasia.[82] Some squamous cell carcinomas may present with hypercalcemia; but are unrelated to Epstein–Barr virus infection.[83] Survival at five-year followup is poor.[82] The pathologic characteristics are similar to those of squamous cell carcinoma arising in the bladder (see **Chapter 14** for further discussion).

Tumor of the Urethra

This category includes epithelial and nonepithelial neoplasms of the male and female urethra between from the urinary bladder and the urethral meatus, and tumors arising in the accessory glands (Cowper and Littre glands as well as Skene glands in the female) (**Figs. 28-43** and **28-44**; **Table 28-3**). Epithelial tumors of the urethra are rare and three to four times more common in women than in men. Urethral carcinomas occurring in men are strikingly different in clinical and pathologic features than tumors in women. This difference seems to be attributable to the distinct differences in the anatomy and histology of the urethra in both genders. Congenital diverticulum as well as acquired strictures of the female urethra contribute to the female preponderance of carcinomas. Columnar and mucinous adenocarcinomas are thought to arise from glandular metaplasia, whereas cribriform adenocarcinoma that shows PSA-positive staining seems to originate from Skene glands.[18]

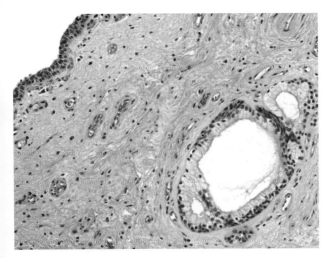

Figure 28-43   Normal urethra. Note the Littre glands.

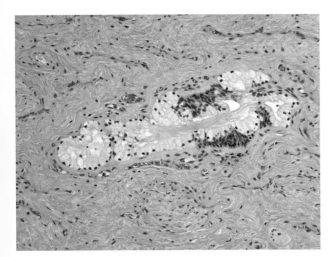

Figure 28-44   Littre glands of the urethra.

Benign Epithelial Tumors of the Urethra

Benign epithelial tumors are exquisitely rare in the urethra of either gender. Tumors occurring in males are similar to those in the female urethra. Some reports of squamous papilloma, villous adenoma, condyloma acuminatum, and urothelial papilloma of the urethra are available but are rare overall (**Figs. 28-45** to **28-49**).[84] Other tumors, including leiomyoma, neurofibroma, paraganglioma, inverted papilloma, and nephrogenic adenoma, have also been reported in the urethra.[85–87] Inflammatory or fibrovascular polyps are noted occasionally in the urethra. The histological features are identical to neoplasms described in the urinary bladder and other sites. Villous adenoma of the urethra is often associated with tubulovillous adenoma and adenocarcinoma of the rectum.[88,89]

Table 28-3   WHO Histological Classification of the Tumors of the Urethra

Epithelial tumors
  Benign
    Squamous papilloma
    Villous adenoma
    Urothelial papilloma, including inverted papilloma
  Malignant
    Primary
      Squamous cell carcinoma
      Urothelial carcinoma
      Adenocarcinoma
      Clear cell carcinoma
      Nonclear cell carcinoma
    Enteric
      Colloid (mucinous) carcinoma
      Signet ring cell carcinoma
      Adenocarcinoma, not otherwise specified
      Adenosquamous carcinoma
      Neuroendocrine carcinoma
      Undifferentiated carcinoma
    Secondary
Nonepithelial tumors
  Benign
    Leiomyoma
    Hemangioma
    Glomangiomyoma
  Malignant
    Malignant melanoma
    Non-Hodgkin lymphoma
    Plasmocytoma
Tumor-like lesions
  Fibroepithelial polyp
  Prostatic polyp
  Caruncle
  Condyloma acuminatum
  Nephrogenic adenoma (metaplasia)
Tumors of accessory glands
  Malignant
    Carcinoma of Skene, Littré, and Cowper glands

Carcinoma of the Urethra

General Features

Tumors involving the distal urethra and meatus are most common and appear as exophytic nodular, infiltrative, or papillary lesions with frequent ulceration (**Figs. 28-50** and **28-51**).[90–95] Tumors involving the proximal urethra that are urothelial exhibit macroscopic diversity with cases showing papillary growth, erythematous or white plaque-like, or the nodular/infiltrative growth of invasive carcinoma.[90–95] Adenocarcinomas are often large infiltrative or expansile neoplasms that may have an exophytic surface.[95–100] They can be mucinous, gelatinous, or cystic. These tumors may

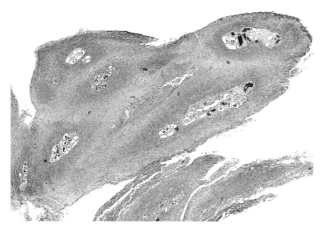

Figure 28-45   Squamous papilloma of the urethra.

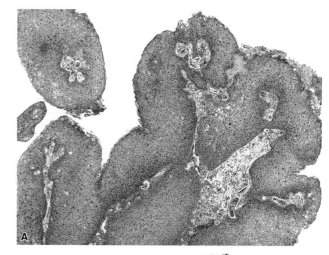

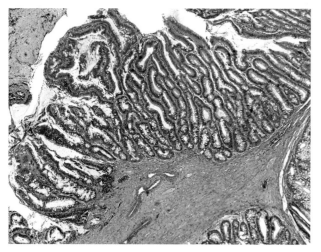

Figure 28-46   Villous adenoma of the urethra.

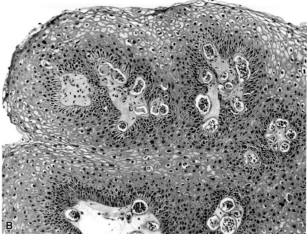

Figure 28-48   Condyloma acuminatum of the urethra (A and B).

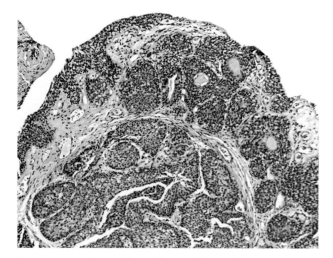

Figure 28-47   Inverted papilloma of the urethra.

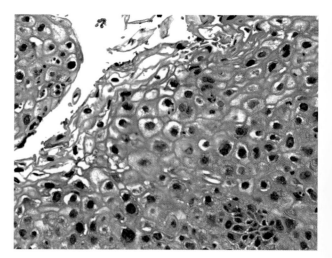

Figure 28-49   Condyloma acuminatum of the urethra.

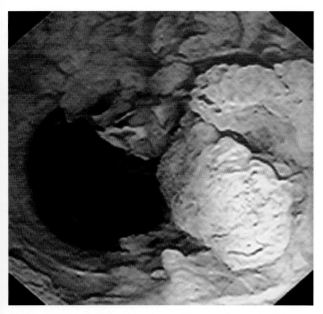

Figure 28-50 Cystoscopic view of low grade urothelial carcinoma arising from the urethra. (Photo courtesy of Dr. Koch.)

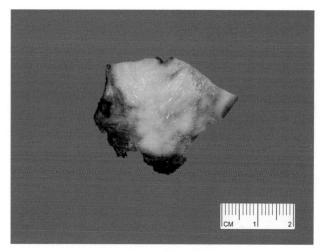

Figure 28-51 Gross appearance of urethral urothelial carcinoma.

occur within a urethral diverticulum.[95–100] Other tumors may occur in the penile urethra, bulbomembranous urethra, or the prostatic urethra, which often determines the gross and histological appearance. These tumors grow as ulcerative, nodular, papillary, cauliflower-like, or ill-defined lesions. Histologically, there are some differences between female and male urethral carcinomas, mainly because of its different anatomic location. Distal urethral and meatus tumors are squamous cell carcinomas (70%), and tumors of the proximal urethra are urothelial carcinomas (20%) or adenocarcinomas (10%).[90–100]

Urothelial neoplasms may be noninvasive, papillary low grade or high grade urothelial carcinoma, urothelial CIS, or invasive urothelial carcinoma (**Figs. 28-52** and **28-53**).[91,94] CIS may involve suburethral glands, focally or extensively, a fact that should not be mistaken as invasion. Deeply invasive carcinomas are high grade, with or without a papillary component, and characterized by irregular nests, sheets, or cords of cells with a desmoplastic and/or inflammatory response. Tumors may exhibit squamous, glandular differentiation or unusual morphologic variations (nested, microcystic, micropapillary, clear cell, or plasmacytoid) (**Fig. 28-54**).[66] A small cell carcinoma or sarcomatoid carcinoma component is rarely seen.[97] In the penile and bulbomembranous urethra, about 75% of carcinomas are squamous cell carcinoma, followed by urothelial carcinomas (usually, prostatic urethra and, less commonly, bulbomembranous and penile urethra), adenocarcinomas (usually, bulbomembranous urethra), or undifferentiated carcinoma.[64,90–100] Urothelial carcinoma

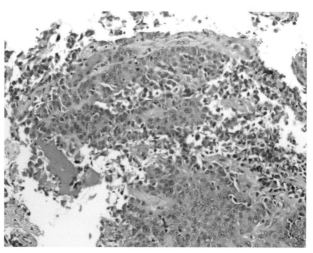

Figure 28-52 High grade papillary urothelial carcinoma of the urethra.

may involve the prostatic urethra, exhibiting the same grade and histological spectrum described in the female urethra.[91] It may be synchronous or metachronous to bladder neoplasia. A feature unique to prostatic urethral urothelial cancers is the frequent proclivity of high grade tumors to extend into the prostatic ducts and acini in a pagetoid fashion.[91] In these cases (CK7+/CK20+), the differential diagnosis with Paget disease of the vulva (CK7+/CK20−) extending through the urethra is mandatory, as it is with melanoma extending from the urethra (HMB45+/Melan A+). Rare cases of prostatic ductal adenocarcinoma arising in periurethral ducts may mimic high grade papillary urothelial carcinoma, a pitfall that should be avoided since therapy is significantly different in prostatic tumors (**Fig. 28-55**). Immunohistochemical evaluation can be of help in difficult cases.

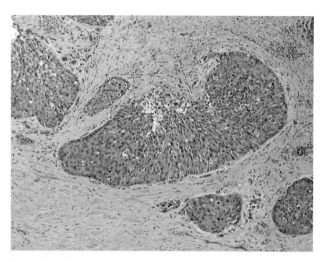

Figure 28-53 Invasive urothelial carcinoma of the urethra.

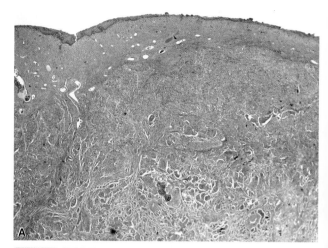

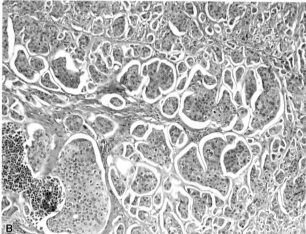

Figure 28-54 Micropapillary variant of urothelial carcinoma of the urethra (A and B).

Urothelial tumors are graded as outlined in the urinary bladder (see also **Chapter 9**).[64,101,102] There is a separate TNM staging system for urothelial carcinomas arising from the prostatic urethra (**Table 28-4**).[1] The overall prognosis is relatively poor.[90–100] Tumor stage and location are important prognostic factors. In females and males, proximal tumors have better overall survival than distal tumors (51% for proximal versus 6% for distal in females and 50% for proximal versus 20% for distal tumors in males, five-year survival). In both genders, high pT tumor stage and the presence of lymph node metastasis are adverse prognostic parameters.

A number of tumor-like conditions enter the differential diagnosis of urethral carcinoma including nephrogenic metaplasia (nephrogenic adenoma), fibroepithelial and prostatic polyps, condyloma acuminatum, and caruncle.[94]

Squamous Cell Carcinoma of the Urethra

Squamous cell carcinomas of the urethra span the range from well-differentiated (including the rare verrucous carcinoma) to moderately differentiated (most common) to poorly differentiated.[90–100] Squamous cell carcinomas are similar in histology to invasive squamous cell carcinomas at other sites (**Figs. 28-56 to 28-58**). Squamous cell carcinomas are usually graded following similar carcinomas in other organs—well, moderately, and poorly differentiated carcinomas using the classic criteria of degree of differentiation.

Squamous cell carcinoma of the urethra is associated with high risk human papillomavirus (HPV) infection in female and male patients.[77,78] HPV16 or HPV18 may be detected in up to 60% of urethral carcinomas in women. In men, about 30% of squamous cell carcinomas test positive for HPV16; tumors in the bulbar urethra are usually negative. Some HPV16-positive tumors may have a more favorable prognosis. Low risk HPV (HPV6 or HPV11) infection

plays a crucial role in the etiology of condyloma acuminatum of the urethra. The association of urothelial carcinoma with HPV, both in the urethra and the urinary bladder, remains controversial. The variable reported incidence may be related to geographical or demographic issues.[103]

Adenocarcinoma of the Urethra

Adenocarcinoma of the female urethra may be seen in two patterns, clear cell adenocarcinoma (approximately 40%) and nonclear cell adenocarcinoma (approximately 60%), the latter frequently exhibiting similar patterns as in other portions of the urinary tract (enteric, mucinous, signet ring cell, or adenocarcinoma not otherwise specified). Clear cell adenocarcinomas are usually characterized by pattern heterogeneity within the same neoplasm with solid, tubular, tubulocystic, or papillary patterns (**Figs. 28-59** and **28-60**).[90–100] The cytologic features vary from low grade (resembling nephrogenic adenoma focally) to high grade (more frequently). Necrosis, mitotic activity, and extensive infiltrative growth are commonly observed. The relationship to

Table 28-4   TNM Classification of Tumors of the Urethra (2010 Revision)

T: Primary tumor	
TX	Primary tumor cannot be assessed
T0	No evidence of primary tumor
Urethra (male and female)	
Ta	Noninvasive papillary, polypoid, or verrucous carcinoma
Tis	Carcinoma in situ
T1	Tumor invades subepithelial connective tissue
T2	Tumor invades any of the following: corpus spongiosum, prostate, periurethral muscle
T3	Tumor invades any of the following: corpus cavernosum, beyond prostatic capsule, anterior vagina, bladder neck
T4	Tumor invades other adjacent organs
Urothelial (transitional cell) carcinoma of prostate (prostatic urethra)	
Tis pu	Carcinoma in situ, involvement of prostatic urethra
Tis pd	Carcinoma in situ, involvement of prostatic ducts
T1	Tumor invades subepithelial connective tissue
T2	Tumor invades any of the following: prostatic stroma, corpus spongiosum, periurethral muscle
T3	Tumor invades any of the following: corpus cavernosum, beyond prostatic capsule, bladder neck (extraprostatic extension)
T4	Tumor invades other adjacent organs (invasion of bladder)
N: Regional lymph nodes	
NX	Regional lymph nodes cannot be assessed
N0	No regional lymph node metastasis
N1	Metastasis in a single lymph node 2 cm or less in greatest dimension
N2	Metastasis in a single lymph node more than 2 cm in greatest dimension, or in multiple nodes
M: Distant metastasis	
M0	No distant metastasis
M1	Distant metastasis

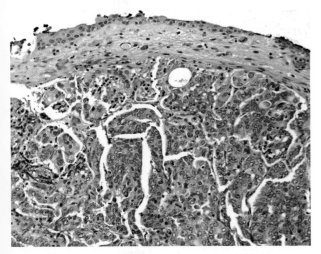

Figure 28-55   Prostatic adenocarcinoma involving the urethra.

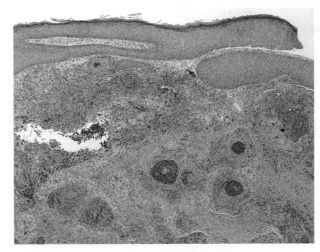

Figure 28-56   Squamous cell carcinoma of the urethra. Note the overlying keratinizing squamous metaplasia.

nephrogenic adenoma remains uncertain. Adenocarcinomas are usually graded following criteria similar to carcinomas in other organs—well, moderately, and poorly differentiated carcinomas using the classic criteria of degree of differentiation.

Bulbourethral gland carcinomas may show a mucinous, papillary, adenoid cystic, acinar, or tubular architecture. Female periurethral gland adenocarcinomas are clear cell or mucinous and often show PSA immunoexpression.

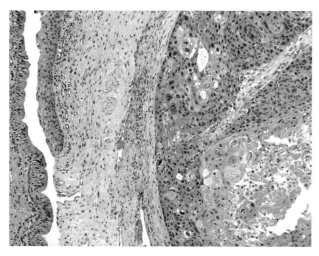

Figure 28-57   Squamous cell carcinoma of the urethra.

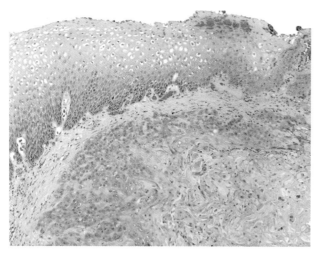

Figure 28-58   Squamous cell carcinoma of the urethra.

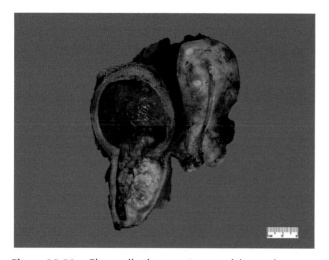

Figure 28-59   Clear cell adenocarcinoma of the urethra.

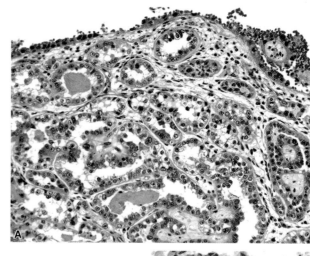

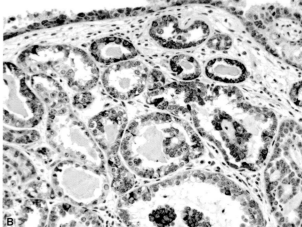

Figure 28-60   Clear cell adenocarcinoma of the urethra (A and B). Immunostaining of α-methylacyl-CoA racemase (AMACR) is positive (B).

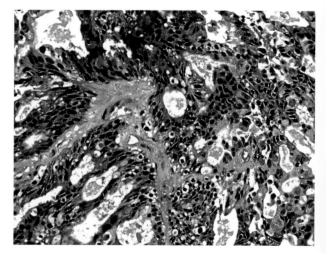

Figure 28-61   Metastatic colon adenocarcinoma involving the urethra.

Metastatic adenocarcinoma, especially from a colorectal primary, should be ruled out before making a definite diagnosis of urethral adenocarcinoma (**Fig. 28-61**).

Soft Tissue Tumors

Renal Pelvis and Ureter

Rare examples of nonepithelial tumors and tumor-like conditions arising in the renal pelvis and/or ureter have been described, including leiomyoma, neurofibroma, fibrous histiocytoma, hemangioma, lipoma, hibernoma, or glomus tumor.[26,104–110] Malignant soft tissue tumors include leiomyosarcoma and, less frequently, rhabdomyosarcoma, osteosarcoma, fibrosarcoma, angiosarcoma, malignant schwannoma, and Ewing sarcoma. Gastrointestinal stromal tumor-like lesions as well as myofibroblastic proliferations may also occur.[105–111] Fibroepithelial polyp with prominent pseudosarcomatous stroma enters the differential diagnosis as well.[111]

Urethra

Rare examples of soft tissue tumors arising in the urethra have been described.[112–114] Benign tumors include leiomyoma with similar morphology and immunoprofile as in other organs; in female patients, leiomyoma may show expression of estrogen receptors. Leiomyoma may occur as a part of diffuse leiomyomatosis syndrome (esophageal and rectal leiomyoma).[112–114] Hemangioma has also been described.

Miscellaneous Tumors

Few cases of ureteric pheochromocytoma have been reported. Pelvic and ureteric carcinoid is similarly rare and

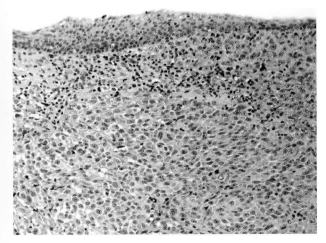

Figure 28-62   Malignant melanoma of the urethra.

must be differentiated from metastatic disease.[26,105–111] Small cell carcinoma of the renal pelvis is a rarity observed in elderly patients.[26,61] These aggressive tumors usually contain foci of urothelial carcinoma and have a typical neuroendocrine immunohistochemical profile. Renal pelvic and ureteric lymphomas are usually associated with systemic disease, while localized pelvic plasmacytoma has been reported.[115] Wilms tumor confined to the renal pelvis or extending into the ureter and cases of malignant melanoma of the renal pelvis may be seen rarely in the literature.[26,104]

A curious case of tumor-like lesion of the renal pelvis composed of Liesegang rings has been reported.[116] Malignant melanoma has also been described in the male and

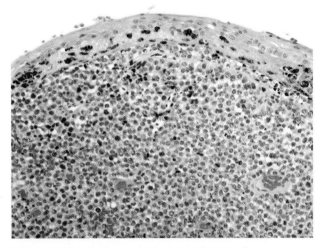

Figure 28-63   Malignant melanoma of the urethra.

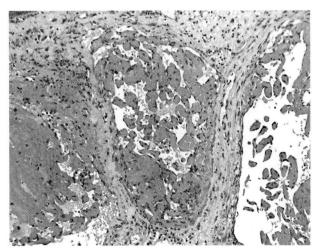

Figure 28-64   Intravascular papillary endothelial hyperplasia of the urethra.

female urethra, with some cases of amelanotic melanoma mimicking urethral carcinoma (**Figs. 28-62** and **28-63**).[117] Primary non-Hodgkin lymphoma and plasmacytoma have

also been described.[112] Carcinoid tumor may occur in the urethra. Other rare lesions have also been noted in the urethra (**Fig. 28-64**).

REFERENCES

1. Edge S, B, Byrd DR, Compton CC, Fritz AG, Greene FL, Trotti A. American Joint Committee on Cancer Staging Manual, 7th ed. New York: Springer, 2010.
2. Bonsib SM, Cheng L. Renal pelvis and ureter. In: Bostwick DG, Cheng L, eds. Urologic Surgical Pathology, 2nd ed. Philadelphia: Elsevier/Mosby, 2008;173–94.
3. Davis CJ. The microscopic pathology of Peyronie's disease. *J Urol* 1997;157:282–4.
4. Corradi D, Maestri R, Palmisano A, Bosio S, Greco P, Manenti L, Ferretti S, Cobelli R, Moroni G, Dei Tos AP, Buzio C, Vaglio A. Idiopathic retroperitoneal fibrosis: clinicopathologic features and differential diagnosis. *Kidney Int* 2007;72:742–53.
5. Vaglio A, Salvarani C, Buzio C. Retroperitoneal fibrosis. *Lancet* 2006;367:241–51.
6. Zen Y, Onodera M, Inoue D, Kitao A, Matsui O, Nohara T, Namiki M, Kasashima S, Kawashima A, Matsumoto Y, Katayanagi K, Murata T, Ishizawa S, Hosaka N, Kuriki K, Nakanuma Y. Retroperitoneal fibrosis: a clinicopathologic study with respect to immunoglobulin G4. *Am J Surg Pathol* 2009;33:1833–9.
7. Miyajima N, Koike H, Kawaguchi M, Zen Y, Takahashi K, Hara N. Idiopathic retroperitoneal fibrosis associated with IgG4-positive-plasmacyte infiltrations and idiopathic chronic pancreatitis. *Int J Urol* 2006;13:1442–4.
8. Miura H, Miyachi Y. IgG4-related retroperitoneal fibrosis and sclerosing cholangitis independent of autoimmune pancreatitis. A recurrent case after a 5-year history of spontaneous remission. *JOP* 2009;10:432–7.
9. Gill J, Taylor G, Carpenter L, Lewis C, Chiu W. A case of hyperIgG4 disease or IgG4-related sclerosing disease presenting as retroperitoneal fibrosis, chronic sclerosing sialadenitis and mediastinal lymphadenopathy. *Pathology* 2009;41:297–300.
10. Kikuno N, Sato H, Ryoji O. Case of IgG4-related retroperitoneal fibrosis with concomitant rheumatoid arthritis. *Int J Urol* 2010;17:1011–2.
11. Marumo K, Tatsuno S, Noto K. Elevated serum IgG4 may predict sensitivity to steroid therapy in retroperitoneal fibrosis. *Int J Urol* 2009;16:427.
12. Matsushita M, Fukui T, Uchida K, Nishio A, Okazaki K. Atypical retroperitoneal fibrosis associated with biliary stricture: IgG4-related sclerosing disease? *Scand J Gastroenterol* 2009;44:1146–7.
13. Okazaki K, Uchida K, Fukui T. Recent advances in autoimmune pancreatitis: concept, diagnosis, and pathogenesis. *J Gastroenterol* 2008;43:409–18.
14. Yamamoto H, Yamaguchi H, Aishima S, Oda Y, Kohashi K, Oshiro Y, Tsuneyoshi M. Inflammatory myofibroblastic tumor versus IgG4-related sclerosing disease and inflammatory pseudotumor: a comparative clinicopathologic study. *Am J Surg Pathol* 2009;33:1330–40.
15. Zen Y, Nakanuma Y. IgG4-related disease: a cross-sectional study of 114 cases. *Am J Surg Pathol* 2010;34:1812–9.
16. Al-Khawaja M, Tan PH, MacLennan GT, Lopez-Beltran A, Montironi R, Cheng L. Ureteral endometriosis: clinicopathological and immunohistochemical study of 7 cases. *Hum Pathol* 2008;39:954–9.
17. Conces MR, Williamson SR, Montironi R, Lopez-Beltran A, Scarpelli M, Cheng L. Urethral caruncle: clinicopathologic features and evidence supporting etiology as an IgG4-associated disease (submitted).
18. Halat S, Eble JN, Grignon DG, Lacy S, Montironi R, MacLennan GT, Lopez-Beltran A, Tan PH, Baldridge LA, Cheng L. Ectopic prostatic tissue: histogenesis and histopathologic characteristics. *Histopathology* 2011;58:750–8.
19. Iczkowski KA, Sweat SD, Bostwick DG. Subepithelial pelvic hematoma of the kidney clinically mimicking cancer: report of six cases and review of the literature. *Urology* 1999;53:276–9.
20. Lopez-Beltran A, Sauter G, Gasser T, Hartmann A, Schmitz-Dräger BJ, Helpap B, Ayala AG, Tamboli P, Knowles MA, Sidransky D, Cordon-Cardo C, Jones PA, Cairns P, Simon R, Amin MB. Urothelial tumors: infiltrating urothelial carcinoma. In: Eble JN, Sauter G, Epstein JI, Sesterhenn I, eds. World Health Organization Classification of Tumors. Pathology and Gentics of Tumors of the Urinary System and Male Genital Organs. Lyon, France: IARC Press, 2004.
21. Lopez-Beltran A, Maclennan GT, de la Haba-Rodriguez J, Montironi R, Cheng L. Research advances in apoptosis-mediated cancer therapy: a review. *Anal Quant Cytol Histol* 2007;29:71–8.
22. Lopez-Beltran A, Perez-Seoane C, Montironi R, Hernandez-Iglesias T, Mackintosh C, de Alava E. Primary primitive neuroectodermal tumour of the urinary bladder: a clinico-pathological study emphasising immunohistochemical, ultrastructural and molecular analyses. *J Clin Pathol* 2006;59:775–8.

23. Bostwick DG, Ramnani D, Cheng L. Diagnosis and grading of bladder cancer and associated lesions. *Urol Clin North Am* 1999;26:493–507.

24. Bostwick DG, Mikuz G. Urothelial papillary (exophytic) neoplasms. *Virchows Arch* 2002;441:109–16.

25. Jemal A, Siegel R, Ward E, Murray T, Xu J, Smigal C, Thun MJ. Cancer statistics, 2006. *CA Cancer J Clin* 2006;56:106–30.

26. Busby JE, Brown GA, Tamboli P, Kamat AM, Dinney CP, Grossman HB, Matin SF. Upper urinary tract tumors with nontransitional histology: a single-center experience. *Urology* 2006;67:518–23.

27. Perez-Montiel D, Wakely PE, Hes O, Michal M, Suster S. High grade urothelial carcinoma of the renal pelvis: clinicopathologic study of 108 cases with emphasis on unusual morphologic variants. *Mod Pathol* 2006;19:494–503.

28. Langner C, Hutterer G, Chromecki T, Leibl S, Rehak P, Zigeuner R. Tumor necrosis as prognostic indicator in transitional cell carcinoma of the upper urinary tract. *J Urol* 2006;176:9104.

29. Holmang S, Johansson SL. Impact of diagnostic and treatment delay on survival in patients with renal pelvic and ureteral cancer. *Scand J Urol Nephrol* 2006;40:479–84.

30. Holmang S, Johansson SL. Urothelial carcinoma of the upper urinary tract: comparison between the WHO/ISUP 1998 consensus classification and WHO 1999 classification system. *Urology* 2005;66:274–8.

31. Olgac S, Mazumdar M, Dalbagni G, Reuter VE. Urothelial carcinoma of the renal pelvis: a clinicopathologic study of 130 cases. *Am J Surg Pathol* 2004;28:1545–52.

32. Holmang S, Johansson SL. Synchronous bilateral ureteral and renal pelvic carcinomas: incidence, etiology, treatment and outcome. *Cancer* 2004;101:741–7.

33. Park S, Hong B, Kim CS, Ahn H. The impact of tumor location on prognosis of transitional cell carcinoma of the upper urinary tract. *J Urol* 2004;171:621–5.

34. Kirkali Z, Tuzel E. Transitional cell carcinoma of the ureter and renal pelvis. *Crit Rev Oncol Hematol* 2003;47:155–69.

35. Sung MT, Eble JN, Wang M, Tan PH, Lopez-Beltran A, Cheng L. Inverted papilloma of the urinary bladder: a molecular genetic appraisal. *Mod Pathol* 2006;19:1289–94.

36. Sauter G, Algaba, F, Amin, MB, Busch, C, Cheville, J, Gasser, T, Grignon, D, Hofstaedter, F, Lopez-Beltran, A, and Epstein, JI. Non-invasive urothelial neoplasias. In: Eble JN, Sauter G, Epstein JI, Sesterhenn IA, eds. WHO Classification of Non-invasive Papillary Urothelial Tumors. In World Health Organization Classification of Tumors. Pathology and Gentics of Tumors of the Urinary System and Male Genital Organs, Lyon, France: IARCC Press, 2004.

37. Cameron KM, Lupton CH. Inverted papilloma of the lower urinary tract. *Br J Urol* 1976;48:567–77.

38. Darras J, Inderadjaja N, Vossaert P. Synchronous inverted papilloma of bladder and renal pelvis. *Urology* 2005;65:798.

39. Guo CC, Fine SW, Epstein JI. Noninvasive squamous lesions in the urinary bladder: a clinicopathologic analysis of 29 cases. *Am J Surg Pathol* 2006;30:883–91.

40. Perez-Montiel D, Hes O, Michal M, Suster S. Micropapillary urothelial carcinoma of the upper urinary tract: clinicopathologic study of five cases. *Am J Clin Pathol* 2006;126:86–92.

41. Bermejo JL, Eng C, Hemminki K. Cancer characteristics in Swedish families fulfilling criteria for hereditary nonpolyposis colorectal cancer. *Gastroenterology* 2005;129:1889–99.

42. Brock KE, Gridley G, Brown LM, Yu MC, Schoenberg JB, Lynch CF, McLaughlin JK. Dietary factors and cancers of the renal pelvis and ureter. *Cancer Epidemiol Biomarkers Prev* 2006;15:1051–3.

43. Chow WH, Lindblad P, Gridley G, Nyren O, McLaughlin JK, Linet MS, Pennello GA, Adami HO, Fraumeni JF Jr. Risk of urinary tract cancers following kidney or ureter stones. *J Natl Cancer Inst* 1997;89:1453–7.

44. Azemar MD, Comperat E, Richard F, Cussenot O, Roupret M. Bladder recurrence after surgery for upper urinary tract urothelial cell carcinoma: frequency, risk factors, and surveillance. *Urol Oncol* 2011;29:130–6.

45. Catto JW, Yates DR, Rehman I, Azzouzi AR, Patterson J, Sibony M, Cussenot O, Hamdy FC. Behavior of urothelial carcinoma with respect to anatomical location. *J Urol* 2007;177:1715–20.

46. Langner C, Hutterer G, Chromecki T, Rehak P, Zigeuner R. Patterns of invasion and histological growth as prognostic indicators in urothelial carcinoma of the upper urinary tract. *Virchows Arch* 2006;448:604–11.

47. Lopez-Beltran A. Immunohistochemical markers in evaluation of urinary and bladder tumors. *Anal Quant Cytol Histol* 2007;29:121–2.

48. Lopez-Beltran A, Cheng L. Histologic variants of urothelial carcinoma: differential diagnosis and clinical implications. *Hum Pathol* 2006;37:1371–88.

49. Lopez-Beltran A, Bassi P, Pavone-Macaluso M, Montironi R. Handling and pathology reporting of specimens with carcinoma of the urinary bladder, ureter, and renal pelvis. *Eur Urol* 2004;45:257–66.

50. Jones TD, Wang M, Eble JN, MacLennan GT, Lopez-Beltran A, Zhang S, Cocco A, Cheng L. Molecular evidence supporting field effect in urothelial carcinogenesis. *Clin Cancer Res* 2005;11:6512–9.

51. Roig JM, Amerigo J, Velasco FJ, Gimenez A, Guerrero E, Soler JL, Gonzalez-Campora R. Lymphoepithelioma-like carcinoma of ureter. *Histopathology* 2001;39:106–7.

52. Lopez-Beltran A, Escudero AL, Cavazzana AO, Spagnoli LG, Vicioso-Recio L. Sarcomatoid transitional cell carcinoma of the renal pelvis. A report of five cases with clinical, pathological, immunohistochemical and DNA ploidy analysis. *Pathol Res Pract* 1996;192:1218–24.

53. Leroy X, Leteurtre E, De La Taille A, Augusto D, Biserte J, Gosselin B. Microcystic transitional cell carcinoma: a report of 2 cases arising in the renal pelvis. *Arch Pathol Lab Med* 2002;126:859–61.

54. Kobayashi M, Hashimoto S, Hara Y, Kobayashi Y, Nakamura S, Tokue A, Shimizu H. [Squamous carcinoma with pseudosarcomatous stroma of the renal pelvis and ureter: a case report]. *Hinyokika Kiyo* 1994;40:55–9.

55. Kotliar SN, Wood CG, Schaeffer AJ, Oyasu R. Transitional cell carcinoma exhibiting clear cell features. A differential diagnosis for clear cell adenocarcinoma of the urinary tract. *Arch Pathol Lab Med* 1995;119:79–81.

56. Fukunaga M, Ushigome S. Lymphoepithelioma-like carcinoma of the renal pelvis: a case report with immunohistochemical analysis and in situ hybridization for the Epstein-Barr viral genome. *Mod Pathol* 1998;11:1252–6.

57. Thiel DD, Igel TC, Wu KJ. Sarcomatoid carcinoma of transitional cell origin confined to renal pelvis. *Urology* 2006;67:622 e9–11.

58. Holmang S, Thomsen J, Johansson SL. Micropapillary carcinoma of the renal pelvis and ureter. *J Urol* 2006;175:463–7.

59. Baydar D, Amin MB, Epstein JI. Osteoclast-rich undifferentiated carcinomas of the urinary tract. *Mod Pathol* 2006;19:161–71.

60. Hes O, Curik R, Mainer K, Michal M. Urothelial signet-ring cell carcinoma of the renal pelvis with collagenous spherulosis: a case report. *Int J Surg Pathol* 2005;13:375–8.

61. Shimasaki N, Inoue K, Nishigawa H, Kuroda N, Shuin T. Combined small cell carcinoma and sarcomatoid squamous cell carcinoma in the renal pelvis. *Int J Urol* 2005;12:686–9.

62. Acikalin MF, Kabukcuoglu S, Can C. Sarcomatoid carcinoma of the renal pelvis with giant cell tumor-like features: case report with immunohistochemical findings. *Int J Urol* 2005;12:199–203.

63. Shiga Y, Kawai K, Shimazui T, Iijima T, Noguchi M, Akaza H. Case of alpha-fetoprotein-producing transitional cell carcinoma of the renal pelvis. *Int J Urol* 2004;11:117–8.

64. Lopez-Beltran A. Bladder cancer: clinical and pathological profile. *Scand J Urol Nephrol Suppl* 2008:95–109.

65. Wang X, MacLennan GT, Zhang S, Montironi R, Lopez-Beltran A, Tan PH, Foster S, Baldridge LA, Cheng L. Sarcomatoid carcinoma of the upper urinary tract: clinical outcome and molecular characterization. *Hum Pathol* 2009;40:211–7.

66. Lopez-Beltran A, Requena MJ, Luque RJ, Alvarez-Kindelan J, Quintero A, Blanca AM, Rodriguez ME, Siendones E, Montironi R. Cyclin D3 expression in primary Ta/T1 bladder cancer. *J Pathol* 2006;209:106–13.

67. Onishi T, Franco OE, Shibahara T, Arima K, Sugimura Y. Papillary adenocarcinoma of the renal pelvis and ureter producing carcinoembryonic antigen, carbohydrate antigen 19–9 and carbohydrate antigen 125. *Int J Urol* 2005;12:214–6.

68. Lopez-Beltran A, Luque RJ, Alvarez-Kindelan J, Quintero A, Merlo F, Carrasco JC, Requena MJ, Montironi R. Prognostic factors in stage T1 grade 3 bladder cancer survival: the role of G1-S modulators (p53, p21Waf1, p27Kip1, Cyclin D1, and Cyclin D3) and proliferation index (Ki67-MIB1). *Eur Urol* 2004;45:606–12.

69. Langner C, Hutterer G, Chromecki T, Winkelmayer I, Rehak P, Zigeuner R. pT classification, grade, and vascular invasion as prognostic indicators in urothelial carcinoma of the upper urinary tract. *Mod Pathol* 2006;19:272–9.

70. Zigeuner R, Shariat SF, Margulis V, Karakiewicz PI, Roscigno M, Weizer A, Kikuchi E, Remzi M, Raman JD, Bolenz C, Bensalah K, Capitanio U, et al. Tumour necrosis is an indicator of aggressive biology in patients with urothelial carcinoma of the upper urinary tract. *Eur Urol* 2009;57:575–81.

71. Tsai YS, Tzai TS, Chow NH, Wu CL. Frequency and clinicopathologic correlates of ErbB1, ErbB2, and ErbB3 immunoreactivity in urothelial tumors of upper urinary tract. *Urology* 2005;66:1197–202.

72. Kamijima S, Tobe T, Suyama T, Ueda T, Igarashi T, Ichikawa T, Ito H. The prognostic value of p53, Ki–67 and matrix metalloproteinases MMP–2 and MMP–9 in transitional cell carcinoma of the renal pelvis and ureter. *Int J Urol* 2005;12:941–7.

73. Miyata Y, Kanda S, Nomata K, Eguchi J, Kanetake H. Expression of cyclooxygenase-2 and EP4 receptor in transitional cell carcinoma of the upper urinary tract. *J Urol* 2005;173:56–60.

74. Simon R, Jones PA, Sidransky D, Cordon-Cardo C, Cairns P, Amin MB, Gasser T, Knowles MA. Genetics and predictive factors of non-invasive urothelial neoplasias. In: Eble JN, Sauder G, Epstein JI, Sesterhenn IA, eds. WHO Classification of Non-invasive Papillary Urothelial Tumors. In World Health Organization Classification of Tumors. Pathology and Gentics of Tumors of the Urinary System and Male Genital Organs, Lyon, France: IARCC Press, 2004.

75. Hartmann A, Schlake G, Zaak D, Hungerhuber E, Hofstetter A, Hofstaedter F, Knuechel R. Occurrence of chromosome 9 and p53 alterations in multifocal dysplasia and carcinoma in situ of human urinary bladder. *Cancer Res* 2002;62:809–18.

76. Ericson KM, Isinger AP, Isfoss BL, Nilbert MC. Low frequency of defective mismatch repair in a population-based series of upper urothelial carcinoma. *BMC Cancer* 2005;5:23.

77. Maloney KE, Wiener JS, Walther PJ. Oncogenic human papillomaviruses are rarely associated with squamous cell carcinoma of the bladder: evaluation by differential polymerase chain reaction. *J Urol* 1994;151:360–4.

78. Wiener JS, Walther PJ. A high association of oncogenic human papillomaviruses with carcinomas of the female urethra: polymerase chain reaction-based analysis of multiple histological types. *J Urol* 1994;151:49–53.

79. Lopez-Beltran A, Nogales F, Donne CH, Sayag JL. Adenocarcinoma of the urachus showing extensive calcification and stromal osseous metaplasia. *Urol Int* 1994;53:110–3.

80. Nogales FF, Andujar M, Beltran AL, Martinez JL, Zuluaga A. Adenocarcinoma of the renal pelvis. A report of two cases. *Urol Int* 1994;52:172–5.

81. Torres Gomez FJ, Torres Olivera FJ. [Renal pelvis mucinous carcinoma. Case report]. *Arch Esp Urol* 2006;59:300–2.

82. Talwar N, Dargan P, Arora MP, Sharma A, Sen AK. Primary squamous cell carcinoma of the renal pelvis masquerading as pyonephrosis: a case report. *Indian J Pathol Microbiol* 2006;49:418–20.

83. Ng KF, Chuang CK, Chang PL, Chu SH, Wallace CG, Chen TC. Absence of Epstein-Barr virus infection in squamous cell carcinoma of upper urinary tract and urinary bladder. *Urology* 2006;68:775–7.

84. Reuter VE. Urethra. In: Bostwick DG, Cheng L, eds. Urologic Surgical Pathology, 2nd ed. Philadelphia: Elsevier/Mosby, 2008:595–614.

85. Boyle M, Gaffney EF, Thurston A. Paraganglioma of the prostatic urethra. A report of three cases and a review of the literature. *Br J Urol* 1996;77:445–8.

86. Fine SW, Chan TY, Epstein JI. Inverted papillomas of the prostatic urethra. *Am J Surg Pathol* 2006;30:975–9.

87. Sung MT, Maclennan GT, Lopez-Beltran A, Montironi R, Cheng L. Natural history of urothelial inverted papilloma. *Cancer* 2006;107:2622–7.

88. Cheng L, Montironi R, Bostwick DG. Villous adenoma of the urinary tract: a report of 23 cases, including 8 with coexistent adenocarcinoma. *Am J Surg Pathol* 1999;23:764–71.

89. Noel JC, Fayt I, Aguilar SF. Adenosquamous carcinoma arising in villous adenoma from female vulvar urethra. *Acta Obstet Gynecol Scand* 2006;85:373–6.

90. Kuroda N, Shiotsu T, Ohara M, Hirouchi T, Mizuno K, Miyazaki E. Female urethral adenocarcinoma with a heterogeneous phenotype. *APMIS* 2006;114:314–8.

91. Achiche MA, Bouhaoula MH, Madani M, Azaiez M, Chebil M, Ayed M. [Primary transitional cell carcinoma of the bulbar urethra]. *Prog Urol* 2005;15:1145–8.

92. Shalev M, Mistry S, Kernen K, Miles BJ. Squamous cell carcinoma in a female urethral diverticulum. *Urology* 2002;59:773.

93. Hruby G, Choo R, Lehman M, Herschorn S, Kapusta L. Female clear cell adenocarcinoma arising within a urethral diverticulum. *Can J Urol* 2000;7:1160–3.

94. Velazquez EF, Soskin A, Bock A, Codas R, Cai G, Barreto JE, Cubilla AL. Epithelial abnormalities and precancerous lesions of anterior urethra in patients with penile carcinoma: a report of 89 cases. *Mod Pathol* 2005;18:917–23.

95. Yvgenia R, Ben Meir D, Sibi J, Koren R. Mucinous adenocarcinoma of posterior urethra. Report of a case. *Pathol Res Pract* 2005;201:137–40.

96. Cimentepe E, Bayrak O, Unsal A, Koc A, Ataoglu O, Balbay MD. Urethral adenocarcinoma mimicking urethral caruncle. *Int Urogynecol J Pelvic Floor Dysfunct* 2006;17:96–8.

97. Jayamohan Y, Urs L, Rowland RG, Woolums S, Lele SM. Periurethral carcinosarcoma: a report of 2 cases with a review of the literature. *Arch Pathol Lab Med* 2005;129:e91–3.

98. Stein JP, Clark P, Miranda G, Cai J, Groshen S, Skinner DG. Urethral tumor recurrence following cystectomy and urinary diversion: clinical and pathological characteristics in 768 male patients. *J Urol* 2005;173:1163–8.

99. Wiedemann A, Muller H, Jaussi J, Rabs U. [Mesonephric carcinoma of the urethra. A case report]. *Urologe A* 2005;44:396–400.

100. Kato H, Kobayashi S, Islam AM, Nishizawa O. Female para-urethral adenocarcinoma: histological and immunohistochemical study. *Int J Urol* 2005;12:117–9.

101. Maclennan GT, Kirkali Z, Cheng L. Histologic grading of noninvasive papillary urothelial neoplasms. *Eur Urol* 2007;51:889–98.

102. Copp HL, Wong IY, Krishnan C, Malhotra S, Kennedy WA. Clinical presentation and urachal remnant pathology: implications for treatment. *J Urol* 2009;182:1921–4.

103. Lopez-Beltran A, Escudero AL. Human papillomavirus and bladder cancer. *Biomed Pharmacother* 1997;51:252–7.

104. Nagahara A, Kawagoe M, Matsumoto F, Tohda A, Shimada K, Yasui M, Inoue M, Kawa K, Hamana K, Nakayama M. Botryoid Wilms' tumor of the renal pelvis extending into the bladder. *Urology* 2006;67:845 e15–7.

105. Ferrero Doria R, Garcia Victor F, Moreno Perez F, Gasso Matoses M, Diaz Calleja E. [Cavernous haemangioma as the cause of ureteral pyelic junction obstruction]. *Arch Esp Urol* 2005;58:960–3.

106. Kapusta LR, Weiss MA, Ramsay J, Lopez-Beltran A, Srigley JR. Inflammatory myofibroblastic tumors of the kidney: a clinicopathologic and immunohistochemical study of 12 cases. *Am J Surg Pathol* 2003;27:658–66.

107. Ho PH, Chen SY, Hsueh C, Lai MW, Chao HC, Chang PY. Inflammatory myofibroblastic tumor of renal pelvis presenting with prolonged fever and abdominal pain in children: report of 1 case and review of literature. *J Pediatr Surg* 2005;40:e35–7.

108. Hirsch MS, Dal Cin P, Fletcher CD. ALK expression in pseudosarcomatous myofibroblastic proliferations of the genitourinary tract. *Histopathology* 2006;48:569–78.

109. Peyromaure M, Mao K, Comperat E, de Pinieux G, Beuzeboc P, Zerbib M. [Leiomyosarcoma of the renal pelvis]. *Prog Urol* 2005;15:538–9.

110. Herawi M, Parwani AV, Edlow D, Smolev JK, Epstein JI. Glomus tumor of renal pelvis: a case report and review of the literature. *Hum Pathol* 2005;36:299–302.

111. Parada D, Moreira O, Gledhill T, Luigii JC, Paez A, Pardo M. Cellular pseudosarcomatous fibroepithelial stromal polyp of the renal pelvis. *APMIS* 2005;113:70–4.

112. Dell'Atti C, Missere M, Restaino G, Carlino S, Cucci E, Ciuffreda M, Sallustio G. Primary lymphoma of the female urethra. *Rays* 2005;30:269–72.

113. Ozel B, Ballard C. Urethral and paraurethral leiomyomas in the female patient. *Int Urogynecol J Pelvic Floor Dysfunct* 2006;17:93–5.

114. Daneshmand S. Adenomatous polyp of the verumontanum causing bladder outlet obstruction. *ScientificWorldJournal* 2004;4 (Suppl 1):89–91.

115. Bozas G, Tassidou A, Moulopoulos LA, Constandinidis C, Bamias A,

Dimopoulos MA. Non-Hodgkin's lymphoma of the renal pelvis. *Clin Lymphoma Myeloma* 2006;6:404–6.

116. Vizcaino JR, Macedo-Dias JA, Teixeira-de-Sousa JM, Silva RM,

Carpenter S. Pseudotumour of renal pelvis: Liesegang rings mimicking a solid neoplasm of the renal pelvis. *Histopathology* 2005;47:115–7.

117. Sanchez-Ortiz R, Huang SF, Tamboli

P, Prieto VG, Hester G, Pettaway CA. Melanoma of the penis, scrotum and male urethra: a 40-year single institution experience. *J Urol* 2005;173:1958–65.

Chapter 29

Molecular Determinants of Tumor Recurrence

Bladder Pathology, First Edition. Liang Cheng, Antonio Lopez-Beltran, David G. Bostwick.
© 2012 Wiley-Blackwell. Published 2012 by John Wiley & Sons, Inc.

Overview

Urinary bladder cancer is a heterogeneous disease with diverse morphologic and clinical manifestations.[1-3] Clinical and pathological parameters are widely used to predict clinical outcome, but these parameters have limited utility for an individual patient. Three major risks for patients after initial management of tumor include recurrence, progression into higher grade and higher stage tumors, and metastasis. These risks are well known for each stage of the disease, but are not sufficiently quantifiable for prospectively assessing the risk in individual patients.

Tumor recurrence is a major clinical concern for patients with urothelial carcinoma of the urinary bladder (**Table 29-1**). The incidence of tumor recurrence for a bladder cancer patient ranges from 50% to 90%, and 25% of cancers that recur ultimately progress to invasive cancers.[3-9] Despite radical cystectomy and systemic therapy, 50% of patients with advanced stage bladder cancer will eventually die from metastasis.[8,10-13]

Eighty percent of patients with urothelial bladder cancer suffer from recurrence within one to two years of initial treatment. Traditional morphological analysis is of limited utility for identifying cases in which recurrence will occur. Reliable parameters for tumor recurrence risk would be valuable when advising patients about surveillance measures and aggressiveness of therapy. Molecular and genetic analyses offer new perspectives on the prediction of bladder tumor recurrence (**Table 29-2**).[4,5,11,14-17]

Table 29-1   Clinical Impact of Molecular Prediction of Recurrence

High grade urothelial cancers are less likely to be completely excised by transurethral resection and, therefore, are more likely to recur.
Eighty percent of urothelial bladder cancers recur. These recurred tumors tend to have grade and stage progression.
Routine clinical and pathological parameters are widely used to predict patients' clinical outcomes, but these parameters are of limited utility for predicting tumor recurrence.
Recently discovered molecular alterations in bladder cancer have shown potential for predicting tumor recurrence.
Bladder cancer is often a multifocal disease with anatomically separate tumors arising simultaneously or sequentially. Recent molecular analyses of multifocal bladder tumors suggest that there is a field effect of transforming agents influencing the entire urothelial surface.
Cancer stem cells may be the cellular seeds of tumor recurrence. Tumor progression and field cancerization may be important mechanisms for these recurrence events.

Table 29-2   Use of Molecular Markers to Predict Tumor Recurrence

A gene expression signature of a urothelial cancer could be used to predict tumor recurrence. Molecular signature of tumor could be at the chromosomal, allelic, or genomic level.
FGFR3 and *TP53* mutations are findings that consistently define low and high grade bladder cancers, respectively.
Genetic alterations determined by loss of heterozygosity and fluorescence in situ hybridization analysis could classify patients according to probability of bladder tumor recurrence.
Global assessment by gene expression profiling could potentially identify other markers useful in the clinical setting.
Aberrant promoter hypermethylation is an important mechanism for inactivation of tumor suppressor genes, their regulators and downstream factors. Histone modification may also play a role in the bladder cancer recurrence. Epigenetic alteration of certain gene promoters is associated with increased or decreased risk of tumor recurrence.
Multiple markers provide a global assessment to more definitively predict clinical tumor behavior. A combined biomarker approach is a powerful tool for predicting tumor recurrence.

Molecular Pathways Linked to Tumor Recurrence

The molecular changes may additionally prove useful for developing preventive and therapeutic strategies for bladder cancer.[4,5,11,14-24] Two major molecular pathways have been identified in bladder cancer: the fibroblast growth factor receptor 3 (*FGFR3*)- and *TP53*-associated pathways (**Table 29-3**). These two pathways are characterized by different genomic, epigenetic, and gene expression alterations. Their outcomes correlate with the markedly different clinical and pathologic features of both relatively indolent low grade cancers and aggressive high grade cancers. As such, these molecular findings are potentially useful for counseling patients and for assessing risk of recurrence and biological aggressiveness of a patient's tumor (see also **Chapters 30 to 34**).

FGFR3 Mutation is Associated with a Low Risk of Recurrence

As noted previously, it seems likely that bladder carcinomas arise through at least two separate mechanisms.[4,5,11,14-24] *FGFR3* mutation is strongly associated with low recurrence rates in superficial papillary bladder cancers.[15,25-27] Van Rhijn et al. analyzed 72 bladder cancer patients and

Table 29-3 Divergent Carcinogenesis Pathways of Bladder Cancer

FGFR3 and *TP53* gene mutations define two distinct tumorigenesis pathways of bladder cancer.

FGFR3 mutations are frequently found in exons 7, 10, and 15; *TP53* mutations are frequently found in exons 5, 7, 8, and 10.

FGFR3 and *TP53* mutations with changes in associated downstream factors, alterations of apoptosis pathways, modifications of cell adhesion molecules, and changes in epigenetic control tumor suppressor regulators and chromosomal rearrangements have been proposed as components of tumor recurrence panels.

FGFR3 mutations are associated with low recurrence rates of superficial, low grade papillary urothelial carcinoma.

TP53 mutation is associated with high cancer grade, invasive biologic behavior, and enhanced risk of recurrence.

About 5% of bladder cancers carrying both *FGFR3* and *TP53* mutations. This may represent a third pathway leading to high grade carcinoma.

found *FGFR3* mutation in 34 of 53 pTaG1–2 bladder cancers.[28] None of the 19 patients with higher stage tumors had *FGFR3* mutations. A 12-month followup study on 57 patients with superficial bladder cancer revealed that 61% of the patients in the wild type *FGFR3* group developed recurrence, compared with only 20% of patients in the mutant group. The per year recurrence rate was 4.7-fold lower for tumors with *FGFR3* mutation than for tumors with wild type *FGFR3* gene.[28]

Hernandez et al. performed a large prospective study to evaluate the frequency and prognostic value of *FGFR3* mutations in 747 patients with nonmuscle-invasive bladder tumors.[29] They correlated *FGFR3* mutations with recurrence, progression, and cancer-associated mortality.[29] The median prospective followup time was 62.6 months. *FGFR3* exon 7 and 10 mutations were analyzed by direct sequencing. They found that *FGFR3* mutations were more common among low malignant potential neoplasms (77%) and TaG1/TaG2 tumors (61%/58%) than among TaG3 tumors (34%) and T1G3 tumors (17%). In the multivariate analysis of all noninvasive tumors, mutations were paradoxically associated with increased risk of recurrence. However, in the stratified analyses, only patients with TaG1 tumors had a significantly higher risk of recurrence, but recurrence did not lead to worse outcomes in these patients.[29] The results strongly support the notion that *FGFR3* mutations characterize a subgroup of bladder cancers with good prognosis, but that patients with mutant TaG1 tumors may have a higher risk of recurrence.

Increased FGFR3 protein expression is also found in papillary neoplasm with low malignant potential (PUNLMP). Barbisan et al. studied 80 PUNLMP cases

and demonstrated that 81% of the 41 nonrecurring tumors showed strong FGFR3 expression compared to only 56% of the 39 recurrent cases. Strong expression of FGFR3 predicted the nonrecurrence of PUNLMP.[30]

FGFR3 mutations were also found in inverted papillomas of bladder.[24] Lott et al. analyzed 20 cases of inverted papilloma of the urinary tract. Mutations of the *FGFR3* (exon 7, 10, and 15) and *TP53* genes were evaluated by DNA sequencing.[24] Point mutations of the *FGFR3* gene were identified in 45% (9/20) of inverted papillomas, with four cases exhibiting mutations at multiple exons. Seven cases had exon 7 mutations at R248C, S249T, L259L, P260P, and V266M. Two cases had exon 10 and 15 mutations at A366D, H412H, E627D, D641N, and H643. Five of the exon 15 mutation cases had N653H. The most frequent mutation was identified at R248C. None of the inverted papillomas exhibited mutations in *TP53*. During a mean followup of 78 months, none of these patients had recurrence or developed urothelial carcinoma. These findings support the concept that low grade and low stage urothelial neoplasms arise in a background of molecular changes that are distinctly different from the molecular changes of high grade and high stage urothelial cancers.[24]

TP53 Mutation is Associated with a High Risk of Recurrence

Numerous studies have indicated that *TP53* mutations are strongly associated with high tumor grade, invasive behavior, risk of recurrence, and adverse clinical outcome. As discussed above, *TP53* mutations are typically mutually exclusive of *FGFR3* mutations.[18,26,31] Studies of primary and recurrent urothelial cancers for *TP53* mutation at exons 5 to 8 found that *TP53* mutations occur predominantly in highly malignant, invasive tumors. High grade primary tumors and their metachronous recurrences usually harbor the same *TP53* mutation, indicating a common clonal origin.[32]

In the evaluation of *TP53* genetic status on 75 noninvasive urothelial carcinoma cases, Ecke et al. found that the overall tumor recurrence rate was 76% (57/75). Tumor recurrence frequency was 69% (34/49) in patients with wild type *TP53*, and 89% (23/26) in patients with *TP53* mutations. The progression-free survival was significantly shorter in patients with *TP53* mutations, and the frequency of tumor progression was significantly higher in mutated compared to wild type tumors.[33] The results suggest that *TP53* mutation predicts patients at a higher risk of tumor recurrence and progression.

Hernandez et al. performed a followup study on 119 patients with stage T1 grade 3 urothelial carcinoma.[34] They examined the correlation between *TP53* or *FGFR3* mutations and tumor recurrence. *FGFR3* mutations were detected in 17% of tumors, and *TP53* mutations were found in 66% of these high grade tumors. The combined mutation distribution (*FGFR3/TP53*) was as follows: wt/wt (35%), mut/wt (8%), wt/mut (49%), and mut/mut (9%). This pattern of genomic defects is drastically different from that of low grade superficial urothelial carcinomas. These T1G3 tumors may be at the crossroads of the two main bladder cancer molecular pathways and may represent a third genesis with activation of both pathways concurrently.[34]

TP53 mutations have long been proposed as a predictor of patients' clinical outcomes. Nonetheless, reported research works have shown conflicting results, ranging from independent determinant,[35,36] to association with patients' clinical outcomes but not independently predictive,[37] to unrelated to outcome in patients with bladder cancer.[38,39] It is noteworthy that Malats et al.[38] reviewed 168 publications from 117 studies to evaluate the predictive power of *TP53* mutation as a marker of bladder cancer recurrence, progression, and mortality. They found that 27% of studies that assessed *TP53* overexpression as a predictor recurrence by multivariate tests showed a significant association. The mean values in these studies for progression and mortality were 50% and 29%, respectively. The authors suggested that in studies that used Cox models, the findings could be overestimates because of publication and reporting bias. The results showed that after 10 years of research, evidence is still not sufficient to conclude whether or not changes in *TP53* act as markers of outcome in patients with bladder cancer. More studies are needed to provide sufficient data to clarify this issue.

Gene Expression Signature to Predict Bladder Cancer Recurrence

High-throughput DNA microarrays allow identification of the most prevalent and relevant alteration patterns in bladder tumors. Clusters of differentially expressed genes identify biomarkers to discriminate differences in histopathology or in clinical outcome. Those profiles may also identify potential therapeutic targets. Gene expression signatures to predict aggressive tumor behavior at the earliest clinical stages are urgently needed not only to select current treatment, but also to identify targets for developing future treatments.[4,5,14]

Gene expression profiling provides a global view of functional DNA alterations. Combining this understanding of the genotype with longitudinal studies of the clinical phenotype for each tumor will open a new window on clinical outcome. Array-based molecular profiling technology enables the physician to obtain a more complete picture of gene expression networks and thus to improve the prediction of recurrence risk. Specific bladder tumor subtypes have distinct gene expression profiles.

Dyrskjot et al.[40] report the identification of clinically relevant subclasses of bladder carcinoma using expression microarray analysis of 40 bladder cancers. To delineate non-recurring Ta tumors from frequently recurring Ta tumors, the expression patterns in 31 tumors were analyzed. In an independent series, the validation study confirmed the clinical utility of molecular classifiers to predict the recurrence risk for patients initially diagnosed with nonmuscle-invasive bladder cancer. The authors also built a 32-gene molecular classifier using a cross-validation approach that was able to classify benign and muscle-invasive tumors. The genetic classification correlated closely with pathological staging in an independent test set of 68 tumors.

It has been suggested that the origin and progression of bladder carcinoma result from accumulation of specific genetic or epigenetic alterations, often termed genetic signatures. Studies in bladder cancer have established links between specific expression patterns and clinical outcome. Gene expression profiles could also help select not only genes associated with tumor recurrence, but also expression associated with invasion and progression. To identify bladder cancers with a high risk of intravesical recurrence after transurethral bladder tumor resection, Ito et al. studied 20 invasive and 22 superficial human bladder tumors from 34 patients with known outcomes.[41] Microarray cDNA hybridization identified 25 genes whose expression was associated with recurrence, including *PAK1*. *PAK1* expression was also associated with recurrence in a validation set of 86 bladder cancers. In these tumors, high *PAK1* expression was associated with nearly threefold greater risk of recurrence at 24 months than the risk in tumors with median or decreased expression. High PAK1 protein expression assessed by immunohistochemistry was an independent factor associated with recurrence in multivariate analysis.[41] The authors postulate that *PAK1* actively promotes recurrence of bladder urothelial carcinoma.

DNA microarray expression profiling may also identify genes underlying clinical heterogeneity of bladder cancer. In another cDNA array study, 40 cases of superficial low grade bladder carcinoma, including 20 recurrent and 20 nonrecurrent cases, were evaluated.[42] Genes identified in the array included matrix metalloproteinase, oncogenes and cell cycle-related genes. By this analysis, matrix metalloproteinase-1, -2, -9, -12, and -15, transforming growth factor-β1, vascular endothelial growth factor, and *fos* were upregulated in recurrent cases. Overexpression of matrix metalloproteinase-1 and -12, transforming growth factor-β1, vascular endothelial growth factor, and *fos* predicted recurrence even for superficial low grade bladder cancer.[42] In another study, a two-way clustering algorithm classified tumor samples according to clinical outcome as superficial, invasive, or metastasizing.[43]

Gene expression profiling of human bladder cancers affords a window into the causes of cancer recurrence and progression and identifies patients with distinct clinical phenotypes.

Combined Biomarkers as Predictors of Tumor Recurrence

Evolution in the research of bladder cancer recurrence has moved from a single marker or pathway to multiple markers and global assessment for prediction of clinical tumor behavior (see also **Chapters 33** and **34** for further discussion). Although markers such as Ki67 directly indicate high proliferation activity and are significantly related to tumor recurrence, they are unreliable for assessing individual risk.[44–46] High expression of vascular endothelial growth factor and high microvessel density are associated with early recurrence of nonmuscle-invasive bladder cancer.[47,48] Combined markers or pathways may predict recurrence risk more accurately and precisely than prediction by any single marker.

Identifying a central theme for predicting cancer recurrence has been a focus of many researchers. For the last decade, research efforts have resulted in a long list of potential molecular markers for bladder cancer recurrence. Mutations of *FGFR3* and *TP53* genes, alterations of apoptosis pathways, modifications of cell adhesion molecules, changes in epigenetic control of tumor suppressor regulators, and chromosomal rearrangements have been put forward as recurrence predictors. Some molecular markers hold considerable promise to assess the risk of recurrence, and only a few studies have analyzed the performance of multiple molecular markers concurrently. Van Rhijn et al. investigated 286 bladder urothelial cancer patients for *FGFR3* status and expression levels of MIB1, p53, and p27Kip1.[27] *FGFR3* mutations were detected in 172 (60%) of 286 cancers. *FGFR3* mutations were detected in 88% of grade 1 cancers, but detected only in 16% of grade 3 cancers. Aberrant expression patterns of MIB1, p53, and p27Kip1 were found in 5%, 2%, and 3% of grade 1 tumors but in 85%, 60%, and 56% of grade 3 tumors. In multivariate analysis with recurrence rate, progression, and disease-specific survival as endpoints, the combination of *FGFR3* and MIB1 proved independently significant for all endpoints. The authors suggested that the *FGFR3* mutation combining with MIB1, p53, and p27Kip1 could provide a new, simple, and highly reproducible tool for making clinical decisions in bladder cancer patients.

Yurakh et al. investigated 84 patients with bladder cancer by detection of homozygous deletion of p14ARF, p15INK4B, p16INK4A, loss of heterozygosity (LOH) of the locus 9p21, *TP53* mutations, and by measuring immunohistochemical expression of p53, p16, p14, p21, p27, pRb, Ki67, MDM2, and cyclin D1 proteins in relation to overall survival, recurrence-free survival, and progression-free survival.[49] Recurrence-free survival was shorter in cases with p14ARF, p15INK4B, p16INK4A homozygous deletion, low p14 expression, and high Ki67 index. Homozygous deletions of 9p21 and downregulation of p14 are independent prognostic factors for early recurrence of bladder cancer.[49] Chatterjee et al. investigated the combined effects of p53, p21, and pRb alterations for predicting bladder cancer progression from 164 patients with invasive or high grade recurrent urothelial carcinoma.[36] After stratifying by stage, the authors found that these altered proteins remained significantly associated with time to recurrence and overall survival. Analysis of molecular determinants in combination provides more reliable prognostic information than does any single determinant alone. However, even combined molecular markers still have false-positive and false-negative results for some cases.

Shariat et al. analyzed 191 patients with pTa to pT3N0M0 urothelial bladder cancers using the combined biomarker approach (**Figs. 29-1** and **29-2**).[50] All patients were treated with radical cystectomy and bilateral lymphadenectomy, and this cohort had a median followup of 3.1 years. The combined immunohistochemical biomarkers included p53, pRb, p21, p16, and cyclin E1. When used together, these markers improved the power to predict bladder cancer recurrence compared to established prediction tools.[50] Univariate analyses indicated that the number of altered biomarkers had a greater predictive accuracy for disease recurrence than did pathological stage, lymphovascular invasion, patient age, or coexisting carcinoma in situ (CIS). The predictive power and accuracy of altered biomarkers for tumor recurrence increased as the number of altered biomarkers increased. Regression coefficients in the full multivariate model revealed that patients with three and four to five altered biomarkers were 3.8 and 11.2 times more likely to experience disease recurrence than were patients bearing zero to two altered biomarkers.[50] Risk of recurrence and cancer-specific mortality were more strongly associated with the increasing number of altered biomarkers than with increasing T stage.

Altered molecular mechanisms of apoptosis also play an important role in the carcinogenesis of urothelium. Allowing neoplastic cells to survive longer and acquire resistance to harmful stresses is a prerequisite for tumor progression. Combined apoptosis biomarkers were investigated for the ability to predict bladder cancer recurrence. A recent study of multiple apoptosis markers BCL-2, CASP3, p53, and survivin, found that simultaneously altered apoptosis markers are associated independently with increased risk of recurrence.[51] There appears to be a cooperative effect of BCL-2, CASP3, p53, and survivin on bladder cancer progression as well as recurrence.[51] Immunoperoxidase

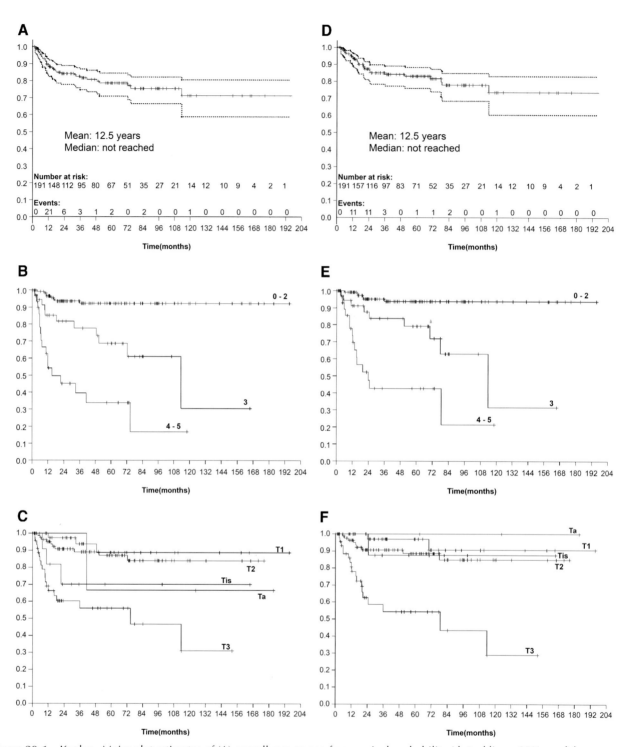

Figure 29-1 Kaplan–Meier plot estimates of (A) overall recurrence-free survival probability (dotted lines, 95% confidence intervals); (B) recurrence-free survival probability stratified according to the number of altered biomarkers; (C) recurrence-free survival probability stratified according to pathologic stage; (D) overall bladder cancer-specific survival probability (dotted lines, 95% confidence intervals); (E) bladder cancer-specific survival probability stratified according to the number of altered biomarkers; (F) the overall bladder cancer-specific survival probability stratified according to pathologic stage. (From Ref. 50; with permission.)

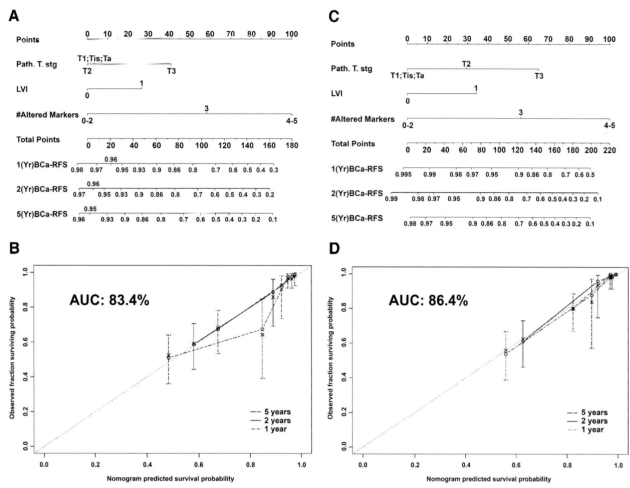

Figure 29-2   (A) Postoperative nomogram predicting one-, two-, and five-year risk of disease recurrence in patients with pTa-3 N0M0 urothelial carcinoma of the bladder treated with radical cystectomy and bilateral lymphadenectomy. Instructions for physicians: Locate the patient's T stage on the sexaxis. Draw a straight line up to the pointsaxis to determine how many points toward recurrence the patient should receive. Repeat this process for each of the remaining axes, drawing a straight line each time to the points axis. Sum the points received for each predictive variable and locate this number on the totalpointsaxis. Draw a straight line down from the total points axis to one of the recurrence-free prediction axes for the patient's specific risk of remaining free from recurrence for one, two, and five years. (B) Calibration plot of the postoperative nomogram predicting risk of disease recurrence after radical cystectomy and bilateral lymphadenectomy. (C) Postoperative nomogram predicting one-, two-, and five-year risk of cancer-specific survival in patients with pTa-3 N0M0 urothelial carcinoma of the bladder treated with radical cystectomy and bilateral lymphadenectomy. (D) Calibration plot of the postoperative nomogram predicting risk of cancer-specific survival after radical cystectomy and bilateral lymphadenectomy. (From Ref. 50; with permission.)

staining for these four apoptosis-related markers in tissue microarrays from 226 consecutive bladder tumors showed altered expression in 32% to 64% of the cases. These alterations were associated with a 1.7-fold to 2.7-fold increase in risk of recurrence, and with a 2.0-fold to 3.2-fold increase in risk of cancer-specific mortality during the 37-month median followup. Assessment of combined apoptosis markers provides prognostic information that could help to identify the patient with a high risk of disease recurrence.

Epigenetic Alterations as Predictors of Tumor Recurrence

Promoter CpG island methylation is a key regulator of gene transcription and a guardian of genomic stability (see also **Chapters 32** and **34**).[52–54] Alterations in DNA methylation patterns are frequently detected in human tumors. Hypermethylation of normally unmethylated CpG islands in the promoter regions of tumor suppressor genes causes loss of gene expression. In bladder carcinoma, promoter region hypermethylation and decreased expression of tumor suppressor genes such as *RUNX3*, *p16*, and *E-cadherin* have been reported.[55] Aberrant promoter hypermethylation of other genes, such as *hMLH1*, *MGMT*, *VHL*, *DAPK*, and *GSTP1*, has also been observed.[56] There is increasing evidence for a role of epigenetic gene silencing in superficial bladder cancer tumorigenesis.[57,58] Analysis of the methylation status of 20 cancer-associated genes (*p14ARF*, *p16*, *STAT1*, *SOCS1*, *DR3*, *DR6*, *PIG7*, *BCL2*, *hTERT*, *BAX*, *EDNRB*, *DAPK*, *RASSF1A*, *FADD*, *TMS-1*, *E-cadherin*, *ICAM1*, *TIMP3*, *MLH1*, *COX2*) in primary nonmuscle-invasive bladder carcinoma showed increased tumor recurrence with the methylation of *SOCS1*, *STAT1*, *BCL2*, *DAPK*, or *E-cadherin*. *TIMP3* methylation is associated with improved recurrence-free survival.[59] Hypermethylation of these gene promoters was observed in 7% of patients in the nonrecurrence group and 28% of patients in the recurrence group. The recurrence rate for 24-month followup was 88% for hypermethylation of *DAPK* and 28% for nonmethylation of *DAPK*. The results suggest that hypermethylation of *DAPK* might be a useful marker to predict recurrence of non-muscle-invasive bladder cancers.[59] These findings were validated by another group.[60] Further, hypermethylation of *DAPK* predicted recurrence for superficial bladder cancer in 88% of cases.[60]

Epigenetic silencing of tumor suppressor genes by promoter hypermethylation has been shown for multiple genes in bladder cancer. Christoph et al. evaluated the methylation status of 110 bladder cancer patients for four *TP53* target genes: *APAF1*, *CASP8*, *DAPK1*, and *IGFBP3*.[57] The investigators found that the methylation levels of two tumor suppressor genes, *APAF1* and *IGFBP3*, were able to separate tumors with high recurrence risk from low risk tumors, not only for pTa and pT1, but also for muscle-invasive urothelial carcinomas.[57]

Histone modifications are linked to DNA replication, transcription, and repair. The phosphorylation of histone H2AX at serine 139 (γ-H2AX) is associated with DNA breaks. Cheung et al. studied the expression of γ-H2AX using a polyclonal antibody directed against the aberrant protein.[61] A retrospective assessment of 60 patients with bladder cancer using this antibody found that recurrence was more likely to develop in γ-H2AX-negative than in γ-H2AX-positive cases. These results indicate epigenetic alterations may have an important role in the mechanism of bladder tumor recurrence.[61]

Other Genomic Alterations as Predictors of Tumor Recurrence

Microsatellite markers and chromosomal deletions are also promising for bladder cancer screening, diagnosing, and possibly predicting recurrence. Such irreversible DNA alterations have been called genomic signatures. Previous studies have shown that microsatellite analysis can be helpful in the screening and diagnosis of bladder urothelial tumors.[62–64] However, results regarding the prediction of recurrence, progression, and survival with microsatellite analysis in urothelial carcinomas are conflicting and unresolved. Invasive bladder cancer commonly shows losses of chromosomes 2q, 5q, 8p, 9p, 9q, 10q, 11p, 18q, and Y.[4,5,14,16,22,23,54,65–77] LOH at 9p21 significantly correlates with reduced recurrence-free interval. A low 9p21 index (mean 9p signal per cell <0.9) appears to indicate a significantly lower recurrence-free survival.[78]

Edwards et al. conducted a study of 109 primary and recurrent bladder cancers from 47 patients to explore genetic alterations of three loci (*INK4A* at 9p21, *DBC1* at 9q32–33, and *TSC1* at 9q34) on chromosome 9 as predictors of recurrence.[79] The risk of recurrence was significantly higher in patients with deleted 9q34 than in those who retained the 9q34 region.[79]

LOH at 9p and 9q34 has also been reported by other researchers in bladder cancer for selecting a subset of patients with a high risk of recurrence.[80,81] Simoneau et al. studied 139 Ta or T1 bladder tumors for LOH at 28 chromosome 9 microsatellite loci.[81] LOH at one or more loci was detected in 67 (48%) of the 139 tumors. Followup of 163 patients for eight years demonstrated that any LOH on chromosome 9 was associated with an elevated risk of recurrence. However, four regions were associated with a particularly high risk of recurrence. Tumors with deletions in 9ptr–p22, 9q22.3, 9q33, and 9q34 had earlier recurrence than those without deletions.[81] This finding is not surprising, since deletion of a chromosome 9 allele is an early event in urothelial transformation that does not distinguish the two tumorigenesis pathways.[11]

Fornari et al. analyzed LOH of 13 microsatellite loci on 10 different chromosomal arms from 59 patients with recurrent bladder cancer and 25 patients with no history of recurrence at the time of the study.[82] The median followup period was 23 months for the 59 patients and 25 months for the 25 patients.[82] The authors found that LOH at 11p is associated with tumor recurrence in patients with noninvasive urothelial carcinoma. Other investigators have confirmed that LOH of D11S490 or D17S928 is associated with bladder cancer recurrence.[80]

Numerical and structural alterations of chromosomes are common in urothelial carcinoma. However, it is difficult to ascertain whether a given aberration is the cause or the consequence of urothelial carcinogenesis. It is also unclear whether certain alterations are associated with a specific urothelial tumorigenesis pathway, or whether chromosomal alterations in general predict clinical outcome.

UroVysion, a multitarget fluorescence in situ hybridization (FISH) test, detects numerical alterations of chromosomes 3, 7, and 17, and deletion of 9p21 (see **Chapter 32** for further discussion).[4,17,23,54,75] Gofrit et al. studied 64 patients with non-muscle-invasive bladder cancer to evaluate whether UroVysion could predict tumor recurrence.[83] All the patients were followed for at least 6 months after their initial UroVysion testing. Abnormal UroVysion results were observed in 40 patients (62.5%). After a median followup of 13.5 months, 21 patients (33%) developed tumor recurrence (Ta in 13 patients, T1 in five patients, and Tis in three patients). Recurrent tumors developed in 45% of the patients with abnormal UroVysion test compared with 12.5% of the patients with a normal result. An abnormal UroVysion test result preceded the diagnosis of tumor recurrence in 18/21 (86%) cases, including all high grade tumor recurrences.[83] Most FISH-positive patients who develop recurrent urothelial carcinoma will do so within one year.[84]

Serum Markers to Predict Bladder Cancer Recurrence

Very few studies have explored serum markers as predictors of tumor recurrence. Serum markers associated with bladder cancer recurrence would be useful to assess recurrence risk and to monitor the patient for tumor recurrence. Zhao et al. used an enzyme-linked immunosorbent assay (ELISA) to compare plasma levels of angiogenin in 209 patients with bladder carcinoma and in 208 healthy control participants who were matched according to age, gender,

and ethnicity.[85] Patients who had recurrent bladder cancer had significantly higher plasma angiogenin levels than those who were without recurrence. Elevated plasma level of angiogenin may serve as an indicator of the risk of bladder carcinoma.[85]

Implications of Field Effect and Cancer Stem Cells in the Recurrence of Bladder Cancer

Human urothelial carcinoma appears to arise from a field change that affects the entire urothelial cell population (see also **Chapter 34**).[52–54] Evidence of field cancerization comes from studies of multifocal bladder tumors, colocalized phenotypically distinct bladder cancers, and bladder precursor lesions. Cancer is formed through clonal expansion of one or few cancer stem cells (CSCs). Each CSC and its lineage possesses a particular set of genetic, epigenetic, and phenotypic biological features.[32,86,87] Jones et al. examined 58 tumors from 21 patients who underwent surgical excision for multifocal urothelial carcinoma.[54] All patients had two to four separate foci of urothelial carcinoma in the urinary tract. LOH assays for three polymorphic microsatellite markers on chromosomes 9p21 and 17p13, and X chromosome inactivation analyses on urothelial tumors from the 11 female patients showed concordance in only three patients. The results suggest that each of the coexisting tumors of multifocal urothelial carcinoma has a unique clonal signature. Each tumor arises independently from a transformed progenitor cell distributed by carcinogenic influences throughout the affected field.[54] According to this "field effect" theory for urothelial carcinogenesis,[54] transforming factors affect a large area and induce CSCs distributed throughout the field.

The modern cancer model hypothesis is based on the observation that only a minority of cells can form new tumors. Cancer is formed through clonal expansion of one or a few CSCs.[14,88–90] Each CSC and its lineage possess a unique set of genetic, epigenetic, and phenotypic biological features.[32,86,87] The recurrence of a bladder cancer may originate from the CSCs remaining in the shared field after the primary cancer was surgically removed. Evidence suggests that CSCs may play a key role in the initiation, recurrence, and progression of bladder cancer.

Urothelial cancer recurrence occurs in many cases after the tumor has been eradicated by surgical removal, chemotherapy, or radiation. Relapse may now be attributed to incomplete CSC elimination in the shared field outside the primary tumor.[91] Recent developments indicate that most current therapies eliminate differentiated cells, which are more sensitive to therapy than are CSCs.[89,90] Proliferation and clonal expansion of fugitive CSCs results in the establishment of new neoplasms wherever the surviving cells find a favorable niche.

Marker Validation and Experimental Bias

The twenty-first century has begun with great effort and numerous publications generated through molecular studies. However, marker validation and clinically experience are required before proposed markers become clinical relevant. Publication bias should be ruled out before any prognostic association is considered established. Dyrskjot et al. studied 404 bladder cancers and found an 88-gene progression signature, which predicted progression independently from standard clinical risk variables.[92] A 52-gene stage signature correctly classified tumor stage, and a 68-gene CIS signature accurately detected CIS in the specimens. However, no RNA microarray profile or combination of signatures could accurately predict recurrence. This negative study result included a 26-gene recurrence predication set, which showed changes in patients with medium and high recurrence rates.[93] Published marker systems must still be repeated with large samples at multiple institutions with independent data sets.

At this time, many potential biomarkers for recurrence are still investigative and need to be validated as independent predictors of outcome in prospective studies.

Future Perspective and Molecular Markers for Early Detection of Bladder Cancer

With accumulating molecular knowledge of bladder cancer, we are about to bridge the gap between genetic findings and clinical outcomes (see also **Chapter 34**).[4] Assessment of key genetic pathways and expression profiles should establish a set of molecular markers to predict the likelihood of tumor recurrence and progressive transformation. *FGFR3* and *TP53* mutation pathways, which correlate with low and high grade bladder cancer, respectively, provide not only tools for bladder cancer diagnosis and prognosis, but also handles for potential therapeutic interventions. Therapies targeting *FGFR3, TP53*, or their key downstream pathways could become new options for bladder cancer management.

Prevention is the most effective method for cancer management. At this time, however, it is unclear whether distinct carcinogens cause the two different urothelial carcinogenesis pathways. We have yet to learn how carcinogens may mediate the "field cancerization" often observed with bladder tumors. Ascertaining why certain highly frequent genetic mutations occur in urothelial tumor classes may shed light on their underlying carcinogenic mechanisms, but may also contribute to the development of new preventive and therapeutic strategies.

Currently, urine cytology is the most widely used method for bladder cancer recurrence after initial diagnosis. Diagnostic cytologic criteria are largely based on cell morphology, and accuracy is hampered by the element of subjectivity (see **Chapter 30** for further discussion). Cytology is highly effective in detecting high grade cancers, but its sensitivity and specificity in detecting low grade urothelial carcinoma are poorer. Accumulated knowledge in the molecular processes involved in carcinogenesis has resulted in the development of many new markers for diagnosis, surveillance, and prognostication of bladder cancer. Of these, UroVysion, BTA *stat*/BTA-TRAK, NMP22, and ImmunoCyt/uCyt are currently available testing methods that are used relatively widely and have been approved for clinical use by the U.S. Food and Drug Administration (see **Chapters 30, 31,** and **32** for further discussion).

REFERENCES

1. Cheng L, Neumann RM, Weaver AL, Cheville JC, Leibovich BC, Ramnani DM, Scherer BG, Nehra A, Zincke H, Bostwick DG. Grading and staging of bladder carcinoma in transurethral resection specimens. Correlation with 105 matched cystectomy specimens. *Am J Clin Pathol* 2000;113:275–9.
2. Cheng L, Neumann RM, Nehra A, Spotts BE, Weaver AL, Bostwick DG. Cancer heterogeneity and its biologic implications in the grading of urothelial carcinoma. *Cancer* 2000;88:1663–70.
3. Cheng L, Lopez-Beltran A, MacLennan GT, Montironi R, Bostwick DG. Neoplasms of the urinary bladder. In: Bostwick DG, Cheng L, eds. Urologic Surgical Pathology, 2nd ed. Philadelphia: Elsevier/Mosby, 2008; 259–352.
4. Cheng L, Zhang S, Maclennan GT, Williamson SR, Lopez-Beltran A, Montironi R. Bladder cancer: translating molecular genetic insights into clinical practice. *Hum Pathol* 2011;42:455–81.
5. Cheng L, Davidson DD, Maclennan GT, Williamson SR, Zhang S, Koch MO, Montironi R, Lopez-Beltran A. The origins of urothelial carcinoma. *Expert Rev Anticancer Ther* 2010;10:865–80.
6. Raghavan D, Shipley WU, Garnick MB, Russell PJ, Richie JP. Biology and management of bladder cancer. *N Engl J Med* 1990;322:1129–38.

7. Grossman HB, Soloway M, Messing E, Katz G, Stein B, Kassabian V, Shen Y. Surveillance for recurrent bladder cancer using a point-of-care proteomic assay. *JAMA* 2006;295:299–305.

8. Jacobs BL, Lee CT, Montie JE. Bladder cancer in 2010: How far have we come? *CA Cancer J Clin* 2010;60:244–72.

9. Bostwick DG, Cheng L. Urologic Surgical Pathology, 2nd ed. Philadelphia: Elsevier/Mosby, 2008.

10. Black PC, Brown GA, Dinney CP. Molecular markers of urothelial cancer and their use in the monitoring of superficial urothelial cancer. *J Clin Oncol* 2006;24:5528–35.

11. Wu XR. Urothelial tumorigenesis: a tale of divergent pathways. *Nature Rev Cancer* 2005;5:713–25.

12. Cheng L, Weaver AL, Leibovich BC, Ramnani DM, Neumann RM, Sherer BG, Nehra A, Zincke H, Bostwick DG. Predicting the survival of bladder carcinoma patients treated with radical cystectomy. *Cancer* 2000;88:2326–32.

13. Cheng L, Neumann RM, Weaver AL, Spotts BE, Bostwick DG. Predicting cancer progression in patients with stage T1 bladder carcinoma. *J Clin Oncol* 1999;17:3182–7.

14. Cheng L, Zhang D. Molecular Genetic Pathology. New York: Humana Press/Springer, 2008.

15. Cheng L, Zhang S, Davidson DD, MacLennan GT, Koch MO, Montironi R, Lopez-Beltran A. Molecular determinants of tumor recurrence in the urinary bladder. *Future Oncol* 2009;5:843–57.

16. Cheng L, Zhang S, Alexander R, MacLennan GT, Hodges KB, Harrison BT, Lopez-Beltran A, Montironi R. Sarcomatoid carcinoma of the urinary bladder: the final common pathway of urothelial carcinoma dedifferentiation. *Am J Surg Pathol* 2011;35:e34–46.

17. Lacy S, Lopez-Beltran A, MacLennan GT, Foster SR, Montironi R, Cheng L. Molecular pathogenesis of urothelial carcinoma: the clinical utility of emerging new biomarkers and future molecular classification of bladder cancer. *Anal Quant Cytol Histol* 2009;31:5–16.

18. van Rhijn BW, van der Kwast TH, Vis AN, Kirkels WJ, Boeve ER, Jobsis AC, Zwarthoff EC. FGFR3 and P53 characterize alternative genetic pathways in the pathogenesis of urothelial cell carcinoma. *Cancer Res* 2004;64:1911–4.

19. Wallerand H, Bakkar AA, de Medina SG, Pairon JC, Yang YC, Vordos D, Bittard H, Fauconnet S, Kouyoumdjian JC, Jaurand MC, Zhang ZF, Radvanyi F, Thiery JP, Chopin DK. Mutations in TP53, but not FGFR3, in urothelial cell carcinoma of the bladder are influenced by smoking: contribution of exogenous versus endogenous carcinogens. *Carcinogenesis* 2005;26:177–84.

20. Bakkar AA, Wallerand H, Radvanyi F, Lahaye JB, Pissard S, Lecerf L, Kouyoumdjian JC, Abbou CC, Pairon JC, Jaurand MC, Thiery JP, Chopin DK, de Medina SG. FGFR3 and TP53 gene mutations define two distinct pathways in urothelial cell carcinoma of the bladder. *Cancer Res* 2003;63:8108–12.

21. Sung MT, Lopez-Beltran A, Eble JN, MacLennan GT, Tan PH, Montironi R, Jones TD, Ulbright TM, Blair JE, Cheng L. Divergent pathway of intestinal metaplasia and cystitis glandularis of the urinary bladder. *Mod Pathol* 2006;19:1395–401.

22. Sung MT, Eble JN, Wang M, Tan PH, Lopez-Beltran A, Cheng L. Inverted papilloma of the urinary bladder: a molecular genetic appraisal. *Mod Pathol* 2006;19:1289–94.

23. Sung MT, Wang M, MacLennan GT, Eble JN, Tan PH, Lopez-Beltran A, Montironi R, Harris JJ, Kuhar M, Cheng L. Histogenesis of sarcomatoid urothelial carcinoma of the urinary bladder: evidence for a common clonal origin with divergent differentiation. *J Pathol* 2007;211:420–30.

24. Lott S, Wang M, MacLennan GT, Lopez-Beltran A, Montironi R, Sung M-T, Tan P-H, Cheng L. FGFR3 and TP53 mutation analysis in inverted urothelial papilloma: incidence and etiological considerations. *Mod Pathol* 2009;22:627–32.

25. van Rhijn BW, Lurkin I, Radvanyi F, Kirkels WJ, van der Kwast TH, Zwarthoff EC. The fibroblast growth factor receptor 3 (FGFR3) mutation is a strong indicator of superficial bladder cancer with low recurrence rate. *Cancer Res* 2001;61:1265–8.

26. van Rhijn BW, Burger M, Lotan Y, Solsona E, Stief CG, Sylvester RJ, Witjes JA, Zlotta AR. Recurrence and progression of disease in non-muscle-invasive bladder cancer: from epidemiology to treatment strategy. *Eur Urol* 2009;56:430–42.

27. van Rhijn BW, Lurkin I, Chopin DK, Kirkels WJ, Thiery JP, van der Kwast TH, Radvanyi F, Zwarthoff EC. Combined microsatellite and FGFR3 mutation analysis enables a highly sensitive detection of urothelial cell carcinoma in voided urine. *Clin Cancer Res* 2003;9:257–63.

28. van Rhijn BW, Lurkin I, Radvanyi F, Kirkels WJ, van der Kwast TH, Zwarthoff EC. The fibroblast growth factor receptor 3 (FGFR3) mutation is a strong indicator of superficial bladder cancer with low recurrence rate. *Cancer Res* 2001;61:1265–8.

29. Hernandez S, Lopez-Knowles E, Lloreta J, Kogevinas M, Amoros A, Tardon A, Carrato A, Serra C, Malats N, Real FX. Prospective study of FGFR3 mutations as a prognostic factor in nonmuscle invasive urothelial bladder carcinomas. *J Clin Oncol* 2006;24:3664–71.

30. Barbisan F, Santinelli A, Mazzucchelli R, Lopez-Beltran A, Cheng L, Scarpelli M, van der Kwast T, Montironi R. Strong immunohistochemical expression of fibroblast growth factor receptor 3, superficial staining pattern of cytokeratin 20, and low proliferative activity define those papillary urothelial neoplasms of low malignant potential that do not recur. *Cancer* 2008;112:636–44.

31. Shariat SF, Ashfaq R, Sagalowsky AI, Lotan Y. Predictive value of cell cycle biomarkers in nonmuscle invasive bladder transitional cell carcinoma. *J Urol* 2007;177:481–7.

32. Dahse R, Gartner D, Werner W, Schubert J, Junker K. P53 mutations as an identification marker for the clonal origin of bladder tumors and its recurrences. *Oncol Rep* 2003;10:2033–7.

33. Ecke TH, Sachs MD, Lenk SV, Loening SA, Schlechte HH. TP53 gene mutations as an independent marker for urinary bladder cancer progression. *Int J Mol Med* 2008;21:655–61.

34. Hernandez S, Lopez-Knowles E, Lloreta J, Kogevinas M, Jaramillo R, Amoros A, Tardon A, Garcia-Closas R, Serra C, Carrato A, Malats N, Real FX. FGFR3 and Tp53 mutations in T1G3 transitional bladder carcinomas: independent distribution and lack of association with prognosis. *Clin Cancer Res* 2005;11:5444–50.

35. George B, Datar RH, Wu L, Cai J, Patten N, Beil SJ, Groshen S, Stein J, Skinner D, Jones PA, Cote RJ. p53 gene and protein status: the role of p53 alterations in predicting outcome in patients with bladder cancer. *J Clin Oncol* 2007;25:5352–8.

36. Chatterjee SJ, Datar R, Youssefzadeh D, George B, Goebell PJ, Stein JP, Young L, Shi SR, Gee C, Groshen S, Skinner DG, Cote RJ. Combined effects of p53, p21, and pRb expression in the progression of bladder transitional cell carcinoma. *J Clin Oncol* 2004;22:1007–13.

37. Lopez-Knowles E, Hernandez S, Kogevinas M, Lloreta J, Amoros A, Tardon A, Carrato A, Kishore S, Serra C, Malats N, Real FX. The p53 pathway and outcome among patients with T1G3 bladder tumors. *Clin Cancer Res* 2006;12:6029–36.

38. Malats N, Bustos A, Nascimento CM, Fernandez F, Rivas M, Puente D, Kogevinas M, Real FX. P53 as a prognostic marker for bladder cancer: a meta-analysis and review. *Lancet Oncol* 2005;6:678–86.

39. Frank I, Cheville JC, Blute ML, Lohse CM, Karnes RJ, Weaver AL, Sebo TJ, Nehra A, Zincke H. Prognostic value of p53 and MIB–1 in transitional cell carcinoma of the urinary bladder with regional lymph node involvement. *Cancer* 2004;101:1803–8.

40. Dyrskjot L, Thykjaer T, Kruhoffer M, Jensen JL, Marcussen N, Hamilton-Dutoit S, Wolf H, Orntoft TF. Identifying distinct classes of bladder carcinoma using microarrays. *Nat Genet* 2003;33:90–6.

41. Ito M, Nishiyama H, Kawanishi H, Matsui S, Guilford P, Reeve A, Ogawa O. P21-activated kinase 1: a new molecular marker for intravesical recurrence after transurethral resection of bladder cancer. *J Urol* 2007;178:1073–9.

42. Choi YD, Cho NH, Ahn HS, Cho KS, Cho SY, Yang WJ. Matrix metalloproteinase expression in the recurrence of superficial low grade bladder transitional cell carcinoma. *J Urol* 2007;177:1174–8.

43. Modlich O, Prisack HB, Pitschke G, Ramp U, Ackermann R, Bojar H, Vogeli TA, Grimm MO. Identifying superficial, muscle-invasive, and metastasizing transitional cell carcinoma of the bladder: use of cDNA array analysis of gene expression profiles. *Clin Cancer Res* 2004;10:3410–21.

44. Margulis V, Shariat SF, Ashfaq R, Sagalowsky AI, Lotan Y. Ki-67 is an independent predictor of bladder cancer outcome in patients treated with radical cystectomy for organ-confined disease. *Clin Cancer Res* 2006;12:7369–73.

45. Gontero P, Casetta G, Zitella A, Ballario R, Pacchioni D, Magnani C, Muir GH, Tizzani A. Evaluation of p53 protein overexpression, Ki67 proliferative activity and mitotic index as markers of tumour recurrence in superficial transitional cell carcinoma of the bladder. *Eur Urol* 2000;38:287–96.

46. Helpap B, Schmitz-Drager BJ, Hamilton PW, Muzzonigro G, Galosi AB, Kurth KH, Lubaroff D, Waters DJ, Droller MJ. Molecular pathology of non-invasive urothelial carcinomas (part I). *Virchows Arch* 2003;442:309–16.

47. Inoue K, Kamada M, Slaton JW, Fukata S, Yoshikawa C, Tamboli P, Dinney CP, Shuin T. The prognostic value of angiogenesis and metastasis-related genes for progression of transitional cell carcinoma of the renal pelvis and ureter. *Clin Cancer Res* 2002;8:1863–70.

48. Crew JP, O'Brien T, Bradburn M, Fuggle S, Bicknell R, Cranston D, Harris AL. Vascular endothelial growth factor is a predictor of relapse and stage progression in superficial bladder cancer. *Cancer Res* 1997;57:5281–5.

49. Yurakh AO, Ramos D, Calabuig-Farinas S, Lopez-Guerrero JA, Rubio J, Solsona E, Romanenko AM, Vozianov AF, Pellin A, Llombart-Bosch A. Molecular and immunohistochemical analysis of the prognostic value of cell-cycle regulators in urothelial neoplasms of the bladder. *Eur Urol* 2006;50:506–15; discussion 515.

50. Shariat SF, Karakiewicz PI, Ashfaq R, Lerner SP, Palapattu GS, Cote RJ, Sagalowsky AI, Lotan Y. Multiple biomarkers improve prediction of bladder cancer recurrence and mortality in patients undergoing cystectomy. *Cancer* 2008;112:315–25.

51. Karam JA, Lotan Y, Karakiewicz PI, Ashfaq R, Sagalowsky AI, Roehrborn CG, Shariat SF. Use of combined apoptosis biomarkers for prediction of bladder cancer recurrence and mortality after radical cystectomy. *Lancet Oncol* 2007;8:128–36.

52. Davidson DD, Cheng L. "Field cancerization" in the urothelium of the bladder. *Anal Quant Cytol Histol* 2006;28:337–8.

53. Cheng L, Gu J, Ulbright TM, MacLennan GT, Sweeney CJ, Zhang S, Sanchez K, Koch MO, Eble JN. Precise microdissection of human bladder carcinomas reveals divergent tumor subclones in the same tumor. *Cancer* 2002;94:104–10.

54. Jones TD, Wang M, Eble JN, MacLennan GT, Lopez-Beltran A, Zhang S, Cocco A, Cheng L. Molecular evidence supporting field effect in urothelial carcinogenesis. *Clin Cancer Res* 2005;11:6512–9.

55. Kim WJ, Quan C. Genetic and epigenetic aspects of bladder cancer. *J Cell Biochem* 2005;95:24–33.

56. Tada Y, Wada M, Taguchi K, Mochida Y, Kinugawa N, Tsuneyoshi M, Naito S, Kuwano M. The association of death-associated protein kinase hypermethylation with early recurrence in superficial bladder cancers. *Cancer Res* 2002;62:4048–53.

57. Christoph F, Weikert S, Kempkensteffen C, Krause H, Schostak M, Miller K, Schrader M. Regularly methylated novel pro-apoptotic genes associated with recurrence in transitional cell carcinoma of the bladder. *Int J Cancer* 2006;119:1396–402.

58. Dominguez G, Carballido J, Silva J, Silva JM, Garcia JM, Menendez J, Provencio M, Espana P, Bonilla F. p14ARF promoter hypermethylation in plasma DNA as an indicator of disease recurrence in bladder cancer patients. *Clin Cancer Res* 2002;8:980–5.

59. Friedrich MG, Chandrasoma S, Siegmund KD, Weisenberger DJ, Cheng JC, Toma MI, Huland H, Jones PA, Liang G. Prognostic relevance of methylation markers in patients with non-muscle invasive bladder carcinoma. *Eur J Cancer* 2005;41:2769–78.

60. Tada Y, Wada M, Taguchi K, Mochida Y, Kinugawa N, Tsuneyoshi M, Naito S, Kuwano M. The association of death-associated protein kinases hypermethylation with early recurrence in superficial bladder cancers. *Cancer Res* 2002;62:4048–53.

61. Cheung WL, Albadine R, Chan T, Sharma R, Netto GJ. Phosphorylated H2AX in noninvasive low grade urothelial carcinoma of the bladder: correlation with tumor recurrence. *J Urol* 2009;181:1387–92.

62. Lopez-Beltran A, Alvarez-Kindelan J, Luque RJ, Blanca A, Quintero A, Montironi R, Cheng L, Gonzalez-Campora R, Requena MJ. Loss of heterozygosity at 9q32-33 (DBC1 locus) in primary non-invasive papillary urothelial neoplasm of low malignant potential and low grade urothelial carcinoma of the bladder and their associated normal urothelium. *J Pathol* 2008;215:263–72.

63. van Tilborg AA, de Vries A, de Bont M, Groenfeld LE, Zwarthoff EC. The random development of LOH on chromosome 9q in superficial bladder cancers. *J Pathol* 2002;198:352–8.

64. Stoehr R, Zietz S, Burger M, Filbeck T, Denzinger S, Obermann EC, Hammerschmied C, Wieland WF, Knuechel R, Hartmann A. Deletions of chromosomes 9 and 8p in histologically normal urothelium of patients with bladder cancer. *Eur Urol* 2005;47:58–63.

65. Wu XR. Urothelial tumorigenesis: a tale of divergent pathways. *Nat Rev Cancer* 2005;5:713–25.

66. Dalbagni G, Presti J, Reuter V, Fair WR, Cordon-Cardo C. Genetic alterations in bladder cancer. *Lancet* 1993;342:469–71.

67. Knowles MA, Elder PA, Williamson M, Cairns JP, Shaw ME, Law MG. Allelotype of human bladder cancer. *Cancer Res* 1994;54:531–8.

68. Rosin MP, Cairns P, Epstein JI, Schoenberg MP, Sidransky D. Partial allelotype of carcinoma in situ of the human bladder. *Cancer Res* 1995;15:5213–6.

69. Cheng L, MacLennan GT, Pan CX, Jones TD, Moore CR, Zhang S, Gu J, Patel NB, Kao C, Gardner TA. Allelic loss of the active X chromosome during bladder carcinogenesis. *Arch Pathol Lab Med* 2004;128:187–90.

70. Cheng L, MacLennan GT, Zhang S, Wang M, Pan CX, Koch MO. Laser capture microdissection analysis reveals frequent allelic losses in papillary urothelial neoplasm of low malignant potential of the urinary bladder. *Cancer* 2004;101:183–8.

71. Cheng L, Jones TD, McCarthy RP, Eble JN, Wang M, MacLennan GT, Lopez-Beltran A, Yang XJ, Koch MO, Zhang S, Pan CX, Baldridge LA. Molecular genetic evidence for a common clonal origin of urinary bladder small cell carcinoma and coexisting urothelial carcinoma. *Am J Pathol* 2005;166:1533–9.

72. Jones TD, Wang M, Eble JN, MacLennan GT, Lopez-Beltran A, Zhang S, Cocco A, Cheng L. Molecular evidence supporting field effect in urothelial carcinogenesis. *Clin Cancer Res* 2005;11:6512–9.

73. Jones TD, Carr MD, Eble JN, Wang M, Lopez-Beltran A, Cheng L. Clonal origin of lymph node metastases in bladder carcinoma. *Cancer* 2005;104:1901–10.

74. Sung MT, Zhang S, MacLennan GT, Lopez-Beltran A, Montironi R, Wang M, Tan PH, Cheng L. Histogenesis of clear cell adenocarcinoma in the urinary tract: evidence of urothelial origin. *Clin Cancer Res* 2008;14:1947–55.

75. Jones TD, Zhang S, Lopez-Beltran A, Eble JN, Sung MT, MacLennan GT, Montironi R, Tan PH, Zheng S, Baldridge LA, Cheng L. Urothelial carcinoma with an inverted growth pattern can be distinguished from inverted papilloma by fluorescence in-situ hybridization, immunohistochemistry, and morphologic analysis. *Am J Surg Pathol* 2007;31:1861–7.

76. Cheng L, Bostwick DG, Li G, Zhang S, Vortmeyer AO, Zhuang Z. Conserved genetic findings in metastatic bladder cancer: a possible utility of allelic loss of chromosomes 9p21 and 17p13 in diagnosis. *Arch Pathol Lab Med* 2001;125:1197–9.

77. Houskova L, Zemanova Z, Babjuk M, Melichercikova J, Pesl M, Michalova K. Molecular cytogenetic characterization and diagnostics of bladder cancer. *Neoplasma* 2007;54:511–6.

78. Kawauchi S, Sakai H, Ikemoto K, Eguchi S, Nakao M, Takihara H, Shimabukuro T, Furuya T, Oga A, Matsuyama H, Takahashi M, Sasaki K. 9p21 index as estimated by dual-color fluorescence in situ hybridization is useful to predict urothelial carcinoma recurrence in bladder washing cytology. *Hum Pathol* 2009;40:1783–9.

79. Edwards J, Duncan P, Going JJ, Watters AD, Grigor KM, Bartlett JM. Identification of loci associated with putative recurrence genes in transitional cell carcinoma of the urinary bladder. *J Pathol* 2002;196:380–5.

80. Edwards J, Duncan P, Going JJ, Grigor KM, Watters AD, Bartlett JM. Loss of heterozygosity on chromosomes 11 and 17 are markers of recurrence in TCC of the bladder. *Br J Cancer* 2001;85:1894–9.

81. Simoneau M, LaRue H, Aboulkassim TO, Meyer F, Moore L, Fradet Y. Chromosome 9 deletions and recurrence of superficial bladder cancer: identification of four regions of prognostic interest. *Oncogene* 2000;19:6317–23.

82. Fornari D, Steven K, Hansen AB, Jepsen JV, Poulsen AL, Vibits H, Horn T. Transitional cell bladder tumor: predicting recurrence and progression by analysis of microsatellite loss of heterozygosity in urine sediment and tumor tissue. *Cancer Genet Cytogenet* 2006;167:15–19.

83. Gofrit ON, Zorn KC, Silvestre J, Shalhav AL, Zagaja GP, Msezane LP, Steinberg GD. The predictive value of multi-targeted fluorescent in-situ hybridization in patients with history of bladder cancer. *Urol Oncol* 2008;26:246–9.

84. Nguyen CT, Litt DB, Dolar SE, Ulchaker JC, Jones JS, Brainard JA. Prognostic significance of nondiagnostic molecular changes in urine detected by UroVysion fluorescence in situ hybridization

during surveillance for bladder cancer. *Urology* 2009;73:347–50.

85. Zhao H, Grossman HB, Delclos GL, Hwang LY, Troisi CL, Chamberlain RM, Chenoweth MA, Zhang H, Spitz MR, Wu X. Increased plasma levels of angiogenin and the risk of bladder carcinoma: from initiation to recurrence. *Cancer* 2005;104:30–5.

86. Denzinger S, Mohren K, Knuechel R, Wild PJ, Burger M, Wieland WF, Hartmann A, Stoehr R. Improved clonality analysis of multifocal bladder tumors by combination of histopathologic organ mapping, loss of heterozygosity, fluorescence in situ hybridization, and p53 analyses. *Hum Pathol* 2006;37:143–51.

87. Duggan BJ, Gray SB, McKnight JJ, Watson CJ, Johnston SR, Williamson KE. Oligoclonality in bladder cancer: the implication for molecular therapies. *J Urol* 2004;171:419–25.

88. Jordan CT, Guzman ML, Noble M. Cancer stem cells. *N Engl J Med* 2006;355:1253–61.

89. Pan CX, Zhu W, Cheng L. Implications of cancer stem cells in the treatment of cancer. *Future Oncol* 2006;2:723–31.

90. Cheng L, Zhang S, Davidson DD, Montironi R, Lopez-Beltran A. Implications of cancer stem cells for cancer therapy. In: Bagley R, G, Teicher BA, eds. Cancer Drug Discovery and Development: Stem Cells and Cancer. New York: Humana Press/Springer, 2009.

91. Blagosklonny MV. Why therapeutic response may not prolong the life of a cancer patient: selection for oncogenic resistance. *Cell Cycle* 2005;4:1693–8.

92. Dyrskjot L, Zieger K, Real FX, Malats N, Carrato A, Hurst C, Kotwal S, Knowles M, Malmstrom PU, de la Torre M, Wester K, Allory Y, et al. Gene expression signatures predict outcome in non-muscle-invasive bladder carcinoma: a multicenter validation study. *Clin Cancer Res* 2007;13:3545–51.

93. Schultz IJ, Wester K, Straatman H, Kiemeney LA, Babjuk M, Mares J, Willems JL, Swinkels DW, Witjes JA, Malmstrom PU, de Kok JB. Gene expression analysis for the prediction of recurrence in patients with primary Ta urothelial cell carcinoma. *Eur Urol* 2007;51:416–23.

Chapter 30

Urinary Cytology

Bladder Pathology, First Edition. Liang Cheng, Antonio Lopez-Beltran, David G. Bostwick.
© 2012 Wiley-Blackwell. Published 2012 by John Wiley & Sons, Inc.

Overview

Urinary cytology is useful in the diagnosis of a wide variety of benign and malignant diseases of the bladder, urethra, ureter, and renal pelvis.[1] We focus mainly on diagnostic cytology of the urothelium with special emphasis on bladder diseases. Urine cytology has important limitations; for example, this method is not fully reliable for identification of grade 1 or low grade papillary tumors.[2-9] However, cytology yields good to excellent results in the identification of urothelial carcinoma in situ (CIS) and high grade cancer. The diagnostic accuracy of urinary cytology is high in patients who are symptomatic or are being followed for recurrence after diagnosis and treatment for bladder cancer. The major indications and diagnostic categories for urinary cytology are presented in **Tables 30-1** and **30-2**.[1-49] We recommend always reporting the presence, amount, and preservation of erythrocytes in cytology reports since the test is usually ordered because of hematuria.

Table 30-1 **Major Indications for the Use of Urinary Cytology**

Diagnosis of carcinoma in situ, high grade carcinomas of the bladder

Evaluation of patients with hematuria and urinary tract symptoms

Monitoring of patients at risk for developing bladder cancer

Diagnosis and followup of patients with upper urinary tract cancers

Followup and monitoring of patients with a history of bladder cancer

Followup and monitoring of patients following augmentation cystoplasty

Assessing the effectiveness of various treatment regimens for bladder cancer

Types of Specimens

Most urinary cytology specimens come from voided urine, catheterized urine, bladder washing (barbotage),[39] brushing,[40] and neobladder urine from an ileal conduit or colonic pouch.[41-43] It is critical for interpretation of the specimen to have the collection method specified on the specimen requisition.

Normal Components of the Urinary Cytology Specimens

Superficial (Umbrella) Cells

Regardless of the type of sample and collection technique, superficial urothelial cells are a common component of

Table 30-2 **Major Diagnostic Categories in Urinary Cytology**

Nontumor-associated cytology
  Normal cells/negative for malignant cells
  Benign cellular changes (such as inflammatory changes)
  Unsatisfactory (specify the reason)

Tumor-associated cytology
  Atypical cells present, favor reactive
    Specific type (e.g., lithiasis, chemotherapy, other)
    Nonspecific
  Atypia indeterminate for neoplasia
    Rare single cells and clusters of mildly to moderately atypical urothelial cells; this may represent a reactive process, but neoplasm should be considered; clinical correlation is indicated
    Rare highly atypical urothelial cells, favor a low grade neoplasm; a reactive process cannot be excluded; repeat study and/or further investigation may be indicated
    Severely atypical urothelial cells highly suspicious for carcinoma; clinical correlation is recommended
  Malignant cells present
    Malignant cells present, most compatible with urothelial carcinoma (specify low grade vs. high grade)
    Malignant cells present, most compatible with urothelial carcinoma in situ or high grade urothelial carcinoma
    Malignant cells present, specify urothelial carcinoma, squamous cell carcinoma, adenocarcinoma, small cell carcinoma, sarcomatoid carcinoma, and others
    Malignant cells present, not otherwise specified

the urine sediment. These cells have one or more nuclei that are large. The cells measure up to 30 μm in diameter, comparable to superficial squamous cells (**Figs. 30-1** to **30-4**). Binucleated cells are common. Such cells are often larger than the mononucleated superficial cells, and their nuclei are somewhat smaller. Large multinucleated superficial cells may be the most striking component of the urinary sediment, particularly in washings or brushing specimens from patients with partial bladder outlet obstruction. Multinucleated superficial cells are particularly large, and may be mistaken for giant cells. A common pitfall in diagnosis is misinterpreting large superficial cells as macrophages or tumor cells. The DNA content may be twice that of normal cells (tetraploid nuclei).[44-46] Aneuploidy is a better indicator of malignancy.[4,47-51]

The chromatinic rim of the nucleus is thick and sharply demarcated. The chromatin is finely granular, often with a "salt and pepper" appearance and may contain one or more prominent chromocenters. The structure of the nucleus is better preserved in bladder washings than in voided urine. In women, there may be a sex chromatin body (Barr body)

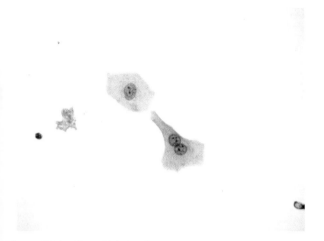

Figure 30-1 Superficial cells.

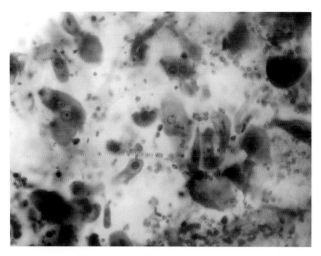

Figure 30-3 Superficial cells.

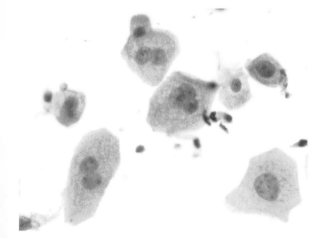

Figure 30-2 Superficial cells. Note the superficial umbrella cells with binucleation, fine nuclear chromatin, and occasional nucleoli.

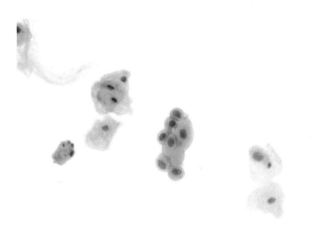

Figure 30-4 Superficial and intermediate cells (in the center) admixed with squamous cells.

attached to the nuclear membrane. The cytoplasm of these cells is usually cyanophilic, often finely granular, and sometimes vacuolated.

Cells from the Deeper Layers of the Urothelium

Epithelial cells smaller than the superficial cells are derived from the deeper layers of the urothelium (Fig. 30-5). These cells often exfoliate in clusters, particularly if the specimen was obtained with an instrument. Single small urothelial cells are observed in voided urine, usually in the presence of inflammation and destruction of the superficial cell layer. The clusters of urothelial cells may be tightly packed and assume a spherical "papillary" configuration with sharp borders. When numerous such clusters are present, they may indicate low grade papillary carcinoma, especially when the background is bloody.[52,53] When the deep cells are removed by an instrument, they often appear in loose clusters. These

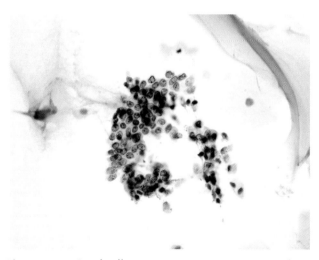

Figure 30-5 Basal cells.

cells are polygonal or elongate, sometimes columnar, and usually display cytoplasmic extensions in contact with other cells. Since only superficial cells exfoliate spontaneously, it may be significant to observe many of these clusters in voided urine without bladder instrumentation. The amount of basophilic cytoplasm in such cells depends on the depth of origin and is more abundant in cells derived from superficial layers. Single cells resemble parabasal squamous cells in size and configuration. These cells are often spherical, particularly in voided urine, but may also show cytoplasmic extensions. The nuclei of the smaller urothelial cells are approximately the same size, measuring about 5 μm in diameter. These nuclei, usually finely granular and benign-appearing, contain one or rarely two small chromocenters. In voided urine, the nuclei may be pale, opaque, or occasionally somewhat darker. Therefore, clustering of cells with high nuclear-to-cytoplasmic ratio may be the only indication in voided urine that intermediate urothelial cells have been shed.

Mucus-containing Epithelial Cells

Occasionally, urine cytology specimens contain mucus-secreting columnar epithelial cells with peripheral nuclei and distended clear cytoplasm. These cells may be ciliated. Such cells derive from cystitis cystica or cystitis glandularis. However, since clear cell prostate carcinoma and prostate cancer may also appear as vacuolated columnar cells, it may be advisable to cystoscope patients with persistent findings of this type in voided specimens.

Squamous Cells

Squamous cells of varying size and different degrees of maturation are common in urine sediment, particularly in

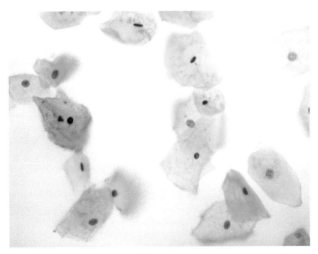

Figure 30-6 Squamous cells with small pyknotic nuclei, uniform "glassy" cytoplasm, polygonal shape, and frequent folded edges.

voided specimens from women (**Fig. 30-6**). Such cells are more abundant in specimens from female patients than those from male patients but less frequent when care is taken to separate the labia minora and retract the foreskin during collection. In women, these cells originate in the squamous epithelium of the vulva and urethra, or in the trigone of the urinary bladder, and are usually glycogenated. Voided urine sediment may also contain squamous cells derived from the vulva, vagina, or uterine cervix. In men, the origin of the squamous cells is the terminal portion of the urethra or, in rare cases, vaginal-type squamous metaplasia. Among the benign squamous cells, there may be superficial cells, intermediate cells, and smaller parabasal cells. Navicular cells are intermediate squamous cells with large cytoplasmic glycogen content and peripheral nuclei; these cells often stain yellow with Papanicolaou stain. Such cells may be observed during pregnancy, early menopause, and sometimes in women or in men receiving hormonal therapy (estrogen therapy) for prostate cancer. In women, the population of squamous cells in the urinary sediment may be used to determine the level of estrogenic activity (the so-called "urocytogram"). Squamous cells may also be anucleated and fully keratinized. The presence of such hyperkeratotic "ghost" cells may be of diagnostic significance, representing urethral stricture, leukoplakia or squamous cell carcinoma of the bladder.[10]

Other Cellular Components

Cells derived from renal tubules may sometimes appear in the urine sediment. These cells are small and usually poorly preserved, with pyknotic, hyperchromatic, condensed, spherical nuclei, and granular eosinophilic cytoplasm. Occasionally, the tubular cells form small clusters or casts. They may be prevalent in urine from patients with acute tubular necrosis. The significance of tubular cells in urine sediment remains uncertain. In patients following kidney transplant, the presence of renal tubular cells may indicate rejection of the allograft.[54] Occasionally, cells of prostatic and seminal vesicle origin may be present in the urinary sediment. Such cells accompany spermatozoa and are common after prostate massage.[55]

Macrophages are often observed in inflammatory reactions of the urinary tract. The cells may be mononucleated or multinucleated, and contain fine cytoplasmic vacuoles, sometimes with phagocytic debris. Erythrocytes are a frequent component of the urinary sediment, particularly in patients with clinical evidence of hematuria.[10] When the erythrocytes appear as ghost cells or have surface membrane blebs (acanthocytes), they may indicate bleeding from the upper urinary tract. Normal urine sediment contains very few lymphocytes or neutrophils. The presence of large numbers of such cells may precede clinical evidence of inflammation.

Figure 30-7   Calcium oxalate crystals.

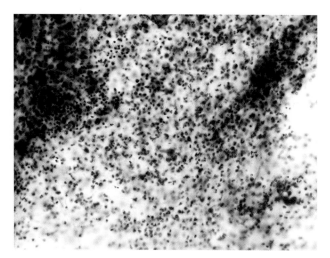

Figure 30-8   Acute cystitis. Note the presence of numerous neutrophils and degenerative cells.

Noncellular Components of the Urinary Sediment

Polygonal transparent crystalline precipitates of urates or calcium oxalate may also be seen in voided urine (**Fig. 30-7**). Their presence results from changes in the acidity of urine after collection, but has no diagnostic significance. Crystals derived from true uric acid are exceedingly rare. Other crystals are very rarely of diagnostic value.[56] Voided urine and occasional specimens obtained by instrumentation may contain contaminants and renal casts.

Inflammatory Lesions

Bacteria

A wide variety of bacteria may affect the epithelium of the urinary tract. Most are coliforms and other gram-negative rods. Cystitis may be acute or chronic. Acute cystitis is usually associated with symptoms that rarely require confirmatory tissue biopsy or cytologic examination. In those cases in which urine is studied, the sediment may contain numerous exfoliated umbrella cells, necrotic material, and inflammatory cells, with a predominance of neutrophils (**Fig. 30-8**). Marked necrosis and inflammation may also occur in the presence of necrotic tumors, particularly high grade urothelial carcinoma and squamous cell carcinoma. Urine with extensive acute inflammation should be examined thoroughly for atypical cells when cultures are negative.

The urinary sediment in chronic cystitis usually contains a background of chronic inflammation with macrophages and erythrocytes.[10] Urothelial cells may be abundant and poorly preserved, occasionally forming small clusters. The cytoplasm in these cells is granular and vacuolated. When the cells degenerate, especially in the presence of blood,

the cytoplasm contains spherical eosinophilic inclusions of no significance. There may be slight nuclear enlargement and hyperchromasia, but the contours of the nuclei are regular and the chromatin texture is finely granular. There may be necrosis of urothelial cells, with nuclear pyknosis and marked cytoplasmic vacuolization. In ulcerative cystitis, large sheets of urothelial cells may be observed.

Interstitial cystitis, a form of chronic cystitis associated with submucosal inflammation, displays nonspecific cytologic changes.[11] Eosinophilic cystitis has a predominance of eosinophils, a pattern seen in patients with allergic disorders, previous biopsies, or following mitomycin C treatment.[57] Granulomatous cystitis may be observed in patients with acquired immunodeficiency syndrome (AIDS) and those receiving treatment for urothelial carcinoma with bacillus Calmette–Guérin (BCG). In such patients, the sediment shows inflammatory cells and may contain fragments of tubercles in the form of clusters of elongate, carrot-shaped epithelioid histiocytes, sometimes accompanied by multinucleated Langhans-type giant cells and reactive atypia of urothelial cells.[58,59] Similar findings may occur in patients with tuberculosis of the bladder.

Fungi

Fungi occasionally affect the lower urinary tract, particularly the urinary bladder, and *Candida albicans* is the most common pathogen (**Fig. 30-9**). *Candida* cystitis is usually seen in pregnant women, diabetics, and those with impaired immunity, such as AIDS patients, those undergoing chemotherapy for cancer, bone marrow transplant recipients, and any patient with a chronic indwelling catheter. In the urinary sediment, the fungi may appear as yeast forms, with small oval bodies, or as pseudohyphae, with

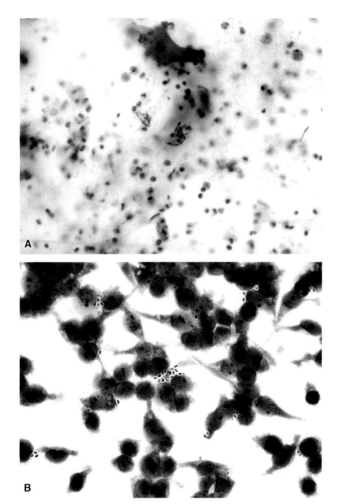

Figure 30-9 *Candida albicans* (A and B). Note the presence of pseudohyphae and budding yeast.

oblong branching nonencapsulated filaments. Other uncommon fungi include *Blastomyces dermatitidis*, *Aspergillus*, and *Zygomycetes* (mucormycosis). A fungus of the species *Alternaria* is a common laboratory contaminant.[11]

Viruses

Several important viruses cause morphologic changes in the urothelial cells, which may be confused with malignancy. The dominant feature of viral infections is the formation of nuclear and cytoplasmic inclusions (**Table 30-3**).

Herpes simplex is an obligate intracellular virus, and florid infection with permissive replication of the virus causes abnormalities in urothelial cells that are readily recognized (**Fig. 30-10**). In the early stages of viral replication, the nuclei of infected cells appear hazy with a ground glass appearance and margination of chromatin. Multinucleation with nuclear molding is commonly observed in such cells. Multiple nuclei are often densely packed, with nuclear molding and tightly fitting contoured nuclei. In later stages

Table 30-3   Characteristic Cytologic Changes Associated with Specific Types of Virus

Cytomegalovirus
   Enlarged cells
   High nuclear-to-cytoplasmic ratio
   Basophilic intranuclear inclusion with "owl eye" appearance; occasionally small, dark intracytoplasmic inclusions

Herpes simplex virus
   Enlarged, multinucleated cells with "ground glass" chromatin
   High nuclear-to-cytoplasmic ratio
   Opaque, structureless chromatin
   Eosinophilic intranuclear inclusion

Polyomavirus
   Enlarged cells
   High nuclear-to-cytoplasmic ratio
   Opaque, structureless chromatin, chromatinic membrane is common
   Nuclei stain with a magenta hue
   Intranuclear inclusion fills almost the entire nuclear area

Papillomavirus
   Perinuclear clear cytoplasmic zones (koilocytosis)
   Nuclear enlargement and homogeneous hyperchromasia

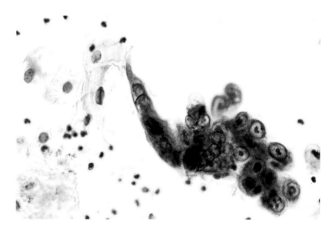

Figure 30-10   Herpes simplex virus infection.

of infection, the viral particles concentrate in the center of the nuclei, forming bright eosinophilic inclusions with a narrow clear zone or halo at the periphery. Infected cells may contain single or multiple nuclei.[11,56] Cytomegalovirus is a virus usually seen in newborn infants with impaired immunity (**Fig. 30-11**). The infection is also common in adults with AIDS. The characteristic changes are readily recognized in the urinary sediment, including large cells with large basophilic nuclear inclusions surrounded by a large peripheral clear zone. There is a distinct outer band of condensed nuclear chromatin.

Polyomavirus infection is widespread, according to serologic studies of adults. The latent virus can become activated and recognized in voided urine sediment.[60-69] One form of polyomavirus, the BK virus, plays a major role in urine cytology because it produces cell abnormalities that are readily confused with cancer. These cells are also known as "decoy cells" because of their similarity to dysplastic urothelial cells (**Fig. 30-12**).[60,61] In permissive infections, the BK virus produces large, homogeneous, basophilic nuclear inclusions that occupy almost the entire volume of the nuclei. Occasionally, a narrow rim of clearing separates the inclusion from the chromatinic rim. The infected cells are often enlarged and usually contain a single nucleus, but binucleation and occasional large multinucleated cells may be seen.[62] The cytologic picture in some cases may be quite dramatic and has led to misdiagnosis of carcinoma.[63] Another rare form of polyomavirus infection of the urine is caused by the JC virus, which is associated with progressive multifocal leukoencephalopathy.

More than 120 types of human papillomavirus are recognized, and types 6 and 11 are associated with condyloma acuminatum. Condylomata may appear in the urethra, and invariably induces koilocytosis, which shed into voided urine. Urothelial carcinoma may also exhibit a low incidence of types 16 and 18 human papillomavirus infections.[70]

Trematodes and Other Parasites

The most important parasitic bladder infection is *Schistosoma haematobium* (*Bilharzia*) (see also **Chapter 2**). There are two important cytologic manifestations of infection with *S. haematobium*: recognition of the ova and of the malignant tumors that may be associated with it.[57] The ova are elongate structures with a thick transparent capsule and a sword-shaped protrusion at the narrow end of the ovum known as the terminal spine. Fresh or calcified ova may be readily recognized in the urinary sediment. The epizootic infectious form of the parasite, known as miracidium, is released in human stool and urine, retaining the shape of the ovum with its terminal spine.

Other common intestinal parasites that also affect the bladder include *Ascaris lumbricoides, Enterobius vermicularis*, and agents of filariasis.

Reactive Changes in Urinary Cytology

A variety of conditions may cause reactive changes in the urothelium (**Table 30-4**). Pertinent clinical history is important in assessing urinary cytology specimens.

Lithiasis

About 40% of patients with calculi have abnormal cytologic findings in voided urine.[52] These patients have numerous large smooth-bordered clusters of benign urothelial cells with an abundance of superficial cells (**Fig. 30-13**). These changes may overlap with the spectrum of findings for low grade urothelial carcinoma, but the cells tend to cluster, with fewer single cells and finer nuclear chromatin.[52] Calculi are abrasive to the mucosa of the renal pelvis, ureter, or urinary bladder. The resulting cytologic specimens closely resemble the effects of instrumentation. Significant atypia of urothelial cells due to lithiasis is uncommon.[1,11] Nonetheless, lithiasis remains a major diagnostic pitfall in urinary cytology interpretation and should always be mentioned on the urine cytology requisition.

Drug Effects

Intravesically administered drugs such as BCG, mitomycin C, and thiotepa are commonly used for treatment of bladder tumors and their recurrence. They may induce cell enlargement or cytoplasmic vacuolization (**Figs. 30-14** and **30-15**). Intravesical chemotherapy contributes to a high rate of false-positive results in urine cytology and should be documented when the specimen is delivered to the lab.[4]

Systemically administered drugs such as the alkylating agents, cyclophosphamide and busulfan, have a marked effect on the urothelium, with significant cytologic abnormalities (**Fig. 30-16**). These drugs may induce changes that include bizarre abnormal urothelial cells with marked nuclear and nucleolar enlargement mimicking poorly differentiated carcinoma.[1,11,71,72] Large doses of cyclophosphamide have been shown to induce urothelial carcinoma, leiomyosarcoma, and carcinosarcoma.[73,74]

Radiation Therapy Effects

Radiation therapy typically induces marked cell enlargement, with bizarre cell shapes and vacuolation of nuclei and cytoplasm. These findings may persist for years after treatment (**Figs. 30-17** and **30-18**).[11,75,76]

Urinary Cytology in Renal Transplant Recipients

The epithelial cells of collecting tubules are well preserved in patients following renal transplantation. When they appear in urine specimens, collecting tubule cells have scant vacuolated cytoplasm with spherical and somewhat opaque nuclei. A feature of impending rejection is the presence of numerous T lymphocytes and erythrocytes in

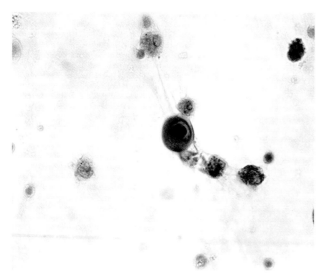

Table 30-4   Differential Diagnosis of Urothelial Atypia

Urinary tract conditions
  Urethral catheterization or cystoscopy
  Urinary calculi
  Chronic cystitis and cystitis glandularis
  Cellular changes due to radiation therapy and
    chemotherapy
  Atypical and/or hyperplastic urothelium
  Neoplasm (grade 1 urothelial carcinoma, low grade
    urothelial carcinoma)

Renal parenchymal conditions
  Acute tubular necrosis
  Papillary necrosis
  Renal infarction
  Acute allograft rejection with ischemic necrosis

Figure 30-11   Cytomegalovirus infection.

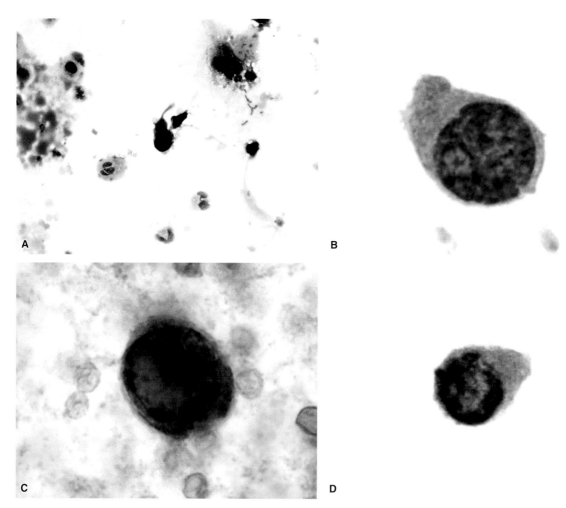

Figure 30-12   Polyomavirus infection (A to D). Note the decoy cells, which may be mistaken for urothelial carcinoma in situ.

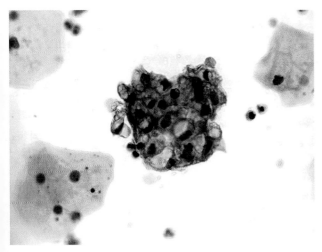

Figure 30-13 Lithiasis. Note the clusters of superficial umbrella cells with smooth contours and cytoplasmic vacuolization.

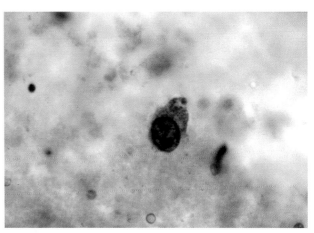

Figure 30-16 Reactive atypia after cyclophosphamide treatment.

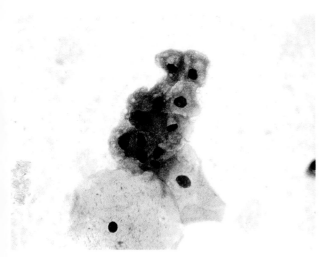

Figure 30-14 Reactive atypia after BCG treatment.

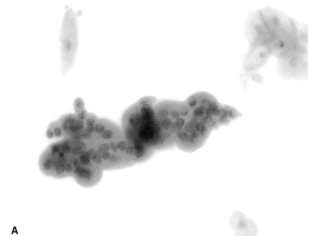

A

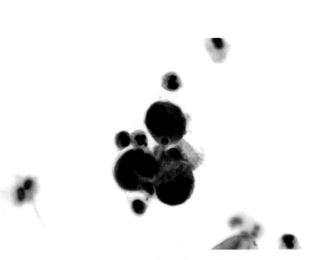

Figure 30-15 Reactive atypia after mitomycin C treatment.

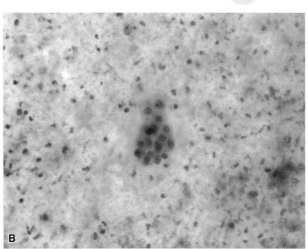

B

Figure 30-17 Reactive atypia after radiation therapy (A and B).

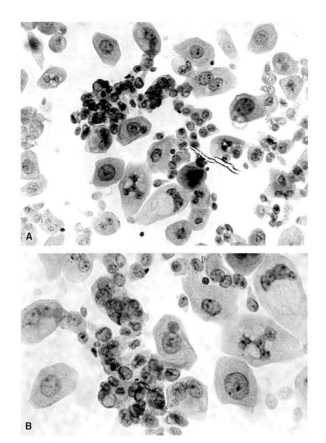

Figure 30-18   Reactive atypia after radiation therapy (A and B).

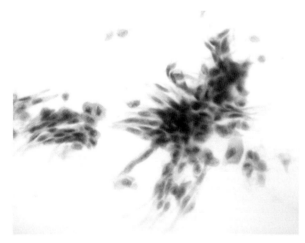

Figure 30-19   Reactive changes. Note the clusters of cells with elongated cytoplasms, caused by ureteral brushing.

the urine. The erythrocytes have a thick outer border and clear center, suggestive of renal origin. In rejection, tissue fragments may also be present, including necrotic renal tubules and hyaline casts.[54]

Other Benign Conditions

Partial or complete keratinization of the squamous epithelium, referred to clinically as leukoplakia, often replaces the urothelium, resulting in a cystoscopic gray-white appearance of the mucosa. In the urinary sediment, anucleated keratinized cells, indicative of hyperkeratosis, may be present. When such cells are identified with bright orangophilia on Papanicolaou stain, further investigation should be undertaken to exclude the possibility of squamous cell carcinoma.[10,11] Cystitis glandularis may shed ciliated and mucus-containing epithelial cells that contain peripheral nuclei and clear cytoplasm. Such cells may be mistaken for adenocarcinoma. Large numbers of macrophages are present in urine samples from patients with malakoplakia, and release of such inflammatory cells usually occurs after biopsy and is detected in the urine stream. The spherical, intracytoplasmic, eosinophilic, or calcified Michaelis–Guttmann bodies in the cytoplasm of the macrophages are usually readily identified and may confirm the diagnosis suspected on biopsy.

A variety of conditions, such as instrumentation, can also be sources of false-positive results (see further discussion below) (**Fig. 30-19**).

Benign Tumors and Tumor-like Processes

There are no unique cell changes characteristic of papilloma, inverted papilloma, or nephrogenic adenoma (nephrogenic metaplasia). Cytologic findings from these processes are, therefore, not specific for an accurate diagnosis of these lesions.[77,78] Condyloma acuminatum of the urinary bladder is uncommon and may be associated with condyloma of the urethra or external genitalia. The characteristic koilocytosis is characterized by squamous cells with large hyperchromatic nuclei and prominent perinuclear clear zones or halos. These changes result from infections by human papillomavirus types 6 and 11. The presence of koilocytes in voided urine sediment in males often indicates a lesion in the bladder or urethra. In women, such cells may also indicate contamination from the lower genital tract. Occasionally, koilocytes may mimic squamous cell carcinoma. Endometrial-type glandular cells in urine sediment have been reported in women with endometriosis.[79]

Cytologic Diagnosis of Dysplasia and Urothelial Carcinoma in Situ

In cases of dysplasia, the only cytologic finding may be the presence of rare atypical urothelial cells.[80] It is difficult,

Table 30-5 Cellular Features of Reactive Atypia, Carcinoma In Situ, and Urothelial Neoplasia

	Reactive Atypia	Carcinoma in Situ	Grade 1 Carcinoma	Grade 2–4 Urothelial Carcinoma
Cells				
Arrangement	Papillary aggregates	Numerous single cells	Papillary and loose clusters	Isolated and loose clusters
Size	Increased	Increased	Increased, uniform	Increased, pleomorphic
Number	Variable	Variable	Often numerous	Variable
Cytoplasm	Vacuolated	Variable maturation	Homogeneous	Variable
Nuclear-to-cytoplasmic ratio	Normal/increased	Increased	Increased	Increased
Nuclei				
Position	Noneccentric	Noneccentric	Eccentric	Eccentric
Size	Enlarged	Enlarged	Enlarged	Variable
Morphology	Uniform within aggregates	Syncytia, cannibalism	Variable within aggregates	Variable
Borders	Smooth	Marked membrane irregularity	Irregular (notches, creases)	Irregular
Chromatin	Dusty-peripheral concentration	Increased chromatin, coarsely granular, evenly distributed	Fine, even	Coarse, uneven
Nucleoli	Often large	Rare nucleoli	Small/absent	Variable
Background	Variable	Clean	Clean	Dirty, tumor diathesis

Table 30-6 Criteria for Cytologic Grading of Urothelial Carcinoma

Morphologic Features	Carcinoma in Situ	Grade 1 Carcinoma	Grade 2 Carcinoma	Grade 3/4 Carcinoma
Background	Clean	Clean	Clean	Dirty, tumor diathesis
Cellular arrangement	Numerous single cells, rare fragments	Large fragments of urothelium	Large fragments of urothelium and single cells	Large fragments and numerous single cells
Nuclear features	Syncytia, cannibalism	Slightly enlarged	Nuclear crowding and overlap	Syncytia, cannibalism
Nuclear membrane	Marked membrane irregularity	Regular, round or oval	Minimal membrane irregularity	Marked membrane irregularity
Chromatin	Increased chromatin, coarsely granular, evenly distributed	Finely granular (vesicular)	Finely granular, evenly distributed	Increased chromatin, coarsely granular, unevenly distributed
Nucleolus	Rare nucleoli	Occasional micronucleoli	Variable micronucleoli	Macronucleoli
Cytoplasmic features	Variable maturation	Cell maturation present	Moderate degree of maturation	Maturation absent, squamoid and/or glandular features

if not impossible, to specifically recognize cellular changes corresponding to dysplasia in cytology specimens.[11] Therefore, the diagnosis of urothelial dysplasia is rarely made based on examination of urine specimens but rare atypical cells similar to CIS may alert the cystoscopist to perform random biopsies for a flat urothelial lesion.

Urothelial CIS is characterized by the presence of malignant cells that are often uniform in size and may be either small or large (**Tables 30-5** and **30-6**).[21,36,72,81–85] Cells shed into the urine from CIS typically exhibit cytologic features of high grade urothelial carcinoma, and consequently, CIS is easier to detect by cytology than urothelial dysplasia. CIS cells are large and often single, with a very high nuclear-to-cytoplasmic ratio and a hyperchromatic nucleus (**Figs. 30-20** to **30-23**). Prominent nucleoli, irregular nuclear outlines, coarse chromatin, mitotic figures, and glandular

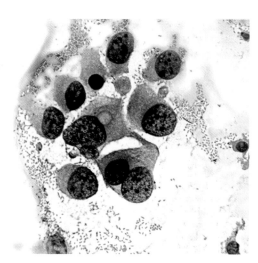

Figure 30-20   Urothelial carcinoma in situ.

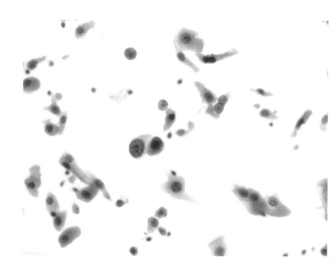

Figure 30-22   Urothelial carcinoma in situ.

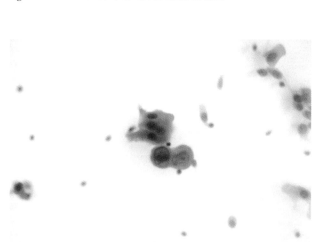

Figure 30-21   Urothelial carcinoma in situ. The nuclei of malignant cells are four to five times larger than the nuclei of normal adjacent urothelial cells.

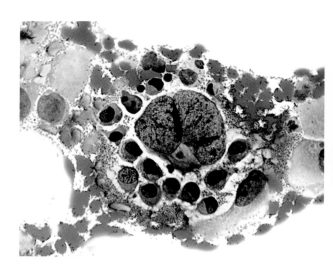

Figure 30-23   Urothelial carcinoma in situ, large cell (pleormorphic) variant.

or squamous differentiation may also be present in urine cytology preparations from patients with CIS.

Catheterization or washing specimens may include tissue fragments rather than single cells, in which overlapping nuclei and atypical architectural features are appreciated. Demir et al. note that a cell-in-cell or "cell cannibalism" phenomenon is particularly common in CIS cases (65%).[85] To avoid misdiagnosis, pathologists should be aware of the histologic variation of CIS lesions (see **Chapter 7** for further discussion).

Since CIS is a noninvasive lesion, the background of the specimen is often clean, free of necrotic debris, blood, and heavy inflammation. Occasionally, the cells are heterogeneous and large, particularly after biopsies. When there is prominent inflammation present, it is

often prudent not to attempt separation of CIS from invasive carcinoma. Microinvasive carcinoma may not be recognizable in cytologic samples, particularly when CIS is present. CIS may persist after intravesical therapy such as BCG, causing difficulty distinguishing therapy changes from persistent neoplasia. Cells of persistent or recurrent CIS following BCG therapy may have coarse, distinct chromatin (**Fig. 30-20** and **30-23**) rather than opaque, smudged and featureless (**Fig. 30-14** and **30-15**).

Sensitivity of cytology in detecting CIS varies from 66% to 83%.[81–84] In a study of 592 bladder washing samples, including 50 patients with CIS, the authors found the diagnoses of either "suspicious for high grade neoplasia" or "consistent with high grade neoplasia" to be 70% sensitive and 99% specific for CIS.[81]

Cytologic Diagnosis of Malignancies

Grade 1 Urothelial Carcinoma

Urinary cytology is a commonly used noninvasive method of bladder cancer surveillance. However, accurate cytologic diagnosis of grade 1 urothelial carcinoma is particularly problematic. The recently introduced 2004 World Health Organization (WHO) grading scheme is also a source of confusion for many cytopathologists.[14] We have proposed a new grading system that incorporates features of both the 1973 and 2004 WHO grading systems. The key modifications are (1) elimination of papillary urothelial neoplasm of low malignant potential (PUNLMP); (2) the use of both numerical (grades 1 to 4) and categorical (low grade vs. high grade) schemes for easy interpretation; and (3) subdividing of 2004 WHO high grade urothelial carcinomas into grade 3 and grade 4 carcinomas (see **Chapter 9** for further discussion) (**Fig. 30-24**).[14] In this proposal, grade 1 (low grade) urothelial carcinoma corresponds to PUNLMP in 2004 WHO classification or grade 1 in 1973 WHO classification; grade 2 (low grade)

urothelial carcinoma corresponds to low grade urothelial carcinoma defined by the 2004 WHO classification.[14]

In general, papilloma and grade 1 urothelial carcinoma cannot be diagnosed reliably by urine cytology, despite several investigations of key cytologic findings purported to identify these low grade lesions. It is impossible in cytology specimens to separate grade 1 urothelial carcinoma from papilloma.[78,86] The urothelial cell clusters often show a papillary configuration and are difficult to distinguish from those shed from the normal benign urothelium after palpation, instrumentation, or irritation by calculi and cystitis.[52,53] In voided urine, spontaneously shed complex clusters of morphologically benign urothelial cells may be suggestive of a papillary tumor, provided that trauma can be excluded clinically. Diagnostic features of grade 1 urothelial carcinoma include the presence of tumor fragments with connective tissue stalks or central capillary vessels (**Tables 30-5** and **30-6**) identified on cell block sections.[87] Numerous attempts to define the precise microscopic features of tumor fragments that separate benign urothelial cell clusters from grade 1 urothelial carcinoma have met with limited success.[37] Some authors found that low grade papillary urothelial tumors shed

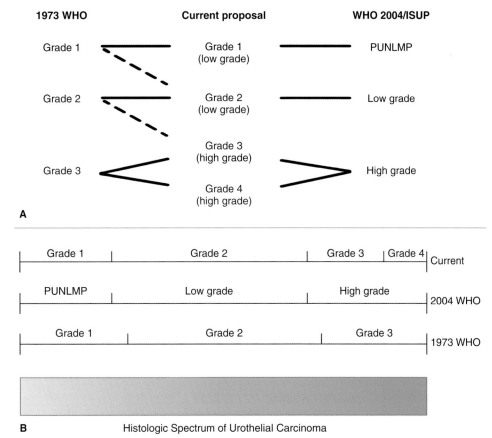

Figure 30-24 Comparison of newly proposed grading system with the 1973 and 2004 WHO grading systems. (From Ref. 14; with permission.)

recognizable cells and clusters in the urinary sediment (**Figs. 30-25** and **30-26**).[88] Characteristic features of these include increased ratio of nucleus to cytoplasm, enlarged and hyperchromatic nuclei, and absence of nucleoli. These features are present in 70% of such tumors but may also be a consequence of minor trauma.[24] Consequently, others report a correct cytologic diagnosis in only 33% of cases.[37] Nevertheless, such clusters may be a sufficient indication for fiberoptic cystoscopy.

Differentiation of grade 1 urothelial carcinoma from instrumentation artifact is suggested by the presence of cell clusters with ragged borders in grade 1 urothelial carcinoma, unlike the smooth borders, tight cohesiveness, and densely stained cytoplasm at the edge of benign cell clusters in the case of instrumentation.[53] Grade 1 urothelial carcinoma can be identified with 45% sensitivity and 98% specificity based on the cytologic criteria of an increased nuclear-to-cytoplasmic ratio, irregular nuclear borders, and cytoplasmic homogeneity.[6] Overall observer accuracy was 76%, with a specificity of 82% for a definitive negative diagnosis and a sensitivity for a definitive positive diagnosis of 96%.[7] In another study,[4] the sensitivity of 90% and specificity of 65% for grade 1 urothelial carcinoma was based on the absence of inflammation, the presence of single and overlapping groups of cells with a high nuclear-to-cytoplasmic ratio, hypochromasia, nuclear grooves and notches, and small nucleoli. Despite these findings, grade 1 urothelial carcinoma is a major source of false-negative results in urine cytology.[4]

Ancillary techniques (see **Chapters 29** to **34** for further discussion) may be valuable for separating benign and neoplastic urothelial cells, including DNA ploidy analysis,[88] immunohistochemical markers,[89] and numeric chromosomal abnormalities detected by fluorescent in situ hybridization (FISH).[90] Digital image analysis may be superior to bladder wash cytology for prediction of tumor recurrence.[91]

Grade 2 (Low Grade) and Grade 3/4 (High Grade) Urothelial Carcinoma

Key diagnostic features are listed in **Tables 30-5** and **30-6**. It may be difficult to separate grade 1 from grade 2 urothelial carcinoma (**Figs. 30-27** to **30-29**) or grade 3/4 (high grade) urothelial carcinoma (**Figs. 30-30** to **30-35**) from urothelial CIS (**Tables 30-5** and **30-6**). Unlike benign urothelial cells, these cells have substantial nuclear and cytoplasmic abnormalities. The principal value of urine cytology is the diagnosis and monitoring of high grade tumors that may not be evident cystoscopically, including CIS and occult invasive carcinoma.[21,92]

In voided urine, low and high grade urothelial carcinoma cells vary in size and shape. The nuclei are enlarged, with coarsely granular chromatin, hyperchromasia, abnormal

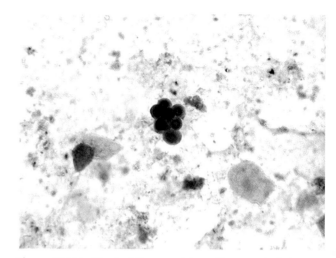

Figure 30-25   Grade 1 (low grade) papillary urothelial carcinoma.

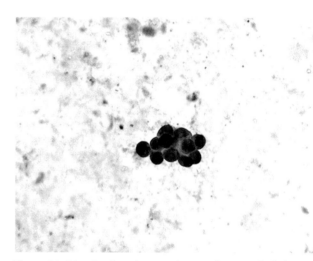

Figure 30-26   Grade 1 (low grade) papillary urothelial carcinoma.

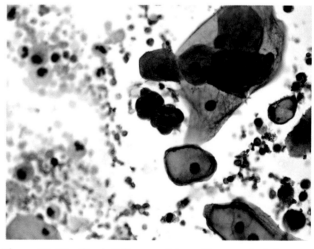

Figure 30-27   Grade 2 (low grade) papillary urothelial carcinoma.

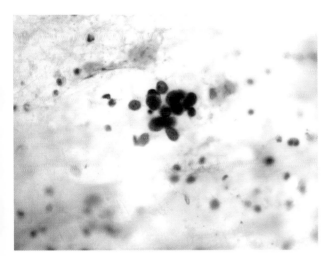

Figure 30-28 Grade 2 (low grade) papillary urothelial carcinoma.

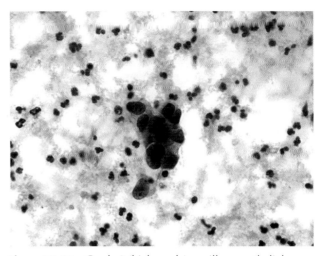

Figure 30-31 Grade 3 (high grade) papillary urothelial carcinoma. Note the dirty background.

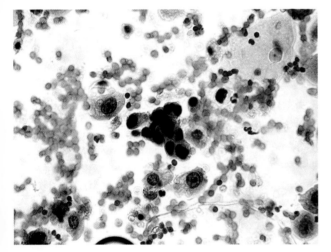

Figure 30-29 Grade 2 (low grade) papillary urothelial carcinoma.

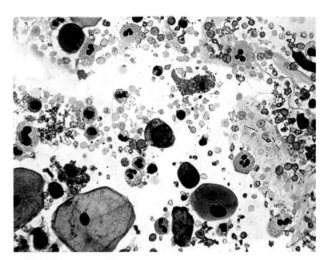

Figure 30-32 Grade 3 (high grade) urothelial carcinoma. Note the dirty background.

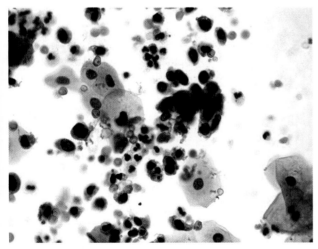

Figure 30-30 Grade 3 (high grade) papillary urothelial carcinoma.

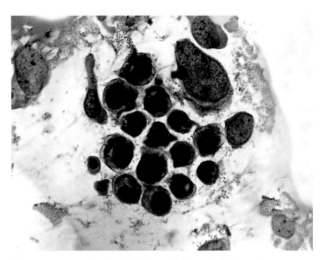

Figure 30-33 Grade 4 (high grade) urothelial carcinoma.

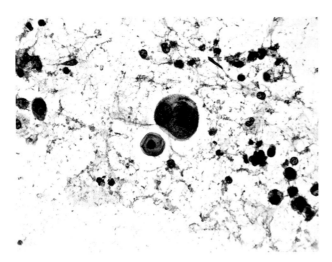

Figure 30-34 Grade 4 (high grade) urothelial carcinoma.

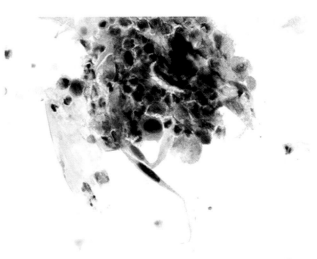

Figure 30-36 Squamous cell carcinoma. Note the spindle cells with nuclear pleomorphism.

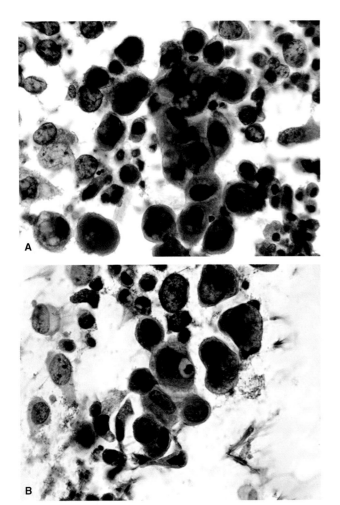

Figure 30-35 Grade 4 (high grade) urothelial carcinoma (A and B). Note the cannibalism (or cytophagocytosis) that is typically associated with high grade urothelial carcinoma.

nuclear contours, and prominent nucleoli. Multinucleated cancer cells and mitotic figures are often readily identified.[93]

In bladder washings, urothelial carcinoma may demonstrate a lower degree of nuclear hyperchromasia, perhaps resulting in more prominent large nucleoli. The cells may be poorly preserved, particularly when there is inflammation or necrosis. A variety of degenerative changes may be seen, including frayed or vacuolated cytoplasm, nonspecific eosinophilic cytoplasmic inclusions, and pyknotic nuclei. In some high grade papillary tumors, the dominant cytologic finding may be the presence of loose groupings of cancer cells, with single tumor cells or small groups of two or three. Papillary tumors of intermediate grade often present a diagnostic challenge.[11,92] In some cases, the majority of cells with irregular nuclear contours are similar to those in grade 1 urothelial carcinoma. Fortunately, in most cases, atypical urothelial cells with irregular nuclear contours are observed, and these alert the clinician to the need for cystoscopic examination.

There appears to be good correlation between urine cytology and biopsy findings, although the results reported vary considerably.[2-9,27,94] Approximately two-thirds of cases of grade 1 urothelial carcinoma/PUNLMP are diagnosed as suspicious or malignant. The sensitivity increases to 80% for grade 2 and 95% for grade 3 urothelial carcinomas. Urothelial CIS can be diagnosed as suspicious or positive in virtually all instances. The overall sensitivity of urine cytology for primary carcinoma of the bladder ranges from 45% to 97%. In Loh et al.'s report, urine cytology predicted 82% of all recurrent tumors in the bladder.[95] Two major drawbacks of urinary cytology are the high rate of false-positive results in patients on intravesical chemotherapy and the high rate of false-negative results in those with grade 1 or low grade urothelial carcinoma.

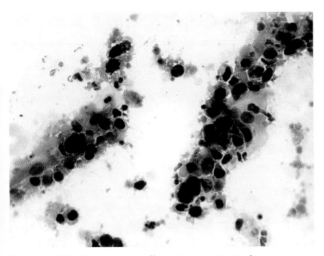

Figure 30-37 Squamous cell carcinoma. Note the keratinized cells with hyperchromatic nuclei and dense brightly stained cytoplasm.

Squamous Cell Carcinoma

Invasive squamous cell carcinoma is common in Africa and the Middle East, particularly in patients infected with *Schistosoma haematobium*. Predominantly squamous tumors, on the other hand, are uncommon in developed countries, accounting for no more than 3% of bladder tumors (see also **Chapter 14**). Squamous cell carcinoma has been observed with increasing frequency in long-term survivors with severe spinal cord injury and neurogenic bladder.

Squamous cell carcinoma may display varying degrees of differentiation. In well-differentiated invasive squamous cell carcinoma, the cytologic findings in voided urine are somewhat characteristic (**Figs. 30-36** and **30-37**). The presence of markedly keratinized cells with thick, yellow or orange cytoplasm on Papanicolaou stain, and large, irregular, often dark pyknotic nuclei are useful. Squamous pearls, characterized by cell aggregates arranged concentrically around a core of keratin, may be observed.[11] The background of the slide often shows evidence of marked necrosis, and ghost cells may be present. A mixture of cancer cells is observed in the urine of patients with poorly differentiated squamous cell carcinoma, including sharply demarcated cells with eosinophilic cytoplasm and large nuclei.[10,11] Most cases are aneuploid.[96]

Adenocarcinoma

In colonic-type adenocarcinoma of the bladder, the urinary sediment contains columnar cancer cells with large, hyperchromatic nuclei and large nucleoli, sometimes in clusters. In poorly differentiated mucus-producing carcinoma, the cancer cells are small, more spherical or cuboidal in shape, and contain large hyperchromatic nuclei, also with prominent nucleoli. The cytoplasm is usually basophilic, scant, and sometimes poorly preserved with "stripped" tumor cell nuclei in the specimen. When there are large cytoplasmic vacuoles containing mucus, the nuclei may be pushed to the periphery of the cell, features diagnostic of signet ring cell carcinoma.[97,98]

In clear cell adenocarcinoma, the cancer cells are large, with abundant finely vacuolated or granular cytoplasm, open vesicular nuclei, and prominent nucleoli. Such cells usually form round "papillary" clusters.[10] Most cases are DNA aneuploid.[99,100]

Neuroendocrine Carcinoma, Including Small Cell Carcinoma

In small cell carcinoma, the cancer cells are small, about four times the size of lymphocytes, and contain compact, pyknotic nuclei, with scant basophilic cytoplasm.[101–103] Nucleoli are not visible. The presence of numerous small clusters of tightly packed tumor cells with nuclear molding may be diagnostically useful.[11] The presence of cell clusters without prominent nucleoli is helpful in differentiating these cells from malignant lymphoma. In lymphoma, the cells do not cluster and usually contain at least a small nucleolus. The demonstration of neuroendocrine differentiation may require immunohistochemical or ultrastructural study.

Rare cases of carcinoid (low grade neuroendocrine carcinoma) and large cell neuroendocrine carcinoma have been diagnosed by urine cytology.[104,105]

Other Malignant Tumors

Urothelial cancer may contain foci with more than one histologic type, including squamous cell carcinoma, adenocarcinoma, small cell carcinoma, sarcomatoid carcinoma, and others (see also **Chapters 12** to **17**). The cytologic findings in such tumors rarely allow the diagnosis of mixed carcinoma. Usually, one cytologic pattern is dominant, although rarely a mixed population of cancer cells may be observed.

Other rare cancers that may be diagnosed by cytology include sarcoma, melanoma,[106] lymphoma,[107] plasmacytoma,[108] yolk sac tumor, and choriocarcinoma. In most cases, urine cytology may not be conclusive, but may suggest the correct diagnosis when immunocytochemical stains are performed or lead to cystoscopy and diagnostic biopsy of malignancy.

Secondary Tumors

Occasionally, a metastatic malignant tumor is observed in the urinary sediment. The most common metastases arise from adjacent or contiguous organs, including the uterine cervix, endometrium, or ovary in women, the prostate in men, and the colon in both genders. Urine cytology in such cases may show squamous cell carcinoma or adenocarcinoma. Clinicopathologic correlation is usually required for diagnosis. Rare cases of lymphoma, leukemia, and melanoma may be diagnosed from urine samples.

Cytology of Anatomic Sites Other Than Urinary Bladder

Primary cancer of the urethra not associated with a bladder tumor is rare. The most common of such urethral primaries are squamous cell carcinoma, adenocarcinoma, and urothelial carcinoma, although all are rare. Other rare cancers of the urethra or upper urinary collecting tract include malignant melanoma and clear cell adenocarcinoma. Cytologic examination of the urethra is commonly used for surveillance after cystectomy for bladder cancer. These examinations may reveal CIS or early invasive carcinoma in the urethral remant.[21]

Urine cytology is usually diagnostic in urothelial carcinoma of the renal pelvis and ureter, particularly when the cancers are high grade. In low grade urothelial malignancies, the same diagnostic problems are encountered as in the bladder.[109] The cytologist should bear in mind that normal superficial and intermediate cells of the upper tract urothelium tend to be smaller and have higher nuclear-to-cytoplasmic ratio than corresponding cells in the bladder when examined in cytologic preparations.

Urine cytology is generally unsatisfactory for detection of renal cell carcinoma. When malignant cells are present from large or medullary tumors, they are large cells with clear or vacuolated cytoplasm and distinct nucleoli.

Prostatic adenocarcinoma may yield cells in voided urine spontaneously or after prostatic massage, particularly if the carcinoma is high grade. The cancer cells in urine sediment are usually small, often spherical or columnar. Small cell clusters may be observed. The cells usually have basophilic cytoplasm and open vesicular nuclei with prominent nucleoli. Prostatic massage is not considered useful for the early detection of prostate carcinoma.

Sources of Diagnostic Pitfalls

A frequent error in urine cytology is overdiagnosis of benign cellular changes as malignant (Table 30-7; see also the previous section for discussion). Knowledge of these benign changes is fundamental to the practice of cytology.

Table 30-7 Major Diagnostic Pitfalls in Lower Urinary Tract Cytology

Underdiagnosis of low grade urothelial carcinoma as benign
Overdiagnosis of normal and degenerated urothelium as malignant
Overdiagnosis of human polyomavirus infection as malignant
Overdiagnosis of effects of cyclophosphamide as malignant

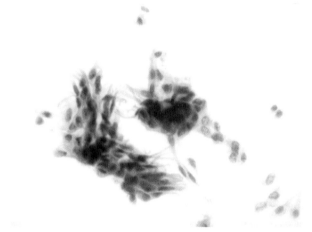

Figure 30-38 Reactive changes after instrumentation. This ureteral washing specimen shows aggregates and sheets of elongated urothelial cells with dense cytoplasm and enlarged nuclei; however, the nuclei are relatively uniform. The background is clean.

Trauma or Instrumentation

The normal urothelium tends to exfoliate when abraded or traumatized appearing in the form of tissue fragments that are round or oval, commonly as papillary clusters (Figs. 30-38 and 30-39). Vigorous palpation, catheterization, or any form of instrumentation may result in the formation of such epithelial clusters. When present in large numbers, these clusters are easily misinterpreted as papillary carcinoma although the background often shows lubricant and scant blood with this instrumentation artifact.[30,53,110] Another important source of error is the presence of numerous superficial urothelial cells (umbrella cells) that may be mistaken for cancer cells because of their large nuclei and variable nuclear features.[72] The nuclear-to-cytoplasmic ratio of these umbrella cells, however, is usually low. Simple bladder distension or chronic bladder outlet obstruction appears sufficient to release these umbrella cells into voided urine.

Cell Preservation

Cells in voided urine sediment, particularly in the first morning voiding, are often poorly preserved, compounding

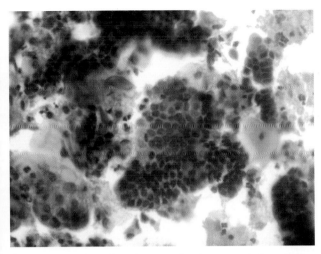

Figure 30-39 Reactive changes after instrumentation. Cells are arranged in papillary aggregate configuration that may be mistaken for papillary urothelial carcinoma.

the diagnostic difficulty. The diagnosis of cancer in voided urine should be avoided unless the findings are unequivocal and well-preserved tumor cells are present.[11]

Human Polyomavirus

Polyomavirus forms large intranuclear inclusions that may mimic cancer cell nuclei. However, the inclusions are homogeneous and lack the coarse granularity of chromatin

seen in cancer.[62] This is an important source of diagnostic errors that can contribute to costly and lengthy patient investigations.

Lithiasis

As mentioned previously, calculi anywhere in the lower urinary tract may act as abrasive instruments, dislodging epithelial fragments that may be quite large with papillary appearances mimicking low grade papillary carcinoma.[52] The presence of numerous superficial cells may also create diagnostic difficulty, due to reactive nuclear abnormalities (**Fig. 30-13**).[4,11,72] A history of bladder outlet obstruction, flank pain, or radiographic diagnosis of stone on noncontrast CT may prevent this error.

Drugs and Other Therapeutic Procedures

Urine cell changes may result from a wide variety of inciting agents, including chemotherapeutic agents, radiotherapy, and other interventions. Intravesical chemotherapy is responsible for a high rate of false-positive results.[4] A further source of diagnostic difficulty may be synchronous infection with polyomavirus in patients who are immunocompromised.[11] It should be remembered that urothelial carcinoma or sarcoma may develop in patients receiving cyclophosphamide for treatment of lymphoma.[73,74]

REFERENCES

1. Koss LG, Melamed MR. Koss' Diagnostic Cytology and Its Histopathologic Bases. Philadelphia: Lippincott Williams & Wilkins, 2005.
2. Tetu B. Diagnosis of urothelial carcinoma from urine. *Mod Pathol* 2009;22(Suppl 2):S53–9.
3. Bastacky S, Ibrahim S, Wilczynski SP, Murphy WM. The accuracy of urinary cytology in daily practice. *Cancer* 1999;87:118–28.
4. Maier U, Simak R, Neuhold N. The clinical value of urinary cytology: 12 years of experience with 615 patients. *J Clin Pathol* 1995;48:314–7.
5. Raab SS, Grzybicki DM, Vrbin CM, Geisinger KR. Urine cytology discrepancies: frequency, causes, and outcomes. *Am J Clin Pathol* 2007;127:946–53.
6. Raab SS, Lenel JC, Cohen MB. Low grade transitional cell carcinoma of

the bladder. Cytologic diagnosis by key features as identified by logistic regression analysis. *Cancer* 1994;74:1621–6.
7. Raab SS, Slagel DD, Jensen CS, Teague MW, Savell VH, Ozkutlu D, Lenel JC, Cohen MB. low grade transitional cell carcinoma of the urinary bladder: application of select cytologic criteria to improve diagnostic accuracy [corrected]. *Mod Pathol* 1996;9:225–32.
8. Lokeshwar VB, Soloway MS. Current bladder tumor tests: Does their projected utility fulfill clinical necessity? *J Urol* 2001;165:1067–77.
9. Turco P, Houssami N, Bulgaresi P, Troni GM, Galanti L, Cariaggi MP, Cifarelli P, Crocetti E, Ciatto S. Is conventional urinary cytology still reliable for diagnosis of primary

bladder carcinoma? Accuracy based on data linkage of a consecutive clinical series and cancer registry. *Acta Cytol* 2011;55:193–6.
10. Fracchia JA, Motta J, Miller LS, Armenakas NA, Schumann GB, Greenberg RA. Evaluation of asymptomatic microhematuria. *Urology* 1995;46:484–9.
11. Koss LG. Errors and pitfalls in cytology of the lower urinary tract. *Monogr Pathol* 1997:60–74.
12. Ooms EC, Veldhuizen RW. Cytological criteria and diagnostic terminology in urinary cytology. *Cytopathology* 1993;4:51–4.
13. Potts SA, Thomas PA, Cohen MB, Raab SS. Diagnostic accuracy and key cytologic features of high grade transitional cell carcinoma in the upper urinary tract. *Mod Pathol* 1997;10:657–62.

14. Cheng L, MacLennan GT, Lopez-Beltran A. Histologic grading of urothelial carcinoma: A reappraisal. *Hum Pathol* 2012 (in press).

15. Messing EM, Teot L, Korman H, Underhill E, Barker E, Stork B, Qian J, Bostwick DG. Performance of urine test in patients monitored for recurrence of bladder cancer: a multicenter study in the United States. *J Urol* 2005;174:1238–41.

16. Berlac PA, Holm HH. Bladder tumor control by abdominal ultrasound and urine cytology. *J Urol* 1992;147:1510–2.

17. Chow NH, Tzai TS, Cheng HL, Chan SH, Lin JS. Urinary cytodiagnosis: Can it have a different prognostic implication than a diagnostic test? *Urol Int* 1994;53:18–23.

18. Koss LG, Deitch D, Ramanathan R, Sherman AB. Diagnostic value of cytology of voided urine. *Acta Cytol* 1985;29:810–6.

19. Schwalb DM, Herr HW, Fair WR. The management of clinically unconfirmed positive urinary cytology. *J Urol* 1993;150:1751–6.

20. Curry JL, Wojcik EM. The effects of the current World Health Organization/International Society of Urologic Pathologists bladder neoplasm classification system on urine cytology results. *Cancer* 2002;96:140–5.

21. Gamarra MC, Zein T. Cytologic spectrum of bladder cancer. *Urology* 1984;23:23–6.

22. Papanicolaou GN. Cytology of the urine sediment in neoplasms of the urinary tract. *J Urol* 1947;57:375–9.

23. Orandi A, Orandi M. Urine cytology in the detection of bladder tumor recurrence. *J Urol* 1976;116:568–9.

24. Murphy WM, Soloway MS, Jukkola AF, Crabtree WN, Ford KS. Urinary cytology and bladder cancer. The cellular features of transitional cell neoplasms. *Cancer* 1984;53:1555–65.

25. Ajit D, Dighe S, Desai S. Has urine cytology a role to play in the era of fluorescence in situ hybridization? *Acta Cytol* 2010;54:1118–22.

26. Boon ME, Blomjous CE, Zwartendijk J, Heinhuis RJ, Ooms EC. Carcinoma in situ of the urinary bladder. Clinical presentation, cytologic pattern and stromal changes. *Acta Cytol* 1986;30:360–6.

27. Brimo F, Vollmer RT, Case B, Aprikian A, Kassouf W, Auger M. Accuracy of urine cytology and the significance of an atypical category. *Am J Clin Pathol* 2009;132:785–93.

28. Broghamer WL Jr, Parker JE, Harty JI, Gilkey CM. Cytohistologic correlation of urothelial lesions secondary to photodynamic therapy. *Acta Cytol* 1989;33:881–6.

29. Cant JD, Murphy WM, Soloway MS. Prognostic significance of urine cytology on initial followup after intravesical mitomycin C for superficial bladder cancer. *Cancer* 1986;57:2119–22.

30. Chu YC, Han JY, Han HS, Kim JM, Suh JK. Cytologic evaluation of low grade transitional cell carcinoma and instrument artifact in bladder washings. *Acta Cytol* 2002;46:341–8.

31. Deshpande V, McKee GT. Analysis of atypical urine cytology in a tertiary care center. *Cancer* 2005;105:468–75.

32. Highman WJ. Transitional carcinoma of the upper urinary tract: a histological and cytopathological study. *J Clin Pathol* 1986;39:297–305.

33. Highman WJ. Flat in situ carcinoma of the bladder: cytological examination of urine in diagnosis, follow up, and assessment of response to chemotherapy. *J Clin Pathol* 1988;41:540–6.

34. Kern WH. The cytology of transitional cell carcinoma of the urinary bladder. *Acta Cytol* 1975;19:420–8.

35. Sedlock DJ, MacLennan GT. Urine cytology in the evaluation of upper tract urothelial lesions. *J Urol* 2004;172:2406.

36. Rosa B, Cazin M, Dalian G. Urinary cytology for carcinoma in situ of the urinary bladder. *Acta Cytol* 1985;29:117–24.

37. Wiener HG, Vooijs GP, van't Hof-Grootenboer B. Accuracy of urinary cytology in the diagnosis of primary and recurrent bladder cancer. *Acta Cytol* 1993;37:163–9.

38. Nabi G, Greene DR, O'Donnell M. How important is urinary cytology in the diagnosis of urological malignancies? *Eur Urol* 2003;43:632–6.

39. Matzkin H, Moinuddin SM, Soloway MS. Value of urine cytology versus bladder washing in bladder cancer. *Urology* 1992;39:201–3.

40. Bian Y, Ehya H, Bagley DH. Cytologic diagnosis of upper urinary tract neoplasms by ureteroscopic sampling. *Acta Cytol* 1995;39:733–40.

41. Malmgren RA, Soloway MS, Chu EW, Del Vecchio PR, Ketcham AS. Cytology of ileal conduit urine. *Acta Cytol* 1971;15:506–9.

42. Ajit D, Dighe SB, Desai SB. Cytology of lleal conduit urine in bladder cancer patients: diagnostic utility and pitfalls. *Acta Cytol* 2006;50:70–3.

43. Watarai Y, Satoh H, Matubara M, Asakawa K, Kamaguchi H, Nagai S, Murase Y, Yokoyama M, Kimura G, Tamura K, Sugisaki Y. Comparison of urine cytology between the ileal conduit and Indiana pouch. *Acta Cytol* 2000;44:748–51.

44. Amberson JB, Laino JP. Image cytometric deoxyribonucleic acid analysis of urine specimens as an adjunct to visual cytology in the detection of urothelial cell carcinoma. *J Urol* 1993;149:42–5.

45. Kline MJ, Wilkinson EJ, Askeland R, Given RW, Stephen C, Hendricks JB. DNA tetraploidy in Feulgen-stained bladder washings assessed by image cytometry. *Anal Quant Cytol Histol* 1995;17:129–34.

46. Biesterfeld S, Gerres K, Fischer-Wein G, Bocking A. Polyploidy in non-neoplastic tissues. *J Clin Pathol* 1994;47:38–42.

47. Katz RL, Sinkre PA, Zhang HH, Kidd L, Johnston D. Clinical significance of negative and equivocal urinary bladder cytology alone and in combination with DNA image analysis and cystoscopy. *Cancer* 1997;81:354–64.

48. Liu J, Katz R, Shin HJ, Johnston DA, Zhang HZ, Caraway NP. Use of mailed urine specimens in diagnosing urothelial carcinoma by cytology and DNA image analysis. *Acta Cytol* 2005;49:157–62.

49. Pritchett TR, Kanzler AW, Nichols PW, Bakke AC, Hechinger MK, Skinner DG, Parker JW. A simple and practical technic for detecting cancer cells in urine and urinary bladder washings by flow cytometry. *Am J Clin Pathol* 1985;84:191–6.

50. Tribukait B, Gustafson H, Esposti P. Ploidy and proliferation in human bladder tumors as measured by flow-cytofluorometric DNA-analysis and its relations to histopathology and cytology. *Cancer* 1979;43:1742–51.

51. Koss LG, Wersto RP, Simmons DA, Deitch D, Herz F, Freed SZ. Predictive value of DNA measurements in bladder washings. Comparison of flow cytometry, image cytophotometry, and cytology in patients with a past history of urothelial tumors. *Cancer* 1989;64:916–24.

52. Highman W, Wilson E. Urine cytology in patients with calculi. *J Clin Pathol* 1982;35:350–6.

53. Kannan V, Bose S. Low grade transitional cell carcinoma and instrument artifact. A challenge in urinary cytology. *Acta Cytol* 1993;37:899–902.

54. Roberti I, Reisman L, Burrows L, Lieberman KV. Urine cytology and urine flow cytometry in renal transplantation—a prospective double blind study. *Transplantation* 1995;59:495–500.

55. Rupp M, O'Hara B, McCullough L, Saxena S, Olchiewski J. Prostatic carcinoma cells in urine specimens. *Cytopathology* 1994;5:164–70.

56. Marcussen N, Schumann J, Campbell P, Kjellstrand C. Cytodiagnostic urinalysis is very useful in the differential diagnosis of acute renal failure and can predict the severity. *Ren Fail* 1995;17:721–9.

57. Eltoum IA, Suliaman SM, Ismail BM, Ismail AI, Ali MM, Homeida MM. Evaluation of eosinophiluria in the diagnosis of schistosomiasis hematobium: a field-based study. *Am J Trop Med Hyg* 1992;46:732–6.

58. Betz SA, See WA, Cohen MB. Granulomatous inflammation in bladder wash specimens after intravesical bacillus Calmette-Guérin therapy for transitional cell carcinoma of the bladder. *Am J Clin Pathol* 1993;99:244–8.

59. Schwalb MD, Herr HW, Sogani PC, Russo P, Sheinfeld J, Fair WR. Positive urinary cytology following a complete response to intravesical bacillus Calmette-Guerin therapy: pattern of recurrence. *J Urol* 1994;152:382–7.

60. Crabbe JG. "Comet" or "decoy" cells found in urinary sediment smears. *Acta Cytol* 1971;15:303–5.

61. Koss LG. On decoy cells. *Acta Cytol* 2005;49:233–4.

62. Koss LG, Sherman AB, Eppich E. Image analysis and DNA content of urothelial cells infected with human polyomavirus. *Anal Quant Cytol* 1984;6:89–94.

63. Seftel AD, Matthews LA, Smith MC, Willis J. Polyomavirus mimicking high grade transitional cell carcinoma. *J Urol* 1996;156:1764.

64. Filie AC, Wilder AM, Brosky K, Kopp JB, Miller KD, Abati A. Urinary cytology associated with human polyomavirus and indinavir therapy in HIV-infected patients. *Am J Clin Pathol* 2002;117:922–6.

65. Herawi M, Parwani AV, Chan T, Ali SZ, Epstein JI. Polyoma virus-associated cellular changes in the urine and bladder biopsy samples: a cytohistologic correlation. *Am J Surg Pathol* 2006;30:345–50.

66. Hashida Y, Yunis EJ. Polyomavirus inclusions in urinary cytology. *Am J Clin Pathol* 1981;75:767.

67. Thamboo TP, Jeffery KJ, Friend PJ, Turner GD, Roberts IS. Urine cytology screening for polyoma virus infection following renal transplantation: the Oxford experience. *J Clin Pathol* 2007;60:927–30.

68. Semple K, Lovchik J, Drachenberg C. Identification of polyoma BK virus in kidney transplant recipients by shell vial cell culture assay and urine cytology. *Am J Clin Pathol* 2006;126:444–7.

69. Kipp BR, Sebo TJ, Griffin MD, Ihrke JM, Halling KC. Analysis of polyomavirus-infected renal transplant recipients' urine specimens: correlation of routine urine cytology, fluorescence in situ hybridization, and digital image analysis. *Am J Clin Pathol* 2005;124:854–61.

70. Lopez-Beltran A, Escudero AL, Carrasco-Aznar JC, Vicioso-Recio L. Human papillomavirus infection and transitional cell carcinoma of the bladder. Immunohistochemistry and in situ hybridization. *Pathol Res Pract* 1996;192:154–9.

71. Forni AM, Koss LG, Geller W. Cytological study of the effect of cyclophosphamide on the epithelium of the urinary bladder in man. *Cancer* 1964;17:1348–55.

72. Murphy WM. Current status of urinary cytology in the evaluation of bladder neoplasms. *Hum Pathol* 1990;21:886–96.

73. Travis LB, Curtis RE, Boice JD Jr, Fraumeni JF Jr. Bladder cancer after chemotherapy for non-Hodgkin's lymphoma. *N Engl J Med* 1989;321:544–5.

74. Wall RL, Clausen KP. Carcinoma of the urinary bladder in patients receiving cyclophosphamide. *N Engl J Med* 1975;293:271–3.

75. Macfarlane EW, Ceelen GH, Taylor JN. Urine cytology after treatment of bladder tumors. *Acta Cytol* 1964;8:288–92.

76. Loveless KJ. The effects of radiation upon the cytology of benign and malignant bladder epithelia. *Acta Cytol* 1973;17:355–60.

77. Stilmant MM, Siroky MB. Nephrogenic adenoma associated with intravesical bacillus Calmette-Guérin treatment: a report of 2 cases. *J Urol* 1986;135:359–61.

78. Wolinska WH, Melamed MR, Klein FA. Cytology of bladder papilloma. *Acta Cytol* 1985;29:817–22.

79. Schneider V, Smith MJ, Frable WJ. Urinary cytology in endometriosis of the bladder. *Acta Cytol* 1980;24:30–3.

80. Murphy WM, Soloway MS. Urothelial dysplasia. *J Urol* 1982;127:849–54.

81. Garbar C, Mascaux C, Wespes E. Is urinary tract cytology still useful for diagnosis of bladder carcinomas? A large series of 592 bladder washings using a five-category classification of different cytological diagnoses. *Cytopathology* 2007;18:79–83.

82. Halling KC, King W, Sokolova IA, Meyer RG, Burkhardt HM, Halling AC, Cheville JC, Sebo TJ, Ramakumar S, Stewart CS, Pankratz S, O'Kane DJ, Seelig SA, Lieber MM, Jenkins RB. A comparison of cytology and fluorescence in situ hybridization for the detection of urothelial carcinoma. *J Urol* 2000;164:1768–75.

83. Gudjonsson S, Isfoss BL, Hansson K, Domanski AM, Warenholt J, Soller W, Lundberg LM, Liedberg F, Grabe M, Mansson W. The value of the UroVysion assay for surveillance of non-muscle-invasive bladder cancer. *Eur Urol* 2008;54:402–8.

84. Moonen PM, Merkx GF, Peelen P, Karthaus HF, Smeets DF, Witjes JA. UroVysion compared with cytology and quantitative cytology in the surveillance of non-muscle-invasive bladder cancer. *Eur Urol* 2007;51:1275–80.

85. Demir MA, Ryd W, Aldenborg F, Holmang S. Cytopathological expression of different types of urothelial carcinoma in situ in urinary bladder washings. *BJU Int* 2003;92:906–10.

86. Renshaw AA, Nappi D, Weinberg DS. Cytology of grade 1 papillary transitional cell carcinoma. A comparison of cytologic, architectural and morphometric criteria in cystoscopically obtained urine. *Acta Cytol* 1996;40:676–82.

87. Green LK, Meistrich H. Dramatically increased specificity and sensitivity in detecting low grade papillary TCC via a combination of cytospin and cell blocking techniques. *Mod Pathol* 1995;8:40A.

88. Sack MJ, Artymyshyn RL, Tomaszewski JE, Gupta PK. Diagnostic value of bladder wash cytology, with special reference to low grade urothelial neoplasms. *Acta Cytol* 1995;39:187–94.

89. Panosian KJM, Lopez-Beltran A, Croghan G. An immunohistochemical evaluation of urinary bladder cytology utilizing monoclonal antibodies. *World J Urol* 1989;7:73–79.

90. Cajulis RS, Haines GK 3rd, Frias-Hidvegi D, McVary K, Bacus JW. Cytology, flow cytometry, image analysis, and interphase cytogenetics by fluorescence in situ hybridization in the diagnosis of transitional cell carcinoma in bladder washes: a comparative study. *Diagn Cytopathol* 1995;13:214–24.

91. Van der Poel HG, Boon ME, van Stratum P, Ooms EC, Wiener H, Debruyne FM, Witjes JA, Schalken JA, Murphy WM. Conventional bladder wash cytology performed by four experts versus quantitative image analysis. *Mod Pathol* 1997;10:976–82.

92. Rife CC, Farrow GM, Utz DC. Urine cytology of transitional cell neoplasms. *Urol Clin North Am* 1979;6:599–612.

93. Shenoy UA, Colby TV, Schumann GB. Reliability of urinary cytodiagnosis in urothelial neoplasms. *Cancer* 1985;56:2041–5.

94. Zein T, Wajsman Z, Englander LS, Gamarra M, Lopez C, Huben RP, Pontes JE. Evaluation of bladder washings and urine cytology in the diagnosis of bladder cancer and its correlation with selected biopsies of the bladder mucosa. *J Urol* 1984;132:670–1.

95. Loh CS, Spedding AV, Ashworth MT, Kenyon WE, Desmond AD. The value of exfoliative urine cytology in combination with flexible cystoscopy in the diagnosis of recurrent transitional cell carcinoma of the urinary bladder. *Br J Urol* 1996;77:655–8.

96. Shaaban AA, Tribukait B, el-Bedeiwy AF, Ghoneim MA. Characterization of squamous cell bladder tumors by flow cytometric deoxyribonucleic acid analysis: a report of 100 cases. *J Urol* 1990;144:879–83.

97. Kim SS, Choi YD, Nam JH, Kwon DD, Juhng SW, Choi C. Cytologic features of primary signet ring cell carcinoma of the bladder: a case report. *Acta Cytol* 2009;53:309–12.

98. Bardales RH, Pitman MB, Stanley MW, Korourian S, Suhrland MJ. Urine cytology of primary and secondary urinary bladder adenocarcinoma. *Cancer* 1998;84:335–43.

99. Tribukait B. Clinical DNA flow cytometry. *Med Oncol Tumor Pharmacother* 1984;1:211–8.

100. Hausdorfer GS, Chandrasoma P, Pettross BR, Carriere CA. Cytologic diagnosis of mesonephric adenocarcinoma of the urinary bladder. *Acta Cytol* 1985;29:823–6.

101. Rollins S, Schumann GB. Primary urinary cytodiagnosis of a bladder small-cell carcinoma. *Diagn Cytopathol* 1991;7:79–82.

102. Yamaguchi T, Imamura Y, Shimamoto T, Kawada T, Nakayama K, Tokunaga S, Yasuda M. Small cell carcinoma of the bladder. Two cases diagnosed by urinary cytology. *Acta Cytol* 2000;44:403–9.

103. McRae S, Garcia BM. Cytologic diagnosis of a primary pure oat cell carcinoma of the bladder in voided urine. A case report. *Acta Cytol* 1997;41:1279–83.

104. Rudrick B, Nguyen GK, Lakey WH. Carcinoid tumor of the renal pelvis: report of a case with positive urine cytology. *Diagn Cytopathol* 1995;12:360–3.

105. Oshiro H, Gomi K, Nagahama K, Nagashima Y, Kanazawa M, Kato J, Hatano T, Inayama Y. Urinary cytologic features of primary large cell neuroendocrine carcinoma of the urinary bladder: a case report. *Acta Cytol* 2010;54:303–10.

106. Khalbuss WE, Hossain M, Elhosseiny A. Primary malignant melanoma of the urinary bladder diagnosed by urine cytology: a case report. *Acta Cytol* 2001;45:631–5.

107. Tanaka T, Yoshimi N, Sawada K, Takami T, Sugie S, Etori F, Kachi H, Mori H. Ki–1-positive large cell anaplastic lymphoma diagnosed by urinary cytology. A case report. *Acta Cytol* 1993;37:520–4.

108. Mokhtar GA, Yazdi H, Mai KT. Cytopathology of extramedullary plasmacytoma of the bladder: a case report. *Acta Cytol* 2006;50:339–43.

109. Gourlay W, Chan V, Gilks CB. Screening for urothelial malignancies by cytologic analysis and flow cytometry in a community urologic practice: a prospective study. *Mod Pathol* 1995;8:394–7.

110. Kapur U, Venkataraman G, Wojcik EM. Diagnostic significance of 'atypia' in instrumented versus voided urine specimens. *Cancer* 2008;114:270–4.

Chapter 31

Evaluation of Hematuria and Urinalysis

Bladder Pathology, First Edition. Liang Cheng, Antonio Lopez-Beltran, David G. Bostwick.
© 2012 Wiley-Blackwell. Published 2012 by John Wiley & Sons, Inc.

Evaluation of Hematuria and Urinalysis

Overview

Hematuria is the most common symptom of urinary tract disease, present in about 21% of the U.S. population, including 2% of children.[1-19] It is defined as excretion of three or more red blood cells per high power field in 10 mL to 15 mL of well-mixed freshly voided centrifuged urine, preferably documented on up to three separate occasions.[2] Up to 3% of healthy adults excrete small numbers of red blood cells (up to two red blood cells per high power field or the equivalent of 1000 red blood cells/mL), so it is important in such cases to avoid overdiagnosis of hematuria.

Red blood cells in the urine result from trauma or spontaneous response to a multitude of causes or conditions throughout the urinary tract. This spontaneous process of diapedesis or oozing of red and white blood cells through the vessel walls may result from a variety of causes for increased vascular permeability. The vessels are usually preserved except with glomerular hematuria, in which there is damage to the endothelial cells and glomerular basement membranes. Hematuria may be occult (not visible by the naked eye; usually discovered incidentally during laboratory studies accompanying routine physical examination), gross (usually obvious to the patient), or associated with blood clots. Gross hematuria often presents as an abnormal color ranging from pink to bright red or dark red. As little as 1 mL of blood/L creates a noticeable change in the color of urine. Hematuria may be asymptomatic or symptomatic and transient or persistent. It is often associated with other findings, such as proteinuria, hypertension, edema, or other physical findings. A through history and physical examination should always be performed with attention to family history, pain symptoms, and chronic medical conditions.

Hematuria may occur anywhere along the urinary tract. There are many causes, including anatomic abnormalities, calculi, medications, urinary tract infection, vigorous exercise, foreign bodies, trauma, hemoglobinopathies, coagulopathies, glomerulonephritis, benign prostatic hyperplasia, and malignancy (**Tables 31-1 and 31-2**).[6] Only a small percentage of hematuria cases identified by screening, however, are ultimately attributable to bladder cancer.[20] It is critical that the source of persistent hematuria be identified, according to the Best Practice Policy of the American Urologic Association.[2] There is no "safe" level of hematuria, and the patient with persistent painless hematuria should undergo urologic workup, including urinalysis, urine culture, imaging studies (**Fig. 31-1**), urine chemistry and serum panels, urine cytology, and molecular assays (see **Chapters 8, 29, 30, 32, 33, and 34** for further discussion). Cohen et al. recommend that patients with nonglomerular hematuria undergo imaging and—depending on the presence or absence of detectable lesions—subsequent urine cytology.[4] For those at high risk for bladder cancer, fiberoptic cystoscopy should be performed, even in the absence of abnormal cytology or imaging studies. Risk factors for bladder cancer that may require fiberoptic cystoscopy include smoking, prolonged heavy phenacetin use, male gender, greater than 50 years of age, *Schistosoma* exposure, frequent urinary tract infections, and exposure to industrial chemicals or dyes.

Laboratory Investigation

Routine urinalysis combines macroscopic reagent strip (dipstick) testing with microscopic examination of the sediment to detect chemical and structural disorders of the urinary tract. Dipstick examination has about 90% sensitivity to detect three or more red blood cells or the equivalent amount of free hemoglobin or myoglobin.[7] The degree of hematuria bears no relation to the seriousness of the underlying disease, so hematuria should be considered a symptom of serious disease until proven otherwise.[5]

The dipstick test and confirmatory tests for protein, glucose, and bilirubin are standardized and easy to perform, but there is a great deal of inconsistency in the performance of the microscopic examination. Procedures are not standardized, and variables include the amount of urine examined, the method of processing, the method of evaluation and reporting, and the technical ability of the individual performing the examination. Unfortunately, most abnormal urinalyses are not pursued clinically, except perhaps to obtain repeat of the test, often with progression of treatable disease that could have been prevented.[14] One study demonstrated 100% sensitivity (17 cases) of hemoglobin dipstick for urothelial carcinoma in situ (CIS) (**Figs. 31-2 and 31-3**).[21] Specificity, however, is much less.

Microscopic examination is often performed only if the dipstick test is abnormal, but this approach should be discouraged. Exclusive reliance on the dipstick test significantly decreases the sensitivity of urinalysis for detection of serious and treatable disease. The combination of dipstick and microscopic examination greatly improves detection of urinary tract disease, and is recommended. Molecular methods, such as the UroVysion fluorescence in situ hybridization (FISH) test, is helpful in detecting malignant urothelial cells (**Fig. 31-4**; see **Chapters 29, 32, 33, and 34** for further discussion).

Dysmorphic Red Blood Cells Indicate Glomerular Disease

Red blood cells of glomerular origin are referred to as "dysmorphic" (abnormal and misshapen), whereas red blood

646

Table 31-1 Possible Causes of Lower Urinary Tract and Renal Parenchymal Hematuria

Possible Causes for Lower Tract Bleeding	Possible Causes for Upper Tract (Renal) Bleeding

Tumors (urethra, bladder, prostate, ureters, renal pelvis)	Primary glomerulopathies
	  IgA nephrology
	  Postinfectious glomerulonephritis
	  Membranoproliferative glomerulonephritis
	  Focal glomerular sclerosis

Obstructive uropathy	
Benign prostatic hyperplasia	

Lithiasis (stones)	Secondary glomerulopathy
	  Lupus nephritis
	  Henoch–Schönlein syndrome

Infections (cystitis, prostatitis, schistosomiasis, tuberculosis, condyloma acuminatum)	Vasculitis (polyarteritis nodosa)
	  Wegner granulomatosis
	  Hemolytic uremic syndrome

Systemic bleeding disorders or coagulopathy	Essential mixed cryoglobulinemia Interstitial nephritis
Trauma	

Radiation therapy	Familial conditions
	  Hereditary nephritis (Alport syndrome)
	  Renal tumors (renal cell carcinoma)

Instrumentation	Vascular disorders (malignant hypertension)
	  Sickle cell trait or disease
	  Metabolic disorders (hypercalcuria)

Vigorous exercise	Polycystic kidney
Menstrual contamination	

Endometriosis	Infections
	  Pyelonephritis (acute or chronic)
	  Tuberculosis
	  Cytomegalovirus
	  BK polyomavirus

	Nephrolithiasis Light chain immunoglobulinopathy (multiple myeloma) Diabetes mellitus Amyloidosis

cells leaking though vessels in the renal tubules and in the lower urinary tract are "isomorphic" (normal size and shape, smooth cell membranes, and uniform hemoglobin content). There are two defining features of dysmorphic red blood cells: each "target" cell should have a clear and distinct central inclusion of heme pigment surrounded by a clear zone. Other dysmorphic erythrocytes have one or several abnormal outpouchings ("blebs") of the red cell membrane caused by osmotic shock as the red blood cell travels through the nephron.

Most investigators agree that the presence of even one dysmorphic red blood cell in urine is clinically significant, and some debate on this point persists. The presence of dysmorphic red blood cells accompanied by even a small amount of protein is especially significant, indicating a glomerular source of bleeding. The overall percentage of dysmorphism diagnostic of renal hematuria varies between experts from 40% to 80%.[22]

Epithelium of the Lower Urinary Tract and Kidney

Urothelium consists of two distinct layers. The larger cells form a protective surface layer, usually one cell deep, covering the entire urothelial lining. These superficial cells, or umbrella cells, have abundant pale or vacuolated cytoplasm with a large nucleus, fine chromatin, and a round nucleus.

Urothelial (intermediate) cells typically have round to oval nuclei with moderate, homogeneous, predominantly basophilic cytoplasm. Fragments of urothelium are commonly found in catheterized specimens as well as bladder washes (**Fig. 31-5**); however, it is abnormal to see urothelial fragments in spontaneously voided urine, and their presence may be associated with papilloma or low grade urothelial cancer.

Table 31-2   **Selected List of Drugs, Pigments, Diuretics, and Miscellaneous Factors Leading to Hematuria[a]**

Drugs and Medications	Others
Antibiotics	Pigments
Penicillin	Rhabdomyolysis (myoglobin)
Cephalosporin	Hemoglobin (transfusion reaction)
Rifampin	Heme pigment (hemolysis)
Erythromycin	Diuretics
Sulfonamides	Thiazide
Aminoglycosides	Furosemide
Tetracycline	Triamterene
NSAIDs	Chlorthalidone
Acetaminophen	Other
Acetylsalicylic acid	Radiocontrast agents
Naproxen	Cisplatin
Ibuprofen	Heavy metals (gold, cadmium, mercury)
Indomethacin	Organic solvents
Phenylbutazone	
Tolmetin	
Mefenamic acid	
Fenoprofen	
Other drugs	
Captopril	
Cimetidine	
Phenobarbital	
Dilantin	
Interferon	
Lithium	

[a]Possible causes of hematuria, including antibiotics, nonsteroidal antiinflammatory drugs (NSAIDs), anticoagulants, diuretics, anticancer agents, and pigments. Certain foods (beets) may mimic the presence of hematuria.

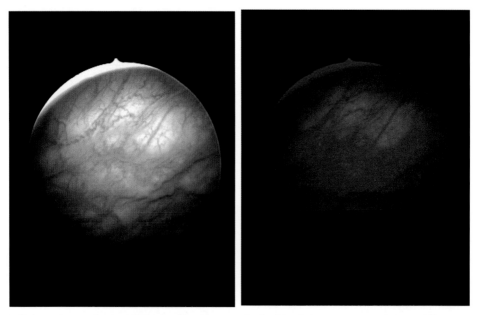

Figure 31-1   Urothelial carcinoma in situ (CIS) visualized by standard white light cystoscopy (left) and fluorescence cystoscopy (right). Sharp (red) appearance of CIS lesion under fluorescence cystoscopy (right panel). These CIS lesions as shown may be difficult to detect using standard white light cystoscopy (left). Hexaminolevulinate causes photoactive porphyrins to accumulate preferentially in rapidly proliferating tumor cells. These porphyrins emit red fluorescence when exposed to blue light. (Photo courtesy of Dr. Montironi.)

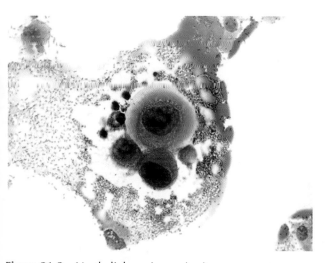

Figure 31-2 Urothelial carcinoma in situ.

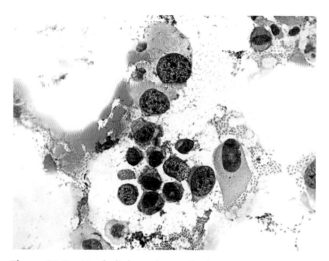

Figure 31-3 Urothelial carcinoma in situ.

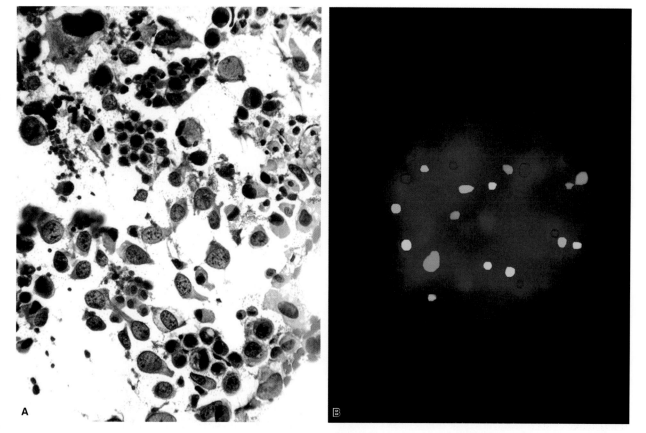

Figure 31-4 (A) High grade urothelial carcinoma. UroVysion fluorescence in situ hybridization (FISH) analysis of urothelial carcinoma (B). Normal urothelial cells have two signals from each probe for CEP3 (red), CEP7 (green), CEP17 (aqua), and 9p21 (gold). Urothelial cancer cell shows gaining of chromosome 3 (red, seven signals), 7 (green, four signals), 17 (aqua, five signals), and chromosome arm 9p21 (gold, five signals.)

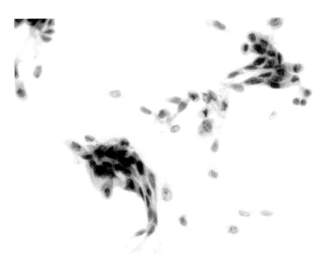

Figure 31-5 Reactive changes after instrumentation from the ureteral washing specimen. Note the sheets of elongated urothelial cells with dense cytoplasm and enlarged nuclei.

Urothelial cells are the most variably sized cells in the urinary sediment. They vary from 20 μm in diameter to the typical "umbrella" cell, whose size may approach 100 μm. Umbrella cells are often multinucleated with reactive nuclei. Cells from the basal urothelium are smaller, round, and display well-defined thickened cytoplasmic membranes. Chromocenters and multiple eosinophilic micronucleoli may be present, especially in cases with accompanying inflammation or in the reparative process after passage of a stone. Occasionally, a large urothelial fragment displays cytoplasmic vacuoles containing neutrophils. Multinucleation, nuclear enlargement, and hyperchromasia can be found in inflammatory processes within the lower urinary tract as well as in urothelial dysplasia and neoplasia, so cytologic atypia should always be confirmed by biopsy or cystoscopic mass resection prior to instituting any additional therapy.

Renal Epithelium

Cells from the convoluted tubular epithelium are the largest cells in the nephron, extending from the entrance to Bowman capsule to the beginning of the loop of Henle. These cells are rarely seen in normal individuals, but are shed in large numbers in cases of renal toxicity and renal ischemia caused by shock and a wide variety of drugs, heavy metals, immunosuppressants, and other toxins.

Proximal and distal tubular cells in urine are easily identified by their large size (20 μm to 60 μm in diameter), irregular elongate or cigar-like appearance, and coarsely granular basophilic cytoplasm. Cytoplasmic borders are indistinct and may be ragged or torn. The granular cytoplasm contains large numbers of mitochondria ultrastructurally. The nuclei are slightly larger than an erythrocyte and may occasionally be double or multiple. Interestingly, proximal and distal tubular cells appear singly, never in fragments or clusters. These cells are often mistaken for small granular casts in unstained bright-field microscopy, but when studied carefully, they are seen to consist of only a single cell. Proximal and distal renal tubular cells slough from their basement membranes and can be found in urine as intact preserved cells or as "ghost" or necrotic forms, which retain their size and cytoplasmic characteristics.

Renal tubular cells lining the proximal and distal loop of Henle are small (12 μm to 18 μm in diameter). Each contains a single slightly eccentric nucleus with coarse and evenly distributed chromatin. There may be an occasional nucleolus, as these cells may be reactive because of metabolic or ischemic stimuli, but they are never multinucleated. The cytoplasm is polygonal to columnar, finely granular, and uniformly basophilic, with distinct borders. Vacuolization may occasionally be seen, especially in reactive states. The cells may phagocytize cast-like material, crystals, and pigments.

Collecting duct cells in urine may be seen in very low numbers in normal individuals, but are significant when found with renal casts and/or as fragments. An abnormal number, greater than one per high power field, may be found in a wide variety of clinical conditions, including shock, trauma, burns, and exposure to toxins. An increased number of collecting duct cells in renal transplant patients heralds clinical rejection by up to 48 hours.

Renal epithelial cell fragments in urine indicate a severe form of renal tubular injury ("ischemic necrosis") and are exclusively from the collecting duct following survival and recovery from shock. This reflects loss of blood flow (ischemic injury) to the renal tubules and subsequent sloughing of entire segments or portions of the renal tubules with regeneration of the lost epithelium. This tubular regeneration is a process similar to "repair" in cervical smears. There are five types of fragments, classified according to morphology: (1) spindle fragments; (2) fragments attached to or surrounding cast material; (3) pavement or "en face" fragments; (4) fragments with reactive cellular or noncellular inclusions [shown are cast-like, crystal, or pigmented (bile) inclusions]; and (5) cylindrical tube-like fragments.

Renal Casts in Urine Sediment

Renal casts are observed in urine sediment from patients with glomerular and renal parenchymal diseases. Casts are composed of Tamm–Horsfall protein and originate in the distal tubules and collecting ducts. In normal individuals, hyaline and rare granular casts may appear due to dehydration, fever, exercise, and other factors. Such casts are considered physiologic. Conversely, nonphysiologic casts made of abnormal urine protein and those that contain cells of various types are easily identified. The type of cells contained within the cast matrix, the width of the cast, and the number of casts are indicative of the severity of the underlying disease. The presence of abnormal amounts of protein, blood, leukocytes, nitrites, and bilirubin all correlate with the various types of casts.

Urolithiasis

About one in 15 people in the industrialized world develops kidney stones. All age groups and both genders are affected, with an apparent genetic predisposition.[23]

Urinary tract calculi are composed of waste products, and hematuria commonly occurs during the earliest stages of stone formation. They form as the result of increased excretion of solutes (calcium oxalate, calcium phosphate, magnesium ammonium phosphate, struvite or triple phosphate, uric acid, cystine), abnormal urine pH, stasis, dehydration, and/or urinary concentration. Once a stone grows to a significant size, the patient may experience symptoms that range from a dull ache to severe pain often equated with the pain of childbirth or abdominal surgery without anesthesia. Stones originate as microscopic grains of mineral debris, enlarging to the size of gravel and later to a large stone.

Stones may occur anywhere along the urinary tract, and many patients pass stones spontaneously. Large calculi require surgical intervention or shockwave extracorporeal lithotripsy to create passable fragments.

Optimal Cytodiagnostic Urinalysis of Hematuria

Optimal cytodiagnostic urinalysis (OCU) includes all of the elements of testing to obtain a comprehensive quantitative evaluation of the urine sediment and correlative physiochemical assessment (Table 31-3). This method incorporates advances in routine urinalysis, including dipstick tests and confirmatory tests such as the SSA test for protein, the Ictotest for bilirubin, and the Clinitest tablet test for glucose. In addition, enhanced cytopreparation improves cell recovery to maximize microscopic visualization and quantitative assessment. Diagnostic interpretation involves correlation of both chemical and microscopic findings, informing the clinician which chemical and morphologic abnormalities

Table 31-3   Six Essential Components of Optimal Cytodiagnostic Urinalysis

Patient history
Physical examination of the urine sample, including color, character, and specific gravity
Chemical examination, consisting of multiparameter reagent dipstick testing and confirmatory chemical tests
Microscopic urine sediment examination using standardized sediment recovery and high contrast transparent Papanicolaou stain
Quantitative microscopic examination to identify clinically important sediment entities and systematically evaluate 10 specific morphologic categories: background, cellularity, epithelial fragments, inclusion-bearing cells, red blood cells, neutrophils, eosinophils, lymphocytes, renal tubular cells, and casts
Diagnostic interpretation, with appropriate recommendations, including possible confirmatory testing and clinical followup

Table 31-4   Advantages of Optimal Cytodiagnostic Urinalysis

Improves visualization of urine sediment entities
Provides for early information on the nature of urinary tract disorders
Allows for cost-effective triaging of patients to appropriate specialists (e.g., urologists, nephrologists)
Provides a noninvasive method of monitoring patients
Optimizes clinicopathologic correlation of results
Standardizes sediment results reporting
Is adaptable to various laboratory sizes and settings
Requires a minimum of equipment and space
Is adaptable to automation
Provides a permanent record of urine sediment findings for review and quality control

are present. OCU also often provides recommendations for future testing and possible treatment considerations. OCU is superior to routine unstained sediment examination for patient management (Table 31-4).

The clinical utility of OCU is its ability to detect various types of mononuclear cells, viral and nonviral inclusions, and precancerous and cancerous cells. It is valuable in the differential diagnosis and monitoring of renal tubular injury for conditions such as acute tubular necrosis, tubulointerstitial inflammation (nephritis), acute renal allograft rejection, and primary or secondary renal lesions. OCU can also help to discriminate inflammatory, infectious, degenerative, or neoplastic conditions of the kidney and the lower urinary tract; to evaluate and monitor immunosuppressed patients; to screen patients with nephrotoxic or carcinogenic exposure; and to eliminate the need for renal biopsy in some cases.[9]

Table 31-5 Correlation of Optimal Cytodiagnostic Urinalysis with Renal Biopsy Findings

Lesion Location	Sensitivity	Specificity	Accuracy	Positive Predictive Value	Negative Predictive Value
Glomerular	0.95	0.85	0.91	0.90	0.92
Tubular	0.80	0.89	0.88	0.57	0.96
Interstitial	0.78	0.87	0.82	0.88	0.76
Tubulointerstitial (combined)	0.91	0.91	0.91	0.95	0.83
Vascular	0.50	0.74	0.64	0.58	0.67

Discrimination of origin of renal cells (glomerular, tubular, interstitial, or vascular cells) by OCU has a high level of intraobserver and interobserver agreement. The interpretation correlates with biopsy findings in 89% of native kidneys and 77% of transplant kidneys. The sensitivity and specificity for the diagnosis of glomerular lesions alone in native and transplant kidneys was 91%, and 85%, respectively. Severity scores also showed good correlation between OCU and renal biopsy results in both native and transplanted kidneys (Table 31-5). The severity scores correlated well with increase in creatinine concentrations. In cases with biopsy-proven glomerular lesions, more severe changes were found by OCU when the biopsy showed proliferative glomerular lesions than when the biopsy showed only normal glomeruli. OCU has an advantage over renal biopsy in that it can be repeated as often as necessary without risk to the patient. Repeated OCU allows observation of progression or regression of a renal disease over time.[24,25]

The accuracy of OCU for localizing the origin and etiology of blood in the urine was studied in 100 consecutive patients with occult hematuria.[15] Thirteen percent of the patients had urological lesions [three had renal tumors (two stage I renal cell carcinomas and one renal angiomyolipoma), two had urothelial bladder cancer, and eight had urinary calculi]. OCU identified both bladder cancers, seven of eight urinary calculi, but none of the renal tumors (probably because a renal tumor must be of significant size and stage and in direct contact with the distal collecting system to shed malignant cells). The presence of dysmorphic red blood cells and red blood casts was strongly suggestive of renal parenchymal disease. The authors found that OCU increased the diagnostic yield and distinguished between bladder and renal origin of microscopic hematuria.

OCU is effective for evaluating patients with asymptomatic hematuria, urological symptoms, and renal lesions. Thirty years of experience has shown that OCU is superior to standard tests such as routine microscopic urinalysis and creatinine as widely practiced. It is an advanced laboratory test that is inexpensive, noninvasive, and easily performed by properly trained technologists and pathologists.

REFERENCES

1. Chan D, Ong A, Schoenberg M. Microscopic hematuria. *N Engl J Med* 2003;349:1292–3.
2. Grossfeld GD, Litwin MS, Wolf JS Jr, Hricak H, Shuler CL, Agerter DC, Carroll PR. Evaluation of asymptomatic microscopic hematuria in adults: the American Urological Association best practice policy—part II: patient evaluation, cytology, voided markers, imaging, cystoscopy, nephrology evaluation, and followup. *Urology* 2001;57:604–10.
3. Grossfeld GD, Litwin MS, Wolf JS, Hricak H, Shuler CL, Agerter DC, Carroll PR. Evaluation of asymptomatic microscopic hematuria in adults: the American Urological Association best practice policy—part I: definition, detection, prevalence, and etiology. *Urology* 2001;57:599–603.
4. Cohen RA, Brown RS. Clinical practice. Microscopic hematuria. *N Engl J Med* 2003;348:2330–8.
5. Thaller TR, Wang LP. Evaluation of asymptomatic microscopic hematuria in adults. *Am Fam Physician* 1999;60:1143–52, 1154.
6. Neiberger RE. The ABC's of evaluating children with hematuria. *Am Fam Physician* 1994;49:623–8.
7. Sutton JM. Evaluation of hematuria in adults. *JAMA* 1990;263:2475–80.
8. Nabi G, Greene D, O'Donnell MO. Suspicious urinary cytology with negative evaluation for malignancy in the diagnostic investigation of haematuria: How to follow up? *J Clin Pathol* 2004;57:365–8.
9. Schumann GB, Colon VF. Urine cytology. Part II: renal cytology. *Am Fam Physician* 1980;21:102–6.
10. Yadin O. Hematuria in children. *Pediatr Ann* 1994;23:474–8, 481–5.
11. Messing EM, Madeb R, Young T, Gilchrist KW, Bram L, Greenberg EB, Wegenke JD, Stephenson L, Gee J, Feng C. Long-term outcome of hematuria home screening for bladder cancer in men. *Cancer* 2006;107:2173–9.
12. Golin AL, Howard RS. Asymptomatic microscopic hematuria. *J Urol* 1980;124:389–91.

13. Chiong E, Gaston KE, Grossman HB. Urinary markers in screening patients with hematuria. *World J Urol* 2008;26:25–30.
14. Ritchie CD, Bevan EA, Collier SJ. Importance of occult haematuria found at screening. *Br Med J (Clin Res Ed)* 1986;292:681–3.
15. Fracchia JA, Motta J, Miller LS, Armenakas NA, Schumann GB, Greenberg RA. Evaluation of asymptomatic microhematuria. *Urology* 1995;46:484–9.
16. Jaffe JS, Ginsberg PC, Gill R, Harkaway RC. A new diagnostic algorithm for the evaluation of microscopic hematuria. *Urology* 2001;57:889–94.
17. Nakamura K, Kasraeian A, Iczkowski KA, Chang M, Pendleton J, Anai S, Rosser CJ. Utility of serial urinary cytology in the initial evaluation of the patient with microscopic hematuria. *BMC Urol* 2009;9:12.

18. Ripley TL, Havrda DE, Blevins S, Culkin D. Early evaluation of hematuria in a patient receiving anticoagulant therapy and detection of malignancy. *Pharmacotherapy* 2004;24:1638–40.
19. Yun EJ, Meng MV, Carroll PR. Evaluation of the patient with hematuria. *Med Clin North Am* 2004;88:329–43.
20. Lokeshwar VB, Soloway MS. Current bladder tumor tests: Does their projected utility fulfill clinical necessity? *J Urol* 2001;165:1067–77.
21. Halling KC, King W, Sokolova IA, Karnes RJ, Meyer RG, Powell EL, Sebo TJ, Cheville JC, Clayton AC, Krajnik KL, Ebert TA, Nelson RE, et al. A comparison of BTA stat, hemoglobin dipstick, telomerase and Vysis UroVysion assays for the detection of urothelial carcinoma in urine. *J Urol* 2002;167:2001–6.

22. Dinda AK, Saxena S, Guleria S, Tiwari SC, Dash SC, Srivastava RN, Singh C. Diagnosis of glomerular haematuria: role of dysmorphic red cell, G1 cell and bright-field microscopy. *Scand J Clin Lab Invest* 1997;57:203–8.
23. Amato M, Lusini ML, Nelli F. Epidemiology of nephrolithiasis today. *Urol Int* 2004;72 Suppl 1:1 5.
24. Marcussen N, Schumann J, Campbell P, Kjellstrand C. Cytodiagnostic urinalysis is very useful in the differential diagnosis of acute renal failure and can predict the severity. *Ren Fail* 1995;17:721–9.
25. Marcussen N, Schumann JL, Schumann GB, Parmar M, Kjellstrand C. Analysis of cytodiagnostic urinalysis findings in 77 patients with concurrent renal biopsies. *Am J Kidney Dis* 1992;20:618–28.

Chapter 32

Urine-based Biomarkers

Overview

Urine cytology is an important tool in the diagnosis and management of urothelial malignancy. However, urine cytology has a low sensitivity for the detection of bladder cancer, and is particularly insensitive for low grade tumors; thus, there is a need for superior methods of initial diagnosis and, subsequently, for detection of recurrence or progression.

There has been substantial progress in recent years exploiting urine specimens to increase sensitivity and specificity for detecting urothelial carcinoma. New methods provide more accurate information to assist urologists in the management of bladder cancer. These efforts have been stimulated and supplemented by expansion in our understanding of the molecular and genetic alterations underlying urothelial carcinoma.[1–4] Many new biomarkers are now available, and some are touted as superior to urine cytology for select patient cohorts.[4–6] One large study compared the sensitivity and specificity of commercially available tests and determined the predictive value of many urine biomarkers (**Table 32-1**).[4]

Proprietary markers include UroVysion, ImmunoCyt, BTA (bladder tumor antigen), NMP22 (nuclear matrix protein 22), and hemoglobin dipstick. Nonproprietary markers include DNA ploidy, proliferation markers, apoptosis markers, oncogene markers, gene methylation profiles, growth factors, mitogen receptors, cell adhesion markers, telomerase activation, cycloxygenase-2 expression, vascular endothelial growth factors, multidrug resistance proteins, and a wide variety of other markers (see also **Chapters 29**, **33**, and **34**).[5,7–93]

Most studies provide sensitivity and specificity data. Low sensitivity indicates numerous false-negative results (delayed diagnosis of cancer), and low specificity indicates numerous false-positive results (presumptive overdiagnosis of cancer, leading to unnecessary investigation such as cystoscopy).[94] Different studies may not be comparable, owing to such issues as patient selection, ascertainment bias, limited number of patients, limited length of followup, lack of central pathology review, sample variation with different techniques, variance in endpoints, and different thresholds for test result reporting.[95] Decision analysis models indicate that the use of urine-based cancer markers may be cost-effective when alternating with cystoscopy and/or cytology.[96]

The clinical utility of current cell-based biomarkers in human bladder neoplasia, with emphasis on improvement over urine cytology to identify bladder cancer (diagnosis) and to predict outcome for individual patients (prognosis), is discussed in this chapter. (**Table 32-2**). Tissue-based biomarkers and prognostic factors are discussed in the next chapter (**Chapter 33**).

UroVysion Fluorescence in Situ Hybridization Test

Use of the fluorescence in situ hybridization (FISH) assay on voided urine specimens (UroVysion, Vysis, Downers Grove, Illinois) is a useful adjunct to urinary cytology. UroVysion is the first U.S. Food and Drug Administration (FDA)-sanctioned FISH test to detect bladder cancer. The test was first approved by the FDA in 2001[26] to monitor patients with bladder cancer for tumor recurrence and was subsequently approved to assess patients with hematuria (gross and microscopic) for bladder cancer.[97] UroVysion is a multicolor, multitargeted FISH assay using chromosome enumeration probes (CEP) for chromosomes 3, 7, and 17, and a locus-specific indicator probe for 9p21, which are labeled with red, green, aqua, and gold fluorophores, respectively (**Figs. 32-1** and **32-2**).[10,23–26,97] Polysomy of one or more of these three chromosomes or deletion of the 9p21 locus detects common abnormalities in urothelial neoplasia (**Table 32-3**).

For the UroVysion FISH test, a minimum of 25 morphologically abnormal cells are analyzed. Morphologically abnormal cells are defined by large nuclear size, irregular nuclear shape, patchy DAPI staining, and clustering. The signal distribution for these abnormal cells showing either three or more signals or one or more of the following (CEP 3 red, CEP 7 green, or CEP 17 aqua) or a homozygous loss of 9p21 (i.e., no signals for LSI 9p21 yellow) is recorded. Analysis continues until either four or more cells show gains of multiple chromosomes, or 12 or more cells show homozygous loss of 9p21. If no polysomy or deletion of 9p21 is found, counting continues until the entire sample is analyzed. The total number of chromosomally abnormal cells (i.e., cells with gains of multiple chromosomes or homozygous loss of 9p21) is determined and results are reported as positive or negative. Results at or near the cutoff point (four cells with gains of multiple chromosomes or 12 cells with homozygous loss of 9p21) should be interpreted with caution. The specimen slide should be reenumerated by another technician to verify the results. If the results are still equivocal, the test should be repeated with a fresh specimen slide.

The UroVysion FISH test markedly improved the sensitivity of urine cytology, from 58% to a sensitivity of 81%, with a specificity of 96%, similar to the specificity of cytology (98%).[23] It was superior to the BTA test, urine hemoglobin dipstick, and telomerase in comparative analyses.[23,26] This method can be used successfully on destained routinely processed cytology slides.[98,99] The UroVysion test is very helpful in distinguishing low grade papillary urothelial carcinoma from benign conditions such as reactive changes from instrumentations (**Figs. 32-3** to **32-5**; see **Chapters 30** and **31** for further discussion).

Table 32-1 Selected Urine Markers Used for Bladder Cancer Detection[a]

Markers	Sensitivity	(Range %)	Specificity	(Range %)	PPV (%)	NPV (%)	Comments
Cytology[5,32]	60	(46–76)	83	(67–99)	77	88	Low sensitivity for low grade tumors
[b]UroVysion[7,12,13,262]	78	(69–87)	81	(66–95)	68	71	High specificity, low sensitivity for low grade tumors
[b]BTA[5,7,9]	61	(32–89)	66	(50–82)	63	67	Sensitivity depends on tumor grade; specificity is low in patients with benign bladder conditions
[b]NMP22[5,7,33,67,262]	71	(56–85)	90	(85–94)	57	60	High false-negative rate, affected by hematuria and intravesical BCG treatment
[b]ImmunoCyt[5,7,16,262]	57	(29–84)	79	(73–85)	72	74	Sensitive to detect low grade tumors, low sensitivity for recurrence
UBC[9,263–265]	70	(36–79)	82	(88–93)	52	60	Low sensitivity, not used alone
[b]FDP[9,265,266]	67	(41–93)	85	(77–94)	26	99	Levels tend to be proportional to the tumor grade and stage
Telomerase[9,40,267]	72	(53–91)	73	(46–99)	93	73	Lack of standardized sample processing
CYFRA21–1[9,268–270]	87	(74–99)	68	(57–78)	56	70	False positive may happen in urinary stones, infection, and intravesical BCG treatment
Microsatellite LOH[271,272]	90	(81–91)	88	(79–96)	—	—	High sensitivity in both low- and high grade UC; persistent leukocyturia may affect the results
Cytokeratin 20[32,146,273]	65	(82–87)	90	(55–70)	86	65	Cutoff values yet to be defined
HA-HAase[146,274]	83	(78–83)	78	(78–91)	64	91	High sensitivity to detect low and high grade and stage tumors
TPS[9]	65	(50–80)	79	(63–95)	—	—	Correlate with tumor size, low sensitivity, and specificity for recurrence
MUC7[275]	69	(62–76)	87	(94–96)	97	56	Expression affected by tumor grade but not by tumor volume

[a]PPV, positive predictive value; NPV, negative predictive value; NMP22, nuclear matrix protein 22; BTA, bladder tumor antigen; FDP, urinary fibrinogen degradation products; UBC, urinary bladder cancer ELISA; CYFRA21–1, cytokeratin–19 fragment ELISA; LOH, loss of heterozygosity; HA-HAase, hyaluronic acid and hyaluronidase; TPS, urine tissue-polypeptide-specific antigen; MUC7, mucin 7; BCG, Bacillus Calmette–Guérin; UC, urothelial carcinoma.
[b]U.S. Food and Drug Administration–approved/cleared urine markers.

Table 32-2 Major Indications for the Use of Urine-based Biomarkers

Surveillance and followup of patients with history of bladder cancer

Evaluation of gross/microscopic hematuria

Reflex test for atypical urinary cytology results

Assessment of therapeutic responses

Screening of selected patients at high risk of developing bladder cancer

Detection of urothelial neoplasia in the upper urinary tract

In a prospective multicenter randomized blinded study to evaluate the clinical utility of UroVysion for monitoring patients with hematuria, 497 patients were enrolled from 23 centers. In the 473 (95%) study patients, FISH and cytology results were both considered interpretable.[97] All patients had gross or microscopic hematuria, and none had a prior history of bladder cancer. Bladder cancer was diagnosed histologically in 50 patients (10%) and ureteral cancer was diagnosed in one. FISH assay detected 69% of cases with urothelial cancer and cytology detected 38%. When low grade, low stage (TaG1) tumors were excluded, FISH detected 25 of 30 cancers (84%), while cytology detected only 15 (50%). Based on these data, UroVysion was approved by the FDA for use in patients with hematuria.[97] Subsequent studies using UroVysion probes have resulted in proposals for the use of this methodology in various clinical situations. UroVysion may be helpful for followup of known bladder cancer, for further evaluation of suspicious urine cytology findings, for post-bacillus Calmette–Guérin (BCG) followup, or as a general adjunct to urinary cytology. The overall sensitivity of UroVysion varies between 69% and 87%, but is significantly lower for low grade and low stage tumors.[12,13] Schlomer et al. studied 108 patients with no history of cancer and 108

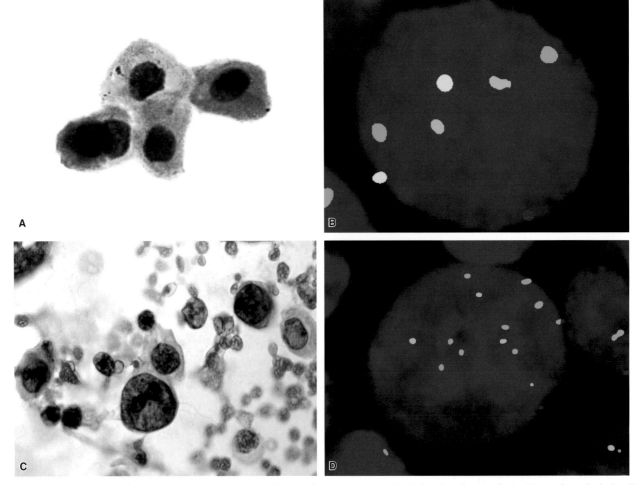

Figure 32-1 Detection of urothelial carcinoma by UroVysion fluorescence in situ hybridization analysis. Normal urothelial cells (A) show two signals from each probe for CEP3 (red), CEP7 (green), CEP17 (aqua), and 9p21 (gold) (B). Malignant urothelial cells (C) demonstrate gaining of chromosomes as indicated by seven red (CEP3), nine green (CEP7), four aqua (CEP17), and loss of 9p21 as indicated by the absence of yellow signals (9p21). (From Ref. 4; with permission.)

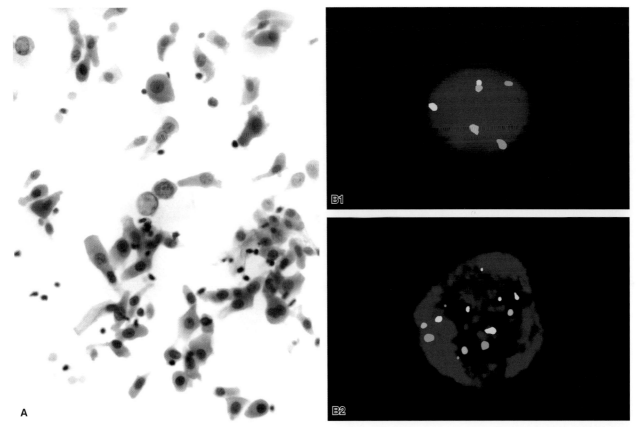

Figure 32-2 Urothelial carcinoma in situ (CIS) (A) detected by UroVysion fluorescence in situ hybridization analysis (B1 and B2). Normal urothelial cells (B1) show two signals from each probe for CEP3 (red), CEP7 (green), CEP17 (aqua), and 9p21 (gold) (B). CIS cells show gaining of chromosome 17 (five aqua) and arm 9p21 (six gold), while chromosomes 3 (red) and 7 (green) show normal disomic profiles (two red and two green signals, respectively).

who underwent cystoscopy for cancer surveillance.[14] The results showed that UroVysion had a positive predictive value of 100% in patients with cystoscopically visible lesions. In patients with equivocal cystoscopy and no prior cancer history, the positive predictive value was 100% since there were no false-negative results. Moreover, UroVysion detected 100% of cancers in patients with negative cystoscopy.[14]

The UroVysion performed extremely well in patients receiving BCG intravesical treatment. Test results are in agreement with the gold standard of cystoscopy and histology was 92%, indicating that the test results are unaffected by BCG treatment.[100] Thus, FISH assay (UroVysion) combines the ease of cytology with many of the advantages over cystoscopy. It is, therefore, a valuable complementary method to cytology for the diagnosis and followup of patients with urothelial carcinoma. UroVysion is also useful for prediction of tumor recurrence,[18,101] for grading,[19] and for prognostication.[16,17]

In a clinical study including 64 patients with biopsy-proven bladder carcinoma, positive UroVysion results were observed in 40 patients (62.5%). Tumor recurrence

developed in 45% of the patients with positive UroVysion tests, compared with 12.5% of the patients with normal assay after a median followup of 13.5 months.[18] A positive UroVysion predicted tumor recurrence in 18/21 cases (86%), including all high grade recurrences. To establish independent prognostic factors for superficial bladder cancer recurrence, Mian et al. studied 75 urine specimens using UroVysion. FISH negative, or 9p21−/CEP3+, cases were associated with a low risk of recurrence. On the other hand, CEP 7+/17+ tumor cells on the UroVysion study were associated with a high risk of recurrence. Nine (33%) patients with a low risk pattern recurred after a mean followup of 30 months, but 18 (67%) patients with a high risk pattern developed recurrence within 18 months. Thus, UroVysion patterns may predict the risk of recurrence and disease-free survival of such patients.[16]

Bladder cancer is a heterogeneous malignancy with divergent clinical manifestations and a wide variety of chromosomal aberrations. Houskova studied 128 urine samples by UroVysion assay and correlated the result with histological grades of the tumors. UroVysion testing was positive in 64% of grade 1 tumors, 64% of grade 2

Table 32-3   UroVysion Interpretation in Urinary Cytology Specimens[a]

Cells with gains (i.e., three or more copies) of two or more of the four probes in the same cell are referred to as "polysomic" cells

Definition of "morphologically abnormal cells"
  Large nuclear size
  Irregular nuclear shape
  "Patchy" DAPI staining
  Cell clusters (do not count overlapping cells in clusters)

At least 25 well-preserved cells should be evaluated
  Begin with those cells that appear morphologically abnormal. If few morphologically abnormal cells are present, select the largest cells or those with the largest nuclei
  If morphologically abnormal cells are not readily apparent, the entire sample should be scanned and nuclei representing the most morphologically abnormal cells should be scored first

Recording the chromosome patterns in morphologically abnormal cells
  Gain (i.e., three or more signals) of two or more of chromosomes 3 (red), 7 (green), or 17 (aqua), or
  Loss of both copies of LSI 9p21
  If surrounding cells show abnormal chromosome patterns, as described above, these cells should be recorded, even if they are not morphologically abnormal
  If chromosomes 3, 7, or 17 show the loss of both chromosomes, consider the cell to be uninterpretable due to hybridization failure
  Cells with nondiploid counts having at least one signal for each of the four probes but not fitting the criteria specified above should be included, along with the diploid cells, in the overall total number of morphologically abnormal cells viewed

Record the total number of morphologically abnormal cells viewed (diploid and abnormal)
  If, after 25 morphologically abnormal cells have been analyzed, any of the following criteria have been met, stop analysis if:
    ≥ 4 of the 25 cells show gains for two or more chromosomes (3, 7, or 17) in the same cell, or
    ≥ 12 of the 25 cells have zero 9p21 signals
  Otherwise, continue analysis until either
    Four cells with gain for multiple chromosomes have been detected, or
    12 cells with zero 9p21 signals have been detected, or
    The entire sample has been analyzed

[a]Modified from UroVysion Bladder Cancer Kit package insert.

tumors, and 92% of grade 3 tumors, indicating that it may be useful as a grading tool.[19]

UroVysion is particularly attractive because it is an objective, quantitative assessment of urothelial cell abnormalities. Diagnosis of urothelial carcinoma in situ (CIS) is especially challenging, since lesions are not always cystoscopically identifiable, and biopsies are not taken from the abnormal urothelium. In the study by Gudjonsson et al., UroVysion identified 100% of CIS cases (five patients), two of whom were not identified by cystoscopy.[20] Similarly, Halling et al. found 100% sensitivity for 17 cases of CIS, and a statistically significant advantage in sensitivity compared to cytology.[24] Sarosdy and colleagues found 100% sensitivity for CIS in seven of seven cases, compared to 33% by urine cytology.[26] Blinded studies of CIS, however, are limited in the literature. More extensive investigations of CIS may reveal clinical circumstances for which this method is particularly useful. For example, applying the UroVysion assay to paraffin-embedded biopsy samples, Schwarz and colleagues found polysomy of one or more chromosomes in 91% of CIS cases (30/33) and deletion of 9p21 in 74% (22/31), leading the authors to propose this technique as

an aid for resolution of histologically challenging biopsies as well as cytologic samples.[28]

In a recent analysis of 1006 consecutive urine specimens from 600 patients at the M.D. Anderson Cancer Center, the sensitivity for detection of bladder cancer for UroVysion and cytology was 58% and 39%, respectively. The specificity for detection of bladder cancer for UroVysion and cytology was 66% and 84%, respectively.[102]

Bladder Tumor Antigen

BTA *stat* is a point of care (qualitative) latex agglutination immunoassay using two monoclonal antibodies to detect human complement factor H-related protein in the urine. Factor H is a soluble glycoprotein regulator of complement activation that appears to have an immunoprotective effect for tumor cells. These high molecular weight basement membrane complexes are produced when cancer cells become invasive and cause proteolytic degradation of the external lamina supporting urothelium. These complexes are frequently released into urine when urothelial

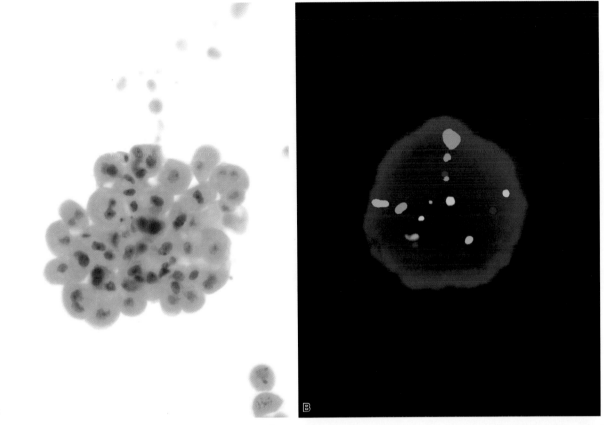

Figure 32-3   Low grade papillary urothelial carcinoma (A) detected by UroVysion fluorescence in situ hybridization (B) analysis. Urothelial cancer cell with malignant UroVysion pattern as indicated by three red (CEP3), four green (CEP7), three aqua (CEP17), and three gold signals.

neoplasms become invasive or remodeled the urothelial architecture. BTA *stat* testing is rapid, easily performed, and readily interpretable in a clinician's office. A recent modification of the test (BTA TRAK test) is a quantitative standard enzyme-linked immunosorbent assay (ELISA), allowing quantitation of immunoenzymatic results giving superior sensitivity and specificity over the qualitative BTA *stat* test.[9,23,103,104,116–124] Similar to urine cytology, both tests have higher sensitivity for detection of high grade lesions.[30]

The specificity of the BTA test for monitoring patients with a history of urothelial carcinoma varies from 40% to 70%, significantly greater than 17% to 32% with cytology alone. The sensitivity is similar with 90% to 96% for cytology and 100% for BTA, respectively.[9,23,105,106,116–124] Interestingly, cytology was more predictive that the BTA test in patients with carcinoma in situ,[104,107,129,130] so the utility of the BTA test appears to be greatest in followup of patients with low grade papillary tumors.[9,108,131,132] This test is now commonly used as an adjunct to cystoscopy and is being investigated as a possible screening test in high-risk patients.[9,104] The tests can be falsely positive in patients with inflammation, infection, or benign hematuria.[109]

Despite high sensitivity, the use of BTA TRAK and BTA *stat* is limited due to its low specificity.[110,111] This test was a significant improvement over cytology for the detection of urothelial carcinoma,[112,113] with sensitivity results reportedly twice those of cytology.[112] These high sensitivity levels demonstrate the usefulness of BTA in the diagnosis and followup of bladder cancer[114] and have suggested a possible prognostic significance.[115]

The BTA test was useful for detecting both primary and recurrent tumors (sensitivity, 90% and 74%, respectively),[125] and identified tumors that could not be visualized by routine cystoscopy.[126] However, photodynamic diagnosis with 5-aminolevulinic acid (ALA) cystoscopic fluorescence was slightly superior to the BTA test for cancer detection.[127]

In a multicenter study, BTA detected 82% of primary cancers, a sensitivity rate much higher than that of cytology (30%).[128] The BTA test showed sensitivity of 82% and specificity of 89% for detection of upper urinary tract cancer, greater than the usual accuracy of ureteral washing cytology and voided urine cytology in this clinical setting.[113] This test is now often used as an adjunct to cystoscopy for bladder cancer, and is being investigated

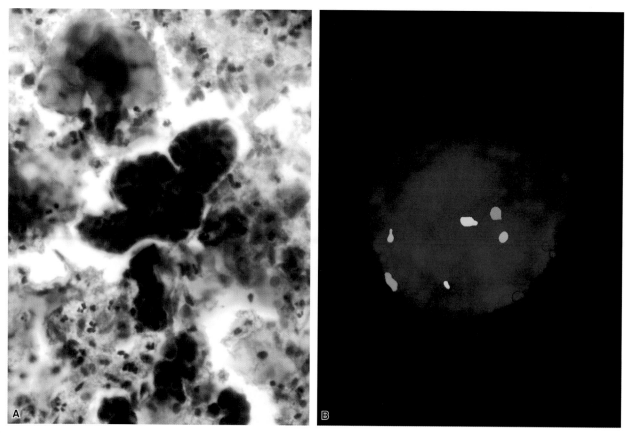

Figure 32-4 UroVysion fluorescence in situ hybridization analysis in a catheterized urine specimen from an 80-year-old male. There are numerous cells in papillary aggregate configurations (A). It is difficult to distinguish benign reactive urothelial cells after instrumentation from low grade papillary urothelial carcinoma. The normal UroVysion pattern (B) confirms the benign nature of these cells.

as a possible screening test in high risk patients.[130] BTA was found useful in identifying patients at high risk for recurrence.[120,131] However, others have found that BTA provides "no additional information" beyond that from cytology and hematuria anaylsis.[124]

In a 2002 study, Halling et al. found 94% sensitivity of BTA *stat* for pT1 to pT4 and pTis lesions, with overall specificity of 78%. Sensitivity of the test improved with grade from 50% (grade 1) to 72% (grade 2) and 91% (grade 3).[23] Schroeder and colleagues found a somewhat lower overall sensitivity of 53%.[32] With regard to urothelial CIS, the two cases of primary CIS in Schroeder et al.'s series were not identified by BTA *stat*. Similarly, Sarosdy et al. found that BTA demonstrated 50% sensitivity, with greater than 70% sensitivity for grade 2 to 3 lesions.[26] As a screening modality, BTA *stat* is associated with false-positive results that are usually caused by inflammatory conditions in the urinary tract.

Multiple recent reports have found that the sensitivity and specificity of BTA were comparable to those of voided urine cytology, but the false-positive rate showed that this test would best be used only as an adjunct to cytology rather than as an independent screening device.[133–135] Conversely, another study[136] found that the false-positive rate was only in 2% of a screened population. False-positive rates were higher in cases with gross hematuria,[137] urinary tract calculi (90%), positive urine cultures,[120] and prostatic hyperplasia (73%).[138] The specificity of BTA was lower in patients who received intravesical treatment. The specificity was 81%, 71%, and 65% in patients without, with past, or with present intravesical treatments, respectively. The difference between those with no treatment and present instillation treatments was significant ($P = 0.023$); however, the differences between those with no treatment and past instillations ($P = 0.076$) and between those with past and present instillations ($P = 0.558$) were not significant. Intravesical treatment appeared to exhibit an adverse effect on BTA testing, so the test should not be used in such patients.[139]

For tumor detection, BTA was superior to the NMP22 test in some reports[135,140–143] but not in others.[144] BTA had a sensitivity of 70% to 89% for detecting bladder

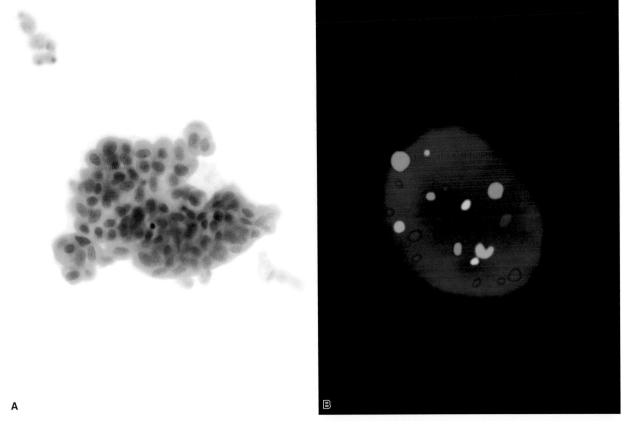

Figure 32-5   low grade papillary urothelial carcinoma detected by UroVysion FISH analysis. It is difficult to separate low grade papillary urothelial carcinoma from benign reactive urothelial cells (especially after instrumentation) (A). Abnormal chromosomal patterns in these cells indicate their malignant nature (B).

cancer, while NMP22 had a sensitivity of only 67% to 69%.[143] The specificity was also higher for BTA at 71% to 79%, compared to 65% to 70% for NMP22.[140,143] Conversely, Giannopoulos et al. found that NMP22 was more specific.[145] BTA *stat* was less efficient and inferior to the hyaluronic acid–hyaluronidase test in a prospective study of recurrence in 225 cancer patients over a four-year period. Sensitivity and specificity were 74% versus 63% and 61% versus 94% for the hyaluronidase test and BTA *stat*, respectively.[146]

Nuclear Matrix Protein 22

NMP22 is a nuclear matrix protein usually present in very low quantities in the urine of normal individuals, but with greatly elevated levels in the urine of patients with bladder cancer.[4,5,81] The commercial NMP22 assay is a quantitative sandwich ELISA test using two antibodies, recognizing two epitopes. It is rapid, easily performed, readily interpretable, and available in many clinical laboratories. It is also simple, noninvasive, and cost-effective.[147] NMP22 had a sensitivity

of 71% and a specificity of 90% for urothelial carcinoma in patients with microscopic hematuria, greater than respective values of 60% and 83% for urine cytology.[2,4,119,144,148,149] The sensitivity of NMP22 in patients with a history of bladder cancer was 59% to 100%.[150,151] NMP22 had a sensitivity to detect malignancy of 100% in invasive disease and 70% overall.[152–154]

NMP22 at a cutoff value of 6 units/mL was also significantly more sensitive in detecting bladder cancer (sensitivity of 83% in pTa cases and 98% in pT1 cases) than urine cytology (20% in pTa and 64% in pT1).[155] This difference in sensitivity was also found in patients stratified according to cancer grade; NMP22 was positive in 86%, 97%, and 90% of grade 1, grade 2, and grade 3 tumors, respectively, while urine cytology was positive in 38%, 44%, and 80%, respectively.[156] The optimal reference range for detecting recurrent cancer was 6.4 units/mL in one study, with higher results indicating a greater likelihood of recurrence.[151] Other authors used different cutoff points for positive and negative tests, limiting comparability; Chahal found that the optimum threshold was 4.75 U/mL from the receiver operating characteristics curve, with a sensitivity of 42%, specificity of 85%, positive predictive value of 39%, and negative predictive value of 89%.[157] Poulakis and colleagues found that the optimal cutoff point on the receiver operating characteristics curve was 8.25 U/mL. They reported a sensitivity of 85% and specificity of 68%, a significantly lower specificity than urine cytology (96%).[122] Oge et al. used a cutoff point of 10 U/mL, and found an overall sensitivity and specificity of 72% and 73%, respectively.[158] Using the same threshold, Friedrich et al. found a sensitivity of 69% and specificity of 65% for the detection of cancer, considerably lower than the BTA *stat* test and Lewis X antigen.[143] Boman and colleagues found a "disappointingly low sensitivity" (65%) for detection of recurrence for cancers of small size and low grade.[142] Chahal and colleagues noted that urinary NMP22 was "at best supportive only" as a diagnostic marker.[157] However, the sensitivity and specificity of NMP22, reported by Grossman et al., were 56% and 85%, respectively, compared to 16% and 99% for cytology.[33]

The NMP22 test may allow lengthening of the interval between followup cystoscopies in patients with low risk cancer. NMP22 was effective at predicting tumor status at followup cystoscopy.[152,159] One study suggested that this test may be useful for prescreening cystoscopy.[160] Urinary tract infections and calculi must be excluded, owing to interference with the test.[135,159,161,162] Pyuria and hematuria significantly affect the level of urinary NMP22 and could lead to false-positive results,[162] but the majority of those followed for bladder cancer correlated with recurrences.[122] Prior transurethral resection also lowered the accuracy of the test,[158] as did urinary diversion.[163]

A nomogram has been developed to better predict the probability of urothelial cancer recurrence and progression using the NMP22 test.[70] However, the reliability of the test is uncertain due to the reported variability in the diagnostic performance of the test at different institutions.[43,71] Some studies found that the BTA test was more sensitive than NMP22,[140,141] but NMP22 may be more specific.[145] However, another report found NMP22 to be superior.[144]

ImmunoCyt

The ImmunoCyt technique employs three fluorescent-tagged monoclonal antibodies against three urothelial carcinoma antigens: specifically, two cytoplasmic mucin-related proteins (M344 and 19A211), and high molecular weight carcinoembryonic antigen (CEA).[4,5,164] Cells showing green fluorescence are positive for bladder cancer mucins, while red fluorescent cells are positive for glycosylated CEA.

This urine test had a cumulative 90% specificity and up to 96% sensitivity in cancer detection in 1493 cases, and invariably identified all high grade cancers.[165] Pfister et al. confirmed the high sensitivity of ImmunoCyt testing.[166] A multicenter study, however, showed that the overall sensitivity of cytology alone, ImmunoCyt alone, and the two methods combined was 23%, 81%, and 81%, respectively.[167] The specificity of cytology alone, ImmunoCyt alone, and of the two methods combined, was 93%, 75%, and 73%, respectively.[167] Importantly, the immunocytochemical test could detect 71% of small (less than 1 cm) tumors.[167] Because of its high sensitivity for detecting small tumors, even those of low histological grade, and its high negative predictive value, this test may have a role for decreasing the frequency of cystoscopic examinations and for monitoring patients with low risk bladder cancer.[4,17,31,168] In another study, ImmunoCyt (76%) had a sensitivity superior to that of cytology (21%) and UroVysion (13%).[169] The specificity was 63%, 97%, and 90%, respectively, for cytology, ImmunoCyt, and UroVysion.[169]

The sensitivity was as high as 100% when ImmunoCyt was combined with urine cytology for the detection of CIS. The combination of cytology and ImmunoCyt also raised the detection of grade 3 cancer from 75% to 94%, and the detection of low grade low stage tumors from 50% to 90%.[170] A Swedish hospital-based study found a sensitivity of 100% and a specificity of 69% for recurrence in a consecutive prospective series of histologically proven bladder cancers.[171] Conversely, a Dutch study of 104 patients followed for recurrent urothelial carcinoma revealed an area under the receiver operating characteristic curve of only up to 60%, although this may have resulted from high level of interobserver variability.[172] ImmunoCyt showed a specificity of 79% for grade 1, 84% for grade 2, and 92% for grade 3 tumors.[17]

Schmitz-Dräger et al. showed that the combination of cystoscopy and ImmunoCyt testing provided 100% sensitivity in bladder cancer detection, while combining cystoscopy and cytology marginally improved on the sensitivity of cystoscopy alone.[35] The major advantage of ImmunoCyt over other tests is its sensitivity for detecting both low and high grade tumors.[17] Lodde et al. reported that the sensitivity of testing voided urine from 37 patients was 50% for cytologic analysis, 75% for ImmunoCyt, and 87% for both methods combined.[15,173]

Similar to UroVysion, the ImmunoCyt technique identified 100% (five cases) of CIS patients in a study by Messing et al. It demonstrated particularly high sensitivity (when used in combination with cytology) for CIS or grade 3 tumors. These two histologic diagnoses were combined in the authors' review of the literature.[167]

The combination of urine cytology and ImmunoCyt significantly increased the detection rate for upper urinary tract cancer when compared with cytology alone, thereby providing an improvement for clinical management of patients at great risk (about 29%) of cancer recurrence.[15,173]

Urinary Bladder Cancer Antigen

The urine antigen ELISA test of IDL Biotech (Sollentona, Sweden) showed 64% sensitivity (at 73% specificity) for bladder cancer in patients with hematuria, lower than that observed with BTA *stat* (78%) and NMP 22 (75%), but higher than flow cytometry (61%).[119] False-positive results were observed in seven of 65 samples from patients with bladder cancer receiving intravesical BCG, usually owing to urinary tract infection.[159,161] A recent report found that the combination of urinary bladder cancer and DNA/cytokeratin flow cytometry increased sensitivity to 89%.[161] Using a cutoff point of 1 for urinary bladder cancer to provide the same specificity as BTA *stat* for identifying new cancers provided a lower sensitivity for urinary bladder cancer (60%) than for BTA *stat* (75%) or NMP22 (65%).[142]

Hemoglobin Dipstick

The specificity and sensitivity of hemoglobin dipstick for cancer screening and detection of recurrence in voided urine samples of patients prior to cystoscopy was 54% to 74% and 50% to 51%, respectively, well below that of most other commercially available tests.[121,144]

Other Urine Biomarkers

Other markers are also being evaluated for their utility in detecting cancer cells in urine sediment, including epigenetic markers,[38,90,174] telomerase,[40,175] microRNAs, and survivin (see also **Chapters 33 and 34**).[4,78,176]

Ancillary Studies

Flow Cytometry/DNA Ploidy Analysis

Voided urine is generally not adequate for flow cytometry, so cell samples for this test must be obtained by vigorous flushing of the bladder through a soft rubbery catheter five to 10 times with saline solution or during cystoscopy by lavage (barbotage). Subpopulations of bladder epithelial cells can be identified by interactive digital image analysis. The diagnosis of cancer is strongly suspected in cases with an aneuploid stemline or 16% or more of cells with hyperdiploid DNA (greater than 2C DNA content). A specimen is less likely to be malignant if no aneuploid stemline is detected and if fewer than 11% of the cells are hyperdiploid.

If 11% to 16% of the cells measured are hyperdiploid and no ancuploid stemline is detected, the samples are considered suspicious. Recurrent cancer can be detected by using combined urine cytology and image analysis.[177,178]

DNA ploidy analysis correlates with cancer grade and stage in urothelial carcinoma of the bladder and upper urinary tract, in urinary tract squamous cell carcinoma, and in bladder adenocarcinoma. At present, it remains a research tool in most laboratories. Most cases of World Health Organization (WHO) grade 1 carcinoma are diploid, whereas high grade carcinoma (WHO grade 3 carcinoma), including CIS, is usually aneuploid.[179–183] low grade carcinoma (WHO grade 2 carcinoma) is equally likely to be diploid and nondiploid.[184]

Ploidy results were strongly correlated with cancer invasion. Diploid cancer was usually confined to the lamina propria, whereas muscle-invasive cancer tended to be aneuploid.[182,185,186] About one-half of aneuploid low grade carcinomas were tetraploid, and very few tetraploid cancers were deeply invasive, suggesting that tetraploid low grade carcinoma was less likely than aneuploid cancer to invade the wall of the bladder. Tetraploidy may be an intermediate stage in the development of invasive aneuploid cancers.[187] CIS with two aneuploid peaks was more likely than CIS with a single peak to progress to invasive cancer.[188] Adjacent urothelium often shared the same DNA ploidy abnormality as cancer,[189] suggesting that aneuploid cancer arises from global aneuploid epithelial abnormalities.[182] The significance of the S phase fraction in the prognosis of bladder cancers is uncertain, although two reports found that it was better than DNA ploidy as a predictor of progression in patients with cancer treated by intravesical chemotherapy.[190,191]

DNA ploidy as assessed by flow cytometry increased the predictive value of urine cytology for cancer in untreated patients,[192] although this claim was refuted in another study.[119] It was also of value in patients with both low and high stage cancer, and after treatment with intravesical or systemic chemotherapy. However, since DNA flow cytometry requires a large number of cells, it may not be as effective for detecting small aneuploid tumors, which are usually present in cases of primary urothelial CIS.[193] DNA content according to computer-based image analysis was at least as sensitive as flow cytometry for detecting malignant cells, and was superior in hypocellular specimens.[194] When combined with cytology, DNA image cytometry provided a sensitivity of 68% and specificity of 100%.[195] DNA content was predictive of recurrence in papillary urothelial carcinoma after controlling for grade and stage.[183,196]

DNA ploidy patterns of urothelial carcinoma of the renal pelvis and ureter are similar to those in the bladder.[181] Patients with an aneuploid cancer have a poorer prognosis than those with a diploid cancer.[181,185,186,197]

Well-differentiated squamous cell carcinoma was usually diploid, whereas moderately and poorly differentiated carcinomas were usually aneuploid.[198] DNA ploidy was predictive of survival after radical cystectomy in patients with schistosomiasis-associated squamous cell carcinoma.[199] Most cases of primary adenocarcinoma of the urinary bladder are aneuploid.

Digital Image Analysis

Some investigators believe that digital image analysis was superior to flow cytometry for DNA ploidy analysis in specimens with low cellularity, with sensitivities of 91% and 71%, respectively.[200] Furthermore, image analysis was superior to cytologic examination for prediction of tumor recurrence after normal findings at cystoscopic examination, and was equivalent to cytology for detection of high grade lesions.[201] Combined cytologic evaluation and digital image analysis may be a reliable method of detecting recurrent bladder cancer in patients with urinary diversions and can be used to regularly monitor these high-risk patients.[202] Computer-assisted quantitative morphological parameters can be an effective tool to distinguish reactive renal tubular cells from low grade urothelial carcinoma cells in voided urine.[203] Among five nuclear morphometric parameters, including nuclear area, perimeter, roundness factor, maximum length, and linear factor, linear factor was most important in differentiating reactive renal tubular cells in renal disease from low grade urothelial carcinoma cells.[203]

Despite the apparent utility of digital image analysis for evaluation of urinary cells and bladder tissues, this methodology is no longer in use in most institutions, owing to the high technical complexity and significant labor cost of the test.

Immunohistochemistry and Enzyme-linked Immunosorbent Assay

Numerous protein-based biomarkers have been evaluated in urine samples (see also **Chapters 33 and 34**).[4,93] Immunostaining with cytokeratin 20 was potentially useful in detecting urothelial carcinoma in urine samples.[204] The proliferation marker Ki67 and reactivity to the URO series, reported by Panosian and colleagues, of monoclonal antibodies have been detected in urine cytology specimens.[205] Immunostaining against blood group antigens and other tumor markers have been investigated for clinical use in urinary cytology.[206–210] Deletion of A, B, and H blood group antigens is associated with biochemical and structural changes of glycoprotein and glycolipid components of the cell surface during neoplastic transformation. Blood group reactivity is decreased in high grade and aggressive tumors. Carcinoembryonic antigen immunostaining has

been used for evaluation of exfoliated urothelial cancer cells. These immunostain-based assays may have potential for clinical use in selected cases.

Urinary concentration of soluble cytokeratin 19 fragments, measured by the immunoradiometric CYFRA 21-1 assay, with a cutoff point concentration of 4.9 μg/L resulted in a sensitivity of 79% and a specificity of 89%, up to threefold greater than the sensitivity for cytology in detecting grade 1 carcinoma.[211] However, false-positive results were encountered with calculi, infections, and previous BCG immunotherapy. Cytokeratin 20 is expressed in neoplastic urothelial cells, but apparently not in normal urothelium, and mRNA extraction from urine samples of patients with bladder cancer revealed a sensitivity of 91% and a specificity of 67%.[212]

Progression marker T138 detected a surface antigen that together with the cancer stage, was an independent predictor of metastases.[165] The glycosaminoglycan hyaluronic acid promotes cell migration and adhesion, and levels in the urine, when measured by ELISA, are elevated threefold to fivefold in patients with urothelial carcinoma.[213]

Molecular Genetic Studies

Remarkable progress has been made in understanding the molecular basis of urothelial carcinogenesis.[1] These scientific discoveries have been translated successfully into clinical practice samples (see also **Chapters 29, 31, 33, and 34**).[4,93] Molecular analysis of urine samples is becoming routine practice. A number of molecular platforms have been utilized in the analysis of urine samples. FISH is useful for investigating numeric chromosomal abnormalities (see the earlier discussion of UroVysion FISH).[4,10,23,24,200,214] FISH revealed abnormalities of chromosomes 8 and 12 in 83% of 26 bladder tumors of all grades.[200]

Microsatellite analysis studies have shown that allelic imbalances of 2q, 3p, 4p, 5q, 8p, 9p, 9q, 10q, 11p, 13q, 17p, and 18q (which are known sites of tumor suppressor genes) are common in urothelial neoplasms.[1,3,4,19,60,215–246] In microsatellite analysis, normal patient cells (buccal mucosa or peripheral blood) are compared to urine cytology cells. Polymerase chain reaction (PCR) is performed, and then electrophoretically separated loci (the predetermined most commonly altered loci, such as 3p, 8p, 9p, 11p, 17p, and 18q) can delineate if loss of heterozygosity (LOH) or microsatellite instability (MSI) is present.[46,247–252] However, urinary leukocytes can interfere with the results (which would not be useful in patients that have received BCG therapy). Squamous epithelium can also interfere with results.[215–217]

Other chromosomal imbalances in bladder carcinoma have been found by comparative genomic hybridization[253–256] or a novel method of detecting polymorphic microsatellite markers in urine samples with a high sensitivity for bladder cancer recurrence.[248] Allelic deletion fingerprinting using microsatellite primers from chromosomes 3, 4, 8, 11, 14, and 17 was positive in 88% of tumors, including 69% of incipient tumors initially classified as benign by cytology.[252] Denaturing gradient gel electrophoresis of urine DNA samples from patients with T1 bladder cancer had 69% sensitivity and 100% specificity for recurrence.[249] LOH study of 24 microsatellite markers to detect bladder cancer revealed a sensitivity of 96% and a specificity of 100%.[250]

Microsatellite analysis of urine samples has been investigated for the surveillance of bladder cancer patients after treatment. van der Aa et al. evaluated 228 patients by analyzing 20 microsatellite markers located on 10 chromosomes.[46] Cross-sectional sensitivity and specificity of microsatellite analysis for detection of a recurrence were 58% (49/84) and 73% (531/731), respectively. The two-year risk of developing a recurrence reached 83% if microsatellite results were persistently positive, and declined to 22% when microsatellite analysis was persistently negative. The data suggest that microsatellite alteration is a strong predictor for tumor recurrences.[46]

In a single nucleotide polymorphism (SNP) analysis using HuSNP chips, Hoque et al. found that 31 of 31 (100%) urine DNA samples from patients with bladder tumors had 24 or more SNP DNA alterations, but such alterations were not identified in nine normal control subjects. Their findings suggest that the HuSNP chip is a valuable tool for the detection of bladder cancer.[257]

Efforts to develop DNA methylation markers in urine sediments for detection of bladder cancer are also under way.[4,38,90,91,251,258–261] In a study of Yu et al. using methylation-specific PCR, 59 tumor-associated genes were profiled in three bladder cancer cell lines, a small cohort of cancer biopsies, and in urine sediments. Twenty-one candidate genes were then profiled in urine sediments

from 132 bladder cancer patients, 23 age-matched patients with noncancerous urinary lesions, six with neurologic diseases, and seven healthy volunteers. Cancer-specific hypermethylation was identified in 15 genes, and analysis of urine sediments for an 11-gene set showed a positive correlation with existing bladder cancer in 92% of bladder cancer cases.[38] A methylation panel comprising *GDF15, TMEFF2*, and *VIM* can detect tumor cells accurately with 94% sensitivity and 100% specificity.[90] The sensitivity of methylation analysis in voided urine samples of cancer was greater than that of urine cytology (91% vs. 46%, respectively).[261]

Studies of the methylation status of Wnt antagonist genes in 54 transitional cell carcinoma and corresponding normal bladder mucosa biopsies showed that the methylation levels of Wnt antagonists were significantly higher in bladder tumors than in normal bladder mucosa. The overall sensitivity was 77%, and the specificity was 67%.[91] In patients with bladder cancer, 81% of the methylation-specific PCR results had identical methylation patterns in samples of tumor- and urine-derived DNA. Urine DNAs derived from normal controls typically showed no aberrant methylation of the Wnt antagonist genes. Thus, analysis of methylation status of Wnt antagonist genes could serve as an excellent epigenetic biomarker panel for urinary cytology.[91]

In a gene expression analysis of 576 urine samples, Mengual and colleagues identified a 12+2 gene expression signature that is useful for bladder cancer diagnosis and prediction of tumor aggressiveness.[92] Overall, this gene set panel had 98% sensitivity and 99% specificity in discriminating between bladder cancer and normal control samples and 79% sensitivity and 92% specificity in predicting tumor aggressiveness.[92] Identification of a gene expression signature in urine sample will further improve the detection and monitoring of patients with bladder cancer (see **Chapter 34** for further discussion).[4]

REFERENCES

1. Cheng L, Davidson DD, MacLennan GT, Williamson SR, Zhang S, Koch MO, Montironi R, Lopez-Beltran A. The origins of urothelial carcinoma. *Expert Rev Anticancer Ther* 2010;10:865–80.
2. Cheng L, Zhang S, Davidson DD, MacLennan GT, Koch MO, Montironi R, Lopez-Beltran A. Molecular determinants of tumor recurrence in the urinary bladder. *Future Oncol* 2009;5:843–57.
3. Cheng L, Zhang D. Molecular Genetic Pathology. New York: Humana Press/Springer, 2008.
4. Cheng L, Zhang S, Maclennan GT, Williamson SR, Lopez-Beltran A, Montironi R. Bladder cancer: translating molecular genetic insights into clinical practice. *Hum Pathol* 2011;42:455–81.
5. Tetu B. Diagnosis of urothelial carcinoma from urine. *Mod Pathol* 2009;22 (Suppl 2):S53–9.
6. Proctor I, Stoeber K, Williams GH. Biomarkers in bladder cancer. *Histopathology* 2010;57:1–13.
7. Kaufman DS, Shipley WU, Feldman AS. Bladder cancer. *Lancet* 2009;374:239–49.
8. Dinney CP, McConkey DJ, Millikan RE, Wu X, Bar-Eli M, Adam L, Kamat AM, Siefker-Radtke AO, Tuziak T, Sabichi AL, Grossman HB, Benedict WF, Czerniak B. Focus on bladder cancer. *Cancer Cell* 2004;6:111–6.

9. van Rhijn BW, van der Poel HG, van der Kwast TH. Urine markers for bladder cancer surveillance: a systematic review. *Eur Urol* 2005;47:736–48.

10. Bubendorf L, Grilli B, Sauter G, Mihatsch MJ, Gasser TC, Dalquen P. Multiprobe FISH for enhanced detection of bladder cancer in voided urine specimens and bladder washings. *Am J Clin Pathol* 2001;116:79–86.

11. Habuchi TMM, Droller MJ, Hemstreet GP 3rd, Grossman HB, Schalken JA, Schmitz-Drager BJ, Murphy WM, Bono AV, Goebell P, Getzenberg RH, Hautmann SH, Messing E, Fradet Y, Lokeshwar VB. Prognostic markers for bladder cancer: International Consensus Panel on bladder tumor markers. *Urology* 2005;66:64–74.

12. Lokeshwar VB, Habuchi T, Grossman HB, Murphy WM, Hautmann SH, Hemstreet GP 3rd, Bono AV, Getzenberg RH, Goebell P, Schmitz-Drager BJ, Schalken JA, Fradet Y, Marberger M, Messing E, Droller MJ. Bladder tumor markers beyond cytology: International Consensus Panel on bladder tumor markers. *Urology* 2005;66:35–63.

13. Moonen PM, Merkx GF, Peelen P, Karthaus HF, Smeets DF, Witjes JA. UroVysion compared with cytology and quantitative cytology in the surveillance of non-muscle-invasive bladder cancer. *Eur Urol* 2007;51:1275–80.

14. Schlomer BJ, Ho R, Sagalowsky A, Ashfaq R, Lotan Y. Prospective validation of the clinical usefulness of reflex fluorescence in situ hybridization assay in patients with atypical cytology for the detection of urothelial carcinoma of the bladder. *J Urol* 2010;183:62–7.

15. Lodde M, Mian C, Comploj E, Palermo S, Longhi E, Marberger M, Pycha A. uCyt+ test: alternative to cystoscopy for less-invasive followup of patients with low risk of urothelial carcinoma. *Urology* 2006;67:950–4.

16. Mian C, Lodde M, Comploj E, Lusuardi L, Palermo S, Mian M, Maier K, Pycha A. Multiprobe fluorescence in situ hybridisation: prognostic perspectives in superficial bladder cancer. *J Clin Pathol* 2006;59:984–7.

17. Mian C, Maier K, Comploj E, Lodde M, Berner L, Lusuardi L, Palermo S, Vittadello F, Pycha A. uCyt+/ImmunoCyt in the detection of recurrent urothelial carcinoma: an update on 1991 analyses. *Cancer* 2006;108:60–5.

18. Gofrit ON, Zorn KC, Silvestre J, Shalhav AL, Zagaja GP, Msezane LP, Steinberg GD. The predictive value of multi-targeted fluorescent in-situ hybridization in patients with history of bladder cancer. *Urol Oncol* 2008;26:246–9.

19. Houskova L, Zemanova Z, Babjuk M, Melichercikova J, Pesl M, Michalova K. Molecular cytogenetic characterization and diagnostics of bladder cancer. *Neoplasma* 2007;54:511–6.

20. Gudjonsson S, Isfoss BL, Hansson K, Domanski AM, Warenholt J, Soller W, Lundberg LM, Liedberg F, Grabe M, Mansson W. The value of the UroVysion assay for surveillance of non-muscle-invasive bladder cancer. *Eur Urol* 2008;54:402–8.

21. Liedberg F, Anderson H, Chebil G, Gudjonsson S, Hoglund M, Lindgren D, Lundberg LM, Lovgren K, Ferno M, Mansson W. Tissue microarray based analysis of prognostic markers in invasive bladder cancer: Much effort to no avail? *Urol Oncol* 2008;26:17–24.

22. Kipp BR, Halling KC, Campion MB, Wendel AJ, Karnes RJ, Zhang J, Sebo TJ. Assessing the value of reflex fluorescence in situ hybridization testing in the diagnosis of bladder cancer when routine urine cytological examination is equivocal. *J Urol* 2008;179:1296–301.

23. Halling KC, King W, Sokolova IA, Meyer RG, Burkhardt HM, Halling AC, Cheville JC, Sebo TJ, Ramakumar S, Stewart CS, Pankratz S, O'Kane DJ, Seelig SA, Lieber MM, Jenkins RB. A comparison of cytology and fluorescence in situ hybridization for the detection of urothelial carcinoma. *J Urol* 2000;164:1768–75.

24. Halling KC, King W, Sokolova IA, Meyer RG, Burkhardt HM, Halling AC, Cheville JC, Sebo TJ, Ramakumar S, Stewart CS, Pankratz S, O'Kane DJ, Seelig SA, Lieber MM, Jenkins RB. A comparison of cytology and fluorescence in situ hybridization for the detection of urothelial carcinoma. *J Urol* 2000;164:1768–75.

25. Sokolova IA, Halling KC, Jenkins RB, Burkhardt HM, Meyer RG, Seelig SA, King W. The development of a multitarget, multicolor fluorescence in situ hybridization assay for the detection of urothelial carcinoma in urine. *J Mol Diagn* 2000;2:116–23.

26. Sarosdy MF, Schellhammer P, Bokinsky G, Kahn P, Chao R, Yore L, Zadra J, Burzon D, Osher G, Bridge JA, Anderson S, Johansson SL, Lieber M, Soloway M, Flom K. Clinical evaluation of a multi-target fluorescent in situ hybridization assay for detection of bladder cancer. *J Urol* 2002;168:1950–4.

27. Ferreira CS, Papamichael K, Guilbault G, Schwarzacher T, Gariepy J, Missailidis S. DNA aptamers against the MUC1 tumour marker: design of aptamer-antibody sandwich ELISA for the early diagnosis of epithelial tumours. *Anal Bioanal Chem* 2008;390:1039–50.

28. Schwarz S, Rechenmacher M, Filbeck T, Knuechel R, Blaszyk H, Hartmann A, Brockhoff G. Value of multicolour fluorescence in situ hybridisation (UroVysion) in the differential diagnosis of flat urothelial lesions. *J Clin Pathol* 2008;61:272–7.

29. Hautmann SH, Lokeshwar VB, Schroeder GL, Civantos F, Duncan RC, Gnann R, Friedrich MG, Soloway MS. Elevated tissue expression of hyaluronic acid and hyaluronidase validates the HA-HAase urine test for bladder cancer. *J Urol* 2001;165:2068–74.

30. Lokeshwar VB, Soloway MS. Current bladder tumor tests: Does their projected utility fulfill clinical necessity? *J Urol* 2001;165:1067–77.

31. Hautmann S, Toma M, Lorenzo Gomez MF, Friedrich MG, Jaekel T, Michl U, Schroeder GL, Huland H, Juenemann KP, Lokeshwar VB. Immunocyt and the HA-HAase urine tests for the detection of bladder cancer: a side-by-side comparison. *Eur Urol* 2004;46:466–71.

32. Schroeder GL, Lorenzo-Gomez MF, Hautmann SH, Friedrich MG, Ekici S, Huland H, Lokeshwar V. A side by side comparison of cytology and biomarkers for bladder cancer detection. *J Urol* 2004;172:1123–6.

33. Grossman HB, Messing E, Soloway M, Tomera K, Katz G, Berger Y, Shen Y. Detection of bladder cancer using a point-of-care proteomic assay. *JAMA* 2005;293:810–6.

34. Goebell PJ, Groshen SL, Schmitz-Drager BJ. Guidelines for development of diagnostic markers in bladder cancer. *World J Urol* 2008;26:5–11.

35. Schmitz-Drager B, Tirsar LA, Schmitz-Drager C, Dorsam J, Bismarck E, Ebert T. Immunocytology in the assessment of patients with painless gross haematuria. *BJU Int* 2008;101:455–8.

36. Schmitz-Drager BJ, Fradet Y, Grossman HB. Bladder cancer markers in patient management: the current perspective. *World J Urol* 2008;26:1–3.

37. Schmitz-Drager BJ, Tirsar LA, Schmitz-Drager C, Dorsam J, Mellan Z, Bismarck E, Ebert T. Immunocytology in the assessment of patients with asymptomatic hematuria. *World J Urol* 2008;26:31–7.

38. Yu J, Zhu T, Wang Z, Zhang H, Qian Z, Xu H, Gao B, Wang W, Gu L, Meng J, Wang J, Feng X, Li Y, Yao X, Zhu J. A novel set of DNA methylation markers in urine sediments for sensitive/specific detection of bladder cancer. *Clin Cancer Res* 2007;13:7296–304.

39. Eissa S, Ali-Labib R, Swellam M, Bassiony M, Tash F, El-Zayat TM. Noninvasive diagnosis of bladder cancer by detection of matrix metalloproteinases (MMP–2 and MMP–9) and their inhibitor (TIMP–2) in urine. *Eur Urol* 2007;52:1388–96.

40. Eissa S, Swellam M, Ali-Labib R, Mansour A, El-Malt O, Tash FM. Detection of telomerase in urine by 3 methods: evaluation of diagnostic accuracy for bladder cancer. *J Urol* 2007;178:1068–72.

41. Lotan Y, Bensalah K, Ruddell T, Shariat SF, Sagalowsky AI, Ashfaq R. Prospective evaluation of the clinical usefulness of reflex fluorescence in situ hybridization assay in patients with atypical cytology for the detection of urothelial carcinoma of the bladder. *J Urol* 2008;179:2164–9.

42. Kausch I, Bohle A. Molecular aspects of bladder cancer III. Prognostic markers of bladder cancer. *Eur Urol* 2002;41:15–29.

43. Karakiewicz PI, Shariat SF, Palapattu GS, Gilad AE, Lotan Y, Rogers CG, Vazina A, Gupta A, Bastian PJ, Perrotte P, Sagalowsky AI, Schoenberg M, Lerner SP. Nomogram for predicting disease recurrence after radical cystectomy for transitional cell carcinoma of the bladder. *J Urol* 2006;176:1354–61; discussion 1361–2.

44. Margulis V, Shariat SF, Ashfaq R, Sagalowsky AI, Lotan Y. Ki–67 is an independent predictor of bladder cancer outcome in patients treated with radical cystectomy for organ-confined disease. *Clin Cancer Res* 2006;12:7369–73.

45. Khaled HM, Bahnassy AA, Raafat AA, Zekri AR, Madboul MS, Mokhtar NM. Clinical significance of altered nm23-H1, EGFR, RB and p53 expression in bilharzial bladder cancer. *BMC Cancer* 2009;9:32.

46. van der Aa MN, Zwarthoff EC, Steyerberg EW, Boogaard MW, Nijsen Y, van der Keur KA, van Exsel AJ, Kirkels WJ, Bangma C, van der Kwast TH. Microsatellite analysis of voided-urine samples for surveillance of low grade non-muscle-invasive urothelial carcinoma: feasibility and clinical utility in a prospective multicenter study (Cost-Effectiveness of followup of Urinary Bladder Cancer trial [CEFUB]). *Eur Urol* 2009;55:659–67.

47. Hoque MO, Lee CC, Cairns P, Schoenberg M, Sidransky D. Genome-wide genetic characterization of bladder cancer: a comparison of high-density single-nucleotide polymorphism arrays and PCR-based microsatellite analysis. *Cancer Res* 2003;63:2216–22.

48. Hoque MO, Lee J, Begum S, Yamashita K, Engles JM, Schoenberg M, Westra WH, Sidransky D. High-throughput molecular analysis of urine sediment for the detection of bladder cancer by high-density single-nucleotide polymorphism array. *Cancer Res* 2003;63:5723–6.

49. Byun HM, Wong HL, Birnstein EA, Wolff EM, Liang G, Yang AS. Examination of IGF2 and H19 loss of imprinting in bladder cancer. *Cancer Res* 2007;67:10753–8.

50. Urakami S, Shiina H, Enokida H, Kawakami T, Kawamoto K, Hirata H, Tanaka Y, Kikuno N, Nakagawa M, Igawa M, Dahiya R. Combination analysis of hypermethylated Wnt-antagonist family genes as a novel epigenetic biomarker panel for bladder cancer detection. *Clin Cancer Res* 2006;12:2109–16.

51. Yates DR, Rehman I, Abbod MF, Meuth M, Cross SS, Linkens DA, Hamdy FC, Catto JW. Promoter hypermethylation identifies progression risk in bladder cancer. *Clin Cancer Res* 2007;13:2046–53.

52. Catto JW, Miah S, Owen HC, Bryant H, Myers K, Dudziec E, Larre S, Milo M, Rehman I, Rosario DJ, Di Martino E, Knowles MA, Meuth M, Harris AL, Hamdy FC. Distinct microRNA alterations characterize high- and low grade bladder cancer. *Cancer Res* 2009;69:8472–81.

53. Catto JW, Azzouzi AR, Rehman I, Feeley KM, Cross SS, Amira N, Fromont G, Sibony M, Cussenot O, Meuth M, Hamdy FC. Promoter hypermethylation is associated with tumor location, stage, and subsequent progression in transitional cell carcinoma. *J Clin Oncol* 2005;23:2903–10.

54. Catto JW, Azzouzi AR, Amira N, Rehman I, Feeley KM, Cross SS, Fromont G, Sibony M, Hamdy FC, Cussenot O, Meuth M. Distinct patterns of microsatellite instability are seen in tumours of the urinary tract. *Oncogene* 2003;22:8699–706.

55. Dyrskjot L, Ostenfeld MS, Bramsen JB, Silahtaroglu AN, Lamy P, Ramanathan R, Fristrup N, Jensen JL, Andersen CL, Zieger K, Kauppinen S, Ulhoi BP, Kjems J, Borre M, Orntoft TF. Genomic profiling of microRNAs in bladder cancer: miR–129 is associated with poor outcome and promotes cell death in vitro. *Cancer Res* 2009;69:4851–60.

56. Dyrskjøt L, Zieger K, Real FX, Malats N, Carrato A, Hurst C, Kotwal S, Knowles M, Malmström PU, de la Torre M, Wester K, Allory Y, Vordos D, Caillault A, Radvanyi F, Hein AM, Jensen JL, Jensen KM, Marcussen N, Orntoft TF. Gene expression signatures predict outcome in non-muscle-invasive bladder carcinoma: a multicenter validation study. *Clin Cancer Res* 2007;13:3545–51.

57. Grossman HB, Blute ML, Dinney CP, Jones JS, Liou LS, Reuter VE, Soloway MS. The use of urine-based biomarkers in bladder cancer. *Urology* 2006;67:62–4.

58. Grossman HB, Soloway M, Messing E, Katz G, Stein B, Kassabian V, Shen Y. Surveillance for recurrent bladder cancer using a point-of-care proteomic assay. *JAMA* 2006;295:299–305.

59. Adam L, Zhong M, Choi W, Qi W, Nicoloso M, Arora A, Calin G, Wang H, Siefker-Radtke A, McConkey D, Bar-Eli M, Dinney C. miR–200 expression regulates epithelial-to-mesenchymal transition in bladder cancer cells and reverses resistance to epidermal growth factor receptor therapy. *Clin Cancer Res* 2009;15:5060–72.

60. Wu XR. Urothelial tumorigenesis: a tale of divergent pathways. *Nat Rev Cancer* 2005;5:713–25.

61. Hutterer GC, Karakiewicz PI, Zippe C, Lüdecke G, Boman H, Sanchez-Carbayo M, Casella R, Mian C, Friedrich MG, Eissa S, Akaza H, Serretta V, Hedelin H, Rupesh R, Miyanaga N, Sagalowsky AI, Perrotte P, Lotan Y, Marberger MJ, Shariat SF. Urinary cytology and nuclear matrix protein 22 in the detection of bladder cancer recurrence other than transitional cell carcinoma. *BJU Int* 2008;101:561–5.

62. Bolenz C, Shariat SF, Karakiewicz PI, Ashfaq R, Ho R, Sagalowsky AI, Lotan Y. Human epidermal growth factor receptor 2 expression status provides independent prognostic information in patients with urothelial carcinoma of the urinary bladder. *BJU Int* 2010;106:1216–22.

63. Karam JA, Lotan Y, Ashfaq R, Sagalowsky AI, Shariat SF. Survivin expression in patients with non-muscle-invasive urothelial cell carcinoma of the bladder. *Urology* 2007;70:482–6.

64. Karam JA, Lotan Y, Karakiewicz PI, Ashfaq R, Sagalowsky AI, Roehrborn CG, Shariat SF. Use of combined apoptosis biomarkers for prediction of bladder cancer recurrence and mortality after radical cystectomy. *Lancet Oncol* 2007;8:128–36.

65. Margulis V, Lotan Y, Shariat SF. Survivin: a promising biomarker for detection and prognosis of bladder cancer. *World J Urol* 2008;26:59–65.

66. Karakiewicz PI, Shariat SF, Palapattu GS, Perrotte P, Lotan Y, Rogers CG, Amiel GE, Vazina A, Gupta A, Bastian PJ, Sagalowsky AI, Schoenberg M, Lerner SP. Precystectomy nomogram for prediction of advanced bladder cancer stage. *Eur Urol* 2006;50:1254–60.

67. Shariat SF, Marberger MJ, Lotan Y, Sanchez-Carbayo M, Zippe C, Ludecke G, Boman H, Sawczuk I, Friedrich MG, Casella R, Mian C, Eissa S, et al. Variability in the performance of nuclear matrix protein 22 for the detection of bladder cancer. *J Urol* 2006;176:919–26; discussion 926.

68. Shariat SF, Ashfaq R, Sagalowsky AI, Lotan Y. Predictive value of cell cycle biomarkers in nonmuscle invasive bladder transitional cell carcinoma. *J Urol* 2007;177:481–7.

69. Shariat SF, Zlotta AR, Ashfaq R, Sagalowsky AI, Lotan Y. Cooperative effect of cell-cycle regulators expression on bladder cancer development and biologic aggressiveness. *Mod Pathol* 2007;20:445–59.

70. Shariat SF, Zippe C, Lüdecke G, Boman H, Sanchez-Carbayo M, Casella R, Mian C, Friedrich MG, Eissa S, Akaza H, Sawczuk I, Serretta V, Huland H, Hedelin H, Rupesh R, Miyanaga N, Sagalowsky AI, Wians F Jr, Roehrborn CG, Lotan Y, Perrotte P, Benayoun S, Marberger MJ, Karakiewicz PI. Nomograms including nuclear matrix protein 22 for prediction of disease recurrence and progression in patients with Ta, T1 or CIS transitional cell carcinoma of the bladder. *J Urol* 2005;173:1518–25.

71. Shariat SF, Karakiewicz PI, Palapattu GS, Amiel GE, Lotan Y, Rogers CG, Vazina A, Bastian PJ, Gupta A, Sagalowsky AI, Schoenberg M, Lerner SP. Nomograms provide improved accuracy for predicting survival after radical cystectomy. *Clin Cancer Res* 2006;12:6663–76.

72. Shariat SF, Karakiewicz PI, Ashfaq R, Lerner SP, Palapattu GS, Cote RJ, Sagalowsky AI, Lotan Y. Multiple biomarkers improve prediction of bladder cancer recurrence and mortality in patients undergoing cystectomy. *Cancer* 2008;112:315–25.

73. Shariat SF, Karam JA, Lerner SP. Molecular markers in bladder cancer. *Curr Opin Urol* 2008;18:1–8.

74. Shariat SF, Karam JA, Margulis V, Karakiewicz PI. New blood-based biomarkers for the diagnosis, staging and prognosis of prostate cancer. *BJU Int* 2008;101:675–83.

75. Shariat SF, Karam JA, Raman JD. Urine cytology and urine-based markers for bladder urothelial carcinoma detection and monitoring: developments and future prospects. *Biomark Med* 2008;2:165–80.

76. Shariat SF, Margulis V, Lotan Y, Montorsi F, Karakiewicz PI. Nomograms for bladder cancer. *Eur Urol* 2008;54:41–53.

77. Shariat SF, Bolenz C, Godoy G, Fradet Y, Ashfaq R, Karakiewicz PI, Isbarn H, Jeldres C, Rigaud J, Sagalowsky AI, Lotan Y. Predictive value of combined immunohistochemical markers in patients with pT1 urothelial carcinoma at radical cystectomy. *J Urol* 2009;182:78–84.

78. Shariat SF, Karakiewicz PI, Godoy G, Karam JA, Ashfaq R, Fradet Y, Isbarn H, Montorsi F, Jeldres C, Bastian PJ, Nielsen ME, Muller SC, Sagalowsky AI, Lotan Y. Survivin as a prognostic marker for urothelial carcinoma of the bladder: a multicenter external validation study. *Clin Cancer Res* 2009;15:7012–9.

79. Shariat SF, Lotan Y, Karakiewicz PI, Ashfaq R, Isbarn H, Fradet Y, Bastian PJ, Nielsen ME, Capitanio U, Jeldres C, Montorsi F, Muller SC, Karam JA, Heukamp LC, Netto G, Lerner SP, Sagalowsky AI, Cote RJ. p53 predictive value for pT1–2N0

disease at radical cystectomy. *J Urol* 2009;182:907–13.

80. Shariat SF, Youssef RF, Gupta A, Chade DC, Karakiewicz PI, Isbarn H, Jeldres C, Sagalowsky AI, Ashfaq R, Lotan Y. Association of angiogenesis related markers with bladder cancer outcomes and other molecular markers. *J Urol* 2010;183:1744–50.

81. Shariat SF, Savage C, Chromecki TF, Sun M, Scherr DS, Lee RK, Lughezzani G, Remzi M, Marberger MJ, Karakiewicz PI, Vickers AJ. Assessing the clinical benefit of nuclear matrix protein 22 in the surveillance of patients with nonmuscle-invasive bladder cancer and negative cytology: a decision-curve analysis. *Cancer* 2011;117:2892–7.

82. Svatek RS, Karam J, Karakiewicz PI, Gallina A, Casella R, Roehrborn CG, Shariat SF. Role of urinary cathepsin B and L in the detection of bladder urothelial cell carcinoma. *J Urol* 2008;179:478–84.

83. Lotan Y, Capitanio U, Shariat SF, Hutterer GC, Karakiewicz PI. Impact of clinical factors, including a point-of-care nuclear matrix protein–22 assay and cytology, on bladder cancer detection. *BJU Int* 2009;103:1368–74.

84. Margulis V, Lotan Y, Karakiewicz PI, Fradet Y, Ashfaq R, Capitanio U, Montorsi F, Bastian PJ, Nielsen ME, Muller SC, Rigaud J, Heukamp LC, Netto G, Lerner SP, Sagalowsky AI, Shariat SF. Multi-institutional validation of the predictive value of Ki–67 labeling index in patients with urinary bladder cancer. *J Natl Cancer Inst* 2009;101:114–9.

85. Svatek RS, Herman MP, Lotan Y, Casella R, Hsieh JT, Sagalowsky AI, Shariat SF. Soluble Fas—a promising novel urinary marker for the detection of recurrent superficial bladder cancer. *Cancer* 2006;106:1701–7.

86. Tilki D, Singer BB, Shariat SF, Behrend A, Fernando M, Irmak S, Buchner A, Hooper AT, Stief CG, Reich O, Ergun S. CEACAM1: a novel urinary marker for bladder cancer detection. *Eur Urol* 2010;57:648–54.

87. Lotan Y. Role of biomarkers to predict outcomes and response to therapy. *Urol Oncol* 2010;28:97–101.

88. Lotan Y, Shariat SF, Schmitz-Drager BJ, Sanchez-Carbayo M, Jankevicius F, Racioppi M, Minner SJ, Stohr B, Bassi PF, Grossman HB. Considerations on implementing diagnostic markers into clinical decision making in bladder cancer. *Urol Oncol* 2010;28:441–8.

89. Robinson VL, Porter M, Messing E, Fradet Y, Kamat AM, Lotan Y. BCAN Think Tank session 2: Molecular detection of bladder cancer: the path to progress. *Urol Oncol* 2010;28:334–7.

90. Costa VL, Henrique R, Danielsen SA, Duarte-Pereira S, Eknaes M, Skotheim RI, Rodrigues A, Magalhaes JS, Oliveira J, Lothe RA, Teixeira MR, Jeronimo C, Lind GE. Three epigenetic biomarkers, GDF15, TMEFF2, and VIM, accurately predict bladder cancer from DNA-based analyses of urine samples. *Clin Cancer Res* 2010;16:5842–51.

91. Urakami S, Shiina H, Enokida H, Kawakami T, Kawamoto K, Hirata H, Tanaka Y, Kikuno N, Nakagawa M, Igawa M, Dahiya R. Combination analysis of hypermethylated Wnt-antagonist family genes as a novel epigenetic biomarker panel for bladder cancer detection. *Clin Cancer Res* 2006;12:2109–16.

92. Mengual L, Burset M, Ribal MJ, Ars E, Marin-Aguilera M, Fernandez M, Ingelmo-Torres M, Villavicencio H, Alcaraz A. Gene expression signature in urine for diagnosing and assessing aggressiveness of bladder urothelial carcinoma. *Clin Cancer Res* 2010;16:2624–33.

93. Caraway NP, Katz RL. A review on the current state of urine cytology emphasizing the role of fluorescence in situ hybridization as an adjunct to diagnosis. *Cancer Cytopathol* 2010;118:175–83.

94. Droller MJ. Current concepts of tumor markers in bladder cancer. *Urol Clin North Am* 2002;29:229–34.

95. Albert PS, McShane LM, Shih JH. Latent class modeling approaches for assessing diagnostic error without a gold standard: with applications to p53 immunohistochemical assays in bladder tumors. *Biometrics* 2001;57:610–9.

96. Lotan Y, Roehrborn CG. Cost-effectiveness of a modified care protocol substituting bladder tumor markers for cystoscopy for the followup of patients with transitional cell carcinoma of the bladder: a decision analytical approach. *J Urol* 2002;167:75–9.

97. Sarosdy MF, Kahn PR, Ziffer MD, Love WR, Barkin J, Abara EO, Jansz K, Bridge JA, Johansson SL, Persons DL, Gibson JS. Use of a multitarget fluorescence in situ hybridization assay to diagnose bladder cancer in patients with hematuria. *J Urol* 2006;176:44–7.

98. Mezzelani A, Dagrada G, Alasio L, Sozzi G, Pilotti S. Detection of bladder cancer by multitarget multicolour FISH: comparative analysis on archival cytology and paraffin-embedded tissue. *Cytopathology* 2002;13:317–25.

99. Skacel M, Pettay JD, Tsiftsakis EK, Procop GW, Biscotti CV, Tubbs RR. Validation of a multicolor interphase fluorescence in situ hybridization assay for detection of transitional cell carcinoma on fresh and archival thin-layer, liquid-based cytology slides. *Anal Quant Cytol Histol* 2001;23:381–7.

100. Kipp BR, Karnes RJ, Brankley SM, Harwood AR, Pankratz VS, Sebo TJ, Blute MM, Lieber MM, Zincke H, Halling KC. Monitoring intravesical therapy for superficial bladder cancer using fluorescence in situ hybridization. *J Urol* 2005;173:401–4.

101. Whitson J, Berry A, Carroll P, Konety B. A multicolour fluorescence in situ hybridization test predicts recurrence in patients with high-risk superficial bladder tumours undergoing intravesical therapy. *BJU Int* 2009;104:336–9.

102. Caraway NP, Khanna A, Fernandez RL, Payne L, Bassett RL Jr, Zhang HZ, Kamat A, Katz RL. Fluorescence in situ hybridization for detecting urothelial carcinoma: a clinicopathologic study. *Cancer Cytopathol* 2010;118:259–68.

103. Ellis WJ, Blumenstein BA, Ishak LM, Enfield DL. Clinical evaluation of the BTA TRAK assay and

comparison to voided urine cytology and the Bard BTA test in patients with recurrent bladder tumors. The Multi Center Study Group. *Urology* 1997;50:882–7.

104. Leyh H, Treiber U, Thomas L, et al. Results of a European multicenter tria comparing the BTA TRAK test to urine cytology in patients suspected of having bladder cancer (Abstract). *J Urol* 1998;159:244.

105. Raitanen MP, Marttila T, Nurmi M, Ala-Opas M, Nieminen P, Aine R, Tammela TL; Finnbladder Group. Human complement factor H related protein test for monitoring bladder cancer. *J Urol* 2001;165:374–7.

106. Ishak LM, Ellis WJ. A comparison of the BTA stat and the BTA TRAK assays: two new tests for the detection of recurrent bladder cancer (BC) in urine (Abstract). *J Urol* 1998;159:245.

107. Landman J, Chang Y, Kavaler E, Droller MJ, Liu BC. Sensitivity and specificity of NMP–22, telomerase, and BTA in the detection of human bladder cancer. *Urology* 1998;52:398–402.

108. Van der Poel HG, Van Balken MR, Schamhart DH, Peelen P, de Reijke T, Debruyne FM, Schalken JA, Witjes JA. Bladder wash cytology, quantitative cytology, and the qualitative BTA test in patients with superficial bladder cancer. *Urology* 1998;51:44–50.

109. van Rhijn BW, van der Poel HG, van der Kwast TH. Urine markers for bladder cancer surveillance: a systematic review. *Eur Urol* 2005;47:736–48.

110. Tetu B. Diagnosis of urothelial carcinoma from urine. *Mod Pathol* 2009;22 Suppl 2:S53–9.

111. Vrooman OP, Witjes JA. Molecular markers for detection, surveillance and prognostication of bladder cancer. *Int J Urol* 2009;16:234–43.

112. Sozen S, Biri H, Sinik Z, Kupeli B, Alkibay T, Bozkirli I. Comparison of the nuclear matrix protein 22 with voided urine cytology and BTA stat test in the diagnosis of transitional cell carcinoma of the bladder. *Eur Urol* 1999;36:225–9.

113. Walsh IK, Keane PF, Ishak LM, Flessland KA. The BTA stat test: a tumor marker for the detection of

upper tract transitional cell carcinoma. *Urology* 2001;58:532–5.

114. Gutierrez Banos JL, del Henar Rebollo Rodrigo M, Antolin Juarez FM, Garcia BM. Usefulness of the BTA STAT Test for the diagnosis of bladder cancer. *Urology* 2001;57:685–9.

115. Raitanen MP; FinnBladder Group. The role of BTA stat Test in follow-up of patients with bladder cancer: results from FinnBladder studies. *World J Urol* 2008;26:45–50.

116. Raitanen MP, Kaasinen E, Lukkarinen O, Kauppinen R, Viitanen J, Liukkonen T, Tammela TL; Finnbladder Group. Analysis of false-positive BTA STAT test results in patients followed up for bladder cancer. The Bard BTA stat test in monitoring of bladder cancer. *Urology* 2001;57:680–4.

117. Ishak L, Ellis WJ. A comparison of the BTA stat and the BTA TRAK assay: two new tests for the detection of recurrent bladder cancer (BC) in urine. *J Urol* 1998;159:245.

118. Irani J, Desgrandchamps F, Millet C, Toubert ME, Bon D, Aubert J, Le Duc A. BTA stat and BTA TRAK: A comparative evaluation of urine testing for the diagnosis of transitional cell carcinoma of the bladder. *Eur Urol* 1999;35:89–92.

119. Boman H, Hedelin H, Jacobsson S, Holmang S. Newly diagnosed bladder cancer: the relationship of initial symptoms, degree of microhematuria and tumor marker status. *J Urol* 2002;168:1955–9.

120. Quek P, Chin CM, Lim PH. The role of BTA stat in clinical practice. *Ann Acad Med Singapore* 2002;31:212–6.

121. Halling KC, King W, Sokolova IA, Karnes RJ, Meyer RG, Powell EL, Sebo TJ, Cheville JC, Clayton AC, Krajnik KL, Ebert TA, Nelson RE, et al. A comparison of BTA stat, hemoglobin dipstick, telomerase and Vysis UroVysion assays for the detection of urothelial carcinoma in urine. *J Urol* 2002;167:2001–6.

122. Poulakis V, Witzsch U, De Vries R, Altmannsberger HM, Manyak MJ, Becht E. A comparison of urinary nuclear matrix protein–22 and bladder tumour antigen tests with

voided urinary cytology in detecting and following bladder cancer: the prognostic value of false-positive results. *BJU Int* 2001;88:692–701.

123. Raitanen MP, Aine R, Kylmala T, Kallio J, Liukkonen T, Tammela T. The dilemma of suspicious urine cytology in patients being followed for bladder cancer. *Ann Chir Gynaecol* 2001;90:256–9.

124. Fernandez Gomez JM, Garcia Rodriguez J, Escaf Barmadah S, Raigoso P, Rodriguez Martinez JJ, Allende MT, Casasola Chamorro J, Rodriguez Faba O, Martin Benito JL, Regadera Sejas FJ. [Urinary BTA-TRAK in the followup of superficial transitional-cell bladder carcinoma]. *Arch Esp Urol* 2002;55:41–9.

125. Pode D, Shapiro A, Wald M, Nativ O, Laufer M, Kaver I. Noninvasive detection of bladder cancer with the BTA stat test. *J Urol* 1999;161:443–6.

126. Raitanen MP, Leppilahti M, Tuhkanen K, Forssel T, Nylund P, Tammela T. Routine followup cystoscopy in detection of recurrence in patients being monitored for bladder cancer. *Ann Chir Gynaecol* 2001;90:261–5.

127. Lipinski M, Jeromin L. Comparison of the bladder tumour antigen test with photodynamic diagnosis in patients with pathologically confirmed recurrent superficial urinary bladder tumours. *BJU Int* 2002;89:757–9.

128. Raitanen MP, Marttila T, Kaasinen E, Rintala E, Aine R, Tammela TL. Sensitivity of human complement factor H related protein (BTA stat) test and voided urine cytology in the diagnosis of bladder cancer. *J Urol* 2000;163:1689–92.

129. Landman J, Chang Y, Kavaler E, Droller MJ, Liu BC. Sensitivity and specificity of NMP–22, telomerase, and BTA in the detection of human bladder cancer. *Urology* 1998;52:398–402.

130. Leyh H, Hall R, Mazeman E, Blumenstein BA. Comparison of the Bard BTA test with voided urine and bladder wash cytology in the diagnosis and management of cancer of the bladder. *Urology* 1997;50:49–53.

131. Raitanen MP, Kaasinen E, Luukkarinen O, Kauppinen R, Viitanen J, Liukkonen T, Tammela TL. Analysis of false-positive BTA STAT test results in patients followed up for bladder cancer. *Urology* 2001;57:680–4.

132. Van der Poel HG, Van Balken MR, Schamhart DH, Peelen P, de Reijke T, Debruyne FM, Schalken JA, Witjes JA. Bladder wash cytology, quantitative cytology, and the qualitative BTA test in patients with superficial bladder cancer. *Urology* 1998;51:44–50.

133. Nasuti JF, Gomella LG, Ismial M, Bibbo M. Utility of the BTA stat test kit for bladder cancer screening. *Diagn Cytopathol* 1999;21:27–9.

134. Gibanel R, Ribal MJ, Filella X, Ballesta AM, Molina R, Alcaraz A, Alcover JB. BTA TRAK urine test increases the efficacy of cytology in the diagnosis of low grade transitional cell carcinoma of the bladder. *Anticancer Res* 2002;22:1157–60.

135. Ohtani M, Iwasaki A, Shiraiwa H. [Urinary tumor marker for urothelial cancer]. *Gan To Kagaku Ryoho* 2001;28:1933–7.

136. Raitanen MP, Tammela TL. Specificity of human complement factor H-related protein test (Bard BTA stat Test). *Scand J Urol Nephrol* 1999;33:234–6.

137. Oge O, Kozaci D, Gemalmaz H. The BTA stat test is nonspecific for hematuria: an experimental hematuria model. *J Urol* 2002;167:1318–9; discussion 1319–20.

138. Wald M, Halachmi S, Amiel G, Madjar S, Mullerad M, Miselevitz I, Moskovitz B, Nativ O. Bladder tumor antigen stat test in non-urothelial malignant urologic conditions. *Isr Med Assoc J* 2002;4:174–5.

139. Raitanen MP, Hellstrom P, Marttila T, Korhonen H, Talja M, Ervasti J, Tammela TL. Effect of intravesical instillations on the human complement factor H related protein (BTA stat) test. *Eur Urol* 2001;40:422–6.

140. Oge O, Atsu N, Sahin A, Ozen H. Comparison of BTA stat and NMP22 tests in the detection of bladder cancer. *Scand J Urol Nephrol* 2000;34:349–51.

141. Giannopoulos A, Manousakas T, Gounari A, Constantinides C, Choremi-Papadopoulou H, Dimopoulos C. Comparative evaluation of the diagnostic performance of the BTA stat test, NMP22 and urinary bladder cancer antigen for primary and recurrent bladder tumors. *J Urol* 2001;166:470–5.

142. Boman H, Hedelin H, Holmang S. Four bladder tumor markers have a disappointingly low sensitivity for small size and low grade recurrence. *J Urol* 2002;167:80–3.

143. Friedrich MG, Hellstern A, Hautmann SH, Graefen M, Conrad S, Huland E, Huland H. Clinical use of urinary markers for the detection and prognosis of bladder carcinoma: a comparison of immunocytology with monoclonal antibodies against Lewis X and 486p3/12 with the BTA STAT and NMP22 tests. *J Urol* 2002;168:470–4.

144. Saad A, Hanbury DC, McNicholas TA, Boustead GB, Morgan S, Woodman AC. A study comparing various noninvasive methods of detecting bladder cancer in urine. *BJU Int* 2002;89:369–73.

145. Giannopoulos A, Manousakas T, Mitropoulos D, Botsoli-Stergiou E, Constantinides C, Giannopoulou M, Choremi-Papadopoulou H. Comparative evaluation of the BTAstat test, NMP22, and voided urine cytology in the detection of primary and recurrent bladder tumors. *Urology* 2000;55:871–5.

146. Lokeshwar VB, Schroeder GL, Selzer MG, Hautmann SH, Posey JT, Duncan RC, Watson R, Rose L, Markowitz S, Soloway MS. Bladder tumor markers for monitoring recurrence and screening comparison of hyaluronic acid-hyaluronidase and BTA-stat tests. *Cancer* 2002;95:61–72.

147. Zippe C, Pandrangi L, Agarwal A. NMP22 is a sensitive, cost-effective test in patients at risk for bladder cancer. *J Urol* 1999;161:62–5.

148. Carpinito GA, Rukstalis DB, Pandrangi LV, et al. Prospective multi-center study of NMP22 and cytology in patients with hematuria. *J Urol* 1998;159:245.

149. Miyanaga N, Akaza H, Tsukamoto T, Ishikawa S, Noguchi R, Ohtani M, Kawabe K, Kubota Y, Fujita K, Obata K, Hirao Y, Kotake T, Ohmori H, Kumazawa J, Koiso K. Urinary nuclear matrix protein 22 as a new marker for the screening of urothelial cancer in patients with microscopic hematuria. *Int J Urol* 1999;6:173–7.

150. Ludecke G, Farkas P, Edler M, et al. Nuclear matrix protein 22 (NMP22): A tumor marker in primary diagnosis and follow up of bladder cancer. *J Urol* 1998;159:244.

151. Stampfer DS, Carpinito GA, Rodriguez-Villanueva J, Willsey LW, Dinney CP, Grossman HB, Fritsche HA, McDougal WS. Evaluation of NMP22 in the detection of transitional cell carcinoma of the bladder. *J Urol* 1998;159:394–8.

152. Soloway MS, Briggman V, Carpinito GA, Chodak GW, Church PA, Lamm DL, Lange P, Messing E, Pasciak RM, Reservitz GB, Rukstalis DB, Sarosdy MF, Stadler WM, Thiel RP, Hayden CL. Use of a new tumor marker, urinary NMP22, in the detection of occult or rapidly recurring transitional cell carcinoma of the urinary tract following surgical treatment. *J Urol* 1996;156:363–7.

153. Paoluzzi M, Cuttano MG, Mugnaini P, Salsano F, Giannotti P. Urinary dosage of nuclear matrix protein 22 (NMP22) like biologic marker of transitional cell carcinoma (TCC): a study on patients with hematuria. *Arch Ital Urol Androl* 1999;71:13–8.

154. Lee KH. Evaluation of the NMP22 test and comparison with voided urine cytology in the detection of bladder cancer. *Yonsei Med J* 2001;42:14–8.

155. Gutierrez Banos JL, Rebollo Rodrigo MH, Antolin Juarez FM, Martin Garcia B. NMP 22, BTA stat test and cytology in the diagnosis of bladder cancer: a comparative study. *Urol Int* 2001;66:185–90.

156. Del Nero A, Esposito N, Curro A, Biasoni D, Montanari E, Mangiarotti B, Trinchieri A, Zanetti G, Serrago MP, Pisani E. Evaluation of urinary level of NMP22 as a diagnostic marker for stage pTa-pT1 bladder cancer: comparison with urinary cytology and BTA test. *Eur Urol* 1999;35:93–7.

157. Chahal R, Darshane A, Browning AJ, Sundaram SK. Evaluation of the clinical value of urinary NMP22 as a marker in the screening and surveillance of transitional cell carcinoma of the urinary bladder. *Eur Urol* 2001;40:415–20; discussion 421.

158. Oge O, Atsu N, Kendi S, Ozen H. Evaluation of nuclear matrix protein 22 (NMP22) as a tumor marker in the detection of bladder cancer. *Int Urol Nephrol* 2001;32:367–70.

159. Sanchez-Carbayo M, Urrutia M, Gonzalez de Buitrago JM, Navajo JA. Utility of serial urinary tumor markers to individualize intervals between cystoscopies in the monitoring of patients with bladder carcinoma. *Cancer* 2001;92:2820–8.

160. Witjes JA, van der Poel HG, van Balken MR, Debruyne FM, Schalken JA. Urinary NMP22 and karyometry in the diagnosis and followup of patients with superficial bladder cancer. *Eur Urol* 1998;33:387–91.

161. Sanchez-Carbayo M, Ciudad J, Urrutia M, Navajo JA, Orfao A. Diagnostic performance of the urinary bladder carcinoma antigen ELISA test and multiparametric DNA/cytokeratin flow cytometry in urine voided samples from patients with bladder carcinoma. *Cancer* 2001;92:2811–9.

162. Atsu N, Ekici S, Oge OO, Ergen A, Hascelik G, Ozen H. False-positive results of the NMP22 test due to hematuria. *J Urol* 2002;167:555–8.

163. Ishii T, Okadome A, Takeuchi F, Hiratsuka Y. Urinary levels of nuclear matrix protein 22 in patients with urinary diversion. *Urology* 2001;58:940–2.

164. Williamson SR, Montironi R, Lopez-Beltran A, MacLennan GT, Davidson DD, Cheng L. Diagnosis, evaluation and treatment of carcinoma in situ of the urinary bladder: the state of the art. *Crit Rev Oncol Hematol* 2010;76:112–26.

165. Fradet Y. Phenotypic characterization of bladder cancer. *Eur Urol* 1998;33:5–6.

166. Pfister C, Chautard D, Devonec M, Perrin P, Chopin D, Rischmann P, Bouchot O, Beurton D, Coulange C, Rambeaud JJ. Immunocyt test improves the diagnostic accuracy of urinary cytology: results of a French multicenter study. *J Urol* 2003;169:921–4.

167. Messing EM, Teot L, Korman H, Underhill E, Barker E, Stork B, Qian J, Bostwick DG. Performance of urine test in patients monitored for recurrence of bladder cancer: a multicenter study in the United States. *J Urol* 2005;174:1238–41.

168. Tetu B, Tiguert R, Harel F, Fradet Y. ImmunoCyt/uCyt+ improves the sensitivity of urine cytology in patients followed for urothelial carcinoma. *Mod Pathol* 2005;18:83–9.

169. Sullivan PS, Nooraie F, Sanchez H, Hirschowitz S, Levin M, Rao PN, Rao J. Comparison of ImmunoCyt, UroVysion, and urine cytology in detection of recurrent urothelial carcinoma: a "split-sample" study. *Cancer* 2009;117:167–73.

170. Fradet Y. Recent advances in the management of superficial bladder tumors. *Can J Urol* 2002;9:1544–50.

171. Olsson H, Zackrisson B. ImmunoCyt a useful method in the followup protocol for patients with urinary bladder carcinoma. *Scand J Urol Nephrol* 2001;35:280–2.

172. Vriesema JL, Atsma F, Kiemeney LA, Peelen WP, Witjes JA, Schalken JA. Diagnostic efficacy of the ImmunoCyt test to detect superficial bladder cancer recurrence. *Urology* 2001;58:367–71.

173. Lodde M, Fradet Y. The detection of genetic markers of bladder cancer in urine and serum. *Curr Opin Urol* 2008;18:499–503.

174. Yu J, Zhu T, Wang Z, Zhang H, Qian Z, Xu H, Gao B, Wang W, Gu L, Meng J, Wang J, Feng X, Li Y, Yao X, Zhu J. A novel set of DNA methylation markers in urine sediments for sensitive/specific detection of bladder cancer. *Clin Cancer Res* 2007;13:7296–304.

175. Eissa S, Swellam M, Ali-Labib R, Mansour A, El-Malt O, Tash FM. Detection of telomerase in urine by 3 methods: evaluation of diagnostic accuracy for bladder cancer. *J Urol* 2007;178:1068–72.

176. Shariat SF, Lotan Y, Saboorian H, Khoddami SM, Roehrborn CG, Slawin KM, Ashfaq R. Survivin expression is associated with features of biologically aggressive prostate carcinoma. *Cancer* 2004;100:751–7.

177. Mora LB, Nicosia SV, Pow-Sang JM, Ku NK, Diaz JI, Lockhart J, Einstein A. Ancillary techniques in the followup of transitional cell carcinoma: a comparison of cytology, histology and deoxyribonucleic acid image analysis cytometry in 91 patients. *J Urol* 1996;156:49–54; discussion 54–5.

178. de la Roza GL, Hopkovitz A, Caraway NP, Kidd L, Dinney CP, Johnston D, Katz RL. DNA image analysis of urinary cytology: prediction of recurrent transitional cell carcinoma. *Mod Pathol* 1996;9:571–8.

179. Shiina H, Urakami S, Shirakawa H, Shigeno K, Himeno Y, Mizutani M, Igawa M, Ishibe T. Evaluation of the argyrophilic nucleolar organizer region, nuclear DNA content and mean nuclear area in transitional cell carcinoma of bladder using a quantitative image analyzer. *Eur Urol* 1996;29:99–105.

180. van Velthoven R, Petein M, Oosterlinck WJ, Raviv G, Janssen T, Roels H, Pasteels JL, Schulman C, Kiss R. The additional predictive value contributed by quantitative chromatin pattern description as compared to DNA ploidy level measurement in 257 superficial bladder transitional cell carcinomas. *Eur Urol* 1996;29:245–51.

181. al-Abadi H, Nagel R. Deoxyribonucleic acid content and survival rates of patients with transitional cell carcinoma of the bladder. *J Urol* 1994;151:37–42.

182. Lee SE, Park MS. Prognostic factors for survival in patients with transitional cell carcinoma of the bladder: evaluation by histopathologic grade, pathologic stage and flow-cytometric analysis. *Eur Urol* 1996;29:193–8.

183. Pantazopoulos D, Ioakim-Liossi A, Karakitsos P, Aroni K, Kakoliris S, Kanavaros P, Kyrkou KA. DNA content and proliferation activity in superficial transitional cell carcinoma of the bladder. *Anticancer Res* 1997;17:781–6.

184. Nakopoulou L, Constantinides C, Papandropoulos J, Theodoropoulos G, Tzonou A, Giannopoulos A, Zervas A, Dimopoulos C. Evaluation of overexpression of p53 tumor suppressor protein in superficial and invasive transitional cell bladder cancer: comparison with DNA ploidy. *Urology* 1995;46:334–40.

185. Lopez-Beltran A, Croghan GA, Croghan I, Matilla A, Gaeta JF. Prognostic factors in bladder cancer. A pathologic, immunohistochemical, and DNA flow-cytometric study. *Am J Clin Pathol* 1994;102:109–14.

186. Lopez-Beltran A, Croghan GA, Croghan I, Huben RP, Mettlin C, Gaeta JF. Prognostic factors in survival of bladder cancer. *Cancer* 1992;70:799–807.

187. Bucci B, Pansadoro V, De Paula F, Florio A, Carico E, Zupi G, Vecchione A. Biologic characteristics of T1 papillary bladder cancer. Flow cytometric study of paraffin-embedded material. *Anal Quant Cytol Histol* 1995;17:121–8.

188. Norming U, Tribukait B, Gustafson H, Nyman CR, Wang NN, Wijkstrom H. Deoxyribonucleic acid profile and tumor progression in primary carcinoma in situ of the bladder: a study of 63 patients with grade 3 lesions. *J Urol* 1992;147:11–5.

189. Norming U, Nyman CR, Tribukait B. Comparative flow cytometric deoxyribonucleic acid studies on exophytic tumor and random mucosal biopsies in untreated carcinoma of the bladder. *J Urol* 1989;142:1442–7.

190. deVere White R, Deitch AD, Daneshmand S, et al. Predictors of outcome in bladder transitional cell carcinoma (TCC) treated by intravesical chemotherapy. *J Urol* 1998;159:145.

191. Turkolmez K, Baltaci S, Beduk Y, Muftuoglu YZ, Gogus O. DNA ploidy and S-phase fraction as predictive factors of response and outcome following neoadjuvant methotrexate, vinblastine, epirubicin and cisplatin (M-VEC) chemotherapy for invasive bladder cancer. *Scand J Urol Nephrol* 2002;36:46–51.

192. Barlandas-Rendon E, Muller MM, Garcia-Latorre E, Heinschink A. Comparison of urine cell characteristics by flow cytometry and cytology in patients suspected of having bladder cancer. *Clin Chem Lab Med* 2002;40:817–23.

193. Bakhos R, Shankey TV, Flanigan RC, Fisher S, Wojcik EM. Comparative analysis of DNA flow cytometry and cytology of bladder washings: review of discordant cases. *Diagn Cytopathol* 2000;22:65–9.

194. Slaton JW, Dinney CP, Veltri RW, Miller CM, Liebert M, O'Dowd GJ, Grossman HB. Deoxyribonucleic acid ploidy enhances the cytological prediction of recurrent transitional cell carcinoma of the bladder. *J Urol* 1997;158:806–11.

195. Planz B, Synek C, Deix T, Bocking A, Marberger M. Diagnosis of bladder cancer with urinary cytology, immunocytology and DNA-image-cytometry. *Anal Cell Pathol* 2001;22:103–9.

196. Rotterud R, Skomedal H, Berner A, Danielsen HE, Skovlund E, Fossa SD. TP53 and p21WAF1/CIP1 behave differently in euploid versus aneuploid bladder tumours treated with radiotherapy. *Acta Oncol* 2001;40:644–52.

197. Lopez-Beltran A, Escudero AL, Vicioso L, Munoz E, Carrasco JC. Human papillomavirus DNA as a factor determining the survival of bladder cancer patients. *Br J Cancer* 1996;73:124–7.

198. Shaaban AA, Tribukait B, el-Bedeiwy AF, Ghoneim MA. Characterization of squamous cell bladder tumors by flow cytometric deoxyribonucleic acid analysis: a report of 100 cases. *J Urol* 1990;144:879–83.

199. Elsobky E, El-Baz M, Gomha M, Abol-Enein H, Shaaban AA. Prognostic value of angiogenesis in schistosoma-associated squamous cell carcinoma of the urinary bladder. *Urology* 2002;60:69–73.

200. Cajulis RS, Haines GK 3rd, Frias-Hidvegi D, McVary K, Bacus JW. Cytology, flow cytometry, image analysis, and interphase cytogenetics by fluorescence in situ hybridization in the diagnosis of transitional cell carcinoma in bladder washes: a comparative study. *Diagn Cytopathol* 1995;13:214–24.

201. Van der Poel HG, Boon ME, van Stratum P, Ooms EC, Wiener H, Debruyne FM, Witjes JA, Schalken JA, Murphy WM. Conventional bladder wash cytology performed by four experts versus quantitative image analysis. *Mod Pathol* 1997;10:976–82.

202. Caraway NP, Khanna A, Payne L, Kamat AM, Katz RL. Combination of cytologic evaluation and quantitative digital cytometry is reliable in detecting recurrent disease in patients with urinary diversions. *Cancer* 2007;111:323–9.

203. Ohsaki H, Hirakawa E, Kagawa K, Nakamura M, Kiyomoto H, Haba R. Value of computer-assisted quantitative nuclear morphometry for differentiation of reactive renal tubular cells from low grade urothelial carcinoma. *Cytopathology* 2010;21:334–8.

204. Golijanin D, Shapiro A, Pode D. Immunostaining of cytokeratin 20 in cells from voided urine for detection of bladder cancer. *J Urol* 2000;164:1922–5.

205. Panosian KJM, Lopez-Beltran A, Croghan G, Gaeta JF, Gamarra M. An immunohistochemical evaluation of urinary bladder cytology utilizing monoclonal antibodies. *World J Urol* 1989;7:173–9.

206. Sheinfeld J, Reuter VE, Melamed MR, Fair WR, Morse M, Sogani PC, Herr HW, Whitmore WF, Cordon-Cardo C. Enhanced bladder cancer detection with the Lewis X antigen as a marker of neoplastic transformation. *J Urol* 1990;143:285–8.

207. Sheinfeld J, Reuter VE, Sarkis AS, Cordon-Cardo C. Blood group antigens in normal and neoplastic urothelium. *J Cell Biochem Suppl* 1992;16I:50–5.

208. Sheinfeld J, Reuter VE, Fair WR, Cordon-Cardo C. Expression of blood group antigens in bladder cancer: current concepts. *Semin Surg Oncol* 1992;8:308–15.

209. Witjes JA, Umbas R, Debruyne FM, Schalken JA. Expression of markers for transitional cell carcinoma in normal bladder mucosa of patients with bladder cancer. *J Urol* 1995;154:2185–9.

210. Golijanin D, Sherman Y, Shapiro A, Pode D. Detection of bladder tumors by immunostaining of the Lewis X antigen in cells from voided urine. *Urology* 1995;46:173–7.

211. Nisman B, Barak V, Shapiro A, Golijanin D, Peretz T, Pode D. Evaluation of urine CYFRA 21–1 for the detection of primary and recurrent bladder carcinoma. *Cancer* 2002;94:2914–22.

212. Klein A, Zemer R, Buchumensky V, Klaper R, Nissenkorn I. Expression of cytokeratin 20 in urinary cytology of patients with bladder carcinoma [see comments]. *Cancer* 1998;82:349–54.

213. Lokeshwar VB, Obek C, Soloway MS, Block NL. Tumor-associated hyaluronic acid: a new sensitive and specific urine marker for bladder cancer [published erratum appears in Cancer Res 1998 Jul 15;58(14):3191]. *Cancer Res* 1997;57:773–7.

214. Skacel M, Fahmy M, Brainard JA, Pettay JD, Biscotti CV, Liou LS, Procop GW, Jones JS, Ulchaker J, Zippe CD, Tubbs RR. Multitarget fluorescence in situ hybridization assay detects transitional cell carcinoma in the majority of patients with bladder cancer and atypical or negative urine cytology. *J Urol* 2003;169:2101–5.

215. Dalbagni G, Presti J, Reuter V, Fair WR, Cordon-Cardo C. Genetic alterations in bladder cancer. *Lancet* 1993;342:469–71.

216. Knowles MA, Elder PA, Williamson M, Cairns JP, Shaw ME, Law MG. Allelotype of human bladder cancer. *Cancer Res* 1994;54:531–8.

217. Rosin MP, Cairns P, Epstein JI, Schoenberg MP, Sidransky D. Partial allelotype of carcinoma in situ of the human bladder. *Cancer Res* 1995;15:5213–6.

218. Cheng L, MacLennan GT, Pan CX, Jones TD, Moore CR, Zhang S, Gu J, Patel NB, Kao C, Gardner TA. Allelic loss of the active X chromosome during bladder carcinogenesis. *Arch Pathol Lab Med* 2004;128:187–90.

219. Cheng L, MacLennan GT, Zhang S, Wang M, Pan CX, Koch MO. Laser capture microdissection analysis reveals frequent allelic losses in papillary urothelial neoplasm of low malignant potential of the urinary bladder. *Cancer* 2004;101:183–8.

220. Cheng L, Jones TD, McCarthy RP, Eble JN, Wang M, MacLennan GT, Lopez-Beltran A, Yang XJ, Koch MO, Zhang S, Pan CX, Baldridge LA. Molecular genetic evidence for a common clonal origin of urinary bladder small cell carcinoma and coexisting urothelial carcinoma. *Am J Pathol* 2005;166:1533–9.

221. Cheng L, Gu J, Ulbright TM, MacLennan GT, Sweeney CJ, Zhang S, Sanchez K, Koch MO, Eble JN. Precise microdissection of human bladder cancers reveals divergent tumor subclones in the same tumor. *Cancer* 2002;94:104–10.

222. Jones TD, Carr MD, Eble JN, Wang M, Lopez-Beltran A, Cheng L. Clonal origin of lymph node metastases in bladder carcinoma. *Cancer* 2005;104:1901–10.

223. Sung MT, Eble JN, Wang M, Tan PH, Lopez-Beltran A, Cheng L. Inverted papilloma of the urinary bladder: a molecular genetic appraisal. *Mod Pathol* 2006;19:1289–94.

224. Sung MT, Wang M, MacLennan GT, Eble JN, Tan PH, Lopez-Beltran A, Montironi R, Harris JJ, Kuhar M, Cheng L. Histogenesis of sarcomatoid urothelial carcinoma of the urinary bladder: evidence for a common clonal origin with divergent differentiation. *J Pathol* 2007;211:420–30.

225. Sung MT, Zhang S, MacLennan GT, Lopez-Beltran A, Montironi R, Wang M, Tan PH, Cheng L. Histogenesis of clear cell adenocarcinoma in the urinary tract: evidence of urothelial origin. *Clin Cancer Res* 2008;14:1947–55.

226. Jones TD, Zhang S, Lopez-Beltran A, Eble JN, Sung MT, MacLennan GT, Montironi R, Tan PH, Zheng S, Baldridge LA, Cheng L. Urothelial carcinoma with an inverted growth pattern can be distinguished from inverted papilloma by fluorescence in-situ hybridization, immunohistochemistry, and morphologic analysis. *Am J Surg Pathol* 2007;31:1861–7.

227. Cheng L, Zhang S, Alexander R, MacLennan GT, Hodges KB, Harrison BT, Lopez-Beltran A, Montironi R. Sarcomatoid carcinoma of the urinary bladder: the final common pathway of urothelial carcinoma dedifferentiation. *Am J Surg Pathol* 2011;35:e34–46.

228. Cheng L, Bostwick DG, Li G, Zhang S, Vortmeyer AO, Zhuang Z. Conserved genetic findings in metastatic bladder cancer: a possible utility of allelic loss of chromosomes 9p21 and 17p13 in diagnosis. *Arch Pathol Lab Med* 2001;125:1197–9.

229. Jones TD, Wang M, Eble JN, MacLennan GT, Lopez-Beltran A, Zhang S, Cocco A, Cheng L. Molecular evidence supporting field effect in urothelial carcinogenesis. *Clin Cancer Res* 2005;11:6512–9.

230. Prat E, Bernues M, Caballin MR, Egozcue J, Gelabert A, Miro R. Detection of chromosomal imbalances in papillary bladder tumors by comparative genomic hybridization. *Urology* 2001;57:986–92.

231. Simon R, Burger H, Brinkschmidt C, Bocker W, Hertle L, Terpe HJ. Chromosomal aberrations associated with invasion in papillary superficial bladder cancer. *J Pathol* 1998;185:345–51.

232. Richter J, Wagner U, Schraml P, Maurer R, Alund G, Knonagel H, Moch H, Mihatsch MJ, Gasser TC, Sauter G. Chromosomal imbalances are associated with a high risk of progression in early invasive (pT1) urinary bladder cancer. *Cancer Res* 1999;59:5687–91.

233. Simon R, Burger H, Semjonow A, Hertle L, Terpe HJ, Bocker W. Patterns of chromosomal imbalances in muscle invasive bladder cancer. *Int J Oncol* 2000;17:1025–9.

234. Bruch J, Wohr G, Hautmann R, Mattfeldt T, Bruderlein S, Moller P, Sauter S, Hameister H, Vogel W, Paiss T. Chromosomal changes during progression of transitional cell carcinoma of the bladder and delineation of the amplified interval on chromosome arm 8q. *Genes Chromosomes Cancer* 1998;23:167–74.

235. Natrajan R, Louhelainen J, Williams S, Laye J, Knowles MA. High-resolution deletion mapping of 15q13.2-q21.1 in transitional cell carcinoma of the bladder. *Cancer Res* 2003;63:7657–62.

236. Shaw ME, Knowles MA. Deletion mapping of chromosome 11 in carcinoma of the bladder. *Genes Chromosomes Cancer* 1995;13:1–8.

237. Tsai YC, Nichols PW, Hiti AL, Williams Z, Skinner DG, Jones PA. Allelic losses of chromosomes 9, 11, and 17 in human bladder cancer. *Cancer Res* 1990;50:44–7.

238. Houskova L, Zemanova Z, Babjuk M, Melichercikova J, Pesl M, Michalova K. Molecular cytogenetic characterization and diagnostics of bladder cancer. *Neoplasma* 2007;54:511–6.

239. Sandberg AA, Berger CS. Review of chromosome studies in urological tumors. II. Cytogenetics and molecular genetics of bladder cancer. *J Urol* 1994;151:545–60.

240. Miyao N, Tsai YC, Lerner SP, Olumi AF, Spruck CH 3rd, Gonzalez-Zulueta M, Nichols PW, Skinner DG, Jones PA. Role of chromosome 9 in human bladder cancer. *Cancer Res* 1993;53:4066–70.

241. Seripa D, Parrella P, Gallucci M, Gravina C, Papa S, Fortunato P, Alcini A, Flammia G, Lazzari M, Fazio VM. Sensitive detection of transitional cell carcinoma of the bladder by microsatellite analysis of cells exfoliated in urine. *Int J Cancer* 2001;95:364–9.

242. Hartmann A, Schlake G, Zaak D, Hungerhuber E, Hofstetter A, Hofstaedter F, Knuechel R. Occurrence of chromosome 9 and p53 alterations in multifocal dysplasia and carcinoma in situ of human urinary bladder. *Cancer Res* 2002;62:809–18.

243. Cairns P, Shaw ME, Knowles MA. Initiation of bladder cancer may involve deletion of a tummor suppressor gene on chromosome 9. *Oncogene* 1993;8:1083–5.

244. Linnenbach AJ, Pressler LB, Seng BA, Kimmel BS, Tomaszewski JE, Malkowicz SB. Characterization of chromosome 9 deletions in transitional cell carcinoma by microsatellite assay. *Hum Mol Genet* 1993;2:1407–11.

245. Hartmann A, Schlake G, Zaak D, Hungerhuber E, Hofstetter A, Hofstaedter F, Knuechel R. Occurrence of chromosome 9 and p53 alterations in multifocal dysplasia and carcinoma in situ of human urinary bladder. *Cancer Res* 2002;62:809–18.

246. Lacy S, Lopez-Beltran A, MacLennan GT, Foster SR, Montironi R, Cheng L. Molecular pathogenesis of urothelial carcinoma: the clinical utility of emerging new biomarkers and future molecular classification of bladder cancer. *Anal Quan Cytol Histol* 2009;31:5–16.

247. Seripa D, Parrella P, Gallucci M, Gravina C, Papa S, Fortunato P, Alcini A, Flammia G, Lazzari M, Fazio VM. Sensitive detection of transitional cell carcinoma of the bladder by microsatellite analysis of cells exfoliated in urine. *Int J Cancer* 2001;95:364–9.

248. Utting M, Werner W, Dahse R, Schubert J, Junker K. Microsatellite analysis of free tumor DNA in urine, serum, and plasma of patients: a minimally invasive method for the detection of bladder cancer. *Clin Cancer Res* 2002;8:35–40.

249. Curigliano G, Ferretti G, Flamini G, Goldhirsch A, de Braud F, Calabro MG, Mandaly M, Nole F, De Pas T, D'Addessi A, Cittadini A. Diagnosis of T1 bladder transitional cell carcinoma by denaturing gradient gel electrophoresis urinalysis. *Anticancer Res* 2001;21:3015–20.

250. Neves M, Ciofu C, Larousserie F, Fleury J, Sibony M, Flahault A, Soubrier F, Gattegno B. Prospective evaluation of genetic abnormalities and telomerase expression in exfoliated urinary cells for bladder cancer detection. *J Urol* 2002;167:1276–81.

251. Hoque MO, Begum S, Topaloglu O, Chatterjee A, Rosenbaum E, Van Criekinge W, Westra WH, Schoenberg M, Zahurak M, Goodman SN, Sidransky D. Quantitation of promoter methylation of multiple genes in urine DNA and bladder cancer detection. *J Natl Cancer Inst* 2006;98:996–1004.

252. Larsson PC, Beheshti B, Sampson HA, Jewett MA, Shipman R. Allelic deletion fingerprinting of urine cell sediments in bladder cancer. *Mol Diagn* 2001;6:181–8.

253. Kallioniemi A, Kallioniemi OP, Citro G, Sauter G, DeVries S, Kerschmann R, Caroll P, Waldman F. Identification of gains and losses of DNA sequences in primary bladder cancer by comparative genomic hybridization. *Genes Chromosomes Cancer* 1995;12:213–9.

254. Voorter C, Joos S, Bringuier PP, Vallinga M, Poddighe P, Schalken J, du Manoir S, Ramaekers F, Lichter P, Hopman A. Detection of chromosomal imbalances in transitional cell carcinoma of the bladder by comparative genomic hybridization. *Am J Pathol* 1995;146:1341–54.

255. Richter J, Jiang F, Gorog JP, Sartorius G, Egenter C, Gasser TC, Moch H, Mihatsch MJ, Sauter G. Marked genetic differences between stage pTa and stage pT1 papillary bladder cancer detected by comparative genomic hybridization. *Cancer Res* 1997;57:2860–4.

256. Fadl-Elmula I, Kytola S, Leithy ME, Abdel-Hameed M, Mandahl N, Elagib A, Ibrahim M, Larsson C, Heim S. Chromosomal aberrations in benign and malignant bilharzia-associated bladder lesions analyzed by comparative genomic hybridization. *BMC Cancer* 2002;2:5.

257. Hoque MO, Lee J, Begum S, Yamashita K, Engles JM, Schoenberg M, Westra WH, Sidransky D. High-throughput molecular analysis of urine sediment for the detection of bladder cancer by high-density single-nucleotide polymorphism array. *Cancer Res* 2003;63:5723–6.

258. Chan MW, Chan LW, Tang NL, Tong JH, Lo KW, Lee TL, Cheung HY, Wong WS, Chan PS, Lai FM, To KF. Hypermethylation of multiple genes in tumor tissues and voided urine in urinary bladder cancer patients. *Clin Cancer Res* 2002;8:464–70.

259. Friedrich MG, Weisenberger DJ, Cheng JC, Chandrasoma S, Siegmund KD, Gonzalgo ML, Toma MI, Huland H, Yoo C, Tsai YC, Nichols PW, Bochner BH, Jones PA, Liang G. Detection of methylated apoptosis-associated genes in urine sediments of bladder cancer patients. *Clin Cancer Res* 2004;10:7457–65.

260. Vinci S, Giannarini G, Selli C, Kuncova J, Villari D, Valent F, Orlando C. Quantitative methylation analysis of BCL2, hTERT, and DAPK promoters in urine sediment for the detection of non-muscle-invasive urothelial

carcinoma of the bladder: a prospective, two-center validation study. *Urol Oncol* 2011;29:150–6.

261. Chan MW, Chan LW, Tang NL, Tong JH, Lo KW, Lee TL, Cheung HY, Wong WS, Chan PS, Lai FM, To KF. Hypermethylation of multiple genes in tumor tissues and voided urine in urinary bladder cancer patients. *Clin Cancer Res* 2002;8:464–70.

262. Horstmann M, Patschan O, Hennenlotter J, Senger E, Feil G, Stenzl A. Combinations of urine-based tumour markers in bladder cancer surveillance. *Scand J Urol Nephrol* 2009;43:461–6.

263. Babjuk M, Soukup V, Pesl M, Kostirova M, Drncova E, Smolova H, Szakacsova M, Getzenberg R, Pavlik I, Dvoracek J. Urinary cytology and quantitative BTA and UBC tests in surveillance of patients with pTapT1 bladder urothelial carcinoma. *Urology* 2008;71:718–22.

264. May M, Hakenberg OW, Gunia S, Pohling P, Helke C, Lubbe L, Nowack R, Siegsmund M, Hoschke B. Comparative diagnostic value of urine cytology, UBC-ELISA, and fluorescence in situ hybridization for detection of transitional cell carcinoma of urinary bladder in routine clinical practice. *Urology* 2007;70:449–53.

265. Schroeder GL, Lorenzo-Gomez MF, Hautmann SH, Friedrich MG, Ekici S, Huland H, Lokeshwar V. A side by side comparison of cytology and

biomarkers for bladder cancer detection. *J Urol* 2004;172:1123–6.

266. Ramakumar S, Bhuiyan J, Besse JA, Roberts SG, Wollan PC, Blute ML, O'Kane DJ. Comparison of screening methods in the detection of bladder cancer. *J Urol* 1999;161:388–94.

267. Eissa S, Labib RA, Mourad MS, Kamel K, El-Ahmady O. Comparison of telomerase activity and matrix metalloproteinase–9 in voided urine and bladder wash samples as a useful diagnostic tool for bladder cancer. *Eur Urol* 2003;44:687–94.

268. Gkialas I, Papadopoulos G, Iordanidou L, Stathouros G, Tzavara C, Gregorakis A, Lykourinas M. Evaluation of urine tumor-associated trypsin inhibitor, CYFRA 21–1, and urinary bladder cancer antigen for detection of high grade bladder carcinoma. *Urology* 2008;72:1159–63.

269. Nisman B, Barak V, Shapiro A, Golijanin D, Peretz T, Pode D. Evaluation of urine CYFRA 21–1 for the detection of primary and recurrent bladder carcinoma. *Cancer* 2002;94:2914–22.

270. Fernandez-Gomez J, Rodriguez-Martinez JJ, Barmadah SE, Garcia Rodriguez J, Allende DM, Jalon A, Gonzalez R, Alvarez-Mugica M. Urinary CYFRA 21.1 is not a useful marker for the detection of recurrences in the followup of superficial bladder cancer. *Eur Urol* 2007;51:1267–74.

271. Schneider A, Borgnat S, Lang H, Regine O, Lindner V, Kassem M, Saussine C, Oudet P, Jacqmin D, Gaub MP. Evaluation of microsatellite analysis in urine sediment for diagnosis of bladder cancer. *Cancer Res* 2000;60:4617–22.

272. van Rhijn BW, Smit M, van Geenen D, Wijnmaalen A, Kirkels WJ, van der Kwast TH, Kuenen-Boumeester V, Zwarthoff EC. Surveillance with microsatellite analysis of urine in bladder cancer patients treated by radiotherapy. *Eur Urol* 2003;43:369–73.

273. Soyuer I, Tokat F, Tasdemir A. Significantly increased accuracy of urothelial carcinoma detection in destained urine slides with combined analysis of standard cytology and CK–20 immunostaing. *Acta Cytol* 2009;53:357–60.

274. Hautmann S, Toma M, Lorenzo Gomez MF, Friedrich MG, Jaekel T, Michl U, Schroeder GL, Huland H, Juenemann KP, Lokeshwar VB. Immunocyt and the HA-HAase urine tests for the detection of bladder cancer: a side-by-side comparison. *Eur Urol* 2004;46:466–71.

275. Pu XY, Wang ZP, Chen YR, Wang XH, Wu YL, Wang HP. The value of combined use of survivin, cytokeratin 20 and mucin 7 mRNA for bladder cancer detection in voided urine. *J Cancer Res Clin Oncol* 2008;134:659–65.

Chapter 33

Tissue-based Biomarkers

Overview

Urothelial carcinoma is the fifth most common cancer in industrialized countries, accounting for approximately 5% of all cancers.[1,2] The associated risk factors for bladder cancer include tobacco smoking, aromatic amine exposure, arsenic exposure, chronic infection with *Schistosoma* species, radiation therapy, and exposure to alkylating agents.[3-5]

Low grade papillary tumors comprise approximately 80% of bladder tumors. These tumors most commonly present as superficial, exophytic, or papillary lesions. Most patients (75%) present with pTis, pTa, or pT1 tumors, 20% present with pT2 tumors, and 5% present with metastatic tumors. It has been suggested that these tumors arise from normal urothelium through a urothelial hyperplastic change, such as a papilloma, with subsequent angiogenetic responses and further growth. Although these tumors have a high rate of recurrence, their inherent capacity to become invasive is quite low. Most of these tumors are treated by intravesical chemotherapy, and the five-year survival rate is approximately 90%. Progression has been reported to occur in 10% to 20% of cases. Up to 50% of pT1 tumors may progress.[6] There is an urgent need for biomarkers that can distinguish tumor with potential to progress and metastasize.[7-14]

In recent years, tremendous advances have been made in the discovery of new markers that are associated with alterations at the molecular level and have clinical relevance in the areas of diagnosis, tumor classification, prognosis, and prediction of an individual patient's response to treatment (**Table 33-1**). However, much remains to be learned about how these and to other biomarkers can be used efficiently to improve the management of bladder cancer (see also **Chapters 29, 32, and 34**).

Proliferation Markers

Proliferating cell nuclear antigen (PCNA) is a nonhistone nuclear protein that acts as an accessory of DNA polymerase. Its expression is maximal during the S phase and is closely linked to the cell cycle. The PCNA labeling index in bladder cancer varies from 5% to 92%, and is predictive of cancer recurrence,[15-17] response to radiation therapy,[18] and survival.[19] Diploid urothelial cancer with a PCNA labeling index below 30% of cells did not recur, whereas aneuploid cancer with PCNA index greater than 30% usually recurred.[20] PCNA expression correlated with nuclear morphometric findings in bladder cancer cells[21] as well as Ki67 results.[22] Also, the ratio of apoptosis, seen in 90% of Ta and T1 bladder cancers) to PCNA was greater in patients without recurrence.[23]

Table 33-1 Select Molecular Markers in Bladder Cancer

Proliferation markers
  Proliferating cell nuclear antigen (PCNA)
  Ki67/MIB1
Apoptosis markers
  BCL2
  BAX
  Caspase 3 (CASP3)
  Survivin
  Others
Tumor suppressor genes, oncogenes, mutator genes, and
    cell cycle regulators
  TP53
  p21 (WAF1/Cip1/CDKN1A)
  p16 (INK4/CDKN2A/MTS1)
  p15 (INK4B)
  p27 (Kip1)
  Retinoblastoma gene (Rb)
  TSC1
  Fragile histine triad gene (FHIT)
  PTEN
  TP63
  HER2 (ERBB2)
  HRAS
  MDM2
  MYC
  Cyclins D1 and D3 (CCND1 and CCND3)
  Others
Growth factors and receptors
  Fibroblast growth factor 3 (FGFR3)
  Epidermal growth factor receptor (EGFR)
  Vascular endothelial growth factor (VEGF)
  Acidic fibroblast growth factor
  Basic fibroblast growth factor (bFGF)
  Others
Cell adhesion markers
  E-cadherin
  Integrins
  CD44
  F and G actin
  Others
Vessel density
  Microvessel density
  Lymph vessel density
Telomerase
Miscellaneous protein markers
  Multidrug resistance proteins
  Cyclooxygenase 2 (COX2)
  Gelsolin
  Autocrine motility factor
  Luminal epithelial antigen (LEA.135)
  Androgen receptor
  Estrogen receptor
  Urokinase-type plasminogen activator factor
  Surface glycoprotein T138

(continued)

Table 33-1 (*Continued*)

Hyaluronic acid
Transforming growth factor (TGF) β1
Glyoxalase system enzymes
FEZ1/LTS1 tumor suppressor gene
STK15/BTAK/AuroraA gene product
Peroxisome proliferator-activated receptor gamma
Tissue polypeptide-specific antigen
Thymidylate synthase
Thymidine phosphorylase (platelet-derived endothelial
   cell growth factor)
Dihydropyrimidine dehydrogenase
Matrix metalloproteinase 1 (MMP1)
Tissue inhibitor of metalloproteinase (TIMP)1
Proline-directed protein kinase F(A)
Clusterin
Osteonectin
Ku protein
Caveolin 1 (CAV1)
Glycolipids and glycosyltransferases GM3 synthase
Hypoxia inducible factor (HIF) 2 alpha
S100 calcium-binding protein A4 (S100A4)
Bladder cancer–associated protein (bc10)
Cathepsins
MAGEA4 protein
Oxygen-regulated protein (ORP150)
Hepatoma upregulated protein (HURP)
Others
Urine-based markers (proprietary commercial markers)
   (see **Chapter 32** for further discussion)
   ImmunoCyt
   BTA
   NMP22
   UBC antigen
   Fluorescence in situ hybridization (FISH) and UroVysion
   Hemoglobin dipstick
DNA ploidy
   See **Chapter 32** for further discussion
Loss of heterozygosity and microsatellite instability
   See **Chapters 29** and **34** for further discussion
Methylation markers
   See **Chapter 34** for further discussion
microRNAs
   See **Chapter 34** for further discussion

Ki67 is a monoclonal antibody that recognizes a human nuclear antigen expressed in the S, G1, G2, and M phases of the cell cycle. Ki67 expression, measured as the proportion of immunoreactive cell nuclei in frozen tissue specimens, correlates with cancer grade and stage.[24-27] A number of investigators have reported a prognostic role for Ki67 index in advanced urothelial carcinoma of the urinary bladder.[28-30] Lymph node metastases had Ki67 expression that was similar to that in the primary cancer.[31] Also, Ki67 expression is predictive of a recurrence of urothelial carcinoma,[32-35] but not always by multivariate analysis.[27,36] Margulis et al. assessed Ki67 expression in 713 urothelial carcinoma patients treated with radical cystectomy and bilateral lymphadenectomy at six centers. Bladder cancer recurred in 318 (44.6%) of these patients. Using a cutoff of $\geq$20% of tumor cells Ki67-labeled cells, the Ki67 positivity was significantly associated with increased probability of disease recurrence.[28]

MIB1 is a monoclonal antibody that is the equivalent of Ki67 displaying immunoreactivity in formalin-fixed paraffin-embedded sections. Its expression is significantly associated with p53 expression[37]; in a multivariate analysis of 62 patients followed for recurrent grade 1 cancer, MIB1 immunopositivity was the only significance predictor of recurrence and cancer-specific survival when compared with p53, HER2, and BCL2 expression.[38] Patients with a labeling index greater than 30% had a worse prognosis than did those with a lower index.[22] The labeling index was increased with greater depth of muscle invasion.[39]

Apoptosis Markers

BCL2 is a protooncogene that encodes a mitochondrial membrane protein blocking apoptosis without influencing cell proliferation. *BCL2* immunoreactivity was observed in benign and dysplastic urothelium and in up to 80% of cases of urothelial carcinoma,[40,41] but was negative in CIS.[27,37,42,43] Expression decreased with higher stage and higher grade cancer,[27,37,44] although this has been disputed.[40] Expression did not correlate with prognosis for surgically treated patients, regardless of age.[45] For those treated with curative radiotherapy, *BCL2* immunoreactivity correlated with recurrence and shortened survival.[46]

Wild type *TP53* leads to apoptotic cell death, whereas mutant *TP53* inhibits apoptotic death, similar to *BCL2* (see the discussion below). Thus, it is interesting to note that *BCL2* is expressed more frequently in low grade low stage urothelial cancer, whereas mutant *TP53* is more frequent in high grade and high stage cancer. One possible explanation is that mutant *TP53* prolongs survival of cells with established genetic defects, allowing them to become more unstable and clinically aggressive; conversely, *BCL2* may be an early event that prolongs the survival of cells, allowing them to acquire initial genetic defects without abrogating DNA proofreading and repair mechanisms.[27]

Other apoptosis markers include the proapoptosis protein, BAX, that appears to be an independent predictor of survival[40]; however, this marker and two others (FAS receptor and caspase 3) did not correlate with apoptotic rate of bladder cancer.[47] Most cancers were immunoreactive for BAX (52% to 73%) and BCL–XL (81%), but not for BCL-XS (29%).[40,46] Expression of BCL-XL and BCL-XS correlated with high grade and advanced stage.[40] Survivin, a caspase inhibitor, is another promising biomarker in bladder cancer.[48-53]

Tumor Suppressor Genes

TP53 and Cell Cycle Regulators

TP53

p53 is a 53-kDa DNA-binding phosphoprotein coded for by a tumor suppressor gene located on the short arm of chromosome 17 (17p13.1) (Table 33-2). It is the gatekeeper of the G1/S phase of the cell cycle and acts as a tumor suppressor.[54] This transcription factor regulates cell growth and inhibits cells from entering the S phase. p53 also regulates antiapoptotic genes such as BAX. Loss or mutation of this gene results in unregulated and aberrant growth with reduced apoptosis of cells whose proliferation would normally be kept under control.

The half-life of wild type TP53 is estimated to be between 20 minutes and 30 minutes, whereas, due to decreased degradation, mutant TP53 has a much longer half-life, estimated to be approximately 24 hours. Mutations in TP53 most frequently involve exons 5 to 11. Approximately 95% of mutations occur between exons 5 through 8 in the region of the DNA-binding domain, otherwise known as the hot spot region of the TP53 gene. Mutations in TP53 are usually missense substitutions that cluster in one particular region of the gene product between amino acids 130 and 290, involving residues 117 to 142, 171 to 181, 239 to 258, and 270 to 286. These regions are highly conserved among species, and are probably necessary for normal TP53 function. The region encompassing codons 280 and 285 are a hot spot for TP53 mutations rich in purines, which seem to be a target for chemical carcinogens.[55] p53 codon 72 polymorphism and homozygosity for arginine at residue 72 was associated with increased risk of bladder cancer,[56] although this was disputed by others.[57]

Loss of heterozygosity (LOH) of the TP53 locus occurs in many human cancers.[58] Therefore, TP53 probably contributes to human carcinogenesis when its normal allele is deleted or inactivated. Transforming activity in the heterozygous state may be due to formation of an oligomeric complex between mutant and wild type TP53. In cells transformed with mutant TP53 gene, the altered protein complex remains in the cytoplasm and wild type TP53 is degraded.

Mutated TP53 genes can cooperate with RAS genes to transform primary cultured fibroblasts in the presence of endogenous wild type p53 protein.[59] In some cancers, deletion of chromosome 17 loci occurs concurrently with other chromosomal abnormalities, suggesting that TP53 mutation

is a late event in carcinogenesis. Cancer cell aneuploidy, reflecting chromosomal instability, may play a role in the selection of cancer cells with TP53 gene mutations. This process could lead to loss of the remaining wild type allele and inactivation of the growth control function of the normal p53 protein.[60]

In approximately 50% of bladder tumors, especially those in the advanced stages of disease, missense mutations in the TP53 tumor suppressor gene are found.[61] Mutations of TP53 are very common (>50%) in high grade invasive tumors and in flat carcinoma in situ (CIS). Therefore, tumors with TP53 mutations to have a poorer prognosis and a higher recurrence rate than those without the mutation. A comparison of the survival of bladder cancer patients with wild type TP53 versus those with mutant TP53 showed a significant decreased survival time in those patients with mutant TP53 (median survival 12 months vs. 51 months for wild type TP53).[62,63] Not surprisingly, tumors with p21 mutations are also associated with poorer prognosis and higher recurrence rates.

p53 protein can be inactivated by viral proteins such as the E6 protein of human papillomavirus (HPV) 16. HPV is detected in occasional cases of papillary noninvasive and invasive cancer (12% in one study), and the presence of HPV correlates with higher stage and grade.[56,64-71] TP53 mutations are rarely observed in patients with HPV-positive cancer, suggesting separate etiologic pathways.[72]

Mutations of TP53 or functional inactivation with intact TP53 genes are common in many human cancers, causing loss of normal growth regulation. Mutations result in prolonged half-life and accumulation of the p53 protein to a level that makes it detectable immunohistochemically in cancer cell nuclei. Overexpression of p53 protein is associated with a poor prognosis in a variety of cancers, and appears to precede loss of chromosome 9 in CIS as a precursor of invasive bladder cancer.[73]

Most antibodies for p53 require antigen retrieval procedures when used with deparaffinized formalin-fixed sections. Staining results may vary due to differences in fixation, specimen pretreatment, and antibody binding sites. Immunohistochemical methods rely on the accumulation of p53 protein in cells with TP53 missense mutations. The cause of this is not known with certainty, and immunoreactivity is usually but not always indicative of TP53 mutation.[31] Wild type p53 protein may accumulate in the setting of p53 activation, including hypoxia and DNA damage. In addition, not all TP53 missense mutations result in protein accumulation and may cause false-negative immunohistochemical results. Finally, there may be a gradient of TP53 inactivation that varies according to the site and extent of the mutation. Nonetheless, there is a strong positive correlation of immunoreactivity and TP53 mutations.[59,74] Benign urothelium rarely displays p53 staining, whereas expression in carcinoma is

Table 33-2 Select Mutations in Urothelial Neoplasms

Gene(s)	Chromosome Location	Frequency in Bladder Neoplasms	Mechanism(s)
P16INK4	9p21	>50%	Inactivation of CDKN2 leading to uncontrolled cell cycle signaling pathways
FGFR3	4p16.3 Exons 7, 10, 15	74% pTa 21% pT1 16% > pT2 >40% overall	Activation of RAS-MAPK pathway
ERBB2 (HER2)	17q23	37–50%, especially >pT2	Encodes for receptor protein tyrosine kinase
TP53	17p13 Exons 5–8	50% high grade or invasive carcinomas	Regulation of antiapoptotic genes
MDM2	12q14	4–6%	Regulation of protein degradation
EGFR1	7p12.3–p12.1	30–50% invasive carcinomas	Tyrosine kinase
HRAS	13q14.1–q14.2	30–40%	Oncogene
RB1	13q14.1–14.2	>50% high grade urothelial carcinomas	Increased cell proliferation
FHIT	3p	25–60%	Tumor suppressor gene
SFRP1	8p	25–30%	Tumor suppressor gene
PTEN	10q23	≥50%	Tumor suppressor gene
DBC1	9q32–33	>50%	Tumor suppressor gene
PTCH (Gorlin syndrome)	9q22	>50%	Tumor suppressor gene
TSC1	9q34	12–34%	Tumor suppressor gene

observed in 18% to 78% of cases.[75–78] Different cutoff points have been used for positive and negative staining, including 0% of cells,[79,80] 10% of cells,[27,78,81] and 20% of cells.[37,75,77,82,83] Intratumoral variance is reflected in the heterogeneous expression of staining. In one study, the investigators found no difference in expression between the central cancer and the invasive front.[31]

The cellular urine sediment may be used for genetic analysis of TP53 mutations.[84,85] However, comparison of TP53 mutations in microdissected cancer correlates poorly with mutations observed in urine and blood.[86] Lymph node metastases have expression similar to that in the primary cancer.[31]

TP53 alterations in urothelial carcinoma may result in increased sensitivity to chemotherapeutic agents that damage DNA, including doxorubicin and ciplatin.[87,88] In patients with TP53 mutations, adjuvant chemotherapy resulted in a threefold decreased risk of recurrence and a 2.6-fold increased chance of survival with a median followup of about 9 years.[87] Patients without TP53 mutations derived no survival advantage with chemotherapy. These results suggest that patients at greatest risk of progression and death (those with TP53 mutations) may also derive the maximum benefit from adjuvant chemotherapy, and that TP53 status may identify such patients. Nonetheless, the response of tumors with TP53 mutations to various therapies, including chemotherapeutic agents, radiation therapy, and DNA-damaging agents (including cisplatin

and doxorubicin) has been variable in the literature.[89–92] TP53 status was not predictive of initial clinical response to BCG therapy in T1 cancer treated by transurethral resection, regardless of grade.[93,94]

In urothelial carcinoma, nuclear p53 protein immunoreactivity correlated with high grade,[27,95–99] high stage,[27,95,97,99–102] vascular invasion,[95] cancer recurrence and progression,[45,82,96,103–107] decreased survival,[75,82,104,105,108–111] and TP53 mutations, including 17p deletion and 17 polysomy.[27,37,75,83,98,112–114] Immunoreactivity had independent prognostic significance in many reports,[75,80,82,108,115,116] but this has been disputed refuted.[27,76,79,96,99,100,106,117–120] Stage T1 bladder carcinoma with more than 20% p53 immunoreactive cells had a higher progression rate than that of cancer with fewer stained cells (21% vs. 3% progression per year, respectively).[115] Similarly, CIS with more than 20% p53 immunoreactive cells had a higher progression rate than cases with fewer stained cells (86% vs. 16% per year, respectively).[75,116,121–123] Conversely, one study showed that cancer grade and stage were the only independent predictive factors for patient survival when p53 and BCL2 were included in the analysis.[27]

The predictive value of p53 may be increased when combined with other factors. p53 immunoreactivity and DNA aneuploidy are closely associated, and, when found in combination, predict a very poor outcome for patients with invasive cancer[100]; conversely, another study found no correlation of p53 expression and DNA ploidy status.[101]

About 65% of cases of CIS contain *TP53* mutations,[124,125] considerably greater than the 28% to 33% of cases of atypia and dysplasia.[126] This high frequency of mutations is similar to that in invasive urothelial carcinoma, and may explain on a genetic basis the great propensity for CIS to progress.[124] Moreover, germline transmission of *TP53* mutations occurs in cancer-prone families, including those with Li–Fraumeni syndrome.[127] In one study, *TP53* gene mutations were present in 11 of 18 invasive bladder cancers, and the most common mutation was single-base-pair substitution.[128] Missense mutations were present in seven of 11 cases, and nonsense mutations in three. Mutations of *TP53* are also detectable in urine sediment[128] and may be predictive of progression.[129] In a study of 25 bladder cancers from 23 patients, the incidence of *TP53* mutations was significantly higher in muscle-invasive than nonmuscle-invasive cancer (58% vs. 8%, respectively).[112] high grade bladder cancer contains diverse *TP53* mutations in 36% to 51% of cases.[59,130] These molecular studies confirm the immunohistochemical observations of p53 protein expression in bladder carcinoma.

The identification of mutations of *p21* and *p16* genes in urothelial carcinoma and other human cancers indicates that similar biologic effects can be due to alterations of different genes in the *TP53* regulatory pathway (see the discussion below).[131,132]

p21 (WAF1/Cip1/CDKN1A)

p53 induces *TP53*-dependent genes. A prototype of this class of genes, *p21* (*WAF1/Cip1/CDKN1A*), encodes a 21-kDa protein that inhibits cyclin-dependent kinases responsible for initiation of the G1 phase of the cell cycle. Tumors with loss of *TP53* function show downregulation of *p21*, which is a downstream target of *TP53*. Mutations in the *TP53* gene result in failure to stimulate *p21*, with subsequent loss of inhibition of cyclin-dependent kinase complexes and initiation of G1.[58] The discovery of p53-dependent cyclin-dependent kinase inhibitors linked this gene to the basic enzyme mechanisms operative in cell cycle regulation.

The *p21* gene is transcriptionally activated by *TP53* and mediates *TP53*-dependent G1 arrest following DNA damage (see *TP53*, above). Although there was no apparent association of *TP53* and p21 expression, *p21*-positive cancers in patients receiving cisplatinum-based systemic chemotherapy had greater survival than that of *p21*-negative cancers (60 months vs. 23 months, respectively).[106] Similarly, *p21* expression predicted cancer-specific survival in patients with muscle-invasive cancer treated by radiation therapy.[46,111] The combination of *p21* and *TP53* improved prediction of survival in patients with muscle-invasive cancer treated by radiation

therapy; those with p21+TP53+ cancer had the best survival, whereas those with p21−TP53+ had the worst prognosis.[133]

p16 (INK4/CDKN2A/MTS1)

The *p16* gene, present on chromosome 9, is abnormal in up to 60% of cases of squamous cell carcinoma associated with schistosomiasis, but only 18% of cases of urothelial carcinoma.[134–136] Moreover, anomalies of *p16* and *TP53* are mutually exclusive, suggesting a complementary role in the pathogenesis of bladder cancer.[135] Synchronous *TP53* and *nm23-H1* detection correlates with poor patient survival,[137] although *nm23-H1* by itself predicts only extent of cancer invasion and recurrence.[138]

Expression of the protooncogene *p16* was observed in 40% to 51% of bladder cancers, compared with absence in benign urothelium.[139] Decreased expression correlates with increasing grade, stage, and poor prognosis,[139,140] although the opposite was also reported by some investigators.[139,141] A recent study found that *p16* expression is significantly higher in muscle-invasive cancer that follows Ta or T1 primary cancer compared with cancer presenting at first diagnosis as muscle invasive.[142]

p15 (INK4B/CDKN2B)

The gene encodes a cyclin-dependent kinase inhibitor on chromosome 9p21. Messenger RNA (mRNA) expression is present in benign urothelium, is decreased in superficial cancer, and is heterogeneous in muscle-invasive cancer.[143]

Retinoblastoma Gene

The retinoblastoma (*RB*) gene on chromosome 13p14 encodes a 105-kDa protein that regulates transcription in all adult cells (Table 33-2). The normal gene product suppresses expression of genes required for cell cycle progression. Cyclin and cyclin-dependent kinases inactivate the *RB* gene product by phosphorylation. pRB can be inactivated by the protein corresponding to the open reading frame E6 of HPV16 without mutation of the *RB* gene.[144] Loss of function of the *p16* gene, which encodes the p16 protein, is an upstream enabler of *RB*, maintaining the pRB in its active or hypophosphorylated state. Absence of *p16* correlates with functional inactivation of the RB protein, perhaps accounting for the equal prognosis in patients with *RB1* absence or overexpression in some studies since *p16* deficient cells may be abundant pRB that is inactivated by phosphorylation.[145]

Any mutation of the *RB* gene may lead to decreased inhibition of the *E2F* transcription factor family of transcription factors, which leads to an increase in cell proliferation. It has been found that over 50% of high grade urothelial carcinomas have mutations in both *TP53* and *RB*.[146,147]

$E2F3$ is amplified in approximately 14% of invasive bladder cancers.[148]

pRB is expressed in all human tissues. Mutational inactivation of *RB* gene and reduction of pRB expression occurs in retinoblastoma and other cancers.[149] The two main alterations of RB in human cancer are deletion and mutation. Major deletions of large segments of the gene result in the absence of a properly functioning gene product.[149] Mutations, including nucleotide substitutions that alter gene function, create improper initiation signals, more splicing sites, shift stop codons, or make amino acid substitutions, or will destabilize transcription, produce a truncated gene product or otherwise corrupt the mRNA. These changes cause absence of a functional pRB protein.[150] *RB* alterations in bladder cancer usually appear to be subtle point mutations rather than major deletions. *RB* gene is one of the major genetic factors responsible for development and progression of high grade muscle-invasive bladder cancer.[144] Loss of *RB* function occurs in 30% of high grade papillary and nonpapillary urothelial carcinomas. Loss of *RB* correlates with LOH at the *RB* gene locus, which correlates with high grade tumor and muscle invasion. Lymph node metastases have pRB expression that is similar to that in the primary cancer.[31]

Altered expression of pRB is associated with decreased survival of patients with urothelial carcinoma.[150] Benign urothelial mucosa and noninvasive urothelial carcinoma have pRB immunoreactivity in most cells.[151] Immunohistochemical detection of pRB appears to be a useful marker of cancer progression, but is not routinely used.[144,152,153] Allelic deletions for *RB* and *LMYC* in urine sediment were observed in 32% of cases of CIS and 20% of bladder cancers, but the correlation between cancer tissue and urine sediment was not strong.[154]

TSC1

The *TSC1* gene (tuberous sclerosis complex) encodes the protein hamartin and is mutated in patients with tuberous sclerosis. *TSC1* is located on 9q34.[155] LOH studies have shown that 34% of bladder cancers, especially Ta tumors, have mutations in this gene[156]; other investigators have reported *TSC1* gene mutation frequency rates of 11% to 13% in urothelial carcinomas.[155,157,158]

FHIT

The fragile histidine triad (*FHIT*) gene is located on the short arm of chromosome 3 (3p14.2) and has decreased protein expression in bladder tumors. Loss of the *FHIT* gene has been identified in 25% to 60% of bladder cancers, and this finding is more common in higher stage cancers. Patients whose cancers show this loss of expression are found to have poorer prognoses as well as decreased survival.[159–161]

PTEN

PTEN (phosphatase and tensin homolog deleted on chromosome 10) is located on 10q23, which is a common region of LOH in high grade and high stage urothelial carcinoma.[158,162–164] Loss of *PTEN* causes PI3 kinase activation (acts in the same way as *TSC1*). Tsuruta et al. reported 53% of primary bladder cancers exhibited decreased or absent expression of PTEN protein in either the cytoplasm or nucleus of tumor cells.[165] In advanced bladder cancers, PTEN protein was reduced significantly (particularly in the nucleus) in 94% of cases, and this decrease in PTEN correlated with disease stage and grade.[165] *PTEN* expression did not correlate with patient survival.[166] Reduced *PTEN* expression relates to aggressiveness of bladder tumors. The alteration of *PTEN* expression was significantly different according to tumor stage and grade.[167] However, *PTEN* expression was not significantly correlated with disease recurrence, progression, and recurrence- or progression-free survival.[167]

p63

P63 is a member of the *TP53* gene family that is present in normal urothelium but lost in most invasive cancers.[168] p63 (−/−) mice fail to complete urothelial differentiation.[168]

Growth Factors and Receptors

Fibroblast Growth Factor Receptor 3

Fibroblast growth factor receptor (*FGFR*) 3 is a crucial gene in embryonic development, cell growth, differentiation, proliferation, and angiogenesis.[169] *FGFR* is composed of four active components, designated as *FGFRs 1* to *4*; these are high-affinity cell surface-associated receptors, encoded on 4p16.3.[170] Each component is composed of an extracellular domain made up of an amino-terminal hydrophobic signal peptide with three immunoglobulin-like domains to which fibroblast growth factors bind, a hydrophobic transmembrane domain, and an intracellular tyrosine kinase domain. *FGFR3* mutations are known most commonly for causing autosomal-dominant skeletal dysplasia syndromes such as achondroplasia and hypochondroplasia.[169,171] A mutation in *FGFR3* (especially in exons 7, 10, and 15) may be one of the earliest genetic alterations in the transformation from normal urothelium to malignant urothelium, as evidenced by the fact that mutations in *FGFR3* have also been identified in urothelial papillomas.[172] Mutations are most commonly found in low grade and low stage tumors. Eight point mutations (missense) have been identified in urothelial carcinomas that cause substitutions in the extracellular, transmembrane, and/or cytoplasmic domains of the receptor.[172–175] Recent studies show that 74% of pTa tumors, 21% pT1 tumors, 16% of tumors >pT2, and 0% of carcinomas in situ harbor this mutation.[173,174,176] It has been reported that more than 40% of patients with urothelial carcinoma harbor mutations in *FGFR3* and that absence of this mutation in other tumor sites may indicate that *FGFR3* mutations are quite specific for urothelial tumors.

It is postulated that a mutation in *FGFR3* results in activation of the *RAS-MAPK* pathway; however, such activation has not been found in all *FGFR3*-mutated tumors.[177,178] Yet *RAS* mutations are associated with approximately 15% of bladder tumors. Mutations of *PIK3CA*, the α-catalytic subunit of PI3 kinase, is also been found to be associated with low grade and low stage tumors (but not as strongly associated as *FGFR3* mutations). Reports indicate that this mutation is demonstrable in approximately 20% of Ta tumors, and it coexists with *FGFR3* mutations in about 26% of such tumors. More studies are needed to clarify the relationships between *FGFR3* and other genetic abnormalities in the genesis and progression of bladder tumors.[179]

Real-time PCR detects *FGFR3* expression and other FGFR expressions in urothelium. Different isoforms of *FGFR3* have been identified. Most common of these are *FGFR3b* (which may inhibit FGF-stimulated proliferation) and *FGFR3c* (the mesenchymal isoform). In many tumors an isoform switch occurs between *FGFR3b* and *FGFR3c*, and this may indicate a possible autocrine or paracrine pathway that thereby stimulates *FGFR3* signaling in tumors.

Both *HRAS* (discussed below) and *FGFR3* mutations are found in approximately 30% and 70%, respectively, of low grade urothelial carcinoma, and this pattern may indicate that activation of the RTK-RAS pathway is responsible for the transformation of cells that occurs in low grade tumors.[178,180] However, to date, no investigation has found whether the two mutations can exist simultaneously within the same tumor.[180]

Point mutations of the *FGFR3* gene are present in up to 88% of low grade cancers, and these bear no relation to patient age or clinical status.[181,182] Remarkably, one report found that about 75% of papillomas also contain mutations, representing the first genetic defect found in urothelial papilloma.[181]

Epidermal Growth Factor Receptor

Epidermal growth factor receptor (EGFR) is a tyrosine kinase, similar to *FGFR3*. It is encoded by a protooncogene located on chromosome 7p13. EGFR is a transmembrane, growth-regulating 170-kDa glycoprotein. The extracellular domain represents the ligand-binding site and is a receptor for epidermal growth factor (EGF) and transforming growth factor α (TGFA). Binding of EGF to its receptor results in downregulation by endocytosis of the normal receptor and stimulation of tyrosine kinase.[183,184] Amplification of EGFR is identified in 5% of urothelial carcinomas with protein overexpression in 23% of tumors, which is associated with a poorer prognosis and more aggressive tumor behavior.[185,186] Failure of ubiquitination may explain the accumulation of cytoplasmic EGFR in some tumor cells.[186a] Some studies have indicated that EGFR is overexpressed in as many as 30% to 50% of invasive bladder cancers.[187] Currently, phase I trials are under way in patients with solid tumors, other than urothelial carcinomas, exploiting two sites of targeted therapy: monoclonal antibodies specifically directed against the extracellular domain of the receptor, and small molecule blockade of tyrosine kinase within the intracellular domain of the receptor. Gefitinib has been studied recently in lung cancers, and the resulting studies indicate that it inhibits DNA synthesis and decreases cell proliferation, especially in cancers that harbor mutations in EGFR1.[188–190] Overexpression of EGFR and *ERBB2* are associated with invasive tumors and a worse prognosis.[191,192]

EGFR is present in many cells, including the basal cell layer of normal urothelium.[193] Staining is predominantly membranous. EGFR immunoreactivity is present in about 50% of bladder cancers, with increased expression in stage T2 to T4 cancers (71% of cases).[194] Staining is most at the advancing edge of the invasive cancer.[194]

EGFR immunoreactivity correlates with bladder cancer recurrence, shorten time to recurrence, and shorten survival,[194,195] although there are some conflicting results.[196] The strong association between EGFR immunoreactivity and the proliferation index (using bromodeoxyuridine staining) in bladder cancer suggests that this receptor may be involved in tumor promotion and proliferation.[194] Furthermore, the combination of increased EGFR immunoreactivity with loss of blood group antigen and spontaneous expression of the T antigen suggests that defective glycosylation is involved in urothelial carcinogenesis and is associated with increasing stage.[197] EGFR immunoreactivity may be related to expression of c-jun oncoprotein.[198]

Vascular Endothelial Growth Factor

Vascular endothelial growth factor (VEGF) and, to a lesser extent, basic fibroblast growth factor (see below) are the primary inducers of angiogenesis in bladder cancer cells.[199] VEGF mRNA and protein levels are higher in cancer than in benign urothelium,[200,201] and high VEGF expression level predicts a poor prognosis.[202–204] However, urinary VEGF does not correlate with cancer stage, size, or grade.[203] An inhibitor of VEGF, thrombospondin 1, appears to play a key role in angiogenesis; its downregulation is associated with the switch from an antiangiogenic to an angiogenic phenotype which occurs early in urothelial carcinoma.[199]

Acidic Fibroblast Growth Factor

Acidic fibroblast growth factor is a monomeric 16-kDa protein originally purified from normal brain and widely distributed in normal human tissues.[194] It is present in most cases of urothelial carcinoma, and the intensity and frequency of immunoreactivity around tumor cell correlate with the grade and stage of the carcinoma.

Basic Fibroblast Growth Factor

Basic fibroblast growth factor is one of a family of nine fibroblast growth factors that all have a strong affinity for heparin and are functional ligands for FGFRs with have intrinsic tyrosine kinase activity. Basic fibroblast growth factor is present in the basal lamina of the normal urothelium, in normal muscle, and around blood vessels, but in only 13% of cases of urothelial carcinoma.[205] Basic fibroblast growth factor is a potent angiogenic factor and is an independent predictor of bladder tumor recurrence when present.[206]

Oncogenes

ERBB2 (HER2)

*ERBB*2 (*HER2*), found on 17q23,[186,207,208] encodes yet another protein receptor tyrosine kinase. As with breast cancers, urothelial carcinoma shows amplification of this protein. Immunohistochemical analysis shows that 37% to 50% of bladder cancers overexpress the HER2 protein, especially advanced-stage tumors (>pT2); consequently, the *ERBB*2 gene may be a potential future therapeutic target in bladder cancer.[209,210] Other studies have shown that *ERBB*2 overexpression occurs in 10% to 50% of invasive bladder cancers. *ERBB3* and *ERBB4* have also been linked to low grade noninvasive papillary tumors.[186,207,208,211]

The *HER2* protooncogene is present as a single-copy gene in normal cells, present on chromosome 17q12–21.32. It encodes a protein in the cytoplasmic membrane that has an external (*HER1*) component, a transmembrane component, and an internal (*HER2*) 185-kDa cytoplasmic component.[212] *HER2* has tyrosine kinase activity and is 85% homologous with EGFR.[212] The transmembrane segment is not as closely related to EGFR and the extracellular domain shares only 40% homology with EGFR.

HER2 immunoreactivity in urothelial carcinoma is usually present on the cell membrane,[193] although cytoplasmic reactivity has also been reported.[213] Stained cells are distributed diffusely, with no preference for superficial or basal cells of the tumor or normal urothelium. The frequency of HER2 protein expression varied from 2% to 65% in the normal and inflamed urothelium, and was present in 19% of cases of dysplasia and 64% of cases of

CIS.[214] Immunoreactivity increased with urothelial cancer stage[215] and recurrence,[140,196,212] although some reports found no correlation of *HER2* staining and outcome.[216,217] A recent report revealed that *HER2* expression independently predicts cancer-related survival.[218] A prospective study of patients with high grade muscle-invasive urothelial carcinoma treated by paclitaxel-based chemotherapy found *HER2* expression in 71% of high stage urothelial carcinomas. There was a lower risk of cancer death with *HER2* expression, suggesting a possible association between chemosensitivity and *HER2* expression.[219]

HRAS

Most investigators find *HRAS* mutations (causing constitutive activation) on codons 12, 13, and 61 in 30% to 40% of bladder cancers. Reported mutation rates vary from 0% to 84%. Transgenic mice studies have suggested that the *HRAS* oncogene could be associated with the transformation of benign urothelium to urothelial hyperplasia and subsequently to low grade noninvasive papillary tumors.[220–224] Currently available data in humans, however, do not support a straightforward association between *RAS* mutations and either superficial or invasive urothelial cancer.

The human *RAS* gene family, including *HRAS*, *KRAS*, and *NRAS*, is a prototype of cellular genes whose mutations or overexpression often lead to malignant transformation.[225] These genes encode a group of closely related 21-kDa proteins (p21). RAS p21 binds guanine nucleotides with high affinity and has guanosine triphosphatase activity. The protein is anchored to the cytoplasmic surface of the cell membrane and is a transducer for signals affecting cell proliferation.[225]

Two mechanisms may explain how *RAS* genes transform cells. One involves a single nucleotide mutation in codons 12, 13, 29, and 61, resulting in an amino acid substitution of the gene product *p21* that reduces the enzyme activity of the GTP binding domain. The second mechanism involves overexpression of the *RAS* gene product.

Mutations of *RAS* genes are the most frequent genetic alterations in urothelial cancer.[225] These mutations usually involve codon 12, and, less frequently, codon 13 or 61 of *HRAS*. Sporadically, the *KRAS* gene is also affected. The elimination of functional *HRAS* gene in human bladder cancer cell line T24 by an antisense oligonucleotide inhibited cell proliferation indicating that mutant *HRAS* is essential to the high proliferation of this tumor culture. *HRAS* mutations occur in about 50% of urinary bladder cancers.[226] G-T substitution in the second nucleotide of codon 12 of the *HRAS* gene results in replacement of glycine for valine in the gene product *p21* and is a dominant mutation in human bladder cancer.[227,228] *HRAS* gene codon 12 mutations occur more frequently in high grade aneuploid bladder carcinoma than in low grade diploid papillary carcinoma, but there is no definitive correlation with cancer grade or stage. Similar results have been obtained with *p21* by immunohistochemistry; *p21* overexpression correlates with DNA ploidy status, but not with grade and stage.[229] *c-HRAS* gene polymorphisms have been found in bladder cancer, but *c-HRAS* genotyping appears to be of limited value in the clinical management of patients.[230] *KRAS* mutations were observed in 29% of patients but their clinical significance has not been prospectively investigated.[231]

MDM2

The *MDM2* gene, located on chromosome 12q14, encodes an oncoprotein that interacts with p53 and causes degradation of the protein. *MDM2* cannot function as a degradation mechanism when there are contact mutations in *TP53*.

TP53 mutations may be either contact mutation, that prevent p53 from acting as a transcription factor for the *MDM2* gene, or structural mutations that cause nuclear aggregation due to protein unfolding. These unfolded p53 proteins may be seen in immunohistochemical imaging. Both of the *TP53* mutation mechanisms have been described in bladder cancers. Wild type p53 can activate the protooncogene nuclear protein *MDM2*.[103,232]

Overexpression of *MDM2* is inversely associated with high grade tumors.[233,234] This protein is increased in 67% of cases of noninvasive and early invasive (pT1) bladder cancer, but is present in only 27% of muscle-invasive carcinoma cases. Approximately 4% to 6% of all bladder cancers have amplification of *MDM2*, although some available data show no clear correlation between *MDM2* status and tumor grade or stage.[235–238]

MYC

Increase in *MYC/CCND1* copy number may occur prior to muscle invasion in bladder cancer[239] and is correlated with grade.[240] However, there is no correlation between MYC protein overexpression and *MYC* gene amplification indicating that expression controls may be effective even when multiple gene copies are present.[240] *MYC* copy gains, however, correlated with *TP53* deletions and DNA ploidy.[240] *MYC* is an independent predictor of progression-free and cancer-specific survival.[166]

Cyclin D1 and D3

Cyclin D1 is a nuclear protein encoded by the *CCND1* gene on chromosome 11q13 that has been identified as the *PRAD1* protooncogene and the most likely candidate for the *BCL1* protooncogene. It is a nuclear protein expressed early in the cell cycle of dividing cells. Cyclin D1 binds to cyclin-dependent kinases and displays specific and periodic expression during cell cycle progression, suggesting an important role in growth regulation. It interacts with pRB and other cell cycle-related proteins, such as PCNA and

p21. Benign and dysplastic urothelium, including inverted papilloma, do not express cyclin D1.[241]

Conflicting results have been obtained with immunohistochemical studies of cyclin D1 expression. One study identified nuclear cyclin D1 only in stage Ta and T1 papillary urothelial cancer, but not in invasive cancer or nonpapillary cancer. In some studies, there was a marked decline with cancer grade and progression.[139,241,242] There was an inverse correlation of cyclin D1 expression with PCNA and p53 expression, suggesting that cyclin D1 plays a role in negatively controlling cellular proliferation and allowing cancer differentiation. Conversely, other studies found no correlation of cyclin D1 expression with grade and stage, although cyclin D1 immunoreactive cancers recurred more rapidly than unreactive cancer.[243,244] Overexpression of cyclin D1 mRNA was found in 81% of nonmuscle invasive cancer and 38% of muscle-invasive cancer.[245] For comparison, about 10% to 15% of bladder cancer have amplification of the 11q13 region, so influences beside gene dose must contribute to the level of cyclin D1.[245] The cumulative results indicate that genetic alterations in cyclin D1 are probably early events in urothelial carcinogenesis. Some of the differences in outcome may result from polymorphisms of the cyclin D1 gene; the variant A allele was associated with increased risk of bladder cancer in Japanese patients.[246] The combination of low cyclin D1, low p27 (Kip1), and high Ki67 expression was most predictive of recurrence.[35]

More recently, cyclin D3 deregulation has been reported in bladder cancer.[247,248] Cyclin D3, another G1-S phase regulator, and tumor proliferation were investigated by immunohistochemistry and measured by the grid-counting method. To validate the immunohistochemical expression, cyclin D3 was also quantitated by Western blotting in selected cases. Cyclin D3 overexpression was related to larger tumor size (>5 cm; $P < 0.0001$) and high tumor proliferation (>10%; Ki67 labeling index; $P = 0.025$). Mean cyclin D3 expression levels increased with 2004 World Health Organization (WHO) grade for stage Ta ($P = 0.035$, ANOVA) and stage T1 ($P = 0.047$, t test) tumors. Cyclin D3 was not related to other clinicopathological parameters, G1-S phase modulators, or 9p21 LOH. Cox multivariate analysis selected cyclin D3 as an independent predictor of progression-free survival [$P = 0.0012$, relative risk (RR) = 5.2366] together with tumor size ($P = 0.0115$, RR = 4.4442) and cyclin D1 ($P = 0.0065$, RR = 3.3023). Cyclin D3 expression had the highest risk ratio.[247]

Cell Adhesion Markers

E-cadherin

E-cadherin is the epithelial member of the cadherin molecule family, a group of transmembrane glycoproteins of 80 kDa to 120 kDa molecular weight with 723 to 748 amino acids involved in intercellular adhesion. They have extracellular, membranous, and cytoplasmic domains, and the extracellular domain contains the binding site for calcium that protects the molecule from proteolysis.[249-251] The cytoplasmic domain forms complexes with catenins and cytoplasmic elements.

The normal human urothelium displays intense homogeneous immunohistochemical membranous staining at cell borders of E-cadherin in 88% of cells.[252-254] The luminal membrane of superficial cells is devoid of staining, as are parts of the cell in contact with the basement membrane. Staining was present in 93% of cells of CIS, 21% to 98% of low-stage cancers, and 45% to 76% of invasive cancers.[249,252,255]

The inverse correlation of E-cadherin expression with cancer stage indicates that it plays a role in invasion.[252,256] Expression of E-cadherin was identical in the primary cancer and lymph node metastases.[31] There was also a strong correlation between E-cadherin expression and survival; conversely, the presence of normal E-cadherin staining appeared to indicate a good prognosis, even if the cancer was high stage.[253,257,258] High ratio of matrix metalloproteinase 9 to E-cadherin expression correlated with microvessel density and predicted a poor prognosis.[258] Serum concentration of E-cadherin correlated with cancer grade, number of cancers at presentation, and cancer recurrence, but not with immunoreactivity in tissue sections.[259]

CpG hypermethylation plays a pivotal role in *E-cadherin* gene inactivation in cancer, with 63% to 84% of malignant cases showing methylation of the promoter region, compared with only 0% to 24% of benign urothelium.[260,261] Two sites, nucleotide (nt) 892 and nt 940, showed 100% methylation in all cancer samples.[260]

Integrins

The integrins are a family of adhesion molecules that are transmembrane heterodimers of noncovalently linked α and β subunits. There are at least eight different subfamilies of integrins, each with a common β subunit capable of combining with various α subunits. Integrins function as receptors for extracellular molecules, and can be segregated broadly into those that bind primarily to major constituents of the basement membrane (collagens and laminin), those that bind primarily to the extracellular matrix proteins (fibrinogen, fibronectin, and thrombospondin), and those that function as cell adhesion molecules (found primarily on lymphocytes).[262] Normal urothelium does not express α 1, α 4, or α 5 subunits, but shows cell membrane staining for α 2 and α 3 that is stronger in the basal cell layer than in luminal cells. There is progressive loss of α 2 β 1 expression and, to a lesser extent, α 3 β 1, in progression from Ta and T1 cancer to T2-3 cancer.[262] In normal urothelium, the

α 6 β 4 integrin colocalizes with type VII collagen at the junction of the basal cell and the lamina propria.[262] In noninvasive bladder cancers, integrin expression is present on the suprabasal and basal cells, type VII collagen remains bound at the hemidesmosomal basal cell anchoring complex. This finding suggests that the anchoring complex in low stage cancer is normal or only slightly altered, whereas in 83% of invasive cancers, loss of integrin or type VII collage, or loss of both, indicates attachment abnormalities.[262]

CD44

CD44 (PgP-1, ECM III, Hermes antigen) designates a family of cell surface glycoproteins involved in cell–cell and cell–matrix interactions present chiefly in epithelial cells.[263] The normal urothelium expresses CD44, but greater expression is present in early noninvasive papillary urothelial carcinoma, and there is progressive loss with greater invasion.[138,264-266] *CD44v* aberrant gene product overexpression correlated with invasive extent and cancer recurrence in a small series.[138] CD44 protein isoforms and mRNA species were also detectable in exfoliated cancer cells in urine specimens.[267-269] The ratio of CD44v8-10 to standard CD44 in urine samples predicts invasion and disease-free survival.[269] Soluble CD44 protein is detectable in serum, with lower levels in men having bladder cancer than in matched healthy controls.[270]

F and G Actin

Alterations in actin polymerization are linked to the phenotype of bladder cancer and may be useful as a marker of early invasion and progression.[88] Such alterations result from activation of oncogenic actin signaling pathways (e.g., *RAS* and *SRC*) or inactivation of actin-binding tumor suppressor proteins (e.g., E-cadherin, gelsolin, and others).

The amounts of the cytoskeletal proteins, F actin, and its precursor, G actin, are markers for decreased differentiation and risk for bladder cancer.[271,272] The differentiation-related changes occur early in carcinogenesis, and can be reversed in vitro by treatment with retinoid or other differentiation-promoting agents.[273]

Vessel Density

Microvessel Density

Angiogenesis is an essential component of cancer growth, and it is measured indirectly by counting the number of small blood vessels to create the microvessel density score (number of blood vessels per unit area).[206] All studies of microvessel density in bladder cancer to date have been retrospective, and comparison is often difficult, owing to differences in methods of microvessel density measurement, patient populations, and outcome variables.[206,274] Standards have recently been proposed to facilitate confirmation of the suggested predictive value of microvessel density in bladder cancer and other cancers.[275,276]

Lymph node metastases had microvessel density similar to that in the primary cancer.[31] Increased microvessel density in urothelial carcinoma was predictive of lymph node metastases,[277] recurrence, and poor survival.[278,279] This parameter appeared to be an independent prognostic factor.[258,278,279] Similar results were found in patients with schistosomiasis-associated adenocarcinoma of the bladder.[280] However, other reports found no correlation of microvessel density with recurrence or progression.[120]

Lymph Vessel Density

Lymph vessel density can be distinguished immunohistochemically using D2-40 antibody, a specific lymphatic endothelial cell marker.[281] Fernandez and colleagues performed a double immunostaining for D2-40 and the proliferation marker Ki67 in 108 patients with muscle-invasive bladder cancer.[282] Peritumoral vessels were observed in 97% of cases and intratumoural vessels in 60% of cases. Higher intratumoral lymph vessel density correlated significantly with poor histological differentiation. Higher peritumoral lymph vessel density was associated with lymph node metastasis. However, lymph vessel density had no impact on survival. These findings suggest that lymphangiogenesis may contribute to tumor dissemination and thus provide a potential target for bladder cancer therapy.[282]

Telomerase

The chromosome ends, referred to as telomeres, shorten progressively with each normal cell division, ultimately resulting in destruction of ability to duplicate the chromosome. Telomere shortening acts as a biologic clock to induce cell senescence and death, and is reversed by telomerase, a DNA polymerase that repairs the ends of chromosomes, thereby prolonging cell life and replicative potential. The presence or increased expression of telomerase has been implicated in the immortality and growth advantage of cancer cells in a variety of organs, including the urinary bladder.[283]

Benign urothelium displays little or no telomerase activity, whereas virtually every cancer expressed high levels, according to studies of tissue extracts.[284,285] An in situ hybridization assay confirmed these results recently in formalin-fixed paraffin-embedded tissues.[286]

The majority of urine samples with cancer cells contained telomerase activity, whereas most benign samples did not.[287–292] Analysis of telomerase activity in urine samples using PCR-based amplification in the Telomeric Repeat Amplification Protocol (TRAP) assay revealed a superior combination of sensitivity and specificity (74% to 84% and 69% to 93%, respectively) when compared with cytology.[292–294] However, comparison of the TRAP assay with the BTA *stat* test and NMP22 has yielded conflicting results.[295–297] A recent comparative analysis from one of the same centers revealed poor sensitivity (46%) and specificity (74%) compared to other markers.[298] Telomerase activity did not correlate with cancer stage, grade, multifocality, or cancer recurrence.[285,286]

Miscellaneous Markers

Multidrug Resistance Proteins

There is a significant correlation of P-glycoprotein/multidrug resistance 1 (MDR1) and multidrug resistance proteins 1 and 3 (MRP1 and MRP3, respectively) with resistance to doxorubicin in patients with bladder cancer.[299] The expression of these proteins in residual and recurrent cancer after treatment is much higher than in untreated primary tumors.

Cyclooxygenase 2

Cyclooxygenase 2 (COX2) enzyme expression is greater in urothelial carcinoma than in benign urothelium,[300–303] and the expression of COX2 correlates with the cancer grade.[301] The value of its determination as a marker of response to COX2 inhibitors remains unsettled.

Gelsolin

Gelsolin is a protein that surrounds actin cores in the organization of hemidesmosomes and has a function in the actin polymerization and remodeling of malignant cells.[62,63,304] The gelsolin gene (*GSN*) is located on chromosome 9q33, one of the most frequently deleted loci in urothelial carcinoma. Utilizing sequencing analysis, gene profiling, immunohistochemical analysis, and reversed-phase arrays of various samples of bladder cancers, investigators have shown that patients with low gelsolin expression had shorter survival times than those of patients who had higher levels of gelsolin expression. In fact, those patients that showed mutated *TP53* (vs. wild type *TP53*) also displayed lower levels of gelsolin expression, indicating a function for gelsolin as a possible tumor suppressor. These findings illustrate a strong potential for future therapeutic interventions and possible prevention through the targeting of specific actin signaling pathways.[62,63,304] The data suggest that actin alterations can be linked with bladder cancer development and progression, and specific patterns of remodeling may be associated with separate stages of bladder cancer.

Expression of the cytoskeletal protein gelsolin was decreased in CIS and bladder cancer compared with benign urothelium, and showed strong independent prediction of cancer recurrence and progression.[255]

Others

A variety of other markers have been evaluated in limited series. Autocrine motility factor receptor (*AMFR* or *gp78*) was not expressed by benign urothelium, whereas its expression in urothelial carcinoma was an independent predictor of outcome in patients treated surgically.[257] Expression of the surface glycoprotein luminal epithelial antigen (LEA.135) in immunohistochemical assays showed progressive loss with high grade and high stage cancer.[305] Androgen receptor, a member of the steroid hormone nuclear receptor superfamily, is expressed in the majority of urothelial carcinomas,[306] but not in benign urothelium.[307] Urokinase plasminogen activator is a serine protease whose expression was an independent predictor of survival in node-negative muscle-invasive bladder cancer,[308,309] but not in upper urinary tract carcinoma.[310] The fragile histidine triad (*FHIT*) gene on chromosome 3p14.2 was aberrantly expressed in most primary urothelial cancers.[311]

Estrogen receptors were detected in 12% of superficial bladder cancers, but were not predictive of survival.[312]

Altered expression of *TGFβ1* and its receptors is common in urothelial carcinoma, and overexpression of *TGFβ1* and *TGFβR1* was independently associated with progression and cancer-specific mortality.[313] In another study, *TGFβ1* expression was greater in benign urothelium and low grade tumors than in CIS and high grade tumors; together with interleukin 4, it may induce expression of tenascin-C around foci of stromal invasion.[314]

The glyoxalase enzymes detoxify cytotoxic methylglyoxal and have unchanged or increased expression in invasive bladder cancer compared with benign urothelium (glyoxalase I and glyoxalase II, respectively).[315] The *β3GNT2* member of the glycosyltransferase family is downregulated in invasive cancer compared with noninvasive cancer.[316] *FEZ1/LZTS1* tumor suppressor gene product was found in 37 of 60 primary bladder cancers by immunohistochemistry.[317] Expression of the protein product of the mitotic kinase-encoding gene *STK15/BTAK/*AuroraA was strongly associated with high grade, cancer invasion, and mortality.[318] Peroxisome proliferator-activated receptor gamma was expressed more commonly in papillary tumors than in solid tumors.[319] Tissue polypeptide-specific antigen was shown to correlate with cancer size, stage, and grade, with 95% specificity and

33% sensitivity for cancer diagnosis.[320] Low expression of thymidylate synthase, a critical enzyme in pyrimidine synthesis, and high expression of dihydropyrimidine dehydrogenase, an important pyrimidine salvage enzyme, predicted longer cancer-free survival after surgery.[321] Thymidine phosphorylase level was highest in high grade muscle-invasive cancer[322] and in those with recurrence.[323]

Urinary matrix metalloproteinase 1 (MMP1) correlated with cancer progression and mortality, whereas tissue inhibitor of metalloproteinase-a (TIMP1) did not[324]; however, another report found that patients with high TIMP1 expression had a poorer prognosis than those with low expression.[325] Proline-directed protein kinase F(A) was overexpressed in high grade and high stage urothelial carcinoma, and correlated with recurrence and mortality.[326] High clusterin mRNA expression independently predicted lower recurrence-free survival by multivariate analysis with multiple clinical and pathologic factors.[327] Osteonectin gene expression correlated with matrix metalloproteinase 2 expression and also with cancer grade, stage, and progression.[328] Ku protein is involved in DNA double-stranded break repair, and its expression is greatly increased in cancer compared with benign bladder tissue.[329]

Caveolin 1 immunoreactivity in bladder cancer correlated with grade but not with progression or survival.[330] Glycolipid *GM3* expression was inversely correlated with invasive potential of urothelial carcinoma.[331] Expression of hypoxia inducible factor (*HIF*) 2α/endothelial PAS domain protein 1 was observed in invasive cancer but not in superficial cancer.[332] Calcium-binding protein, S100A4, is more commonly expressed in invasive cancer and metastases, and predicts reduced survival.[333]

A novel gene found by comparison of mRNA expression profiles, (*BLCAP* or *BC10*), is found in noninvasive cancer but downregulated with invasion.[334] Cathepsin L is a cysteine protease that was elevated in urine samples with cancer invasion and high grade cancer; conversely, cathepsins B and H were not increased.[335] Glycosphingolipid sialosyl-Le(x) expression in bladder cancer was predictive of invasion and metastases; no other carbohydrate epitope had prognostic value.[336] MAGEA4 protein was more commonly expressed in squamous cell carcinoma than in adenocarcinoma, sarcomatoid carcinoma, small cell carcinoma, and urothelial carcinoma (46% vs. 27%, 29%, 25%, and 19%, respectively) and was predictive of decreased cancer-specific survival.[337] The 150-kDa oxygen-regulated protein, ORP150, was commonly expressed in bladder cancer, particularly in higher stages; its expression correlated with matrix metalloproteinase 2 expression.[338] A preliminary study of hepatoma upregulated protein (HURP) revealed a sensitivity for malignant versus benign urothelium in tissues of 89% and a specificity of 100%.[339] The authors suggested a potential use for this marker in urine screening to detect urothelial neoplasia.

Combined Biomarkers and Nomograms

Stratification of risk is a key component of decision making in clinical practice, with a variety of factors influencing selection of treatment for a given patient. The current tumor, lymph nodes, and metastases (TNM) staging system continues to be the standard determinant of bladder cancer prognosis after radical cystectomy. However, the heterogeneity of tumor biology and patient characteristics within each prognostic group result in significant variation of outcome within each staging category. Incorporation of molecular variables with the TNM classification might improve the risk prediction for patients.

A nomogram is a graphical representation of a mathematical formula or algorithm that incorporates several predictors, modeled as continuous variables, to predict a particular endpoint.[340] By incorporating all relevant continuous prognostic factors for individual patients, nomograms provide more accurate predictions than models based on risk grouping and generally surpass clinical experts at predicting outcomes.[341]

Molecular markers provide a promising approach for improving the predictive accuracy of current prognostic indices. Risk prediction may be more precise and reliable when several predictive variables are considered simultaneously. Multivariate nomograms, which facilitate the probability of event predictions at specific points after cystectomy, may provide incremental predictive accuracy.[342,343] Calculation of the probability of urothelial carcinoma recurrence risk progression, or metastasis utilizes the knowledge of clinical variables, pathological characteristics and the molecular alterations identified in the patient's tumor. Several postcystectomy nomograms have been developed to aid in predicting the natural outcome of surgically treated bladder cancers and to assist in deciding upon the use of adjuvant therapy after radical cystectomy.[343–349]

Shariat et al. showed that adding a panel of five cell cycle regulators, including p53, pRB, p21, p27, and cyclin E1, improved the predictive accuracy of competing risk nomograms for predicting bladder cancer recurrence and survival after radical cystectomy in a group of patients with pTa–pT3 node-negative urothelial carcinomas. The alteration of cell cycle regulators was detectable in 82% of patients, and 20% of patients had three and 16% had four or five altered biomarkers. Patients with three or more altered biomarkers had a four-ford to 10-fold higher risk of bladder cancer prognosis recurrence and mortality after radical cystectomy.[347]

In another study, Shariat et al. developed nomograms that accurately predicted disease recurrence and progression in patients with Ta, T1, or CIS urothelial carcinoma using a large international cohort.[345] Multivariate logistic regression models targeted histologically confirmed disease recurrence and focused on 2542 patients with bladder urothelial carcinoma from 10 participating centers, 957 with recurrent disease. The authors evaluated nuclear matrix protein 22 (NMP22) testing and traditional cytology, as well as patient age and gender. Tumor grade spanned grade 1 (24%), grade 2 (43%), and grade 3 (33%). Similarly, tumor stage included Ta (45%), T1 and/or CIS (32%), and T2 or greater (23%). The authors identified a bootstrap-corrected predictive accuracy for any urothelial carcinoma recurrence of 0.842. Similarly, values for grade 3 lesions (Ta/T1/CIS) and T2 or higher stage urothelial carcinoma (any grade) were 0.869 and 0.858, respectively. The study found excellent performance characteristics for the nomograms generated predicting urothelial carcinoma recurrence or grade 3 Ta/T1/CIS; however, the nomogram for T2 or higher stage urothelial carcinoma overestimated the probability of recurrence observed. Along these lines, nomograms incorporating traditional staging and predictive information with molecular features may ultimately be used to counsel patients regarding recurrence risks and aid in treatment selection.

Catto et al. have compared the predictive accuracies of neurofuzzy modeling (NFM), artificial neural networks (ANN), and traditional statistical methods, for the behavior of bladder cancer. The authors examined 109 patients with bladder cancer, utilizing p53 and mismatch repair proteins as molecular markers, as well as clinicopathologic information. For each of the methods, models were produced to predict the presence and timing of a tumor relapse. Both of the artificial intelligence methods studied predicted relapse, with an accuracy ranging from 88% to 95%, superior to regular statistical methods.[350]

Impact of Biomarkers on Pathologic Classification of Bladder Tumors

Many investigators have evaluated the associations between tumor mutations, including *FGFR3*, and disease progression and recurrence. However, the most recent data suggest that within Ta bladder tumors, mutation of *FGFR3* confers an increased risk of recurrence. Nevertheless, its presence or absence does not predict progression in any stage or grade of tumor.

A multicenter study evaluating bladder tumors for Ki67 immunostaining status and *FGFR3* mutation status resulted in the categorization of these tumors into three prognostic groups: molecular grade 1 (*FGFR3* mutation with a low Ki67 index), which had the best survival rate, molecular grade 2 (wild type *FGFR3* and low Ki67 index or mutant *FGFR3* and high Ki67 index with intermediate survival), and molecular grade 3 (wild type *FGFR3* and high Ki67 index), which was associated with poor survival.[351–356]

This study alludes to a future potential for classifying bladder tumors based on molecular makeup.

The advancements in molecular genetics of bladder neoplasms may support a future change to the currently proposed 2004 WHO grading system for bladder neoplasms.[357,358] As more is discovered about the molecular profiles of the various entities, perhaps a separate classification scheme, based on these findings, will eventually be used where the specialized testing is available. As many papillomas, papillary urothelial neoplasms of low malignant potential, and low grade papillary urothelial carcinomas show similar genetic profiles, this may eventually change the currently established definitions and once again reorganize the process of bladder tumor diagnosis.[357,358] Establishing the presence of LOH may play a major role in these definitions as well.

Future Perspectives

Considerable effort has been expended by numerous investigators in the search for molecular biomarkers that can reliably help to predict recurrence of bladder cancers. The recognition of two distinct pathways for urothelial carcinogenesis represents a major leap forward in the management of urothelial carcinoma, since this will facilitate the development of more specific novel therapeutic strategies. However, the processes of urothelial carcinogenesis, progression, recurrence, and metastasis may involve other molecular alterations yet to be discovered. At this time, there are no molecular biomarkers with proven utility in predicting recurrence, but several promising candidates have been identified. Bladder tumor recurrence may develop through transformation of cancer stem cells that remain in the shared field affected by global carcinogenetic influences. Improved definition of recurrence-related molecular pathways and genes will lead to new guidelines for clinical management and therapy of bladder urothelial neoplasia. Moreover, understanding the mechanisms underlying bladder urothelial transformation may lead to better prevention and early detection strategies.

REFERENCES

1. Jemal A, Siegel R, Xu J, Ward E. Cancer statistics, 2010. *CA Cancer J Clin* 2010;60:277–300.
2. Jemal A, Bray F, Center MM, Ferlay J, Ward E, Forman D. Global cancer statistics. *CA Cancer J Clin* 2011;61:69–90.
3. Cheng L, Lopez-Beltran A, MacLennan GT, Montironi R, Bostwick DG. Neoplasms of the urinary bladder. In: Bostwick DG, Cheng L, eds. Urologic Surgical Pathology, 2nd ed. Philadelphia: Elsevier/Mosby, 2008;259–352.
4. Eble JN, Sauter G, Epstein JI, Sesterhenn IA, eds. World Health Organization Classification of Tumours: Pathology and Genetics of Tumours of the Urinary System and Male Genital Organs. Lyon, France: IARC Press, 2004.
5. Kirkali Z, Chan T, Manoharan M, Algaba F, Busch C, Cheng L, Kiemeney L, Kriegmair M, Montironi R, Murphy WM, Sesterhenn IA, Tachibana M, Weider J. Bladder cancer: epidemiology, staging and grading, and diagnosis. *Urology* 2005;66:4–34.
6. Cheng L, Neumann RM, Weaver AL, Spotts BE, Bostwick DG. Predicting cancer progression in patients with stage T1 bladder carcinoma. *J Clin Oncol* 1999;17:3182–7.
7. Cheng L, Zhang S, Maclennan GT, Williamson SR, Lopez-Beltran A, Montironi R. Bladder cancer: translating molecular genetic insights into clinical practice. *Hum Pathol* 2011;42:455–81.
8. Soloway MS. Progression and survival in patients with T1G3 bladder tumors. *Urology* 2002;59:631.
9. Mhawech-Fauceglia P, Cheney RT, Schwaller J. Genetic alterations in urothelial bladder carcinoma: an updated review. *Cancer* 2006;106:1205–16.
10. Proctor I, Stoeber K, Williams GH. Biomarkers in bladder cancer. *Histopathology* 2010;57:1–13.
11. Mitra AP, Datar RH, Cote RJ. Molecular pathways in invasive bladder cancer: new insights into mechanisms, progression, and target identification. *J Clin Oncol* 2006;24:5552–64.
12. Dinney CP, McConkey DJ, Millikan RE, Wu X, Bar-Eli M, Adam L, Kamat AM, Siefker-Radtke AO, Tuziak T, Sabichi AL, Grossman HB, Benedict WF, Czerniak B. Focus on bladder cancer. *Cancer Cell* 2004;6:111–6.
13. Jacobs BL, Lee CT, Montie JE. Bladder cancer in 2010: How far have we come? *CA Cancer J Clin* 2010;60:244–72.
14. Raghavan D. Bladder cancer: optimal application of preclinical models to suitable translational questions. *Sci Transl Med* 2010;2:22ps11.
15. Blasco-Olaetxea E, Belloso L, Garcia-Tamayo J. Superficial bladder cancer: study of the proliferative nuclear fraction as a prognostic factor. *Eur J Cancer* 1996;32A:444–6.
16. Chen G, Lin MS, Li RC. Expression and prognostic value of proliferating cell nuclear antigen in transitional cell carcinoma of the urinary bladder. *Urol Res* 1997;25:25–30.

17. Cheng HL, Chow NH, Tzai TS, Tong YC, Lin JS, Chan SH, Yang WH, Chang CC, Lin YM. Prognostic significance of proliferating cell nuclear antigen expression in transitional cell carcinoma of the upper urinary tract. *Anticancer Res* 1997;17:2789–93.

18. Ogura K, Habuchi T, Yamada H, Ogawa O, Yoshida O. Immunohistochemical analysis of p53 and proliferating cell nuclear antigen (PCNA) in bladder cancer: positive immunostaining and radiosensitivity. *Int J Urol* 1995;2:302–8.

19. Shiina H, Igawa M, Nagami H, Yagi H, Urakami S, Yoneda T, Shirakawa H, Ishibe T, Kawanishi M. Immunohistochemical analysis of proliferating cell nuclear antigen, p53 protein and nm23 protein, and nuclear DNA content in transitional cell carcinoma of the bladder. *Cancer* 1996;78:1762–74.

20. Pantazopoulos D, Ioakim-Liossi A, Karakitsos P, Aroni K, Kakoliris S, Kanavaros P, Kyrkou KA. DNA content and proliferation activity in superficial transitional cell carcinoma of the bladder. *Anticancer Res* 1997;17:781–6.

21. Ogura K, Fukuzawa S, Habuchi T, Ogawa O, Yoshida O. Correlation of nuclear morphometry and immunostaining for p53 and proliferating cell nuclear antigen in transitional cell carcinoma of the bladder. *Int J Urol* 1997;4:561–6.

22. Bozlu M, Orhan D, Baltaci S, Yaman O, Elhan AH, Tulunay O, Muftuoglu YZ. The prognostic value of proliferating cell nuclear antigen, Ki–67 and nucleolar organizer region in transitional cell carcinoma of the bladder. *Int Urol Nephrol* 2002;33:59–66.

23. Chen L, Wang X, Mei H, et al. [Apoptosis and expression of PCNA in superficial transitional cell bladder cancer as related to recurrence]. *Zhonghua Wai Ke Za Zhi* 1998;36:484–6.

24. Okamura K, Miyake K, Koshikawa T, Asai J. Growth fractions of transitional cell carcinomas of the bladder defined by the monoclonal antibody Ki–67. *J Urol* 1990;144:875–8.

25. Busch C, Price P, Norton J, Parkins CS, Bailey MJ, Boyd J, Jones CR, A'Hern RP, Horwich A. Proliferation in human bladder carcinoma measured by Ki-67 antibody labelling: its potential clinical importance. *Br J Cancer* 1991;64:357–60.

26. Mulder AH, Van Hootegem JC, Sylvester R, ten Kate FJ, Kurth KH, Ooms EC, Van der Kwast TH. Prognostic factors in bladder carcinoma: histologic parameters and expression of a cell cycle-related nuclear antigen (Ki–67). *J Pathol* 1992;166:37–43.

27. Nakopoulou L, Vourlakou C, Zervas A, Tzonou A, Gakiopoulou H, Dimopoulos MA. The prevalence of bcl–2, p53, and Ki-67 immunoreactivity in transitional cell bladder carcinomas and their clinicopathologic correlates. *Hum Pathol* 1998;29:146–54.

28. Margulis V, Lotan Y, Karakiewicz PI, Fradet Y, Ashfaq R, Capitanio U, Montorsi F, Bastian PJ, Nielsen ME, Muller SC, Rigaud J, Heukamp LC, Netto G, Lerner SP, Sagalowsky AI, Shariat SF. Multi-institutional validation of the predictive value of Ki-67 labeling index in patients with urinary bladder cancer. *J Natl Cancer Inst* 2009;101:114–9.

29. Margulis V, Shariat SF, Ashfaq R, Sagalowsky AI, Lotan Y. Ki-67 is an independent predictor of bladder cancer outcome in patients treated with radical cystectomy for organ-confined disease. *Clin Cancer Res* 2006;12:7369–73.

30. Shariat SF, Youssef RF, Gupta A, Chade DC, Karakiewicz PI, Isbarn H, Jeldres C, Sagalowsky AI, Ashfaq R, Lotan Y. Association of angiogenesis related markers with bladder cancer outcomes and other molecular markers. *J Urol* 2010;183:1744–50.

31. Malmstrom PU, Ren ZP, Sherif A, de la Torre M, Wester K, Thorn M. Early metastatic progression of bladder carcinoma: molecular profile of primary tumor and sentinel lymph node. *J Urol* 2002;168:2240–4.

32. Fontana D, Bellina M, Gubetta L, Fasolis G, Rolle L, Scoffone C, Porpiglia F, Colombo M, Tarabuzzi R, Leonardo E. Monoclonal antibody Ki-67 in the study of the proliferative activity of bladder carcinoma. *J Urol* 1992;148:1149–51.

33. Stavropoulos NE, Ioackim-Velogianni E, Hastazeris K, Kitsiou E, Stefanaki S, Agnantis N. Growth fractions in bladder cancer defined by Ki67: association with cancer grade, category and recurrence rate of superficial lesions. *Br J Urol* 1993;72:736–9.

34. Asakura T, Takano Y, Iki M, Suwa Y, Noguchi S, Kubota Y, Masuda M. Prognostic value of Ki-67 for recurrence and progression of superficial bladder cancer. *J Urol* 1997;158:385–8.

35. Sgambato A, Migaldi M, Faraglia B, De Aloysio G, Ferrari P, Ardito R, De Gaetani C, Capelli G, Cittadini A, Trentini GP. Cyclin D1 expression in papillary superficial bladder cancer: its association with other cell cycle-associated proteins, cell proliferation and clinical outcome. *Int J Cancer* 2002;97:671–8.

36. Blanchet P, Droupy S, Eschwege P, Viellefond A, Paradis V, Pichon MF, Jardin A, Benoit G. Prospective evaluation of Ki-67 labeling in predicting the recurrence and progression of superficial bladder transitional cell carcinoma. *Eur Urol* 2001;40:169–75.

37. Liukkonen TJ, Lipponen PK, Helle M, Jauhiainen KE. Immunoreactivity of bcl-2, p53 and EGFr is associated with tumor stage, grade and cell proliferation in superficial bladder cancer. Finnbladder III Group. *Urol Res* 1997;25:1–7.

38. Pich A, Chiusa L, Formiconi A, Galliano D, Bortolin P, Navone R. Biologic differences between noninvasive papillary urothelial neoplasms of low malignant potential and low grade (grade 1) papillary carcinomas of the bladder. *Am J Surg Pathol* 2001;25:1528–33.

39. Blanes A, Rubio J, Martinez A, Wolfe HJ, Diaz-Cano SJ. Kinetic profiles by topographic compartments in muscle-invasive transitional cell carcinomas of the bladder: role of TP53 and NF1 genes. *Am J Clin Pathol* 2002;118:93–100.

40. Korkolopoulou P, Lazaris A, Konstantinidou AE, Kavantzas N, Patsouris E, Christodoulou P, Thomas-Tsagli E, Davaris P.

Differential expression of bcl-2 family proteins in bladder carcinomas. Relationship with apoptotic rate and survival. *Eur Urol* 2002;41:274–83.

41. Uchida T, Minei S, Gao JP, Wang C, Satoh T, Baba S. Clinical significance of p53, MDM2 and bcl-2 expression in transitional cell carcinoma of the bladder. *Oncol Rep* 2002;9:253–9.

42. Furihata M, Sonobe H, Ohtsuki Y, Yamashita M, Morioka M, Yamamoto A, Terao N, Kuwahara M, Fujisaki N. Detection of p53 and bcl-2 protein in carcinoma of the renal pelvis and ureter including dysplasia. *J Pathol* 1996;178:133–9.

43. Lipponen PK, Aaltomaa S, Eskelinen M. Expression of the apoptosis suppressing bcl-2 protein in transitional cell bladder tumours. *Histopathology* 1996;28:135–40.

44. Posch B, Haitel A, Pycha A, et al. Bcl-2 is a prognostic factor in advanced bladder cancer. *J Urol* 1998;159:246.

45. Asci R, Yildiz L, Sarikaya S, Buyukalpelli R, Yilmaz AF, Kandemir B. p53 and bcl-2 overexpression as associated risk factors in patients 40 years old or less with transitional cell carcinoma of the bladder. *Urol Int* 2001;67:34–40.

46. Ong F, Moonen LM, Gallee MP, ten Bosch C, Zerp SF, Hart AA, Bartelink H, Verheij M. Prognostic factors in transitional cell cancer of the bladder: an emerging role for Bcl-2 and p53. *Radiother Oncol* 2001;61:169–75.

47. Giannopoulou I, Nakopoulou L, Zervas A, Lazaris AC, Stravodimos C, Giannopoulos A, Davaris PS. Immunohistochemical study of pro-apoptotic factors Bax, Fas and CPP32 in urinary bladder cancer: prognostic implications. *Urol Res* 2002;30:342–5.

48. Shariat SF, Lotan Y, Saboorian H, Khoddami SM, Roehrborn CG, Slawin KM, Ashfaq R. Survivin expression is associated with features of biologically aggressive prostate carcinoma. *Cancer* 2004;100:751–7.

49. Karam JA, Lotan Y, Ashfaq R, Sagalowsky AI, Shariat SF. Survivin expression in patients with non-muscle-invasive urothelial cell carcinoma of the bladder. *Urology* 2007;70:482–6.

50. Chen YB, Tu JJ, Kao J, Zhou XK, Chen YT. Survivin as a useful adjunct marker for the grading of papillary urothelial carcinoma. *Arch Pathol Lab Med* 2008;132:224–31.

51. Shariat SF, Ashfaq R, Karakiewicz PI, Saeedi O, Sagalowsky AI, Lotan Y. Survivin expression is associated with bladder cancer presence, stage, progression, and mortality. *Cancer* 2007;109:1106–13.

52. Shariat SF, Karakiewicz PI, Godoy G, Karam JA, Ashfaq R, Fradet Y, Isbarn H, Montorsi F, Jeldres C, Bastian PJ, Nielsen ME, Muller SC, Sagalowsky AI, Lotan Y. Survivin as a prognostic marker for urothelial carcinoma of the bladder: a multicenter external validation study. *Clin Cancer Res* 2009;15:7012–9.

53. Skagias L, Politi E, Karameris A, Sambaziotis D, Archondakis A, Ntinis A, Moreas I, Vasou O, Koutselini H, Patsouris E. Survivin expression as a strong indicator of recurrence in urothelial bladder cancer. Predictive value of nuclear versus cytoplasmic staining. *Anticancer Res* 2009;29:4163–7.

54. Cheng L, Zhang D. Molecular Genetic Pathology. New York: Humana Press/Springer, 2008.

55. Xu X, Stower MJ, Reid IN, Garner RC, Burns PA. A hot spot for p53 mutation in transitional cell carcinoma of the bladder: clues to the etiology of bladder cancer. *Cancer Epidemiol Biomarkers Prev* 1997;6:611–6.

56. Soulitzis N, Sourvinos G, Dokianakis DN, Spandidos DA. p53 codon 72 polymorphism and its association with bladder cancer. *Cancer Lett* 2002;179:175–8.

57. Toruner GA, Ucar A, Tez M, Cetinkaya M, Ozen H, Ozcelik T. P53 codon 72 polymorphism in bladder cancer—no evidence of association with increased risk or invasiveness. *Urol Res* 2001;29:393–5.

58. Miyamoto H, Shuin T, Ikeda I, Hosaka M, Kubota Y. Loss of heterozygosity at the p53, RB, DCC and APC tumor suppressor gene loci in human bladder cancer. *J Urol* 1996;155:1444–7.

59. Cordon-Cardo C, Dalbagni G, Saez GT, Oliva MR, Zhang ZF, Rosai J,

Reuter VE, Pellicer A. p53 mutations in human bladder cancer: genotypic versus phenotypic patterns. *Int J Cancer* 1994;56:347–53.

60. Dalbagni G, Cordon-Cardo C, Reuter V, Fair WR. Tumor suppressor gene alterations in bladder carcinoma. Translational correlates to clinical practice. *Surg Oncol Clin N Am* 1995;4:231–40.

61. Schulz WA. Understanding urothelial carcinoma through cancer pathways. *Int J Cancer* 2006;119:1513–8.

62. Sanchez-Carbayo M, Socci ND, Lozano JJ, Haab BB, Cordon-Cardo C. Profiling bladder cancer using targeted antibody arrays. *Am J Pathol* 2006;168:93–103.

63. Sanchez-Carbayo M, Socci ND, Lozano J, Saint F, Cordon-Cardo C. Defining molecular profiles of poor outcome in patients with invasive bladder cancer using oligonucleotide microarrays. *J Clin Oncol* 2006;24:778–89.

64. LaRue H, Simoneau M, Fradet Y. Human papillomavirus in transitional cell carcinoma of the urinary bladder. *Clin Cancer Res* 1995;1:435–40.

65. Simoneau M, LaRue H, Fradet Y. Low frequency of human papillomavirus infection in initial papillary bladder tumors. *Urol Res* 1999;27:180–4.

66. Shibutani YF, Schoenberg MP, Carpiniello VL, Malloy TR. Human papillomavirus associated with bladder cancer. *Urology* 1992;40:15–7.

67. Lopez-Beltran A, Carrasco-Aznar JC, Reymundo C, et al. Bladder cancer survival in human papillomavirus infection. Immunohistochemistry and in-situ hybridization. In: Olsson CA, ed. Oncogenes and Molecular Genetics of Urological Tumours. London: Churchill Livingstone, 1992.

68. Lopez-Beltran A, Munoz E. Transitional cell carcinoma of the bladder: low incidence of human papillomavirus DNA detected by the polymerase chain reaction and in situ hybridization. *Histopathology* 1995;26:565–9.

69. Lopez-Beltran A, Escudero AL, Carrasco-Aznar JC, Vicioso-Recio L. Human papillomavirus infection and transitional cell carcinoma of the bladder. Immunohistochemistry and in situ hybridization. *Pathol Res Pract* 1996;192:154–9.

70. Lopez-Beltran A, Escudero AL, Vicioso L, Munoz E, Carrasco JC. Human papillomavirus DNA as a factor determining the survival of bladder cancer patients. *Br J Cancer* 1996;73:124–7.

71. Lopez-Beltran A, Escudero AL. Human papillomavirus and bladder cancer. *Biomed Pharmacother* 1997;51:252–7.

72. LaRue H, Simoneau M, Fradet Y. Human papillomavirus in transitional cell carcinoma of the urinary bladder. *Clin Cancer Res* 1995;1:435–40.

73. Hopman AH, Kamps MA, Speel EJ, Schapers RF, Sauter G, Ramaekers FC. Identification of chromosome 9 alterations and p53 accumulation in isolated carcinoma in situ of the urinary bladder versus carcinoma in situ associated with carcinoma. *Am J Pathol* 2002;161:1119–25.

74. Zhang ZF, Sarkis AS, Cordon-Cardo C, Dalbagni G, Melamed J, Aprikian A, Pollack D, Sheinfeld J, Herr HW, Fair WR, Reuter VE, Begg C. Tobacco smoking, occupation, and p53 nuclear overexpression in early stage bladder cancer. *Cancer Epidemiol Biomarkers Prev* 1994;3:19–24.

75. Esrig D, Elmajian D, Groshen S, Freeman JA, Stein JP, Chen SC, Nichols PW, Skinner DG, Jones PA, Cote RJ. Accumulation of nuclear p53 and tumor progression in bladder cancer. *N Engl J Med* 1994;331:1259–64.

76. Burkhard FC, Markwalder R, Thalmann GN, Studer UE. Immunohistochemical determination of p53 overexpression. An easy and readily available method to identify progression in superficial bladder cancer? *Urol Res* 1997;25:S31–5.

77. Caliskan M, Turkeri LN, Mansuroglu B, Toktas G, Aksoy B, Unluer E, Akdas A. Nuclear accumulation of mutant p53 protein: a possible predictor of failure of intravesical therapy in bladder cancer. *Br J Urol* 1997;79:373–7.

78. Sinik Z, Alkibay T, Ataoglu O, Akyol G, Tokucoglu H, Bozkirli I. Correlation of nuclear p53 overexpression with clinical and histopathological features of transitional cell bladder cancer. *Int Urol Nephrol* 1997;29:25–31.

79. Vatne V, Maartmann-Moe H, Hoestmark J. The prognostic value of p53 in superficially infiltrating transitional cell carcinoma. *Scand J Urol Nephrol* 1995;29:491–5.

80. Casetta G, Gontero P, Russo R, Pacchioni D, Tizzani A. p53 expression compared with other prognostic factors in OMS grade-I stage-Ta transitional cell carcinoma of the bladder. *Eur Urol* 1997;32:229–36.

81. Gardiner RA, Walsh MD, Allen V, Rahman S, Samaratunga ML, Seymour GJ, Lavin MF. Immunohistological expression of p53 in primary pT1 transitional cell bladder cancer in relation to tumour progression. *Br J Urol* 1994;73:526–32.

82. Cordon-Cardo C, Zhang ZF, Dalbagni G, Drobnjak M, Charytonowicz E, Hu SX, Xu HJ, Reuter VE, Benedict WF. Cooperative effects of p53 and pRB alterations in primary superficial bladder tumors. *Cancer Res* 1997;57:1217–21.

83. Raitanen MP, Tammela TL, Kallioinen M, Isola J. P53 accumulation, deoxyribonucleic acid ploidy and progression of bladder cancer. *J Urol* 1997;157:1250–3.

84. Friedrich M, Erbersdobler A, Schwalbold H, et al. Detection of loss of heterozygosity (LOH) in the p53-gene among bladder cancer patients in tumor and urinary sediment using a simple polymerase chain reaction (PCR) technique. *J Urol* 1998;159:280.

85. Sachs M, Schlechte HH, Lenk SV, et al. TP 53—Genetic analysis shows monoclonality of primary and recurrent tumor of the urinary bladder. *J Urol* 1998;159:279.

86. Dahse R, Utting M, Werner W, Schimmel B, Claussen U, Junker K. TP53 alterations as a potential diagnostic marker in superficial bladder carcinoma and in patients serum, plasma and urine samples. *Int J Oncol* 2002;20:107–15.

87. Cote RJ, Esrig D, Groshen S, Jones PA, Skinner DG. p53 and treatment of bladder cancer [letter; comment]. *Nature* 1997;385:123–5.

88. Rao J. Targeting actin remodeling profiles for the detection and management of urothelial cancers—a perspective for bladder cancer research. *Front Biosci* 2002;7:e1–8.

89. Lu M, Wikman F, Orntoft TF, Charytonowicz E, Rabbani F, Zhang Z, Dalbagni G, Pohar KS, Yu G, Cordon-Cardo C. Impact of alterations affecting the p53 pathway in bladder cancer on clinical outcome, assessed by conventional and array-based methods. *Clin Cancer Res* 2002;8:171–9.

90. Orntoft TF, Wolf H. Molecular alterations in bladder cancer. *Urol Res* 1998;26:223–33.

91. Stein JP, Ginsberg DA, Grossfeld GD, Chatterjee SJ, Esrig D, Dickinson MG, Groshen S, Taylor CR, Jones PA, Skinner DG, Cote RJ. Effect of p21WAF1/CIP1 expression on tumor progression in bladder cancer. *J Natl Cancer Inst* 1998;90:1072–9.

92. Cordon-Cardo C, Dalbagni G, Saez GT, Oliva MR, Zhang ZF, Rosai J, Reuter VE, Pellicer A. p53 mutations in human bladder cancer: genotypic versus phenotypic patterns. *Int J Cancer* 1994;56:347–53.

93. Lebret T, Becette V, Barbagelatta M, Herve JM, Gaudez F, Barre P, Lugagne PM, Botto H. Correlation between p53 over expression and response to bacillus Calmette-Guérin therapy in a high risk select population of patients with T1G3 bladder cancer. *J Urol* 1998;159:788–91.

94. Pages F, Flam TA, Vieillefond A, Molinie V, Abeille X, Lazar V, Bressac-de Paillerets B, Mosseri V, Zerbib M, Fridman WH, Debre B, Thiounn N. p53 status does not predict initial clinical response to bacillus Calmette-Guérin intravesical therapy in T1 bladder tumors. *J Urol* 1998;159:1079–84.

95. Dalbagni G, Presti JC Jr, Reuter VE, Zhang ZF, Sarkis AS, Fair WR, Cordon-Cardo C. Molecular genetic alterations of chromosome 17 and p53 nuclear overexpression in human bladder cancer. *Diagn Mol Pathol* 1993;2:4–13.

96. Lipponen PK. Over-expression of p53 nuclear oncoprotein in transitional-cell bladder cancer and its prognostic value. *Int J Cancer* 1993;53:365–70.

97. Miyamoto H, Kubota Y, Shuin T, Torigoe S, Hosaka M, Iwasaki Y, Danenberg K, Danenberg PV. Analyses of p53 gene mutations in primary human bladder cancer. *Oncol Res* 1993;5:245–9.

98. Oyasu R, Nan L, Szumel RC, Kawamata H, Hirohashi S. p53 gene mutations in human urothelial carcinomas: analysis by immunohistochemistry and single-strand conformation polymorphism. *Mod Pathol* 1995;8:170–6.

99. Inagaki T, Ebisuno S, Uekado Y, Hirano A, Hiroi A, Shinka T, Ohkawa T. PCNA and p53 in urinary bladder cancer: correlation with histological findings and prognosis. *Int J Urol* 1997;4:172–7.

100. Nakopoulou L, Constantinides C, Papandropoulos J, Theodoropoulos G, Tzonou A, Giannopoulos A, Zervas A, Dimopoulos C. Evaluation of overexpression of p53 tumor suppressor protein in superficial and invasive transitional cell bladder cancer: comparison with DNA ploidy. *Urology* 1995;46:334–40.

101. al-Abadi H, Nagel R, Neuhaus P. Immunohistochemical detection of p53 protein in transitional cell carcinoma of the bladder in correlation to DNA ploidy and pathohistological stage and grade. *Cancer Detect Prev* 1998;22:43–50.

102. Pfister C, Flaman JM, Martin C, Grise P, Frebourg T. Selective detection of inactivating mutations of the tumor suppressor gene p53 in bladder tumors. *J Urol* 1999;161:1973–5.

103. Schmitz-Drager BJ, Kushima M, Goebell P, Jax TW, Gerharz CD, Bultel H, Schulz WA, Ebert T, Ackermann R. p53 and MDM2 in the development and progression of bladder cancer. *Eur Urol* 1997;32:487–93.

104. Lerner SP, Benedict WF, Green A, et al. Molecular staging and prognosis following radical cystectomy using p53 and retinoblastoma protein expression. *J Urol* 1998;159:165.

105. Llopis J, Alcaraz A, Ribal MJ, Solé M, Ventura PJ, Barranco MA, Rodriguez A, Corral JM, Carretero P. p53 expression predicts progression and poor survival in T1 bladder tumours. *Eur Urol* 2000;37:644–53.

106. Jankevicius F, Goebell P, Kushima M, Schulz WA, Ackermann R, Schmitz-Drager BJ. p21 and p53 immunostaining and survival following systemic chemotherapy for urothelial cancer. *Urol Int* 2002;69:174–80.

107. Ikegami S, Yoshimura I, Tsuji A, Seta K, Kimura F, Odajima K, Asano T, Hayakawa M. [Immunohistochemical study of p53 and Ki-67 overexpression in grade 3 superficial bladder tumor in relationship to tumor recurrence and prognosis]. *Nippon Hinyokika Gakkai Zasshi* 2001;92:656–65.

108. Sarkis AS, Bajorin DF, Reuter VE, Herr HW, Netto G, Zhang ZF, Schultz PK, Cordon-Cardo C, Scher HI. Prognostic value of p53 nuclear overexpression in patients with invasive bladder cancer treated with neoadjuvant MVAC. *J Clin Oncol* 1995;13:1384–90.

109. Uchida T, Wada C, Ishida H, Wang C, Egawa S, Yokoyama E, Kameya T, Koshiba K. p53 mutations and prognosis in bladder tumors. *J Urol* 1995;153:1097–104.

110. Tsuji M, Kojima K, Murakami Y, Kanayama H, Kagawa S. Prognostic value of Ki-67 antigen and p53 protein in urinary bladder cancer: immunohistochemical analysis of radical cystectomy specimens. *Br J Urol* 1997;79:367–72.

111. Rotterud R, Skomedal H, Berner A, Danielsen HE, Skovlund E, Fossa SD. TP53 and p21WAF1/CIP1 behave differently in euploid versus aneuploid bladder tumours treated with radiotherapy. *Acta Oncol* 2001;40:644–52.

112. Fujimoto K, Yamada Y, Okajima E, Kakizoe T, Sasaki H, Sugimura T, Terada M. Frequent association of p53 gene mutation in invasive bladder cancer. *Cancer Res* 1992;52:1393–8.

113. Vet JA, Debruyne FM, Schalken JA. Molecular prognostic factors in bladder cancer. *World J Urol* 1994;12:84–8.

114. Vollmer RT, Humphrey PA, Swanson PE, Wick MR, Hudson ML. Invasion of the bladder by transitional cell carcinoma: its relation to histologic grade and expression of p53, MIB-1, c-erb B-2, epidermal growth factor receptor, and bcl-2. *Cancer* 1998;82:715–23.

115. Sarkis AS, Dalbagni G, Cordon-Cardo C, Zhang ZF, Sheinfeld J, Fair WR, Herr HW, Reuter VE. Nuclear overexpression of p53 protein in transitional cell bladder carcinoma: a marker for disease progression. *J Natl Cancer Inst* 1993;85:53–9.

116. Sarkis AS, Dalbagni G, Cordon-Cardo C, Melamed J, Zhang ZF, Sheinfeld J, Fair WR, Herr HW, Reuter VE. Association of p53 nuclear overexpression and tumor progression in carcinoma in situ of the bladder. *J Urol* 1994;152:388–92.

117. Caterino M, Finocchi V, Giunta S, De Carli P, Crecco M. Bladder cancer within a direct inguinal hernia: CT demonstration. *Abdom Imaging* 2001;26:664–6.

118. Peyromaure M, Weibing S, Sebe P, Verpillat P, Toublanc M, Dauge MC, Boccon-Gibod L, Ravery V. Prognostic value of p53 overexpression in T1G3 bladder tumors treated with bacillus Calmette-Guérin therapy. *Urology* 2002;59:409–13.

119. Tiguert R, Bianco FJ Jr, Oskanian P, Li Y, Grignon DJ, Wood DP Jr, Pontes JE, Sarkar FH. Structural alteration of p53 protein in patients with muscle invasive bladder transitional cell carcinoma. *J Urol* 2001;166:2155–60.

120. Reiher F, Ozer O, Pins M, Jovanovic BD, Eggener S, Campbell SC. p53 and microvessel density in primary resection specimens of superficial bladder cancer. *J Urol* 2002;167:1469–74.

121. Watanabe R, Tomita Y, Nishiyama T, Tanikawa T, Sato S. Correlation of p53 protein expression in human urothelial transitional cell cancers with malignant potential and patient survival. *Int J Urol* 1994;1:43–8.

122. Terrell RB, Cheville JC, See WA, Cohen MB. Histopathological features and p53 nuclear protein staining as predictors of survival and tumor recurrence in patients with transitional cell carcinoma of the renal pelvis. *J Urol* 1995;154:1342–7.

123. Glick SH, Howell LP, White RW. Relationship of p53 and bcl-2 to prognosis in muscle-invasive transitional cell carcinoma of the bladder. *J Urol* 1996;155:1754–7.

124. Schmitz-Drager BJ, van Roeyen CR, Grimm MO, Gerharz CD, Decken K, Schulz WA, Bultel H, Makri D, Ebert T, Ackermann R. p53 accumulation in precursor lesions and early stages of bladder cancer. *World J Urol* 1994;12:79–83.

125. Spruck CH 3rd, Ohneseit PF, Gonzalez-Zulueta M, Esrig D, Miyao N, Tsai YC, Lerner SP, Schmutte C, Yang AS, Cote R, Dubeau L, Nichols PW, Hermann GG, Steven K, Horn T, Skinner DG, Jones PA. Two molecular pathways to transitional cell carcinoma of the bladder. *Cancer Res* 1994;54:784–8.

126. Hodges KB, Lopez-Beltran A, Davidson DD, Montironi R, Cheng L. Urothelial dysplasia and other flat lesions of the urinary bladder: clinicopathologic and molecular features. *Hum Pathol* 2010;41:155–62.

127. Schulte PA. The role of genetic factors in bladder cancer. *Cancer Detect Prev* 1988;11:379–88.

128. Sidransky D, Von Eschenbach A, Tsai YC, Jones P, Summerhayes I, Marshall F, Paul M, Green P, Hamilton SR, Frost P, Vogelstein B. Identification of p53 gene mutations in bladder cancers and urine samples. *Science* 1991;252:706–9.

129. Vet JA, Witjes JA, Marras SA, Hessels D, van der Poel HG, Debruyne FM, Schalken JA. Predictive value of p53 mutations analyzed in bladder washings for progression of high-risk superficial bladder cancer. *Clin Cancer Res* 1996;2:1055–61.

130. Lu ML, Wikman F, Orntoft TF, Charytonowicz E, Rabbani F, Zhang Z, Dalbagni G, Pohar KS, Yu G, Cordon-Cardo C. Impact of alterations affecting the p53 pathway in bladder cancer on clinical outcome, assessed by conventional and array-based methods. *Clin Cancer Res* 2002;8:171–9.

131. Patard JJ, Brasseur F, Gil-Diez S, Radvanyi F, Marchand M, Francois P, Abi-Aad A, Van Cangh P, Abbou CC, Chopin D, et al. Expression of MAGE genes in transitional-cell carcinomas of the urinary bladder. *Int J Cancer* 1995;64:60–4.

132. Kinzler KW, Vogelstein B. Life (and death) in a malignant tumour. *Nature* 1996;379:19–20.

133. Qureshi KN, Griffiths TR, Robinson MC, Marsh C, Roberts JT, Lunec J, Neal DE, Mellon JK. Combined p21WAF1/CIP1 and p53 overexpression predict improved survival in muscle-invasive bladder cancer treated by radical radiotherapy. *Int J Radiat Oncol Biol Phys* 2001;51:1234–40.

134. Gonzalez-Zulueta M, Shibata A, Ohneseit PF, Spruck CH 3rd, Busch C, Shamaa M, El-Baz M, Nichols PW, Gonzalgo ML. High frequency of chromosome 9p allelic loss and CDKN2 tumor suppressor gene alterations in squamous cell carcinoma of the bladder. *J Natl Cancer Inst* 1995;87:1383–93.

135. Orlow I, Lacombe L, Hannon GJ, Serrano M, Pellicer I, Dalbagni G, Reuter VE, Zhang ZF, Beach D, Cordon-Cardo C. Deletion of the p16 and p15 genes in human bladder tumors. *J Natl Cancer Inst* 1995;87:1524–9.

136. Warren W, Biggs PJ, el-Baz M, Ghoneim MA, Stratton MR, Venitt S. Mutations in the p53 gene in schistosomal bladder cancer: a study of 92 tumours from Egyptian patients and a comparison between mutational spectra from schistosomal and non-schistosomal urothelial tumours. *Carcinogenesis* 1995;16:1181–9.

137. Nakopoulou LL, Constandinides CA, Tzonou A, Lazaris AC, Zervas A, Dimopoulos CA. Immunohistochemical evaluation of nm23-H1 gene product in transitional cell carcinoma of the bladder. *Histopathology* 1996;28:429–35.

138. Li B, Li Y, Dai Q, Zhu J, Jia J. [CD44v and nm23-H1 gene product expression and its clinical significance in human recurrent bladder cancer]. *Zhonghua Wai Ke Za Zhi* 1998;36:312–3.

139. Yang CC, Chu KC, Chen HY, Chen WC. Expression of p16 and cyclin D1 in bladder cancer and correlation in cancer progression. *Urol Int* 2002;69:190–4.

140. Wang C, Liu X, Wang L, Chen D, Tan Z, Wang Z, Chen T. [p16, p53 and c-erbB-2 gene expression in bladder carcinoma]. *Zhonghua Bing Li Xue Za Zhi* 2000;29:20–3.

141. Friedrich MG, Blind C, Milde-Langosch K, Erbersdobler A, Conrad S, Loning T, Hammerer P, Huland H. Frequent p16/MTS1 inactivation in early stages of urothelial carcinoma of the bladder is not associated with tumor recurrence. *Eur Urol* 2001;40:518–24.

142. Primdahl H, von der Maase H, Sorensen FB, Wolf H, Orntoft TF. Immunohistochemical study of the expression of cell cycle regulating proteins at different stages of bladder cancer. *J Cancer Res Clin Oncol* 2002;128:295–301.

143. Le Frere-Belda MA, Cappellen D, Daher A, Gil-Diez-de-Medina S, Besse F, Abbou CC, Thiery JP, Zafrani ES, Chopin DK, Radvanyi F. p15(INK4b) in bladder carcinomas: decreased expression in superficial tumours. *Br J Cancer* 2001;85:1515–21.

144. Cordon-Cardo C, Wartinger D, Petrylak D, Dalbagni G, Fair WR, Fuks Z, Reuter VE. Altered expression of the retinoblastoma gene product: prognostic indicator in bladder cancer. *J Natl Cancer Inst* 1992;84:1251–6.

145. Benedict WF, Lerner SP, Zhou J, Shen X, Tokunaga H, Czerniak B. Level of retinoblastoma protein expression correlates with p16 (MTS-1/INK4A/CDKN2) status in bladder cancer. *Oncogene* 1999;18:1197–203.

146. Cote RJ, Dunn MD, Chatterjee SJ, Stein JP, Shi SR, Tran QC, Hu SX, Xu HJ, Groshen S, Taylor CR, Skinner DG, Benedict WF. Elevated and absent pRb expression is associated with bladder cancer progression and has cooperative effects with p53. *Cancer Res* 1998;58:1090–4.

147. Grossman HB, Liebert M, Antelo M, Dinney CP, Hu SX, Palmer JL, Benedict WF. p53 and RB expression predict progression in T1 bladder cancer. *Clin Cancer Res* 1998;4:829–34.

148. Oeggerli M, Tomovska S, Schraml P, Calvano-Forte D, Schafroth S, Simon R, Gasser T, Mihatsch MJ, Sauter G. E2F3 amplification and overexpression is associated with invasive tumor growth and rapid tumor cell proliferation in urinary bladder cancer. *Oncogene* 2004;23:5616–23.

149. Ishikawa J, Xu HJ, Hu SX, Yandell DW, Maeda S, Kamidono S, Benedict WF, Takahashi R. Inactivation of the retinoblastoma gene in human bladder and renal cell carcinomas. *Cancer Res* 1991;51:5736–43.

150. Kubota Y, Miyamoto H, Noguchi S, Shuin T, Kitamura H, Xu HJ, Hu SX, Benedict WF. The loss of retinoblastoma gene in association with c-myc and transforming growth factor-beta 1 gene expression in human bladder cancer. *J Urol* 1995;154:371–4.

151. Goodrich DW, Chen Y, Scully P, Lee WH. Expression of the retinoblastoma gene product in bladder carcinoma cells associates with a low frequency of tumor formation. *Cancer Res* 1992;52:1968–73.

152. Lipponen PK, Liukkonen TJ. Reduced expression of retinoblastoma (Rb) gene protein is related to cell proliferation and prognosis in transitional-cell bladder cancer. *J Cancer Res Clin Oncol* 1995;121:44–50.

153. Wright C, Thomas D, Mellon K, Neal DE, Horne CH. Expression of retinoblastoma gene product and p53 protein in bladder carcinoma: correlation with Ki67 index. *Br J Urol* 1995;75:173–9.

154. Primdahl H, von der Maase H, Christensen M, Wolf H, Orntoft TF. Allelic deletions of Rb and L-myc in urine sediments from patients with bladder tumors or carcinoma in situ. *Oncol Rep* 2002;9:551–5.

155. Knowles MA, Habuchi T, Kennedy W, Cuthbert-Heavens D. Mutation spectrum of the 9q34 tuberous sclerosis gene TSC1 in transitional cell carcinoma of the bladder. *Cancer Res* 2003;63:7652–6.

156. Edwards J, Duncan P, Going JJ, Watters AD, Grigor KM, Bartlett JM. Identification of loci associated with putative recurrence genes in transitional cell carcinoma of the urinary bladder. *J Pathol* 2002;196:380–5.

157. Hornigold N, Devlin J, Davies AM, Aveyard JS, Habuchi T, Knowles MA. Mutation of the 9q34 gene TSC1 in sporadic bladder cancer. *Oncogene* 1999;18:2657–61.

158. Platt FM, Hurst CD, Taylor CF, Gregory WM, Harnden P, Knowles MA. Spectrum of phosphatidylinositol 3-kinase pathway gene alterations in bladder cancer. *Clin Cancer Res* 2009;15:6008–17.

159. Wada T, Louhelainen J, Hemminki K, Adolfsson J, Wijkstrom H, Norming U, Borgstrom E, Hansson J, Steineck G. The prevalence of loss of heterozygosity in chromosome 3, including FHIT, in bladder cancer, using the fluorescent multiplex polymerase chain reaction. *BJU Int* 2001;87:876–81.

160. Baffa R, Gomella LG, Vecchione A, Bassi P, Mimori K, Sedor J, Calviello CM, Gardiman M, Minimo C, Strup SE, McCue PA, Kovatich AJ, Pagano F, Huebner K, Croce CM. Loss of FHIT expression in transitional cell carcinoma of the urinary bladder. *Am J Pathol* 2000;156:419–24.

161. Skopelitou AS, Gloustianou G, Bai M, Huebner K. FHIT gene expression in human urinary bladder transitional cell carcinomas. In Vivo 2001;15:169–73.

162. Aveyard JS, Skilleter A, Habuchi T, Knowles MA. Somatic mutation of PTEN in bladder carcinoma. *Br J Cancer* 1999;80:904–8.

163. Cappellen D, Gil Diez de Medina S, Chopin D, Thiery JP, Radvanyi F. Frequent loss of heterozygosity on chromosome 10q in muscle-invasive transitional cell carcinomas of the bladder. *Oncogene* 1997;14:3059–66.

164. Kagan J, Liu J, Stein JD, Wagner SS, Babkowski R, Grossman BH, Katz RL. Cluster of allele losses within a 2.5 cM region of chromosome 10 in high grade invasive bladder cancer. *Oncogene* 1998;16:909–13.

165. Tsuruta H, Kishimoto H, Sasaki T, Horie Y, Natsui M, Shibata Y, Hamada K, Yajima N, Kawahara K, Sasaki M, Tsuchiya N, Enomoto K, Mak TW, Nakano T, Habuchi T, Suzuki A. Hyperplasia and carcinomas in Pten-deficient mice and reduced PTEN protein in human bladder cancer patients. *Cancer Res* 2006;66:8389–96.

166. Schultz L, Albadine R, Hicks J, Jadallah S, DeMarzo AM, Chen YB, Neilsen ME, Gonzalgo ML, Sidransky D, Schoenberg M, Netto GJ. Expression status and prognostic significance of mammalian target of rapamycin pathway members in urothelial carcinoma of urinary bladder after cystectomy. *Cancer* 2010;116:5517–26.

167. Han KS, Jeong IG, Joung JY, Yang SO, Chung J, Seo HK, Kwon KS, Park WS, Lee KH. Clinical value of PTEN in patients with superficial bladder cancer. *Urol Int* 2008;80:264–9.

168. Urist MJ, Di Como CJ, Lu ML, Charytonowicz E, Verbel D, Crum CP, Ince TA, McKeon FD, Cordon-Cardo C. Loss of p63 expression is associated with tumor progression in bladder cancer. *Am J Pathol* 2002;161:1199–206.

169. Wilkie AO, Patey SJ, Kan SH, van den Ouweland AM, Hamel BC. FGFs, their receptors, and human limb malformations: clinical and molecular correlations. *Am J Med Genet* 2002;112:266–78.

170. Johnson DE, Williams LT. Structural and functional diversity in the FGF receptor multigene family. *Adv Cancer Res* 1993;60:1–41.

171. Passos-Bueno MR, Wilcox WR, Jabs EW, Sertie AL, Alonso LG, Kitoh H. Clinical spectrum of fibroblast growth factor receptor mutations. *Hum Mutat* 1999;14:115–25.

172. van Rhijn BW, Montironi R, Zwarthoff EC, Jobsis AC, van der Kwast TH. Frequent *FGFR3* mutations in urothelial papilloma. *J Pathol* 2002;198:245–51.

173. Bakkar AA, Wallerand H, Radvanyi F, Lahaye J-B, Pissard S, Lecerf L, Kouyoumdjian JC, Abbou CC, Pairon JC, Jourand MC, Thiery JP, Chopin DK, Gil Diez de Medina S. *FGFR3* and *TP53* gene mutations define two

distinct pathways in urothelial cell carcinoma of the bladder. *Cancer Res* 2003;63:8108–12.

174. Rieger-Christ KM, Mourtzinos A, Lee PJ, Zagha RM, Cain J, Silverman M, Libertino JA, Summerhayes IC. Identification of fibroblast growth factor receptor 3 mutations in urine sediment DNA samples complements cytology in bladder tumor detection. *Cancer* 2003;98:737–44.

175. Cappellen D, De Oliveira C, Ricol D, Gil Diez de Medina S, Bourdin J, Sastre-Garau X, Chopin D, Thiery JP, Radvanyi F. Frequent activating mutations of *FGFR3* in human bladder and cervix carcinomas. *Nat Genet* 1999;23:18–20.

176. van Rhijn BW, van der Kwast TH, Vis AN, Kirkels WJ, Boeve ER, Jobsis AC, Zwarthoff EC. *FGFR3* and p53 characterize alternative genetic pathways in the pathogenesis of urothelial cell carcinoma. *Cancer Res* 2004;64:1911–4.

177. Hart KC, Robertson SC, Kanemitsu MY, Meyer AN, Tynan JA, Donoghue DJ. Transformation and Stat activation by derivatives of FGFR1, FGFR3, and FGFR4. *Oncogene* 2000;19:3309–20.

178. Jebar AH, Hurst CD, Tomlinson DC, Johnston C, Taylor CF, Knowles MA. *FGFR3* and Ras gene mutations are mutually exclusive genetic events in urothelial cell carcinoma. *Oncogene* 2005;24:5218–25.

179. Lopez-Knowles E, Hernandez S, Malats N, Kogevinas M, Lloreta J, Carrato A, Tardon A, Serra C, Real FX. PIK3CA mutations are an early genetic alteration associated with *FGFR3* mutations in superficial papillary bladder tumors. *Cancer Res* 2006;66:7401–4.

180. Wu XR. Urothelial tumorigenesis: a tale of divergent pathways. *Nat Rev Cancer* 2005;5:713–25.

181. van Rhijn BW, Montironi R, Zwarthoff EC, Jobsis AC, Van Der Kwast TH. Frequent *FGFR3* mutations in urothelial papilloma. *J Pathol* 2002;198:245–51.

182. Kimura T, Suzuki H, Ohashi T, Asano K, Kiyota H, Eto Y. The incidence of thanatophoric dysplasia mutations in *FGFR3* gene is higher in low grade or superficial bladder carcinomas. *Cancer* 2001;92:2555–61.

183. Nakanishi K, Kawai T, Suzuki M, Torikata C. Growth factors and oncogene products in transitional cell carcinoma. *Mod Pathol* 1996;9:292–7.

184. Cheng L, Zhang S, Alexander R, Yao Y, MacLennan GT, Pan CX, Huang J, Wang M, Montironi R, Lopez-Beltran A. The landscape of EGFR pathways and personalized management of non-small-cell lung cancer. *Future Oncol* 2011;7:519–41.

185. Yarden Y, Sliwkowski MX. Untangling the ErbB signalling network. *Nat Rev Mol Cell Biol* 2001;2:127–37.

186. Chow NH, Chan SH, Tzai TS, Ho CL, Liu HS. Expression profiles of ErbB family receptors and prognosis in primary transitional cell carcinoma of the urinary bladder. *Clin Cancer Res* 2001;7:1957–62.

186a. Mizuno E, Iura T, Mukai A, Yoshimori T, Kitamura N, Komada M. Regulation of epidermal growth factor receptor down-regulation by UBPY–mediated deubiquitination at endosomes. *Mol Biol Cell* 2005;16:5163–74.

187. Neal DE, Sharples L, Smith K, Fennelly J, Hall RR, Harris AL. The epidermal growth factor receptor and the prognosis of bladder cancer. *Cancer* 1990;65:1619–25.

188. Janmaat ML, Giaccone G. The epidermal growth factor receptor pathway and its inhibition as anticancer therapy. *Drugs Today (Barc)* 2003;39 Suppl C:61–80.

189. Lynch TJ, Bell DW, Sordella R, Gurubhagavatula S, Okimoto RA, Brannigan BW, Harris PL, Haserlat SM, Supko JG, Haluska FG, Louis DN, Christiani DC, Settleman J, Haber DA. Activating mutations in the epidermal growth factor receptor underlying responsiveness of non-small-cell lung cancer to gefitinib. *N Engl J Med* 2004;350:2129–39.

190. Sordella R, Bell DW, Haber DA, Settleman J. Gefitinib-sensitizing EGFR mutations in lung cancer activate anti-apoptotic pathways. *Science* 2004;305:1163–7.

191. Messing EM. Growth factors and bladder cancer: clinical implications of the interactions between growth factors and their urothelial receptors. *Semin Surg Oncol* 1992;8:285–92.

192. Coogan CL, Estrada CR, Kapur S, Bloom KJ. HER-2/neu protein overexpression and gene amplification in human transitional cell carcinoma of the bladder. *Urology* 2004;63:786–90.

193. Gorgoulis VG, Barbatis C, Poulias I, Karameris AM. Molecular and immunohistochemical evaluation of epidermal growth factor receptor and c-erb-B-2 gene product in transitional cell carcinomas of the urinary bladder: a study in Greek patients. *Mod Pathol* 1995;8:758–64.

194. Sauter G, Haley J, Chew K, Kerschmann R, Moore D, Carroll P, Moch H, Gudat F, Mihatsch MJ, Waldman F. Epidermal-growth-factor-receptor expression is associated with rapid tumor proliferation in bladder cancer. *Int J Cancer* 1994;57:508–14.

195. Turkeri LN, Erton ML, Cevik I, Akdas A. Impact of the expression of epidermal growth factor, transforming growth factor alpha, and epidermal growth factor receptor on the prognosis of superficial bladder cancer. *Urology* 1998;51:645–9.

196. Ravery V, Grignon D, Angulo J, Pontes E, Montie J, Crissman J, Chopin D. Evaluation of epidermal growth factor receptor, transforming growth factor alpha, epidermal growth factor and c-erbB2 in the progression of invasive bladder cancer. *Urol Res* 1997;25:9–17.

197. Pinnock CB, Roxby DJ, Ross JM, Pozza CH, Marshall VR. Ploidy and Tn-antigen expression in the detection of transitional cell neoplasia in non-tumour-bearing patients. *Br J Urol* 1995;75:461–9.

198. Tiniakos DG, Mellon K, Anderson JJ, Robinson MC, Neal DE, Horne CH. c-jun oncogene expression in transitional cell carcinoma of the urinary bladder. *Br J Urol* 1994;74:757–61.

199. Campbell SC, Volpert OV, Ivanovich M, Bouck NP. Molecular mediators of angiogenesis in bladder cancer. *Cancer Res* 1998;58:1298–1304.

200. Brown LF, Berse B, Jackman RW, Tognazzi K, Manseau EJ, Dvorak HF, Senger DR. Increased expression of vascular permeability factor (vascular endothelial growth factor) and its receptors in kidney and bladder carcinomas. *Am J Pathol* 1993;143:1255–62.

201. Wang S, Xia T, Zhang Z, Kong X, Zeng L, Mi P, Xue Z. [Expression of VEGF and tumor angiogenesis in bladder cancer]. *Zhonghua Wai Ke Za Zhi* 2000;38:34–6.

202. Crew JP, O'Brien T, Bradburn M, Fuggle S, Bicknell R, Cranston D, Harris AL. Vascular endothelial growth factor is a predictor of relapse and stage progression in superficial bladder cancer. *Cancer Res* 1997;57:5281–5.

203. Jeon SH, Lee SJ, Chang SG. Clinical significance of urinary vascular endothelial growth factor in patients with superficial bladder tumors. *Oncol Rep* 2001;8:1265–7.

204. Turner KJ, Crew JP, Wykoff CC, Watson PH, Poulsom R, Pastorek J, Ratcliffe PJ, Cranston D, Harris AL. The hypoxia-inducible genes VEGF and CA9 are differentially regulated in superficial vs invasive bladder cancer. *Br J Cancer* 2002;86:1276–82.

205. O'Brien T, Cranston D, Fuggle S, Bicknell R, Harris AL. Two mechanisms of basic fibroblast growth factor-induced angiogenesis in bladder cancer. *Cancer Res* 1997;57:136–40.

206. Shariat SF, Youssef RF, Gupta A, Chade DC, Karakiewicz PI, Isbarn H, Jeldres C, Sagalowsky AI, Ashfaq R, Lotan Y. Association of angiogenesis related markers with bladder cancer outcomes and other molecular markers. *J Urol* 2010;183:1744–50.

207. Coombs LM, Pigott DA, Sweeney E, Proctor AJ, Eydmann ME, Parkinson C, Knowles MA. Amplification and over-expression of c-erbB-2 in transitional cell carcinoma of the urinary bladder. *Br J Cancer* 1991;63:601–8.

208. Sauter G, Moch H, Moore D, Carroll P, Kerschmann R, Chew K, Mihatsch MJ, Gudat F, Waldman F. Heterogeneity of erbB-2 gene amplification in bladder cancer. *Cancer Res* 1993;53:2199–2203.

209. Kruger S, Weitsch G, Buttner H, Matthiensen A, Bohmer T, Marquardt T, Sayk F, Feller AC, Bohle A. HER2 overexpression in muscle-invasive urothelial carcinoma of the bladder: prognostic implications. *Int J Cancer* 2002;102:514–8.

210. Ohta JI, Miyoshi Y, Uemura H, Fujinami K, Mikata K, Hosaka M, Tokita Y, Kubota Y. Fluorescence in situ hybridization evaluation of c-erbB-2 gene amplification and chromosomal anomalies in bladder cancer. *Clin Cancer Res* 2001;7:2463–7.

211. Gardiner RA, Samaratunga ML, Walsh MD, Seymour GJ, Lavin MF. An immunohistological demonstration of c-erbB-2 oncoprotein expression in primary urothelial bladder cancer. *Urol Res* 1992;20:117–20.

212. Mellon JK, Lunec J, Wright C, Horne CH, Kelly P, Neal DE. C-erbB-2 in bladder cancer: molecular biology, correlation with epidermal growth factor receptors and prognostic value. *J Urol* 1996;155:321–6.

213. Tetu B, Fradet Y, Allard P, Veilleux C, Roberge N, Bernard P. Prevalence and clinical significance of HER/2neu, p53 and Rb expression in primary superficial bladder cancer. *J Urol* 1996;155:1784–8.

214. Underwood M, Bartlett J, Reeves J, Gardiner DS, Scott R, Cooke T. C-erbB-2 gene amplification: a molecular marker in recurrent bladder tumors? *Cancer Res* 1995;55:2422–30.

215. Wester K, Sjostrom A, de la Torre M, Carlsson J, Malmstrom PU. HER-2—a possible target for therapy of metastatic urinary bladder carcinoma. *Acta Oncol* 2002;41:282–8.

216. Moch H, Sauter G, Mihatsch MJ, Gudat F, Epper R, Waldman FM. p53 but not erbB-2 expression is associated with rapid tumor proliferation in urinary bladder cancer. *Hum Pathol* 1994;25:1346–51.

217. Wang L, Habuchi T, Takahashi T, Kamoto T, Zuo T, Mitsumori K, Tsuchiya N, Sato K, Ogawa O, Kato T. No association between HER-2 gene polymorphism at codon 655 and a risk of bladder cancer. *Int J Cancer* 2002;97:787–90.

218. Kruger S, Weitsch G, Buttner H, Matthiensen A, Bohmer T, Marquardt T, Sayk F, Feller AC, Bohle A. Overexpression of c-erbB-2 oncoprotein in muscle-invasive bladder carcinoma: relationship with gene amplification, clinicopathological parameters and prognostic outcome. *Int J Oncol* 2002;21:981–7.

219. Gandour-Edwards R, Lara PN Jr, Folkins AK, LaSalle JM, Beckett L, Li Y, Meyers FJ, DeVere-White R. Does HER2/neu expression provide prognostic information in patients with advanced urothelial carcinoma? *Cancer* 2002;95:1009–15.

220. Czerniak B, Cohen GL, Etkind P, Deitch D, Simmons H, Herz F, Koss LG. Concurrent mutations of coding and regulatory sequences of the Ha-ras gene in urinary bladder carcinomas. *Hum Pathol* 1992;23:1199–1204.

221. Fitzgerald JM, Ramchurren N, Rieger K, Levesque P, Silverman M, Libertino JA, Summerhayes IC. Identification of H-ras mutations in urine sediments complements cytology in the detection of bladder tumors. *J Natl Cancer Inst* 1995;87:129–33.

222. Knowles MA, Williamson M. Mutation of H-ras is infrequent in bladder cancer: confirmation by single-strand conformation polymorphism analysis, designed restriction fragment length polymorphisms, and direct sequencing. *Cancer Res* 1993;53:133–9.

223. Buyru N, Tigli H, Ozcan F, Dalay N. Ras oncogene mutations in urine sediments of patients with bladder cancer. *J Biochem Mol Biol* 2003;36:399–402.

224. Mo L, Zheng X, Huang HY, Shapiro E, Lepor H, Cordon-Cardo C, Sun TT, Wu XR. Hyperactivation of Ha-ras oncogene, but not Ink4a/Arf deficiency, triggers bladder tumorigenesis. *J Clin Invest* 2007;117:314–25.

225. Barbacid M. ras genes. *Annu Rev Biochem* 1987;56:779–827.

226. Knowles MA, Williamson M. Mutation of H-ras is infrequent in bladder cancer: confirmation by single-strand conformation polymorphism analysis, designed restriction fragment length polymorphisms, and direct sequencing. *Cancer Res* 1993;53:133–9.

227. Czerniak B, Cohen GL, Etkind P, Deitch D, Simmons H, Herz F, Koss LG. Concurrent mutations of coding and regulatory sequences of the Ha-ras gene in urinary bladder carcinomas. *Hum Pathol* 1992;23:1199–204.

228. Cerutti P, Hussain P, Pourzand C, Aguilar F. Mutagenesis of the H-ras protooncogene and the p53 tumor suppressor gene. *Cancer Res* 1994;54:1934s–8s.

229. Olsson CA, ed. Oncogenes and Molecular Genetics of Urological Tumours London: Churchill Livingstone, 1992.

230. Bittard H, Descotes F, Billerey C, Lamy B, Adessi GR. A genotype study of the c-Ha-ras-1 locus in human bladder tumors. *J Urol* 1996;155:1083–8.

231. Ayan S, Gokce G, Kilicarslan H, Ozdemir O, Yildiz E, Gultekin EY. K-RAS mutation in transitional cell carcinoma of urinary bladder. *Int Urol Nephrol* 2001;33:363–7.

232. Lianes P, Orlow I, Zhang ZF, Oliva MR, Sarkis AS, Reuter VE, Cordon-Cardo C. Altered patterns of MDM2 and *TP53* expression in human bladder cancer [see comments]. *J Natl Cancer Inst* 1994;86:1325–30.

233. Korkolopoulou P, Christodoulou P, Kapralos P, Exarchakos M, Bisbiroula A, Hadjiyannakis M, Georgountzos C, Thomas-Tsagli E. The role of p53, MDM2 and c-erb B-2 oncoproteins, epidermal growth factor receptor and proliferation markers in the prognosis of urinary bladder cancer. *Pathol Res Pract* 1997;193:767–75.

234. Simon R, Struckmann K, Schraml P, Wagner U, Forster T, Moch H, Fijan A, Bruderer J, Wilber K, Mihatsch MJ, Gasser T, Sauter G. Amplification pattern of 12q13-q15 genes (MDM2, CDK4, GLI) in urinary bladder cancer. *Oncogene* 2002;21:2476–83.

235. Habuchi T, Kinoshita H, Yamada H, Kakehi Y, Ogawa O, Wu WJ, Takahashi R, Sugiyama T, Yoshida O. Oncogene amplification in urothelial cancers with p53 gene mutation or MDM2 amplification. *J Natl Cancer Inst* 1994;86:1331–5.

236. Schmitz-Drager BJ, Kushima M, Goebell P, Jax TW, Gerharz CD, Bultel H, Schulz WA, Ebert T, Ackermann R. p53 and MDM2 in the development and progression of bladder cancer. *Eur Urol* 1997;32:487–93.

237. Pfister C, Moore L, Allard P, Larue H, Lacombe L, Tetu B, Meyer F, Fradet Y. Predictive value of cell cycle markers p53, MDM2, p21, and Ki-67 in superficial bladder tumor recurrence. *Clin Cancer Res* 1999;5:4079–84.

238. Tuna B, Yorukoglu K, Tuzel E, Guray M, Mungan U, Kirkali Z. Expression of p53 and mdm2 and their significance in recurrence of superficial bladder cancer. *Path Res Pract* 2003;199:323–8.

239. Watters AD, Latif Z, Forsyth A, Dunn I, Underwood MA, Grigor KM, Bartlett JM. Genetic aberrations of c-myc and CCND1 in the development of invasive bladder cancer. *Br J Cancer* 2002;87:654–8.

240. Mahdy E, Pan Y, Wang N, Malmstrom PU, Ekman P, Bergerheim U. Chromosome 8 numerical aberration and C-MYC copy number gain in bladder cancer are linked to stage and grade. *Anticancer Res* 2001;21:3167–73.

241. Lee CC, Yamamoto S, Morimura K, Wanibuchi H, Nishisaka N, Ikemoto S, Nakatani T, Wada S, Kishimoto T, Fukushima S. Significance of cyclin D1 overexpression in transitional cell carcinomas of the urinary bladder and its correlation with histopathologic features. *Cancer* 1997;79:780–9.

242. Tut VM, Braithwaite KL, Angus B, et al. Cyclin D1 expression in transitional cell carcinoma (TCC) of the bladder. Correlation with WAF1, P53 and Ki67. *J Urol* 1998;159:281.

243. Proctor AJ, Coombs LM, Cairns JP, Knowles MA. Amplification at chromosome 11q13 in transitional cell tumours of the bladder. *Oncogene* 1991;6:789–95.

244. Shin KY, Kong G, Kim WS, Lee TY, Woo YN, Lee JD. Overexpression of cyclin D1 correlates with early recurrence in superficial bladder cancers. *Br J Cancer* 1997;75:1788–92.

245. Bringuier PP, Tamimi Y, Schuuring E, Schalken J. Expression of cyclin D1 and EMS1 in bladder tumours; relationship with chromosome 11q13 amplification. *Oncogene* 1996;12:1747–53.

246. Wang L, Habuchi T, Takahashi T, Mitsumori K, Kamoto T, Kakehi Y, Kakinuma H, Sato K, Nakamura A, Ogawa O, Kato T. Cyclin D1 gene polymorphism is associated with an increased risk of urinary bladder cancer. *Carcinogenesis* 2002;23:257–64.

247. Lopez-Beltran A, Requena MJ, Luque RJ, Alvarez-Kindelan J, Quintero A, Blanca AM, Rodriguez ME, Siendones E, Montironi R. Cyclin D3 expression in primary Ta/T1 bladder cancer. *J Pathol* 2006;209:106–13.

248. Lopez-Beltran A, Ordonez JL, Otero AP, Blanca A, Sevillano V, Sanchez-Carbayo M, Munoz E, Cheng L, Montironi R, de Alava E. Cyclin D3 gene amplification in bladder carcinoma in situ. *Virchows Arch* 2010;457:555–61.

249. Lipponen PK, Eskelinen MJ. Reduced expression of E-cadherin is related to invasive disease and frequent recurrence in bladder cancer. *J Cancer Res Clin Oncol* 1995;121:303–8.

250. Cheng L, Nagabhushan M, Pretlow TP, Amini SB, Pretlow TG. E-cadherin expression in primary and metastatic prostate cancer. *Am J Pathol* 1996;148:1375–80.

251. Shariat SF, Pahlavan S, Baseman AG, Brown RM, Green AE, Wheeler TM, Lerner SP. E-cadherin expression predicts clinical outcome in carcinoma in situ of the urinary bladder. *Urology* 2001;57:60–5.

252. Sun W, Herrera GA. E-cadherin expression in urothelial carcinoma in situ, superficial papillary transitional cell carcinoma, and invasive transitional cell carcinoma. *Hum Pathol* 2002;33:996–1000.

253. Ross JS, del Rosario AD, Figge HL, Sheehan C, Fisher HA, Bui HX. E-cadherin expression in papillary

transitional cell carcinoma of the urinary bladder. *Hum Pathol* 1995;26:940–4.

254. Ross JS, Cheung C, Sheehan C, del Rosario AD, Bui HX, Fisher HA. E-cadherin cell-adhesion molecule expression as a diagnostic adjunct in urothelial cytology. *Diagn Cytopathol* 1996;14:310–5.

255. Rao J, Seligson D, Visapaa H, Horvath S, Eeva M, Michel K, Pantuck A, Bekkdegrun A, Palotie A. Tissue microarray analysis of cytoskeletal actin-associated biomarkers gelsolin and E-cadherin in urothelial carcinoma. *Cancer* 2002;95:1247–57.

256. Wakatsuki S, Watanabe R, Saito K, Saito T, Katagiri A, Sato S, Tomita Y. Loss of human E-cadherin (ECD) correlated with invasiveness of transitional cell cancer in the renal pelvis, ureter and urinary bladder. *Cancer Lett* 1996;103:11–7.

257. Otto T, Bex A, Schmidt U, Raz A, Rubben H. Improved prognosis assessment for patients with bladder carcinoma. *Am J Pathol* 1997;150:1919–23.

258. Inoue K, Kamada M, Slaton JW, Fukata S, Yoshikawa C, Tamboli P, Dinney CP, Shuin T. The prognostic value of angiogenesis and metastases-related genes for progression of transitional cell carcinoma of thre renal pelvis and ureter. *Clin Cancer Res* 2002;8:1863–70.

259. Griffiths TR, Brotherick I, Bishop RI, White MD, McKenna DM, Horne CH, Shenton BK, Neal DE, Mellon JK. Cell adhesion molecules in bladder cancer: soluble serum E-cadherin correlates with predictors of recurrence. *Br J Cancer* 1996;74:579–84.

260. Ribeiro-Filho LA, Franks J, Sasaki M, Shiina H, Nojima D, Arap S, Carroll P, Enokida H, Nakagawa M, Yonezawa S, Dahiya R. CpG hypermethylation of promoter region and inactivation of E-cadherin gene in human bladder cancer. *Mol Carcinog* 2002;34:187–98.

261. Chan MW, Chan LW, Tang NL, Tong JH, Lo KW, Lee TL, Cheung HY, Wong WS, Chan PS, Lai FM, To KF. Hypermethylation of multiple genes in tumor tissues and voided urine in

urinary bladder cancer patients. *Clin Cancer Res* 2002;8:464–70.

262. Liebert M, Washington R, Wedemeyer G, Carey TE, Grossman HB. Loss of co-localization of alpha 6 beta 4 integrin and collagen VII in bladder cancer. *Am J Pathol* 1994;144:787–95.

263. Cohen MB, Griebling TL, Ahaghotu CA, Rokhlin OW, Ross JS. Cellular adhesion molecules in urologic malignancies. *Am J Clin Pathol* 1997;107:56–63.

264. Sugino T, Gorham H, Yoshida K, Bolodeoku J, Nargund V, Cranston D, Goodison S, Tarin D. Progressive loss of CD44 gene expression in invasive bladder cancer. *Am J Pathol* 1996;149:873–82.

265. Ross JS, del Rosario AD, Bui HX, Kallakury BV, Okby NT, Figge J. Expression of the CD44 cell adhesion molecule in urinary bladder transitional cell carcinoma. *Mod Pathol* 1996;9:854–60.

266. Stavropoulos NE, Filliadis I, Ioachim E, Michael M, Mermiga E, Hastazeris K, Nseyo UO. CD44 standard form expression as a predictor of progression in high risk superficial bladder tumors. *Int Urol Nephrol* 2001;33:479–83.

267. Sugiyama M, Woodman A, Sugino T, Crowley S, Ho K, Smith J, Matsumura Y, Tarin D. Non-invasive detection of bladder cancer by identification of abnormal CD44 proteins in exfoliated cancer cells in urine. *Clin Mol Pathol* 1995;48:M142–7.

268. Muller M, Heicappell R, Habermann F, Kaufmann M, Steiner U, Miller K. Expression of CD44V2 in transitional cell carcinoma of the urinary bladder and in urine. *Urol Res* 1997;25:187–92.

269. Miyake H, Eto H, Arakawa S, Kamidono S, Hara I. Over expression of CD44V8-10 in urinary exfoliated cells as an independent prognostic predictor in patients with urothelial cancer. *J Urol* 2002;167:1282–7.

270. Lein M, Jung K, Weiss S, Schnorr D, Loening SA. Soluble CD44 variants in the serum of patients with urological malignancies. *Oncology* 1997;54:226–30.

271. Rao JY, Hemstreet GP 3rd, Hurst RE, Bonner RB, Min KW, Jones PL.

Cellular F-actin levels as a marker for cellular transformation: correlation with bladder cancer risk. *Cancer Res* 1991;51:2762–7.

272. Hemstreet GP 3rd, Rao J, Hurst RE, Bonner RB, Waliszewski P, Grossman HB, Liebert M, Bane BL. G-actin as a risk factor and modulatable endpoint for cancer chemoprevention trials. *J Cell Biochem Suppl* 1996;25:197–204.

273. Rao JY, Hurst RE, Bales WD, Jones PL, Bass RA, Archer LT, Bell PB, Hemstreet GP 3rd. Cellular F-actin levels as a marker for cellular transformation: relationship to cell division and differentiation. *Cancer Res* 1990;50:2215–20.

274. Streeter EH, Harris AL. Angiogenesis in bladder cancer—prognostic marker and target for future therapy. *Surg Oncol* 2002;11:85–100.

275. Vermeulen PB, Gasparini G, Fox SB, Toi M, Martin L, McCulloch P, Pezzella F, Viale G, Weidner N, Harris AL, Dirix LY. Quantification of angiogenesis in solid human tumours: an international consensus on the methodology and criteria of evaluation. *Eur J Cancer* 1996;32A:2474–84.

276. Weidner N. Intratumoral vascularity as a prognostic factor in cancers of the urogenital tract. *Eur J Cancer* 1996;32A:2506–12.

277. Jaeger TM, Weidner N, Chew K, Moore DH, Kerschmann RL, Waldman FM, Carroll PR. Tumor angiogenesis correlates with lymph node metastases in invasive bladder cancer. *J Urol* 1995;154:69–71.

278. Dickinson AJ, Fox SB, Persad RA, Hollyer J, Sibley GN, Harris AL. Quantification of angiogenesis as an independent predictor of prognosis in invasive bladder carcinomas. *Br J Urol* 1994;74:762–6.

279. Bochner BH, Cote RJ, Weidner N, Groshen S, Chen SC, Skinner DG, Nichols PW. Angiogenesis in bladder cancer: relationship between microvessel density and tumor prognosis. *J Natl Cancer Inst* 1995;87:1603–12.

280. El-Sobky E, Gomha M, El-Baz M, Abol-Enein H, Shaaban AA. Prognostic significance of tumour angiogenesis in schistosoma-associated

adenocarcinoma of the urinary bladder. *BJU Int* 2002;89:126–32.

281. Cheng L, Bishop E, Zhou H, Maclennan GT, Lopez-Beltran A, Zhang S, Badve S, Baldridge LA, Montironi R. Lymphatic vessel density in radical prostatectomy specimens. *Hum Pathol* 2008;39:610–5.

282. Fernandez MI, Bolenz C, Trojan L, Steidler A, Weiss C, Alken P, Grobholz R, Michel MS. Prognostic implications of lymphangiogenesis in muscle-invasive transitional cell carcinoma of the bladder. *Eur Urol* 2008;53:571–8.

283. Muller M. Telomerase: its clinical relevance in the diagnosis of bladder cancer. *Oncogene* 2002;21:650–5.

284. Lin Y, Miyamoto H, Fujinami K, Uemura H, Hosaka M, Iwasaki Y, Kubota Y. Telomerase activity in human bladder cancer. *Clin Cancer Res* 1996;2:929–32.

285. Kyo S, Kunimi K, Uchibayashi T, Namiki M, Inoue M. Telomerase activity in human urothelial tumors. *Am J Clin Pathol* 1997;107:555–60.

286. Fagelson JE, Rathi A, Miura N, et al. Detection of telomerase expression by in situ hybridization: A promising new technique in the evaluation of bladder cancer. *J Urol* 1998;159:283.

287. Muller M, Heine B, Heicappell R, Emrich T, Hummel M, Stein H, Miller K. Telomerase activity in bladder cancer, bladder washings and in urine. *Int J Oncol* 1996;9:1169–73.

288. Kinoshita H, Ogawa O, Kakehi Y, Mishina M, Mitsumori K, Itoh N, Yamada H, Terachi T, Yoshida O. Detection of telomerase activity in exfoliated cells in urine from patients with bladder cancer. *J Natl Cancer Inst* 1997;89:724–30.

289. Landman J, Kavaler E, Droller MJ, Liu BC. Applications of telomerase in urologic oncology. *World J Urol* 1997;15:120–4.

290. Yoshida K, Sugino T, Tahara H, Woodman A, Bolodeoku J, Nargund V, Fellows G, Goodison S, Tahara E, Tarin D. Telomerase activity in bladder carcinoma and its implication for noninvasive diagnosis by detection of exfoliated cancer cells in urine. *Cancer* 1997;79:362–9.

291. Fedriga R, Gunelli R, Nanni O, Bacci F, Amadori D, Calistri D. Telomerase activity detected by quantitative assay in bladder carcinoma and exfoliated cells in urine. *Neoplasia* 2001;3:446–50.

292. Wu WJ, Liu LT, Huang CH, Chang SF, Chang LL. Telomerase activity in human bladder tumors and bladder washing specimens. *Kaohsiung J Med Sci* 2001;17:602–9.

293. Neves M, Ciofu C, Larousserie F, Fleury J, Sibony M, Flahault A, Soubrier F, Gattegno B. Prospective evaluation of genetic abnormalities and telomerase expression in exfoliated urinary cells for bladder cancer detection. *J Urol* 2002;167:1276–81.

294. Fukui T, Nonomura N, Tokizane T, Sato E, Ono Y, Harada Y, Nishimura K, Takahara S, Okuyama A. Clinical evaluation of human telomerase catalytic subunit in bladder washings from patients with bladder cancer. *Mol Urol* 2001;5:19–23.

295. Landman J, Chang Y, Kavaler E, Droller MJ, Liu BC. Sensitivity and specificity of NMP-22, telomerase, and BTA in the detection of human bladder cancer. *Urology* 1998;52:398–402.

296. Saad A, Hanbury DC, McNicholas TA, Boustead GB, Morgan S, Woodman AC. A study comparing various noninvasive methods of detecting bladder cancer in urine. *BJU Int* 2002;89:369–73.

297. Ramakumar S, Bhuiyan J, Besse JA, Roberts SG, Wollan PC, Blute ML, O'Kane DJ. Comparison of screening methods in the detection of bladder cancer. *J Urol*. 1999;161:388–94.

298. Halling KC, King W, Sokolova IA, Karnes RJ, Meyer RG, Powell EL, Sebo TJ, Cheville JC, Clayton AC, Krajnik KL, Ebert TA, Nelson RE, et al. A comparison of BTA stat, hemoglobin dipstick, telomerase and Vysis UroVysion assays for the detection of urothelial carcinoma in urine. *J Urol* 2002;167:2001–6.

299. Tada Y, Wada M, Migita T, Nagayama J, Hinoshita E, Mochida Y, Maehara Y, Tsuneyoshi M, Kuwano M, Naito S. Increased expression of multidrug resistance-associated proteins in bladder cancer during clinical course and drug resistance to doxorubicin. *Int J Cancer* 2002;98:630–5.

300. Sweeney CJ, Marshall MS, Barnard DS, Heilman DK, Billings SD, Cheng L, Marshall SJ, Yip-Schneider MT. Cyclo-oxygenase-2 expression in primary cancers of the lung and bladder compared to normal adjacent tissue. *Cancer Detect Prev* 2002;26:238–44.

301. El-Sheikh SS, Madaan S, Alhasso A, Abel P, Stamp G, Lalani EN. Cyclooxygenase-2: a possible target in schistosoma-associated bladder cancer. *BJU Int* 2001;88:921–7.

302. Mohammed SI, Knapp DW, Bostwick DG, Foster RS, Khan KN, Masferrer J, Woerner B, Snyder PW, Koki AT. Expression of cyclooxygenase-2 (COX-2) in human invasive transitional cell carcinoma (TCC) of the urinary bladder. *Cancer Res* 1999;59:5647–50.

303. Shariat SF, Kim JH, Ayala GE, Kho K, Wheeler TM, Lerner SP. Cyclooxygenase-2 is highly expressed in carcinoma in situ and T1 transitional cell carcinoma of the bladder. *J Urol* 2003;169:938–42.

304. Sanchez-Carbayo M, Socci ND, Richstone L, Corton M, Behrendt N, Wulkfuhle J, Bochner B, Petricoin E, Cordon-Cardo C. Genomic and proteomic profiles reveal the association of gelsolin to *TP53* status and bladder cancer progression. *Am J Pathol* 2007;171:1650–8.

305. Jones HL, Delahunt B, Bethwaite PB, Thornton A. Luminal epithelial antigen (LEA.135) expression correlates with tumor progression for transitional carcinoma of the bladder. *Anticancer Res* 1997;17:685–7.

306. Zhuang YH, Blauer M, Tammela T, Tuohimaa P. Immunodetection of androgen receptor in human urinary bladder cancer. *Histopathology* 1997;30:556–62.

307. Ruizeveld de Winter JA, Trapman J, Vermey M, Mulder E, Zegers ND, van der Kwast TH. Androgen receptor expression in human tissues: an immunohistochemical study. *J Histochem Cytochem* 1991;39:927–36.

308. Hofmann R, Krusmann, Lehmer S, Hartung R. Prognostic factors for muscle invasive bladder cancer. *J Urol* 1998;159:246.

309. Seddighzadeh M, Steineck G, Larsson P, Wijkstrom H, Norming U, Onelov E, Linder S. Expression of UPA and UPAR is associated with the clinical course of urinary bladder neoplasms. *Int J Cancer* 2002;99:721–6.

310. Nakanishi K, Kawai T, Torikata C, Aurues T, Ikeda T. Urokinase-type plasminogen activator, its inhibitor, and its receptor in patients with upper urinary tract carcinoma. *Cancer* 1998;82:724–32.

311. Baffa R, Gomella LG, Strup SE, et al. Pathologic role of the FHIT gene in transitional cell carcinoma of the bladder. *J Urol* 1998;159:278.

312. Basakci A, Kirkali Z, Tuzel E, Yorukoglu K, Mungan MU, Sade M. Prognostic significance of estrogen receptor expression in superficial transitional cell carcinoma of the urinary bladder. *Eur Urol* 2002;41:342–5.

313. Kim JH, Shariat SF, Kim IY, Menesses-Diaz A, Tokunaga H, Wheeler TM, Lerner SP. Predictive value of expression of transforming growth factor-beta(1) and its receptors in transitional cell carcinoma of the urinary bladder. *Cancer* 2001;92:1475–83.

314. Booth C, Harnden P, Selby PJ, Southgate J. Towards defining roles and relationships for tenascin-C and TGFbeta-1 in the normal and neoplastic urinary bladder. *J Pathol* 2002;198:359–68.

315. Mearini E, Romani R, Mearini L, Antognelli C, Zucchi A, Baroni T, Porena M, Talesa V. Differing expression of enzymes of the glyoxalase system in superficial and invasive bladder carcinomas. *Eur J Cancer* 2002;38:1946.

316. Gromova I, Gromov P, Celis JE. A novel member of the glycosyltransferase family, beta 3 Gn-T2, highly downregulated in invasive human bladder transitional cell carcinomas. *Mol Carcinog* 2001;32:61–72.

317. Vecchione A, Ishii H, Baldassarre G, Bassi P, Trapasso F, Alder H, Pagano F, Gomella LG, Croce CM, Baffa R. FEZ1/LZTS1 is down-regulated in high grade bladder cancer, and its restoration suppresses tumorigenicity in transitional cell carcinoma cells. *Am J Pathol* 2002;160:1345–52.

318. Sen S, Zhou H, Zhang RD, Yoon DS, Vakar-Lopez F, Ito S, Jiang F, Johnston D, Grossman HB, Ruifrok AC, Katz RL, Brinkley W, Czerniak B. Amplification/overexpression of a mitotic kinase gene in human bladder cancer. *J Natl Cancer Inst* 2002;94:1320–9.

319. Possati L, Rocchetti R, Talevi S, Beatrici V, Margiotta C, Ferrante L, Calza R, Sagrini D, Ferri A. The role of peroxisome proliferator-activated receptor gamma in bladder cancer in relation to angiogenesis and progression. *Gen Pharmacol* 2000;35:269–75.

320. Boman H, Hedelin H, Holmang S. Urine tissue-polypeptide-specific antigen (TPS) as a marker for bladder cancer. *Scand J Urol Nephrol* 2001;35:270–4.

321. Mizutani Y, Wada H, Yoshida O, Fukushima M, Bonavida B, Kawauchi A, Miki T. Prognostic significance of a combination of thymidylate synthase and dihydropyrimidine dehydrogenase activities in grades 1 and 2 superficial bladder cancer. *Oncol Rep* 2002;9:289–92.

322. Iizumi T, Hariu K, Sato M, Sato S, Shimizu H, Tomomasa H, Umeda T. Thymidine phosphorylase and dihydropyrimidine dehydrogenase in bladder cancer. *Urol Int* 2002;68:122–5.

323. Li S, Nomata K, Sawase K, Noguchi M, Kanda S, Kanetake H. Prognostic significance of platelet-derived endothelial cell growth factor/thymidine phosphorylase expression in stage pT1 G3 bladder cancer. *Int J Urol* 2001;8:478–82.

324. Durkan GC, Nutt JE, Rajjayabun PH, Neal DE, Lunec J, Mellon JK. Prognostic significance of matrix metalloproteinase-1 and tissue inhibitor of metalloproteinase-1 in voided urine samples from patients with transitional cell carcinoma of the bladder. *Clin Cancer Res* 2001;7:3450–6.

325. Yano A, Nakamoto T, Hashimoto K, Usui T. Localization and expression of tissue inhibitor of metalloproteinase-1 in human urothelial cancer. *J Urol* 2002;167:729–34.

326. Hsueh SF, Lai MT, Yang CC, Chung YC, Hsu CP, Peng CC, Fu HH, Cheng YM, Chang KJ, Yang SD. Association of overexpressed proline-directed protein kinase F(A) with chemoresistance, invasion, and recurrence in patients with bladder carcinoma. *Cancer* 2002;95:775–83.

327. Miyake H, Gleave M, Kamidono S, Hara I. Overexpression of clusterin in transitional cell carcinoma of the bladder is related to disease progression and recurrence. *Urology* 2002;59:150–4.

328. Yamanaka M, Kanda K, Li NC, Fukumori T, Oka N, Kanayama HO, Kagawa S. Analysis of the gene expression of SPARC and its prognostic value for bladder cancer. *J Urol* 2001;166:2495–9.

329. Stronati L, Gensabella G, Lamberti C, Barattini P, Frasca D, Tanzarella C, Giacobini S, Toscano MG, Santacroce C, Danesi DT. Expression and DNA binding activity of the Ku heterodimer in bladder carcinoma. *Cancer* 2001;92:2484–92.

330. Rajjayabun PH, Garg S, Durkan GC, Charlton R, Robinson MC, Mellon JK. Caveolin-1 expression is associated with high grade bladder cancer. *Urology* 2001;58:811–4.

331. Kawamura S, Ohyama C, Watanabe R, Satoh M, Saito S, Hoshi S, Gasa S, Orikasa S. Glycolipid composition in bladder tumor: a crucial role of GM3 ganglioside in tumor invasion. *Int J Cancer* 2001;94:343–7.

332. Xia G, Kageyama Y, Hayashi T, Hyochi N, Kawakami S, Kihara K. Positive expression of HIF-2alpha/EPAS1 in invasive bladder cancer. *Urology* 2002;59:774–8.

333. Davies BR, O'Donnell M, Durkan GC, Rudland PS, Barraclough R, Neal DE, Mellon JK. Expression of S100A4 protein is associated with metastasis and reduced survival in human bladder cancer. *J Pathol* 2002;196:292–9.

334. Gromova I, Gromov P, Celis JE. bc10: A novel human bladder cancer-associated protein with a conserved genomic structure downregulated in invasive cancer. *Int J Cancer* 2002;98:539–46.

335. Staack A, Koenig F, Daniltchenko D, Hauptmann S, Loening SA, Schnorr

D, Jung K. Cathepsins B, H, and L activities in urine of patients with transitional cell carcinoma of the bladder. *Urology* 2002;59:308–12.

336. Numahata K, Satoh M, Handa K, Saito S, Ohyama C, Ito A, Takahashi T, Hoshi S, Orikasa S, Hakomori SI. Sialosyl-Le(x) expression defines invasive and metastatic properties of bladder carcinoma. *Cancer* 2002;94:673–85.

337. Kocher T, Zheng M, Bolli M, Simon R, Forster T, Schultz-Thater E, Remmel E, Noppen C, Schmid U, Ackermann D, Mihatsch MJ, Gasser T, Heberer M, Sauter G, Spagnoli GC. Prognostic relevance of MAGE-A4 tumor antigen expression in transitional cell carcinoma of the urinary bladder: a tissue microarray study. *Int J Cancer* 2002;100:702–5.

338. Asahi H, Koshida K, Hori O, Ogawa S, Namiki M. Immunohistochemical detection of the 150-kDa oxygen-regulated protein in bladder cancer. *BJU Int* 2002;90:462–6.

339. Chiu AW, Huang YL, Huan SK, Wang YC, Ju JP, Chen MF, Chou CK. Potential molecular marker for detecting transitional cell carcinoma. *Urology* 2002;60:181–5.

340. Kattan MW. Nomograms. Introduction. *Semin Urol Oncol* 2002;20:79–81.

341. Specht MC, Kattan MW, Gonen M, Fey J, Van Zee KJ. Predicting nonsentinel node status after positive sentinel lymph biopsy for breast cancer: clinicians versus nomogram. *Ann Surg Oncol* 2005;12:654–9.

342. Shariat SF, Tilki D. Bladder cancer: nomogram aids clinical decision making after radical cystectomy. *Nat Rev Urol* 2010;7:182–4.

343. Karakiewicz PI, Shariat SF, Palapattu GS, Gilad AE, Lotan Y, Rogers CG, Vazina A, Gupta A, Bastian PJ, Perrotte P, Sagalowsky AI, Schoenberg M, Lerner SP. Nomogram for predicting disease recurrence after radical cystectomy for transitional cell carcinoma of the bladder. *J Urol* 2006;176:1354–61.

344. Shariat SF, Karakiewicz PI, Palapattu GS, Amiel GE, Lotan Y, Rogers CG, Vazina A, Bastian PJ, Gupta A, Sagalowsky AI, Schoenberg M, Lerner SP. Nomograms provide improved accuracy for predicting survival after radical cystectomy. *Clin Cancer Res* 2006;12:6663–76.

345. Shariat SF, Zippe C, Ludecke G, Boman H, Sanchez-Carbayo M, Casella R, Mian C, Friedrich MG, Eissa S, Akaza H, Sawczuk I, Serretta V, et al. Nomograms including nuclear matrix protein 22 for prediction of disease recurrence and progression in patients with Ta, T1 or CIS transitional cell carcinoma of the bladder. *J Urol* 2005;173:1518–25.

346. Shariat SF, Karakiewicz PI, Palapattu GS, Amiel GE, Lotan Y, Rogers CG, Vazina A, Bastian PJ, Gupta A, Sagalowsky AI, Schoenberg M, Lerner SP. Nomograms provide improved accuracy for predicting survival after radical cystectomy. *Clin Cancer Res* 2006;12:6663–76.

347. Shariat SF, Karakiewicz PI, Ashfaq R, Lerner SP, Palapattu GS, Cote RJ, Sagalowsky AI, Lotan Y. Multiple biomarkers improve prediction of bladder cancer recurrence and mortality in patients undergoing cystectomy. *Cancer* 2008;112:315–25.

348. Shariat SF, Margulis V, Lotan Y, Montorsi F, Karakiewicz PI. Nomograms for bladder cancer. *Eur Urol* 2008;54:41–53.

349. Shariat SF, Tilki D. Bladder cancer: nomogram aids clinical decision making after radical cystectomy. *Nat Rev Urol* 2010;7:182–4.

350. Catto JW, Linkens DA, Abbod MF, Chen M, Burton JL, Feeley KM, Hamdy FC. Artificial intelligence in predicting bladder cancer outcome: a comparison of neuro-fuzzy modeling and artificial neural networks. *Clin Cancer Res* 2003;9:4172–7.

351. Tomlinson DC, L'Hote CG, Kennedy W, Pitt E, Knowles MA. Alternative splicing of fibroblast growth factor receptor 3 produces a secreted isoform that inhibits fibroblast growth factor-induced proliferation and is repressed in urothelial carcinoma cell lines. *Cancer Res* 2005;65:10441–9.

352. Chodak GW, Hospelhorn V, Judge SM, Mayforth R, Koeppen H, Sasse J. Increased levels of fibroblast growth factor-like activity in urine from patients with bladder or kidney cancer. *Cancer Res* 1988;48:2083–8.

353. Chopin DK, Caruelle JP, Colombel M, Palcy S, Ravery V, Caruelle D, Abbou CC, Barritault D. Increased immunodetection of acidic fibroblast growth factor in bladder cancer, detectable in urine. *J Urol* 1993;150:1126–30.

354. Gravas S, Bosinakou I, Kehayas P, Giannopoulos A. Urinary basic fibroblast growth factor in bladder cancer patients. Histopathological correlation and clinical potential. *Urol Int* 2004;73:173–7.

355. O'Brien T, Cranston D, Fuggle S, Bicknell R, Harris AL. Two mechanisms of basic fibroblast growth factor-induced angiogenesis in bladder cancer. *Cancer Res* 1997;57:136–40.

356. van Rhijn BW, Vis AN, van der Kwast TH, Kirkels WJ, Radvanyi F, Ooms EC, Chopin DK, Boeve ER, Jobsis AC, Zwarthoff EC. Molecular grading of urothelial cell carcinoma with fibroblast growth factor receptor 3 and MIB-1 is superior to pathologic grade for the prediction of clinical outcome. *J Clin Oncol* 2003;21:1912–21.

357. Maclennan GT, Kirkali Z, Cheng L. Histologic grading of noninvasive papillary urothelial neoplasms. *Eur Urol* 2007;51:889–98.

358. Jones TD, Cheng L. Papillary urothelial neoplasm of low malignant potential: evolving terminology and concepts. *J Urol* 2006;175:1995–2003.

Chapter 34

Molecular Pathology of Bladder Cancer

Overview

Conventional clinical and pathological parameters are widely used to grade and stage tumors and to predict the clinical outcome of bladder cancer; the predictive ability of these parameters is limited, and there is no index that could allow prospective assessment of risk for an individual patient. In the last decade, a wide range of candidate biomarkers representing key pathways in carcinogenesis have been reported to be potentially useful diagnostic and prognostic markers, and as potential therapeutic targets.[1-7]

Recent studies have suggested that urothelial carcinogenesis occurs as a "field effect" that can involve any number of sites in the bladder mucosa.[3,5,7-10] Accumulating evidence supports the notion that resident urothelial stem cells in the affected field are transformed into cancer stem cells (CSCs) by acquiring genetic alterations that lead to tumor formation through clonal expansion. Both initial and recurrent tumors are derived from cancer stem cells in the affected field via two distinct molecular pathways. These provide a genetic framework for understanding urothelial carcinogenesis, tumor recurrence, and progression.

Fibroblast growth factor receptor 3 (*FGFR3*) and *TP53* mutations are key to the two genetic pathways in urothelial carcinogenesis. *FGFR3* appears to be the most frequently mutated oncogene in bladder cancer and its mutation is strongly associated with low tumor grade, early stage, and low recurrence rate, which confers a favorable overall prognosis. In contrast, *TP53* mutations are associated with higher tumor grade, more advanced stage, and more frequent tumor recurrences. These molecular findings offer the potential to characterize individual urothelial neoplasms more completely than by histologic evaluation alone.

Areas in which molecular pathology may prove valuable include prediction of tumor recurrence, molecular staging of bladder cancer, detection of lymph node metastasis, exposure of circulating cancer cells, identification of therapeutic targets, and prediction of response to therapy. With accumulating molecular knowledge of bladder cancer, we are closer to bridging the gap between molecular findings and clinical outcomes. Assessment of key genetic pathways and expression profiles could ultimately establish a set of molecular markers to predict the biological nature of tumors and to establish new standards for molecular tumor grading, classification, prognostication, and individualized therapy (**Fig. 34-1**).

FGFR3 and *TP53* Mutations Define Two Key Pathways in Urothelial Carcinogenesis

Current studies indicate that bladder epithelial carcinomas arise through at least two separate mechanisms: the *FGFR3*- and *TP53*-associated pathways.[2-7,11-18] Tumors derived from these two pathways present as heterogeneous groups with distinct phenotypes and genotypes, and with drastically different biological behaviors and clinical outcomes. There are two classes of urothelial carcinoma that harbor distinctive genetic defects: low grade noninvasive tumors are characterized by activating mutations in *FGFR3*, but high grade urothelial carcinomas are characterized by genetic or epigenetic alterations in the *TP53* gene[11,19] or in a *TP53* regulation gene, such as *p16*.[20] *FGFR3* mutations are usually present in low grade papillary carcinomas with limited genetic instability, whereas high grade urothelial carcinomas are characterized by *TP53* mutation (**Fig. 34-2; Tables 34-1 and 34-2**).[11,13,21-28]

FGFR3 Pathway

FGFR3 mutations were discovered in individuals with thanatophoric dysplasia and hypochondroplasia.[29,30] These mutations seem to mediate opposing signals in different tissues, acting as a negative regulator of growth in bone and as a transforming oncogene in several epithelial tumor types.[29,30] Expression of a mutated, constitutively activated *FGFR3* gene in bladder and cervical cancer was reported in 1999.[31]

FGFR3 is a member of four highly conserved and structurally related tyrosine kinase receptor genes. It is located at chromosome 4p16.3 and is composed of 19 exons spanning 16.5 kb. It encodes an 806 amino acid protein belonging to the fibroblast growth factor receptor family. The protein consists of an extracellular region, composed of three immunoglobulin-like domains, a single hydrophobic transmembrane segment, and a cytoplasmic tyrosine kinase domain.[32] The extracellular portion of the protein interacts with fibroblast growth factors and initiates cascades of downstream signals, ultimately influencing cell growth, migration, differentiation, and angiogenesis.[32] Alternative splicing between exon 8 and 9 creates two different variants of the juxtamembrane Ig-like domain, isoforms *FGFR3b* and *FGFR3c*. These alternative mRNA splicing forms are tissue specific. *FGFR3b* is the expression form of epithelial cells and *FGFR3c* is expressed predominantly in mesenchymal cells.[31]

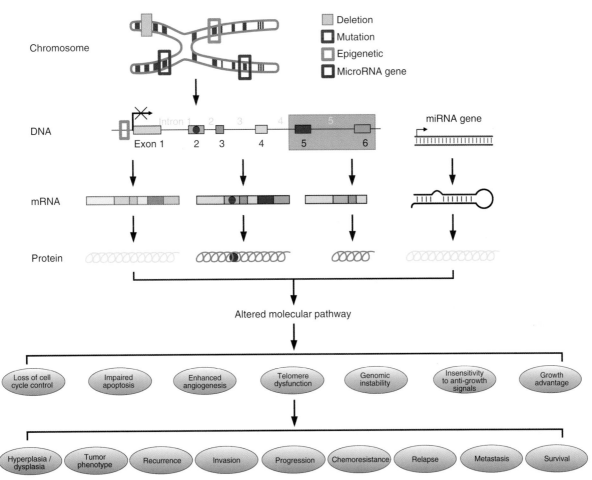

Figure 34-1 Molecular mechanisms of urothelial carcinogenesis. Molecular alterations contributing to urothelial carcinogenesis can be structural or functional chromosomal alterations. The deletion of chromosome fragments, gene mutations, epigenetic alterations and recently reported microRNA alterations, are among the most common factors associated with carcinogenesis, and biological behavior affect downstream pathways further through loss of cell-cycle control, impaired apoptosis, enhanced angiogenesis, telomere dysfunction, genomic instability, insensitive to antigrowth signals, and growth advantages. (From Ref. 7; with permission.)

The signal transduction pathways for *FGFR3* receptors are shared by many receptor tyrosine kinases. Mutations between the IgII and IgIII domains (exon 7) are by far the most common, accounting for 50% to 80% of all mutations of *FGFR3*. Mutations affecting the transmembrane domain (exon 10) account for 15% to 40%, and those affecting tyrosine kinase 2 domain (exon 15) account for 5% to 10%.[2] Mutations located at exons 5 and 10 often create a novel cysteine, which might be responsible for receptor dimerization and tyrosine kinase phosphorylation in the absence of ligand, resulting in constitutive activation.

FGFR3 activation triggers several downstream kinase pathways. The most important is the *RAS* cell cycle regulation pathway, which induces mitogenic signals and plays a central role in the proliferation and renewal of epithelial cells. Therefore, *FGFR3* and *RAS* mutations seem to be mutually exclusive, as both may be alternative avenues to a similar phenotype.[33,34] Alternatively, activated *FGFR3* activates phosphatidylinositol 3-kinase (*PI3-K*), which generates specific inositol lipids for regulation of cell growth, proliferation, survival, differentiation, and cytoskeletal changes. Activated *FGFR3* can also trigger the signal transducer and activator of transcription (*STAT*) pathway and interacts with proline-rich tyrosine kinase 2 (*PYK2*), leading to further *STAT* pathway activation. Experiments indicate that mutations of the *FGFR3* gene kinase domain can transform NIH3T3 cells as shown by focus formation in culture.[35] Knockdown of the S294C mutation *FGFR3* appears to be the most frequently mutated oncogene in bladder cancer.[30,31,36]

FGFR3 appears to be the most frequently mutated oncogene in bladder cancer. Over 70% of low grade noninvasive papillary urothelial neoplasms harbor *FGFR3* mutations, strongly implying that *FGFR3*-activating mutation is one of

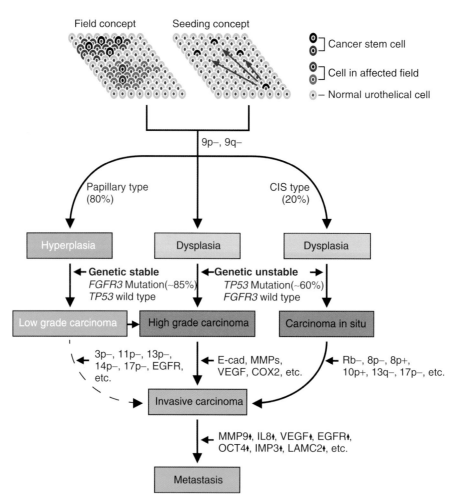

Figure 34-2 Proposed pathways of urothelial carcinogenesis, progression, and metastasis. It is proposed that urothelial carcinoma originates from cancer stem cells (CSCs) in the affected field or that tumor cells are distributed in the urothelium through a migration-seeding mechanism. CSCs acquire genetic alterations, leading to tumor initiation by clonal expansion. CSCs are the source of tumor recurrences as well as synchronous or metachronous multifocal tumors. Two distinct pathways are involved in the initial tumorigenesis in cancer stem cells. Papillary neoplasms are thought to develop through intermediate steps of hyperplasia or dysplasia, whereas high grade flat lesions are believed to evolve through dysplasia/carcinoma in situ. Papillary tumors account for about 80% of all urothelial carcinomas. They are characterized by activating mutations of *FGFR3* and wild type *TP53*, and, in general, they are genetically stable. However, these tumors may possibly gain further genetic alterations, leading to progression and metastasis (dashed line). High grade flat lesions account for about 20% of urothelial carcinomas and are characterized by loss of function mutations of *TP53* and intrinsic genetic instability. These two pathways provide a genetic framework for understanding urothelial cancers and their clinical behavior. (From Ref. 7; with permission.)

the key genetic events underlying the genesis of low grade urothelial tumors.[2–7,14–18] Such mutations in urothelial carcinoma are frequently found in exons 7, 10, and 15. Ranked by frequency, *FGFR3* mutations are found on exon 7 codon 249 (63%), exon 10 codon 375 (18%), exon 7 codon 248 (9%), and exon 10 codon 372 (6%).[37] Mutation of *FGFR3* is strongly associated with low recurrence rates in superficial papillary bladder cancers (see also **Chapters 29** and **33**).[5,25,36,38–40]

It is postulated that mutation in *FGFR3* results in activation of the RAS–MAPK pathway. Such activation, however, has not been proven in all *FGFR3*-mutated tumors.[33,41] Most *FGFR3* mutations are known to result in constitutive activation of the receptor. Evidence suggests that *FGFR3* mutations give a growth advantage to affected cells, but that cell cycle regulation and apoptosis mechanisms remain intact. This may explain the differences between indolent and aggressive urothelial cancers, the lat-

Table 34-1 Divergent Molecular Pathways in Urothelial Carcinogenesis

	FGFR3 Mutation	TP53 Mutation
Chromosome loci	4p16.3	17p13.1
Exons frequently involved by mutations	7, 10, 15	5, 7, 8
Gene type	Oncogene	Tumor suppressor gene
Mutation type	Activating mutation	Loss of function mutation
Molecular mechanisms	Kinase activation	Failure of cell cycle regulation, DNA repair, apoptosis
Key genes involved	Ras, STAT1, PI3K, cyclin D1	Rb, p21, BAX, Bcl-2, and TSP1
Clinical impact		
Histologic grade	Low grade	High grade
Invasion	Low risk	High risk
Pathologic stage	Low stage	High stage
Recurrence	Low risk	High risk
Progression	Low risk	High risk
Overall prognosis	Favorable	Unfavorable

Table 34-2 FGFR3 and TP53 Mutation Status in Relation to Tumor Grade, Pathology Stage, Recurrence, Progression, and Overall Survival of the Patients[1-9]

	FGFR3		TP53	
	Wt[a] (%)	Mu[a] (%)	Wt (%)	Mu (%)
Grade				
G1	18	82	93	7
G2	35	65	70	30
G3	78	22	51	58
Stage				
pTa	23	77	89	11
pT1	63	37	49	51
≥ pT2	8	20	44	56
Recurrence	67	33	42	58
Progression	63	37	44	56
Overall survival	25	75	70	30

[a]Wt, wild type; Mu, mutant.

ter bearing *TP53* mutations that cause impaired apoptosis and genetic instability. The reported frequency of *FGFR3* mutation in pTa tumors is 70% to 80% and there are several specific missense mutations associated with these tumors.[42-44] These mutations are significantly associated with tumors of low grade, early stage, and low recurrence rate.[36,43,44] Urothelial cancer bearing *FGFR3* mutation confers a better overall prognosis than cancer bearing *TP53* mutation. *TP53* mutations indicate a worse prognosis and higher recurrence rate.[11,13,26,36,40,45] Conversely, *FGFR3* mutation is detectable in only 10% to 20% of invasive tumors. This suggests strongly that *FGFR3*-activating mutation is a key genetic event in the genesis of low grade noninvasive papillary bladder tumors and that this event confers no added risk of *TP53* mutation.[13,36,45] Activating *FGFR3* mutations are found most frequently in grade 1 tumors (80%), and low grade tumors show a strong correlation with *FGFR3* expression (Tables 34-1 and 34-2).[46]

TP53 Pathway

Alterations of the *TP53* tumor suppressor gene play a crucial role in the carcinogenesis of many tumors, including bladder urothelial cancers. The *TP53* gene, located at the short arm of chromosome 17 (17p13.1), spans 19.2 kb and is composed of 11 exons. *TP53* encodes a 393 amino

acid protein (p53) which regulates the cell cycle, DNA repair, and apoptosis. The N-terminus of p53 contains several functional domains. The activation domain 1 (amino acids 1 to 42) activates transcription of downstream factors. Activation domain 2 (amino acids 43 to 63) regulates apoptotic activity. The proline-rich domain (amino acids 80 to 94) is also important in apoptosis. The DNA-binding domain (amino acids 100 to 300) activates downstream transactivation of other genes. The nuclear localization signaling domain (amino acids 316 to 325) and the homo-oligomerization domain (amino acids 307 to 355) are essential for the structure and homing of p53.

TP53 mutations in cancers are usually missense, loss of function mutations occurring in the DNA-binding domain. These impair the binding of p53 to its target DNA, reducing transcriptional activation of downstream genes. Mutant forms of p53 can also dimerize with wild type p53, blocking its function. *TP53* mutations induce a series of downstream effects, including decreased expression of p21. This important downstream target of p53 is downregulated in the majority of urothelial carcinomas with *TP53* mutations.

TP53 mutations are strongly associated with high tumor grade, invasive behavior, risk of recurrence, and adverse clinical outcome. *TP53* mutations are generally mutually exclusive of *FGFR3* mutations,[11,47] and the rate of *TP53* mutation is twofold higher in high grade urothelial cancers than in low grade tumors. However, when assessing high grade nonmuscle-invasive tumors, *FGFR3* and *TP53* mutations are not categorically mutually exclusive.[48] These findings are interesting and suggest that doubly mutant T1G3 tumors are either at the crossroads of the two main molecular pathways or represent progression from low grade papillary tumors to high grade tumors by acquisition of *TP53* mutations.

Third Pathway?

Mutations in the *FGFR3* and *TP53* genes usually define two independent and distinct pathways in superficial papillary and invasive flat urothelial carcinomas.[2] However, Lindgren et al. found that 5% of bladder cancers carry both *FGFR3* and *TP53* mutations.[46] This led to a proposal that there may be a third pathway leading to high grade carcinoma.[49] Others have suggested that this may represent the progression of low grade papillary carcinomas by acquired *TP53* mutation.[50]

Understanding Urothelial Carcinogenesis: Methodological Considerations

Multistep carcinogenesis refers to the accumulation of sequential genetic alterations, resulting in the progressive disruption of the regulatory circuits controlling normal cellular proliferation and differentiation. Tumorigenesis is a complex process with multiple molecular alterations occurring in various sequences and combinations. Each of these alterations confers to the various abilities of the cells, such as self-sufficient growth, insensitivity to anti-growth signals, evasion of apoptosis, unlimited replication potential, sustained angiogenesis, and the development of invasion and metastasis.[51] The major pathways of carcinogenesis involve the inactivation of tumor suppressor genes and/or activation of oncogenes. Evidence suggests that urothelial carcinomas develop through divergent pathways, and they often exhibit a variety of distinct biological and morphological characteristics.[2-7]

Current approaches to the discovery of genetic alterations in urothelial carcinomas can be subdivided into those that are pathway oriented and those that involve global genetic/expression profiling. The molecular pathways in urothelial carcinogenesis can be roughly categorized into four different levels: (1) chromosomal-level alterations including numerical and/or structural anomalies of chromosomes; (2) gene-level alterations including genetic mutation, fragment deletion, amplification, or abnormal epigenetic changes; (3) expression alterations; and (4) protein-level alterations including increased or decreased protein concentration, tumor-associated proteins, and fusion proteins (**Fig. 34-3**).

Numerical Chromosomal Alterations

Numerical chromosome aberrations represent changes in copy number of various genetic regions. A variety of chromosomal aberrations are identified in bladder tumors.

These aberrations can be detected by multicolor interphase fluorescence in situ hybridization (FISH), single nucleotide polymorphism analysis (SNP), or comparative genomic hybridization (CGH). The most frequently observed copy number aberrations in bladder cancer have been identified on chromosomes 1–5, 8–9, 13, 14, 17, 19, and Y (see also **Chapters 8, 29, 32,** and **33**).[3,4,6-9,16,17,52-80]

Numerical chromosomal changes have been used widely for bladder cancer screening, diagnosis, and prognostication. In patients with high risk superficial bladder tumors undergoing intravesical therapy, a positive UroVysion test after treatment is highly predictive of recurrence, even in a multivariate model (see also **Chapter 32**).[81] Recurrent tumors developed in 45% of the patients with abnormal UroVysion tests compared with 13% of patients with normal UroVysion assays after a median followup of 15 months.[82] Apart from prediction of recurrence, numerical chromosomal alterations have been proposed for use in categorizing bladder cancer into high or low risk groups.[83] The clinical applications of SNP and CGH are limited since these are not readily compatible with many routine pathology practice settings.

Structural Chromosomal Alterations and Allelic Imbalance

Structural alterations involve gains, losses, translocations, or more complicated rearrangements of chromosomes, resulting in the alteration of DNA copy number at the chromosome locus level. Structural chromosomal alterations may also involve gene regulatory regions, leading to locus overexpression or underexpression. These alterations can be detected by cytogenetics, FISH, restriction fragment length polymorphisms (RFLP), microsatellite polymorphism analysis, SNP, and CGH.[4,84,85]

Microsatellite analysis studies the deletion or instability of gene alleles, via loss of heterozygosity (LOH) and microsatellite instability analysis. LOH represents the loss of a DNA fragment in one allele of a gene, frequently a tumor suppressor gene, in which the other allele has already been inactivated by mutation. Thus, LOH results in complete inactivation of a tumor suppressor gene, leading to cell transformation. LOH analysis can be done in a locus-specific fashion or in a global fashion through SNP. A global analysis may provide information on whole genome alterations in gene copy number. There is a high correlation of LOH and FISH methods for the study of urothelial carcinogenesis.[76] LOH at some microsatellite loci is significantly associated with clinical outcomes,[86-91] including tumor recurrence-free survival[89,90] and progression-free survival.[90]

Allelic losses of chromosome 2q, 3p, 4p, 5q, 8p, 9p, 9q, 10q, 11p, 13q, 17p, and 18q are relatively common in urothelial neoplasms.[3,4,6-9,16,17,52-80]

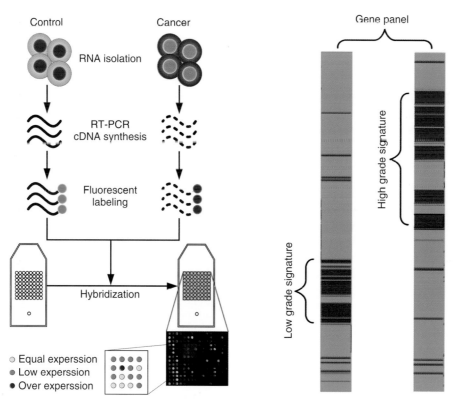

Figure 34-3 The principle of gene expression profile analysis. The basis of this analysis is the differential expression of certain genes between normal and tumor cells. mRNA is isolated from normal or cancerous tissue, fluorescence-labeled, mixed, and hybridized to a microarray. The expression levels of the genes can be quantified as equal, downregulated or upregulated, and represented by different colors, such as yellow, green, or red. Specific expression patterns of individual tumors can be correlated with clinical phenotypes such as grade, stage, response to treatment, and clinical outcome, as demonstrated on the right panel. (From Ref. 7; with permission.)

Chromosome 9

Chromosome 9 alterations are the most common cytogenetic abnormalities in all stages and grades of urothelial carcinoma, as indicated by FISH studies, CGH, and array-based CGH.[1,54,77,92–95] Studies have indicated that more than 50% of bladder tumors display LOH at chromosome 9. It appears likely that small deletions become more frequent, leading to eventual coalescence and further tumor progression, even with loss of an entire chromosome in some patients. Noninvasive papillary urothelial carcinomas typically exhibit loss of either all or part of chromosome 9. Invasive tumors also have high numbers of gains and losses of other chromosomes.

Chromosome 9 frequently shows LOH in some of the earliest stages of urothelial tumorigenesis, as proven by cytogenetics, LOH analysis, CGH (comparative genomic hybridization), and array CGH.[3,76,79,80] Over 50% of bladder tumors have been found to have LOH of chromosome 9, regardless of stage and grade.[71,77,78] Both 9q and 9p losses are present in low grade noninvasive papillary tumors and urothelial hyperplasia. Adjacent normal-appearing urothelium harbors the same LOH of chromosome 9 as the tumor

does, indicating that somehow LOH of chromosome 9 plays a pivotal role in the transformation from benign urothelium to tumor.[3,79,80] However, loss of chromosome 9 does not bias tumor progression toward either tumor development pathway (see the discussion above).[3,79]

The regions commonly lost on chromosome 9 include 9p21 [*CDKN2A/ARF* locus, which encodes for *p16* and *p14ARF*. These are key cell cycle regulators, which interact with retinoblastoma (*RB*) and *TP53*, respectively], and the loci often lost are 9q22 (*PTCH*, the Gorlin syndrome gene), 9q32–33 (*DBC1*), and 9q34 (*TSC1*).[96–98] A loss at 9p21 inactivates *CDKN2A* (*p16*), which encodes for two spliced products, *INK4A* and *ARF*. These products induce cell cycle arrest through the *RB* and *TP53* signaling pathways, respectively.[99,100] In many cases, the locus is homozygously deleted, and this cancellation has been associated with tumors of both higher grade and higher stage. However, there is some discordance between studies, as one recent study of homozygous deletion found no association with tumor grade and stage.[80]

Several studies have compared chromosome 9 loss and *FGFR3* mutations by LOH analysis. Chromosome 9 loss usually occurs prior to *FGFR3* mutation in the development of malignant tumors. *FGFR3* mutations, however, tend to be detected only in those tumors with a papillary-type configuration, as compared to those in flat dysplasia and CIS.[80] Primary CIS and CIS that occur in association with a papillary tumor may follow different developmental pathways. In primary CIS, chromosome 9 loss is infrequent, whereas CIS that was identified in association with papillary tumor has frequent losses of chromosome 9.[101]

Chromosome 8

Mutations and deletions in the short arm of chromosome 8 may occur in bladder tumors, resulting in decreased expression of the secreted frizzled-related protein 1 (*sFRP1*) gene, with resulting diminished signaling within cells. The *sFRP1* gene may be a tumor suppressor gene regulating the Wnt/β-catenin contact growth inhibition pathway. Immunohistochemistry techniques have shown that loss of sFRP1 protein expression is associated with a higher stage and grade of tumors and a decreased patient survival rate.[102] Some studies have reported a *sFRP1* gene mutation frequency rate of 25% to 30% in urothelial carcinomas.[103]

DNA Sequence Aberrations

DNA sequence aberrations (point mutations) are alterations in the DNA sequence that may lead to production of nonfunctional or truncated proteins, or modification of DNA methylation sites. Mutation analysis has identified hundreds of candidate genes mutations that may have functional roles in various human cancers.[11,104]

Such sequence alterations can be detected by DNA sequencing, utilizing sequence-specific termination of the DNA synthesis reaction with modified nucleotide substrates. Thus, clinicopathologic features of a tumor may be associated with even a single nucleotide mutation. Gene mutations frequently associated with bladder cancer include loss of function mutations of *TP53* and activation mutations of *FGFR3*, which characterize alternative genetic pathways in urothelial pathogenesis.[11] Tumors derived from these pathways present as heterogeneous lesions with distinct phenotypes and genotypes, and with drastically different biological behaviors and clinical outcomes (**Tables 34-1** and **34-2**).[11,26,105]

Microsatellite Instability

Microsatellite instability indicates that tumor cells accumulate genomic errors in these regions at a much higher rate than other sequences in the genome because of defective DNA repair mechanisms. These errors appear as gains or losses of gene loci and can be detected by examining the size of microsatellite repeat fragments, because the numbers of repeats in some microsatellites can change due

to defective DNA repair.[106] Microsatellite instability has been evaluated as a prognostic marker and associated with increased tumor stage and grade.[107]

Epigenetic Alteration and Gene Methylation

DNA methylation of cytosine–guanine dinucleotide (CpG) islands involves the addition of a methyl moiety to the cytosine-5 position at a gene promoter region (see also **Chapters 29** and **32**).[4,7,108,109] This cytosine chemical modification alters gene function without changing the base sequence of DNA and has been recognized as a common alternative mechanism for gene inactivation, especially during the early stages of tumor development. There is growing evidence that methylation plays a pivotal role in the function of key gene promoters, blocking transcriptional activation. As such, alterations in this essential epigenetic mechanism may play a role in carcinogenesis.[110] Several techniques have been developed to analyze the DNA methylation pattern, including methylation-specific PCR, methylation sequencing, and methylation-sensitive endonuclease digestion followed by electrophoretic separation.

Many tumor suppressor genes contain CpG islands and show evidence of methylation-specific gene silencing associated with neoplasia. Hypermethylation of CpG islands is associated with transcriptional repression, whereas hypomethylation may lead to increased gene activity or chromosomal instability. Numerous studies have shown that epigenetically inactivated tumor suppressor genes are associated with carcinogenesis, higher tumor grade,[111] more advanced staging,[111,112] early recurrence,[113,114] progression,[115,116] and adverse clinical outcome.[117–124] Methylation of CDH1 and FHIT predicted poor survival.[125]

The findings of Jones also suggest that mutations in the form of C → T transitions at methylated CpG sites are a common result of hydrolytic deamination of 5-methylcytosine. These C → T transitions commonly produce mutations in tumor suppressor genes such as *TP53*.[126]

The methylation status in a number of genes, including *E-cadherin, RASSF1a, RARB, MGMT, p16, p14, DAPK, PTEN, CD44, TP53, WT1, BCL2*, and *hTERT*, has been particularly associated with bladder cancer. The link between aberrant DNA methylation and urothelial carcinogenesis has been well established. Aberrant hypermethylation of the promoter region of *hMlH1*, *O*(6)-methylguanine-DNA-methyltransferase, *p15, p16*, von Hippel–Lindau (*VHL*), *RARB*, and *GSTP1* appear to play an important role in inactivation of these tumor suppressor genes.[113,118] CpG hypermethylation is an important mechanism of *E-cadherin* gene inactivation in cancer.[127]

MicroRNA Deregulation

MicroRNAs (miRNA) are short noncoding RNA molecules that modulate mRNA at the posttranscriptional level. They act as tumor suppressors or oncogenes and appear to be involved in bladder cancer development and progression. The causes of the widespread disruption of miRNA expression in tumor cells are not clear; however, it has been shown that more than one half of the known human miRNAs reside in genomic regions that are prone to alteration in cancer cells.[128] Alterations of miRNA-processing genes/proteins and miRNA gene promoter hypermethylation are both responsible for miRNA downregulation.[129-131] Genome-wide miRNA expression profiling can be analyzed by miRNA microarray, enabling sensitive and specific detection of miRNAs. Alternatively, small-scale miRNA profiling using quantitative RT-PCR may be used to measure the clustered miRNA targets.

Recent evidence suggests that alterations of miRNA expression contribute to urothelial carcinogenesis. Distinct miRNA alterations characterize urothelial carcinoma and target genes in a pathway-specific[132] or tumor phenotype-specific manner, predictive of tumor grade,[132] disease progression, and clinical behavior.[133-136]

Global Analysis of Gene Expression Profiles

The global approach adopts an all-encompassing strategy toward genetic alteration and gene expression by profiling the entire coding genome for alterations at the genomic and transcriptional levels.[4] Genetic and expression profiling can be achieved by CGH, SNP, and microarray-based approaches. These high-throughput strategies are based on the differences between tumor and reference normal DNA or RNA. Global investigation studies focus on panoramic alterations in copy number of chromosomal fragments, changes in gene expression pattern, and, more recently, shift in miRNA profile. In bladder cancer, these techniques have allowed the high-throughput mapping of DNA copy number alterations.[67,137,138] The resulting patterns of copy number alterations have aided in differentiating tumors into biologically and clinically relevant subtypes.

Similarly, it has been suggested that the origin and progression of each bladder carcinoma results from accumulation of specific genetic or epigenetic alterations, the overall pattern of which is termed the genetic signature. In this context, global analysis resolves both whole genome copy number alterations and identifies involvement of specific loci. Thus, whole or partial chromosome gains and losses, amplifications, and heterozygous deletions are easily quantified. The pattern of these alterations may have significant clinical implications in relation to tumorigenesis, progression, and metastasis.[3,5-7,137,139-142] Such genetic signatures could also be used to classify urothelial carcinoma according to stage, grade, biological behavior, and clinical outcome.[143-162]

Gene expression profiling provides a global view of gene expression levels in comparison to normal cells of same tissue. Commonly used methods include cDNA microarray and quantitative PCR. The cost-effectiveness endpoint of one investigation was to generate limited gene panels that can identify presence or absence of cancer, tumor grade, tumor stage, and clinical outcome.[137,163-165] Translation of the expression pattern of a gene panel into clinical phenotype with followup for each tumor may facilitate more accurate diagnosis and clinical outcome prediction. Gene expression signatures that predict aggressive tumor behavior at the earliest clinical stages are needed urgently, not only to guide ongoing treatment, but also to identify targets for developing future treatments. Array-based molecular profiling technology enables physicians to obtain a more complete picture of gene expression networks and to correlate clustering of differentially expressed genes with histopathology of various tumors with their clinical outcomes. Expression profile analysis is potentially useful in determining diagnosis,[166] tumor stage,[167-169] tumor grade,[170] presence or absence of CIS,[171,172] risk of recurrence,[173-176] risk of progression,[175,177,178] risk of metastasis,[179,180] and response to chemotherapy.[181,182]

Gene expression profiling of human bladder cancers provides insights into mechanisms underlying cancer progression and helps to categorize patients into distinct clinical subgroups (**Table 34-3**).[137,144,150,151,153,160-162,165-167,171,174,179,180,183-190]

Proteomics and Protein Expression Alterations

Proteomics is the global study of including cellular proteins, similar to genomics, analysis of protein structures and functional alterations in protein activity compared to proteins of normal cells of the same type. Investigations are focused on the quantity of protein production and on modifications of proteins, since these proteins represent the metabolic pathways of cells. In recent years, five major proteomic technology platforms have been employed: two-dimensional gel electrophoresis (2DE), surface-enhanced laser desorption/ionization (SELDI), liquid chromatography mass spectrometry (LC-MS), capillary electrophoresis coupled to mass spectroscopy (CE-MS), and protein arrays.[191] Proteomic studies reportedly have utility in bladder cancer diagnosis,[192-194] surveillance for recurrence,[195,196] prediction of invasive behavior,[197,198] and prediction of outcome.[197,199]

Many protein biomarkers have been investigated for their role in the development and progression of bladder carcinomas. These markers include the products of oncogenes, tumor suppressor genes, cell cycle regulators, growth factors, and cell adhesion molecules.[200-203] Some

Table 34-3 Selected Gene Expression Profiling Studies in Bladder Cancer[a]

Ref.	Year	Patient Number/Tissue	Gene Panel Size	Methodology	Endpoint	Key Findings
Dubosq et al.[160]	2011	47/FF	110	RT-PCR	Recurrence	3-gene panel predicted early recurrence
Smith et al.[162]	2011	341/FFPE	20	Microarray	Nodal staging	Identified the patients with high risk of nodal positive cancer
Lindgren et al.[153]	2010	144/FF	150	Microarray and array CGH	Grading, staging, and survival	Distinguish low vs high grade tumor; distinguished Ta/Ta from T2 cancer; predict cancer-specific and metastasis-free survival
Birkhahn et al.[144]	2010	177/FF	24	qRT-PCR	Recurrence and progression	24-gene panel predicted tumor recurrence and progression
Kim et al.[150]	2010	80/FF	24	Microarray	Recurrence and progression	12-gene expression predicted recurrence; 12-gene expression predicted progression
Kim et al.[151]	2010	272/FF	42/97	Microarray	Recurrence and progression	42-gene correlated recurrence; 97 genes correlated with progression
Kim et al.[161]	2010	128/FF	4	RT-PCR	Progression	4-gene panel predicted progression
Mengual et al.[190]	2009	79/FF	8	Microarray	Histological grading	8-gene panel classified low and high grade tumors
Mitra et al.[189]	2009	58/FF	4	qRT-PCR	Recurrence and survival	4-gene panel defined prognostically distinct tumors
Rosser et al.[166]	2009	46/BW	14	Microarray	Diagnosis	46-gene panel confirmed 76% of cancer
Als et al.[182]	2007	124/FF	55	Microarray	Response to treatment	Gene panel predicted response to treatment, and five-year overall survival
Dyrskjot et al.[172]	2007	404/FF	52/88	Microarray	Pathologic stage, progression, and cancer-specific survival	52-gene panel correlated with pathological stage; 88-gene panel correlated with cancer-specific survival
Schultz et al.[174]	2007	44/FF	23	qRT PCR	Tumor recurrence	23-gene panel predicted the risk of recurrence in stage Ta tumor
Takata et al.[181]	2007	22/FF	14	Microarray	Response to M-VAC chemotherapy	14-gene panel predicted 79% of M-VAC response and 100% of nonresponse cases
Sanchez-Carbayo et al.[180]	2006	294/FF	174	Microarray	Lymph node metastasis overall survival	Gene expression profile predicted the lymph node metastasis and overall survival
Mitra et al.[179]	2006	60/FFPE	70	qRT-PCR	Lymph node metastasis	70-gene panel predicted lymph node metastasis with an accuracy of 81%
Aaboe et al.[170]	2005	147/FF	230	Microarray	Diagnosis, histological grading	Expression patterns differentiated normal and tumor, and low- vs. high grade tumors
Blaveri et al.[137]	2005	98/FFPE	2464	Array CGH	Histological grade, pathological stage	DNA copy number alterations patterns predicted the tumor grade and pathological stage
Dyrskjot et al.[177]	2005	29/FF	45	Microarray	Tumor progression	45-gene panel identified patients with high risk of progression
Wild et al.[183]	2005	67/FF	225	Microarray	Overall survival	Gene panel predicted progression-free survival
Dyrskjot et al.[171]	2004	41/FF	16	Microarray	Presence of CIS	16-gene classifier identified CIS with an accuracy of 80%
Modlich et al.[164]	2004	34/FF	41	Microarray	Pathological stage, metastasis	41-gene panel classified UC into superficial, invasive, and metastatic UC
Dyrskjot et al.[165]	2002	40/FF	32	Microarray	Muscle invasion, tumor recurrence	32-gene panel classified tumors with high risk of progression

[a]UC, urothelial carcinoma; CIS, carcinoma in situ; M-VAC, methotrexate, vinblastine, doxorubicin, and cisplatin; FF, fresh frozen tissue; BW, bladder wash specimen; FFPE, formalin-fixed

of these protein factors hold considerable promise in the assessment of tumor grading, staging, progression, and prognostication. Important candidates include p53, Rb, p21, p27, Ki67, and E-cadherin.[204,205]

Combined Biomarkers and Nomograms

See also **Chapters 29** and **32** for further discussion.

Cancer Stem Cells and Urothelial Carcinogenesis

CSCs comprise 1% to 4% of the viable cells in a malignant neoplasm. These cells proliferate through asymmetric differentiation and can diversify into heterogeneous cancer cell lineages.[5,206-212] The asymmetric differentiation concept infers that following cell division, one daughter cell retains the capacity to divide again, and the other daughter cell possesses genetic plasticity, allowing phenotypic variation in the offspring. When tumors arise from CSCs or progenitor cells, a specific set of genomic, epigenomic, and microenvironmental niche alterations is essential for continued clonal expansion. Therefore, each CSC and its progeny possess a unique set of genetic, epigenetic, and phenotypic features. Urothelial CSCs may be endowed with either *FGFR3* mutation or *TP53* mutations. Although purified bladder CSCs have not yet been isolated, many studies have observed putative stem cell-like cell populations in bladder cancer. These bladder CSCs appear to be present in urothelial carcinoma and can be identified by their properties of colony formation, self-renewal, high proliferation rate, and expression of stem cell-related genes (**Fig. 34-2**).[3,7,207,208,213-215] Genetic alterations of tumor stromal cells assist CSCs in their niche, promoting cancer development and progression.[216]

Ben-Porath et al. reported an embryonic stem cell-like gene expression signature from bladder cancers.[214] Overexpression of some of these CSC genes appeared to correlate with an adverse clinical outcome in a microarray study of 105 bladder cancers.[215] Yang and Cheng studied nine cases of human bladder cancer using DNA array and immunohistochemistry panels for 28 stem cell surface markers, including EMA and CD44v6. EMA− cells and CD44v6+ cells showed properties of colony formation, self-renewal, and proliferation, which are characteristic of CSCs. These authors concluded that persistence of bladder CSCs accounts for most recurrences of human bladder cancer.[213] Atlasi et al. investigated the expression of OCT4, a progenitor cell marker, in 32 bladder cancers. They found that OCT4 is highly expressed in 97% of the tumors examined,[217] suggesting the existence of transformed progenitor cells in bladder cancer. In support

of this, She et al. showed that a side population of cells (putative stem cells isolated from bladder cancer) can both self-renew and differentiate into nonside population cells.[218] These investigators further proved that these cells have colony-forming and tumor-initiating ability,[218] consistent with CSCs. Hoechst 33342 is the classical method to detect CSCs based on the ability of stem cells to efflux chemical dyes. Using Hoechst 33342, Oates et al. isolated side population cells from urological cancers. These side population cells possess enhanced colony-forming ability and increased proliferation rate.[219]

More recently, Chan et al. described the isolation and characterization of a tumor-initiating cell subpopulation in primary human bladder cancer based on protein expression.[220] Bladder tumor-initiating cells are characterized by their ability to induce xenograft tumors in vivo that recapitulate the heterogeneity of the original tumor. Molecular analysis of more than 300 bladder cancer specimens revealed heterogeneity among activated oncogenic pathways in tumor-initiating cells (80% Gli1, 45% Stat3, 10% Bmi-1, and 5% β-catenin) and a unique bladder tumor-initiating cell gene signature was identified by gene chip analysis.[220] It is suggested that differences in CSC genetic signatures are is responsible for the variation observed in the clinical course of bladder carcinomas, even within identical clinical and pathological groups.

CSCs gain growth advantages and develop into an expanding clonal patch with genetically altered daughter cells.[221] The subsequent clonal expansion gradually displaces the normal epithelium to form a field. The growth advantage of this genetically altered clonal unit is the driving force of the urothelial oncogenic process. Tumor development at distant sites within the bladder is probably the result of cancer precursors in the affected mucosal field. Multifocality or concomitant CIS, a highly dysplastic flat precursor lesion, may also indicate field disease.[3,8,9,222,223]

Precursor Lesions of Bladder Cancer

See **Chapters 6** and **7** for further discussion.

Multifocal Bladder Tumors and Field Effects

Modern carcinogenesis models suggest that malignancy represents clonal expansion of one or a few CSCs in the fields affected.[3,4,7,224-226] Development of multifocal tumors in the same patient, either synchronously or metachronously, is characteristic of urothelial malignancy.[8,56,210,223,227–231] Two theories have been proposed to explain this frequency of urothelial tumor multifocality. The monoclonal theory suggests that multiple tumors arise from a single transformed cell, which proliferates and spreads throughout the urothelium either by intraluminal implantation or by intraepithelial migration. The second theory, the field effect theory, explains tumor multifocality as a development secondary to a field cancerization effect; in this scenario, chemical carcinogens cause independent initiating alterations at different sites in the urothelial lining, leading to multiple genetically unrelated tumors.

The clonal origin of multifocal bladder carcinomas is clinically important for understanding patterns of early tumor development and for planning treatment and surgical strategies.[9,10,56,210,216,222,232,233] The mechanisms of multifocality also influence test design for genetic detection of recurrent or residual tumor cells in post-treatment urine samples. However, there is currently no consensus concerning whether multifocal urothelial carcinoma is of monoclonal or oligoclonal origin. Many studies have suggested a monoclonal origin for multifocal bladder cancers,[234–245] but other studies have shown an independent origin for some multicentric urothelial tumors using similar methods.[79,236,239,243,244,246–251] A recent study suggests that both field cancerization and monoclonal tumor spread may coexist in the same patient.[8] In this study, molecular evidence supporting an oligoclonal origin for multifocal urothelial carcinomas in the majority of cases was found, consistent with the field cancerization theory for multicentric urothelial carcinogenesis. This finding is clinically important because molecular tumor development and spread must be considered to develop sufficient treatment and surgical strategies, and when molecular diagnostic techniques are to be used in the detection of recurrent or residual disease.

Evidence of field cancerization comes from studies on head and neck tumors. Multifocal bladder carcinomas are postulated to arise in the same manner. In the field cancerization process, simultaneous or sequential tumors result from numerous independent mutational events at different sites in the urothelium. These independent transformations are a consequence of external cancer-causing influences. In support of the field effect theory is the frequent finding of genetic instability in normal-appearing bladder mucosa in patients with bladder cancer in adjacent urothelium.[252,253] Premalignant changes, such as dysplasia or CIS, are often found in urothelial mucosa distant from an invasive bladder cancer. Many genetic comparisons and mapping studies of urothelial atypia in cystectomy specimens have supported the concepts of oligoclonality and field cancerization in the development of multifocal urothelial tumors, especially in early stage disease. Since the monoclonal and oligoclonal theories of urothelial tumor multifocality are not mutually exclusive, various theories have been proposed to combine the two mechanisms. One proposal is that oligoclonality is more common in early lesions, with progression to higher stages leading to the overgrowth of one clone and pseudomonoclonality.[244,254] Thus, early or preneoplastic lesions may arise independently with a specific clone undergoing more successful malignant transformation, and subsequently spreading through the urothelium by either an intraluminal or intraepithelial dissemination. Although tumor multifocality seems to be an oligoclonal phenomenon in the majority of cases, there is undeniable support for the monoclonal hypothesis in some cases.[8] Another possibility is that large areas of urothelium are predisposed by genetic instability to transforming events. When a malignant clone develops in this field, it triggers full transformation in other parts of the mucosa by paracrine or inflammatory mediators.

Selected Applications

Early Detection of Urothelial Carcinoma

See **Chapters 29, 30, 31, 32,** and **33** for further discussion.

Molecular Grading

See **Chapter 9** for further discussion.

Molecular Staging

Tumor staging is critical in predicting the disease course of an affected person.[255] The most common tool that clinicians use to predict bladder cancer outcomes is the American Joint Committee on Cancer tumor, lymph nodes, and metastases (TNM) staging system, which offers general outcome estimates based on classic pathologic criteria.[256] However, the predictive accuracy of TNM staging alone is limited. Therefore, nomograms combining molecular markers and classic pathologic criteria, as described in the preceding section, were developed to improve prediction of clinical outcomes after cystectomy.

Reported studies to date indicate that expression and genome profiling of bladder cancers allow reasonably good correlations between molecular findings and pathologic stage. Stage pTa bladder carcinomas are characterized by genetic stability, since they commonly lack TP53 mutations. Their chromosomal changes are limited predominantly to chromosome 9, whereas the majority of pT1 urothelial carcinomas show increased genetic instability with chromosomal changes in 17p, 13q, and 8p.[257]

FGFR3 and *TP53* mutations are frequently found in superficial papillary and invasive disease, respectively. Bakkar et al. used denaturing high-performance liquid chromatography and sequencing to screen for *FGFR3* and *TP53* mutations in 81 newly diagnosed urothelial carcinomas, including 31 pTa, 1 CIS, 30 pT1, and 19 pT2–T4 urothelial carcinomas. *FGFR3* mutations were associated with low stage tumors, whereas *TP53* mutations were associated with high stage tumors. In pTa tumors, *FGFR3* mut/*TP53* wt (68%) was the most prevalent genotype. The next most prevalent genotype was *FGFR3* wt/*TP53* wt, found in 29% of tumors. In pT1 tumors, *FGFR3* wt/*TP53* wt was the most frequent genotype (50%), followed by *FGFR3* mut/*TP53* wt (27%) and *FGFR3* wt/*TP53* mut (20%). In pT2–p14 tumors, the *FGFR3* wt/*TP53* wt genotype accounted for 53% of cases, and *FGFR33* wt/*TP53* mut was observed in 42% tumors.[13] These results demonstrated significant overlap with the TNM stages, and molecular staging subcategorized patients more accurately. Molecular staging, because it reflects malignancy inducing changes more directly and predicts tumor behavior more closely, may be more useful than traditional staging methods. Similar findings were reported by Dyrskjot et al., who correlated clinical stage with expression microarray analysis in 40 cases of bladder cancer. Hierarchical cluster analysis identified three main stages: Ta, T1, and T2 to T4, with the Ta tumors further classified into subgroups. The expression classifier correctly staged 84% of the Ta tumors, 50% of the T1 tumors, and 74% of the T2–T4 tumors.[169]

Chromosomal instability could also potentially be used as a staging parameter. An array-based CGH study by Blaveri et al. demonstrated significantly elevated copy numbers and increased genomic instability with increments in stage. Molecular staging was successful in 71% of cases, suggesting that identification of genomic instability independently enhances the accuracy of molecular staging of bladder cancer.[137]

Expression microarray analysis could further classify bladder tumors into more homogeneous and clinically relevant molecular expression subgroups. Blaveri et al. characterized the global mRNA array patterns of 80 bladder tumors, nine bladder cancer cell lines, and three normal bladder samples by gene expression profile. Unsupervised hierarchical clustering successfully classified the samples into two subgroups containing superficial (pTa and pT1) versus muscle-invasive (pT2–pT4) tumors. Supervised classification had a 91% success rate, separating superficial from muscle-invasive tumors based on expression of a gene panel. Tumors could also be classified into transitional versus squamous subtypes (89% success rate) and good versus bad prognosis (78% success rate).[168]

More recently, Simonetti et al. reported that polysomy 17 was related to the stage of bladder cancer. FISH results demonstrated polysomy 17 in 8/32 of Ta tumors, 14/18 of T1 tumors, and 13/13 of T2–T4 tumors.[257] miRNAs are thought to play roles in cancer development, differentiation, and progression. Specific groups of miRNAs are differentially expressed in various cancers and may influence tumor

phenotype and behavior. However, the specific role of miRNAs in the metastatic process is largely unknown. In a study of miRNAs in bladder cancer, Veerla et al. performed miRNA profiling on 34 urothelial carcinomas.[129] Unsupervised hierarchical clustering using expression information for 300 miRNAs produced three major clusters of tumors, corresponding to Ta, T1, and T2–T3 tumors. miR-452 was shown to be overexpressed in node-positive tumors.

Molecular Detection of Lymph Node Metastasis

Approximately 25% of patients undergoing radical cystectomy with pelvic lymph node dissection are found to have lymph node metastases.[259,260] The presence of lymph node metastases is predictive of poor clinical outcome. Molecular markers enable the detection of micrometastatic disease with high sensitivity and specificity, and could potentially guide therapeutic decision making. Seraj et al. analyzed lymph nodes from 19 cystectomy cases for the presence of uroplakin II (UPII) mRNA and found that 17% of pT2N0 tumors had molecularly positive lymph nodes, and 67% of lymph nodes from pT3–4N0 bladder cancers were also molecularly positive. When molecular findings are taken into consideration, 25% of microscopically negative lymph nodes appear to harbor metastases.[261] Other investigators have reported similar findings. Retz et al. found that 29% of microscopically negative lymph nodes from 17 cystectomy specimens showed positivity for MUC7, whereas lymph nodes from 20 control specimens were MUC7 negative.[262] Wu et al. studied 19 cystectomy specimens with lymphadenectomy, performing RT-PCR analysis for UPII and cytokeratin (CK) 20 mRNA on the bladder primary tumor, on microscopically identified lymph node metastases, and on microscopically negative lymph nodes. The UPII and CK20 mRNA detection rates were 100% and 68%, respectively, in bladder cancer tissues, 94% and 57% in microscopically visible lymph node metastases, and 10% and 0% in microscopically negative lymph nodes. Further in vitro studies illustrated the sensitivity of RT-PCR analysis for UPII and CK20 mRNA, with detection of as few as 50 and 500 HT1197 bladder cancer cells, respectively.[263] In another study, histopathology detected 29 positive lymph nodes, expression of CK19 detected a total of 49 positive lymph nodes, and expression of UPII detected a total of 98 positive lymph nodes among 760 lymph nodes from 40 patients.[264]

A study using RT-PCR by Marin-Aguilera et al. analyzed the expression of FXYD3 and KRT20 in histologically negative lymph nodes from 102 bladder cancer patients. They found that their combined expression differentiated between positive lymph nodes and normal controls with 100% sensitivity and specificity. The expression of both genes identified urothelial tumor cells in 21% of patients with histologically negative lymph nodes.[265]

Molecular Detection of Circulating Cancer Cells

Circulating tumor cells (CTCs) originate from the primary tumor, migrate to distant body sites through the bloodstream, and, at times, establish new colonies at these sites, eventually growing into detectable metastases. The presence of CTCs in whole blood before and during radical cystectomy has been evaluated as a parameter for determining the need for adjuvant or perioperative chemotherapy, but the results and conclusions gained from these studies have been contradictory and inconclusive.[266,267] It is notable that mobilization of tumor cells from the primary site is necessary but not sufficient to produce distant metastases.

Attempts at molecular detection of CTCs in the blood have been hampered by a paucity of molecules specific to urothelial cancer. Immunodetection relies on antibodies specifically chosen to attach to bladder cancer cells, such as certain cytokeratins, uroplakin, or MUC7. A major concern is that such detection methods may lack sufficient sensitivity and specificity for bladder cancer tumor cells.

Using the CellSearch system, Gallagher et al. analyzed peripheral blood from 33 patients with metastatic bladder carcinomas. Fourteen of 33 patients had a positive assay, with 10 patients (31%) having five or more CTCs. The number of CTCs detected in patients with two or more metastatic sites was significantly higher than the number detected in patients with fewer metastatic sites. The authors concluded that CTC numbers may be useful indicators of metastasis risk.[268]

In another CellSearch study of metastatic and nonmetastatic urothelial cancers, circulating urothelial cancer cells were detected in eight of 14 patients with distant metastasis, but none were detected in patients with nonmetastatic urothelial cancers, further suggesting that CTCs correlate with an increased risk of metastasis.[269]

Currently, the use of PCR-based technologies to detect CTCs in the blood is a field of intense investigation. Several bladder cancer cell markers, such as UPII,[270] CK20, EGFR,[271] and MUC7,[272] have been analyzed as candidate detection molecules. The sensitivity of these techniques is well documented, but their specificity for diagnostic purposes remains debatable. Peripheral blood of 62 patients was studied by nested RT-PCR assay for uroplakins (UP) Ia, Ib, II, III, and for EGFR. The combination of UPIa/UPII detected 75% of the CTCs, with a specificity of 50%.[273] In the study of Kinjo et al., MUC7 positivity was detected in all bladder cancer cell lines, in 11 of 29 (38%) peripheral blood samples from patients with Ta and T1 bladder cancer, and in seven of nine (78%) patients with advanced stage bladder cancer ($\geq$ T2).[274] These findings suggest that amplification techniques may be useful for combining markers and for eliminating subjective bias from immunodetection methods.

Molecular Classification

Most carcinomas that arise in the epithelium lining the urinary tract are purely urothelial. However, urothelial carcinoma tends to exhibit remarkable morphologic plasticity and frequently demonstrates divergent morphology with glandular, squamous, small cell, neuroendocrine, lymphoepithelioma-like, sarcomatoid, or other elements.[275] Different histologic grades are often observed in the same tumor.[276] Accurately distinguishing the various morphologic subtypes from one another is sometimes difficult, but clinically important because optimum treatment may vary from one tumor morphologies type to another. A number of unusual bladder tumors have been shown to be histogenetically of urothelial origin: sarcomatoid carcinoma,[7,17,277] clear cell adenocarcinoma,[60] lipoid carcinoma,[278] and plasmacytoid urothelial carcinoma.[279,280] These additional components may exhibit biologic behavior different from that of the underlying urothelial carcinoma. However, in some such cases, differential diagnostic considerations must include the possibility of direct extension of a contiguous cancer of another organ or metastasis from a distant cancer. Clearly, this distinction is important for prognostic and therapeutic reasons.

The relationship between urothelial carcinoma and associated divergent elements has been investigated recently. Urothelial carcinomas with divergent differentiation are relatively uncommon, and the histogenesis of these divergent components is incompletely understood. Two principal theories have been proposed to account for their development. One theory is that they develop initially as monoclonal proliferations derived from a single multipotent undifferentiated CSC, subsequently diverging into morphologically distinct components. As a part of the CSC theory, this concept is based on the premise that only 1% to 4% of tumor cells are capable of initiating and sustaining neoplastic growth and forming a tumor and that progenitor cells from these are the source of divergent elements. The second theory proposes that the two dissimilar components are similar only in their location and synchrony, developing independently from two separate CSCs of different histologic types. Histologic support for the divergence theory focused on identification of a "transition zone" between the histologically dissimilar areas to indicate evolution from a monoclonal origin.

In recent years, a number of molecular investigations have focused on ascertaining the true relationship between urothelial carcinoma and its various putative divergent elements.[6,7] Armstrong et al. studied a series of 17 sarcomatoid carcinomas using single-strand conformation polymorphism, DNA sequencing, and p53 immunohistochemistry to clarify their clonal origin.[277] The results showed that five of the 17 sarcomatoid urothelial carcinomas contained *TP53* point mutations in exons 5 and 8. In each of these five cases, the *TP53* point mutations were identical in both the epithelial and sarcomatoid components. Despite conspicuous divergence at the phenotypic level, the sarcomatoid and carcinomatoid elements of this uncommon tumor apparently develop from a common progenitor cell. The study of Sung et al. supported this notion.[17] Cumulative evidence suggests that sarcomatoid carcinoma represents the final common pathway of urothelial carcinoma dedifferentiation.[6] This understanding of phenotypic plasticity implies a new understanding of the relationship between grade, subtype, cancer recurrence and progression.

More recently, Cheng et al. examined five polymorphic microsatellite markers in 20 patients with small cell carcinoma of the urinary bladder and concurrent urothelial carcinoma. A nearly identical pattern of allelic loss was observed in the two tumor types in all cases, with an overall frequency of allelic loss of 90% (18 of 20 cases). Three patients showed different allelic loss patterns in the two tumor types at a single locus; however, the LOH patterns at the remaining loci were identical. Moreover, the same pattern of nonrandom X chromosome inactivation was present in both carcinoma components in the four female cases analyzed. Concordant genetic alterations and X chromosome inactivation between small cell carcinoma and coexisting urothelial carcinoma suggest that both tumor components originate from the same cells in the urothelium but may subsequently undergo genetic divergence.[58]

cDNA microarrays containing human gene elements were used to characterize the global gene expression patterns in 74 urothelial carcinomas, six squamous cell carcinomas, nine bladder cancer cell lines, and three normal bladder controls. Prediction analysis for microarrays classified five of six squamous cell carcinoma and 42 of 47 urothelial carcinomas correctly for an overall success rate of 89%.[168] Such data may open new understanding of acquired or concurrent divergent phenotypes.

In contrast, numerical chromosomal alterations do not efficiently separate urothelial and nonurothelial tumors (see **Chapters 29, 30,** and **32**). Reid-Nicholson et al. using UroVysion FISH analyzed 31 nonurothelial bladder carcinomas, 12 pure urothelial carcinomas, and two urothelial carcinomas with squamous differentiation. The study found that 11% of squamous carcinomas and 79% of primary and secondary adenocarcinomas were UroVysion-positive, compared to 75% of urothelial carcinomas.[281] It is unclear at this time whether urothelial adenocarcinoma and squamous cell carcinoma arise by clonal evolution or by unrelated events.

Targeted Therapy

In the management of bladder cancer, there is considerable interest in targeted therapy,[7,282–287] due to the poor overall response to cytotoxic chemotherapy in patients with metastatic disease.[288] The goal of "personalized medicine," prescribing the appropriate treatment regimen for each patient's tumor, may be achievable by selecting specific sets of biomarkers based on their ability to predict effective therapy according to the knowledge of urothelial carcinogenesis. Identifying markers that predict patients at risk for recurrence or progression after radical cystectomy is a high priority; identifying molecular biomarkers that have potential to identify specific therapeutic targets might be most beneficial even if only a few patients qualify for each specific therapy. The increasing availability of novel targeted therapies offers the possibility of individualized treatment for bladder cancer patients.

FGFR3 may be useful as a target for future therapeutic strategies, since it is a tyrosine kinase receptor. *S249C* is a mutation that induces disulfide bonding in the extracellular domain of *FGFR3b*, which then autophosphorylates the intracellular kinase domain and causes increased and prolonged activation of the *FGFR3* receptor.[289–293] When this mutation was knocked down by *FGFR3* shRNA, an inhibition of proliferation was found specific to tumor cells. Additionally, the tumor cell line MGH-U3 expresses Y375C mutant *FGFR3*, and when these cells were treated with the small molecule inhibitor SU5402 or siRNAs, there is reduced receptor phosphorylation, reduced proliferation, and reduced colony formation in soft agarose. Other target molecules include SU6668, PD173074, and CHIR-258.[289–293] In the experimental therapeutics for multiple myeloma (another disease in which mutations of *FGFR3* occur), human single-chain Fv antibody fragments have been isolated that inhibit *FGFR3* signaling and halt cell proliferation.[289–293] Similar studies of bladder tumors have discovered that similar antibody fragments (particularly those to *FGFR3c*) block proliferation of epithelial tumor cells (specifically those of tumor cell line RT112, which inherently expresses high levels of *FGFR3*).

Als and colleagues performed Affymetrix GeneChip expression profiling analysis on 30 patients with bladder cancer. Fifty-five genes that correlated with survival time after chemotherapy were identified. Increased expression of two proteins, emmprin and survivin, was identified as an independent prognostic marker for poor outcome. The significance of the proteins was validated by subsequent studies of 124 patients treated with cytotoxic chemotherapy. The median survivals were 18.7 and 9.7 months, and the five-year survivals were 23% and 15% for emmprin-negative tumors versus emmprin-positive tumors, respectively. The median survival time for survivin was 18.4 months versus 9.8 months, and the five-year survivals were 28% and 5% for negative and positive tumors, respectively.[182]

The results of a study of 35 patients with high risk nonmuscle-invasive bladder cancer treated with bacillus

Calmette–Guérin (BCG) mitomycin C, anthracyclines, and gemcitabine after transurethral bladder tumor resection found that response to specific therapies correlates with the molecular characteristics of each tumor. In the study of Gazzaniga et al., molecular chemosensitivity profiles were constructed according to the BCL2/BAX ratio, survivin expression, and the expression status of MRP1-MRP2, hENT-dCK, and $\alpha 5\beta 1$ integrin. The chemosensitivity test accurately predicted response to treatment in 96% of patients.[294]

In the study of Takata and colleagues, 22 patients with bladder cancer were investigated to predict the efficacy of combined methotrexate, vinblastine, doxorubicin, and cisplatin (M-VAC) neoadjuvant chemotherapy for invasive bladder cancers. A 14-gene profile predicted clinical response correctly in 19 of 22 tested cases. The group of patients with positive predictive scores had significantly longer survival times than those with negative scores.[186]

In summary, current pathology practice, diagnosis, and surveillance for bladder cancer are heavily dependent upon cystoscopy with biopsy, urine cytology, and a few select biomarker studies. It is critical that all of these methods should be regarded as complementary rather than competitive or self-determining. The real challenge for researchers who are seeking clinically relevant molecular biomarkers in bladder cancer is to apply knowledge derived from molecular studies to clinical practice. With accumulating molecular knowledge of bladder cancer, we are closer to the goal of bridging the gap between molecular findings and clinical outcomes. However, prospective multicenter validation studies of large patient groups will be necessary to provide high-quality evidence. An important step forward would be consensus on a valid risk assessment based on the molecular biomarker status of bladder cancer, derived from routine paraffin embedded surgical pathology specimens. Assessment of key genetic pathways and expression profiles may ultimately establish a set of molecular markers to predict the risk of tumor recurrence and progression, to establish new standards for molecular tumor grading, classification, and prognostication, and to direct targeted therapy selection in cases of advanced urothelial carcinoma.

REFERENCES

1. Dinney CP, McConkey DJ, Millikan RE, Wu X, Bar-Eli M, Adam L, Kamat AM, Siefker-Radtke AO, Tuziak T, Sabichi AL, Grossman HB, Benedict WF, Czerniak B. Focus on bladder cancer. *Cancer Cell* 2004;6:111–6.
2. Wu XR. Urothelial tumorigenesis: a tale of divergent pathways. *Nat Rev Cancer* 2005;5:713–25.
3. Cheng L, Davidson DD, Maclennan GT, Williamson SR, Zhang S, Koch MO, Montironi R, Lopez-Beltran A. The origins of urothelial carcinoma. *Expert Rev Anticancer Ther* 2010;10:865–80.
4. Cheng L, Zhang D. Molecular Genetic Pathology. New York: Humana Press/Springer, 2008.
5. Cheng L, Zhang S, Davidson DD, MacLennan GT, Koch MO, Montironi R, Lopez-Beltran A. Molecular determinants of tumor recurrence in the urinary bladder. *Future Oncol* 2009;5:843–57.
6. Cheng L, Zhang S, Alexander R, MacLennan GT, Hodges KB, Harrison BT, Lopez-Beltran A, Montironi R. Sarcomatoid carcinoma of the urinary bladder: the final common pathway of urothelial carcinoma dedifferentiation. *Am J Surg Pathol* 2011;35:e34–46.
7. Cheng L, Zhang S, MacLennan GT, Williamson SR, Lopez-Beltran A, Montironi R. Bladder cancer: translating molecular genetic insights into clinical practice. *Hum Pathol* 2011;42:455–81.
8. Jones TD, Wang M, Eble JN, MacLennan GT, Lopez-Beltran A, Zhang S, Cocco A, Cheng L. Molecular evidence supporting field effect in urothelial carcinogenesis. *Clin Cancer Res* 2005;11:6512–9.
9. Jones TD, Carr MD, Eble JN, Wang M, Lopez-Beltran A, Cheng L. Clonal origin of lymph node metastases in bladder carcinoma. *Cancer* 2005;104:1901–10.
10. Cheng L, Gu J, Ulbright TM, MacLennan GT, Sweeney CJ, Zhang S, Sanchez K, Koch MO, Eble JN. Precise microdissection of human bladder carcinomas reveals divergent tumor subclones in the same tumor. *Cancer* 2002;94:104–10.
11. van Rhijn BW, van der Kwast TH, Vis AN, Kirkels WJ, Boeve ER, Jobsis AC, Zwarthoff EC. FGFR3 and p53 characterize alternative genetic pathways in the pathogenesis of urothelial cell carcinoma. *Cancer Res* 2004;64:1911–4.
12. Wallerand H, Bakkar AA, de Medina SG, Pairon JC, Yang YC, Vordos D, Bittard H, Fauconnet S, Kouyoumdjian JC, Jaurand MC, Zhang ZF, Radvanyi F, Thiery JP, Chopin DK. Mutations in TP53, but not FGFR3, in urothelial cell carcinoma of the bladder are influenced by smoking: contribution of exogenous versus endogenous carcinogens. *Carcinogenesis* 2005;26:177–84.
13. Bakkar AA, Wallerand H, Radvanyi F, Lahaye JB, Pissard S, Lecerf L, Kouyoumdjian JC, Abbou CC, Pairon JC, Jaurand MC, Thiery JP, Chopin DK, de Medina SG. FGFR3 and TP53 gene mutations define two distinct pathways in urothelial cell carcinoma of the bladder. *Cancer Res* 2003;63:8108–12.
14. Lacy S, Lopez-Beltran A, MacLennan GT, Foster SR, Montironi R, Cheng L. Molecular pathogenesis of urothelial carcinoma: the clinical utility of emerging new biomarkers and future molecular classification of bladder cancer. *Anal Quant Cytol Histol* 2009;31:5–16.

15. Sung MT, Lopez-Beltran A, Eble JN, MacLennan GT, Tan PH, Montironi R, Jones TD, Ulbright TM, Blair JE, Cheng L. Divergent pathway of intestinal metaplasia and cystitis glandularis of the urinary bladder. *Mod Pathol* 2006;19:1395–401.

16. Sung MT, Eble JN, Wang M, Tan PH, Lopez-Beltran A, Cheng L. Inverted papilloma of the urinary bladder: a molecular genetic appraisal. *Mod Pathol* 2006;19:1289–94.

17. Sung MT, Wang M, MacLennan GT, Eble JN, Tan PH, Lopez-Beltran A, Montironi R, Harris JJ, Kuhar M, Cheng L. Histogenesis of sarcomatoid urothelial carcinoma of the urinary bladder: evidence for a common clonal origin with divergent differentiation. *J Pathol* 2007;211:420–30.

18. Lott S, Wang M, MacLennan GT, Lopez-Beltran A, Montironi R, Sung M-T, Tan P-H, Cheng L. FGFR3 and TP53 mutation analysis in inverted urothelial papilloma: Incidence and etiological considerations. *Mod Pathol* 2009;22:627–32.

19. Kouidou S, Malousi A, Maglaveras N. Methylation and repeats in silent and nonsense mutations of p53. *Mutat Res* 2006;599:167–77.

20. Marsit CJ, Karagas MR, Danaee H, Liu M, Andrew A, Schned A, Nelson HH, Kelsey KT. Carcinogen exposure and gene promoter hypermethylation in bladder cancer. *Carcinogenesis* 2006;27:112–6.

21. Lin HH, Ke HL, Huang SP, Wu WJ, Chen YK, Chang LL. Increase sensitivity in detecting superficial, low grade bladder cancer by combination analysis of hypermethylation of E-cadherin, p16, p14, RASSF1A genes in urine. *Urol Oncol* 2010;28:597–602.

22. Burger M, van der Aa MN, van Oers JM, Brinkmann A, van der Kwast TH, Steyerberg EC, Stoehr R, Kirkels WJ, Denzinger S, Wild PJ, Wieland WF, Hofstaedter F, Hartmann A, Zwarthoff EC. Prediction of progression of non-muscle-invasive bladder cancer by WHO 1973 and 2004 grading and by FGFR3 mutation status: a prospective study. *Eur Urol* 2008;54:835–43.

23. van Oers JM, Zwarthoff EC, Rehman I, Azzouzi AR, Cussenot O, Meuth M, Hamdy FC, Catto JW. FGFR3 mutations indicate better survival in invasive upper urinary tract and bladder tumours. *Eur Urol* 2009;55:650–7.

24. Junker K, van Oers JM, Zwarthoff EC, Kania I, Schubert J, Hartmann A. Fibroblast growth factor receptor 3 mutations in bladder tumors correlate with low frequency of chromosome alterations. *Neoplasia* 2008;10:1–7.

25. van Rhijn BW, Burger M, Lotan Y, Solsona E, Stief CG, Sylvester RJ, Witjes JA, Zlotta AR. Recurrence and progression of disease in non-muscle-invasive bladder cancer: from epidemiology to treatment strategy. *Eur Urol* 2009;56:430–42.

26. van Rhijn BW, Lurkin I, Radvanyi F, Kirkels WJ, van der Kwast TH, Zwarthoff EC. The fibroblast growth factor receptor 3 (FGFR3) mutation is a strong indicator of superficial bladder cancer with low recurrence rate. *Cancer Res* 2001;61:1265–8.

27. van Rhijn BW, Vis AN, van der Kwast TH, Kirkels WJ, Radvanyi F, Ooms EC, Chopin DK, Boeve ER, Jobsis AC, Zwarthoff EC. Molecular grading of urothelial cell carcinoma with fibroblast growth factor receptor 3 and MIB-1 is superior to pathologic grade for the prediction of clinical outcome. *J Clin Oncol* 2003;21:1912–21.

28. Moonen PM, van Balken-Ory B, Kiemeney LA, Schalken JA, Witjes JA. Prognostic value of p53 for high risk superficial bladder cancer with long-term followup. *J Urol* 2007;177:80–3.

29. Tavormina PL, Shiang R, Thompson LM, Zhu YZ, Wilkin DJ, Lachman RS, Wilcox WR, Rimoin DL, Cohn DH, Wasmuth JJ. Thanatophoric dysplasia (types I and II) caused by distinct mutations in fibroblast growth factor receptor 3. *Nat Genet* 1995;9:321–8.

30. Bellus GA, Spector EB, Speiser PW, Weaver CA, Garber AT, Bryke CR, Israel J, Rosengren SS, Webster MK, Donoghue DJ, Francomano CA. Distinct missense mutations of the FGFR3 lys650 codon modulate receptor kinase activation and the severity of the skeletal dysplasia phenotype. *Am J Hum Genet* 2000;67:1411–21.

31. Cappellen D, De Oliveira C, Ricol D, de Medina S, Bourdin J, Sastre-Garau X, Chopin D, Thiery JP, Radvanyi F. Frequent activating mutations of FGFR3 in human bladder and cervix carcinomas. *Nat Genet* 1999;23:18–20.

32. Jaye M, Schlessinger J, Dionne CA. Fibroblast growth factor receptor tyrosine kinases: molecular analysis and signal transduction. *Biochim Biophys Acta* 1992;1135:185–99.

33. Jebar AH, Hurst CD, Tomlinson DC, Johnston C, Taylor CF, Knowles MA. FGFR3 and Ras gene mutations are mutually exclusive genetic events in urothelial cell carcinoma. *Oncogene* 2005;24:5218–25.

34. Wolff EM, Liang G, Jones PA. Mechanisms of disease: genetic and epigenetic alterations that drive bladder cancer. *Nat Clin Pract Urol* 2005;2:502–10.

35. Webster MK, Donoghue DJ. Enhanced signaling and morphological transformation by a membrane-localized derivative of the fibroblast growth factor receptor 3 kinase domain. *Mol Cell Biol* 1997;17:5739–47.

36. van Rhijn BW, Lurkin I, Chopin DK, Kirkels WJ, Thiery JP, van der Kwast TH, Radvanyi F, Zwarthoff EC. Combined microsatellite and FGFR3 mutation analysis enables a highly sensitive detection of urothelial cell carcinoma in voided urine. *Clin Cancer Res* 2003;9:257–63.

37. van Rhijn BW, Montironi R, Zwarthoff EC, Jobsis AC, van der Kwast TH. Frequent FGFR3 mutations in urothelial papilloma. *J Pathol* 2002;198:245–51.

38. Billerey C, Chopin D, Aubriot-Lorton MH, Ricol D, Gil Diez de Medina S, Van Rhijn B, Bralet MP, Lefrere-Belda MA, Lahaye JB, Abbou CC, Bonaventure J, Zafrani ES, van der Kwast T, Thiery JP, Radvanyi F. Frequent FGFR3 mutations in papillary non-invasive bladder (pTa) tumors. *Am J Pathol* 2001;158:1955–9.

39. van Rhijn BW, Lurkin I, Radvanyi F, Kirkels WJ, van der Kwast TH, Zwarthoff EC. The fibroblast growth factor receptor 3 (FGFR3) mutation is a strong indicator of superficial bladder cancer with low recurrence rate. *Cancer Res* 2001;61:1265–8.

40. Hernandez S, Lopez-Knowles E, Lloreta J, Kogevinas M, Amoros A, Tardon A, Carrato A, Serra C, Malats N, Real FX. Prospective study of FGFR3 mutations as a prognostic factor in nonmuscle invasive urothelial bladder carcinomas. *J Clin Oncol* 2006;24:3664–71.

41. Hart KC, Robertson SC, Kanemitsu MY, Meyer AN, Tynan JA, Donoghue DJ. Transformation and stat activation by derivatives of FGFR1, FGFR3, and FGFR4. *Oncogene* 2000;19:3309–20.

42. Tomlinson DC, Baldo O, Harnden P, Knowles MA. FGFR3 protein expression and its relationship to mutation status and prognostic variables in bladder cancer. *J Pathol* 2007;213:91–8.

43. Bernard-Pierrot I, Brams A, Dunois-Larde C, Caillault A, Diez de Medina SG, Cappellen D, Graff G, Thiery JP, Chopin D, Ricol D, Radvanyi F. Oncogenic properties of the mutated forms of fibroblast growth factor receptor 3b. *Carcinogenesis* 2006;27:740–7.

44. Knowles MA. Role of FGFR3 in urothelial cell carcinoma: biomarker and potential therapeutic target. *World J Urol* 2007;25:581–93.

45. van Rhijn BW, Vis AN, van der Kwast TH, Kirkels WJ, Radvanyi F, Ooms EC, Chopin DK, Boeve ER, Jobsis AC, Zwarthoff EC. Molecular grading of urothelial cell carcinoma with fibroblast growth factor receptor 3 and MIB-1 is superior to pathologic grade for the prediction of clinical outcome. *J Clin Oncol* 2003;21:1912–21.

46. Lindgren D, Liedberg F, Andersson A, Chebil G, Gudjonsson S, Borg A, Mansson W, Fioretos T, Hoglund M. Molecular characterization of early-stage bladder carcinomas by expression profiles, FGFR3 mutation status, and loss of 9q. *Oncogene* 2006;25:2685–96.

47. Shariat SF, Ashfaq R, Sagalowsky AI, Lotan Y. Predictive value of cell cycle biomarkers in nonmuscle invasive bladder transitional cell carcinoma. *J Urol* 2007;177:481–7.

48. Hernandez S, Lopez-Knowles E, Lloreta J, Kogevinas M, Jaramillo R, Amoros A, Tardon A, Garcia-Closas R, Serra C, Carrato A, Malats N, Real FX. FGFR3 and Tp53 mutations in T1G3 transitional bladder carcinomas: independent distribution and lack of association with prognosis. *Clin Cancer Res* 2005;11:5444–50.

49. Knowles MA. Molecular subtypes of bladder cancer: Jekyll and Hyde or chalk and cheese? *Carcinogenesis* 2006;27:361–73.

50. Lopez-Beltran A, Cheng L, Mazzucchelli R, Bianconi M, Blanca A, Scarpelli M, Montironi R. Morphological and molecular profiles and pathways in bladder neoplasms. *Anticancer Res* 2008;28:2893–2900.

51. Hanahan D, Weinberg RA. The hallmarks of cancer. *Cell* 2000;100:57–70.

52. Wu XR. Urothelial tumorigenesis: a tale of divergent pathways. *Nat Rev Cancer* 2005;5:713–25.

53. Dalbagni G, Presti J, Reuter V, Fair WR, Cordon-Cardo C. Genetic alterations in bladder cancer. *Lancet* 1993;342:469–71.

54. Knowles MA, Elder PA, Williamson M, Cairns JP, Shaw ME, Law MG. Allelotype of human bladder cancer. *Cancer Res* 1994;54:531–8.

55. Rosin MP, Cairns P, Epstein JI, Schoenberg MP, Sidransky D. Partial allelotype of carcinoma in situ of the human bladder. *Cancer Res* 1995;15:5213–6.

56. Cheng L, MacLennan GT, Pan CX, Jones TD, Moore CR, Zhang S, Gu J, Patel NB, Kao C, Gardner TA. Allelic loss of the active X chromosome during bladder carcinogenesis. *Arch Pathol Lab Med* 2004;128:187–90.

57. Cheng L, MacLennan GT, Zhang S, Wang M, Pan CX, Koch MO. Laser capture microdissection analysis reveals frequent allelic losses in papillary urothelial neoplasm of low malignant potential of the urinary bladder. *Cancer* 2004;101:183–8.

58. Cheng L, Jones TD, McCarthy RP, Eble JN, Wang M, MacLennan GT, Lopez-Beltran A, Yang XJ, Koch MO, Zhang S, Pan CX, Baldridge LA. Molecular genetic evidence for a common clonal origin of urinary bladder small cell carcinoma and coexisting urothelial carcinoma. *Am J Pathol* 2005;166:1533–9.

59. Jones TD, Wang M, Eble JN, MacLennan GT, Lopez-Beltran A, Zhang S, Cocco A, L C. Molecular evidence supporting field effect in urothelial carcinogenesis. *Clin Cancer Res* 2005;11:6512–9.

60. Sung MT, Zhang S, MacLennan GT, Lopez-Beltran A, Montironi R, Wang M, Tan PH, Cheng L. Histogenesis of clear cell adenocarcinoma in the urinary tract: evidence of urothelial origin. *Clin Cancer Res* 2008;14:1947–55.

61. Jones TD, Zhang S, Lopez-Beltran A, Eble JN, Sung MT, MacLennan GT, Montironi R, Tan PH, Zheng S, Baldridge LA, Cheng L. Urothelial carcinoma with an inverted growth pattern can be distinguished from inverted papilloma by fluorescence in-situ hybridization, immunohistochemistry, and morphologic analysis. *Am J Surg Pathol* 2007;31:1861–7.

62. Cheng L, Bostwick DG, Li G, Zhang S, Vortmeyer AO, Zhuang Z. Conserved genetic findings in metastatic bladder cancer: a possible utility of allelic loss of chromosomes 9p21 and 17p13 in diagnosis. *Arch Pathol Lab Med* 2001;125:1197–9.

63. Houskova L, Zemanova Z, Babjuk M, Melichercikova J, Pesl M, Michalova K. Molecular cytogenetic characterization and diagnostics of bladder cancer. *Neoplasma* 2007;54:511–6.

64. Prat E, Bernues M, Caballin MR, Egozcue J, Gelabert A, Miro R. Detection of chromosomal imbalances in papillary bladder tumors by comparative genomic hybridization. *Urology* 2001;57:986–92.

65. Simon R, Burger H, Brinkschmidt C, Bocker W, Hertle L, Terpe HJ. Chromosomal aberrations associated with invasion in papillary superficial bladder cancer. *J Pathol* 1998;185:345–51.

66. Richter J, Wagner U, Schraml P, Maurer R, Alund G, Knonagel H, Moch H, Mihatsch MJ, Gasser TC, Sauter G. Chromosomal imbalances are associated with a high risk of progression in early invasive (pT1) urinary bladder cancer. *Cancer Res* 1999;59:5687–91.

67. Simon R, Burger H, Semjonow A, Hertle L, Terpe HJ, Bocker W. Patterns of chromosomal imbalances

in muscle invasive bladder cancer. *Int J Oncol* 2000;17:1025–9.

68. Bruch J, Wohr G, Hautmann R, Mattfeldt T, Bruderlein S, Moller P, Sauter S, Hameister H, Vogel W, Paiss T. Chromosomal changes during progression of transitional cell carcinoma of the bladder and delineation of the amplified interval on chromosome arm 8q. *Genes Chromosomes Cancer* 1998;23:167–74.

69. Natrajan R, Louhelainen J, Williams S, Laye J, Knowles MA. High-resolution deletion mapping of 15q13.2-q21.1 in transitional cell carcinoma of the bladder. *Cancer Res* 2003;63:7657–62.

70. Shaw ME, Knowles MA. Deletion mapping of chromosome 11 in carcinoma of the bladder. *Genes Chromosomes Cancer* 1995;13:1–8.

71. Tsai YC, Nichols PW, Hiti AL, Williams Z, Skinner DG, Jones PA. Allelic losses of chromosomes 9, 11, and 17 in human bladder cancer. *Cancer Res* 1990;50:44–7.

72. Houskova L, Zemanova Z, Babjuk M, Melichercikova J, Pesl M, Michalova K. Molecular cytogenetic characterization and diagnostics of bladder cancer. *Neoplasma* 2007;54:511–6.

73. Sandberg AA, Berger CS. Review of chromosome studies in urological tumors. II. Cytogenetics and molecular genetics of bladder cancer. *J Urol* 1994;151:545–60.

74. Miyao N, Tsai YC, Lerner SP, Olumi AF, Spruck CH 3rd, Gonzalez-Zulueta M, Nichols PW, Skinner DG, Jones PA. Role of chromosome 9 in human bladder cancer. *Cancer Res* 1993;53:4066–70.

75. Seripa D, Parrella P, Gallucci M, Gravina C, Papa S, Fortunato P, Alcini A, Flammia G, Lazzari M, Fazio VM. Sensitive detection of transitional cell carcinoma of the bladder by microsatellite analysis of cells exfoliated in urine. *Int J Cancer* 2001;95:364–9.

76. Stoehr R, Zietz S, Burger M, Filbeck T, Denzinger S, Obermann EC, Hammerschmied C, Wieland WF, Knuechel R, Hartmann A. Deletions of chromosomes 9 and 8p in histologically normal urothelium of patients with bladder cancer. *Eur Urol* 2005;47:58–63.

77. Cairns P, Shaw ME, Knowles MA. Initiation of bladder cancer may involve deletion of a tummor suppressor gene on chromosome 9. *Oncogene* 1993;8:1083–5.

78. Linnenbach AJ, Pressler LB, Seng BA, Kimmel BS, Tomaszewski JE, Malkowicz SD. Characterization of chromosome 9 deletions in transitional cell carcinoma by microsatellite assay. *Hum Mol Genet* 1993;2:1407–11.

79. Hartmann A, Schlake G, Zaak D, Hungerhuber E, Hofstetter A, Hofstaedter F, Knuechel R. Occurrence of chromosome 9 and p53 alterations in multifocal dysplasia and carcinoma in situ of human urinary bladder. *Cancer Res* 2002;62:809–18.

80. Lacy S, Lopez-Beltran A, MacLennan GT, Foster SR, Montironi R, Cheng L. Molecular pathogenesis of urothelial carcinoma: the clinical utility of emerging new biomarkers and future molecular classification of bladder cancer. *Anal Quan Cytol Histol* 2009;31:5–16.

81. Whitson J, Berry A, Carroll P, Konety B. A multicolour fluorescence in situ hybridization test predicts recurrence in patients with high-risk superficial bladder tumours undergoing intravesical therapy. *BJU Int* 2009;104:336–9.

82. Gofrit ON, Zorn KC, Silvestre J, Shalhav AL, Zagaja GP, Msezane LP, Steinberg GD. The predictive value of multi-targeted fluorescent in-situ hybridization in patients with history of bladder cancer. *Urol Oncol* 2008;26:246–9.

83. Mian C, Lodde M, Comploj E, Lusuardi L, Palermo S, Mian M, Maier K, Pycha A. Multiprobe fluorescence in situ hybridisation: prognostic perspectives in superficial bladder cancer. *J Clin Pathol* 2006;59:984–7.

84. Knowles MA. Molecular genetics of bladder cancer. *Br J Urol* 1995;75 Suppl 1:57–66.

85. Berger AP, Parson W, Stenzl A, Steiner H, Bartsch G, Klocker H. Microsatellite alterations in human bladder cancer: detection of tumor cells in urine sediment and tumor tissue. *Eur Urol* 2002;41:532–9.

86. Fornari D, Steven K, Hansen AB, Vibits H, Jepsen JV, Poulsen AL, Schwartz M, Horn T. Under-representation of bladder transitional cell tumour 9q, 11p and 14q LOH in urine and impact on molecular diagnosis. *Anticancer Res* 2005;25:4049–52.

87. Edwards J, Duncan P, Going JJ, Grigor KM, Watters AD, Bartlett JM. Loss of heterozygosity on chromosomes 11 and 17 are markers of recurrence in TCC of the bladder. *Br J Cancer* 2001;85:1894–9.

88. Trkova M, Babjuk M, Duskova J, Benesova-Minarikova L, Soukup V, Mares J, Minarik M, Sedlacek Z. Analysis of genetic events in 17p13 and 9p21 regions supports predominant monoclonal origin of multifocal and recurrent bladder cancer. *Cancer Lett* 2006;242:68–76.

89. Bartoletti R, Cai T, Nesi G, Roberta Girardi L, Baroni G, Dal Canto M. Loss of P16 expression and chromosome 9p21 LOH in predicting outcome of patients affected by superficial bladder cancer. *J Surg Res* 2007;143:422–7.

90. Lopez-Beltran A, Alvarez-Kindelan J, Luque RJ, Blanca A, Quintero A, Montironi R, Cheng L, Gonzalez-Campora R, Requena MJ. Loss of heterozygosity at 9q32-33 (DBC1 locus) in primary non-invasive papillary urothelial neoplasm of low malignant potential and low grade urothelial carcinoma of the bladder and their associated normal urothelium. *J Pathol* 2008;215:263–72.

91. Yamamoto Y, Matsuyama H, Kawauchi S, Furuya T, Liu XP, Ikemoto K, Oga A, Naito K, Sasaki K. Biological characteristics in bladder cancer depend on the type of genetic instability. *Clin Cancer Res* 2006;12:2752–8.

92. Halling KC, King W, Sokolova IA, Meyer RG, Burkhardt HM, Halling AC, Cheville JC, Sebo TJ, Ramakumar S, Stewart CS, Pankratz S, O'Kane DJ, Seelig SA, Lieber MM, Jenkins RB. A comparison of cytology and fluorescence in situ hybridization for the detection of urothelial carcinoma. *J Urol* 2000;164:1768–75.

93. Knowles MA. What we could do now: molecular pathology of bladder cancer. *Mol Pathol* 2001;54:215–21.

94. Hovey RM, Chu L, Balazs M, DeVries S, Moore D, Sauter G, Carroll PR, Waldman FM. Genetic alterations in primary bladder cancers and their metastases. *Cancer Res* 1998;58:3555–60.

95. Stoehr R, Zietz S, Burger M, Filbeck T, Denzinger S, Obermann EC, Hammerschmied C, Wieland WF, Knuechel R, Hartmann A. Deletions of chromosomes 9 and 8p in histologically normal urothelium of patients with bladder cancer. *Eur Urol* 2005;47:58–63.

96. Knowles MA, Habuchi T, Kennedy W, Cuthbert-Heavens D. Mutation spectrum of the 9q34 tuberous sclerosis gene TSC1 in transitional cell carcinoma of the bladder. *Cancer Res* 2003;63:7652–6.

97. Hornigold N, Devlin J, Davies AM, Aveyard JS, Habuchi T, Knowles MA. Mutation of the 9q34 gene TSC1 in sporadic bladder cancer. *Oncogene* 1999;18:2657–61.

98. Adachi H, Igawa M, Shiina H, Urakami S, Shigeno K, Hino O. Human bladder tumors with 2-hit mutations of tumor suppressor gene TSC1 and decreased expression of p27. *J Urol* 2003;170:601–4.

99. Baud E, Catilina P, Bignon YJ. p16 involvement in primary bladder tumors: analysis of deletions and mutations. *Int J Oncol* 1999;14:441–5.

100. Orlow I, Lacombe L, Hannon GJ, Serrano M, Pellicer I, Dalbagni G, Reuter VE, Zhang ZF, Beach D, Cordon-Cardo C. Deletion of the p16 and p15 *genes* in human bladder tumors. *J Natl Cancer Inst* 1995;87:1524–9.

101. Hopman AH, Kamps MA, Speel EJ, Schapers RF, Sauter G, Ramaekers FC. Identification of chromosome 9 alterations and p53 accumulation in isolated carcinoma in situ of the urinary bladder versus carcinoma in situ associated with carcinoma. *Am J Pathol* 2002;161:1119–25.

102. Stoehr R, Wissmann C, Suzuki H, Knuechel R, Krieg RC, Klopocki E, Dahl E, Wild P, Blaszyk H, Sauter G, Simon R, Schmitt R, Zaak D, Hofstaedter F, Rosenthal A, Baylin SB, Pilarsky C, Hartmann A. Deletions of chromosome 8p and loss of sFRP1 expression are progression markers of papillary bladder cancer. *Lab Invest* 2004;84:465–78.

103. Knowles MA, Shaw ME, Proctor AJ. Deletion mapping of chromosome 8 in cancers of the urinary bladder using restriction fragment length polymorphisms and microsatellite polymorphisms. *Oncogene* 1993;8:1357–64.

104. Boulalas I, Zaravinos A, Karyotis I, Delakas D, Spandidos DA. Activation of RAS family *genes* in urothelial carcinoma. *J Urol* 2009;181:2312–9.

105. Malats N, Bustos A, Nascimento CM, Fernandez F, Rivas M, Puente D, Kogevinas M, Real FX. p53 as a prognostic marker for bladder cancer: a meta-analysis and review. *Lancet Oncol* 2005;6:678–86.

106. de la Chapelle A. Microsatellite instability. *N Engl J Med* 2003;349:209–10.

107. Vaish M, Mandhani A, Mittal RD, Mittal B. Microsatellite instability as prognostic marker in bladder tumors: a clinical significance. *BMC Urol* 2005;5:2.

108. Cote RJ, Laird PW, Datar RH. Promoter hypermethylation: a new therapeutic target emerges in urothelial cancer. *J Clin Oncol* 2005;23:2879–81.

109. Abbosh PH, Wang M, Eble JN, Lopez-Beltran A, Maclennan GT, Montironi R, Zheng S, Pan CX, Zhou H, Cheng L. Hypermethylation of tumor-suppressor gene CpG islands in small-cell carcinoma of the urinary bladder. *Mod Pathol* 2008;21:355–62.

110. Jones PA, Gonzalgo ML. Altered DNA methylation and genome instability: A new pathway to cancer? *Proc Natl Acad Sci U S A* 1997;94:2103–5.

111. Jarmalaite S, Jankevicius F, Kurgonaite K, Suziedelis K, Mutanen P, Husgafvel-Pursiainen K. Promoter hypermethylation in tumour suppressor *genes* shows association with stage, grade and invasiveness of bladder cancer. *Oncology* 2008;75:145–51.

112. Urakami S, Shiina H, Enokida H, Kawakami T, Kawamoto K, Hirata H, Tanaka Y, Kikuno N, Nakagawa M, Igawa M, Dahiya R. Combination analysis of hypermethylated Wnt-antagonist family *genes* as a novel epigenetic biomarker panel for bladder cancer detection. *Clin Cancer Res* 2006;12:2109–16.

113. Tada Y, Wada M, Taguchi K, Mochida Y, Kinugawa N, Tsuneyoshi M, Naito S, Kuwano M. The association of death-associated protein kinases hypermethylation with early recurrence in superficial bladder cancers. *Cancer Res* 2002;62:4048–53.

114. Friedrich MG, Chandrasoma S, Siegmund KD, Weisenberger DJ, Cheng JC, Toma MI, Huland H, Jones PA, Liang G. Prognostic relevance of methylation markers in patients with non-muscle invasive bladder carcinoma. *Eur J Cancer* 2005;41:2769–78.

115. Yates DR, Rehman I, Abbod MF, Meuth M, Cross SS, Linkens DA, Hamdy FC, Catto JW. Promoter hypermethylation identifies progression risk in bladder cancer. *Clin Cancer Res* 2007;13:2046–53.

116. Catto JW, Azzouzi AR, Rehman I, Feeley KM, Cross SS, Amira N, Fromont G, Sibony M, Cussenot O, Meuth M, Hamdy FC. Promoter hypermethylation is associated with tumor location, stage, and subsequent progression in transitional cell carcinoma. *J Clin Oncol* 2005;23:2903–10.

117. Kim WJ, Kim EJ, Jeong P, Quan C, Kim J, Li QL, Yang JO, Ito Y, Bae SC. RUNX3 inactivation by point mutations and aberrant DNA methylation in bladder tumors. *Cancer Res* 2005;65:9347–54.

118. Chan MW, Chan LW, Tang NL, Tong JH, Lo KW, Lee TL, Cheung HY, Wong WS, Chan PS, Lai FM, To KF. Hypermethylation of multiple *genes* in tumor tissues and voided urine in urinary bladder cancer patients. *Clin Cancer Res* 2002;8:464–70.

119. Catto JW, Azzouzi AR, Rehman I, Feeley KM, Cross SS, Amira N, Fromont G, Sibony M, Cussenot O, Meuth M, Hamdy FC. Promoter hypermethylation is associated with tumor location, stage, and subsequent progression in transitional cell carcinoma. *J Clin Oncol* 2005;23:2903–10.

120. Yates DR, Rehman I, Abbod MF, Meuth M, Cross SS, Linkens DA, Hamdy FC, Catto JW. Promoter hypermethylation identifies progression risk in bladder cancer. *Clin Cancer Res* 2007;13:2046–53.

121. Kim WJ, Kim YJ. Epigenetic biomarkers in urothelial bladder cancer. *Expert Rev Mol Diagn* 2009;9:259–69.

122. Kim YK, Kim WJ. Epigenetic markers as promising prognosticators for bladder cancer. *Int J Urol* 2009;16:17–22.

123. Costa VL, Henrique R, Danielsen SA, Duarte-Pereira S, Eknaes M, Skotheim RI, Rodrigues A, Magalhaes JS, Oliveira J, Lothe RA, Teixeira MR, Jeronimo C, Lind GE. Three epigenetic biomarkers, GDF15, TMEFF2, and VIM, accurately predict bladder cancer from DNA-based analyses of urine samples. *Clin Cancer Res* 2010;16:5842–51.

124. Wilhelm-Benartzi CS, Koestler DC, Houseman EA, Christensen BC, Wiencke JK, Schned AR, Karagas MR, Kelsey KT, Marsit CJ. DNA methylation profiles delineate etiologic heterogeneity and clinically important subgroups of bladder cancer. *Carcinogenesis* 2010;31:1972–6.

125. Maruyama R, Toyooka S, Toyooka KO, Harada K, Virmani AK, Zochbauer-Muller S, Farinas AJ, Vakar-Lopez F, Minna JD, Sagalowsky A, Czerniak B, Gazdar AF. Aberrant promoter methylation profile of bladder cancer and its relationship to clinicopathological features. *Cancer Res* 2001;61:8659–63.

126. Jones PA. DNA methylation errors and cancer. *Cancer Res* 1996;56:2463–7.

127. Ribeiro-Filho LA, Franks J, Sasaki M, Shiina H, Li LC, Nojima D, Arap S, Carroll P, Enokida H, Nakagawa M, Yonezawa S, Dahiya R. CpG hypermethylation of promoter region and inactivation of E-cadherin gene in human bladder cancer. *Mol Carcinog* 2002;34:187–98.

128. Lagos-Quintana M, Rauhut R, Lendeckel W, Tuschl T. Identification of novel *genes* coding for small expressed RNAs. *Science* 2001;294:853–8.

129. Veerla S, Lindgren D, Kvist A, Frigyesi A, Staaf J, Persson H, Liedberg F, Chebil G, Gudjonsson S, Borg A, Mansson W, Rovira C, Hoglund M. MiRNA expression in urothelial carcinomas: important roles of miR-10a, miR-222, miR-125b, miR-7 and miR-452 for tumor stage and metastasis, and frequent homozygous losses of miR 31. *Int J Cancer* 2009;124:2236–42.

130. Thomson JM, Newman M, Parker JS, Morin-Kensicki EM, Wright T, Hammond SM. Extensive post-transcriptional regulation of microRNAs and its implications for cancer. *Genes Dev* 2006;20:2202–7.

131. Li X, Chen J, Hu X, Huang Y, Li Z, Zhou L, Tian Z, Ma H, Wu Z, Chen M, Han Z, Peng Z, Zhao X, Liang C, Wang Y, Sun L, Chen J, Zhao J, Jiang B, Yang H, Gui Y, Cai Z, Zhang X. Comparative mRNA and microRNA expression profiling of three genitourinary cancers reveals common hallmarks and cancer-specific molecular events. *PLoS One* 2011;6:e22570.

132. Catto JW, Miah S, Owen HC, Bryant H, Myers K, Dudziec E, Larre S, Milo M, Rehman I, Rosario DJ, Di Martino E, Knowles MA, Meuth M, Harris AL, Hamdy FC. Distinct microRNA alterations characterize high- and low grade bladder cancer. *Cancer Res* 2009;69:8472–81.

133. Dyrskjot L, Ostenfeld MS, Bramsen JB, Silahtaroglu AN, Lamy P, Ramanathan R, Fristrup N, Jensen JL, Andersen CL, Zieger K, Kauppinen S, Ulhoi BP, Kjems J, Borre M, Orntoft TF. Genomic profiling of microRNAs in bladder cancer: miR-129 is associated with poor outcome and promotes cell death in vitro. *Cancer Res* 2009;69:4851–60.

134. Yang H, Dinney CP, Ye Y, Zhu Y, Grossman HB, Wu X. Evaluation of genetic variants in microRNA-related *genes* and risk of bladder cancer. *Cancer Res* 2008;68:2530–7.

135. Dudziec E, Miah S, Choudhry HM, Owen HC, Blizard S, Glover M, Hamdy FC, Catto JW. Hypermethylation of CpG islands and shores around specific microRNAs and mirtrons is associated with the phenotype and presence of bladder cancer. *Clin Cancer Res* 2011;17:1287–96.

136. Wiklund ED, Bramsen JB, Hulf T, Dyrskjot L, Ramanathan R, Hansen TB, Villadsen SB, Gao S, Ostenfeld MS, Borre M, Peter ME, Orntoft TF, Kjems J, Clark SJ. Coordinated epigenetic repression of the miR-200 family and miR-205 in invasive bladder cancer. *Int J Cancer* 2011;128:1327–34.

137. Blaveri E, Brewer JL, Roydasgupta R, Fridlyand J, DeVries S, Koppie T, Pejavar S, Mehta K, Carroll P, Simko JP, Waldman FM. Bladder cancer stage and outcome by array-based comparative genomic hybridization. *Clin Cancer Res* 2005;11:7012–22.

138. Hoque MO, Lee CC, Cairns P, Schoenberg M, Sidransky D. Genome-wide genetic characterization of bladder cancer: a comparison of high-density single-nucleotide polymorphism arrays and PCR-based microsatellite analysis. *Cancer Res* 2003;63:2216–22.

139. Cheng L, Zhang S, Alexander R, Yao Y, MacLennan GT, Pan CX, Huang J, Wang M, Montironi R, Lopez-Beltran A. The landscape of EGFR pathways and personalized management of non-small-cell lung cancer. *Future Oncol* 2011;7:519–41.

140. Tuziak T, Jeong J, Majewski T, Kim MS, Steinberg J, Wang Z, Yoon DS, Kuang TC, Baggerly K, Johnston D, Czerniak B. High-resolution whole-organ mapping with SNPs and its significance to early events of carcinogenesis. *Lab Invest* 2005;85:689–701.

141. Obermann EC, Junker K, Stoehr R, Dietmaier W, Zaak D, Schubert J, Hofstaedter F, Knuechel R, Hartmann A. Frequent genetic alterations in flat urothelial hyperplasias and concomitant papillary bladder cancer as detected by CGH, LOH, and FISH analyses. *J Pathol* 2003;199:50–7.

142. Kallioniemi A, Kallioniemi OP, Citro G, Sauter G, DeVries S, Kerschmann R, Caroll P, Waldman F. Identification of gains and losses of DNA sequences in primary bladder cancer by comparative genomic hybridization. *Genes Chromosomes Cancer* 1995;12:213–9.

143. Bartsch G, Mitra AP, Cote RJ. Expression profiling for bladder cancer: strategies to uncover prognostic factors. *Expert Rev Anticancer Ther* 2010;10:1945–54.

144. Birkhahn M, Mitra AP, Williams AJ, Lam G, Ye W, Datar RH, Balic M, Groshen S, Steven KE, Cote RJ. Predicting recurrence and progression of noninvasive papillary bladder cancer at initial presentation based on quantitative gene expression profiles. *Eur Urol* 2010;57:12–20.

145. Catto JW, Abbod MF, Wild PJ, Linkens DA, Pilarsky C, Rehman I, Rosario DJ, Denzinger S, Burger M, Stoehr R, Knuechel R, Hartmann A, Hamdy FC. The application of artificial intelligence to microarray data: identification of a novel gene signature to identify bladder cancer progression. *Eur Urol* 2010;57:398–406.

146. Chin JL. In search of the perfect crystal ball for Ta urothelial cancer. *Eur Urol* 2010;57:21–2.

147. Costa VL, Henrique R, Danielsen SA, Duarte-Pereira S, Eknaes M, Skotheim RI, Rodrigues A, Magalhaes JS, Oliveira J, Lothe RA, Teixeira MR, Jeronimo C, Lind GE. Three epigenetic biomarkers, GDF15, TMEFF2, and VIM, accurately predict bladder cancer from DNA-based analyses of urine samples. *Clin Cancer Res* 2010;16:5842–51.

148. Hutchinson L. Bladder cancer: Gene-expression signature in urine indicates aggressive disease. *Nat Rev Urol* 2010;7:364.

149. Hutchinson L. Diagnosis: Gene-expression signature in urine diagnoses aggressive bladder cancer. *Nat Rev Clin Oncol* 2010;7:355.

150. Kim YJ, Ha YS, Kim SK, Yoon HY, Lym MS, Kim MJ, Moon SK, Choi YH, Kim WJ. Gene signatures for the prediction of response to bacillus Calmette-Guérin immunotherapy in primary pT1 bladder cancers. *Clin Cancer Res* 2010;16:2131–7.

151. Kim WJ, Kim EJ, Kim SK, Kim YJ, Ha YS, Jeong P, Kim MJ, Yun SJ, Lee KM, Moon SK, Lee SC, Cha EJ, Bae SC. Predictive value of progression-related gene classifier in primary non-muscle invasive bladder cancer. *Mol Cancer* 2010;9:3.

152. Lauss M, Ringner M, Hoglund M. Prediction of stage, grade, and survival in bladder cancer using genome-wide expression data: a validation study. *Clin Cancer Res* 2010;16:4421–33.

153. Lindgren D, Frigyesi A, Gudjonsson S, Sjodahl G, Hallden C, Chebil G, Veerla S, Ryden T, Mansson W, Liedberg F, Hoglund M. Combined gene expression and genomic profiling define two intrinsic molecular subtypes of urothelial carcinoma and gene signatures for molecular grading and outcome. *Cancer Res* 2010;70:3463–72.

154. Marsit CJ, Houseman EA, Christensen BC, Gagne L, Wrensch MR, Nelson HH, Wiemels J, Zheng S, Wiencke JK, Andrew AS, Schned AR, Karagas MR, Kelsey KT. Identification of methylated *genes* associated with aggressive bladder cancer. *PLoS One* 2010;5:e12334.

155. McConkey DJ, Lee S, Choi W, Tran M, Majewski T, Siefker-Radtke A, Dinney C, Czerniak B. Molecular genetics of bladder cancer: emerging mechanisms of tumor initiation and progression. *Urol Oncol* 2010;28:429–40.

156. Mengual L, Burset M, Ribal MJ, Ars E, Marin-Aguilera M, Fernandez M, Ingelmo-Torres M, Villavicencio H, Alcaraz A. Gene expression signature in urine for diagnosing and assessing aggressiveness of bladder urothelial carcinoma. *Clin Cancer Res* 2010;16:2624–33.

157. Neely LA, Rieger-Christ KM, Neto BS, Eroshkin A, Garver J, Patel S, Phung NA, McLaughlin S, Libertino JA, Whitney D, Summerhayes IC. A microRNA expression ratio defining the invasive phenotype in bladder tumors. *Urol Oncol* 2010;28:39–48.

158. Senchenko VN, Krasnov GS, Dmitriev AA, Kudryavtseva AV, Anedchenko EA, Braga EA, Pronina IV, Kondratieva TT, Ivanov SV, Zabarovsky ER, Lerman MI. Differential expression of CHL1 gene during development of major human cancers. *PLoS One* 2010;6:e15612.

159. Wilhelm-Benartzi CS, Koestler DC, Houseman EA, Christensen BC, Wiencke JK, Schned AR, Karagas MR, Kelsey KT, Marsit CJ. DNA methylation profiles delineate

etiologic heterogeneity and clinically important subgroups of bladder cancer. *Carcinogenesis* 2010;31:1972–6.

160. Dubosq F, Ploussard G, Soliman H, Turpin E, Latil A, Desgrandchamps F, de The H, Mongiat-Artus P. Identification of a three-gene expression signature of early recurrence in non-muscle-invasive urothelial cell carcinoma of the bladder. *Urol Oncol* 2012 (in press).

161. Kim WJ, Kim SK, Jeong P, Yun SJ, Cho IC, Kim IY, Moon SK, Um HD, Choi YH. A four-gene signature predicts disease progression in muscle invasive bladder cancer. *Mol Med* 2011;17:478–85.

162. Smith SC, Baras AS, Dancik G, Ru Y, Ding KF, Moskaluk CA, Fradet Y, Lehmann J, Stockle M, Hartmann A, Lee JK, Theodorescu D. A 20-gene model for molecular nodal staging of bladder cancer: development and prospective assessment. *Lancet Oncol* 2011;12:137–43.

163. Sanchez-Carbayo M, Socci ND, Lozano JJ, Li W, Charytonowicz E, Belbin TJ, Prystowsky MB, Ortiz AR, Childs G, Cordon-Cardo C. Gene discovery in bladder cancer progression using cDNA microarrays. *Am J Pathol* 2003;163:505–16.

164. Modlich O, Prisack HB, Pitschke G, Ramp U, Ackermann R, Bojar H, Vogeli TA, Grimm MO. Identifying superficial, muscle-invasive, and metastasizing transitional cell carcinoma of the bladder: use of cDNA array analysis of gene expression profiles. *Clin Cancer Res* 2004;10:3410–21.

165. Dyrskjot L, Thykjaer T, Kruhoffer M, Jensen JL, Marcussen N, Hamilton-Dutoit S, Wolf H, Orntoft TF. Identifying distinct classes of bladder carcinoma using microarrays. *Nat Genet* 2003;33:90–6.

166. Rosser CJ, Liu L, Sun Y, Villicana P, McCullers M, Porvasnik S, Young PR, Parker AS, Goodison S. Bladder cancer-associated gene expression signatures identified by profiling of exfoliated urothelia. *Cancer Epidemiol Biomarkers Prev* 2009;18:444–53.

167. Modlich O, Prisack HB, Pitschke G, Ramp U, Ackermann R, Bojar H, Vogeli TA, Grimm MO. Identifying superficial, muscle-invasive, and metastasizing transitional cell carcinoma of the bladder: use of cDNA array analysis of gene expression profiles. *Clin Cancer Res* 2004;10:3410–21.

168. Blaveri E, Simko JP, Korkola JE, Brewer JL, Baehner F, Mehta K, Devries S, Koppie T, Pejavar S, Carroll P, Waldman FM. Bladder cancer outcome and subtype classification by gene expression. *Clin Cancer Res* 2005;11:4044–55.

169. Marsit CJ, Koestler DC, Christensen BC, Karagas MR, Houseman EA, Kelsey KT. DNA methylation array analysis identifies profiles of blood-derived DNA methylation associated with bladder cancer. *J Clin Oncol* 2011;29:1133–9.

170. Aaboe M, Marcussen N, Jensen KM, Thykjaer T, Dyrskjot L, Orntoft TF. Gene expression profiling of noninvasive primary urothelial tumours using microarrays. *Br J Cancer* 2005;93:1182–90.

171. Dyrskjot L, Kruhoffer M, Thykjaer T, Marcussen N, Jensen JL, Moller K, Orntoft TF. Gene expression in the urinary bladder: a common carcinoma in situ gene expression signature exists disregarding histopathological classification. *Cancer Res* 2004;64:4040–8.

172. Dyrskjot L, Zieger K, Real FX, Malats N, Carrato A, Hurst C, Kotwal S, Knowles M, Malmstrom PU, de la Torre M, Wester K, Allory Y, et al. Gene expression signatures predict outcome in non-muscle-invasive bladder carcinoma: a multicenter validation study. *Clin Cancer Res* 2007;13:3545–51.

173. Schultz IJ, De Kok JB, Witjes JA, Babjuk M, Willems JL, Wester K, Swinkels DW, Tjalsma H. Simultaneous proteomic and genomic analysis of primary Ta urothelial cell carcinomas for the prediction of tumor recurrence. *Anticancer Res* 2007;27:1051–8.

174. Schultz IJ, Wester K, Straatman H, Kiemeney LA, Babjuk M, Mares J, Willems JL, Swinkels DW, Witjes JA, Malmstrom PU, de Kok JB. Gene expression analysis for the prediction of recurrence in patients with primary Ta urothelial cell carcinoma. *Eur Urol* 2007;51:416–23.

175. Birkhahn M, Mitra AP, Williams AJ, Lam G, Ye W, Datar RH, Balic M, Groshen S, Steven KE, Cote RJ. Predicting recurrence and progression of noninvasive papillary bladder cancer at initial presentation based on quantitative gene expression profiles. *Eur Urol* 2010;57:12–20.

176. Mitra AP, Bartsch CC, Cote RJ. Strategies for molecular expression profiling in bladder cancer. *Cancer Metastasis Rev* 2009;28:317–26.

177. Dyrskjot L, Zieger K, Kruhoffer M, Thykjaer T, Jensen JL, Primdahl H, Aziz N, Marcussen N, Moller K, Orntoft TF. A molecular signature in superficial bladder carcinoma predicts clinical outcome. *Clin Cancer Res* 2005;11:4029–36.

178. Wild PJ, Herr A, Wissmann C, Stoehr R, Rosenthal A, Zaak D, Simon R, Knuechel R, Pilarsky C, Hartmann A. Gene expression profiling of progressive papillary noninvasive carcinomas of the urinary bladder. *Clin Cancer Res* 2005;11:4415–29.

179. Mitra AP, Almal AA, George B, Fry DW, Lenehan PF, Pagliarulo V, Cote RJ, Datar RH, Worzel WP. The use of genetic programming in the analysis of quantitative gene expression profiles for identification of nodal status in bladder cancer. *BMC Cancer* 2006;6:159.

180. Sanchez-Carbayo M, Socci ND, Lozano J, Saint F, Cordon-Cardo C. Defining molecular profiles of poor outcome in patients with invasive bladder cancer using oligonucleotide microarrays. *J Clin Oncol* 2006;24:778–89.

181. Takata R, Katagiri T, Kanehira M, Tsunoda T, Shuin T, Miki T, Namiki M, Kohri K, Matsushita Y, Fujioka T, Nakamura Y. Predicting response to methotrexate, vinblastine, doxorubicin, and cisplatin neoadjuvant chemotherapy for bladder cancers through genome-wide gene expression profiling. *Clin Cancer Res* 2005;11:2625–36.

182. Als AB, Dyrskjot L, von der Maase H, Koed K, Mansilla F, Toldbod HE, Jensen JL, Ulhoi BP, Sengelov L, Jensen KM, Orntoft TF. Emmprin and survivin predict response and survival following cisplatin-containing chemotherapy in patients with advanced bladder cancer. *Clin Cancer Res* 2007;13:4407–14.

183. Wild PJ, Herr A, Wissmann C, Stoehr R, Rosenthal A, Zaak D, Simon R, Knuechel R, Pilarsky C, Hartmann A. Gene expression profiling of progressive papillary noninvasive carcinomas of the urinary bladder. *Clin Cancer Res* 2005;11:4415–29.

184. Zaravinos A, Lambrou GI, Boulalas I, Delakas D, Spandidos DA. Identification of common differentially expressed genes in urinary bladder cancer. *PLoS One* 2011;6:e18135.

185. Aaboe M, Marcussen N, Jensen KM, Thykjaer T, Dyrskjot L, Orntoft TF. Gene expression profiling of noninvasive primary urothelial tumours using microarrays. *Br J Cancer* 2005;93:1182–90.

186. Takata R, Katagiri T, Kanehira M, Shuin T, Miki T, Namiki M, Kohri K, Tsunoda T, Fujioka T, Nakamura Y. Validation study of the prediction system for clinical response of M-VAC neoadjuvant chemotherapy. *Cancer Sci* 2007;98:113–7.

187. Riester M, Taylor J, Feifer A, Koppie TM, Rosenberg J, Downey RJ, Bochner BH, Michor F. Combination of a novel gene expression signature with a clinical nomogram improves the prediction of survival in high-risk bladder cancer. Clin Cancer Res. 2012 Jan 6. [Epub ahead of print]

188. Putluri N, Shojaie A, Vasu VT, Vareed SK, Nalluri S, Putluri V, Thangjam GS, Panzitt K, Tallman CT, Butler C, Sana TR, Fischer SM, Sica G, Brat DJ, Shi H, Palapattu GS, Lotan Y, Weizer AZ, Terris MK, Shariat SF, Michailidis G, Sreekumar A. Metabolomic profiling reveals potential markers and bioprocesses altered in bladder cancer progression. *Cancer Res* 2011;71:7376–86.

189. Mitra AP, Pagliarulo V, Yang D, Waldman FM, Datar RH, Skinner DG, Groshen S, Cote RJ. Generation of a concise gene panel for outcome prediction in urinary bladder cancer. *J Clin Oncol* 2009;27:3929–37.

190. Mengual L, Burset M, Ars E, Lozano JJ, Villavicencio H, Ribal MJ, Alcaraz A. DNA microarray expression profiling of bladder cancer allows identification of noninvasive diagnostic markers. *J Urol* 2009;182:741–8.

191. Schiffer E, Mischak H, Zimmerli LU. Proteomics in gerontology: current applications and future aspects—a mini-review. *Gerontology* 2009;55:123–37.

192. Goodison S, Rosser CJ, Urquidi V. Urinary proteomic profiling for diagnostic bladder cancer biomarkers. *Expert Rev Proteomics* 2009;6:507–14.

193. Grossman HB, Messing E, Soloway M, Tomera K, Katz G, Berger Y, Shen Y. Detection of bladder cancer using a point-of-care proteomic assay. *JAMA* 2005;293:810–6.

194. Feldman AS, Banyard J, Wu CL, McDougal WS, Zetter BR. Cystatin B as a tissue and urinary biomarker of bladder cancer recurrence and disease progression. *Clin Cancer Res* 2009;15:1024–31.

195. Grossman HB, Soloway M, Messing E, Katz G, Stein B, Kassabian V, Shen Y. Surveillance for recurrent bladder cancer using a point-of-care proteomic assay. *JAMA* 2006;295:299–305.

196. Shirodkar SP, Lokeshwar VB. Potential new urinary markers in the early detection of bladder cancer. *Curr Opin Urol* 2009;19:488–93.

197. Barboro P, Rubagotti A, Orecchia P, Spina B, Truini M, Repaci E, Carmignani G, Romagnoli A, Introini C, Boccardo F, Carnemolla B, Balbi C. Differential proteomic analysis of nuclear matrix in muscle-invasive bladder cancer: potential to improve diagnosis and prognosis. *Cell Oncol* 2008;30:13–26.

198. Kawanishi H, Matsui Y, Ito M, Watanabe J, Takahashi T, Nishizawa K, Nishiyama H, Kamoto T, Mikami Y, Tanaka Y, Jung G, Akiyama H, Nobumasa H, Guilford P, Reeve A, Okuno Y, Tsujimoto G, Nakamura E, Ogawa O. Secreted CXCL1 is a potential mediator and marker of the tumor invasion of bladder cancer. *Clin Cancer Res* 2008;14:2579–87.

199. Moreira JM, Ohlsson G, Gromov P, Simon R, Sauter G, Celis JE, Gromova I. Bladder cancer associated protein: a potential prognostic biomarker in human bladder cancer. *Mol Cell Proteomics* 2009.

200. Caliskan M, Turkeri LN, Mansuroglu B, Toktas G, Aksoy B, Unluer E, Akdas A. Nuclear accumulation of mutant p53 protein: a possible predictor of failure of intravesical therapy in bladder cancer. *Br J Urol* 1997;79:373–7.

201. Gardiner RA, Walsh MD, Allen V, Rahman S, Samaratunga ML, Seymour GJ, Lavin MF. Immunohistological expression of p53 in primary pT1 transitional cell bladder cancer in relation to tumour progression. *Br J Urol* 1994;73:526–32.

202. Tsuji M, Kojima K, Murakami Y, Kanayama H, Kagawa S. Prognostic value of Ki-67 antigen and p53 protein in urinary bladder cancer: immunohistochemical analysis of radical cystectomy specimens. *Br J Urol* 1997;79:367–72.

203. Wright C, Thomas D, Mellon K, Neal DE, Horne CH. Expression of retinoblastoma gene product and p53 protein in bladder carcinoma: correlation with Ki67 index. *Br J Urol* 1995;75:173–9.

204. Soini Y, Turpeenniemi -Hujanen, T, Kamel D, Autio-Harmainen H, Risteli J, Risteli L, Nuorva K, Pääkkö P, Vähäkangas K. p53 immunohistochemistry in transitional cell carcinoma and dysplasia of the urinary bladder correlates with diease progression. *Br J Cancer* 1993;68:1029–35.

205. Brewster S, Oxley J, Trivella M, Abbott C, Gillatt D. Preoperative p53, bcl-2, CD44, and E-cadherin immunohistochemistry as predictors of biochemical relapse after radical prostatectomy. *J Urol* 1999;161:1238–43.

206. Cheng L, Alexander RE, Zhang S, Pan CX, MacLennan GT, Lopez-Beltran A, Montironi R. Clinical and therapeutic implications of cancer stem cell biology. *Exp Rev Anticancer Ther* 2011;11:1131–43.

207. Pan CX, Zhu W, Cheng L. Implications of cancer stem cells in the treatment of cancer. *Future Oncol* 2006;2:723–31.

208. Cheng L, Zhang S, Davidson DD, Montironi R, Lopez-Beltran A. Implications of cancer stem cells for cancer therapy. In: Bagley RG, Teicher BA, eds. Cancer Drug Discovery and Develepment: Stem Cells and Cancer. New York: Humana Press/Springer, 2009;252–62.

209. Jordan CT, Guzman ML, Noble M. Cancer stem cells. *N Engl J Med* 2006;355:1253–61.

210. Davidson DD, Cheng L. Field cancerization in the urothelium of the bladder. *Anal Quant Cytol Histol* 2006;28:337–8.

211. Dimov I, Visnjic M, Stefanovic V. Urothelial cancer stem cells. *ScientificWorldJournal* 2010;10:1400–15.

212. Chan KS, Volkmer JP, Weissman I. Cancer stem cells in bladder cancer: a revisited and evolving concept. *Curr Opin Urol* 2010;20:393–7.

213. Yang YM, Chang JW. Bladder cancer initiating cells (BCICs) are among EMA-CD44v6+ subset: novel methods for isolating undetermined cancer stem (initiating) cells. *Cancer Invest* 2008;26:725–33.

214. Ben-Porath I, Thomson MW, Carey VJ, Ge R, Bell GW, Regev A, Weinberg RA. An embryonic stem cell-like gene expression signature in poorly differentiated aggressive human tumors. *Nat Genet* 2008;40:499–507.

215. Sanchez-Carbayo M, Socci ND, Lozano J, Saint F, Cordon-Cardo C. Defining molecular profiles of poor outcome in patients with invasive bladder cancer using oligonucleotide microarrays. *J Clin Oncol* 2006;24:778–89.

216. Paterson RF, Ulbright TM, MacLennan GT, Zhang S, Pan CX, Sweeney CJ, Moore CR, Foster RS, Koch MO, Eble JN, Cheng L. Molecular genetic alterations in the laser-capture-microdissected stroma adjacent to bladder carcinoma. *Cancer* 2003;98:1830–6.

217. Atlasi Y, Mowla SJ, Ziaee SA, Bahrami AR. OCT-4, an embryonic stem cell marker, is highly expressed in bladder cancer. *Int J Cancer* 2007;120:1598–1602.

218. She JJ, Zhang PG, Wang ZM, Gan WM, Che XM. Identification of side

population cells from bladder cancer cells by DyeCycle Violet staining. *Cancer Biol Ther* 2008;7.1663–8.

219. Oates JE, Grey BR, Addla SK, Samuel JD, Hart CA, Ramani V, Brown MD, Clarke NW. Hoechst 33342 side population identification is a conserved and unified mechanism in urological cancers. *Stem Cells Dev* 2009.

220. Chan KS, Espinosa I, Chao M, Wong D, Ailles L, Diehn M, Gill H, Presti J Jr, Chang HY, van de Rijn M, Shortliffe L, Weissman IL. Identification, molecular characterization, clinical prognosis, and therapeutic targeting of human bladder tumor-initiating cells. *Proc Natl Acad Sci U S A* 2009;106:14016–21.

221. Braakhuis BJ, Tabor MP, Kummer JA, Leemans CR, Brakenhoff RH. A genetic explanation of Slaughter's concept of field cancerization: evidence and clinical implications. *Cancer Res* 2003;63:1727–30.

222. Cheng L, Cheville JC, Neumann RM, Bostwick DG. Natural history of urothelial dysplasia of the bladder. *Am J Surg Pathol* 1999;23:443–7.

223. Cheng L, Cheville JC, Neumann RM, Bostwick DG. Flat intraepithelial lesions of the urinary bladder. *Cancer* 2000;88:625–31.

224. Paterson RF, Ulbright TM, MacLennan GT, Zhang S, Pan C, Sweeney C, Moore CR, Foster RS, Koch MO, Eble JN, Cheng L. Molecular genetic alterations in the laser-capture microdissected stroma adjacent to bladder carcinoma. *Cancer* 2003;98:1830–6.

225. Jordan CT, Guzman ML, Noble M. Cancer stem cells. *N Engl J Med* 2006;355:1253–61.

226. Davidson DD, Cheng L. "Field cancerization" in the urothelium of the bladder. *Anal Quant Cytol Histol* 2006;28:337–8.

227. Koss LG, Tiamson EM, Robbins MA. Mapping cancerous and precancerous bladder changes. A study of the urothelium in ten surgically removed bladders. *JAMA* 1974;227:281–6.

228. Weinstein RS. Origin and dissemination of human urinary bladder carcinoma. *Semin Oncol* 1979;6:149–56.

229. Lutzeyer W, Rubben H, Dahm H. Prognostic parameters in superficial bladder cancer: an analysis of 315 cases. *J Urol* 1982;127:250–52.

230. Kiemeney LA, Witjes JA, Heijbroek RP, Verbeek AL, Debruyne FM. Predictability of recurrent and progressive disease in individual patients with primary superficial bladder cancer. *J Urol* 1993;150:60–4.

231. Mazzucchelli R, Barbisan F, Stramazzotti D, Montironi R, Lopez-Beltran A, Scarpelli M. Chromosomal abnormalities in macroscopically normal urothelium in patients with bladder pT1 and pT2a urothelial carcinoma: a fluorescence in situ hybridization study and correlation with histologic features. *Anal Quant Cytol Histol* 2005;27:143–51.

232. Kirkali Z, Chan T, Manoharan M, Algaba F, Busch C, Cheng L, Kiemeney L, Kriegmair M, Montironi R, Murphy WM, Sesterhenn IA, Achibana M, Weider J. Bladder cancer: epidemiology, staging and grading, and diagnosis. *Urology*. 2005;66:4–34.

233. Droller MJ. Bladder cancer: state-of-the-art care. *CA Cancer J Clin* 1998;48:269–84.

234. Sidransky EA, Frost P, von Eschenbach A, Oyasu R, Preisinger AC, Vogelstein B. Clonal origin of bladder cancer. *N Engl J Med* 1992;326:737–40.

235. Habuchi T, Takahashi R, Yamada H, Kakehi Y, Sugiyama T, Yoshida O. Metachronous multifocal development of urothelial cancers by intraluminal seeding. *Lancet* 1993;342:1087–8.

236. Miyao N, Tsai YC, Lerner SP, Olumi AF, Spruck CHI, Goñzalez-Zulueta M, Nichols PW, Skinner DG, Jones PA. Role of chromosome 9 in human bladder cancer. *Cancer Res* 1993;53:4066–70.

237. Xu X, Stower MJ, Reid IN, Garner RC, Burns PA. Molecular screening of multifocal transitional cell carcinoma of the bladder using p53 mutations as biomarkers. *Clin Cancer Res* 1996;2:1795–800.

238. Chern HD, Becich MJ, Persad RA, Romkes M, Smith P, Collins C, Li YH, Branch RA. Clonal analysis of human recurrent superficial bladder cancer by immunohistochemistry of P53 and retinoblastoma proteins. *J Urol* 1996;156:1846–9.

239. Takahashi T, Kakehi Y, Mitsumori K, Akao T, Terachi T, Kato T, Ogawa O, Habuchi T. Distinct microsatellite alterations in upper urinary tract tumors and subsequent bladder tumors. *J Urol* 2001;165:672–7.

240. Takahashi T, Habuchi T, Kakehi Y, Mitsumori K, Akao T, Terachi T, Yoshida O. Clonal and chronological genetic analysis of multifocal cancers of the bladder and upper urinary tract. *Cancer Res* 1998;58:5835–41.

241. Li M, Cannizzaro LA. Identical clonal origin of synchronous and metachronous low grade, noninvasive papillary transitional cell carcinomas of the urinary tract. *Hum Pathol* 1999;30:1197–1200.

242. Fadl-Elmula I, Gorunova L, Mandahl N, Elfving P, Lundgren R, Mitelman F, Heim S. Cytogenetic monoclonality in multifocal uroepithelial carcinomas: evidence of intraluminal tumour seeding. *Br J Cancer* 1999;81:6–12.

243. Hartmann A, Rosner U, Schlake G, Dietmaier W, Zaak D, Hofstaedter F, Knuechel R. Clonality and genetic divergence in multifocal low grade superficial urothelial carcinoma as determined by chromosome 9 and p53 deletion analysis. *Lab Invest* 2000;80:709–18.

244. Hafner C, Knuechel R, Zanardo L, Dietmaier W, Blaszyk H, Cheville J, Hofstaedter F, Hartmann A. Evidence for oligoclonality and tumor spread by intraluminal seeding in multifocal urothelial carcinomas of the upper and lower urinary tract. *Oncogene* 2001;20:4910–5.

245. Simon R, Eltze E, Schafer KL, Burger H, Semjonow A, Hertle L, Dockhorn-Dworniczak B, Terpe HJ, Bocker W. Cytogenetic analysis of multifocal bladder cancer supports a monoclonal origin and intraepithelial spread of tumor cells. *Cancer Res* 2001;61:355–62.

246. Goto K, Konomoto T, Hayashi K, Kinukawa N, Naito S, Kumazawa J, Tsuneyoshi M. p53 mutations in multiple urothelial carcinomas: a molecular analysis of the development of multiple carcinomas. *Mod Pathol* 1997;10:428–37.

247. Spruck CH III, Ohneseit PF, Gonzalez-Zulueta M, Esrig D, Miyao N, Tsai YC, Lerner SP, Schmutte C, Yang AS, Cote R, Dubeau L, Nichols PW, Hermann GG, Steven K, Horn T, Skinner DG, Jones PA. Two molecular pathways to transitional cell carcinoma of the bladder. *Cancer Res* 1994;54:784–8.

248. Petersen I, Ohgaki H, Ludeke BI, Kleihues P. p53 mutations in phenacetin-associated human urothelial carcinomas. *Carcinogenesis* 1993;14:2119–22.

249. Hartmann A, Moser K, Kriegmair M, Hofstetter A, Hofstaedter F, Knuechel R. Frequent genetic alterations in simple urothelial hyperplasias of the bladder in patients with papillary urothelial carcinoma. *Am J Pathol* 1999;154:721–7.

250. Yoshimura I, Kudoh J, Saito S, Tazaki H, Shimizu N. p53 gene mutation in recurrent superficial bladder cancer. *J Urol* 1995;153:1711–5.

251. Stoehr R, Hartmann A, Hiendlmeyer E, Murle K, Wieland W, Knuechel R. Oligoclonality of early lesions of the urothelium as determined by microdissection-supported genetic analysis. *Pathobiology* 2000;68:165–72.

252. Cianciulli AM, Leonardo C, Guadagni F, Marzano R, Iori F, De Nunzio C, Franco G, Merola R, Laurenti C. Genetic instability in superficial bladder cancer and adjacent mucosa: an interphase cytogenetic study. *Hum Pathol* 2003;34:214–21.

253. Junker K, Boerner D, Schulze W, Utting M, Schubert J, Werner W. Analysis of genetic alterations in normal bladder urothelium. *Urology* 2003;62:1134–8.

254. Hafner C, Knuechel R, Stoehr R, Hartmann A. Clonality of multifocal urothelial carcinomas: 10 years of molecular genetic studies. *Int J Cancer* 2002;101:1–6.

255. Cheng L, Montironi R, Davidson DD, Lopez-Beltran A. Staging and reporting of urothelial carcinoma of the urinary bladder. *Mod Pathol* 2009;22 (Suppl 2):S70–95.

256. Edge SB, Byrd DR, Compton CC, Fritz AG, Greene FL, Trotti A. American Joint Committee on Cancer Staging Manual, 7th ed. New York: Springer, 2010.

257. Zieger K, Dyrskjot L, Wiuf C, Jensen JL, Andersen CL, Jensen KM, Orntoft TF. Role of activating fibroblast growth factor receptor 3 mutations in the development of bladder tumors. *Clin Cancer Res* 2005;11:7709–19.

258. Simonetti S, Russo R, Ciancia G, Altieri V, De Rosa G, Insabato L. Role of polysomy 17 in transitional cell carcinoma of the bladder: immunohistochemical study of HER2/neu expression and fish analysis of c-erbB-2 gene and chromosome 17. *Int J Surg Pathol* 2009;17:198–205.

259. Vazina A, Dugi D, Shariat SF, Evans J, Link R, Lerner SP. Stage specific lymph node metastasis mapping in radical cystectomy specimens. *J Urol* 2004;171:1830–4.

260. Karl A, Carroll PR, Gschwend JE, Knuchel R, Montorsi F, Stief CG, Studer UE. The impact of lymphadenectomy and lymph node metastasis on the outcomes of radical cystectomy for bladder cancer. *Eur Urol* 2009;55:826–35.

261. Seraj MJ, Thomas AR, Chin JL, Theodorescu D. Molecular determination of perivesical and lymph node metastasis after radical cystectomy for urothelial carcinoma of the bladder. *Clin Cancer Res* 2001;7:1516–22.

262. Retz M, Lehmann J, Szysnik C, Zwank S, Venzke T, Roder C, Kalthoff H, Basbaum C, Stockle M. Detection of occult tumor cells in lymph nodes from bladder cancer patients by MUC7 nested RT-PCR. *Eur Urol* 2004;45:314–9.

263. Wu X, Kakehi Y, Zeng Y, Taoka R, Tsunemori H, Inui M. Uroplakin II as a promising marker for molecular diagnosis of nodal metastases from bladder cancer: comparison with cytokeratin 20. *J Urol* 2005;174:2138–42.

264. Kurahashi T, Hara I, Oka N, Kamidono S, Eto H, Miyake H. Detection of micrometastases in pelvic lymph nodes in patients undergoing radical cystectomy for locally invasive bladder cancer by real-time reverse transcriptase-PCR for cytokeratin 19 and uroplakin II. *Clin Cancer Res* 2005;11:3773–7.

265. Marin-Aguilera M, Mengual L, Burset M, Oliver A, Ars E, Ribal MJ, Colomer D, Mellado B, Villavicencio H, Algaba F, Alcaraz A. Molecular lymph node staging in bladder urothelial carcinoma: impact on survival. *Eur Urol* 2008;54:1363–72.

266. Veltri RW, Makarov DV. Nucleic acid-based marker approaches to urologic cancers. *Urol Oncol* 2006;24:510–27.

267. Guzzo TJ, McNeil BK, Bivalacqua TJ, Elliott DJ, Sokoll LJ, Schoenberg MP. The presence of circulating tumor cells does not predict extravesical disease in bladder cancer patients prior to radical cystectomy. *Urol Oncol* 2012;30:44–8.

268. Gallagher DJ, Milowsky MI, Ishill N, Trout A, Boyle MG, Riches J, Fleisher M, Bajorin DF. Detection of circulating tumor cells in patients with urothelial cancer. *Ann Oncol* 2009;20:305–8.

269. Naoe M, Ogawa Y, Morita J, Omori K, Takeshita K, Shichijyo T, Okumura T, Igarashi A, Yanaihara A, Iwamoto S, Fukagai T, Miyazaki A, Yoshida H. Detection of circulating urothelial cancer cells in the blood using the CellSearch System. *Cancer* 2007;109:1439–45.

270. Li SM, Zhang ZT, Chan S, McLenan O, Dixon C, Taneja S, Lepor H, Sun TT, Wu XR. Detection of circulating uroplakin-positive cells in patients with transitional cell carcinoma of the bladder. *J Urol* 1999;162:931–5.

271. Gazzaniga P, Gandini O, Giuliani L, Magnanti M, Gradilone A, Silvestri I, Gianni W, Gallucci M, Frati L, Agliano AM. Detection of epidermal growth factor receptor mRNA in peripheral blood: a new marker of circulating neoplastic cells in bladder cancer patients. *Clin Cancer Res* 2001;7:577–83.

272. Okegawa T, Kinjo M, Horie S, Nutahara K, Higashihara E. Detection of mucin 7 gene expression in exfoliated cells in urine from patients with bladder tumor. *Urology* 2003;62:182–6.

273. Osman I, Kang M, Lee A, Deng FM, Polsky D, Mikhail M, Chang C, David DA, Mitra N, Wu XR, Sun TT, Bajorin DF. Detection of circulating cancer cells expressing uroplakins and epidermal growth factor receptor in bladder cancer patients. *Int J Cancer* 2004;111:934–9.

274. Kinjo M, Okegawa T, Horie S, Nutahara K, Higashihara E. Detection of circulating MUC7-positive cells by reverse transcription-polymerase chain reaction in bladder cancer patients. *Int J Urol* 2004;11:38–43.

275. Cheng L, Lopez-Beltran A, MacLennan GT, Montironi R, Bostwick DG. Neoplasms of the urinary bladder. In: Bostwick DG, Cheng L, eds. Urologic Surgical Pathology, 2nd ed. Philadelphia: Elsevier/Mosby, 2008;259–352.

276. Cheng L, Neumann RM, Nehra A, Spotts BE, Weaver AL, Bostwick DG. Cancer heterogeneity and its biologic implications in the grading of urothelial carcinoma. *Cancer* 2000;88:1663–70.

277. Armstrong AB, Wang M, Eble JN, MacLennan GT, Montironi R, Tan PH, Lopez-Beltran A, Zhang S, Baldridge LA, Spartz H, Cheng L. TP53 mutational analysis supports monoclonal origin of biphasic sarcomatoid urothelial carcinoma (carcinosarcoma) of the urinary bladder. *Mod Pathol* 2009;22:113–8.

278. Lopez-Beltran A, Amin MB, Oliveira PS, Montironi R, Algaba F, McKenney JK, de Torres I, Mazerolles C, Wang M, Cheng L. Urothelial carcinoma of the bladder, lipid cell variant: clinicopathologic findings and LOH analysis. *Am J Surg Pathol* 2010;34:371–6.

279. Lopez-Beltran A, Requena MJ, Montironi R, Blanca A, Cheng L. Plasmacytoid urothelial carcinoma of the bladder. *Hum Pathol* 2009;40:1023–8.

280. Nigwekar P, Tamboli P, Amin MB, Osunkoya AO, Ben-Dor D. Plasmacytoid urothelial carcinoma: detailed analysis of morphology with clinicopathologic correlation in 17 cases. *Am J Surg Pathol* 2009;33:417–24.

281. Reid-Nicholson MD, Ramalingam P, Adeagbo B, Cheng N, Peiper SC, Terris MK. The use of Urovysion fluorescence in situ hybridization in the diagnosis and surveillance of non-urothelial carcinoma of the bladder. *Mod Pathol* 2009;22:119–27.

282. Wallerand H, Bernhard JC, Culine S, Ballanger P, Robert G, Reiter RE, Ferriere JM, Ravaud A. Targeted therapies in non-muscle-invasive bladder cancer according to the signaling pathways. *Urol Oncol* 2011;29:4–11.

283. Iyer G, Milowsky MI, Bajorin DF. Novel strategies for treating relapsed/refractory urothelial carcinoma. *Expert Rev Anticancer Ther* 2010;10:1917–32.

284. Pan CX, Zhang H, Lara PN, Cheng L. Small-cell carcinoma of the urinary bladder: diagnosis and management. *Expert Rev Anticancer Ther* 2006;6:1707–13.

285. Black PC, Agarwal PK, Dinney CP. Targeted therapies in bladder cancer—an update. *Urol Oncol* 2007;25:433–8.

286. Chen M, Cassidy A, Gu J, Delclos GL, Zhen F, Yang H, Hildebrandt M, Lin J, Ye Y, Chamberlain RM, Dinney CP, Wu X. Genetic variations in PI3K-AKT-mTOR pathway and bladder cancer risk. *Carcinogenesis* 2009;30:2047–52.

287. Pant-Purohit M, Lopez-Beltran A, Montironi R, MacLennan GT, Cheng L. Small cell carcinoma of the urinary bladder. *Histol Histopathol* 2010;25:217–21.

288. Jacobs BL, Lee CT, Montie JE. Bladder cancer in 2010: How far have we come? *CA Cancer J Clin* 2010;60:244–72.

289. Laird AD, Vajkoczy P, Shawver LK, Thurnher A, Liang C, Mohammadi M, Schlessinger J, Ullrich A, Hubbard SR, Blake RA, Fong TA, Strawn LM, Sun L, Tang C, Hawtin R, Tang F, Shenoy N, Hirth KP, McMahon G, Cherrington JM. SU6668 is a potent antiangiogenic and antitumor agent that induces regression of established tumors. *Cancer Res* 2000;60:4152–60.

290. Mohammadi M, McMahon G, Sun L, Tang C, Hirth P, Yeh BK, Hubbard SR, Schlessinger J. Structures of the tyrosine kinase domain of fibroblast growth factor receptor in complex with inhibitors. *Science* 1997;276:955–60.

291. Paterson JL, Li Z, Wen XY, Masih-Khan E, Chang H, Pollett JB, Trudel S, Stewart AK. Preclinical studies of fibroblast growth factor receptor 3 as a therapeutic target in multiple myeloma. *Br J Haematol* 2004;124:595–603.

292. Grand EK, Chase AJ, Heath C, Rahemtulla A, Cross NC. Targeting FGFR3 in multiple myeloma: inhibition of t(4;14)-positive cells by SU5402 and PD173074. *Leukemia* 2004;18:962–6.

293. Trudel S, Li ZH, Wei E, Wiesmann M, Chang H, Chen C, Reece D, Heise C, Stewart AK. CHIR-258, a novel, multitargeted tyrosine kinase inhibitor for the potential treatment of t(4;14) multiple myeloma. *Blood* 2005;105:2941–8.

294. Gazzaniga P, Gradilone A, de Berardinis E, Sciarra A, Cristini C, Naso G, di Silverio F, Frati L, Agliano AM. A chemosensitivity test to individualize intravesical treatment for non-muscle-invasive bladder cancer. *BJU Int* 2009;104:184–8.

Index

Bladder Pathology, First Edition. Liang Cheng, Antonio Lopez-Beltran, David G. Bostwick.
© 2012 Wiley-Blackwell. Published 2012 by John Wiley & Sons, Inc.

Index

Index

Index

Index

Index

Index

Index

James L. Sanderson
Pathology